In Cupboard

Cold vapor steamer—high output type

Enema bag

Douche bag or other douching equipment

Chemical enema in plastic squeeze bottle

Electric heating pad

Vinegar (white)

Hydrogen peroxide—3% solution

Home first-aid kit

In First-Aid Kit (for Home and Car)

Adhesive dressings (Band-Aid type)—
assorted sizes

2"x2" sterile gauze pads—1 dozen,
individually wrapped

4"x4" sterile gauze pads—½ dozen,
individually wrapped

2"x4" "nonstick" sterile pads (Telfa or
other)—½ dozen

2" gauze roller bandage—1 roll

4" gauze roller bandage—1 roll

1" and 2" adhesive tape—1 roll each

2" and 4" elastic (Ace) bandage

1 triangular bandage (1 sq. yard muslin
folded diagonally)

1 pair bandage scissors

1 pair pointed tweezers

1 snakebite kit with rubber suction cup
and tourniquet

Sunburn ointment

Small bottle germicidal soap

First-aid manual

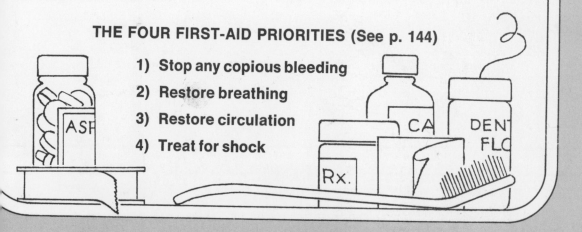

THE FOUR FIRST-AID PRIORITIES (See p. 144)

1) **Stop any copious bleeding**
2) **Restore breathing**
3) **Restore circulation**
4) **Treat for shock**

LADIES' HOME JOURNAL FAMILY MEDICAL GUIDE

LADIES' HOME

JOURNAL

FAMILY MEDICAL GUIDE

Alan E. Nourse, M.D.

HARPER & ROW, PUBLISHERS

New York, Evanston, San Francisco, London

1817

Drawings by Joy Goodwin

The anatomical drawings at the beginning of this book reprinted by permission of A. J. Nystrom & Co.

FIRST EDITION

Designed by Sidney Feinberg

Library of Congress Cataloging in Publication Data

Nourse, Alan Edward.
  Ladies' home journal family medical guide.
  1. Medicine, Popular I. The Ladies' home journal.
II. Title. III. Title. Family medical guide.
[DNLM: 1. Medicine—Popular works. WB 120 N933L
1973]
RC81.N646   616   72-9099
ISBN 0-06-013223-X

The author is indebted to the following institutions and individuals for supplying the X-rays reproduced in this volume:

To Overlake Memorial Hospital, Bellevue, Washington, for Plates 3a, 3b, 4b, 5b, 8a, 8b, 12a, 12b, 14a, 14b, 15, 18, 19, 20, 21, 22a, 22b, 25, 26, 28, 31, 33, 34, 36, 38 and 39. To Issaquah Medical Clinic, Issaquah, Washington, for Plates 1a, 1b, 3c, 4a, 5a, 6a, 10, 16, 32, 37a and 37b. To the Department of Radiology, Virginia Mason Medical Center, Seattle, Washington, for Plates 6b, 9a, 9b, 7a, 7c, 17 and 27. To Clinton M. Furuya, M.D., for Plate 13. To George Hadden, M.D., for Plate 11. To David B. Hurlbut, M.D., for Plates 24, 30, 35a and 35b. To G. Hugh Lawrence, M.D., for Plates 23, 29a and 29b. To James H. Seeley, M.D., for Plates 2a and 2b. To Clinton M. Furuya, M.D., and David B. Hurlbut, M.D., for Plate 37. Inset photo, Plate 39, courtesy of Clinton M. Furuya, M.D., and David B. Hurlbut, M.D.

To Carl Brandt
for reasons too numerous to detail

CONTENTS

Acknowledgments xi

I   THE EVOLUTION OF MODERN HEALTH CARE

   1. Early Medicine: A Crescendo of Discovery   3
   2. The Twentieth-Century Health Care Explosion   11

II   THE HEALTHY BODY AND HOW IT WORKS

   3. The Building Blocks: Cells and Tissues   19
   4. Support and Mobility: The Musculoskeletal System   25
   5. Motivation and Moderation: The Nervous System   42
   6. Protection and Appearance: The Cutaneous System   55
   7. Exchange, Filtration and Secretion: The Lungs, Kidneys and Endocrines   62
   8. The River of Life: The Cardiovascular System   75
   9. The Fuels of Life: Digestion and Metabolism   84
  10. Conspiracy Against Death: Reproduction and Preservation   92

III   EMERGENCIES, FIRST AID AND HOME HEALTH CARE

  11. When Seconds May Save Lives: The Serious Emergencies   103
  12. Minor Injuries and Other Emergencies   124
  13. Temperature, Fever and Febrile Illnesses   148
  14. Home Health Care   157

IV PATTERNS OF ILLNESS: THE INFECTIOUS DISEASES

15. The Causes of Infection   169
16. The "Childhood Rash" Diseases   178
17. The Preventable Killers of Childhood   185
18. A Rogues' Gallery of Other Childhood Infections   191
19. "Strep" and "Staph"—The Omnipresent Invaders   204
20. Tuberculosis, Pneumonia and Other Bacterial Infections   211
21. The Variable Viral and Rickettsial Infections   224
22. The Venereal Diseases—Ancient Plague, Modern Threat   243
23. Intestinal Infections and Parasites   253
24. Malaria and Other Parasitic Infections   262
25. Leprosy, Bubonic Plague and Other Uncommon Infections and Parasitic Diseases   271

V PATTERNS OF ILLNESS: THE MUSCULOSKELETAL SYSTEM

26. Muscle and Tendon Diseases   281
27. Fractures and Other Bone Disorders   294
28. Arthritis and Other Joint Diseases   310

VI PATTERNS OF ILLNESS: THE NERVOUS SYSTEM

29. The Symptoms of Nervous System Disease   335
30. Major Nervous System Disorders   352

VII PATTERNS OF ILLNESS: THE CUTANEOUS SYSTEM

31. The Skin and Connective Tissue   381
32. Care and Disorders of the Teeth and Gums   415
33. The Special Sensory Organs: Eyes, Ears and Nose   424
34. Diseases of the Breast   444

VIII PATTERNS OF ILLNESS: THE RESPIRATORY TRACT

35. Respiration and Life   455
36. Chest Injuries, Mechanical Obstructions and Respiratory Tract Infections   464

37. Hay Fever, Asthma and Emphysema 490
38. Tumors of the Respiratory Tract 498

IX PATTERNS OF ILLNESS: THE CARDIOVASCULAR SYSTEM

39. Disorders of the Blood and Blood-Forming Organs 511
40. Hemorrhage and Shock 533
41. Congenital Anomalies of the Heart and Blood Vessels 542
42. Inflammatory Diseases of the Heart and Blood Vessels 556
43. When the Heart Fails 573
44. Hypertension—The Silent Destroyer 582
45. Atherosclerosis and Coronary Artery Disease 592

X PATTERNS OF ILLNESS: THE DIGESTIVE TRACT

46. Digestive Function and Disease 609
47. Inflammatory Diseases of the Digestive System 630
48. Peptic Ulcer Disease and Intestinal Cancers 648
49. Diseases of the Pancreas, Liver and Gall Bladder 660

XI PATTERNS OF ILLNESS: THE ENDOCRINE GLANDS

50. The Mighty Midgets 681
51. The Major Endocrine Gland Diseases 690

XII PATTERNS OF ILLNESS: THE URINARY AND GENITAL SYSTEMS

52. Diseases and Disorders of the Urinary System 713
53. Disorders of the Male Genital Organs 734
54. Disorders of the Female Genital System 745

XIII PATTERNS OF ILLNESS: THE MIND AND MENTAL ILLNESS

55. Emotional Conflict and Our Mental Defenses 769
56. Disorders of the Mind 778

XIV THE TRYING TIMES OF LIFE

57. Progressing Through Pregnancy 811
58. The New Baby 850

59. The Childhood Years 867

60. Adolescence and How to Live with It 899

61. The Prime Years 909

62. The Hazards of Middle Age 926

63. Aging and Death 944

XV **OUR MODERN MEDICAL RESOURCES**

64. The Medical History and Physical Examination 961

65. Laboratory Tests, X-Rays and Other Diagnostic Aids 968

66. The Doctor's Training 983

67. The Many Kinds of Doctors 991

68. Our Modern Hospitals and Auxiliary Medical Services 1001

69. Medical Costs and How to Meet Them 1011

Glossary 1023

Index 1047

ACKNOWLEDGMENTS

Any book of this magnitude and complexity invariably benefits from the contributions of many people other than the author, from the time the idea is born to the time the finished book is published. In this work I am particularly indebted to John Mack Carter for his enthusiasm and support of the project from the time of its inception; to Carl D. Brandt, whose efforts and encouragement over the years made the writing possible; to Steven M. Spencer for his criticism of early fragments of the manuscript; and to M. S. Wyeth, Jr., for his extraordinary patience and confidence in guiding the book to its ultimate publication.

In addition, I am enduringly grateful to David B. Hurlbut, M.D., F.A.C.S., for his reading and professional criticism of the vast bulk of the manuscript, especially those portions related to surgery, and for his invaluable assistance in assembling the X-rays for reproduction; to Janice Nielson Phelps, M.D., for her consideration of portions of the manuscript dealing with pediatric care; to J. O. Borgen, M.D., for his criticism of sections concerned with obstetrics and gynecology; to Eugen Halar, M.D., for his help with segments related to bone, muscle and joint disorders; and to John H. Walker, M.D., and Kenneth D. Moores, M.D., for their generous assistance in preparing and reviewing the X-ray reproductions included in the book. Although any errors of fact or medical interpretation remain the sole responsibility of the author, the number of such errors has surely been minimized with the indispensable assistance of these and other medical colleagues. I am further grateful to the Department of Medical Illustration and Photography of the Virginia Mason Medical Center, Seattle, Washington, and to Charles Wood, Paul Macapia and Dean Auve for their efforts in supplying negatives and prints of the X-rays for reproduction.

In the matter of organizing, editing, cutting, amplifying, refining and rewriting early drafts of the manuscript, I could scarcely have achieved the final form of the book without the expert aid and guidance of my editor Burton K. Beals, whose real creative contribution has gone far beyond the normal bounds of editorial craftsmanship. Finally, I am indebted to Doris M. Vinnedge for her incomparable assistance in researching, copyreading and manuscript preparation throughout the years that the work was in progress.

ALAN E. NOURSE, M.D.
North Bend, Washington

LADIES' HOME JOURNAL FAMILY MEDICAL GUIDE

NAMES OF PARTS

1. Trachea (windpipe)
2. Left common carotid artery
3. Right common carotid artery
4. Aortic arch
5. Left bronchus and bronchial artery
6. Esophagus (gullet) and diaphragm
7. Hepatic veins
8. Adrenal (suprarenal) gland
9. Right kidney, cut away
10. Left kidney
11. Ureter
12. Urinary bladder
13. Kidney vessels
14. Quadrate muscle
15. Greater psoas muscle
16. Inguinal ring

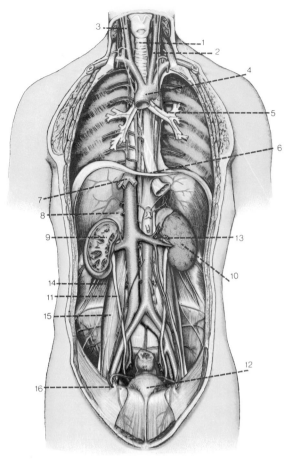

VISCERA OF CHEST AND ABDOMEN

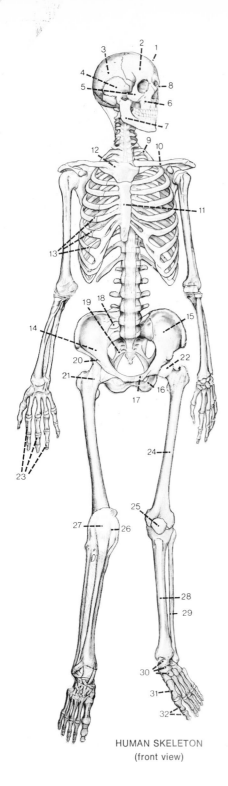

BONES, JOINTS AND LIGAMENTS

1. Skull
2. Frontal bone
3. Parietal bone
4. Temporal bone
5. Zygomatic arch (Cheekbone)
6. Maxilla
7. Mandible (jawbone)
8. Nasal bones
9. First rib
10. Clavicle (collar bone)
11. Sternum (breastbone)
12. Sternoclavicular joint
13. Ribs
14. Pelvis
15. Ilium
16. Ischium
17. Pubic bone (pubis)
18. Sacroiliac joint
19. Ligaments of sacrum and ischium
20. Inguinal (Poupart's) ligament
21. Iliofemoral ligament
22. Head of the femur
23. Phalanges of the fingers
24. Femur (thigh bone)
25. Patella (knee cap)
26. Capsule of the knee joint
27. Tendon of quadriceps muscle
28. Tibia (shin bone)
29. Fibula
30. Tarsals (ankle bones)
31. Metatarsals (foot bones)
32. Phalanges of the toes

HUMAN SKELETON
(front view)

BONES, JOINTS AND LIGAMENTS

33. Occipital bone
34. Seventh cervical vertebra
35. First thoracic vertebra
36. Twelfth ("floating") rib
37. Scapula (shoulder blade)
38. Capsule of the shoulder joint
39. Humerus
40. Ulna
41. Radius
42. Carpals (wrist bones)
43. Metacarpals (hand bones)
44. Phalanges (finger bones)
45. Capsule of elbow joint
46. Wrist joint
47. Pelvis
48. Capsule of hip joint
49. Great trochanter of femur
50. Skull

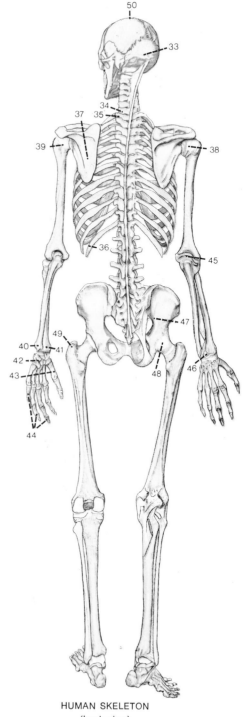

HUMAN SKELETON
(back view)

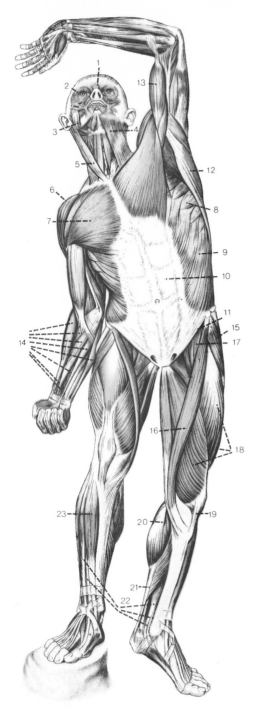

MUSCLES, TENDONS AND LIGAMENTS

1. Frontal
2. Orbicular of eye
3. Masseter
4. Platysma
5. Sternocleido-mastoid
6. Deltoid
7. Greater pectoral
8. Serratus magnus
9. External oblique of abdomen
10. Rectus abdominis sheath
11. Inguinal (Poupart's) ligament
12. Latissimus dorsi (broadest muscle of the back)
13. Biceps
14. Flexors, pronators and abductors of the wrist, hand and fingers
15. Tensor of broad fascia of thigh
16. Sartorius
17. Iliac
18. Four heads of the quadriceps
19. Tendon of the quadriceps
20. Gastrocnemius
21. Achilles tendon
22. Flexors and extensors of foot and toes
23. Anterior tibial

MUSCLES
(front view)

MUSCLES, TENDONS AND LIGAMENTS

24. Occipital
25. Latissimus dorsi (broadest of the back)
26. Trapezius
27. Layered muscles of the back
28. Spine of scapula
29. Deltoid
30. Extensors and adductors of wrist, hand and fingers
31. Dorsal ligament of wrist
32. Gluteus maximus
33. Tensor of broad fascia of thigh
34. Great lateral of thigh (one of quadriceps)
35. Biceps femoris
36. Semitendinous
37. Great adductor of thigh
38. Soleus
39. Flexors and extensors of foot and toes
40. Anterior tibial
41. Gastrocnemius
42. Achilles tendon

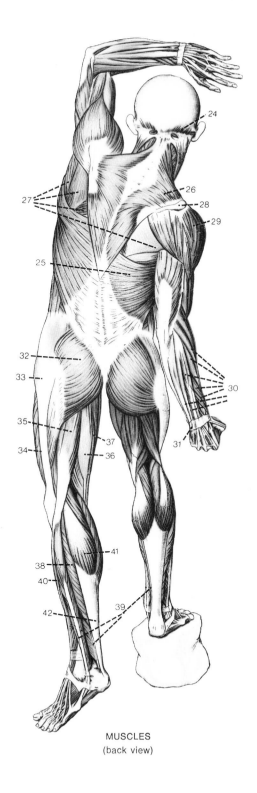

MUSCLES
(back view)

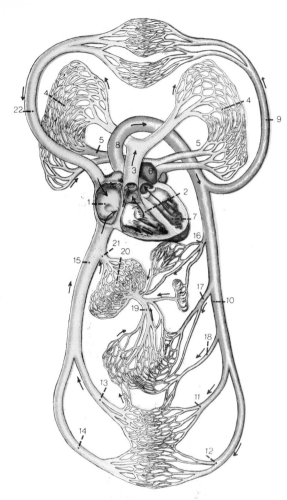

SCHEMA OF CIRCULATION

NAMES OF PARTS

1. Right auricle
2. Right ventricle
3. Pulmonary artery
4. Pulmonary capillaries
5. Pulmonary veins
6. Left auricle
7. Left ventricle
8. Aortic arch
9. Arteries of head and upper limbs
10. Descending aorta
11. Internal iliac artery
12. Arteries of lower limbs
13. Internal iliac vein
14. Veins of lower limbs
15. Inferior vena cava
16. Celiac trunk
17. Superior mesenteric artery
18. Inferior mesenteric artery
19. Portal circulation
20. Capillaries of liver
21. Hepatic veins
22. Superior vena cava

Note: The blood coming into the right auricle (1) passes to the right ventricle (2) and thence through the pulmonary artery (3) to the lung capillaries (4), which join to form the pulmonary veins (5) that carry blood back into the left auricle (6). From here the blood passes to the left ventricle (7) and into the aorta (8), which transports it to various parts of the organism. Notice the vessels to the head and upper extremities (9), to the lower extremities (12), and to the abdomen (17, 18). Blood passes from abdominal organs via the portal system (19) through the liver capillaries (20). Finally the capillaries fuse to form veins (15, 22) that carry blood back to the right auricle.

NAMES OF PARTS   (Figs. 1, 2, 3 and 4)

23. Left common carotid
24. Ascending aorta and arch
25. Pulmonary artery, divides into right and left branches
26. Superior and inferior vena cava
27. Right ventricle
28. Interventricular septum
29. Papillary muscles
30. Semilunar valve
31. Left auricle
32. Right pulmonary vein
33. Left pulmonary vein
34. Bicuspid valve
35. Left ventricle
36. Aortic valve
37. Apex of heart

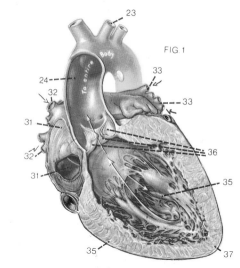

1. THE HEART
Posterior Coronal Section
(showing l. auricle and l. ventricle)

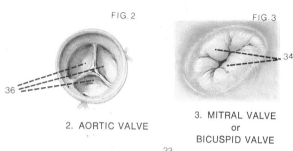

2. AORTIC VALVE

3. MITRAL VALVE
or
BICUSPID VALVE

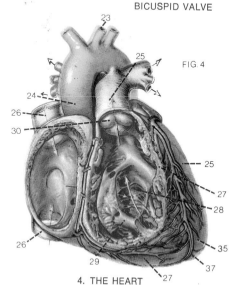

4. THE HEART
Anterior Coronal Section
(showing interior of r. auricle and r. ventricle)

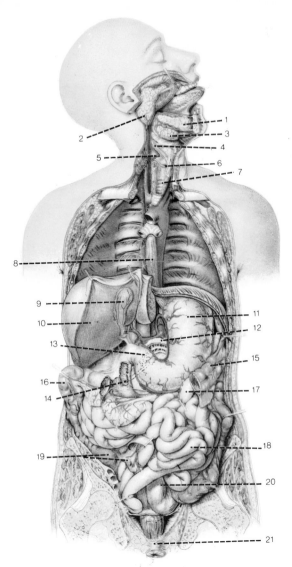

NAMES OF PARTS

1. Sublingual salivary gland
2. Parotid salivary gland
3. Submandibular salivary gland
4. Epiglottis
5. Pharynx
6. Vocal cords
7. Larynx
8. Esophagus (gullet)
9. Gall bladder
10. Liver
11. Stomach
12. Pancreas
13. Pylorus
14. Orifice of bile and pancreatic ducts
15. Splenic flexure of colon
16. Hepatic flexure of colon
17. Jejunum
18. Ileum
19. Cecum and appendix
20. Sigmoid flexure of colon
21. External anal sphincter muscle

ALIMENTARY CANAL

THE EVOLUTION OF MODERN HEALTH CARE

1. Early Medicine: A Crescendo of Discovery   3

2. The Twentieth-Century Health Care Explosion   11

For the vast majority of Americans today a high quality of health care is taken for granted. Our physicians are among the best trained in the world, our hospitals among the best equipped, our nurses among the most proficient. It is easy to forget that the many services and facilities have not always been available. Even as little as 200 years ago, the finest physician had very little sound scientific knowledge upon which to base his practice. Nursing as a highly skilled profession is barely 100 years old, and the modern hospital bears very little resemblance to the hospitals of even 30 or 40 years ago. The comprehensive health care available today is the end result of a painfully slow evolutionary process of discovery and experiment which began centuries ago, but which has only recently accelerated to become a veritable explosion of medical knowledge.

Thanks to this spiraling accumulation of knowledge it is now possible not only to cure many illnesses which were long thought incurable, but to take positive steps to prevent disease before it occurs. The evolution of modern health care is an exciting story in itself; but even more exciting is the realization that today, for the first time in human history, continuing good health is an attainable goal for every American family.

Early Medicine: A Crescendo of Discovery

The United States of America is probably the most health-conscious nation that has ever existed in the world. The evidence of this is everywhere around us. Of the more than 200 million people in this country, all but a tiny fraction consult a physician, visit a medical clinic, emergency room or hospital, or participate in a school health program at least some time every year. More than 300,000 practicing physicians minister to our health needs, aided by multitudes of registered nurses, pharmacists, practical nurses, nurse's aides, physical therapists, occupational therapists and other paramedical workers. Eight thousand or more new physicians are graduated from our medical schools every year, proceeding to train for a career in the field of medicine which may include general practice, a wide variety of medical specialties, research, public health service or hospital administration. Our public health services on both the federal and the local levels work tirelessly to maintain basic standards of hygiene throughout the nation, detect and fight outbreaks of infectious disease and perform many other tasks designed to protect the health of the public at large. As a result, immunizations against many illnesses are available to everyone at minimal cost, public supplies of food are clean and safe, and virtually all communities of any size have unlimited supplies of potable drinking water and safe sewage disposal facilities. In the year 1969 there were over 7,000 major hospitals in the United States with a total of 1,650,000 beds, and those beds were used; over 30.5 million inpatients were admitted to hospitals for treatment in that year

alone, and more than $22 billion were spent for both inpatient and outpatient hospital services, an average cost of $110 for every man, woman and child in the country. In the same year almost 380,000 patients were admitted to state and county mental hospitals, almost three times the number admitted in 1955. When we add to these costs the amounts spent annually for doctors' services, for prescription and nonprescription drugs, the annual expenditures for medical research and the public funds spent for health care for the poor or aged, we find that more than 5 percent of our total gross national income is spent each year for health protection and health services of one sort or another, both from our private pocketbooks and from public tax funds.

Of course it is a well-publicized fact that the cost of these health services has been rising dramatically year by year. Not so well publicized is the fact that public demand for these services, and use of them, is rising even more dramatically. Our health-consciousness as a nation is reflected as well in more subtle ways. The public press is filled with news and information about health care, the control of disease, and the prevention of illness. Even minor advances of medical research become headline news stories. We are constantly reminded in print of areas in which health care standards do not measure up to acceptable levels, and in recent years we have been involved in a great national debate about health care. The substance of that debate is not whether health care should be available to everyone, but rather how the cost of such care can best be met and how the health services needed can best be supplied. At the same time certain of the massive health care problems of the nation—obesity, for example, or our infant mortality rate, which compares unfavorably to many other highly developed nations—have become matters of nationwide public concern. Although the level of health care is high, we are increasingly aware that it is by no means as high as it could and should be.

In such a climate of concern it is easy to imagine that public interest in the problem of health care has always been high. Indeed, it might be difficult for many Americans today to remember a time when health care of high quality was not readily available. Yet even within the last 50 years in this country the availability and quality of health care facilities have undergone a staggering revolution. The facilities that we may now take for granted have not always existed by any means, nor did they appear miraculously overnight. They are the result of a long process of scientific and social evolution which had its beginnings in the dim reaches of human history, and which progressed in a pattern of slow acceleration over many centuries. If we are to see the health care facilities available to us today in any kind of perspective, we must first look briefly at the long succession of men and events that led to their development.

The Earliest Physicians

Some millions of years ago, a particular group of giant apes evolved a higher level of intelligence than their animal brothers, came down from the forests, and formed into hunting bands that roamed the plains of south-central Africa. For the first time these creatures began to use weapons and tools. Gradually a primitive spoken language developed; later symbols and pictographs were used as a means of communicating ideas, and division of labor began. Hardy young males became the hunters for the tribe, swift runners became messengers, and the particularly clever and experienced males planned the hazardous business of the hunt. And, although there are no written records for proof, it is probable that certain of these prehuman creatures became particularly adept at repairing injured bodies and

healing illnesses—the first physicians, long before the dawn of history.

Little is known about these primitive doctors except what can be learned from bones found in ancient midden heaps. Doubtless their healing capabilities were extremely limited, but then, so were the types of illnesses they had to deal with. In those violent days, few lived to be more than fifteen or twenty years old, far too short a time for degenerative diseases to begin to appear. Death at childbirth must have been commonplace, and those infections and illnesses that did occur were undoubtedly regarded with fear and superstition. However, fossil evidence has been found to indicate that the basic principles of fracture care were learned very early. It is also probable that a few herbs and other natural drugs were discovered and used to help relieve pain or promote healing of wounds and infections. By the time the first written records of human civilization appear, the primitive physician was already considered an important member of his society.

The Physician in Egypt

We do have records of the work of physicians in the earliest Egyptian civilizations, and certain kinds of disease other than injuries or fractures were clearly recognized some 4,000 years or more B.C. For example, a "falling sickness," probably epilepsy, was familiar to the Egyptians and regarded in some eras as a mark of divinity, perhaps because it was so unexplainable and unpredictable. There are also indirect evidences that the Egyptians knew and recognized angina pectoris, the kind of chest pain that arises from arteriosclerosis of the arteries in the heart, and that death from coronary thrombosis occurred. Among the archaeological artifacts of the early Egyptian civilizations are a variety of stone or metal burrs and drills known as trephines which were used to make holes through the skull; and judging from the number of skulls showing evidence of having been so drilled, some Egyptian physicians must have been very enthusiastic about this procedure, whatever the ailment they were seeking to treat.

One of the earliest medical textbooks known is also Egyptian; the Papyrus of Ebers, edited by

Georg Moritz Ebers in 1874, is believed to have been written around 1570 B.C., but was probably copied from manuscripts a thousand years older. This ancient document described a variety of medical and surgical treatments used as early as 2600 to 2200 B.C. The physicians of those times, however, were invariably members of the aristocracy, retained by the courts of the pharaohs and other nobles, and consulted only by the wealthy in society. No health care of any sort was available to the masses of peasants and slaves other than pathetic fragments of "folk medicine" learned by trial and error and passed down from family to family.

Indeed, at the very best the health care provided by early physicians in the Egyptian civilizations, and later in the civilizations which arose in Babylon and Persia, bore little resemblance to the scientific health care we know today. All forms of medical treatment involved a strange mixture of folklore, mythology, magic, stargazing, practical experience and educated guesswork. Virtually nothing was known about the actual structure of the human body, or of the changes that occur as a result of illness. Even what little was known or discovered was rarely connected with health care or the work of physicians. In the later Egyptian civilizations, for example, intricate embalming techniques were evolved to make possible the physical preservation of the bodies of dead kings and noblemen; those early embalmers must have developed a certain practical knowledge of human anatomy, and it is highly probable that the secret of the circulation of the blood was discovered in this way as early as 2000 B.C. But if so, it was never recorded, and was ultimately lost until William Harvey approached the problem scientifically some 3,600 years later. It remained for the great civilization which arose in Greece during the last few centuries before Christ to lay the first truly scientific groundwork for health care that would persist to the present time.

The Earliest Medical Schools

Many of the enduring roots of the arts and sciences, mathematics, philosophy and politics which were to become permanent parts of West-

ern civilization evolved in the civilization of ancient Greece which superseded the early civilizations in Egypt and the Middle East. For the first time a great many kinds of illness and injury were recognized as diagnosable and even treatable, and on the island of Kos a group of priest-physicians who identified their healing skills with the god Asklepios founded the first formal medical school at a temple dedicated to him, extending their influence far and wide throughout the civilized world. It was quite different, of course, from the medical schools of today, but it attracted many young men who came there to learn what was known of the arts of diagnosis and treatment. These young doctors served their teachers at a sort of hospital-infirmary where sick people from all over the civilized world congregated to consult with the physicians and oracles, take healing mineral baths, and recover from their illnesses. Diagnosis and treatment at the time were closely related to the supposedly divine predictions of the oracles, and the physicians themselves depended far more on divine intervention for the success of their treatments than on actual knowledge of the structure and function of the body. Even so, the medical school on the island of Kos, and another on the nearby peninsula of Knidos, were active in the 6th century B.C. and had become an important element in Greek life 200 years later.

It was at that time that a young man who was born on the island of Kos about 460 B.C. emerged to take one of the first and greatest steps toward a really scientific approach to the study of medicine, a man whose observations, practice, writings and teachings laid the foundation for the great wave of medical discovery that would finally reach its crest more than 2,000 years later. This brilliant young Greek physician was, of course, Hippocrates. He studied what was then known about medicine according to the traditions of the day, by means of discussion, debate with his teachers and philosophical argument. But he was also an extremely astute observer of the varying symptoms of different illnesses, and was perhaps the first physician in history to become convinced that certain kinds of illness were invariably accompanied by certain specific symptoms, and that by recognizing the symptoms and observing the physical changes of an illness, a physician could identify what the illness was and often predict quite accurately the course it would take. For example, Hippocrates observed one type of illness which always seemed to manifest itself first by coughing and increasing shortness of breath. After a time the victim would develop a bluish pallor of the skin of the face, and the physician could hear changes in the sounds of breathing if he placed his ear to the victim's chest. Hippocrates even found that in such situations the physician could often elicit a strange splashing sound when he struck the victim's chest, as if the chest were filled with fluid. He also noted that this illness was invariably accompanied by feverishness and increasing thirst, and that after a period of some 10 to 12 days from the beginning of symptoms the victim would either die or else begin to improve rapidly, with the fever breaking and disappearing quite suddenly. Hippocrates did not know what caused this train of events, but he meticulously set down his observations and wrote the first accurate medical description of the course of pneumococcal pneumonia ever to be recorded in medical literature.

Even the great Hippocrates had his limitations, however. Like other medical practitioners in those days, he rejected the idea of dissecting human cadavers to learn about the structure of the body, although there were no particular restrictions preventing such a practice. Also, like his colleagues, he regarded surgical treatment of illness as beneath his dignity, a matter to be left in the hands of slaves while he concentrated on treating illnesses with herbs, mineral baths and other conservative methods. Such surgery that was done at all was performed either by household servants or by itinerant "stonecutters" who traveled about the country removing foreign bodies from wounds, for example, or using crude surgical procedures for the removal of kidney or bladder stones, work that was always painful and often fatal because of the infection that almost inevitably followed.

Hippocrates' greatness lay not only in his careful observations, but in his teaching about the changes that occurred in the body with illness, and especially in his prolific medical writings, which were preserved and passed down through the centuries. In the course of a long and active life he founded a great school of medicine, but one of his most important contributions, in addition to his influence as a teacher, was his recognition that a sort of sacred trust must exist between physicians and the patients they treat. It was Hippocrates who first wrote down and taught the standards that should govern the physician's activities and his relationship to his patients, a code which even today remains the underlying basis of modern medical ethics, the so-called Hippocratic Oath.

The Medicine of Galen's Day

Gradually the influence of Greek medicine spread all over the known world. A great school and library of medicine developed at Alexandria in Egypt, for example, and Arabian physicians carried the knowledge of Greek medicine to centers of civilization in the Middle East and Persia. As Greek civilization declined, the value of Greek medicine was recognized by the powerful and ambitious Romans, whose prospective physicians studied medicine with Greek tutors and used Greek medical textbooks. The Romans, however, were far better administrators than innovators; they continued the work the Greek physicians had begun, but for the most part they did little to add to medical knowledge. A singular exception was in the work of one of history's most brilliant medical men, a young man who became world famous as Galen the Physician during the 2nd century A.D.

Galen was actually not a Roman at all, but a Greek born in the city of Pergamon in Asia Minor about the year A.D. 130. He apparently acquired a remarkable knowledge of anatomy as a very young man and began his practice of medicine as a surgeon to the gladiators. Traveling to Rome, he soon became a highly successful and fashionable physician among the upper crust of Roman society, and gathered a school of students and assistants around him. Far more a practical physician than a philosopher, he devoted himself vigorously to finding out *what worked* in the treatment of illness and injury without worrying greatly about *why* it worked.

Furiously energetic, egocentric and contentious, Galen built up a huge practice and a remarkable reputation, often largely on the basis of bluff and blunder; yet he, like Hippocrates, was an acute observer who meticulously wrote down his observations and case histories for future reference. Gradually he developed an immense body of knowledge and theory about human physiology and anatomy, and his teachings and writings were widely disseminated. By the time of his death at the beginning of the 3rd century A.D. he had become the single greatest influence in the world of medicine, and that influence would remain for more than a thousand years.

In some ways his influence was fortunate. In a field of study where the blind were still leading the blind, Galen was unquestionably somewhat less blind than his contemporaries. He wrote voluminously about symptoms, diagnosis and treatment of specific ills, and compiled exhaustive lists of drugs and medicines known in his day. Unfortunately, Galen was not really a scientist as we understand that term today. Much that was valid in his writings was scrambled up indistinguishably with his personal opinions, pet theories and unsupported assumptions. All too often in order to write "authoritatively" about something he did not know or understand, he simply made things up out of whole cloth. Yet throughout the ensuing centuries this strange mixture of the valid and the invalid took on the rigid authority of absolute dogma; no one dared challenge it. Some 1,300 years later when a highly unorthodox alchemist-physician who called himself Paracelsus was invited to become a member of the faculty of a medical school at Basle, he ran head-on into the lingering authority of the long-dead Galen. Condemning all medical teaching that was not based upon actual experience, a wildly unorthodox idea in the early 1500s, Paracelsus is reputed to have held a public burning of Galen's books to dramatize his position.

Even at the height of Roman civilization, however, health care was a matter for the wealthy few in society, while the vast mass of people either had no care at all or were forced to rely on untrained folk doctors. A few practices, to be sure, arose which foreshadowed the concept of public services designed to protect the general health of all the people. The Romans built an intricate system of aqueducts to supply their cities with pure water. They also practiced sanitary sewage disposal methods, and regulations for the slaughtering and handling of meat doubtless had some influence in controlling epidemic outbreaks of intestinal infections. But with the fall of the Roman Empire, these practices were discontinued. Centuries were to pass before even the most basic health care services would again become available to the common man.

Medieval Medicine and the Medical Renaissance

When the Dark Ages enveloped Europe, the theories and practice of medicine came to a virtual standstill; even what little was known of anatomy and physiology was largely forgotten. It was only in the monasteries that medical knowledge was kept alive at all, and there only by virtue of copying and preserving ancient manuscripts. During these many centuries, one of the few lights in the medical darkness was the establishment of a medical school in the town of Salerno in northern Italy in the 9th century A.D., where the teaching and practice of medicine continued.

Fortunately some real progress in medical knowledge was being made in a different part of the world. With the fall of the Roman Empire, the Mohammedan Empire began its gradual rise and spread. Greek and Roman medical works were translated into Arabic, and for several centuries medical teaching blossomed in the Middle East. Arabian and Persian physicians not only studied and taught the ancient texts but also made new and original contributions. Among them was Rhazes, who was born near Tehran in Persia in the middle 800s and who wrote hundreds of books, many of them containing his own clinical descriptions of such diseases as measles and smallpox. Another Persian, Avicenna (980–1037), gathered together medical knowledge derived from both ancient and Arabic writings into a great encyclopedia which became one of the main textbooks of medicine throughout the Middle East and the West until the 17th century. Ultimately their work was carried back to Europe during the Crusades and the great Islamic invasion of North Africa and Spain, ready for the reawakening of knowledge that was to begin in Europe in the 14th and 15th centuries.

Meanwhile, health care as such on the European continent was all but nonexistent. Feudal lords retained astrologers and alchemists in their courts, but the practice of medicine was little more than superstitious ritual. Surgery of any kind was relegated to the hands of traveling stonecutters or barbers. Epidemics of infectious diseases were commonplace and devastating, and the continent was swept time and time again with murderous waves of bubonic plague, an infection so deadly that it frequently took the lives of as many as three-quarters of the people in all the areas it struck.

Then, beginning in the 1300s, a slow but steady series of advances were made. Medieval universities such as the ones at Bologna in Italy, Basle in Switzerland and Montpelier in southern France developed medical faculties who translated textbooks from Greek and Arabic into Latin and began teaching students. Men like Paracelsus (1493–1541) began to emphasize the need for reliance on clinical observation, experience and experiment rather than blind faith in the ancient writings of Galen, an enormous contribution to the medical renaissance. The systematic study of human anatomy by means of dissection of cadavers began in the late 1200s and early 1300s, and this work was splendidly drawn together by Andreas Vesalius, who published in 1543 the first thorough and scientifically accurate textbook of human anatomy, *De Humani Corporis Fabrica* (On the Structure of the Human Body), complete with detailed illustrations that are valid even today. Among other early anatomists, oddly enough, were some of the great artists of the Renaissance, including Michelangelo and Raphael and most particularly Leonardo da Vinci (1452–1519), who himself began the preparation of a textbook of anatomy and physiology in collaboration with a young medical teacher at Padua, but left the work unfinished when his collaborator died.

Gradually the authority of such ancients as Galen and Avicenna was broken. With the awakening of other physical sciences such as astronomy, mathematics and physics, a more scientific method of investigation came into being, and new medical knowledge was more systematically acquired and recorded. It was in this climate that certain of the universities even began to teach surgery as a worthy medical discipline, and the early principles of surgical treatment of wounds were slowly evolved. It was also this climate of investigation which encouraged the monumental work of the English physician William Harvey and led to his discovery of circulation of the blood by 1615, although he did not publish his famous book *De Motu Cordis* (On the Movement of the Heart) until thirteen years later when he had repeated his studies and experiments again and again to satisfy himself that he had made no possible mistake. Harvey was never able to explain all the details of circulation, for he had no way to see the capillary vessels through which blood from the arteries had to pass to reach the veins and thus be returned to the heart. This part of the puzzle was finally supplied by the Italian anatomist Marcello Malpighi, who was born in the year that Harvey's book was published and who was finally able to observe the passage of blood from the arteries to the veins through the capillary vessels in the lung of a frog in 1661 with the aid of a simple single-lensed microscope. It was only twenty years later that the Dutch naturalist Anton van Leeuwenhoek (1632–1723), using a similar microscope designed by himself with a carefully hand-ground lens—really nothing more than a very powerful magnifying glass—began a series of observations that opened the door to a whole previously unsuspected world of microscopic life and eventually led to the great scientific studies of infectious diseases carried out by Pasteur, Koch and many others some 200 years later.

The Age of Medical Discovery

Step by step, as one investigation led to another, the stage was set for the greatest explosion of medical discovery in all history, an explosion which began in the mid-1700s and is still reverberating today.

It is not possible here even to summarize the many breakthroughs that contributed to the vast body of precise medical knowledge that we have today. Some were the work of basic medical research, the seemingly endless labor of identifying thousands of newly discovered microscopic organisms, demonstrating how each was responsible for specific infections, and studying how they were spread and what methods could be devised to protect potential victims. Detailed surgical studies of the human anatomy at last tore away the veils obscuring even the most puzzling structures of the body. A tortuous chain of experiments, both with laboratory animals and with human beings, gradually clarified the mysteries of human physiology and the many strange ways in which the organ systems of the body function both in health and in illness. Equally intricate investigation was required to unravel the complicated biochemical reactions that enter into human metabolism, the "chemistry of life." Other discoveries were in the realm of clinical medicine, discoveries that were made by hard-working physicians and surgeons observing their sick patients, studying the course of their illnesses and doggedly seeking out newer and better ways of diagnosing and treating disease. The English physician Edward Jenner (1749–1823) placed his career and his reputation at stake in 1796 when he performed the first successful vaccination of a young patient against smallpox more than a century before the virus that causes smallpox was even discovered. Ambroise Paré (1517–1590), a French army surgeon who was appalled at the uniformly horrible results that were obtained when gunshot wounds in battle were treated, as was the custom, by immersion in boiling oil, devoted a long and illustrious career to treating surgical patients with gentle and conservative techniques which did much to elevate surgery from a despised handicraft to an honored and respected branch of the healing art. Thomas Sydenham (1624–1689) was an English physician who is seldom heard of today outside of medical histories, yet he dominated the field of clinical medicine in Europe in the 17th century, studied the natural course of multitudes of diseases in more careful detail than anyone before him, and introduced the idea, revolutionary at the time, that many of the effects of disease, however grave, were nothing more than the natural, vigorous effort of the body to destroy or eliminate noxious factors so that self-healing could be possible. Benjamin Rush (1745–1813) of Philadelphia was a great humanitarian and physician who worked vigorously to abolish the chaining and physical torture of the mentally ill in American asylums and was far ahead of his time in teaching simple hygiene and public health measures as a means of preventing infectious diseases. The great English surgeon Joseph Lister (1827–1912) fought down the scorn of his colleagues and almost single-handedly brought about a revolution in surgical techniques that is today the very foundation of modern surgery—the introduction of the antiseptic techniques and procedures which prevent the contamination of surgical wounds with infectious bacteria. Finally, many of these discoveries were in the field of public health, brought about by the growing realization that maintaining high standards of health and sanitation is the responsibility of society as a whole, working together under competent medical direction to achieve safe water supplies, hygienic sewage disposal, the prevention of dangerous infectious illnesses, and the creation of human living conditions that make it difficult for disease to gain a foothold.

Bit by bit this great wave of discovery found its way from research laboratories and clinics into the medical schools and thus into the hands of medical practitioners throughout the Western world. At the same time convulsive social and political changes had the effect of bringing skilled health care to a larger and larger proportion of the general populace. Both the American and the French revolutions helped establish the principle of the equality of all men; rich and poor alike were entitled to certain inalienable rights, among them the right to good health. The prolonged European wars of the 18th and 19th centuries brought medical care to great numbers of men in the field. And ironically, the Industrial Revolution which spawned some of the most inhuman living and working conditions the world has ever known also contributed to the spread of medical care. Industrial medicine, the vigorous pursuit of methods to prevent illness and injury among workingmen on the job and the provision of inexpensive medical services to bring the ill swiftly back to work, was a further powerful influence in bringing health care to the common man.

By the beginning of the 20th century, a great change had been wrought in the attitude of the average man toward the care of his health. For the first time in history people began to realize that illness and disease are not necessarily the natural and inescapable lot of humankind. Hospitals were no longer regarded as places where people went to die and therefore to be avoided at all costs, but rather as places where the duration of illnesses could be shortened by skillful treatment and proper care. Families who had formerly called on the services of a physician only as a desperate last resort began for the first time to seek medical help at the beginning of an illness in hopes of curbing or curing it as quickly as possible. And inevitably, these changing attitudes led to another quite revolutionary idea: that in many cases commonsense precautions and a sensible program of health care can *prevent* many diseases from occurring at all, and postpone the onset of others. It was in this climate of thought that the health care explosion of the 20th century began to take place.

2

The Twentieth-Century Health Care Explosion

In the world of medicine there was nothing magical or mystical about the year 1901, even though it was the first year of a new century and the beginning of a millennium as well. Of course there were all the predictions and speculations one would expect on such an occasion—virtually all of them to fall ridiculously short of the actual march of history that later generations would observe. Perhaps a few romantics in the ranks of medicine paused to reflect that medical knowledge had come a long way in the thousand years just past, but scientists in general are a practical lot, and beyond a fleeting acknowledgment of the start of a new century, most physicians and medical researchers probably went on with their usual activities without much anticipation of the staggering changes the next few decades were destined to bring.

In point of fact, medical knowledge had come a long way indeed during the last thousand years. At the beginning of that time the Western world had witnessed only the first faint stirrings of a scientific revolution that would require centuries to develop full force. What little was known then about human illness and its treatment had been handed down from antiquity, much of it garbled, mistranslated, misunderstood or misinterpreted. As the centuries passed, bits of the truth were slowly and painfully winnowed out of the vast morass of misinformation. To this shaky foundation additional fragments of truth were added a little at a time. Gradually a scientific method of investigation was evolved which made it possible for learned men to test the validity of their assumptions and observations, to move beyond this to the point where they could actually formulate intelligent questions about human disease and then proceed to find answers, make predictions and discover new knowledge. And during the last 200 years of the millennium medical knowledge had begun to accumulate in a swiftly accelerating and ever expanding spiral, reaching into every avenue and byway of human experience with disease.

With the beginning of the 20th century this expanding spiral continued without pause, gathering momentum with every passing year. The Golden Age of discovery had been reached and continues to this day. Diseases that had plagued humans for centuries were at last brought under control as more was learned about the nature of these illnesses and the ways to protect men against them. Public health measures eliminated many plague spots. The science of pharmacology began to flower, bringing forth multitudes of new drugs and medicines with which to fight illness. Previously unheard-of surgical techniques were devised and perfected, vastly expanding the range of illnesses that could be treated with surgery, while a long succession of discoveries in anesthesiology rendered surgical procedures more safe and effective. Widespread application of immunization techniques made it possible virtually to eliminate some of the most dreadful of the infectious diseases: whereas more than 30,000 American soldiers in World War I died in agony of tetanus contracted with their battle wounds, only 12 cases of tetanus were reported among our armed forces during World War II, thanks to the immunization of every GI against tetanus during his first few weeks in service. The discovery of antibiotics, a time-consuming program of research that was actually started in the early 1920s with the study of "bacteriophages"—substances made by certain bacteria which seemed to inhibit the growth of other bacteria—and which came to fruition with Sir Alexander Fleming's almost accidental discovery of penicillin in 1928, completely revolutionized the treatment of multitudes of infectious diseases, most ancient and relentless of all human health hazards. Scores of other discoveries, each basic in some way to the development of the quality of health care that we take for granted today, piled one on top of the other with each passing decade of this century, an awesome progression that still continues.

But it has not been in the area of new medical knowledge alone that the 20th-century health care explosion has been taking place. Since the beginning of the century there has also been an explosion, equally awesome, in the way health care has been provided in the United States, in the numbers of people to whom it has become available and—perhaps most fundamental of all—in our basic attitudes toward the treatment of illness, the availability of health care services, the preservation of general health on an individual basis, and the purposes to which our health care facilities should best be turned, both for our greatest benefit as individuals and for the benefit of our society.

Health Care in America, 1901

To understand the full impact of changes in our attitudes toward medical care in the last several decades, we should consider for a moment just how medicine was practiced in the cities and countrysides of America at the beginning of the 20th century.

Certainly it was far different then from now. Although we were growing in industrial might, America was still predominantly an agricultural country, largely isolated from and indifferent to the social and political storm clouds that were gathering so rapidly abroad. The great universities and clinics of London, Paris, Berlin and Vienna were still the fountainheads of medicine; the American physician who wished to establish a reputation as a specialist was obliged to go abroad for his training if he wanted colleagues or patients to pay serious attention to him.

The majority of doctors in this country at the time did not become specialists. Medical care, for the most part, was provided by general practitioners whose medical school and hospital training, while good enough for the time, was still thoroughly primitive by today's standards. Not that these were not diligent, often selfless men. In rural areas, villages and small cities they were the family doctors of the old school. Many of them practiced in the communities where they grew up. They knew their patients well, often as friends as well as medical consultants, frequently treating three generations in the same family. Usually practicing "solo," they were on call constantly, working long hours in their office dispensaries, devoting hours each day to hospital calls on their patients and thinking nothing of traveling long distances day or night to make house calls.

However limited they may have been in knowledge or skill, they did the best they knew how in all fields of medicine at once, struggling with difficult diagnoses, dispensing medicines, suturing lacerations, setting and treating fractured bones, delivering babies, providing the only pediatric care that was available for children, and performing such surgery as was within their capabilities—and often a good deal that was not. It was only in the gravest of cases that consultation with a specialist was sought, and in most areas of the country the idea that one might consult directly with a surgeon, an obstetrician or an endocrinologist simply never entered a patient's mind. Even in the large cities, where specialists tended to congregate (partly because of better hospital, surgical and laboratory facilities), the patient referrals of 25 general practitioners were needed to keep one specialist in business. Nor was cost, in those days, a serious impediment in seeking medical advice. The family doctor, after a few years of genteel poverty while establishing his practice and paying his medical school debts, was usually comfortably well off, but he was seldom rich, and most of his patients, considering the demands that were made upon him, did not envy him his fees. It was only in cases that required extensive specialty consultation or really prolonged hospital treatment that the cost of medical care became burdensome.

Of course the average American's general attitude toward health care in those days was strikingly different from what it is today. A considerable amount of illness was simply accepted as part of the natural condition and nothing to see a doctor about. Most of the common children's diseases, for example, including such vicious infections as pertussis (whooping cough) or diphtheria, were considered more or less inevitable and were commonly treated at home without medical help unless a victim became gravely ill. Even then the mother knew perfectly well that the doctor would probably have very little to offer, and if a call went out to him it would be a call of desperation in hope of a miracle. Unfortunately, those were not yet the days of medical miracles. Other conditions were stolidly accepted as beyond care: the grandmother with rheumatism, by and large, suffered with it; the farm worker with an inguinal hernia or rupture struggled along with a truss until the hernia became strangulated and took him to the operating table in a life-or-death emergency. And although growing numbers of women in the city went to hospital maternity wards to have their babies, in country areas deliveries were still conducted at home, often with the assistance of local midwives rather than doctors. A great many Americans *never* consulted a doctor, or thought of doing so, even when their lives were plagued repeatedly or continuously with illness, minor or grave.

The New Physician

The status of health care in this country early in the 20th century was limited in its scope as much by widely prevailing attitudes of the people as by the still-narrow capabilities of the doctor. Then, with the end of the First World War and the growing exuberance of the 1920s, a vast revolution began to take place in these attitudes. Like most far-reaching revolutions in the way people feel and think, this one was the result not so much of specific incidents or events as of certain germinal ideas that began to appear. And indeed, in the 40 or 50 years following the end of World War I, there were four such basic yet radical ideas that became widely accepted—ideas which today form the groundwork of our modern attitudes toward health care.

The first of these ideas, perhaps most basic of all, was simply *that proper medical care could actually do something about the course of human illness, that the doctor's work could produce results.* Gradually the impact of the spiraling growth of medical knowledge began to be felt the length and breadth of this country, and it openly challenged the notion that human illness and disease were necessary evils about which nothing could be done. Doctors were learning to *cure* diseases which they previously could only palliate. Concerted attacks upon one medical problem after another had produced not only new knowledge about illness but *solutions.* Means of preventing once-dread diseases were being found. New medicines were coming into use which could turn the progress of an illness, or prevent dangerous complications, or markedly shorten convalescence. New surgical techniques were making it possible to cure certain diseases quickly and easily, diseases which previously had meant prolonged periods of suffering, physical danger or even death.

As these facts became known, many people no longer thought twice about calling a doctor. The wage earner could not afford to be thrown out of work for weeks while he convalesced from an illness; if a doctor could actually do something to shorten that convalescence, and get the man back to work in half the time, then his services were valuable indeed. This thinking extended to hospital care as well; if hospital treatment could help ensure or speed recovery, perhaps hospitalization was not so bad after all. If the new surgical procedures could be performed with fewer risks in a modern hospital operating room than on the kitchen table, perhaps greater effort to reach a hospital would prove worthwhile. If the delivery of babies could be handled more skillfully, comfortably and safely in a hospital, with a far greater degree of protection against the rare but disastrous complications of childbirth, then the "advantages" of home delivery began to look less and less advantageous.

Above all, the old-fashioned family doctor was gradually transformed into an entirely new breed of physician. A few brief years in medical school and his own practical experience were not enough to keep abreast of new medical ideas and techniques; to offer his patients the best and most modern methods of health care, the new physician needed additional years of training, wider clinical experience and an opportunity to study with doctors highly skilled in various medical specialties. He also needed the finest and most modern equipment in his office or surgery, reliable laboratory services within easy reach, frequent and dependable consultation with medical specialists in every field, and a well-equipped and well-managed hospital in which to treat his sicker patients. Like the carpenter first confronted with a power saw, this new physician began to realize *what might be possible* with the aid of the growing body of medical knowledge at his command. For the first time it began to seem that the age-old dream of a world in which illness and disease could be eradicated might actually be coming within reach, and the new physician of the 20th century picked up the challenge.

The New Patient

The second germinal idea which was to help transform our attitudes toward health care arose from the social convulsions that shook the nation and the world during the great depression of the 1930s. Poverty stalked the land, millions were without work, and the country drained its resources to find means to help those who were unable, through no fault of their own, to help themselves—to protect a man from the specter of starvation when he grew too old to work, and to provide humane services, including health care, to the innocent and helpless who might suffer or die without them. In a great wave of social legislation such enduring programs as So-

cial Security and Public Welfare came into being. Hospital facilities and outpatient clinics were vastly expanded to fill the health care needs of those on welfare programs. New county and Public Health Service hospitals were built all over the country; free or low-cost well-baby clinics were established to help care for the children of needy families; public health services throughout the country were expanded, and vast immunization programs were financed for the public benefit.

It was also for the first time, during this period, that the cost of adequate health care became a matter of widespread public concern. The physician suffered along with everyone else during the depression, but at least he had work to do. People with no money and no job found themselves unable to meet the costs of health care they had begun to value and then demand, and although physicians individually, as a matter of professional responsibility, often donated their time and energy generously in manning free clinics and providing care for indigent patients, this work was unmistakably charity. As in so many societies before, it seemed that physician and hospital services were still essentially the privilege of the well-to-do, with the less fortunate left to struggle as best they could. But whereas this notion had once been stoically accepted as inevitable, it was now met with a sense of public outrage. And from this outrage a second germinal idea evolved: *that the maintenance of a sound body and good health with the aid of modern health care facilities is—or should be—a natural right of everyone, not a privilege reserved for those who can afford it.* In short, medical care should be available to all, with society at large undertaking the burden of the cost.

That idea was a far cry from the prevailing attitude toward medical care at the turn of the century. Nor was it by any means accepted by everyone. In fact, it is still a matter of heated debate in our country today, at least in part because no one as yet has been able to think of any acceptable, practical way to implement it. In countries that have tried it—Great Britain, Sweden, parts of Canada, Russia—the results have not been overwhelmingly impressive. In some cases the costs have been staggering, in others the doctors providing the health care have been manifestly unhappy, in still others the quality of health care has been poor. The debate in this country may well continue for years, but there is no question that the idea that every individual has a natural right to enjoy good health, insofar as this can be achieved, has had an overwhelming impact upon our basic attitudes toward health care, for it has made each one of us aware that to a very large extent *good health can be preserved,* given thoughtful attention and the medical resources that exist today.

The New Goal

The third fundamental idea, following naturally from the first two, and coming strongly to public awareness in the past 20 or 30 years, is *that preventive health care is the most valuable health care of all.* Before very much was known about the human body or human illness, the practice of medicine was largely curative, for there was no way then to deal with illness until it had already occurred. Of course, if cure was possible, it was of great value, but obviously knowledgeable health care could be of immensely greater value if it could help prevent the illness in the first place.

Today we know that many human illnesses are completely or partially preventable. This is by no means limited to the infectious diseases that can be prevented by immunization. Many other illnesses have very specific causes that are now clearly understood. We know the natural histories of many diseases in detail; we have come to recognize the signs and symptoms of many diseases when they first appear; and we know that many diseases can be stopped cold, effectively cured, if proper treatment begins early enough. In other diseases in which cure may not be possible, the natural progression of the disease can often be controlled for years.

Indeed, with the wealth of medical knowledge available to us today, with the wealth of laboratory, X-ray and other facilities that enable physicians to diagnose an illness early or to monitor its progress effectively, it is often possible to predict quite accurately what the course of a newly diagnosed disorder will be, and to what degree that course may be altered by various preventive or therapeutic programs of treatment. Further, the physician performing a complete medical history and a thorough physical examination on a healthy young man or woman should be able to outline the *prognostic hazards* his patients may face in the coming years—the kinds of illness that they, as individuals, may be most vulnerable to, and with that knowledge undertake a rational program of preventive observation and maintenance designed to avoid the hazards insofar as possible.

It was doctors themselves, by and large, who first saw the enormous potential of preventive health care and brought this idea to their patients. But even the most vigorous proponent of the idea freely admitted its drawbacks. Many diseases simply could not be predicted in advance. Others could not be detected early enough to do much good. The most highly skilled physician in the world cannot perform miracles, and often the most rational and faithfully executed plan of prevention may prove ineffective. There was always the chance that totally unexpected illness might render a preventive program useless.

But for all of this, out of the idea of preventive medicine, so demonstrably reasonable that no one can argue its merits, emerged a totally new and immensely hopeful concept, a new goal for family health care, entirely attainable with the utilization of our modern medical facilities, far more desirable and far less costly, in the long run, than the old, inadequate goal of attempting to cure disease after it occurs. This new goal—a goal based squarely on the idea of preventive medicine—is very simple: *the maintenance of optimum good health from birth to death.*

The Medical Partnership

The very expression "the maintenance of optimum good health" represented a major change in attitude toward the most effective use of existing medical facilities. The concept of curative medicine was, of course, still extremely important—no one would deny the full resources of medicine to those afflicted with sickness or disease. But here was a change of emphasis which heretofore was virtually unknown. According to this new concept, optimum good health should be the normal condition of life; sickness or disease was the abnormal. What was more, the concept emphasized that optimum good health *could and should be maintained* for as long as possible in every human life. We had the medical knowledge and facilities to do just that; why not use them? Why not use them to their fullest advantage in a way that would do the most good for the most people at the least cost in money, wasted time and human agony?

It was a sound idea, and when seriously applied, it has worked. Its advantages to every family are obvious, particularly today when the cost of medical services, doctors' fees, hospital charges, medical insurance and taxes to pay for "free" or "low-cost" public health facilities becomes greater every year. If a dollar spent to prevent trouble and help maintain optimum good health can save ten dollars treating an illness which might have been prevented or held in control, then that dollar is clearly spent for a bargain.

But the concept of preventive care as a means of maintaining optimum good health necessarily led to one final germinal idea: that ultimately the maintenance of good health is in large part the responsibility not of society, or of the government, or of the doctor or the hospital or the prepaid medical plan, but *of the individual himself*. Preventive health care requires the full utilization of every modern medical facility. But no physician, no matter how great his skill and no matter what facilities are at his command, can do the job alone. He must depend upon the concerned cooperation of the chief benefactor of these medical facilities: the individual patient himself.

If preventive health care is to work effectively, obviously each individual must accept his share of the responsibility. Each individual must recognize the value of maintaining good health and of seeking to prevent illness rather than waiting for it to occur. Each individual should be responsible for learning what he can do himself to maintain his body and his health in good order; he should be aware of the kinds of emergencies that can occur and should be familiar with the first-aid measures necessary to minimize their impact. Above all, each individual should recognize his own responsibility to work with his physician knowledgeably, not only when he is ill but when he is in good health, in order to reduce to the minimum the chances of being overtaken by destructive and preventable illness.

In short, modern preventive health care requires an active partnership between the physician and his patient. The doctor must provide a depth of medical knowledge, a command of medical resources, and the benefits of clinical experience that no one without lengthy medical training can hope to acquire. But the patient can contribute equally in terms of concern, awareness, and basic knowledge of health and disease, with preventive care a matter for his conscious effort and cooperation.

Without such teamwork health care would always remain basically curative, regardless of the medical knowledge accumulated in the future, and the maintenance of optimum good health would remain elusively unattainable. But with modern resources, the active teamwork of doctor and patient can become a virtually unbeatable combination. For the modern American family today it can provide the most powerful and effective health protection that history has ever known.

THE HEALTHY BODY AND HOW IT WORKS

3. The Building Blocks: Cells and Tissues   19

4. Support and Mobility: The Musculoskeletal System   25

5. Motivation and Moderation: The Nervous System   42

6. Protection and Appearance: The Cutaneous System   55

7. Exchange, Filtration and Secretion: The Lungs, Kidneys and Endocrines   62

8. The River of Life: The Cardiovascular System   75

9. The Fuels of Life: Digestion and Metabolism   84

10. Conspiracy Against Death: Reproduction and Preservation   92

3

The Building Blocks: Cells and Tissues

No one knows just when man first appeared and took his place as the dominant creature on this planet. Intelligent, curious and aggressive, he soon outstripped all rivals in the animal kingdom, adapting to life in virtually every climate and condition the planet had to offer. Not once in all the centuries since he first arose has his supremacy on Earth been seriously challenged. To a large extent, his dominion and survival have been possible because of the remarkable nature of his body and the superb brain with which he is equipped. Yet for all its importance, most of us know very little about the structure and function of our single most valuable possession: the human body.

Perhaps it is not surprising that we are oblivious to our bodies so much of the time. Normally, very little is required on our part to keep them operating. Such vital functions as breathing, digestion and heartbeat go on whether we pay attention to them or not. When minor breakdowns occur, they are automatically repaired, often without our even being aware of it. Of course, there are certain things we must do by way of upkeep and maintenance. We must find food, warmth and shelter, but even these jobs have become such an automatic part of our daily lives that we rarely give them a second thought. Usually, it is only when we are injured, when illness strikes, or when some decline in function overtakes us due to fatigue, age or anxiety that we become aware of our bodies at all.

Unfortunately, things *do* go wrong. Injuries of all sorts plagued men from the beginning of time. The ancient Egyptians knew of epilepsy and coronary artery disease, and again and again history records the devastating effects of plagues such as the one that afflicted Athens during the Peloponnesian War. Throughout the ages men have searched for ways to repair injuries and cure disease, usually by a process of trial and error. But bit by bit, starting from the simple observations of early physicians to the most complex revelations of modern medical science, we have acquired a remarkably accurate and useful working knowledge of the way the body is made and the way it functions in health and disease.

What is the body? How is it constructed and how does it perform its everyday activities? We often tend to think of it only in terms of its parts—a sprained ankle, a cut finger, an eye irritated by a speck of dust—but it is much more than a collection of bones here, a bundle of muscles there, a brain, a pair of lungs or a beating heart. Each part must be understood in its relation to every other part, for the body is a *functioning unit* with every part integrated into a supremely logical structure and operating together with other parts to accomplish goals.

As a functioning unit, the body has certain remarkable strengths and, in surprising contrast, some equally remarkable weaknesses and limitations. A mountain climber can fall 500 feet down a slope, smashing ribs, vertebrae, both legs and his skull, and still survive to climb another mountain. Another man, attacked by a submicroscopic virus, may be dead in 48 hours from bulbar poliomyelitis. The human body can adjust to the Arctic cold or the blast-furnace heat of the Arabian desert on the outside, yet an internal fever of eight degrees will permanently destroy vital nerve tissue. Man can survive for days without water or for weeks without food, yet he will die in 20 seconds if some poison such as cyanide suddenly cuts off the supply of oxygen to all of his body's cells simultaneously. He is capable of amazing feats of physical strength, but even a relatively light blow to a strong man's abdomen can rupture the spleen and lead to death from hemorrhage in less than an hour.

One of man's most critical strengths is his ability to use his mind to protect and defend his body, to outwit his enemies instead of outrunning them. This more than anything else sets him apart from other animals. Yet the precious tissue of the human brain is more vulnerable to damage than any other, and unlike other tissues it cannot be repaired. Other curious vulnerabilities—the ease with which our eyes can be injured, for instance—seem to be balanced by special advantages such as our very sensitive finger touch or the fact that our thumbs oppose our fingers.

These strengths and weaknesses result directly from the way the body is constructed and the way it functions. We often speak of the body's structure (or anatomy) and its function (or physiology) as if these were different things. But the two can never really be separated. In order for the body to function as a unit, each part must be complete and do its job properly. Each part in turn depends upon the proper functioning of all the other parts. Thus, oxygen is normally taken up by the lungs, carried to the tissues by blood, and used by the cells there to oxidize fuels—three separate functions of three different body parts. But the cells cannot obtain oxygen if the lungs fail to absorb it properly, or if the flow of blood is obstructed.

In many ways the human body resembles an exceedingly complex machine, precision built from a variety of materials and designed to perform a multitude of tasks. Like a machine, it must have sturdy structural members and some kind of protection from the outside elements. Its most vital working parts must be specially shielded from damage. Like a machine, the body has movable parts, so there has to be a power source to provide energy for motion, along with some arrangement for the transportation of fuel, its utilization and the elimination of waste by-products. It must also have an intricate central control system with built-in facilities for data storage and an efficient mechanism for picking up signals and sending out operational directives. Maintenance is necessary, too. There must be a temperature and humidity control system, for instance, and a janitorial and cleaning service, an efficient self-repair system, a warning and alarm system, a complex pharmaceutical plant, and a dozen other equally critical systems all at work simultaneously.

Many man-made machines can perform some combination of these functions. A relatively complicated machine like an automobile is similar to the human body in many ways, but such a device must be constructed out of hundreds of different parts and materials. The truly remarkable thing about the human body, which is infinitely more complex, is that all its myriad parts are built up from a single basic unit—the living cell—woven together into a mere handful of different structural materials or tissues. In fact, the entire body in all its complexity is constructed of just six basic tissues: *bone, muscle, connective tissue, neurons* (or nerve tissue), *epithelium* (skin and internal membranes) and *blood.*

To understand how such a complex machine can be built from so few materials, we have to begin with a description of the single living cell. There is really no alternative, for the cell is the simplest example there is of a complete and organized unit of life. Probably the first of all living creatures to appear in the warm seas of our planet were one-celled organisms, the ancient ancestors of present-day algae and slime molds. Today we know that certain mysterious protein complexes called viruses are even more primitive, occupying a twilight world between the living and the nonliving, but these tiny entities are not really complete organisms. We are not even sure they are truly alive. For all practical purposes then, the cell is the basic structural unit of all living organisms from the lowly ameba on up. The human body is constructed of hundreds of billions of living cells, and every minute detail of its structure and function is determined by those cells and the reactions that occur within them.

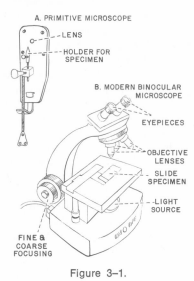

A. PRIMITIVE MICROSCOPE
LENS
HOLDER FOR SPECIMEN
B. MODERN BINOCULAR MICROSCOPE
EYEPIECES
OBJECTIVE LENSES
SLIDE SPECIMEN
LIGHT SOURCE
FINE & COARSE FOCUSING

Figure 3–1.

The cellular nature of living things is such commonplace knowledge today that we forget how recently it was discovered. Until the middle of the 17th century, very few scientists even suspected the existence of living cells. Anton van Leeuwenhoek was not really a scientist at all; we can imagine his surprise when he peered through his primitive "magnifying tube" and discovered that a drop of perfectly clear pond water was actually teeming with tiny creatures invisible to the naked eye—the "animalcules" he later described to the incredulous Royal Society of London. Many of Leeuwenhoek's "animalcules" were common bacteria, but he also described the flat, tile-shaped cells that line the inside of the mouth like pieces of a mosaic, and discovered that a droplet of his own blood was in fact filled with thousands of tiny cell bodies. Today Leeuwenhoek is often called the father of bacteriology, but his first clumsy observations opened the door to a completely new understanding of how all living organisms, including the human body, are made.

In its simplest form the living cell is a tiny transparent blob of fluid contained within a thin membrane or *cell wall*. A cell is so small that as many as 8 million of them may be found in a half-inch cube of tissue in the human body. Within the cell wall the jelly-like fluid which is called *protoplasm* contains a variety of chemical substances dissolved or suspended in it, including inorganic materials like sodium and chloride ions and organic substances such as sugar and protein molecules. Inside the cell, an even tinier island of matter, the *nucleus,* is isolated by another membrane, the *nuclear wall.* The nucleus contains the complex long-chain protein molecules and nucleic acids which together make up the critical life substance of the cell. Among other things, these form the genetic templates or *chromosomes* which determine the nature of the cell and the organism of which it is a part.

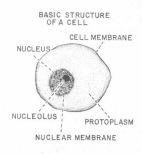

BASIC STRUCTURE OF A CELL
CELL MEMBRANE
NUCLEUS
NUCLEOLUS
PROTOPLASM
NUCLEAR MEMBRANE

Figure 3–2.

There are many characteristics which distinguish this tiny living cell from its nonliving counterparts. Most obvious and striking is the quality of life itself. No one knows precisely why the cells of the human body are alive while crystals of salt or quartz are not, but the life of the cell is clearly related to the complex substances that lie within its nucleus. Part and parcel of this quality of life is the cell's ability to grow in size, to act as a tiny cellular furnace in which fuel materials are burned, and ultimately to reproduce perfect copies of itself.

These fundamental life functions are common to all living cells. But certain cells have special additional capabilities of their own. Some, for instance, can collect and store insoluble calcium salts—the special cells that make up bone tissue. Some cells are immobile, but others can move from place to place, a quality best known in the ameba, but shared by certain of the white blood cells which roam about the body fighting off invading bacteria. Other cells have the curious ability to contract in response to certain stimuli —to draw back when pinched, so to speak— while still others grow tendrils, sometimes as much as four or five feet in length, along which electrochemical impulses can travel at high speeds, much the same as electrons travel along a copper wire. Certain kinds of cells intertwine themselves into fibrous connective tissue networks, sometimes tough and binding like the skin of a sausage, sometimes delicate and filamentous, sometimes as elastic as a rubber band. Other cells can form strong protective linings, secrete special chemicals, or stretch out into thin semipermeable membranes—all functions of epithelial tissue.

The remarkable ability of living cells to take on specialized characteristics is brilliantly illustrated in the earliest stages of the development of the human embryo after conception. Every human body, with its multitude of organs and tissues, ultimately begins its life as a single living cell, the fertilized ovum. This cell is unique among all the body cells because it is formed by the union of two incomplete "germ" cells from the parents, each with only half the genetic material contained by all the other cells. But once two germ cells have fused, the completed or "fertilized" cell has a remarkable potential.

For the first 24 hours after fertilization the cell simply rests, as if gathering strength for the difficult job ahead. Then it begins to grow and divide at a rate far exceeding that of any other tissue. For the first three days or so this growth is little more than carbon-copy reproduction; the new cells are precisely the same as the old and form a round blob of tissue shaped like a hollow ball. But presently a few of the newly formed cells begin to vary from the others. The rudimentary embryo dents in upon itself to become a tiny cuplike structure, and then the cup becomes an elongated pouch. Soon the cells lining the inside of the pouch begin to show quite different characteristics from those on the outside. By the seventh day, still a third kind of cell begins to appear between the inner and outer layers of the pouch, and within ten days the original fertilized ovum has given rise to three well-differentiated layers of tissue, each distinctly different from the others.

At this state of development the human embryo is still ridiculously tiny—less than a quarter of an inch long—yet already the pattern of its future development is set. Each of the three embryonic precursor tissues, called the *ectoderm* (outer layer), the *endoderm* (inner layer) and the *mesoderm* (middle layer), begins to differentiate further, giving rise to the organs of a rudimentary human body. The endoderm elongates to form a primitive gut and then develops tiny air tubes, lungs, liver and other digestive glands. The ectoderm forms a crease along the back of the embryo which later differentiates into the nerve tissue of the spinal cord and brain, while other parts of the ectoderm form the skin, hair, nails and sensory organs. From the mesoderm the connective tissue, muscle and bone develop, as well as the kidneys and the muscular walls of the blood vessels. At the end of three months the fetus is only 2½ inches long, but virtually every detail of differentiation and construction of its body has already taken place, step by step, through variation of the cells in the precursor tissues. The remaining six months of gestation are devoted almost solely to growth and refinement of this new human body to prepare it for life in the outside world.

The simple cell, then, is not so simple after all. The hundreds of billions of cells that make up the human body display a remarkable variety of specialized forms and functions. These variations do not stop with their specialization into the six basic tissues; the cells that make up these tissues are even further specialized. The long, spindly cells bound together in bundles to form the powerful muscle fibers of the leg, for instance, are quite different from the softer and flatter cells of the smooth muscle in the bowel, or from the interlocking meshwork of cells that form the heart muscle. Yet these cells share a characteristic that identifies them all as varying forms of muscle and nothing else—the ability to contract when stimulated and then relax when the stimulus has passed. It is this characteristic which permits muscle tissue of any kind to perform its job, and no other cell or tissue in the body has this unique contractile ability.

Similarly, it is hard to see any relationship between the tough skin on the ball of the foot, the moist inner lining of the lung, and the thick cords of the bile-secreting tissue in the liver. Yet all these varying forms of epithelial tissue have certain vital characteristics in common. Bone tissue may be dense and brittle in one place and spongy in another, while connective tissue may take a dozen different forms to serve different purposes.

SPECIALIZATION OF CELLS

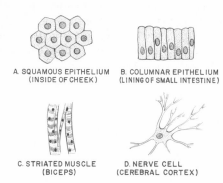

A. SQUAMOUS EPITHELIUM (INSIDE OF CHEEK)

B. COLUMNAR EPITHELIUM (LINING OF SMALL INTESTINE)

C. STRIATED MUSCLE (BICEPS)

D. NERVE CELL (CEREBRAL CORTEX)

Figure 3–3.

It is variations and specializations like these that contribute to the enormous complexity of the body. But cells and tissues, in all their variety, are only the basic building blocks of the human organism. They combine in even greater complexity to form the organ systems that sustain life. Some organs are chiefly formed of a single basic tissue. The skeleton, for example, is primarily bone tissue, while the lung is largely epithelium, although of several different kinds. But the cardiovascular system, including the heart and the vast network of vessels for transporting blood to and from all parts of the body, is constructed of several of the basic tissues: epithelium, which lines the inside of the heart and blood vessels, three different kinds of muscle tissue, tissue to regulate the heart's rhythm and control the rate of blood flow, and connective

tissue which helps hold the heart, the great vessels and the tiny capillaries in their proper places throughout the body. In such a "mixed" organ system, each of the basic tissues has a specific contribution and each must perform its job properly in order for the whole system to work.

Ideally, if all the tissues did their jobs perfectly all the time, the body would suffer no illness, no effects of injury, no wear and tear or breakdown. Unfortunately, nature does not permit such perfection. All of us are vulnerable to malfunctions at one time or another, with ill effects ranging from the annoyance of a common cold to the massive disability of a broken leg or the devastating tissue destruction of a malignant tumor. Sometimes the nature of the malfunction is obvious. When a leg is fractured on a ski slope, it clearly cannot be used to support weight again until the sheared bone heals and hardens. Other malfunctions cannot be detected by simple observation, but examination of tissues under the microscope may reveal changes associated with diseases. Still other malfunctions are even more subtle. We could search every tissue in the body looking for the offender in diabetes mellitus and never find it unless we began to check certain critical biochemical reactions. All the same, we know that malfunctioning tissue cells in the pancreas are the villains, even when we cannot see any physical change in their structure.

Just as the normal functions of a healthy body depend upon the health of its basic tissues, so diseases and malfunctions are always the direct result of breakdowns or disturbances that occur in these basic tissues. Since the body is seldom completely "normal" in all respects, it is not enough to examine its structure and function under normal conditions only. We must also consider the ever present effects of disease, injury or malfunction if we are to see how the body really works. By considering the normal and the abnormal side by side in succeeding chapters we can develop a full picture of the body as a functioning unit, both in sickness and in health. This is, in fact, the way physicians have learned about the nature of human illness over the centuries; and, indeed, this work of discovery is still continuing at an ever increasing pace even today in doctors' offices, laboratories, hospitals and operating rooms all over the world, even though every time a question is answered five new questions seem to arise. Surgeons today are performing operations they would not have dared to perform even ten or fifteen years ago. The modern doctor's office has diagnostic aids available that were undreamed of in our grandfathers' time. Today the physician, the surgeon, the biochemist, the physiologist, the pathologist, the geneticist—even the physicist and the engineer—are working together to challenge the great questions that are still not completely answered: how the body is made, how it works, and why it breaks down with disease and old age.

Modern techniques for studying the body would have astounded the ancient physicians. Today we use X-rays to visualize internal body structures and detect changes in body chemistry by laboratory procedures. Special endoscopic instruments allow us to examine the interior of the stomach, bronchi or bladder by direct visualization. Metabolic tests use such devices as radioactive tracers to untangle the complexities of body chemistry, and pioneering surgeons explore new techniques such as organ transplantation, microscopic surgery of delicate organs and the use of implanted artificial body parts. But twenty years from now, at our present rate of discovery, all these new techniques may seem as primitive as the early microscopes.

Inevitably the study of the human body today has come back once again to the living cells and the basic tissues they comprise. It is here, in the last analysis, that the answers to the great questions will be found—the secrets of cell metabolism, reproduction, and the transfer of identity from generation to generation. And it is here in the years to come that we will witness the next great discoveries in man's continuing battle against disease and death.

4

Support and Mobility: The Musculoskeletal System

Just as the Empire State Building is more than so many miles of steel girders, truckloads of concrete and sheets of plate glass, the human body is more than a collection of bones, a pulsating heart and an intricately connected bundle of nerve cables. Rather, it is a complex living organism in which different tissues make up the various organs, and in which the organs themselves work together in complicated organ systems for the normal maintenance of health and life. Each of these organ systems is delicately attuned to all the rest, and even a minor breakdown or injury in one may well impair the function of the whole body. In many instances such impairment can be deadly. It is not surprising that the heart, the kidneys and the liver are known as "vital organs," for when their proper function ceases and cannot be restored, life itself comes to an end.

One organ system, however, is an odd exception: that remarkable system of bones, joints and muscles which provides the body with both physical support and a wide range of mobility. Strictly speaking, the parts of this so-called *musculoskeletal* system are not "vital" to the body in quite the way that the heart or kidneys are. Bones may be fractured, joints crippled by arthritis, or muscle destroyed by disease without causing death. Even in the tragic case of a paraplegic whose spinal cord has been permanently transected somewhere in the neck, and who is consequently almost totally paralyzed, life can be maintained without the active use of bones, muscles and joints.

But if the musculoskeletal system is not "vital" in terms of life and death, it is enormously important in the way we function from day to day. Taken as a whole, the body has a relatively fixed structure—the heart is always found in the same place, the eyes in another—but many of its parts are plastic in nature. Thanks to the musculoskeletal system, the body has rigid *bone tissue* to form its structural members, but it also has other specialized tissues that permit a remarkably wide degree of mobility as well as additional support. These tissues include soft, contractile *muscle* which is joined to the bone by means of the ropelike *tendons;* smooth *cartilage* that lines the joints and permits them to move without friction; and tough *ligaments* which hold the joints in place.

Working together, these various tissues normally allow an uncanny range of voluntary motion. We are capable of walking, running, jumping, dancing, lying down or standing up according to voluntary directives from the brain. When faced with danger, we may run to escape or turn and fight to defend ourselves. Unlike the jellyfish, which has no fixed structure or form, and which must depend upon winds and tides to carry it from place to place to gather food, we can move according to our own desires in active search of shelter, food, recreation or rest. And although some kinds of movement are physically impossible (try touching your right elbow with your right forefinger, for instance), our control of body motion is almost incredibly fine. The face can smile one moment and frown the next.

The hand can be used gently in patting a puppy or forcefully in pounding on a door. From the most faintly perceptible wink of an eyelid to the massively superb control of a championship swan dive, our muscles, bones and joints function with a degree of smoothness and coordination that has often been compared to the action of a well-oiled machine.

Actually this is a very poor comparison. The fact is that no machine has ever been designed that can hold a candle to the splendid functioning perfection of the human body, simply because no machine can approach the clever structure, coordination and integration of the human musculoskeletal system. It has some weaknesses, to be sure. It is vulnerable to injury, for example, and when injury has caused the fracture of a bone, the rupture of a muscle or the crushing or damaging of a joint surface, function of the system is impaired in the localized region where the injury occurred. Like all living tissue, its proper function depends upon biochemical reactions, and the musculoskeletal system is vulnerable to certain disorders or *dystrophies* due to the breakdown of normal biochemical reactions. The musculoskeletal system and particularly the joints are subject to exaggerated immune reactions and other poorly understood disease processes which can result in long-term chronic change, disability and malfunction. The system is also subject to the normal processes of wear and tear that one might expect of any supporting structure; the hip joint, for example, that continually supports half the weight of a 200-pound man over a period of 30 or 40 years may, eventually, be damaged by wear and tear at a greater rate than it can repair itself, so that finally the structure slowly begins to break down. And finally, like any living tissue, the tissues of the musculoskeletal system are vulnerable to abnormal growth—the development of benign tumors or cancers. (These and other disorders of bones, muscles, and joints are discussed in detail in Part V, "Patterns of Illness: The Musculoskeletal System.")

The remarkable thing, however, is not the wide range of disorders and diseases that can affect this unique organ system, but rather how *few* such disorders occur, and how the body compensates for the disability when they do occur. To understand why this is so, we must look at each of the three basic tissues of the musculoskeletal system in turn—bone, muscle and connective tissue—to see how each makes its special contribution to the support and mobility of the body.

Bone

Toward the end of World War II a number of German war prisoners were treated for battle wounds in Allied field hospitals in Europe. During X-ray examinations, doctors were horrified to discover that some of these men had heavy steel spikes 20 inches long and a half-inch in diameter embedded in the shafts of previously broken thighbones. At first they were indignant at the evidence of such atrocious medical care; *nobody* treated fractures that way, and earlier reports of the use of "intramedullary nails" by a German surgeon named Küntscher had been disregarded. But these soldiers told a strange story. Instead of spending long months hospitalized in traction and still more time walking on crutches as their fractures healed, they insisted that they had been up and about, bearing weight on their broken legs in a matter of weeks, and their fractures seemed well healed in spite of the hardware they were still carrying around. With growing curiosity, American and British doctors began trying out these so-called Küntscher nails in the treatment of fractures of the femur. Today this strange wartime experiment has become the standard treatment in handling many difficult fractures of the long bones of the arm or leg.

There is no better example anywhere of the way a basic tissue is specialized to do its job than in the case of bone. Obviously bone gives the body its support and shape and also makes mobility possible. We know how suddenly and disastrously a fractured bone can put an arm or leg out of commission. On the other hand, bone provides protection as well as support in the "packing crate" construction of the skull or the rib cage.

The most striking characteristic of bone is its hardness, the result of the deposit of insoluble calcium salts in a fibrous cellular matrix. Thus bone has a fixed shape which is not lost even after the body is dead, as we know from the fossil relics of human bones tens of thousands of years old. Along with its hardness, living bone is also amazingly light and strong. The long bones of the limbs, for instance, have a tubular construction that can support enormous weight without damage. Yet for all its strength, the bony tissue in an average-sized man's body weighs little more than 30 pounds. Steel bars or tubes of comparable size and shape would weigh ten times as much.

Bone has certain other unique characteristics. To allow for mobility as well as support, bone ends are molded to "fit together" in different types of *articulations* or joints, permitting motion where it is needed and limiting it where it could be dangerous. These fitted joints are lined and padded with a soft, smooth variation of bony tissues called *cartilage* which provides a slippery articulating surface for moving joints. Cartilage also forms a firm but flexible bone-to-bone connection wherever semirigid "packing crate" construction is necessary. And since broken bone can injure softer tissue, all bones are covered with a tight, fibrous layer of connective tissue called *periosteum,* richly interlaced with nerve fibers. Any injury to this sensitive bone covering sends urgent pain signals to the brain, setting off a warning as clangorous as a midnight burglar alarm.

It is deceptively easy to think of bone and cartilage as a sort of dead material, especially when we examine the dense, hard-packed shafts of the long bones or the tough armor plate of the skull. Nothing could be further from the truth; bone is a tissue made of cells which are very much alive. This fact is dramatically illustrated on X-ray films of bones damaged by bacterial infection, a condition known as osteomyelitis. Because of its deposited calcium, living bone casts a characteristic "skeleton" shadow on an X-ray plate, but a dead area of osteomyelitis can be identified instantly as a radio-opaque island in sharp contrast to the healthy, living bone surrounding it. (*See* Plate 1b.)

Like other basic tissues of the body, bone takes various forms to serve different purposes. The tubular construction of the femur in the thigh is splendidly adapted to heavy weight-bearing. The ulna and radius of the forearm also have tubular construction but are far less sturdy. They serve primarily as levers to permit the delicate, refined movements of the arm and hand. The ribs are curved and laminated like molded plywood staves, while the dense bone plates of the skull have a shock-absorbing layer of spongy bone between them to help protect the delicate matter that lies inside. Similar spongy bone covered with cartilage forms the rounded articulating ends of the long bones.

We can see how perfectly bone meets the varying needs of the body by the many ways in which it is joined together. Compare, for instance, the free mobility of the great ball-and-socket joint of the hip (necessary for both weight-bearing and locomotion) with the fixed immobility of the interlocking suture lines of the skull. In adult life there are no normal circumstances in which the skull needs to expand or contract. Nature cannot risk such flexibility here; the stuff inside is too precious. So the bones of the skull are interlocked at their edges and welded like iron. But these "suture lines" do not close tightly until adulthood. A baby's skull plates are still free to overlap during the process of birth without damage to the brain tissue inside, and remain free to allow for growth of the brain throughout childhood. Only when the brain has reached its mature size do the skull plates finally seal together.

The six bones that join to form the pelvis or "saddle bone" are bound together by fiber and cartilage, forming a heavy bowl to support the contents of the abdomen and provide an anchor for the powerful leg and back muscles. But here the joints are not interlocked as they are in the skull. It might seem more sensible for the pelvis to be made in one solid chunk, but there is a reason for its construction in segments. During the last months of pregnancy these tightly bound joints loosen and separate slightly to permit easier birth of the child.

Other construction details of the bony skeleton show evidence of equally amazing versatility. Like the skull, the rib cage provides rigid protection for vital internal organs, guarding the heart, lungs, liver and spleen from damage. But in

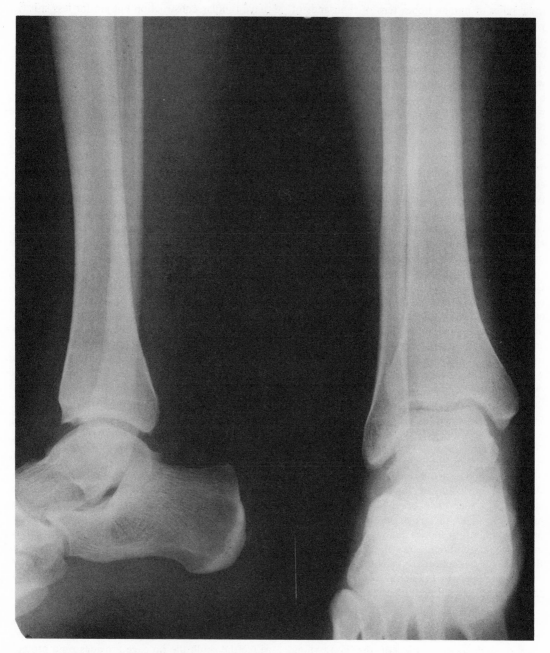

Plate 1a   Normal bone of the ankle and foot. The clean, sharp bone edges and the homogeneous opacity of the bone shaft are characteristic of the X-ray appearance of healthy bone.

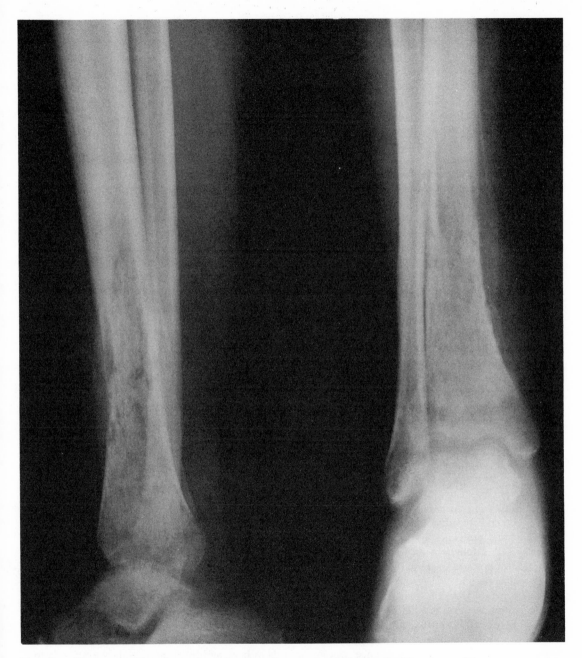

Plate 1b The same patient four years later. Bone is now deeply involved with osteomyelitis, in this case a staphylococcus infection of the bone. Note ragged, irregular bone edges and "motheaten" appearance of bone shaft.

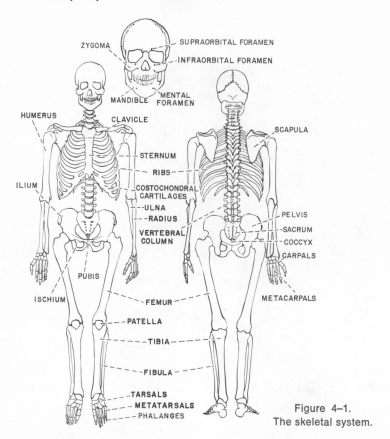

ZYGOMA
SUPRAORBITAL FORAMEN
INFRAORBITAL FORAMEN
MENTAL FORAMEN
MANDIBLE
HUMERUS
CLAVICLE
SCAPULA
STERNUM
RIBS
ILIUM
COSTOCHONDRAL CARTILAGES
ULNA
RADIUS
VERTEBRAL COLUMN
PELVIS
SACRUM
COCCYX
CARPALS
PUBIS
ISCHIUM
METACARPALS
FEMUR
PATELLA
TIBIA
FIBULA
TARSALS
METATARSALS
PHALANGES

Figure 4–1.
The skeletal system.

order for the lungs to inflate with each breath, the "closed cage" of the thorax must expand and contract. Thus, while the barrel-stave ribs are joined quite firmly to the breastbone by cartilage in front, they articulate individually with the vertebrae in back by means of tiny ball-and-socket joints. With each breath the ribs move up and out, allowing for lung expansion without sacrificing their protective function.

Support and protection of body parts are certainly important functions of bone, but mobility is equally important. A remarkable variety of moving joints permits widely differing degrees of body movement. The deep ball-and-socket joint of the hip, which must be solid enough to carry most of the body's weight, allows the leg to move freely in some directions but limits its range in others. Most of us, for instance, cannot turn our feet around backward, no matter how hard we try. In the shoulder, where weight-bearing is far less important, the ball-and-socket joint is more shallow but permits the arm a wide range of rotary motion.

The simple hinge joints of the knees and fingers are sharply limited; they permit movements on only one plane. In contrast the two uppermost vertebrae in the neck (called the *atlas* and the *axis*) combine opposite hingelike movements—up and down, as in nodding the head "yes," and back and forth, as in shaking the head "no." Together they constitute a sort of differential joint that allows a smooth rotary motion of the head. In the elbow an even more intricate differential-type joint is found. Both the ulna and the radius of the forearm articulate with the humerus of the upper arm, but the ulna works primarily as a hinge joint while the radius rotates back and forth, permitting the forearm to twist palm up or palm down. The combined movements of these joints allow us to turn a screw, empty a wastebasket or play a violin—but we cannot bend our elbows back unless we are double-jointed.

THE DIFFERING STRUCTURE
OF BONE

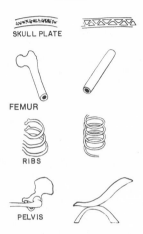

SKULL PLATE

FEMUR

RIBS

PELVIS

Figure 4–2.

In the wrist and the foot there are special "particulate" joints, each made up of many small bones which provide fixed form and strength but also permit limited motion. Finally, there are the flat joints, between the blocklike vertebrae, thickly padded with cartilage, which permit limited flexibility to this pillar of bone that supports the upright weight of the body.

Perhaps more than any other tissue in the body, bone has a definite "life cycle"; that is, it grows and changes in a characteristic fashion with the age of the individual. In the developing fetus some months before birth, all the tissue that will presently become bone is still cartilage; bone gradually forms as compounds of calcium and phosphorus are deposited in certain areas. This bone formation and growth is made possible by two kinds of cells within the cartilage: *osteoblasts* or "bonemakers" and *osteoclasts* or "bone dissolvers," which work together in delicately tuned biochemical balance. In the long bones, osteoblasts are located in the cartilage that forms the knobby ends of the bone, depositing calcium in the center of these knobs of cartilage. In addition, osteoblasts at both ends of

the shaft of these bones deposit calcium along special "growth lines," gradually pushing the cartilage of the knobby ends farther and farther out so that the whole bone lengthens. At the same time osteoclasts are at work dissolving bone in the center of the shafts, hollowing them out, so to speak, but leaving the hard outer shell of the shaft for support, and forming a network of spongy bone in the very center of the knobby ends. Slowly the hollow shafts of the long bones become filled with a fatty material known as *yellow marrow,* while the spongy bone at the ends of the long bones, as well as in the center of the vertebrae, the pelvic bones, the breastbone and the ribs, fills up with blood-enriched *red marrow.*

As a result of this dual process of bone formation and bone destruction, the cartilaginous bone of the fetus and the newborn baby gradually becomes calcified, and these "baby bones" grow steadily longer, thicker and stronger after birth. The rate of this bone growth is primarily controlled by a special growth hormone produced by the pituitary gland, but for normal growth an ample supply of protein in the baby's diet is also essential, together with adequate amounts of vitamins C and D. (*See* p. 857.) The growth process continues steadily for some 15 or more years after birth, often spurting forward at an accelerated rate as the child reaches the age of puberty. Then a point is reached when the process levels off, with the rate of bone destruction just balancing the formation of new bone; from this point on there is no further increase in bone length or diameter, and the individual remains the same height for the next 50 years or so of life. In females this leveling off of the growth process usually comes somewhat earlier than in men, one of the reasons why most women are not only shorter than men but also usually have a somewhat narrower, lighter bone structure.

But because bone ceases to *grow* does not mean that it ceases to *change.* There is continual dissolution of bone as life progresses, neatly matched by continuing formation of new bone cells. Cell by cell, healthy bone is always constantly replacing itself. As old age approaches, there tends to be more decalcification of bone throughout the body than there is replacement of calcium, so the bones become progressively less dense, narrower and more brittle. In addition, after years of weight-bearing, the spongy bone ends in elderly people become somewhat more compacted, and in areas such as the spine, the pads of cartilage between the vertebrae flatten. Thus by the age of fifty-five or so most people normally register some diminution in height, and the very aged seem to shrink perceptibly in size. Because of these changes of bone with age, older people are more vulnerable to fractures than they were in their youth, and when fractures occur, they take much longer to heal than would similar injuries in an adolescent or young adult.

Oddly enough, bone—or more specifically, the red marrow of bone scattered throughout the body—has one truly vital function that has nothing to do with either support or mobility of the body. It is in these centers of red bone marrow that all of the red blood cells, all of the blood platelets and about 60 percent of the white blood cells in the body are produced. This process of blood cell production by specialized "precursor cells" in the red marrow is carried out quite independently of any other bone function, and can even continue when the bone is fractured or when disease has damaged the cartilage-covered bone ends containing the red marrow. Certain kinds of cancer, however, can affect the blood-manufacturing process, most notably leukemia (sometimes spoken of as "bone cancer" but more accurately a cancer of the precursor cells in the red marrow), and various drugs and medicines are capable, on occasion, of depressing blood formation in the bone marrow so severely that a grave form of anemia can result.

For all its strength and versatility, bone tissue has certain singular weaknesses. Precisely because bone is solid and brittle, it is always vulnerable to fracture. Blows, falls or sudden shearing forces can also wrench joints apart; and unlike injury to skin, which may heal in a matter of days, or to muscle, which can be ready for work again within weeks, fractured bone and damaged or dislocated joints may require months to knit. Bone infections are also slow to heal, and when the joints are attacked by arth-

ritis—literally, "inflammation of the joint"—pain and disability may last for months or years of life.

Because bone is the most indestructible of all tissues, the calcium-filled remains of dead bone may be preserved for centuries. Archaeologists have learned much about ancient men from the study of skeletal fragments many tens of thousands of years old. Physical anthropologists apply their knowledge of bone structure to "reconstruct" earlier forms of the human body from such prehistoric relics, deducing from them the size and shape of ancient peoples, the kinds of work they did and the sort of weapons they used. Some workers in this field have turned their knowledge of bone structure to another, more immediate kind of detective work. Skilled at unearthing information from the detailed study of bones and teeth, they have served as consultants in many murder cases and investigations of unidentified bodies. In one famous case a physical anthropologist was asked to help identify a male skeleton discovered long after death at the bottom of a railway embankment in Texas. From a careful examination he was able to reconstruct a picture of the dead man, a young Indian, and provide police authorities with clues from the past that finally brought a murderer to justice for a crime he had committed thirty years before.

Muscle

A single basic tissue—bone—forms the framework on which the rest of the body is constructed. But bone by itself could no more support the body than a skeleton could run, pick apples or chin itself. Bone and muscle tissue must work together to give the body its form, its plasticity and its wide range of smooth and delicate movement. They are a curious team, for bone and muscle are as different from each other as night and day. Unlike hard and brittle bone, muscle tissue is soft and pliable, made up of large, juicy cells with an exceptionally rich blood supply. Unlike bone, muscle is poor at self-repair; when injured it tends to heal by scarring. Both tissues are strong, but muscle has a plastic or elastic strength quite different from the rigid structural strength of bone. A sudden forceful pull of muscle and its tendon can tear off a chunk of bone at the point of attachment.

Muscle resembles other soft tissues of the body in many ways, but it has one unique identifying characteristic: the ability to contract or shorten in length under certain kinds of stimuli, and then to relax when the stimulus has passed. The individual muscle cells are long and thin. When stimulated, they become shorter and fatter, so that a bundle of muscle cells can exert a remarkably powerful pull on anything to which it is attached. When we bite down on a caramel, for instance, the masseter muscles crossing the hinge of the jaw contract with almost unbelievable force. Anyone unwise enough to stick his finger in a year-old baby's mouth can give painful testimony to the remarkable power and tenacity of the jaw muscles.

It is tempting at first to compare this contractile ability of muscle with the elasticity of a rubber band. Actually, the rubber band works just the opposite. It stretches only under stimulus and snaps back passively when released. Muscle contraction, by contrast, is a positive, active function. It is this unique quality of muscle tissue which allows the body to move with a wide range of power or subtlety. Strange as it seems, the clenching of a fist and the blinking of an eye are identical actions of the same kind of tissue. The difference is a matter of size.

All muscle is contractile, but different varieties of muscle contract in different ways to perform very different jobs within the body. *Skeletal muscle*, which responds to voluntary commands and operates the movable parts of the bony framework, is composed of long, stringy bundles of muscle cells bound together in sheaths and attached to bone either directly or by means of tough connective tissue, *tendon.* Skeletal muscle —sometimes called *voluntary muscle,* or "striated" muscle because of its appearance under a microscope—uses the mechanical advantage of the lever and pulley to move legs, arms, fingers and trunk. It is the most powerful kind of muscle, able to exert an enormous concentrated pull, but it also tires most easily. From time to time it must rest and renew its strength; if it is forced

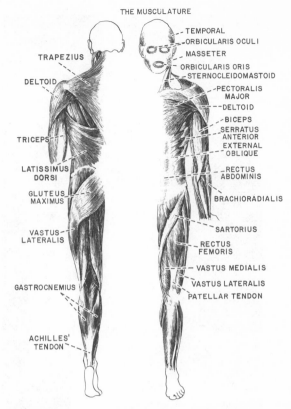

THE MUSCULATURE

Figure 4–3.

to contract repeatedly without rest, it weakens and ultimately stops contracting altogether.

To maintain the body's balance and allow for subtlety of movement, skeletal muscle is usually paired so that one muscle pulls while the opposite one relaxes. When used heavily, it will increase in size or *hypertrophy;* when not used it tends to shrink down or *atrophy,* thus adapting neatly to the actual needs of the body. In general, skeletal muscle is controlled by the will, efficiently obeying our conscious commands, but under certain conditions it can respond by reflex, an important mechanism for self-protection.

Another variety of muscle tissue, called *smooth* or *involuntary muscle,* does not pull and tug on the bony skeleton. It is concerned instead with more subtle forms of activity within the body: the gentle movement of food down the digestive tract, for instance, or the emptying of

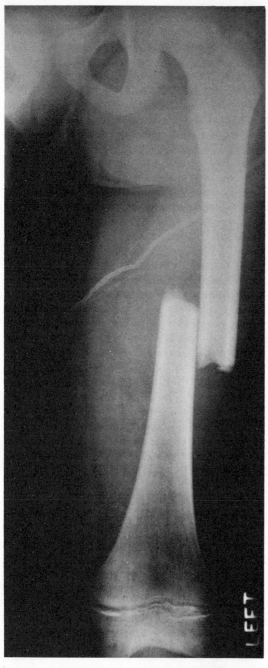

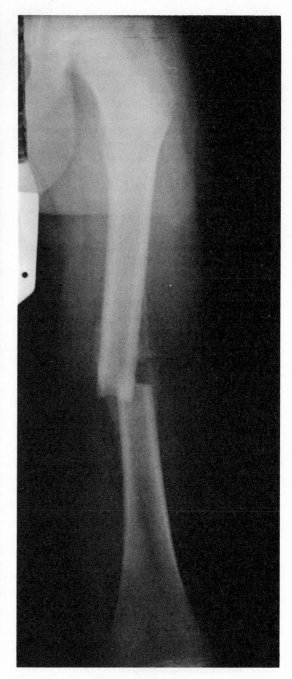

Plate 2a   Complete fracture of the mid-shaft of the femur in a nine-year-old boy, with marked overriding of the fractured bone ends.

Plate 2b   The same patient six weeks later, showing partial healing of the fracture, with callus formation.

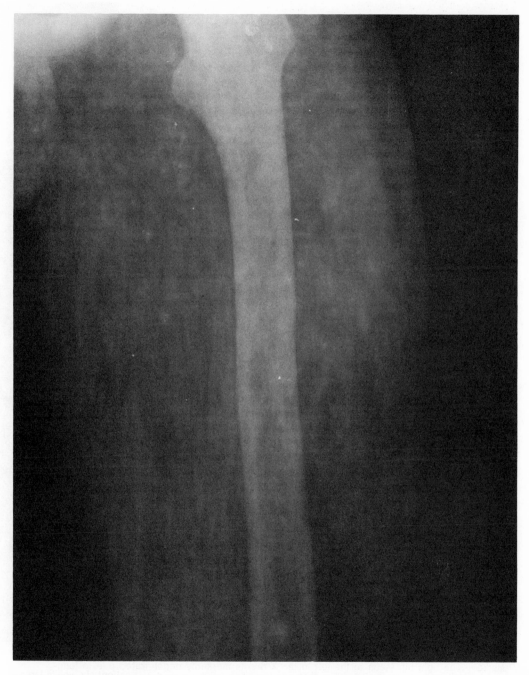

Plate 2c   The same patient five years later, showing complete healing of the bone. Site of the old fracture can hardly be distinguished.

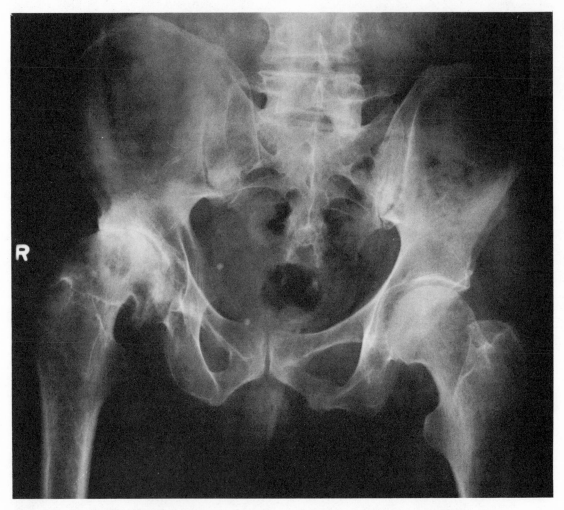

Plate 3a   The right hip (seen to the left in the X-ray) is markedly degenerated due to long-standing rheumatoid arthritis. Left hip is normal. As in all X-rays, the patient's right hand side is seen to the viewer's left and vice versa.

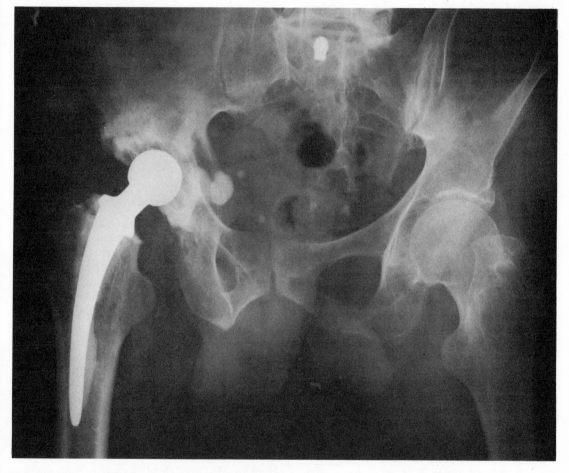

Plate 3b   The same patient with diseased hip replaced surgically with a total hip prosthesis
to restore its function. Bone has been reconstructed to accept the prosthesis, consisting of a metallic ball and a plastic socket.

the urinary bladder by contraction of its muscular wall. Even the flow of blood through the small arteries is regulated by contraction or relaxation of smooth muscle in the vessel walls. Smooth muscle cells are short and fat, arranged in sheets rather than in fibrous bundles. These sheets of muscle line the bowel, the walls of many blood vessels, and the smaller air tubes in the lungs.

In contrast to the straight-line pull of skeletal muscle, smooth muscle contracts in a gentle squeezing motion. It reacts primarily to involuntary stimuli. When we swallow, food is carried down the esophagus by a wave of smooth muscle contraction which, once started, cannot voluntarily be stopped. The presence of the food itself stimulates the peristaltic wave that pushes it downward. Similarly, the action of smooth muscle in the blood vessels is entirely beyond our conscious control, responding to involuntary signals as the need for blood in different tissues increases or decreases.

Since smooth muscle never has to do the heavy labor of skeletal muscle, it is much less powerful. On the other hand, it is less fatigable, resting for spells as it works. And it is less prone to hypertrophy or atrophy. Because it does not work as hard as skeletal muscle, it requires a less abundant flow of blood to supply it with fuel and oxygen. Even so, smooth muscle and skeletal muscle are alike in certain ways. Both respond to injury or irritation by sustained contraction or *spasm* which leads to pain. We are all familiar with the "charley horse" spasm of overworked skeletal muscle and the cramping of smooth muscle that occurs with intestinal flu. Both kinds of muscle heal by scarring, and both lose their function when injury occurs.

Smooth muscle and skeletal muscle together make up 95 percent of all muscle in the body, but certain very special jobs cannot be adequately performed by either. For these tasks there are other kinds of muscle with unique characteristics. The muscle of the heart, for instance, can never stop and rest; it must contract rhythmically from 70 to 90 or more times per minute as long as the body lives. The heart muscle pumps blood with a twisting contraction like the wringing out of a pair of overalls. It has

no origin or insertion, no anchor to the bony skeleton.

The special muscle tissue which performs this essential job resembles both skeletal and smooth muscle in certain ways, yet differs sharply from both. Cardiac muscle fibers are long and thin like skeletal muscle, but respond to involuntary stimuli like smooth muscle. The "clothes-wringing" action of the heart's contraction occurs because the muscle fibers are interlocked in a tight network and wrapped in spiraling sheets

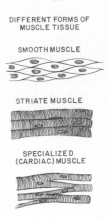

DIFFERENT FORMS OF
MUSCLE TISSUE

SMOOTH MUSCLE

STRIATE MUSCLE

SPECIALIZED
(CARDIAC) MUSCLE

Figure 4–4.

around a fibrous core. This means the heart must work as a unit; if its rhythmic contraction is interrupted by injury or irritation, cardiac arrest may result. The individual muscle fibrils may continue to "fibrillate" or twitch, but they no longer pull together. In such a case death will ensue very promptly if normal rhythmic contraction cannot be reinstated.

Cardiac arrest was a major medical and operating room catastrophe before a pioneering heart surgeon, Dr. Claude S. Beck of Western Reserve University in Cleveland, demonstrated in 1947 that patients with cardiac arrest could literally be brought back from the dead by direct massage of the heart combined with electric shock to the heart muscle. In 1959 Dr. William B. Kouwenhoven and his colleagues at Johns Hopkins Medical School devised an instrument which could jolt a fibrillating heart into normal activity without opening the chest at all. Today modifications of the cardiac defibrillator, sometimes called "shock boxes," are in use in hospitals throughout the world, saving the lives of hundreds of victims of cardiac arrest.

In the uterus another specialized kind of muscle is found, strangely similar to heart muscle. The walls of the uterus contain an interwoven matrix of long, thin muscle fibers which can contract and relax in a rhythmic pattern. But uterine muscle has little function except at one particular time: during pregnancy, especially thoughout the hours of labor prior to the birth of the baby. The muscle of the uterus stretches as the fetus grows, forming a thin sac of interlocking fibers. During labor this muscular network contracts in a slow, forceful rhythm, pushing the baby down the birth canal. But unlike the heart muscle, uterine muscle contraction is prolonged or tetanic, lasting from 30 to 90 seconds followed by a somewhat longer rest period. As labor progresses, the force of the contraction increases and the rest period grows shorter until the baby is born.

The actual working power of the contracting uterus during labor is difficult to believe. When early attempts at indirect measurement suggested a pressure of 25 pounds per square inch on the baby's head at the height of a contraction, the reports met with ridicule. Nobody believed that either mother or baby could tolerate such pressure throughout long hours of labor. But in 1938 direct measurements taken by R. A. Woodbury and his associates proved that uterine muscle could develop a pressure of as much as 45 pounds per square inch on the baby—roughly equivalent to the force required for a strong man to lift a grand piano over his head.

Like the hard-working heart, uterine muscle has an extremely rich blood supply, especially during pregnancy—the reason why dangerous hemorrhages can occur at childbirth. Like skeletal muscle, the muscle of the uterus can tire; uterine inertia can be a serious complication of a greatly prolonged or difficult labor.

A third specialized muscle is found in the diaphragm, a dome-shaped layer of muscle tissue separating the contents of the chest from the abdomen. The diaphragm is actually skeletal muscle, acting like a bellows to help move air in and out of the lungs. But the movement of the diaphragm can be controlled either voluntarily or involuntarily, according to the body's need. It is possible to breathe fast or slowly by conscious effort, but when we fall asleep or pay attention to something else, a complex series of neurochemical reflexes takes over to "tell" the diaphragm to contract and relax.

Regardless of the type of muscle, there is always a direct relationship between the work being done and the blood supply. There is also a relationship between the muscle's size and the work it has to do. After a baby is born, the mother's uterus "involutes" or shrinks back down to the size of a pear within a few weeks. Skeletal muscle paralyzed by poliomyelitis soon begins wasting away unless special efforts are made to exercise it artificially. Those muscle fibers not damaged by the attack can then hypertrophy enough to take over. And we are all familiar with the "shrinking" of the stomach after a few days on a strict diet.

Considering its location in the body we might expect muscle tissue to be highly vulnerable to injury and disability. Strange to say, the opposite is true. Muscle is the most disease-free of any of the basic body tissues, and the least frequently affected by injury. Diseases involving muscle alone are extremely rare; even contusions, tears and strains are relatively infrequent and heal quickly. Probably the most common of all muscle disabilities is the benign overuse myositis which afflicts us the day after we have overtaxed muscles not conditioned to exercise.

Of course muscle suffers like any tissue when its blood supply is cut off. Smooth muscle in the bowel can be destroyed when an abdominal artery is obstructed. If a branch of a coronary artery supplying the heart is blocked by a clot or by advancing atherosclerosis, *infarction* or death of a segment of heart muscle results. If only a minor branch is involved, the undamaged remainder of the heart muscle may be able to carry on, but when a large segment of muscle is damaged death can follow swiftly.

Interestingly enough, many conditions affecting the muscles are actually due to malfunctions of other tissues. In poliomyelitis large bundles of muscle may be paralyzed, but only because the polio virus has destroyed motor nerve cells in the spinal cord. Nothing is wrong with the muscle itself at first except that its signal system has been destroyed. Later, disuse may lead to atrophy and degeneration. In myasthenia gravis a chemical disorder prevents transmission of stimuli across the gap between nerve ending and muscle cell, resulting in a disabling generalized paralysis of skeletal muscle which disappears completely as soon as the chemical defect is corrected with the proper medicine.

Connective Tissue

Bone and muscle tissue together give the body its general shape and permit certain degrees of controlled motion. Still another basic tissue provides a fibrous elastic matrix which holds bone, muscle and other parts of the body together in a fixed, but not rigid, form. This connective tissue pervades all the other tissues and organ systems, unobtrusively binding them together in their normal relationships. It would be hard to find any part of the body that does not have its share of this fibrous binding material. Beneath the skin it is spread out in an elastic network called fascia, tough and resilient in some places, exceedingly delicate in others. Fascia holds in place the "padding" of fat that lies beneath the skin. It also surrounds the skeletal muscles and forms the elastic binder that keeps blood vessels and nerves in their proper positions.

In other places connective tissue forms the tough fibrous capsule that surrounds the bony joints, providing a strong stabilizing jacket of tissue that prevents dislocation and produces the slippery synovial fluid for joint lubrication. Elsewhere, the powerful tendons which slide back and forth in their thin-walled sheaths to move the fingers and toes are made of connective tissue. No fewer than ten such tendons pass side by side through the fibrous carpal tunnel in the wrist, along with three major motor nerves and two major arteries. Connective tissue also forms the fibrous "core" of the heart and the heart valves, the periosteum surrounding the bones, and the slippery sheath lining the lungs and rib cage (the pleura) and covering all the organs within the abdomen (the peritoneum). Because all these connective tissue linings are extremely

rich in pain-sensitive nerve endings, they act as an effective Distant Early Warning system to notify the body of trouble and help fix its location.

Obviously connective tissue must be strong to form a good binding tissue, but it must also be elastic to anchor moving body parts. In some places connective tissue forms a sticky reticulum or network. Elsewhere it provides lubricated sliding surfaces that allow muscles and tendons to glide across each other and prevent internal organs from sticking to one another. When such surfaces do become sticky or scratchy from inflammation, we have the "squeaky" friction rub of acute tendonitis or the pain of pleuritis or peritonitis. Irritation of the peritoneum, in fact, is such a certain sign of trouble going on in the abdomen that the surgeon may be forced to investigate on this basis alone.

We can easily see that widespread disturbances in body function will arise from any condition that causes a thickening or stiffening of connective tissue, reduces its elasticity or destroys its sliding surfaces. Inflammation can bring about all these changes. Localized irritation causes specific localized symptoms, but inflammation is also a common characteristic of a whole family of mysterious and crippling diseases which involve connective tissue in widespread areas of the body—the so-called collagen diseases which afflict four out of every ten people in one form or another sometime in the course of their lives.

Nobody knows the basic cause of these inflammatory diseases, which include rheumatoid arthritis, rheumatic fever and lupus erythematosus. An allergic reaction to certain bacterial poisons has been implicated. So has the body's response to tension. Whatever the cause, these diseases result in widespread damage owing to the scarring that follows the body's attempts to heal inflammation. Because this damage is only partly reversible, the victim's disability tends to increase with each recurrent attack. Rheumatoid arthritis attacks the joints with painful and crippling effects. Lupus erythematosis is an insidious affliction of connective tissue in the skin, joints and internal organs, a chronic, progressive and often fatal disease. Rheumatic fever also involves the joints, but is most dreaded because of its permanent scarring of the heart valves and its tendency to attack children.

The search for weapons against this notorious trio of diseases has led to several major medical and surgical advances within the last 20 years. The discovery of cortisone and related steroid hormones in the 1940s provided an almost miraculous weapon to suppress inflammation in connective tissue and reduce permanent damage from scarring. Even more dramatically, rheumatic heart disease led to the earliest surgical attempts to by-pass or repair damaged heart valves. After surgeon Alfred Blalock and pediatrician Helen Taussig of Baltimore joined forces in 1944 to pioneer heart surgery of congenital defects in children, men like Dr. Charles Bailey of Hahnemann Medical College in Philadelphia forged ahead in the face of scalding criticism to perfect a surgical technique to reopen mitral valves twisted and scarred by rheumatic fever, a procedure that had been regarded as flatly im-possible only two decades before. The early work of these and other courageous innovators actually seems timid and conservative today when hundreds of surgeons are performing heart surgery, inserting completely artificial heart valves, even transplanting entire hearts—but it opened the door to a whole new era of cardiac surgery which has salvaged countless lives that would otherwise surely have been lost.

In the healthy body, then, three basic tissues —bone, muscle and connective tissue—work together to provide support and mobility to the body structure. Each of these tissues plays its part and depends upon the others for its own proper functioning. But body movements, to be useful, must be purposeful and controlled. And other body functions occurring at the same time must be integrated so that they do not conflict with each other. Our complex nervous system works to motivate, moderate and control the many activities of the body, and it too is made up of another basic tissue.

5

Motivation and Moderation: The Nervous System

In this world of modern technology everyone is familiar with the amazing capabilities of highly sophisticated electronic computers. Fast becoming involved in almost every aspect of our lives, computers can handle swiftly and efficiently a staggering variety of tasks that would otherwise require the prolonged labors of armies of mathematicians, engineers, accountants and typists. It is no wonder that these remarkable machines, with their miles of circuitry, their thousands of transistors, their memory storage units and their input and print-out facilities, are often called "giant brains." The term is misleading, however. Giant these machines may be, in some instances —but they are not brains. No matter how startling their capacity to store, retrieve and manipulate great quantities of data, the most sophisticated can barely approach the potential of the dim living brain of the lowly bullfrog. And to compare an electronic computer with a functioning human brain is about as valid as comparing a mechanical doll with a human being simply because they both move.

Even so, there are certain superficial similarities. Like an incredibly complicated, miniaturized electronic computer, the human nervous system functions as an intricate communications and control center for the body. Composed of a single basic tissue which makes up only 3 percent of the total body weight and even at that consists mainly of water, it serves the body as a lookout, as a system for receiving, storing, transmitting and processing information, and as a general headquarters for decision making, strat-

egy, evaluation and direction of all the body's physical, emotional and intellectual activities. It is capable of correcting its own errors and remembering them for future reference. Furthermore, like an electronic computer, the nervous system operates on only one kind of signal, an electrochemical impulse which can be transmitted from one part of the body to another along an interconnecting series of conduits or nerve paths. Just as all data put into a computer must first be translated into "computer language" before it can be used or acted upon, so all data received by the body from either inside or outside sources must be converted into nerve impulses.

Beyond this, however, the comparison with a computer begins to break down. For one thing, the human nervous system is obviously a structure of living tissues, not a machine, and it is far more complex, in both its structure and its function, than any computer ever devised. Perhaps more important, it is capable of an incredible variety of activities that no computer can match, activities that range all the way from the simplest of animal-like instinctive reactions to the most complicated and profound reasoning processes, including the mysterious "intuitive leaps" —still never satisfactorily explained—which have accounted for some of man's most brilliant scientific discoveries.

The part of this remarkable system that is most familiar, the so-called *central nervous system,* is composed of two interconnected structures: the brain itself, enclosed within the skull and protected by three connective tissue membranes known as the *meninges;* and the spinal cord, encased by the semiflexible bony column of the vertebrae and composed of cells that transmit nerve impulses to and from the brain. The less familiar *peripheral nervous system* consists of a network of nerves extending from their origin in the brain or the spinal cord to every part of the body, including the special sense organs, muscle tissue and all of the body's skin surfaces. Part of this peripheral system is a vital auxiliary nerve network known as the *autonomic nervous system,* so called because it works "autonomously" or independently of ordinary voluntary control and provides automatic nervous control for such important and often unconscious body functions as rhythmic breathing, heartbeat, the digestive movements of the gastrointestinal tract and the contraction or dilatation

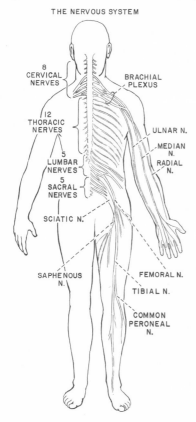

THE NERVOUS SYSTEM

8 CERVICAL NERVES

BRACHIAL PLEXUS

12 THORACIC NERVES

ULNAR N.

MEDIAN N.

5 LUMBAR NERVES

RADIAL N.

5 SACRAL NERVES

SCIATIC N.

SAPHENOUS N.

FEMORAL N.

TIBIAL N.

COMMON PERONEAL N.

Figure 5–1.

of capillary blood vessels to meet the body's changing needs for circulating blood.

The *brain* is in every sense the headquarters of the human nervous system, critical to the functioning of both the central and the peripheral nerve networks. In its overall appearance, the brain is a huge agglomeration of delicate nerve cells and crisscrossing nerve pathways weighing approximately 3¼ pounds in the average mature adult and molded into two symmetrical halves or *hemispheres,* with the nerve cells held together and nourished by specialized nerve tissue known as the *neuroglia,* or just *glial cells.* Superficially one part of the brain looks much like any other part, and for centuries anatomists and physiologists were limited to describing its external appearance and remained totally at sea about its internal structure and its very specialized functions. Today we know that the brain is made up of several segments, each with its own special contribution to the overall operation of the nervous system, with the sections fitted together like a nest of boxes in which each successive part corresponds roughly to a higher stage in our evolutionary development.

The earliest formed, most primitive portion of the brain is little more than a stalk of nerve tissue that is sometimes called the *brain stem* because it extends upward from the spinal cord along the floor of the skull and resembles a thickened stem to which the enlarged, bulbous upper portions of the brain are attached. The lower end of the brain stem, which fuses with the spinal cord below, is known as the *medulla oblongata.* Above this is a slightly widened, rounded area called the *pons* or "bridge," made of nerve fibers which narrow to form the upper end of the brain stem or *midbrain.* These fibers serve as a pedicle by which the brain stem is attached to higher brain centers. The parts of the brain stem, taken together, act as the primitive "life center" of the nervous system; it is here that many involuntary brain functions arise— the sort of activities that are just as vital to the continuing life function of a worm, a toad or a mouse as they are to a man. For example, the medulla contains nerve centers that provide unconscious control of the heartbeat and respiration, and injury to these areas can cause abrupt, permanent cessation of breathing. Special nerve pathways in the pons and midbrain help coordinate varying sensory impressions flowing to the brain and contribute to such functions as smoothly coordinated muscular movement, blinking of the eyes or contraction of the pupils in response to bright light, any of which can go awry if these brain stem areas are damaged or affected by disease. In addition, various parts of the brain stem give rise to twelve pairs of *cranial nerves,* most of which provide for sensory and motor control of structures in and about the head. Among these cranial nerves are the *optic nerves* that connect the retina of the eye with the brain and make vision possible, the *acoustic* or *auditory nerves* to the ears, the *olfactory nerves* with their delicate nerve endings in the nose which provide us with a sense of smell, the *oculomotor nerves* which control the muscles that move our eyes in their sockets, and the *facial nerves* and *trigeminal nerves* which direct movements of the lips and the muscles of facial expression. Loss of one or more of the functions of the cranial nerves may be a vital clue to the neurologist that something has gone wrong somewhere in the area of the brain stem.

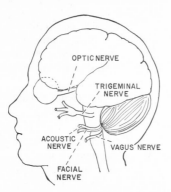

Figure 5–2.

Another important but still primitive part of the brain is the *cerebellum,* composed of two walnut-sized lumps of nerve tissue attached to either side of the brain stem structures and located in the skull just above and behind the ears. Together with the pons and midbrain, the cerebellum is concerned with the coordination of muscular activity, and its other major contribu-

tions include the maintenance of balance and equilibrium while standing or walking (aided by sensory input from the eyes and from the "equilibrium center" located in the middle ear), the

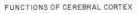

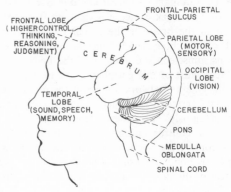

Figure 5–3A.

regulation of voluntary muscular actions such as reaching and grasping, and the interpretation of such deep-seated sensory functions as the body's position sense which ordinarily makes us automatically aware of the relative physical position of various body parts. The victim of a tumor or other disorder of the cerebellum might suffer such symptoms as uncontrolled lurching to one side or the other as he tries to stand or walk, the inability to "connect" properly with an object he reaches for, or the inability to find his nose with his fingertips when his eyes are closed.

With nothing but the brain stem and the cerebellum to serve us we would be simple, stupid, attenuated creatures indeed. But there is still another portion of the brain, a much larger part that evolved later in our natural history, that raises man above any other living creature and has made it possible for him to become the dominant life form on this planet. This part, the *cerebrum,* is bulkier and more massive by far than all the other parts of the brain put together. It is a thick, convoluted mass of nerve tissue which fills the skull from the bony plate just above the eyes in the front to the base of the neck in back, and is divided into two interconnected hemispheres by a deep centerline crease. These cerebral hemispheres are composed of two kinds of nerve tissue that are quite different in appearance: a thick outer layer of gray-colored tissue, made up almost entirely of the cell bodies of nerve cells, called the *cerebral cortex* or "gray matter," and an inner mass of yellowish-white tissue or "white matter" composed of interconnecting nerve fibers interspersed with patches of "gray matter" that form special *ganglia* or "control centers" of nerve cells organized to moderate and integrate the activities of the nerve cells in the cortex.

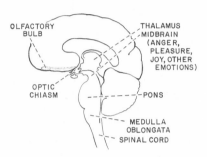

Figure 5–3B.

This inner core of nerve fibers and ganglia, directly connected with the midbrain, was the first part of the cerebrum to evolve, and it contains a number of structures which, like the more primitive parts of the brain stem, help maintain unconscious control of the body's sensory, motor and glandular functions. For example, in this portion of the cerebrum are the *basal ganglia* which are believed to moderate the activities of the motor nerve cells in the cerebral cortex; damage to cells in this area can result in the strange combination of uncontrolled muscle movements and muscular rigidity seen in Parkinson's disease, or in the sudden jerky movements of arms and hands known as chorea that occurs in many children afflicted by rheumatic fever. The *thalamus,* which lies in the same region, acts as a sorting center for such sensory impulses as those relating to touch, pain, heat or cold; in addition, in ways that are still not clearly understood, the thalamus moderates such basic emotions as fear or anger. Disorders of the thalamus often lead to a loss of emotional control and marked personality changes.

Immediately adjacent is the remarkably busy *hypothalamus,* a cluster of nerve centers that control the sex drive or libido, provide a highly effective "thermostat" or temperature-control mechanism for the body, regulate the appetite, help the body interpret all kinds of pleasure sensations, control the waking-sleeping cycle and—oddly enough—also exercise chemical controls such as the regulation of the amount of fluid that is retained in the body. Indeed, nowhere is the close interrelationship between the nervous system and the endocrine glands better illustrated, for it is to the hypothalamus that the *pituitary gland*—the master endocrine gland of them all—is attached, and the posterior part of the pituitary actually arises from the nerve tissue of the hypothalamus in the course of its development. Damage or injury to either the pituitary gland or the hypothalamus can seriously upset the body's fluid balance and result in excessive urine production, a condition known as diabetes insipidus.

But it is the vast mass of nerve cells in the comparatively huge, convoluted cerebral cortex, the most recent part of the brain to evolve in its present enlarged form in human beings, which qualifies our species for its biological name *Homo sapiens*—"man the wise" or "thinking man." It is through the nerve cells in this portion of the brain that most of the voluntary motion of the body is controlled, and most of the sensory data picked up from the outside is received, interpreted, analyzed and channeled for action—visual images, odors, sounds, and the senses of touch, heat and cold, among others. It is also in the cerebral cortex that such higher nervous system functions as memory, thinking, love, sympathy, compassion and the overriding exercise of judgment are carried on.

For convenience anatomists have divided the cerebral cortex into five paired segments or *lobes* according to their location, and neurophysiologists have demonstrated that certain specific brain functions are handled in specific areas of the various lobes and nowhere else. Mentation—the process of thinking—and the exercise of reason and judgment appear to be the function of the *prefrontal* and *frontal lobes* located in the forehead. The prefrontal lobes in particular seem to be the center of intelligence, refined emotions and the individual qualities of personality, for when this area is damaged either by injury or by surgery carried out in an effort to correct certain grave personality disorders, the individual's intelligence and behavior are severely blunted; he becomes tractable but dull and lethargic, a sort of walking vegetable. Control of speech is centered in the frontal lobes, and voluntary motion of all parts of the body is also moderated there. The *parietal lobes* located at the top of the brain receive and channel touch, taste and temperature sensations, and the somatic or "body" senses that do not require any special sensory organs; the *temporal lobes* at the sides of the brain above the ears are primarily concerned with hearing; and the *occipital lobes* located at the back of the brain receive and act upon visual sensations and are so critical to our ability to see that this area of the brain is commonly known as the *visual cortex*. As we might expect, disease or injury in any of these areas will result in sudden or gradual loss of the specific brain functions centered there—an important clue to neurologists in diagnosing the nature or extent of nervous system disorders. A tumor or abscess in the visual cortex, for example, may lead to progressive blindness, while damage to the speech centers in the frontal lobes can cause a form of speech disorder known as *aphasia* ("no speech"), and injury to the sensory cortex of the parietal lobes may result in a loss of touch sensation about the lips or in other parts of the body.

Finally, located almost dead center in the cerebrum is an odd little structure the size of a pea known as the *pineal gland*. No one has any idea what it does or why it is there, but occasionally it will develop a tumor called a pinealoma which can press upon and destroy brain tissue lying around it. In addition, the pineal gland is sometimes of diagnostic importance because it tends to become calcified and thus visible on X-ray examination. A shift of the pineal from its normal midline position may indicate that a brain tumor or abscess is pushing it to one side.

Sometimes more than one part of the brain may contribute to the same job, depending upon the circumstances. For example, we can exercise voluntary (i.e., cerebral) control of our respiration, within certain limits; but if the cerebrum gets hungry enough for oxygen we lose consciousness, and then the involuntary control centers in the medulla take over. In some cases, too, it has been shown that one portion of the brain can take over or *compensate* for loss of an adjacent portion owing to disease or damage, although no one has yet discovered how this miracle of cooperation is accomplished.

Curiously enough, nature has provided us with a remarkable surplus of brain tissue. The two matched hemispheres of the brain are intricately interconnected by multitudes of nerve fibers crossing over from one side to the other. In the lower, more primitive brain centers, the activities of one side of the body are largely controlled by the opposite side of the brain, but in the cerebrum almost all functions are carried out by just one "dominant" hemisphere, the hemisphere on the opposite side from the individual's dominant muscular function, so that the left cerebral hemisphere is usually "dominant" in a right-handed individual and vice versa. The other hemisphere is fully equipped but apparently inactive. Up to a certain point this surplus of brain tissue can be extremely important. If the dominant side of the brain is injured during infancy, the inactive side, which otherwise would remain dormant, may take over the lost functions and restore full normal activity. Unfortunately, this ability to utilize surplus brain tissue seems to be lost as the individual grows older. When an adult suffers injury to the dominant hemisphere of the brain, few if any of the lost functions can be regained, and any recovery at all requires a long and painstaking period of training.

Obviously such a vital and delicate structure as the brain requires extraordinary means of protection to guard it from injury. The skull provides an ideal outer casing to prevent penetrating wounds that might destroy large segments of brain tissue. In addition, the entire brain is covered by three connective tissue membranes, arranged in layers, to supply a different kind of protection. The outer of these three meningeal membranes, called the *dura mater,* is a tough fibrous sheath that coats the interior of the skull. Beneath it is the *arachnoid membrane,* much more delicate, which carries a rich network of capillary blood vessels and multitudes of pain-sensitive nerve endings that give warning signals when pressure or other injury to the arachnoid occurs. The innermost meningeal membrane, the *pia mater,* is even more filamentous, lying in contact with the brain surface.

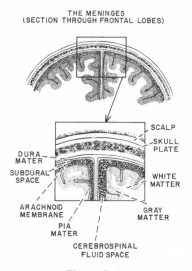

THE MENINGES
(SECTION THROUGH FRONTAL LOBES)

SCALP

SKULL PLATE

DURA MATER

SUBDURAL SPACE

WHITE MATTER

ARACHNOID MEMBRANE

GRAY MATTER

PIA MATER

CEREBROSPINAL FLUID SPACE

Figure 5–4.

All three of these membranes not only ensheath the brain but extend down beyond the brain stem to cover and protect the spinal cord as well. In addition, there is a narrow space between the arachnoid and the pia mater that is filled with a crystal-clear watery liquid, the *cerebrospinal fluid,* that is constantly being exuded in small quantities by the arachnoid. This fluid provides both brain and spinal cord with a sort of watery cushion for additional protection against jolts and jars. Finally, the brain itself is not a solid mass of nerve tissue. Beneath the cerebral cortex and dividing portions of the white matter of the cerebrum are four cavities, also filled with cerebrospinal fluid, known as the *ventricles* of the brain. These ventricles are connected by narrow channels to the fluid-filled space around the brain and spinal cord, so that the pressure of the cerebrospinal fluid outside the brain and spinal cord and within the ventricles is normally

in perfect balance. Any abnormality that disturbs this balance can cause pressure and pain— one source of the distress of headaches. An increase in this pressure can often be measured when a lumbar puncture or "spinal tap" is performed, an invaluable diagnostic aid in detecting nervous system disorders.

The second major structure in the central nervous system is the *spinal cord,* a great conduit of nerve cells and fibers approximately a foot and a half long that provides an efficient transmission system for nerve impulses passing to and from the brain. At the base of the skull, where the cord emerges as a downward extension of the brain stem, it is almost an inch thick; as it passes down through the bony tunnel formed by the vertebrae, *nerve roots* embedded in the cord branch off to form thirty-one pairs of *spinal nerves* that ultimately escape from the vertebral canal through little openings between the vertebrae. At about the level of the midback, the solid substance of the spinal cord tapers to nothing, giving way to the lower of these spinal nerves, which travel on down in a bundle called the *cauda equina* (because it looks so much like a horse's tail) to their appropriate exit points.

Every nerve fiber that enters or leaves the spinal cord has direct connections with special transmitter nerve cells within the cord which lead to and from the brain. In addition, there are also direct connections in the spinal cord between the sensory nerve cells carrying information in from distant parts of the body and the motor nerve cells that control the skeletal muscle. Thus a kind of protective short circuit called the *spinal reflex arc* allows the body to take protective action when threatened even before the threat can be identified and evaluated by the brain, a sort of "survival safeguard" that is a built-in function of the nervous system.

The central nervous system structure is complemented by the network of peripheral nerves that originate in the spinal cord (or in the brain stem, in the case of the cranial nerves) and travel to all parts of the body. Their function is to carry sensory information from the multitudes of distant sensory nerve endings back to the spinal cord and thence to the brain, as well as to carry motor impulses from the brain out to the muscles, causing the muscle cells to contract and various parts of the body to move as a result. In the case of the cranial nerves, with their roots in the brain stem, some are composed only of sensory nerve fibers carrying "incoming

THE REFLEX ARC

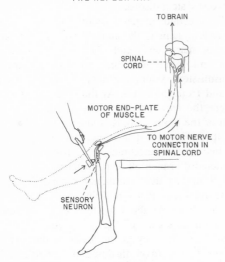

TO BRAIN

SPINAL CORD

MOTOR END-PLATE OF MUSCLE

TO MOTOR NERVE CONNECTION IN SPINAL CORD

SENSORY NEURON

Figure 5–5.

messages" to the brain, some contain only motor nerve fibers to carry "outgoing messages" away from the brain, and some are mixed, made up of both sensory and motor fibers. All thirty-one pairs of spinal nerves, however, contain both sensory and motor fibers, and although many fibers, some sensory and some motor, may be bound together in the same bundle, each individual fiber is capable of carrying either incoming impulses alone or outgoing impulses alone, so that the "messages" never normally get mixed up.

The uppermost eight pairs of spinal nerves emerge from between the cervical vertebrae and are therefore called *cervical nerves*. Once free of the vertebral column, these nerves may either divide and branch into smaller and smaller bundles of fibers to specific nearby areas or else merge together into major *nerve trunks* (bundles containing many nerves together) that travel to distant areas; but ultimately the eight pairs of cervical nerves supply the muscles, bones, joints and skin areas of the neck, the shoulders, the

outer areas of the arms, the wrists, and both hands. The next twelve pairs of spinal nerves, known as the *thoracic nerves* because they emerge from between the thoracic vertebrae, supply the skin, muscle, bone and joints of the entire trunk, front and back, from shoulder level to a line about two inches below the navel, and also provide innervation to the inner surfaces of the arms. Five pairs of *lumbar nerves* emerging from between the lumbar vertebrae, five pairs of *sacral nerves* escaping through little tunnels in the sacrum at the base of the spine, and one pair of *coccygeal nerves* passing out between the sacrum and the coccyx or "tailbone" complete the thirty-one pairs of spinal nerves. These latter supply skin, muscle, bone and joints in the pelvic region of the trunk, the anogenital region, the buttocks and the lower extremities. Among other things, branches of these lower spinal nerves on either side merge to form two of the largest peripheral nerve trunks in the body, the great *femoral nerve* passing down the leg on the inner side from the groin to the foot and measuring almost half an inch in diameter in the upper leg, and the huge *sciatic nerve,* three-quarters of an inch in diameter at its thickest, which extends down the back of the thigh and leg into the foot.

Finally, the autonomic nervous system acts as an auxiliary network of nerve tissue controlled by the brain which provides innervation to the smooth muscle of the blood vessel walls, the gastrointestinal tract, the lungs and the heart, and which also stimulates internal secretions. This auxiliary system is largely concerned with the control of unconscious, involuntary body functions which must be carried on day or night regardless of any conscious awareness or voluntary desire, and as might be expected, its structure is considerably more complicated than the orderly system of spinal nerves. The autonomic system too has sensory nerve fibers leading directly from the various organs to the spinal cord, and motor nerve fibers extending directly from the spinal cord to the organs they control, both connecting with transmitter nerve cells in the cord itself. But in addition, many other motor fibers of the autonomic system do *not* extend directly to the organs they control, but rather converge in special chains of "control centers" or *ganglia* located in the connective tissue that lines the abdomen and thorax just outside the vertebral column on either side, and connected to each other, up and down, like strings of beads. Special nerve cells in these ganglia then send fibers out to form dense nets of nerves known as *plexuses* in the vicinity of the various organs to be controlled. Most familiar of these is the so-called *solar plexus,* a tangled mass of autonomic nerves located in the abdomen behind the stomach; another such network surrounds the testicles and accounts for their extreme sensitivity and for the sense of overwhelming pain and physical sickness that occurs whenever they are traumatized. Finally, the autonomic nervous systems also includes separate nerve trunks such as the *vagus nerve,* one of the cranial nerves that acts as an autonomic nerve, to provide direct, unbroken contact with involuntary control centers in the brain. Complex as this auxiliary arrangement may seem, it serves a vital purpose: even if the spinal cord is massively injured or destroyed, the autonomic nervous system can continue its function unimpaired. It is only when disease or injury affects the brain or the brain stem that these vital involuntary functions are disturbed.

Up until about 80 years ago relatively little was known about the structure and function of the brain and the rest of the nervous system. Part of the trouble was that all nerve tissue looked so much alike—a soft, white, waxy material which did not even stain very well for microscopic examination. Various investigators in the middle and late 1800s were convinced that certain structures in the brain must control specific body functions. The French surgeon Pierre Paul Broca, for example, was able to identify the speech control center in the brain as early as 1861. In the 1870s two German researchers, Gustav Fritsch and Eduard Hitzig, attempted to "map" the function of the entire cerebral cortex, but their methods were crude and their results confusing. Then in the late 1800s the noted British physiologist Sir Charles Scott Sherrington took on the staggering task of identifying specific structures in the nervous system and determining precisely which functions

they performed. Strangely enough, the secret of Sherrington's success lay in working backward— first identifying a particular function and then tracing it to the part of the spinal cord or brain where it seemed to be controlled. Between 1890 and 1910 Sherrington performed a monumental volume of work, removing once and for all the veil of mystery that surrounded the human nervous system and paving the way for the work of thousands who followed him.

Aside from various connective tissues that bind the different parts of the complex nervous system into position, virtually all its tissue is made up of a single kind of cell, the nerve cell or *neuron.* In some areas, such as the brain itself, neurons are packed tightly into solid blocks of nerve tissue. Elsewhere they form short crisscrossing bundles of nerve fibers that connect one block of cells with another, while in still other areas they send out long fibers capable of transmitting nerve impulses to distant parts of the body. But different as they may appear in shape, size and function, all neurons have certain identifying characteristics and capabilities, and all are vulnerable to the same kinds of danger and disability.

Nerve cells can best be classified according to their special functions. First there are the *receptor* or *sensory neurons* which pick up information for transmission to the brain as electrochemical impulses along fibers which make up the *sensory* or *afferent nerves.* Some receive impressions from the outside—visual images or sensations of smell, touch and pain, for instance. Others pick up such internal impressions as pressure changes, shifts in body position or even alterations of body chemistry, translating them into the kind of "nerve impulse" language that can be transmitted and used by the brain.

Second, there are the *motor neurons* which carry decisions and directives from the brain out to the delicate nerve endings in contact with the muscles of the body. These neurons have fibers which make up the *motor* or *efferent nerves* extending from spinal cord to muscle. The impulses they carry literally prod the muscle into activity by setting off certain kinds of chemical reactions at the nerve-muscle junctions.

The cell bodies of both sensory and motor

nerves are located in the spinal cord. Also found there are multitudes of *transmitter neurons* with elongated fibers to carry the sensory nerve impulses to the brain from the eye, ear, skin or internal organs, and to transmit directive impulses back to the motor nerves of the body after the information has been received and processed. In the brain itself there is yet another kind of nerve cell, the masses of tightly packed *control neurons* which form the general headquarters of the nervous system. These cells are constantly in touch with the nerve impulses flowing in from the sensory circuits and out on the motor circuits, and they are also in continuous contact with each other.

All the classes of nerve cells or neurons differ from one another in their structure, location and function, yet they also share certain important identifying characteristics. Except in tightly packed areas of the brain, they all have tendrils or fibers extending from their cell bodies, sometimes for only a fraction of a millimeter, sometimes for as much as five feet. These nerve fibers terminate in either *sensory nerve endings* or *sensory receptors,* in *motor end plates* or in direct cell-to-cell connections, called *synapses,* with other nerve cells. Many of these elongated fibers are coated with a fatty insulating material called *myelin* which seems essential to prevent "grounding" of the nerve impulses being transmitted. In many places they are also surrounded and nourished by the *glial cells,* the special kind of nerve cell that also helps hold the nerve fibers in position.

The major characteristic that distinguishes neurons from other body cells is their strange ability to transmit nerve impulses to distant areas. This transmission is a one-way affair for each neuron; afferent or "input" impulses travel from the sensory nerve endings along one set of fibers and efferent or "output" impulses go out to the motor end plates along another. Although the great nerve trunks in the arms and legs carry fibers going both ways, the signals never seem to get jumbled. No one is quite certain exactly how nerve impulses travel; they are not really electrical, but seem to move as an electrochemical wave which is passed like a hot potato from one molecule to the next along the surface of the nerve fiber. Each molecule in line *depolarizes* or changes its shape, stimulating the next molecule to depolarize; it then promptly *repolarizes* so the impulse cannot run backward. Thus the transmission of a nerve impulse is more like the burning of a trail of renewable gunpowder than the passage of an electrical current.

Whatever the exact mechanism of impulse transmission may be, it consumes energy at an astounding rate. Nerve cells everywhere are hungry for oxygen. They must have a rich and continuous blood supply or they will quickly die. Compared to low-energy tissue like bone, which can get along indefinitely on a skimpy supply of blood, nerve cells in the brain alone use up as much as 40 percent of all the available oxygen in the body. It is believed that a certain number of neurons are permanently destroyed any time that circulation to the brain is slowed down even momentarily.

Nerve tissue is also extremely soft and fragile, easily injured by contusion, cutting and crushing. The central nervous system, the brain and spinal cord, are well protected by the bony armor of the skull and a strong but flexible "coaxial cable" made up of the vertebrae. The nerve trunks of the peripheral system are deeply buried between protective layers of muscle, except in occasional places such as the "funny bone" where the ulnar nerve crosses an exposed bony ridge just beneath the skin at the elbow. Even the major sensory nerve endings in contact with the outside environment are generally well protected. The eyes, for instance, are buried in bony sockets and are equipped with self-adjusting diaphragms—the irises—to shield the retina from too much light. Sound receptors are deeply encased in tiny bony caverns in the skull. Pain and temperature receptors lie unguarded in the skin, but they are so widely distributed that the loss of a few here and there is not important.

Why should nerve tissue be so carefully guarded while bone and muscle tissue is left vulnerable to any shock or blow that may come along? The reason is that nerve cells are so highly specialized that they cannot regenerate. Once a neuron is destroyed it is gone forever; no new ones will take its place. A year-old baby already has all the nerve cells he is ever going to have. Those cells may grow larger and longer, and if the elongated fiber of a motor nerve is cut or separated from its cell body, a new filament may slowly grow out again along the track of the old nerve. But if the nucleus of the cell is destroyed, it is gone. This is the reason why such diseases as poliomyelitis are so serious. When the polio virus destroys motor nerve cells in the spinal cord, the resulting muscle paralysis is permanent, even if the victim ultimately fights off the virus and survives.

One of the most remarkable characteristics of the highly specialized nerve cells is their ability to integrate the thousands of actions and reactions going on in the body at the same time. Most of this activity is beyond our conscious awareness or control. Nerve impulses are transmitted so rapidly that a whole sequence of actions, interpretations and responses can take place before we are even aware that anything has happened. This activity is incredibly complex; although we tend to think that a single stimulus such as pricking a finger with a pin brings about a single specific nervous system response—pulling the finger away with a jerk—the fact is that such a simple stimulus actually triggers a veritable cascade of responses, perhaps thousands of them, all within a fraction of a second. The immediate reflex action is the fastest of these responses, perhaps, but it is followed by a wave of both unconscious and conscious nervous system activity including such a variety of things as a verbal response, a complex mental investigation of the source of the pain stimulus, a series of judgments regarding the seriousness of the injury, a review of the circumstances with storage of the incident in the memory to help protect against recurrences, even a rebalancing of a whole series of emergency biochemical reactions in the body that were initiated by the painful incident. Thus the nervous system not only *motivates* or directs immediate muscular responses; it also *moderates* a complex sequence of mental and physical reactions in order to achieve an appropriate pattern of behavior.

How can a single kind of tissue accomplish such a bewildering complexity of activity within the body? It does so by establishing an electrochemical circuit, beginning with some kind of stimulus at one end and resulting in some kind of motor activity at the other. Each part of this circuit—each individual neuron—is specially constructed to do a particular job. Different sensory nerve endings or sensory receptors, for instance, react to particular kinds of stimuli. The rods and cones in the retina of the eye are sensitive to various wavelengths of light. Special sound receptors in the ear convert mechanical vibrations into electrochemical impulses. In the skin certain raw nerve endings are sensitive to touch, others to pain and still others to heat. All these receptors react to quite specific stimuli; temperature receptors are some 2,000 times more sensitive to radiant heat than pain receptors. But certain stimuli, if strong enough, can excite the wrong receptors. Pressure on the eyeball, for example, can trigger "flashing light" sensations in the retina.

Sensory receptors are specially modified neurons, transmitting their electrochemical messages along different nerve fibers to the spinal cord and thence to the brain. Repeated stimuli may be required to "fire off" a nerve impulse, but once it is fired it will not normally be stopped until it reaches headquarters. An incredible network of receptor neurons provides the body with a sensitive wall of protection, keeping us informed of things going on around us and warning us whenever a detectable threat appears.

"Detectable" is the important word here, however. Our awareness of the world around us, rich as it may be, is limited to those impressions, and only those, for which we have sensory receptors. Certain dangers can sneak past our wall of protection undetected. Overexposure to the sun, for example, may lead to a disabling sunburn, yet the body has no warning of danger until the damage is already done. Foreign proteins to which the body is sensitive can gain access to the bloodstream with no hint of trouble until our allergic defenses swing into action. Similarly, we have no way to detect dangerous or even fatal doses of radiation at the time of exposure; we must rely on man-made warning devices such as exposure badges or Geiger counters.

On May 21, 1946, physicist Louis Slotin was working in a laboratory at Alamogordo, New Mexico, on the assembly of an atom bomb to be tested later at Bikini Atoll. Slotin was engaged in "tickling the dragon's tail," nudging two hemispheres of plutonium toward each other with a screwdriver, when the deadly material accidentally slid close enough together to form the critical mass of an activated bomb. In the violent blue glare of furious radioactivity, Slotin seized the bomb fragments with his bare hands and wrenched them apart with only seconds to spare, saving the lives of seven other men in the laboratory. Ordering the men to keep their places, he calmly recorded the exact positions of his co-workers and the time of the dreadful accident on the blackboard so that the amount of their exposure could be calculated. Then he walked out to the road to wait for an ambulance. As far as his body senses could tell, nothing had happened during that heroic moment, but Slotin knew beyond doubt that he was a walking dead man. Lethally exposed to radiation, he died in agony nine days later, the victim of a destroyer that his nervous system could not detect at all.

The sensory receptors at one end of the nervous system's circuit of reaction have their parallel at the other end in the special motor end plates where nerve comes in contact with muscle —the so-called *myoneural junction.* Here nerve tissue is separated from muscle by two thin cell membranes, with only a tiny bit of body fluid filling the gap between them. Even this minute gap would stop motor nerve impulses as effectively as a mile-wide gulf were it not for certain chemical reactions that take place there. As nerve impulses pile up at the myoneural junction, a chemical known as *acetylcholine* is released. This substance irritates muscle cells, causing them to contract when enough has accumulated. But as soon as the contraction occurs, an enzyme called *cholinesterase* begins breaking down the acetylcholine and clearing it away so that subsequent nerve impulses can set the cycle in motion again. It is this "rechargeable" chemical cycle that permits the conversion of nerve impulse into chemical impulse so that the myoneural junction can be bridged efficiently and muscle action can be stimulated.

Of course, the sensory receptors at one end and the nerve-muscle connections at the other end do not in themselves make a complete nervous system circuit. Impulses from the sensory pickups must reach the brain, and directives from the brain must reach the muscles. The transmitting neurons in the spinal cord provide the vital connecting link between the peripheral nerve endings, both sensory and motor, and the brain, as well as providing a mechanism—the reflex arc—for short-circuiting the brain momentarily when an emergency signal comes through. But ultimately it is the brain itself which must handle the steady flow of incoming impulses, interpret them, evaluate them, think about them, and finally send out the motor messages that will determine what the body does about the information its sensory mechanisms have gathered. Some of this incoming data goes into the brain's memory storage units after being scanned to determine that no action is necessary. Other data is transmitted to a more complex or "higher" center of the brain which is capable of considering, thinking, judging, unraveling puzzling data and finally arriving at decisions for or against action. Only then are these decisions transmitted, by way of the brain's multitudes of interconnecting nerve fibers, to the "output" or motor portions of the brain, where directive impulses arise for transmission down the spinal cord and out along the appropriate motor nerve channels to the particular muscles or other mechanisms (various glands, for instance) which must do the responding. The amazing thing is the incredible speed with which this whole exchange and evaluation of data is accomplished by the central and peripheral systems. And in its own quiet way, the autonomic nervous system carries on its workhorse functions with every bit as much dispatch. It is only when the autonomic nerve centers in the brain are damaged by injury or disease, or when an unguarded blow is received to one of the autonomic nerve crossroads, such as the solar plexus located high in the abdomen, the carotid sinus in the neck overlying the carotid artery, or the sensitive plexus of nerves surrounding the testicles, that the autonomic system falters. Blows to these areas can be truly, if temporarily, debilitating because of all the functions that the autonomic system regulates.

Considering the complexity of structure and

function of the nervous system, it is easy to see how damage or breakdown in one part of the system can cause a disturbance of function at some distant area of the body. Of all nervous system diseases or injuries, those affecting brain tissue itself can be the most devastating as well as the most difficult to diagnose, since the doctor may have only some distant disfunction as a clue, and must then seek to determine as quickly as possible whether the disfunction is due to damage in the brain proper or somewhere more distant in the nervous system. If a muscle ceases to function, for example, the trouble may lie in some disease or injury of the muscle itself, but it may also be due to a breakdown in transmission of nerve signals to the muscle. If the latter is the case, the breakdown might be at the nerve-muscle junction within the muscle cells, or somewhere in the motor nerve fibers running through a peripheral nerve, or in the motor nerve cell body that lies in the spinal cord, or in one of the transmitting neurons in the spinal nerve, or in the part of the brain itself that generates the motor nerve impulse in the first place. Accurate diagnosis of the disorder may depend not just upon examination of the malfunctioning muscle, but on a careful evaluation of the function of the entire nervous system.

And well protected as it is, the nervous system is still vulnerable to many kinds of disease, injury or impairment. Many disabilities of the brain itself are related either to direct destruction of brain tissue by injury or to obstruction of the brain's vital blood supply. A sudden interruption of blood flow to the brain, the so-called stroke, occurs when a blood clot obstructs a cerebral artery. This may lead to partial paralysis or sudden death, even though the brain still obtains some blood from the opposite artery. A more insidious form of destruction to the brain's blood supply occurs when atherosclerosis gradually narrows many small vessels, much the way mineral deposits reduce the diameter of water pipes. This gradual occlusion of arteries supplying the brain can lead to progressive oxygen starvation, with the death of more and more nerve cells every day—probably the major cause of senility and the loss of faculties in the aging.

Viral encephalitis may also destroy cells in all parts of the brain, permanently impairing its function. And finally, growing brain tumors can crowd and crush normal brain tissue and destroy healthy nerve cells. In such cases benign tumors which merely take up space inside the skull can be just as dangerous as cancers which actually invade and destroy brain tissue, except that benign tumors can often be removed with permanent recovery of lost function if they are diagnosed before they have grown too large.

Diseases or injuries affecting neurons in the spinal cord or the peripheral nerve trunks can also cause serious disability or even death. One of the most tragic events in the history of American baseball was the affliction of young Lou Gehrig at the height of his career with a dreadful and disabling disease of the nervous system known as amyotrophic lateral sclerosis. As motor neurons and the muscles they control progressively deteriorated, Gehrig became unable to play his beloved game. Voted the most valuable player of the year in 1936, he died in 1941, victim of a mysterious disorder that is just as poorly understood today as it was then.

In any impairment of nerve tissue, the degree of disability depends upon the part of the nervous system that is afflicted and the nature of the affliction. Anything interrupting the flow of nerve impulses anywhere will cause loss of body function in one area or another. Destruction of the receptor cells in the retina of the eye blocks the reception of visual images and results in permanent blindness. Damage to the auditory nerve, a common toxic side effect of large doses of the antibiotic streptomycin, may prevent the transmission of auditory impulses, resulting in deafness. Any injury crushing or cutting the main nerve trunks in the limbs will block the transmission of nerve impulses to and from the brain. Most damaging of all injuries, perhaps, is the tearing or severing of the spinal cord as a result of dislocation or fracture of the neck vertebrae—the sort of injury that occurs when a diver strikes his head on the bottom or when an athlete loses control on a trampoline. Although heartbeat, respiration and higher brain function are preserved, such an accident can leave the victim permanently paralyzed from the neck down.

Nervous system diseases may affect either sensory or motor nerves separately. The polio virus attacks only the cell bodies of the motor nerves in the spinal cord and brain stem. The spirochete of syphilis, on the other hand, may destroy the sensory nerve cells in the lower part of the spinal cord. In this condition, called *tabes dorsalis,* muscle function of the leg is unimpaired, but such functions as the sense of pressure and position are effectively disconnected. As a result the victim cannot feel where he is placing his feet and develops a characteristic staggering gait. The "demyelinating" diseases such as multiple sclerosis may affect either motor or sensory nerve fibers; often the combined and irregular deterioration of both systems provides an important clue to the diagnosis of this disabling affliction.

Just as the sensory receptors can be impaired, any condition that interferes with the chemical reactions at the myoneural junction can compromise normal motor function and lead to muscle weakness and paralysis. The breakdown of the acetylcholine-cholinesterase reaction in myasthenia gravis has already been mentioned. The Indian arrow poison, curare, made famous by mystery writers, also blocks this reaction at the myoneural junction, causing swift generalized paralysis and death by suffocation. Curiously enough, curare has actually proved a boon to mankind precisely because of its ability to cause widespread temporary paralysis. Surgeons often require profound muscle relaxation in a patient in order to expose internal organs for repair. Today anesthesiologists frequently administer curare-like medicines during surgery for this purpose. Of course, they must also be ready to provide respiration for the patient by artificial means until the curare wears off.

Disorders and diseases of the nervous system are discussed in detail in Part VI, "Patterns of Illness: The Nervous System." But whatever the nature of the injury or disability, destruction of nerve tissue is always extremely serious because it governs every voluntary and involuntary activity of the body. Virtually every animal from the ameba on up has some form of nervous system which grows more complex as the organism becomes more complex. In the human body the nervous system has reached the greatest complexity and the highest level of development of any creature on Earth. The nervous system of every organism motivates and moderates its life activities, but the greater size and complexity of man's nervous system affords him additional advantages. It gives him better memory storage and better capabilities for judgment. It permits him to make quicker, more accurate decisions. It provides him with the ability to reason, to communicate by speech and to moderate his body's primitive fight-or-flight reactions by superimposing such emotional controls as love, joy, understanding, a sense of wonder and a capability for introspection.

6

Protection and Appearance: The Cutaneous System

All the evidence available today indicates that the first cellular life as we know it arose on Earth from the warm, salty ocean—a nutrient broth, so to speak, in which the processes of evolution that led to land-dwelling plants and animals, and ultimately to man, had their beginnings. We know that throughout most of its natural history all life on Earth remained immersed in that saline sea. The reign of the land dwellers has been brief indeed compared to the vast expanse of time in which all life was confined to the sea. And even when life forms finally did move onto the land, they did not leave the sea behind them, for they could never have survived without it. Instead, they brought it with them, and they have kept it with them ever since.

It may seem strange to speak of trees, grasses, birds and land mammals such as men as "ocean dwellers," yet in the strictest sense this is precisely what they are. The simplest sea creatures obtain the dissolved oxygen and nutrients necessary for life directly from the water surrounding them by absorbing these substances through their cell membranes. Taken out of their nutrient broth onto dry land, these creatures would immediately die, unable either to absorb undissolved oxygen from the atmosphere or to withstand the desiccation that would occur owing to evaporation of fluid from their cells. But even a creature as complex as man is composed of fluid-filled cells, all basically similar to the cells of the simplest sea creature. These cells must also obtain their oxygen and nutrients from

a carefully maintained "interior sea" of salty water in which these life-sustaining substances are dissolved: the fluid portion of the blood and the tiny quantities of interstitial fluid surrounding and bathing each living cell in the body.

Without that "interior sea" of nutrient liquid in contact with all the cells and tissues of the body, man too would quickly die. He is able to survive on land, moving about in the dry atmosphere, for only one reason: he, like all other land-dwelling organisms, is equipped with a miraculous protective device—a skin or *integument*—capable of withstanding the drying effects of the atmosphere, thus preserving his "interior sea" and protecting it from evaporation. This integument varies greatly from one kind of organism to another, of course. In beetles or land crabs, it takes the form of a thick, fibrous or bony external skeleton protecting the body fluids within. The cactus is protected by a dense outer layer of horny plant fiber so efficient that the plant can withstand intense outside heat for years at a time with little water and still maintain the necessary fluid inside the cells. In man the integument takes a different form: a delicate but surprisingly substantial movable covering of cells spread over the entire body, impermeable to evaporation and complete with a pliable underlayer of fat and connective tissue which acts as further protection—in short, a highly complex and specialized organ system unlike any other to be found in the body, which is called the *cutaneous system* or, more simply, the skin and its appendages.

The Skin Around Us

People do not ordinarily think of the skin as an organ system like the nervous system or the digestive system, yet it qualifies for the name in exactly the same way. It is a collection of inter-related body organs which, working together, perform certain highly specialized tasks of which other organs are incapable. The cutaneous system has, in fact, an extraordinary variety of functions to perform. The primary task, of course, is to protect and maintain the "interior sea" within the body, to prevent vital fluids held inside from evaporating or leaking out. This means that all the internal tissues of the body must be covered at all times, and it is the skin and underlying tissues that perform that task. It also means that all the body orifices—the mouth, the nostrils, the vagina and the rectum, for example—must have special protection against drying. Technically, none of these orifices actually opens to the true interior of the body at all; that is, they do not lead directly to the unprotected cells and tissues of muscle, connective tissue or lymph channels. Rather, they are either entries to the digestive tract, a tube that passes through the body, or else entries to "cul-de-sacs" or blind pouches such as the vagina or the lungs. The inner surfaces of these tubes and pouches which communicate with the outside are themselves lined with a special kind of cutaneous tissue, the mucous membranes which contain cells that secrete a moist, sticky mucous substance to prevent them from drying. There is, in fact, *no* true interior tissue anywhere in the body that is not protected from exterior exposure by some form of cutaneous lining, at least under normal circumstances.

Because the human body must have a degree of smooth plasticity to permit the expansion of the lungs, the bulging of muscle or the movement of limbs, the cutaneous system must be not only protective but also flexible. The skin cannot dry out and crack on movement. The necessary flexibility is maintained in two ways. First, a pad of fleshy material underlying the outer skin contains quantities of *elastic tissue,* a specialized form of basic connective tissue, which is built into a stretchable subsurface lining that allows the skin to stretch and then regain its shape. Second, the surface of the skin itself is protected from drying and cracking by an oily lubricant called *sebum,* secreted by special *sebaceous glands* located in the outer layers of the skin covering most parts of the body. These "oil-secreting" glands are connected by means of ducts with the *hair follicles,* the tiny organs from which the body hairs grow. Thus the secretion from the sebaceous glands works its way to the surface and covers it with a thin film of oil which helps keep the outer layer of skin supple and soft.

The cutaneous system also provides remarkably efficient insulation from extremes of external heat and cold. The fat pad underlying the skin helps perform that function. In adults of normal weight it varies in thickness from as little as one-sixteenth of an inch under the skin of the back of the hand to as much as half an inch under the skin of the chest or three-quarters of an inch or more under the skin of the abdomen or the buttocks. Only a very few areas—the skin of the upper eyelid, for example—have no significant fat pad at all. Of course in obese individuals the layer of fat under the skin may be many inches thick in places, and there is also some sexual variation in the distribution of subcutaneous fat. Women usually have a somewhat thicker and smoother distribution of this tissue than men, which gives them a less bony and angular appearance. A newborn baby ordinarily has a subcutaneous layer of "baby fat" that gives his arms and legs a characteristic chubby appearance until it is replaced with a more mature fat layer during the second year of life. With advancing maturity the elastic tissue underlying the skin surface tends to stretch and deteriorate, and much of the subcutaneous fat is reabsorbed, ultimately resulting in the looseness and wrinkling of the skin that is seen in old age.

Another protective function of the skin is to shield the body from overexposure to harmful ultraviolet radiation from the sun. Scattered throughout the skin, beneath the outer layer of cells, are cells containing a brownish pigment known as *melanin* which acts as a natural sun screen. Even the fairest-skinned individuals of the Caucasian race in North America or northern Europe have some of this pigment in their skin, and repeated or continuing exposure to sunlight stimulates the formation of more melanin in the process called tanning. In some fair-skinned people, the melanin-containing cells develop in clusters rather than uniformly, forming freckles. In general, the amount of melanin present in the skin is greater among peoples inhabiting, or who once inhabited, hot, semi-tropical or tropical regions of the Earth, which accounts for the darker-colored skin of people from Mediterranean Europe, the mahogany-brown skin of East Indians and skin colors varying from light brown to blue-black among Negroes. These variations of skin color, however, are not a matter of individual body response to immediate living conditions, but rather are determined by the genetic makeup of the individual. Thus the skin of an African Negro will not lighten if he goes to live in Sweden, and the white-skinned Swede will not darken significantly or permanently if he moves to the Congo to live.

There is still another important way in which the cutaneous system guards the body from damage to the cells and tissues within. Thanks to an incredibly complex network of delicate nerve endings located in the skin surface all over the body, the skin is a magnificent sensory organ which keeps us constantly informed of changing conditions outside the body, conditions that might be very dangerous if we had no "early warning system" to tell us about them. Some of these nerve endings are singularly sensitive to heat or cold. Others respond to touch of any kind, while still others are pain receptors that send warning of any contact that may be injurious—a pinprick, a pinch or excessive pressure, for example. In specially sensitive areas of the skin such as the fingertips, there may be a dozen or more of these nerve endings crowded together into an area as small as one-sixteenth of an inch in diameter. Elsewhere the concentration is not quite so great, yet there is no area of the body that does not have an adequate supply of these sensory pickup points. Even on the ball of the foot, which is often coated with a layer of tough dead skin cells one-eighth of an inch thick or

more, sensations of touch, heat or pain are readily detected.

Certain other functions of the cutaneous system have no direct relationship to protection of the tissues within the body, yet are still vital to normal body function. For example, an important part of the body's interior cooling system is centered in the skin. Sweat glands in the skin located all over the body pour out salty perspiration onto the surface in greater or lesser amounts at all times, depending upon the surface temperature. As the perspiration evaporates, the skin surface is cooled, thus cooling the blood that flows in the capillaries just beneath the skin. When the interior of the body becomes over-heated, these capillaries expand, bringing more blood to the cool surface of the body, and the production of sweat is simultaneously increased to produce more cooling of the skin surface. This process is so efficient that the internal body temperature is normally held remarkably stable, close to 98.6° F., even when an enormous excess of internal heat is being generated, as during vigorous physical exercise, or when the outside air temperature is ten or more degrees higher than normal body temperature.

The sweat glands also cause minor irritations and problems. Especially in the hairy region under the arms and in the groin they are unusually numerous and active. Surface bacteria tend to grow in these moist, warm areas and produce an offensive body odor or "BO." Innumerable commercial deodorants may be used to combat this problem, but most contain chemicals that can irritate sensitive skin and often damage clothing as well. In most cases offensive "BO" can be adequately controlled by bathing and changing underclothing daily.

In some creatures the cutaneous system provides an additional insulating layer of fur as protection against the cold. In man the growth of body hair is a vestigial function of the cutaneous system, possibly important at some earlier time in our evolutionary development but no longer particularly useful. Useful or not, each hair follicle is still equipped with a tiny *papillary muscle* that tends to lift the hair up straight on end when we are chilly or frightened, resulting in the familiar "goose pimples." Similarly, our fingernails and toenails are mere vestiges of claws that at one time may have been important to survival but no longer serve any vital purpose.

There is, however, one additional very useful function of this organ system that has nothing to do with physical protection. Mature human females possess *mammary glands,* highly specialized clusters of secreting cells which develop from cells in the skin and subcutaneous tissue at puberty and which are able, under the influence of female sex hormones produced before, during and after childbirth, to manufacture milk for the nurture of the newborn baby.

The Remarkable Structure of the Skin

The cutaneous system is perhaps the most varied of the organ systems in the body, even though, to all outward appearances, it may seem very simple. Its structure is, of course, not simple at all. In fact, during the early development of the embryo, the cutaneous system is one of the first of the organ systems to begin to separate from the other embryonal cells and take on characteristics of its own.

At first all embryonal cells appear much the same, growing by simple cell division from the original fertilized egg. Within two weeks, however, differentiation into three distinct layers of tissue—endoderm, mesoderm and ectoderm—begins to take place. The ectoderm or "outer skin" ultimately differentiates again, developing both into the cutaneous system on the outside and into a groove of special tissues extending the whole length of the embryo, which finally forms the spinal cord and brain on the inside.

The basic surface tissue of the cutaneous system is made up of squamous epithelium called the *epidermis:* flat, tile-shaped cells that form a "pavement" on the surface of the body. The outer layers of these cells are dead or dying, drying up and flaking off continuously, to be replaced by cells lying just beneath in the formative layer of the epithelium—healthy, growing cells that are constantly being formed to replace those on the surface as they are damaged and destroyed. Cells in this formative layer have remarkable regenerative powers. If some are damaged by a cut or scratch, the surrounding cells divide quickly and form a film of new cells over the damaged area. As long as the injury extends no deeper than the epidermis, healing will be complete and featureless, without scarring. It is only when an injury extends into

DIFFERENT KINDS
OF EPITHELIUM

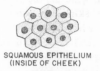

SQUAMOUS EPITHELIUM
(INSIDE OF CHEEK)

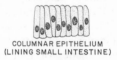

COLUMNAR EPITHELIUM
(LINING SMALL INTESTINE)

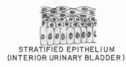

STRATIFIED EPITHELIUM
(INTERIOR URINARY BLADDER)

Figure 6–1.

deeper layers of the skin or the subcutaneous connective tissue, which cannot regenerate as well, that special fibrous cells form during the healing process—a type of cell which, once formed, tends to shrink and pull together in a tough, fibrous strand of tissue which we know as a *scar*. Scar formation represents imperfect healing; in many illnesses in which damaged tissues heal with scarring, the scar itself may cause prolonged or even crippling disability.

Ordinarily we are not particularly aware of the flaking off of the outer layer of epithelial cells, except under special circumstances. When the skin is injured by a sunburn, or rubbed and irritated until a blister of water forms, the outer layer may peel in large chunks, leaving the underlying skin layers exposed. In the scalp area, flakes of desquamated skin are often seen in the hair as *dandruff,* a condition which may be aggravated by inadequate cleansing, excessive dryness or the action of certain kinds of bacteria that live there. Fortunately, even these abnormal circumstances do not bring about excessive wear and tear on the body, thanks to the remarkable regenerative powers of the epidermis.

But there is more to the skin than the surface. Immediately beneath the epidermis is a layer of much thicker epithelial cells forming a "basement membrane" of the skin called the *dermis*. This underlayer of cells is richly supplied with the capillary blood vessels that cause the pinkish tone one sees in fair-skinned people. The phenomenon of *blushing* occurs when emotional states such as embarrassment trigger involuntary nerve impulses that cause the skin capillaries to dilate. Oddly enough, such capillary dilatation is normally confined only to areas of the skin that are ordinarily exposed to view; an embarrassed girl might be even more embarrassed to know that her blush extends only down to the normal neckline of her dress and no further.

It is also in this underlying skin layer that the sensory nerve endings to the skin are found, and here that the melanin pigment is deposited in the cells, sparsely in light-skinned races, moderately to heavily in dark-skinned people. Occasionally a patch of cells containing large amounts of melanin will develop into a small brown or black tumor called a pigmented nevus, more commonly known as a mole. Some moles become as large as several inches in diameter, and most are associated with excessive hair growth in the area. The vast majority of moles are perfectly benign and need not cause worry unless at some time they suddenly begin to enlarge, thicken or bleed. Any such change may indicate that early cancer is developing in the mole, and a doctor should be consulted at once. Usually such cancers, when they occur, can be completely cured by excision of the mole, but on rare occasions an exceedingly dangerous cancer known as malignant melanoma can first develop as an apparently innocent mole. Any kind of change in such a growth should therefore be checked for safety's sake. In addition, most physicians recommend removal of moles that are located in areas where they may be chronically irritated—under a bra strap, for example, or along the belt line.

Finally, it is in the dermis layer that the hair follicles are found as well as the skin's sebaceous and sweat glands. When sebaceous gland outlets at the hair follicles become plugged with surface debris, or inflamed and swollen shut, a condition known as "prickly heat" occurs, most often seen in babies and small children, who are frequently overdressed during extremely warm weather. In adolescents and adults the sebaceous gland ducts may become obstructed with oily sebum mixed with dirt, especially on the face, to form comedones or "blackheads." Among teen-agers in particular, hormonal changes following puberty cause an increase in size and secretion of these sebaceous glands, and the resulting comedones may become infected to form the pus-filled lesions of common acne or pimples. Almost all adolescents suffer from this plague to some degree at one time or another, but the effect can be minimized by fastidious daily cleansing of the affected skin areas to help prevent the blackheads from forming in the first place.

Appearance and Variation

Obviously the human body would have trouble surviving long without the protection of the various physiological functions of the cutaneous system. Yet for practical purposes the one function of the skin and its appendages of which we are most conscious has nothing at all to do with physiology or body function. Because of its location on the surface of the body, it is the skin which contributes the most to our physical appearance and which accounts for the variations in appearance, obvious or subtle, found among individuals and races.

To realize just how important such a thing as outward appearance is to human beings, even though it has nothing to do with physical health or physiological survival, we need only remind ourselves of the millions of dollars spent annually for the cosmetic creams, oils, pigments and dyes designed to accentuate flattering features or to help conceal blemishes and flaws that we consider unsightly or undesirable. Any noticeable abnormality of the skin may cause distress. For instance, the child born with a so-called port wine stain or birthmark—a blotchy purple mark on the skin due to abnormal growth of skin capillaries in certain areas—may suffer lifelong discomfort as a result of his appearance. Even more tragically, physical variations attributable to race, whether they involve skin pigmentation, texture of the hair or other characteristics of the cutaneous system, may set whole groups of individuals completely apart from their fellow men.

Most of these so-called racial characteristics are actually centered in relatively minor group variations in the structure of the cutaneous system. Perhaps the most obvious such variation is skin pigmentation, but differences in the shape of the lips, the nose or other facial features also distinguish the Negroid, Caucasoid and Mongoloid races. Among members of the Mongoloid race, for example, it is a slight fold of skin at the outer corners of the upper eyelids, the *epicanthal fold,* that accounts for the unmistakable almond shape of the eyes. The color, structure and distribution of body hair is another distinguishing racial variation. In the case of Caucasians and Mongoloids hair follicles are circular in cross section, so that hair grows out smoothly, either straight or slightly wavy. In Negroes, however, the follicles are oval in cross section, so that the hair grows tightly curled or kinked. Orientals and Amerinds (native American Indians and Eskimos) generally have far more scanty growth of body hair than Caucasians; the beard of the Oriental man tends to be wispy, while American

GENE–DETERMINED DIFFERENCES IN HAIR

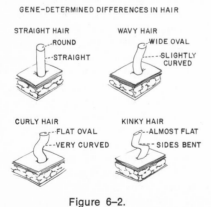

Figure 6–2.

Indians often have little beard at all. As to hair color, Americans usually think of blond, brunette and red hair as fairly common, yet the overwhelming majority of all humans, whatever their race, have either black or dark brown hair. Virtually all Negroes, Orientals, East Indians, Arabs, American Indians and Eskimos, and

most Mediterranean Europeans and Latin Americans have black or brown-black hair except in the rare case of albinos (people born without any skin or hair pigment at all, a genetic abnormality) or in the case of racial admixtures. Naturally blond hair is a native characteristic only in northern Europe and Asia and among Americans of northern European descent. Red hair, on balance around the world, is a rarity indeed, occurring in only a fraction of 1 percent of all human beings.

No one knows why different racial characteristics came into being. They are all transmitted genetically, however, and in our modern world the concept of "pure" racial characteristics has no validity. Although we speak of three basic "racial stocks"—Negroid, Caucasoid and Mongoloid (some throw in a fourth, Australoid, to account for otherwise unclassifiable characteristics of Australian aborigines)—the fact is that *all* these stocks have been so thoroughly intermixed, especially in modern societies, that the distinctions become scientifically meaningless. Fortunately they are becoming more and more meaningless socially as well, as we recognize the absurdity of judging a body—like a book—by its cover. All human beings are singularly alike in their biological form and functions, whatever the minor variations in shape, size or color. We must look elsewhere for the differences and special characteristics that make every human being a unique individual.

The Cutaneous System in Disfunction

Like any other organ system, the cutaneous system is vulnerable to a wide variety of diseases and injuries which can severely impair its normal function. No other organ system is subject to more frequent minor cutting, scraping or bruising. The skin is continually exposed to casual damage from objects in the environment, and to bee stings, insect bites and various other superficial injuries. But none of these generally cause lasting trouble or disturb the function of the system unless infection is introduced through a break in the skin. Often such a complication can be prevented simply by washing a minor skin injury carefully with soap and water and covering it with a clean dressing or bandage to keep dirt out of it until it heals.

Burns are quite a different matter, perhaps the most serious of all common disorders affecting the skin. Even such a minor thing as a "mild" sunburn can cause disruption of the skin's function if it is widespread. More serious burns actually destroy the deeper layers of the skin, as well as the subcutaneous tissue, and can leave large areas of the body denuded—open, weeping wounds, terribly vulnerable to infection, often extremely painful and subject to severe scarring as healing takes place. No burn more serious than a minor scorched finger should ever be ignored. Extensive burns require immediate and continuing expert medical attention and often prolonged hospital care. (*See* p. 119.)

Various kinds of infections can involve portions of the skin as well as other parts of the body. Boils and furuncles are localized infections involving the deep layers of the skin and the subcutaneous connective tissue, usually caused by staphylococcus or streptococcus organisms. Hansen's disease (leprosy), uncommon in America but still afflicting many people in other parts of the world, is a slow-growing infection that destroys skin, nerve endings, connective tissue and bone. It is often first diagnosed because scarring of subcutaneous tissue causes the skin over affected areas to become lumpy and twisted, and because the infection destroys nerve endings, thus causing localized areas of anesthesia in the skin. Tuberculosis is another long-term infection that can affect the skin as well as other organs in the body.

"Dermatitis" is a general term used to describe all varieties of skin inflammations. Some, as noted above, are caused by infectious organisms that gain lodging in the skin. Various insect parasites (chiggers, itch mites, lice, etc.) may also cause dermatitis. Other forms of skin inflammations may arise from causes as variable as malnutrition, chronic chafing, exposure to chemicals, or even emotional upset. Some, such as psoriasis (a skin disease marked by thickening, reddening and scaling of patches of the skin, especially on the knees and elbows), arise from unknown causes.

Perhaps the most common form of dermatitis, suffered at one time or another by virtually everyone, is the swelling, itching and redness that can arise as a result of an allergic reaction, either to some substance contacting the surface of the skin (oil from poison ivy leaves, for instance, or various cosmetics that engender allergic reactions) or to some food or drug that has been taken internally. Contact allergies are usually confined to the areas where the offending substance actually touched the skin. But allergenic foods or medicines can cause more general reactions, owing to an outpouring of a body chemical known as *histamine* into the skin and subcutaneous tissue. This substance causes swelling of the skin tissues, sometimes even the formation of raised red patches called hives, together with intense itching. Such allergic reactions can often be suppressed by administration of medicines known as *antihistamines* which help neutralize the histamine that causes the reaction.

Finally, a number of generalized diseases, fortunately relatively rare, may affect the skin or the underlying connective tissue or both. Among these are lupus erythematosis, a connective tissue disease which is often heralded by an outbreak of the skin in a butterfly-shaped patch across the bridge of the nose and over both cheekbones; dermatomyositis, an inflammatory disease affecting both muscle and skin; and scleroderma, in which the subcutaneous tissue and skin all over the body gradually become thickened and lose their elasticity.

These and other disorders of the skin are discussed in detail in Part VII, "Patterns of Illness: The Cutaneous System." Considering its exposed position in the body, however, the cutaneous system is generally one of the most trouble-free of all the organ systems, and proceeds to carry out its multiple functions throughout life with little but an occasional scratch or bruise to call itself to our attention.

7

Exchange, Filtration and Secretion: The Lungs, Kidneys and Endocrines

When a man dashes for a departing bus he starts a chain of conscious, voluntary acts controlled entirely by his will. He runs, shouts and waves his hand even as he judges how fast the bus is moving, calculates his chances of catching it, and when he misses it wonders how long he will have to wait for the next one. At the same time, activities of a completely different kind are proceeding in his body, quite apart from any voluntary control. These involuntary functions include the circulation of blood, the absorption of oxygen, the digestion of food and the processing of body wastes. All have a critical role in the chain of internal chemical reactions called *metabolism,* and all are carried on in certain vital organs composed largely of epithelium, the fifth of the body's basic tissues. Among these organs are the lungs, the kidneys and the endocrine glands, which together perform three critical epithelial functions—*exchange, filtration* and *secretion.*

The exchange function of epithelial tissue is best illustrated by the lungs, which have a single major job to perform: the transfer of certain gases in and out of the body. Oxygen must be drawn into the blood stream for body use while carbon dioxide in the blood, a by-product of metabolism, must be expelled. Since bubbles of free gas do not circulate in the blood stream, this exchange must involve more than the simple passage of gases back and forth through a sieve. The lungs must manage some kind of *chemical exchange* so that each gas moves in the right direction. To make this possible, the body needs a vast, moist surface area of tissue that is in direct contact with air on one side and with the circulating blood on the other. The epithelium of the lung provides precisely this special kind of surface area.

We can see how efficiently the lung does its job by comparing the oxygen-exhausted venous blood that is pumped into the lungs for aeration with the oxygenated arterial blood flowing back to the heart for distribution to the body tissues. Venous blood is a dark, purplish-black color, almost depleted of oxygen but carrying an overload of dissolved carbon dioxide. In passing through the lung this blood drops off its excess carbon dioxide, becomes 97 percent saturated with oxygen and takes on the bright scarlet color of arterial blood.

How much oxygen and carbon dioxide are actually involved in this exchange? The answer depends upon the body's activity. At complete rest we absorb perhaps a half a pint of oxygen from the air at sea-level pressure every minute, and expel slightly less carbon dioxide at the same time. But when a runner clocks a mile in less than four minutes, his lungs absorb approximately three and a half quarts of oxygen and expel two and a half quarts of carbon dioxide every minute. This amazing exchange is made possible by the masterful engineering of the lungs, which bring a maximum amount of air into contact with a maximum volume of blood in a chest cavity that is seldom as much as two feet square.

Anatomically the lungs are a pair of soft

spongy organs lodged in the bony thorax on either side of the heart. Air is taken in by way of a semirigid pipe called the *trachea,* which divides into two *mainstem bronchi,* each entering one lung. Within the lungs these large air tubes begin branching and rebranching like limbs of a tree, first into smaller *bronchi* and then into even smaller *bronchioles,* each of which finally terminates in clusters of tiny, expansible, thin-walled air sacs called *alveoli* that make up the bulk of the lung. The trachea and the larger bronchi are held open by rings of cartilage to prevent their collapse as air is sucked in; even the smaller bronchioles have spiraling layers of smooth muscle in their walls to help maintain their shape. More important, all these air tubes have an inner lining of tall, columnar epithelial cells kept moist by special mucus-secreting cells.

This protective bronchial lining is of no use for gas exchange. But as the tiniest bronchioles open out into the terminal air sacs, the epithelial lining changes remarkably. Instead of being lined with thick columnar cells, the alveoli are constructed entirely of flat, tile-shaped cells called squamous epithelium stretched out in thin-walled, balloon-like structures which can expand or contract as air is drawn in or out. There may be as many as 600 million of these tiny air sacs in the lungs of an average-sized man. They are so small that a single sac can have a surface area in contact with the air no greater than one hundred-thousandth of a square inch. Yet taken all together they make up a respiratory membrane with an area of *600 square feet*—equal in size to a 30-by-20-foot living room floor.

Of course the air entering these alveolar sacs is, in a sense, still outside the body; somehow oxygen must be drawn from them into the blood stream. In each lung a *pulmonary artery* carrying oxygen-exhausted blood from the heart follows the branching bronchi, dividing into smaller and smaller vessels as the bronchi divide. When the bronchioles expand into terminal alveoli, the blood vessels open into a rich network of tiny *capillaries* surrounding each cluster of sacs. The pulmonary capillaries are barely large enough to allow red blood cells to pass through single file; but like the alveoli themselves, they are made of a single, thin filamentous layer of squamous

epithelium. These two layers of thin, flat cells—capillary and alveolar—lie in direct contact side by side, a microscopically thin double membrane with warmed, moistened air on one side and circulating blood on the other.

It is this double respiratory membrane which permits the diffusion of oxygen from the lung into the blood stream. Once inside the capillary, oxygen is chemically bound by an iron-containing protein material called *hemoglobin* in the red blood cells so that it cannot diffuse back again. This oxygen-loaded hemoglobin gives the aerated blood its rich red color as it is swept back to the heart for distribution to the body cells.

While oxygen is diffusing into the blood stream from the alveoli, dissolved carbon dioxide in the blood is leaking out of the capillaries into the alveolar sacs. Since there is nothing to bind it in the blood, carbon dioxide crosses the respiratory membrane by simple *osmosis.* While some of it is swept out of the lungs with the exhaled air, some goes back into the blood stream again, so that the blood returning to the heart still carries a certain amount of carbon dioxide. This is by no means an accident; although we may think of carbon dioxide solely as a waste material, a small amount dissolved in the blood at all times is essential to the body's chemical balance. It also helps maintain the proper respiratory rate. Certain nerve centers in the brain are exceedingly sensitive to the carbon dioxide concentration in the blood, speeding up the breathing rate when too much is present or slowing it down when carbon dioxide levels drop too low.

The role of carbon dioxide in the maintenance of normal body chemistry was a puzzle to early physiologists, who assumed that this substance was nothing but a useless by-product of metabolism. In the early 1900s the great British physiologist John Scott Haldane was one of the first to suspect carbon dioxide's double role in the body. Individuals who become excited and breathe too fast often experience numbness, dizziness and a kind of muscle cramping called *tetany.* These symptoms had previously been blamed on "oxygen poisoning" due to the rapid breathing, but nobody could see why an excess of oxygen should be "poisonous." Haldane suspected the trouble arose not from taking in too much oxygen but from blowing off too much carbon dioxide. There is a medical school story that Haldane, notorious for experimenting on himself, set out to test this notion by sitting on a stool in a steaming hot shower and panting furiously. By the time he was certain his theory was true, the story goes, his muscles were cramping so uncontrollably that he could neither turn off the water nor get out of the shower, and was nearly *in extremis* by the time he was discovered and rescued. Later experiments (with assistants present) proved that the symptoms of "oxygen poisoning" were in fact a dangerous condition known as respiratory alkalosis, which arises when too much carbon dioxide is driven out of the blood stream by overbreathing.

The epithelial respiratory membrane that performs the exchange of gases in the lungs is remarkably efficient. It absorbs all the oxygen the body requires under normal circumstances and unloads precisely the right amount of carbon dioxide to maintain chemical balance. It is also selective; the tiny molecules of dissolved gases pass through it freely, but the larger protein molecules in the blood are blocked. Because a constant supply of oxygen is utterly critical for the survival of all the body tissues, any impairment of gas exchange through this membrane can quickly lead to oxygen starvation and death. Lack of oxygen or *anoxia* is probably the most extreme hazard that ever threatens the human body. As Haldane once remarked, it can cause not only the stoppage of the machine but the total ruin of the machinery as well.

Unfortunately, a number of conditions do interfere with the body's oxygen supply. When a common cold strikes, watery mucus is secreted in the nose and sinuses and must be cleared out to keep the passageway for air open. In bronchitis, infection causes the lining of the air tubes in the lungs to swell and pour out mucus which obstructs the flow of air to the alveoli. Coughing is the body's method of expelling this sticky stuff, and certain medicines called *expectorants* help make coughing more effective. Prolonged bronchial infection with chronic coughing sometimes leads to a permanent stretching, tearing and scarring of the smooth muscle in the walls

of the smaller bronchi, a condition known as bronchiectasis.

Infection is not the only cause of bronchial obstruction. Every doctor has encountered the child who suddenly begins choking after accidentally inhaling a peanut, a match stick or some other foreign body. When a large air tube is blocked off in this way, the oxygen trapped beyond the obstruction is soon completely absorbed and the affected segment of lung slowly deflates like a leaky balloon, throwing a characteristic wedge-shaped shadow on an X-ray film. This condition is known as atelectasis.

Another kind of obstruction occurs when certain allergic or emotional reactions cause spasm and contraction of the smooth muscle in the bronchioles so that air drawn into the alveoli cannot easily be pushed out again. This is the cause of the sudden attacks of wheezing which occur in asthma. If the condition is prolonged or occurs repeatedly, the alveolar sacs themselves can be stretched until they lose their elasticity to expand and contract with respiratory movements —a condition known as pulmonary emphysema. One of the most bizarre of all human ailments is bullous emphysema, or "disappearing lung disease," in which distended alveoli progressively break down to form great compressed air pockets in the lung, crowding out normal lung tissue. Occasionally one of these pockets will break, causing spontaneous pneumothorax and collapse of a lung. Sometimes the condition must be treated by surgical removal of the damaged lung tissue.

These malfunctions are all related to obstruction of air flow in and out of the lungs. Other diseases affect the alveoli themselves, interfering with the exchange of gases through the respiratory membrane. In pneumonia the alveoli thicken and fill up with a sticky, inflammatory exudate which prevents air from reaching the membrane. If the infection affects only one segment of a lung, it is called lobar pneumonia; but often patchy areas in all the lung segments are affected, as in bronchial and viral pneumonia. In any kind of pneumonia the transfer of oxygen is impaired, and to add insult to injury, high fevers occur, causing the body cells to require more and more oxygen as the supply falls lower and lower. Thirty years ago pneumonia was the number one killer in this country, taking its toll in every age group. Today most forms of the disease can be controlled with antibiotic drugs, but it still remains a serious threat to children and elderly people.

Tuberculosis is a different sort of lung infection. The slow-growing bacteria that cause it can gradually destroy large areas of lung tissue, form cavities and damage blood vessels with subsequent hemorrhage. Tuberculosis cannot be stopped as effectively as pneumonia with antibiotics, but it often can be arrested. World-wide public health efforts are slowly eliminating this disease as a major cause of death.

Other conditions can also impair the oxygenation of blood in the lungs. The lung capillaries not only absorb oxygen but supply the lung tissue itself with fuel and oxygen. When a traveling blood clot or *embolus* obstructs a pulmonary artery, it produces *infarction* and death of a wedge of lung tissue. In certain kinds of heart conditions, fluid seeps out of the capillaries into the alveolar sacs to impair the absorption of oxygen. Embryonic malformations of the heart may shunt venous blood directly back into the general circulation, by-passing perfectly normal lungs and causing the oxygen starvation seen in "blue babies." The utilization of oxygen by the body cells can be blocked by chemicals such as sodium cyanide, the poison taken by Nazi leader Hermann Göring in 1946 in order to cheat the executioner after the Nuremberg trials. Less exotic but just as dangerous is carbon monoxide, which can "masquerade" as oxygen in the blood stream and so completely overload the hemoglobin that it is not free to carry oxygen to the tissues.

Thus any breakdown in the chain of reactions by which oxygen passes through the respiratory membrane in the lung, is carried in the blood stream and is used by the body cells can mean serious illness or even death. Respiratory diseases and disorders are discussed in detail in Part IV, "Patterns of Illness: The Infectious Diseases," and Part VIII, "Patterns of Illness: The Respiratory Tract." But the remarkable fact is not how many things can go wrong but how

efficiently these reactions are handled by epithelial tissue in the normal body and how rarely serious trouble arises.

The lung is not the only organ in which an epithelial membrane plays a vital role in body function. Like the lung, the kidney is utterly necessary for survival, and in many ways they are amazingly similar, both in structure and in function. The kidney also has a membrane which is in direct, if somewhat more circuitous, contact with the outside environment, and like the lung it has an extremely rich blood supply. And the basic "working tissue" of the kidney is a vast thin membrane of epithelium which permits both the exchange and the filtration of substances back and forth through it—in this case, body fluids carrying dissolved chemicals rather than gas molecules.

The importance of proper kidney function has been dramatically demonstrated in recent years by surgical attempts to save lives by kidney transplants and the successful use of artificial kidney machines. At first these machines were used only in operating rooms and during temporary emergencies, but today they are used on a regular basis to sustain the lives of patients with chronic and incurable renal disease. If a kidney machine is not available or if its use is prohibitively expensive, as unfortunately is often the case, patients such as these have no chance for survival.

For such utterly essential organs, the kidneys are small and simple in appearance—dark red, bean-shaped structures, each about the size of a human fist, located in the small of the back on either side of the vertebral column just below the level of the lower ribs. They are protected only by the thick back muscles coursing down either side of the spine and are held in place by a fibrous meshwork of connective tissue. Like the lungs, the kidneys are paired organs, and this pairing provides the body with an important reserve capacity: a person can survive splendidly as long as just one of his kidneys is functioning well.

Each kidney is supplied with blood by a renal artery from the aorta that passes down behind the abdominal cavity, and venous blood returns from the kidneys via the renal veins into the

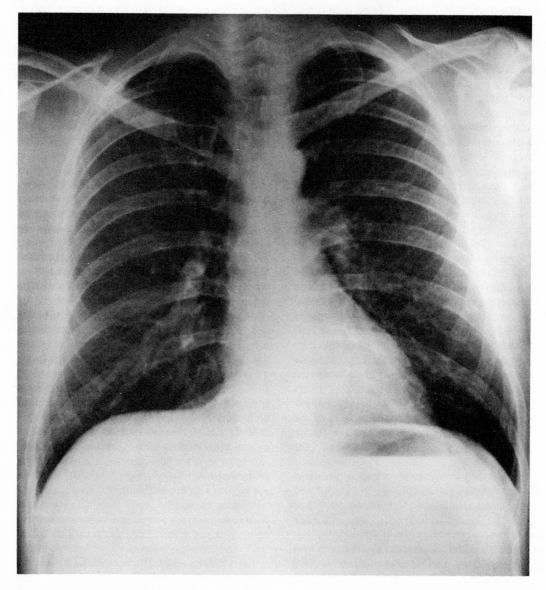

Plate 4a   A normal chest X-ray. The heart shadow in the center of the film appears more dense than the comparatively translucent air-filled lungs on either side.

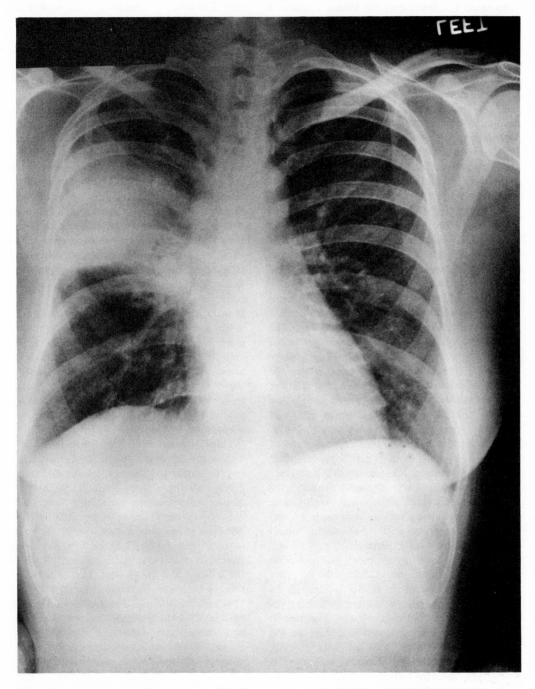

Plate 4b   Lobar pneumonia appears in this film as a dense, cloudy triangular shadow in the middle portion of the right lung. Compare with normal chest film in Plate 4a.

vena cava. The interior of the kidney contains a collecting space for urine, the so-called *kidney pelvis,* leading to a long drainage tube, the *ureter,* which extends down to the urinary *bladder* with its opening to the outside via the *urethra.* Thus the interior of the kidney is actually in direct connection with the exterior of the body by means of this system of drainage tubules.

Why is the kidney so critical to the continued life and health of the body? Essentially, it provides a filter to clear poisonous waste materials from the blood stream. The filtering is accomplished by a remarkable *differential barrier* of epithelium which allows certain substances to pass through it freely in one direction but not in the other. In effect, this barrier membrane traps useless wastes from the blood stream and then refuses them readmission, whereupon they are passed out and discarded in the urine.

Throughout the body living cells are constantly dumping by-products from their cellular metabolism into the blood stream. When the blood enters the kidneys through the renal arteries, it is carried through a special capillary bed which greatly retards its rate of flow. In most tissues the blood capillaries form a fine network around the body cells they supply; by contrast, the capillaries in the kidney wind and twist into tightly packed "knots" called *glomeruli,* very similar in appearance to tiny snarls of fine yarn. The walls of these capillaries are made of simple squamous epithelium, one cell layer thick. As blood passes slowly through the glomeruli, water seeps out into a system of long, convoluted collecting tubules also made of epithelial tissue, carrying with it both useful chemicals and dissolved waste materials.

We still are not sure how much of this fluid is actually filtered into the kidney tubules every day—probably as much as 50 gallons in 24 hours. Obviously the body cannot afford to sacrifice all that fluid or the useful materials it contains, so a second filtration occurs as the original filtrate passes through long twisting miles of kidney tubules. Most of the water is reabsorbed into the blood stream, along with useful substances such as glucose, but useless by-products of protein metabolism such as urea

and uric acid are unable to cross back through the tubular membrane and are carried on out with a small amount of water as *urine.*

It is clear that something more is going on in the kidney tubules than the simple exchange of dissolved substances by osmosis back and forth through a semipermeable membrane. The epithelial cells in the tubules literally pick and choose between substances to be readmitted and waste products to be expelled. This process is dramatically illustrated under certain special conditions. Ordinarily all the glucose that seeps out of the kidney capillaries is retained by the tubules for reabsorption into the blood stream, but if the blood sugar level is too high, as in diabetes mellitus, the tubules reach the limit of their ability to retain the glucose. Any in excess of this limit is "spilled" out into urine—sometimes the first clue that diabetes is present. On the other hand, some foreign materials are expelled by the tubular membrane so vigorously that the blood is cleared of them completely in a single passage through the kidneys. Certain radio-opaque iodine compounds may be seen by X-ray collecting in the kidney pelvis within 60 seconds after injection into a vein, and are completely expelled into the bladder within 30 minutes, making possible a special diagnostic examination of the urinary tract known as an *intravenous pyelogram* (IVP).

Curiously enough, the epithelium of the kidney tubules is the only tissue in the body that has the ability to "identify" useful materials and distinguish them from waste. It is this unique quality which permits the kidney—and only the kidney—to carry on its life-maintaining work. Needless to say, any disturbance in the function of such a specialized tissue will have serious effects on the body. (Diseases and disorders of the kidney and the tissues and organs of the urinary tract are discussed in detail in Part XII, "Patterns of Illness: The Urinary and Genital Systems.") Infection can damage kidney tissue and dangerously interfere with its function. Some kidney infections are readily identified because of high fevers and severe pain, but sometimes the only clue to trouble is the discovery of pus cells and protein in the urine. Of all infections, tuberculosis, which affects the kidney second only to the lung, is probably the most dangerous because it can do irreversible damage before symptoms appear.

Kidney function can also be impaired by any disorder that obstructs the flow of urine into the bladder. Sometimes calcium or uric acid crystals form stones in the kidney which lodge in the ureters leading to the bladder. Such an occurrence may lead to violent pain and prostration until the stone is either passed or removed. Obstructions caused by tumors or abnormal blood vessels crossing the ureter are less dramatic and far less common, but can still result in serious kidney damage.

Of all the kidney diseases, however, the most dangerous are those which directly impair the function of the kidneys by means of inflammatory or degenerative changes in the filtering mechanism itself. One form of inflammatory disease, glomerulonephritis, often afflicts children and seems, like rheumatic fever, to be caused by an acute body reaction following streptococcus infections. The kidney capillaries and connective tissue are seriously damaged, and in some cases the disease may cause either acute sudden shutdown of kidney function or long-term irreparable damage. Another dangerous condition, the so-called nephrotic syndrome, results from degenerative damage to the kidney tubules; this disorder, too, sometimes results in progressive, permanent loss of kidney function. Certain victims of these diseases are among the unfortunate few who may one day have to depend upon regular treatment with an artificial kidney machine to maintain their lives. Finally, injuries involving profound shock or crushing injury to muscles are among a number of disorders that can cause severe and acute renal failure, once a deadly complication which today can often be relieved by the use of the artificial kidney long enough for the causative disorder to be corrected and the kidney to return to normal function.

Quite aside from impairment of the kidney's filtering mechanism, malfunctions of this organ are also dangerous because of the influence the kidney has over other body functions. In 1934 the Cleveland physiologist Harry Goldblatt and his co-workers proved that any conditions reducing blood flow through the kidney could cause an elevation of blood pressure throughout the body, sometimes to extraordinary and dangerous levels. Paradoxically, Goldblatt also noted that the opposite was true: prolonged hypertension from any cause seemed to have a reciprocal damaging effect on blood flow through the kidney. Goldblatt's work opened the door to an understanding of one of the body's most insidious and deadly afflictions. Thanks to his discoveries and the work of dozens of kidney physiologists who followed him, we at last are beginning to unravel the complex interrelationships involving kidney disease, hypertension and heart disease—perhaps the single most complicated and confusing jigsaw puzzle ever tackled by medical researchers.

In addition to their exchange and filtration functions, certain epithelial cells have the ability to manufacture and secrete a variety of complex chemical substances which are vital to normal cellular metabolism. By far the most interesting are the secreting cells that make up the *endocrine glands,* a group of organs which exercise more powerful influence over body chemistry, weight for weight, than any other tissue in the body. Compared to the lung or the kidney these glands seem ridiculously small and unimpressive, tiny bits of tissue tucked away in obscure corners of the body with a total combined weight of perhaps five ounces. Even so, they secrete a variety of complex substances called *hormones* which enter into virtually all the body's biochemical reactions. Because these secretions are absorbed directly into the blood stream by the capillaries running between their cells, the endocrines are often called "ductless glands." Hormones are among the most peculiar chemicals found anywhere in the body. They do not serve as fuel for the cells, nor do they produce any energy themselves. Rather, they seem to act as keys that unlock energy-producing reactions in the tissues. They are not manufactured by the glands in any great quantities, but like the salt in a stew they must be kept in delicate balance or the results may be intolerable.

Most familiar of all the endocrine glands is the *thyroid,* long a standard topic of bridge-table conversation. Located at the base of the throat, straddling the trachea just below the Adam's

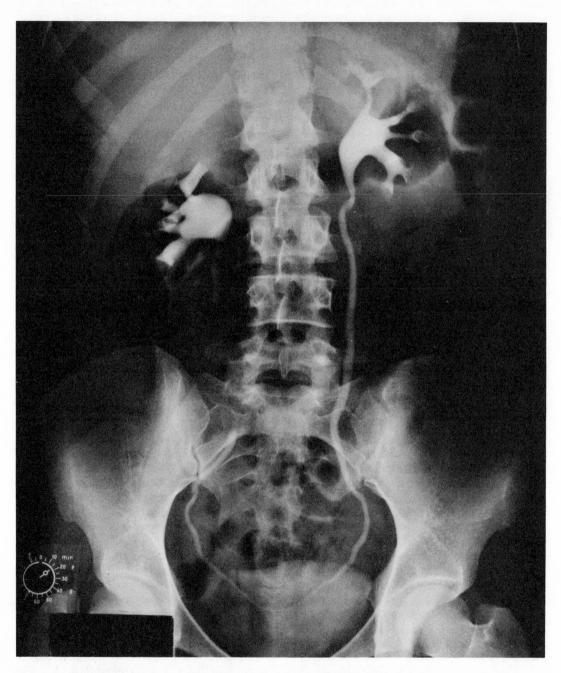

Plate 5a   Normal kidneys as revealed by intravenous pyelogram (IVP). A special radio-opaque
dye, injected into the patient's vein, is excreted by the kidneys and appears as a
shadow outline of the interior of the kidneys and ureters.

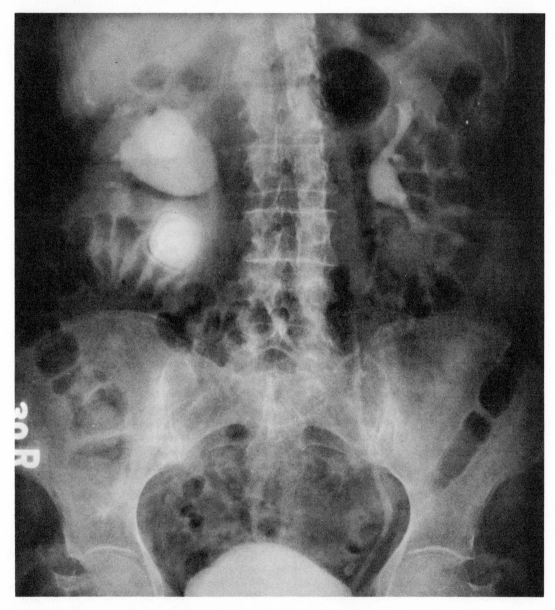

Plate 5b Abnormal IVP. The right kidney (to the left on plate) is obstructed by a huge laminated stone, with resulting hydronephrosis revealed by intravenous pyelogram.
Opposite kidney is normal.

apple, this gland can easily be examined for abnormalities. An enlargement or swelling may even become evident to the casual observer as a goiter. The thyroid produces a hormone called *thyroxin* which must combine with iodine in the blood stream to become active and exercises widespread control over the rate at which fuels

FORMATION OF THYROID HORMONE

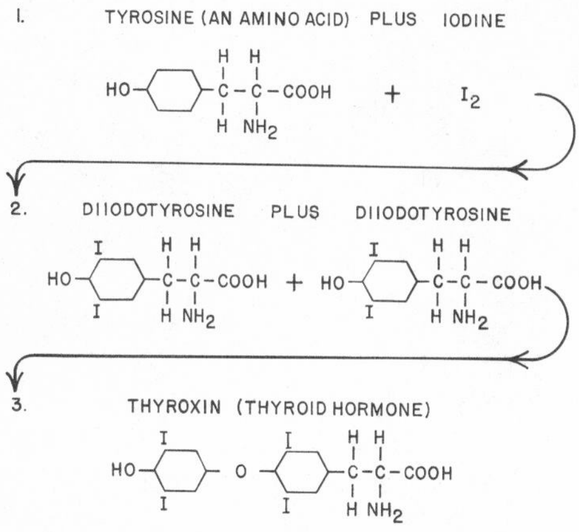

I. TYROSINE (AN AMINO ACID) PLUS IODINE

$$HO-\bigcirc-\underset{\underset{H}{|}}{\overset{\overset{H}{|}}{C}}-\underset{\underset{NH_2}{|}}{\overset{\overset{H}{|}}{C}}-COOH \quad + \quad I_2$$

2. DIIODOTYROSINE PLUS DIIODOTYROSINE

$$HO-\underset{\underset{I}{|}}{\overset{\overset{I}{|}}{\bigcirc}}-\underset{\underset{H}{|}}{\overset{\overset{H}{|}}{C}}-\underset{\underset{NH_2}{|}}{\overset{\overset{H}{|}}{C}}-COOH \quad + \quad HO-\underset{\underset{I}{|}}{\overset{\overset{I}{|}}{\bigcirc}}-\underset{\underset{H}{|}}{\overset{\overset{H}{|}}{C}}-\underset{\underset{NH_2}{|}}{\overset{\overset{H}{|}}{C}}-COOH$$

3. THYROXIN (THYROID HORMONE)

$$HO-\underset{\underset{I}{|}}{\overset{\overset{I}{|}}{\bigcirc}}-O-\underset{\underset{I}{|}}{\overset{\overset{I}{|}}{\bigcirc}}-\underset{\underset{H}{|}}{\overset{\overset{H}{|}}{C}}-\underset{\underset{NH_2}{|}}{\overset{\overset{H}{|}}{C}}-COOH$$

Figure 7–1.

are burned in the body cells. Ultimately thyroxin influences heart rate, speed of respiration, appetite, sexual function and a dozen other reflections of body metabolism. Excessive production of this hormone may speed up metabolic activity to the danger point and lead to the wide variety of disturbing symptoms that characterize hyperthyroidism. Underproduction is even more common and is associated with a general slowing down of metabolism. When thyroxin levels drop too low for too long, a debilitating condition known as hypothyroidism or myxedema occurs.

The thyroid gland is often blamed for a variety of vague symptoms for which it is not in any way responsible. A few years ago it was considered fashionable to take additional thyroid extract even when thyroid function was perfectly normal. This practice is less prevalent today as more and more people (and their doctors) realize that such discouraging conditions as obesity and morning sluggishness, once blamed on the thyroid, are rarely the result of thyroid malfunction.

The main body of the *pancreas* is not an endocrine gland at all. Its job is the secretion of digestive enzymes which are carried to the small intestine through a series of ducts. But scattered throughout this gland are many tiny "islets" of specialized epithelium called *Beta cells* which produce *insulin,* a hormone which helps tissue cells utilize their main fuel, a simple sugar called *glucose.* Certain individuals seem to be born with too few of these insulin-producing cells; early in life they develop a severe and damaging "juvenile" form of diabetes mellitus—"sugar diabetes"—which must be controlled by constant replacement of insulin. More commonly, the Beta cells become depleted or exhausted as a result of aging or disease. When this occurs a somewhat milder form of diabetes appears in maturity or middle age. Insidious in onset, this "adult" form of diabetes may sometimes be treated by diet alone or with special medicines which increase the potency of the insulin the body is still making.

Thanks to the availability of replacement insulin and other medicines, diabetes mellitus today is almost always controllable, and most diabetics can look forward to long and useful lives. But only fifty years ago this disease was as dreaded as cancer is today. Without any means of control, victims of severe diabetes wasted away and died, often suffering from associated blindness, kidney shutdown and heart failure. As early as 1889 it was known that diabetes resulted from some kind of trouble in the pancreas, and in 1907 the German physician Georg Zuelzer prepared a crude pancreatic extract that could lower blood sugar levels in diabetics. Unfortunately, Zuelzer's extract proved so toxic and unpredictable that its use had to be abandoned.

The trouble was that no one really knew what was missing from the pancreas that caused diabetes. Then in 1921 the Canadian surgeon Frederick Grant Banting teamed up with Charles Herbert Best, at that time a twenty-two-year-old medical student at the University of Toronto, and the Scottish physiologist J. J. R. Macleod to isolate and identify the hormone insulin in a series of classic studies that won Banting and Macleod the Nobel prize in 1923. Soon after, James Bertram Collip, an associate, purified the original crude insulin extract, making it safe for use in the treatment of human diabetes. Today we know that diabetes mellitus is a far more complicated condition than Banting and Best suspected, but the work of these men still stands as a great medical breakthrough. It failed to solve the riddle of diabetes completely, but it brought a once deadly killer under firm control.

The *adrenals,* a pair of glands perched on top of the kidneys, have widespread effects throughout the whole body. Actually two endocrines in one, the adrenals produce two completely different classes of hormones. Cells in the central *adrenal medulla* manufacture *epinephrine,* sometimes called adrenalin because it was once thought to be the only adrenal hormone. This substance is a powerful stimulant which speeds up heart rate and respiration, dilates the pupils, sharpens the reflexes and puts the body "on guard" in times of stress. By causing smooth muscle in the blood vessels to contract, it helps maintain blood pressure. It also influences emotional reactions such as anger, fright or nervous tension. When the body suffers a severe injury or hemorrhage, it is epinephrine (along with its first cousin *norepinephrine*) which shores up the blood pressure and heart function, providing us with an extra reserve of strength. However, there are limits to this reserve. Prolonged stress or shock may lead to *adrenal exhaustion;* blood pressure drops and the victim often collapses and dies.

For many years the layers of cells forming the *cortex* or "outer shell" of the adrenal glands were not identified with any particular function. Recently, however, we have learned that the adrenal cortex makes a family of some 30 or more powerful hormones completely unrelated to epinephrine. Because of their distinctive chemical structure, these adrenocortical compounds are called *corticosteroids.* Among the first to be identified were naturally produced *cortisone* and *hydrocortisone,* isolated in 1942. Early extractions of these hormones were a marvel of patience and hard work; one investigator had to process half a ton of beef adrenals in order to secure less than one-tenth of an ounce of relatively pure hydrocortisone. As soon as the remarkable medicinal properties of these

hormones were recognized, however, a whole succession of similar adrenocortical compounds or "cortisone-like" hormones were synthesized in the laboratory, bearing such euphonious names as prednisone, prednisolone, triamcinolone and dexamethasone.

Precisely how these hormones work is still a mystery, but their effects on metabolism are profound. They help regulate the salt content of body fluids and cells, and are involved in protein and carbohydrate chemistry. Because of their ability to suppress inflammation and reduce scarring, they work almost miraculously to relieve pain and retard permanent damage in such conditions as rheumatoid arthritis, glomerulonephritis and rheumatic fever.

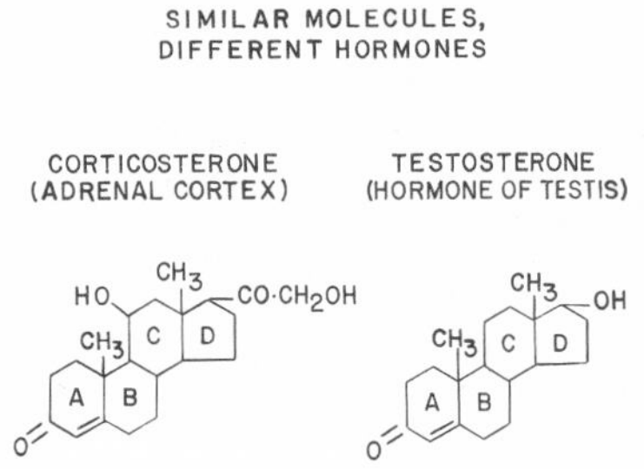

SIMILAR MOLECULES,
DIFFERENT HORMONES

Figure 7–2.

Curiously enough, the adrenocortical hormones are very similar in structure to hormones manufactured by the *gonads,* or "sex glands"— the ovaries in the female and the testes in the male, both part of the body's endocrine system. The hormones secreted by these glands determine the secondary sex characteristics that occur in both male and female at puberty and help regulate the entire reproductive process. The gonads have another equally important role, however: the manufacture of ova in the female and sperm in the male, the union of which makes reproduction possible, and in this function they, like the other endocrine glands, are regulated by the secretions of the tiniest, most mysterious endocrine organ of them all: the *pituitary.*

Like Mighty Mouse, this pea-sized gland is insignificant in appearance but packs a powerful punch. Lodged in a bony pocket in the base of the skull, it produces a hormone that controls body growth, and another called *oxytocin* (or pituitrin) which stimulates the gravid uterus to contract at the end of pregnancy. But the pituitary is called the "master" gland because it also manufactures special hormones that affect the hormone production of other endocrines. One of these, the so-called *thyrotrophic* or *thyroid-stimulating hormone* (TSH), signals the thyroid to manufacture thyroxin. The *adrenocortico-trophic hormone* (ACTH) stimulates production of hormones by the adrenal cortex, and the *follicle-stimulating hormone* (FSH) controls the function of the ovaries, thus indirectly regulating the female cycle of ovulation and menstruation.

Complicated as this "control function" of the pituitary is, it seems doubly complicated because it works both ways. The very hormones that are produced by other glands as a result of pituitary stimulation in turn tend to suppress production of the stimulating hormones in the pituitary. Thus, as the level of thyroxin drops, TSH is poured out to goad the thyroid cells into activity; but as soon as production has been speeded up, the increase in thyroid hormone itself blocks the manufacture of more TSH in the pituitary cells so that thyroid activity slows down again. The net result of this reciprocal control cycle is the maintenance of a remarkably steady balance of thyroid hormone in the blood stream under ordinary circumstances. The control cycles regulating adrenal and ovarian function operate in much the same way.

Obviously, malfunctions of the endocrines can result in a wide variety of disturbances. (These diseases and disorders are discussed in detail in Part XI, "Patterns of Illness: The Endocrine Glands.") Many are relatively easy to diagnose because of distinctive changes that become apparent in the body. Others may cause a multitude of mysterious symptoms that seem completely unrelated to the gland involved. Nevertheless, modern medical research has made great strides in understanding both the complex functions of the endocrine glands and the many hormones they produce. Thus even the most unusual endocrine disorder can now be diagnosed and in most cases effectively treated. It may seem odd that these "mighty midgets" are made up of the same kind of basic tissue that comprises the lungs and kidneys, certainly an indication of the enormous versatility of epithelium. But as various as the structure and functions of these organs are, they share another similarity: they are all intimately involved in basic life functions of the body—the stoking of the metabolic furnace, the disposal of waste materials and the regulation of the body's chemical reactions.

8

The River of Life: The Cardiovascular System

During the first bleak months of the war in the South Pacific, American forces suffered a long succession of defeats, climaxed by the loss of the Philippines and the surrender of more than 11,000 troops on Corregidor. The loss of that fortress island was perhaps the most bitter blow of the war—but Corregidor did not fall for lack of leadership or courage. It fell for lack of supplies. With the Japanese navy in control of the transport lanes of the Pacific, the only alternative to surrender was death.

In a sense, the human body is like an island outpost. Its several complex organ systems, each engaged in vital functions, require continuous and reliable supplies. It needs fuel for combustion in the body cells to provide necessary energy, and it also needs some effective means of evacuating useless by-products after the body's energy-producing chemical reactions have taken place. If these activities are to be accomplished, there must be an efficient system of transport. Like an island, the body depends upon its supply lines for survival.

A simple organism like the ameba has no need for elaborate supply lines. It simply soaks up the food and oxygen it needs through its cell membrane and filters out waste products as they accumulate. Even in more complex creatures each cell may fend for itself in the same way, but in higher organisms a division of labor occurs. A few special cells absorb oxygen for the whole organism, while others take up food materials, filter wastes or manufacture necessary chemicals. With this sort of specialization, vital substances must be carried from one group of cells to another, and a transport system becomes necessary. The more complicated the organism, the more intricate the transport system must be.

The human body requires so much of its transport system that a special kind of tissue is necessary to handle the job. This sixth basic body tissue, the *blood,* differs from the others in a peculiar way. Its cells are not fixed together in masses. Instead, they are suspended in a viscous fluid which is propelled through an intricate system of pipes or blood vessels to all parts of the body, driven continuously by a powerful pump, the heart. Thus the blood circulates through the body on an endless route of pickup and delivery as long as life continues.

Throughout human history men have been puzzled by the strange red fluid in their bodies. Even the most primitive men probably realized their blood was related in some mysterious way to life and death, although they did not understand why or how. When massive bleeding could not be stopped, death would inevitably follow, yet a small blood loss seemed to be harmless or even beneficial. The ancient Greek and Roman physicians knew that the heart pulsated, but it was only three and a half centuries ago that it was learned that blood moved through the body in a closed circuit, driven under a head of pressure by a powerful pump. There still remained the question of how it could flow freely through the blood vessels yet quickly turn to a gel outside the body. Nor did anyone understand why blood transfused from one person to another could be lifesaving in one case and fatal in another. Only within the past half-century have we really begun to grasp the complex structure and behavior of this peculiar fluid tissue.

Blood has several major functions in the body. First and most obvious is the transport of fuels and oxygen to the cells and the return of by-products such as carbon dioxide, urea and uric acid to their special disposal areas. In addition, blood carries within it a mobile army of special cells which can rally at a site of infection to destroy invading microorganisms. Still another function is the maintenance of a balance between the fluid inside the body cells and the fluid outside, either in the blood stream itself or in the spaces between the cells. Other functions include the transport of *antibodies* to help neutralize the effects of foreign protein materials entering the body, and the formation of self-sealing *clots* to prevent severe hemorrhage from broken blood vessels. All these jobs can be managed by the blood only because it is a circulating *fluid tissue* containing several types of specialized cellular components suspended in a viscous protein-rich substrate or *plasma.*

Of all the cellular components of the blood, by far the most numerous are the *erythrocytes,* commonly called "red corpuscles" or simply "red cells," which contain *hemoglobin,* a protein that gives blood its distinctive red color. The red cells are like traveling freight barges which pick up oxygen in the capillaries of the lung and unload it in distant body tissues where it is used in the oxidation of fuel. The oxygen first diffuses through the double respiratory membrane into the blood stream. The hemoglobin in the red cells binds it in chemical combination and then carries it to the *peripheral capillary bed,* a microscopic network of tiny threadlike vessels in contact with the oxygen-hungry cells of bone, muscle, connective, nerve and epithelial tissues all over the body. Here the oxygen is released, and the red cells, relieved of their burden, are swept back to the lungs for another payload while the river of plasma which carries them is busy soaking up carbon dioxide and waste materials from the tissues for disposal.

In the human body the red cells happen to be the sole means by which sufficient oxygen can be carried from the lung to the body tissues. Oxygen is only slightly soluble in plasma; without the binding power of the hemoglobin in the red cells, the blood could barely carry enough dissolved oxygen to supply the tissues for two and a half seconds. Under such conditions the breathless recovery period from a sneeze might well

THE HEMOGLOBIN MOLECULE
(SIMPLIFIED DIAGRAM)

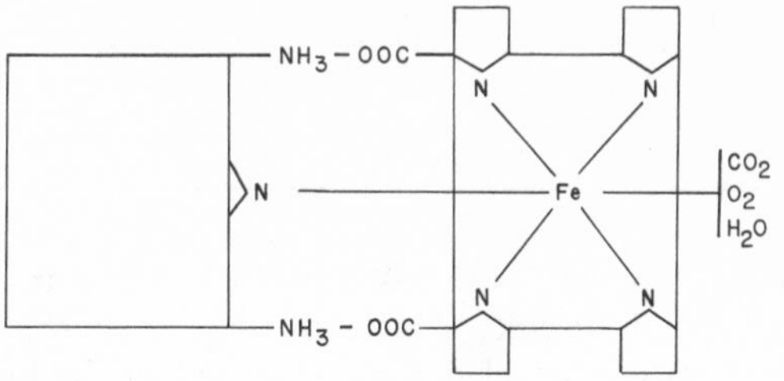

GLOBIN
(COMPLEX BLOOD
PROTEIN)

HEME PIGMENT
(NOTE CENTRAL POSITION
OF IRON ATOM)

Figure 8–1.

prove fatal. But with the hemoglobin-packed red cells in the blood we have about a five-minute reserve supply of oxygen on hand under most conditions—still not very much, but at least a margin that allows for normal body activities.

With such a highly important and specialized job to do, red cells seem to concentrate on it with single-minded vigor; in fact, they are good for little else. Technically they cannot qualify as living cells at all because they lose their nuclei before they leave the bone marrow factories where they are made. They can neither grow nor reproduce like other body cells. Once they have entered the circulation, they simply serve as cargo-carrying hulls, surviving three months or so before they are broken up and replaced.

Ordinarily the body maintains a careful balance between worn-out red cells in the blood stream and new ones produced in the bone marrow because enough hemoglobin must be available to carry oxygen to the body tissues at all times. Normally the red cells contain from 12½ to 15 grams of hemoglobin per 100 cubic centimeters of blood. Minimum body needs can be met with less, but if the hemoglobin level drops much lower than 10 or 11 grams per 100 cc.'s of blood for any reason, the result is a condition called *anemia* (literally, "without blood," a slight exaggeration of the case) and tissues begin to suffer from lack of oxygen.

Anemia may occur for several reasons. It may be the result of hemorrhagic blood loss, abnormal destruction of red cells in the liver and spleen (called *hemolytic anemia*) or failure of the bone marrow to produce sufficient replacement cells (*aplastic anemia*). More commonly, it results from insufficient manufacture of hemoglobin because of inadequate iron in the diet—the so-called nutritional or *iron-deficiency anemia*. Improper absorption of cyanocobalamin (the technical name for vitamin B_{12}) may result in a special kind of anemia called *pernicious* because it was invariably fatal until the cause was discovered and methods for treatment devised.

Whatever the cause, all anemias have the same net result: oxygen transport to body tissues is reduced, metabolism is impaired, and energy production is curtailed. Shortness of breath may develop as the lungs try to draw in more air; the heart speeds up or enlarges, seeking to compensate for the lack of hemoglobin by circulating what little there is faster and faster. At the same time the body works to restore normal oxygen transport by producing more red cells, or manufacturing more hemoglobin, or both at once.

Often an anemia develops so slowly that compensation takes place gradually without any striking symptoms. A severe hemorrhage, however, triggers a swift and dramatic chain reaction. With the loss of two pints of blood, the oxygen available to the cells drops sharply. Energy production falls off and normal body activities become impossible. The victim becomes weak and giddy. He begins to sweat and his heart pounds furiously. If the blood loss is very rapid, his blood pressure sags to dangerous levels and he may pass out or suddenly seem unable to get enough air into his lungs.

The body tries almost immediately to compensate for this sudden blood loss. Reflexes cause the smooth muscle in the arteries all over the body to contract, shoring up sagging blood pressure and combating shock. This process may also clamp down the bleeding blood vessel, helping to stem the hemorrhage. Respiration increases to keep the remaining hemoglobin well saturated with oxygen, and energy-consuming body activities are perforce reduced. The capillaries immediately begin drawing in water and salt from the fluid reservoir between the cells to replace the lost fluid volume of blood. At the same time the bone marrow begins manufacturing new red cells at an accelerated rate.

If the victim has normal body reserves, these compensatory mechanisms can be highly efficient in stemming the hemorrhage by natural means. Within 12 hours the threat of shock is past and much of the fluid volume of the blood has been replaced. In a few days, production of red cells in the bone marrow is in high gear, as evidenced by a sudden increase in number of very young red cells, called *reticulocytes,* in the circulating blood. Two or three months later the red cell count and hemoglobin level will approach normal again, assuming that no further hemorrhage occurs.

Of course, body reserves are severely drained during this recovery period. Today doctors seek to speed up the whole process by administration of additional iron or by transfusion of blood, to restore both hemoglobin and red cells as quickly as possible. As recently as the turn of the century, however, transfusions were not a part of normal medical practice. They had been attempted as early as 1667 when Jean Baptiste Denis (d. 1704), physician to Louis XIV, transfused the blood of a lamb into a dying patient, doubtless hastening his demise. But in spite of later successful transfusions using human blood, the practice was soon abandoned because violent reactions or sudden death so often resulted. It was not until 1901 that the American pathologist Carl Landsteiner discovered that certain blood contained *agglutinins* that made the red cells in other blood samples clump together, plugging up the capillaries of the recipient and causing dangerous or even fatal transfusion reactions. Landsteiner demonstrated that all blood could be classified into three definite groups, the A-B-O system that is still used, laying the groundwork for modern cross-matching techniques that make present-day transfusions so safe and effective. During World War I thousands of severely wounded soldiers were saved by transfusions and the first blood banks were pioneered. Landsteiner's work proved to be so important to the advancement of medicine and surgery that he was awarded the Nobel prize for medicine, rather belatedly, in 1930.

Since compensation begins the moment hemorrhaging occurs, it is tempting to imagine that the body somehow "knows" what is going on and "takes steps" accordingly. Of course, this is not quite true; specialized nerve centers adapted for the purpose simply respond to certain chemical imbalances. Sometimes they over-respond. Red cell production, for instance, is stepped up any time tissues become oxygen-hungry, regardless of the cause. Thus, in certain chronic lung diseases, or when abnormal heart construction allows blood to by-pass the lung, the bone marrow responds to continuously low oxygen levels just as if a shortage of red cells was the problem and turns out excess red cells by the millions, a condition known as *polycythemia* ("many blood cells"). Such overproduction may result in blood so thick it cannot circulate well. In extreme cases, radioactive phosphorus and other medicines have been administered to try to poison the bone marrow and cut down the flow of red cells. Too much of a good thing can be as dangerous as too little.

While red cells or erythrocytes are the most numerous of the blood cells, they are not by any means the only ones. "White cells" or *leucocytes* are also present, with a totally different kind of job to do. True living cells with nuclei, they have the special ability to move freely in and out of the blood stream, wriggling through tiny inter-spaces in the capillary walls into the spaces between the tissue cells. There they engulf and destroy invading bacteria, a process called *phagocytosis*.

Some white cells are manufactured in the bone marrow, others in special lymphoid tissue in various locations in the body. They congregate in enormous numbers wherever bacteria have entered the tissues. Often white cells are themselves destroyed in fighting these invaders, but they form a powerful first line of defense, holding infection in check and blocking the spread of dangerous bacteria through the blood stream. Whenever white cells are mobilized into action, the body compensates by manufacturing more; three times the usual number may appear in the circulating blood in a matter of hours. Such a "rising white cell count" is a help in diagnosing certain kinds of infections. It may, for instance, be a telling clue in the early diagnosis of acute appendicitis.

On the other hand, too many white cells in the blood may be the earliest indication of a grave condition known as leukemia, a cancer of the bone marrow. In this disease huge excesses of half-developed or immature white cells are formed, packing the bone marrow and spilling over into the circulating blood in staggering numbers. Soon the liver, the spleen and other tissues are literally stuffed with white cells as the wild cell production continues. Red cell production in the bone marrow is crowded out and a profound anemia develops, resulting in the watery-appearing "white blood" that gives this disease its name. There is mounting evidence that certain vicious undiscovered viruses may be the cause of leukemia, but in spite of extensive study and many new medicines to combat the disease, leukemia today is still invariably fatal.

In addition to white cells and red cells, there is a third cellular component of the blood—perhaps the strangest one of them all. The *platelets* are nothing more than circulating fragments of certain giant cells called *megakaryocytes* found in the bone marrow. Discovered in 1842, these tiny bits of tissue at first appeared to have no particular function. Then it was observed that people with low platelet counts seemed more vulnerable to bleeding than usual. Gradually, it became clear that platelets had something to do with the blood's clotting mechanism.

Coagulation of blood had long been a puzzle to physiologists, who could not understand how blood could flow freely in the veins under ordinary conditions, yet form a sticky, gelatinous mass both inside and outside the body within moments after a blood vessel was injured or inflamed. Obviously something occurred to alter the blood profoundly—but what? What changes took place, and why were they triggered only when a vessel wall was breached?

After a century of brilliant investigation, we still do not have completely satisfactory answers to these questions. As early as 1768 the English surgeon William Hewson described a substance in fluid blood plasma which solidified into a gel when blood was withdrawn from the body. We know now that Hewson's "coagulable lymph" is a complex blood protein called *fibrinogen* which is changed into long, needle-like crystals of *fibrin* as the blood clots. We also know that the platelets help trigger this conversion. When they touch a rough or "wettable" surface such as a torn or inflamed vessel wall, they become sticky and burst apart, releasing enzymes that enter into a complex biochemical chain reaction. The end result is the conversion of fibrinogen into a network of fibrin that enmeshes red blood cells to form a jelly-like clot.

The cells of the blood are responsible for certain major jobs—oxygen transport and resistance to infection, among others. In blood coagulation both cellular and fluid components play a part. The fluid portion of the blood is, in fact, even more complex than its cellular components. Called *plasma,* it carries the red and white cells to all parts of the body and is a weak solution of salt and water in which a wide variety of substances are dissolved or suspended. Along with sodium and chloride ions, plasma contains other dissolved *electrolytes* such as potassium, calcium and phosphate ions, as well as carbonic acid, lactic acid and acetic acid. The hydrogen ions of these weak "buffer" acids help maintain the body's delicate *acid-base balance.* Any shift toward excessive acidity (as in diabetic acidosis) or excessive alkalinity (which may result from protracted vomiting) can cause profound metabolic changes and even death. Our ability to retain carbon dioxide (as dissolved carbonic acid) or eliminate it (as carbon dioxide) according to body demand gives us a remarkable buffer against sudden shifts in body acidity.

Of course the blood plasma also transports body fuels and building materials to the tissues, including simple sugars such as glucose from carbohydrate foods, amino acids and nucleic acids from the digestion of protein, and various fatty materials called blood *lipids.* Metabolic waste materials such as urea, uric acid and carbon dioxide are also carried by the plasma to the proper disposal areas.

One of the most important functions of blood plasma is the maintenance of the proper balance between the fluid within the capillary blood vessels, the fluid within the tissue cells, and that which lies between the cells in the tissues. Plasma is considerably heavier and more viscous than water because it contains the long-chain molecules of various *blood proteins.* The most familiar of these are *albumin, fibrinogen,* a whole family of *globulins* (including the gamma globulin which helps fight off virus infections) and a number of protein-fat combinations known as *lipoproteins.* These plasma proteins, which are just too big to pass through normal capillary membranes, help maintain an *osmotic pressure balance* between the body fluid outside the capillaries and the volume of blood inside. As with so many other body functions, the importance of this fine balance comes to our attention only when a disturbance occurs. If we sprain an ankle, for instance, the capillaries in the injured area swell with blood. Since blood flow through these engorged capillaries is slow, water leaks out of the plasma into the tissue, producing the swelling that we see. The same thing occurs in an area of localized infection such as a boil. Of all the plasma proteins, albumin seems to be the most responsible for osmotic pressure balance, so if any amount of albumin is lost (as in certain kinds of kidney disease) a generalized *edema* or swelling of all the body tissues comes about.

This does not mean, however, that the water in our cells and blood stream remains stationary under normal circumstances. The body is constantly losing water by way of urine, perspiration and the water vapor in exhaled air. All told, we can lose between three and four quarts of water every day—roughly seven to nine pounds of body weight—without doing any extraordinary work at all. Of course all this water must ultimately be replaced by the fluid and food we eat every day. But because of the continuing cycle of loss and replenishment, there is a constant interchange of fluid between blood stream and tissues. The vast bulk of the water in the body—

something over 70 percent of our body weight—is found either in the plasma (the *intravascular fluid space*) or within the cells (the *intracellular fluid space*). But for water and dissolved metabolites to shift back and forth between these areas, there must also be a third reservoir between the cells and the blood stream—the so-called *extracellular fluid space.*

What is this fluid lying outside the cells, and where does it come from? Essentially it is a watery saline solution containing some plasma proteins. It leaks out of both cells and capillaries continuously to bathe all the tissues and help transport fuels and wastes back and forth. As it moves between the cells, it is pumped along by skeletal muscle activity, draining into a maze of more or less definite channels known as *lymphatics,* through a number of convergence points or *nodes,* and ultimately back into the blood stream through a series of large ducts. This ubiquitous extracellular fluid is generally known as *lymph.*

Many people have trouble understanding the formation of lymph and its sluggish, meandering circulation throughout the body. It can best be described by comparing the body tissues to a swampy lowland area adjacent to a river. The water in the river (the blood stream) moves in one direction in a fixed channel with a noticeable current. When it reaches the lowlands, however, some of the water seeps out into nearby swamps (the extracellular tissue spaces). Here it wanders sluggishly through a series of sloughs, gradually develops a sort of tidal current as it converges into larger and larger channels, and finally drains back into the river again farther downstream. As a result of this flow of water between river and swamp, certain substances from the river are carried into the swamp and left there, while others are picked up and swept back into the river. This same exchange takes place between body tissues, but most important, *the tissues are always kept wet.*

The maintenance of the proper amounts of water in all three fluid spaces is essential to life. Enough food materials can be stored in the body to supply vital needs for weeks in time of emergency, but the loss of water each day is far too great for adequate storage to be possible. Even the body's efforts to conserve water by concentrating the urine and reducing loss from perspiration are not sufficient for long. The body will simply dry out in a few days and "die of thirst" if water is withheld. Thanks to the plasma proteins, however, a critical balance of available water between the blood stream, the lymph and the tissue cells is carefully maintained even under conditions of stress.

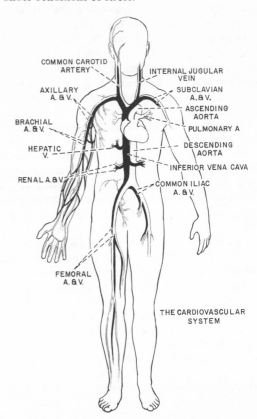

COMMON CAROTID ARTERY

INTERNAL JUGULAR VEIN

AXILLARY A. & V.

SUBCLAVIAN A. & V.

ASCENDING AORTA

BRACHIAL A. & V.

PULMONARY A

HEPATIC V.

DESCENDING AORTA

INFERIOR VENA CAVA

RENAL A. & V.

COMMON ILIAC A. & V.

FEMORAL A. & V.

THE CARDIOVASCULAR SYSTEM

Figure 8–2.

Clearly, this strange fluid tissue we call blood is as important to the body as any other basic tissue, and as different from the others as night from day. To accomplish its work the blood constantly circulates to all parts of the body under a considerable head of pressure, propelled by a great central pump (the *heart*) through a closed system of pipes (the *arteries, capillaries* and *veins*) which all together are called the *cardiovascular system.*

It is amazing that the seemingly obvious concept of continuous circulation of blood should have escaped such brilliant anatomists as Vesalius, who rejected many of Galen's earlier notions of body structure yet accepted his totally erroneous idea that the blood merely washed back and forth in the body like the ocean's tides. It remained for William Harvey (1578–1657), the great English physician and physiologist, to discover the true scheme of the circulation. Harvey was not content to leave his ideas untested. He spent twenty years experimenting until he could prove beyond any shadow of doubt how the blood circulated. Then in 1628 he published his work in a book, *De Motu Cordis,* which remains one of the towering landmarks of medical literature.

The human cardiovascular system is much like a heating plant in which hot water circulates through pipes that can expand or contract according to need, with the water driven by a pump that increases or decreases its speed and capacity as the demand changes. Blood is pushed into the great artery (the *aorta,* about 1½ inches in diameter) and its major branches under high pressure by the rhythmic contractions of the heart. To accommodate the surge of blood with each heartbeat, the great arteries are tough, elastic tubes which actually pulsate as blood is forced into them. We can feel this pulsation at the base of the thumb or in front of the ear where arteries pass close to the surface.

As the major vessels divide into smaller arteries and still smaller *arterioles,* the pressure drops according to the laws of hydrodynamics. Much of the elastic tissue in arteriolar walls is replaced by smooth muscle which regulates the pressure and flow of blood into various tissue areas by contracting or relaxing to narrow or widen the diameter of these vessels. By the time blood reaches the network of tiny, fragile capillaries winding between the tissue cells, its flow is slow, gentle and steady; but the capillaries in an area can dilate and engorge with blood if the arterioles expand. Because the capillary walls are made of a single flat cell layer of epithelium, exchange of dissolved substances between cells and capillaries is easy.

Once blood has passed through the capillary beds it converges into *venules* and then *veins* which ultimately carry it into the *superior* (above the heart) and *inferior* (below the heart) *vena cava* and thence into the heart again. Like all blood vessels, the veins are lined with epithelium, but with no pulsating pressure to withstand, even the larger veins have only thin layers of smooth muscle in their walls. Unlike arteries, however, they are equipped with tiny flaplike valves at regular intervals so that blood can ordinarily move through them in one direction only—toward the heart.

The arteries with their thick layers of elastic tissue and muscle are vulnerable to the deposition of fatty material and calcium, a condition known as *atherosclerosis* that literally "hardens" the vessel walls and reduces their diameter. Veins, on the other hand, develop marked dilatations called *varices* when their valves break down and allow blood to reflux and pool instead of moving on toward the heart. This condition is commonly seen in *varicose veins* in the legs or in *hemorrhoids.* When blood flow through the liver is obstructed, huge varices may form at the base of the esophagus, sometimes leading to hemorrhagic internal bleeding that may be impossible to control.

Essential to the circulation of blood, of course, is the heart itself, constructed of a special kind of interlocking muscle fiber. The contraction of the heart is stimulated by nerve impulses carried from a tiny node of cells called the *cardiac pacemaker* located in the thin-walled upper chamber of the heart, the right atrium, and transmitted to the main heart muscle by way of a curious bundle of neuromuscular cells unlike any other tissue in the body. (*See* Fig. 41–3.) The muscle of the heart is wrapped in spiraling layers attached to a fibrous "skeleton" that also forms the rings and leaflets of the heart valves. As cardiac muscle contracts, it wrings blood out of the heart's collecting chambers into the great arteries; as it relaxes, it allows returning blood to refill those chambers before the next contraction.

In a simple organism that can soak up oxygen from the sea directly into its general blood stream, a two-chamber heart would be sufficient, with a single receiving chamber or *atrium* and a pumping chamber or *ventricle.* Since all the oxygen for the human body is absorbed by a special internal organ, the lung, a completely separate *pulmonary* circulation is needed so that oxygen-exhausted blood returning to the heart can be pumped through the lung for oxygenation before it is returned to the heart for dispersement back to the body tissues. Thus the human heart has two receiving chambers and two pumping chambers working simultaneously. Venous blood is received in the *right atrium* and pumped to the lung by the *right ventricle,* while blood returning from the lung enters the *left atrium* and is pumped out to the body tissues by the *left ventricle.* Since there is ordinarily no opening whatever between the right side of the heart and the left, blood must travel each circuit in succession, first through one and then the other, with the direction of flow controlled by the heart valves. When these valves are damaged (by rheumatic fever or infection, for example) they become *incompetent,* throwing an extraordinary strain on the heart unless they can be repaired.

Obviously, the heart must have great strength and endurance to continue pumping blood day after day for an entire lifetime. It requires more fuel and oxygen than other tissue; in fact, it has the richest supply of freshly oxygenated blood of any single organ in the body, carried to it through the *coronary arteries.* For some reason these vessels are unusually vulnerable to atherosclerosis. Occasionally a branch of a coronary artery will be obstructed on this account, leaving a segment of heart muscle suddenly starved for blood. This condition, called *ischemia,* results in the same sort of pain that occurs when a rubber band is wound around the end of a finger, cutting off circulation, and it occurs for the same reason. If blood from other nearby coronary vessels cannot reach the starved area soon enough, the muscle segment may die—a condition known as *infarction*—disrupting the function of the whole heart and sometimes leading to sudden death. More commonly, the occluded artery is small, so that with proper rest and care the uninjured part of the heart can carry on for the injured muscle segment until it has time to heal.

The heart has an amazing capacity to compensate for trouble elsewhere in the body, too. If tissues temporarily require more fuel and oxygen because of a sudden burst of physical activity, the heart compensates by beating faster, pushing blood more rapidly through the lungs and out to the body cells. Such a short-term increase in its work load causes no permanent change in the heart—it slows down again and "rests" when the demand falls off—but in a condition such as *hypertension* the heart must continually pump blood against increased pressure in the arteries. Under these circumstances the heart muscle thickens and the chambers enlarge. The heart may actually double in size in its effort to compensate for such a strain, but like a tired horse it reaches its final limits sooner or later. If forced for too long to do more than it should, the heart begins to *decompensate* or "fail," beating more and more frantically as its pumping action becomes weaker and less efficient. Blood flow through the lung slows down, making breathing difficult. Fluid begins leaking out of the blood vessels into the body tissues, causing *edema,* and the liver swells and engorges with blood waiting to get back to the heart. These changes, which may take days or weeks to develop, are often spoken of as "congestive heart failure."

Without help, the failing heart is trapped in a vicious circle. The more desperately it struggles to keep up, the less efficient it becomes, until it simply cannot go on. Fortunately, one of the oldest medicines known to man—a powder made from the common foxglove weed—was found by William Withering in 1785 to help the heart recover from failure and "get back on its feet." The leaves of the foxglove contain a potent chemical known as *digitalis* which slows down the heart rate and improves the efficiency of each contraction. Administered today either as pills made from the powdered leaf or as the purified extract, digitalis has proven one of the greatest boons to mankind in the entire history of medicine.

Sometimes the heart is the victim of a congenital malformation that cripples its operation from birth. The walls between the chambers may not close properly, the valves may be abnormally formed, or blood may be shunted from the right side to the left through false passages, by-passing the pulmonary circuit. In recent years many techniques have been devised to diagnose and correct such mistakes of nature.

Like other organ systems in the body, the complex and widespread cardiovascular system is vulnerable to a variety of diseases and injuries. (*See* Part IX, "Patterns of Illness: The Cardiovascular System.") Atherosclerosis, a condition that accompanies the aging process, affects virtually everyone to some degree sooner or later. Sometimes inflammation and roughening of the interior of an artery or vein can lead to formation of a blood clot within the vessel. Such an obstruction, called a *thrombus,* may block circulation to a limb or prevent proper return of blood to the heart. If a portion of a thrombus breaks free and is carried in the blood stream to plug another vessel at some distant site, the moving clot is called an *embolus.* One of the most catastrophic of all disasters to the body occurs when an embolus passes through the heart and lodges in a pulmonary artery feeding the lung, sometimes causing instantaneous death without the slightest warning.

Again, the wall of an artery may be weakened by infection or injury and balloon out to form an *aneurysm* which can rupture internally. Occasionally blood under pressure may split or *dissect* the muscle wall of a great artery. Such conditions were once considered beyond medical help, but today with modern techniques of vascular surgery, a damaged segment of artery can sometimes be removed and replaced with a graft.

One of the remarkable things about the body's network of blood vessels is the reserve it provides in times of trouble. Many vital areas receive blood from more than one artery, and thus cells can still be nourished by way of *collateral circulation* if the major artery is obstructed. Collateral circulation to a limb can sometimes even take over when great vessels like the *femoral artery* to the leg or the *brachial artery* to the arm are destroyed. Elsewhere, the circulatory system is constructed to ensure extraordinary blood flow to vital organs. As much as 40 percent of the blood pumped from the heart is routed to the brain, for instance, where nerve tissue requires unusually large amounts of oxygen. The two great *common carotid arteries* are directly connected at the base of the brain by way of a vascular "traffic circle" called the Circle of Willis, so that blood from one side can supply the other side of the brain directly if necessary.

Finally, certain parts of the body have their own private circulatory systems to handle special jobs. The liver, for instance, must process food materials absorbed into the blood stream from the digestive tract, along with its many other functions. Liver cells receive their own blood supply from the general circulation, but the liver also has a separate and special miniature circulatory system to enable it to do its job. This so-called *portal system* carries blood rich in food materials from the capillaries of the intestine through a large *portal vein* to the liver, where it passes into another capillary bed before entering the general circulation for return to the heart. Such an unusual "capillary to vein to capillary" filtering system is another example of the body's ability to meet and solve a special problem of body function, as well as an illustration of the complexity and versatility of the cardiovascular system.

The Fuels of Life: Digestion and Metabolism

On a June day in 1822 in a town on the Michigan frontier, a young French-Canadian fur trader named Alexis St. Martin suffered a frightful injury. Talking with friends on the porch of a trading post, he was struck broadside by an accidental shotgun blast which tore a hole in his side bigger than a man's fist. A young American army surgeon named William Beaumont was summoned from nearby Fort Mackinac to treat the wounded man, although the case seemed hopeless. Dressing the wound as best he could, the surgeon doubted his patient could live for 36 hours. But like many a patient before him, Alexis St. Martin fooled his doctor. Miraculously, under Beaumont's skillful care, he survived and healed—but a hole remained open into his stomach through the abdominal wall. During his convalescence the two men became fast friends, and it was thus that one of the strangest chapters in the history of medicine came to be written.

Beaumont was only a frontier surgeon, but he realized that his patient presented one of those opportunities that occur only once in a thousand years. No one had ever before been able to study how the living human body digested food, for there was no way to examine the inside of a human stomach and intestine while the process was actually going on. With the cooperation of his patient, Beaumont began a famous series of studies of the human digestive mechanism, while St. Martin went on to marry, father children and lead an otherwise normal life except for the hole into his stomach. In 1833 the surgeon wrote a book summarizing his years of experiment and

observation. His famous patient far outlived him to die at the ripe old age of eighty-three. William Beaumont's monumental work opened the door to the study of one of the most poorly understood of all the vital body functions, and Alexis St. Martin's personal contribution to the knowledge of human physiology has rarely been equaled.

The human body, for all its complex functions, is essentially an energy-producing organism. Whether we are breathing, moving about, growing, digesting our food or just thinking, our bodies produce and use a constant flow of energy. Even during sleep the fires must continue to burn. If that flow of energy were suddenly to stop, the human body would become an inert and lifeless lump of jelly. Where does this energy come from? In ancient times this question preoccupied scientists and philosophers alike. Today we know that special biochemical reactions take place in all the body cells, enabling them to produce heat and energy, to grow, to repair damage and to reproduce themselves. It is this continuous series of reactions which gives the body that mysterious quality we call life.

Just as a gasoline engine must have fuel to provide its energy, our cells must have special organic fuels in order to live. These are obtained from the foods we eat—but steak, vegetables and salad cannot be used directly for fuel. First the body must break them down in the stomach and intestine into fragments, extracting and absorbing the useful parts and casting aside the slag. Then these semirefined fuels must be further reduced or synthesized in the liver and other tissues to obtain the basic combustion materials the cells can use.

Intricate as these processes may be, life itself depends on the *digestion* and *absorption* of food materials, and on the amazing biochemical processes of *synthesis* and *metabolism* that take place within the cells. The study of these fantastically complex body processes, first begun a century and a half ago by an obscure frontier surgeon, still continues today as biochemists and physiologists all over the world seek to unravel the fascinating puzzles of cellular metabolism, the chemistry of life.

In a sense, all of us are experts in the first necessary step in providing our bodies with fuel —gathering in food materials. We are drawn to eating, just as we are drawn to sex, by powerful physical and emotional forces built into our natures: eating is usually a pleasure, especially if the food is well prepared. Tempting aromas and subtle flavors excite our sense of smell and taste; hunger fills us with a sense of vague discomfort until we satisfy it. Even the most creative efforts of a gourmet chef, however, are totally wasted as far as the stomach is concerned. The most delightful dinner, once eaten, is no better prepared for the body's use than a strip of raw fish. It is only after passage through a mechanical and chemical processing machine, remarkably similar to the conveyor belt in a soup factory, that the delights of the dinner table are finally converted into a form the body cells can use for fuel.

The first step in the digestive process is the chopping and grinding of food materials in the mouth, where they are mixed with saliva containing an enzyme that helps initiate the chemical breakdown process. Chewing is aided by the most powerful pair of muscles in the body, the *masseters,* which clamp the jaws together with the strength of a vise. Once food is ground up and moistened, it is swallowed as a semisolid mass and carried on a swift one-way trip down the *esophagus* into the first major chemical processing station, the *stomach.*

Here stronger chemicals are added to the mix, along with more enzymes, and digestion begins in earnest. The muscular walls of the stomach churn and stir the digesting food, storing it for a while in a pouchlike repository and then passing it on a bit at a time into a second processing station, the upper ten inches of the small intestine, called the *duodenum.*

For many years the stomach was given far more credit than it deserved for the digestive work it does. A liberal quantity of dilute hydrochloric acid is secreted by cells lining the stomach—perhaps two and a half quarts a day. Early investigators thought this acid itself had a powerful effect on foods; they could not understand why the digestion that took place so efficiently inside the stomach seemed to slow down and stop as soon as digesting food was removed, acid and all, for examination in a test tube. Today we know that the digestion of most foods is only half started in the stomach, and that certain gastric enzymes, including *pepsin* and *renin,* are responsible for what little digestive work is actually done there. The acid merely provides the right environment for these chemicals to do their work most effectively.

Enzymes have a curious job. They do not actually enter into chemical combination with food materials; rather, they serve to speed up the breakdown of these substances into simpler components by encouraging a process called *hydrolysis* (literally, "loosening with water"). Without the action of enzymes in the stomach and small intestine, the splitting of carbohydrates, proteins and fats would proceed far too slowly to begin to support the body's needs for fuel. But each enzyme works best in its own "ideal climate." Those produced in the stomach can function well only at body temperature in an acid solution. Furthermore, the work they can do is severely limited because they themselves are inactivated by the very breakdown products they help achieve.

Once food is passed into the duodenum the digestive process speeds up remarkably. It is here that the main digestive work is done. Stomach acid is neutralized by alkaline secretions from the pancreas and liver while gastric enzymes are replaced by far more powerful alkaline enzymes. *Trypsin* and *chymotrypsin* from the pancreas attack the peptide bonds of long-chain protein molecules. *Amylase* is a potent starch-splitting enzyme formed in the pancreas, while still another pancreatic enzyme, *lipase,* helps to hydrolyze fats into fatty acids. *Bile salts* from the liver also aid in the breakdown of fats. By the time the digesting food material is moved farther down the canal by the wavelike contractions of smooth muscle in the intestinal walls, it has been converted into a "soup" containing a multitude of particles representing various stages of digestion. Carbohydrates, including the starches and sugars from potatoes, vegetables and fruit, are broken down into simple sugars that can be readily metabolized. Complex proteins from meats, eggs and cheese are split into their component amino acids and nucleic acids, while fats are hydrolyzed into a multitude of fatty acids and lipid-protein combinations the body tissues can use.

In time this soupy material reaches a part of the small intestine called the *jejunum,* quite different in structure from the duodenum. Here the interior of the canal is lined with tiny fingers of epithelium, the intestinal *villi,* which contain a rich network of blood capillaries and lymph vessels. Like a vast, velvety filter this lining absorbs much of the water and the molecule-sized fragments of digested food from the soup as it moves by, leaving larger particles and indigestible debris to be pushed on through the *ileum,* the lower half of the small intestine, and into the large intestine or *colon* for further dehydration and disposal. This absorption is by no means haphazard. Simple sugars and amino acids are taken into the blood capillaries and carried through the portal vein to the liver, where further processing must be done. Most of the hydrolyzed fats, however, are picked up by the lymph vessels and make their way directly into the general circulation. In either case, absorption is an active process involving special chemical reactions in the cells of the intestinal epithelium, thus assuring that all the useful foodstuffs available are efficiently winnowed out as the digesting soup passes through the intestinal tunnel.

No single tissue is responsible for the work done in the digestive tract. In fact, several of the basic tissues have a part to play in the mechanical and chemical preparation of food. Smooth muscle lines the esophagus, stomach and intestine, propelling food down the canal with gentle contractions called *peristalses.* Nerve cells of the autonomic nervous system direct this muscular activity and help control the secretion of digestive juices as well. Some early physiologists thought the physical presence of food in the stomach stimulated the secretion of gastric acid. Others insisted that a chemical response was involved. When still others found convincing evidence that the mere smell of food—or even the thought of it—could start the secretory glands working, all sorts of controversy arose. Of course we now know that all three ideas were right; digestive secretions and intestinal motility are controlled by a long and complex sequence of neurological reactions, some arising from chemical stimuli, some from pressure effects in the intestine and some from the higher brain centers far removed from the digestive tract.

Suppose, for instance, that a person is given an excess of insulin. Along with a sharp lowering of his blood sugar, he will suddenly begin suffering very convincing and uncomfortable hunger sensations. On the other hand, certain nonnutritive bulking substances can be used to "fool" the stomach into feeling full (i.e., "not hungry") even when no food value is present at all. One of the most puzzling of all intestinal diseases, first described in children by the Danish surgeon Harold Hirschsprung in 1886, involves a massive dilatation of the colon. In some cases the bowel would enlarge to almost unbelievable proportions. No one could understand what was blocking the passage of stool in Hirschsprung's disease; no apparent obstruction was present. Only recently have pathologists come up with the answer. A segment of bowel congenitally lacking the proper nerve ganglia acts as an invisible barrier to peristaltic waves moving down the colon. Once this "aganglionic segment" is surgically removed or by-passed, cure of the condition, also known as congenital megacolon, is possible.

Other kinds of tissue also play key roles in the digestive process. For example, such critical secretory organs as the liver and pancreas are composed almost entirely of different kinds of epithelial tissue. Epithelium also forms the absorptive lining of the small intestine and the capillaries around it. But the orderly process of digestion depends upon all the basic tissues doing their job properly at the right time. When they are in good working order the body is assured of a steady supply of usable fuel materials—even when food is not actively being taken in. However, malfunctions do occur, some so minor they cause only transitory discomfort, and some so serious they can cause a massive breakdown of the whole digestive process. (Diseases and disorders of the digestive system are discussed in detail in Part X, "Patterns of Illness: The Digestive Tract.") Among the more serious disorders are those involving malfunction of intestinal motility, or even intestinal obstruction. In addition, the digestive tract is vulnerable to bacterial or viral infections, to a variety of inflammatory diseases that are unrelated to any infective organism, to the formation of peptic ulcers—one of the most widespread of all gastrointestinal diseases in the Western world—and to several forms of cancer. Many of these conditions are purely organic illnesses, but many others also have a strong emotional element which must not be overlooked in diagnosis or treatment. Any or all of these disorders can produce a bewildering variety of symptoms, including such familiar phenomena as heartburn, excessive belching, nausea, vomiting, diarrhea and abdominal pain.

Normal digestive processes of the body also depend upon the proper function of two glandular organs in the abdomen, the pancreas and the liver. In the *pancreas,* a long, soft mass of glandular tissue lying against the back wall of the abdomen behind the stomach and duodenum, two completely different kinds of secretions are formed, one the vital metabolic hormone, *insulin,* that soaks directly into the blood stream, the other the alkaline gastric juices and enzymes which are carried through a series of ducts into the duodenum. In many ways the pancreas behaves as if it were two completely different organs, each functioning quite independently. Thus insulin production may decrease, leading to the development of diabetes mellitus, while the rest of the pancreas continues unimpeded in its normal function of enzyme secretion. On the other hand, pancreatitis (inflamma-

tion of the pancreas) may seriously interfere with the secretion of digestive enzymes while insulin production may continue exactly as if nothing had happened.

Of course some conditions affect the function of all parts of the pancreas, especially if they involve physical destruction of the organ. A form of cancer called carcinoma can rapidly invade and destroy all pancreatic tissue, sometimes reaching an advanced stage before any symptoms other than mild indigestion become evident. In fact, carcinoma of the pancreas may first be suspected when diabetes suddenly appears in a patient who has been complaining of persistent undiagnosed digestive distress.

At least the pancreas has only one general type of function: the secretion of chemical substances. The *liver,* by comparison, has a thoroughly bewildering variety of jobs to do. About the size and weight of a cantaloupe, it lies high in the abdomen on the right side, just beneath the diaphragm, and is protected by the lower edge of the rib cage. The liver is entrusted with so many vital body functions of completely different sorts that disease or injury can cause a multitude of dangerous disfunctions. The cells of the liver are large and many-sided, packed together in clusters with tiny drainage tubules to carry off the secretions that are formed. One of the most obvious functions of liver cells is the manufacture of *bile,* a yellow-green alkaline digestive juice containing bile salts, cholesterol and various pigments from broken-down red blood cells. As bile is formed it is stored and concentrated in a special pouch, the *gall bladder,* located just beneath the liver. Partially digested foods entering the duodenum from the stomach —and especially fats—stimulate the gall bladder to contract and empty its concentrated bile into the intestine through a large duct.

Such an elaborately handled secretion ought to play an important role in the digestive process, but as a matter of fact, digestion can proceed quite nicely without any bile whatever. Of all the functions of the liver, by far the most important is the synthesis and storage of a special body fuel called *glycogen.* The liver can manufacture this "all-purpose food" equally well from simple sugars or amino acids, converting it

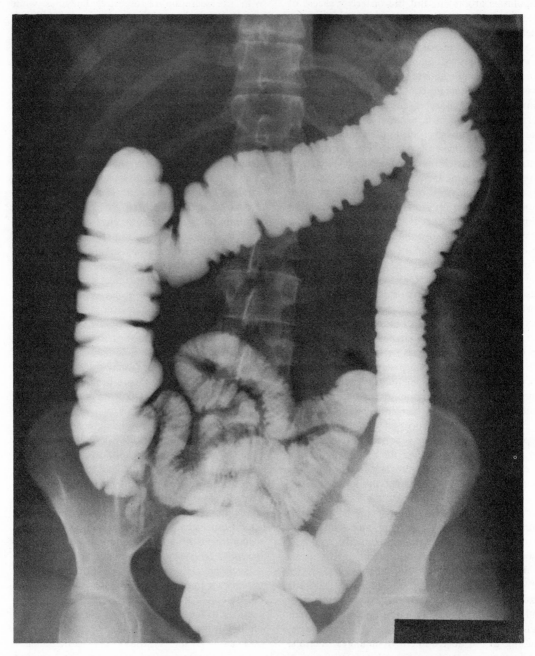

Plate 6a   Normal adult colon X-ray. The entire interior of the colon (large intestine) and a portion of the small intestine are outlined by a radio-opaque suspension of barium sulfate administered as an enema before the film was taken.

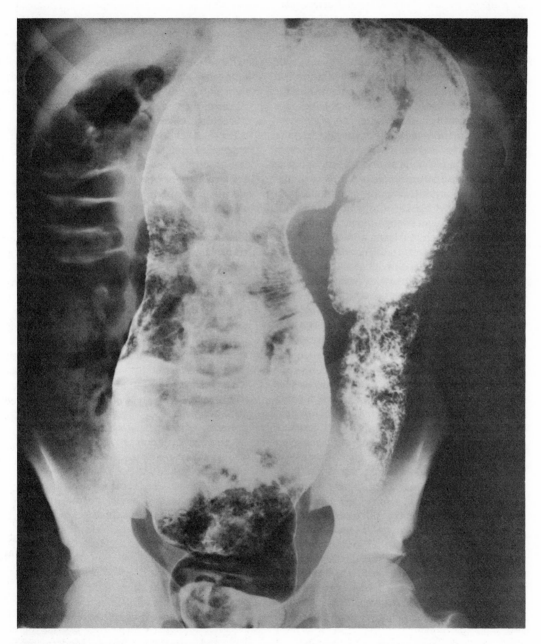

Plate 6b   Congenital megacolon (Hirschprung's disease) in a nineteen-year-old male. Compare the massively enlarged and distended colon with the normal in Plate 6a.

later into glucose for use in the tissues when the need arises. In addition, this living pharmaceutical plant synthesizes fatty acids and esters, certain essential vitamins, the *prothrombin* necessary for blood coagulation, albumin and other plasma proteins, and a wide variety of other body chemicals. It also serves as a storage depot for proteins and amino acids, various fatty fuels, excess supplies of iron and sundry vitamins. Finally, it is capable of detoxifying or rendering harmless a great variety of potentially dangerous chemical substances that find their way into the blood stream.

By entrusting this one organ with such a multitude of functions, it might appear that the body has rather recklessly put a large number of eggs in one basket. And indeed it has; damage to the liver can have devastating effects. But as if to compensate for such recklessness, the body has a vast surplus of liver tissue. We can get along reasonably well with only one-quarter of the liver functioning normally. Furthermore, the liver is remarkably regenerable; damaged areas tend to rebuild themselves by growing new liver cells. Unfortunately this regeneration is often poorly organized, accompanied by scarring and loss of function—a condition called cirrhosis. Thus infectious or serum hepatitis, dangerous virus infections of liver cells, may lead to permanent impairment of all liver functions. Cirrhosis may also occur as a result of the chronic protein starvation that so often accompanies prolonged and excessive use of alcohol—the reason for the popular, but technically erroneous, belief that "alcohol damages the liver."

Because of the double system of blood capillaries within the liver, one from the general circulation and another from the portal system, cancer cells entering the blood stream from distant sites often find their way to the liver. This, in fact, is the reason that careful laboratory studies of liver function are so often employed when a hidden cancer is suspected. But other comparatively rare and obscure conditions can also impair liver function. One of the most dramatic—and alarming—signs of liver damage is the appearance of jaundice, a yellow coloring of the skin and whites of the eyes which occurs when the outflow of bile into the intestine is obstructed and it enters the blood stream instead.

Liver disfunctions of any sort are relatively infrequent. Far more common are disturbances of the gall bladder that arise from inflammation or the formation of stones from cholesterol sediment. Gall bladder disease can be distressing and painful, but often can be cured by the surgical removal of this rather useless little pouch, a procedure known as *cholecystectomy*.

However complex the body's digestive function, it is essentially only a means of converting raw food materials into chemical fuels that can then be used by the cells to produce heat and energy and provide the wherewithal for growth, repair and reproduction. There is no single place in the body where this life-sustaining process does not take place. Every living cell must fend for itself. The final end products of digestion are carried to the tissues everywhere—to bone, to muscle, to the brain, to the heart and lungs, even back to the cells of the liver and the absorptive lining of the intestine. It is within the cells of every tissue in the body that the final conversion of fuel into energy takes place.

This process of fuel combustion, of breaking down certain substances and building up others, involves an incredible variety of extremely complex biochemical reactions which are called collectively *cellular* or *intermediary metabolism*. Virtually all of these reactions are speeded up or retarded by the action of complicated enzyme systems. Many also depend upon hormones as catalysts. Certain reactions occur in long, intricate sequences or *metabolic cycles,* with each step arising from the one previous and each in turn triggering the next. Such cycles may involve dozens of chemical reactions so complex that it seems impossible that anyone could ever have figured them out. And indeed, many have only been partially traced. Many more are not yet understood at all, but biochemists and physiologists have untangled certain of the major chains of reaction, step by step, after decades of brilliant and painstaking work. Modern medical specialists, too, are familiar with these reactions and the disfunctions that may occur. But for our purposes here the exact mechanisms of body metabolism are not important. The really significant point is that such biochemical reactions are taking place constantly, in bewildering variety and at incredible speed in every living cell of the body. Taken together, these metabolic reactions provide the human body with the energy necessary to maintain life. They begin when life begins, and they end only with death.

10

Conspiracy Against Death: Reproduction and Preservation

In recent years electronic engineers have been intrigued by the problem of building machines capable of repairing, protecting or even reproducing themselves according to prearranged commands. Such devices present staggering technical problems. To fill the bill they would need complex control centers, built-in factories for spare parts, mechanisms for the diagnosis of their own troubles, and other "lifelike" capabilities now beyond the capacity of even the most intricate machine.

It is not really surprising that physiologists have often been key collaborators in this line of research, for the living human body is precisely this kind of self-maintaining machine. It has the ability to diagnose its troubles and repair the damage. It manufactures its own spare parts, maintains exceedingly delicate internal chemical balances and protects itself against invading organisms and dangerous foreign materials. But these abilities have their limitations, and like a machine the body tends to age. As parts wear out or break down, its efficiency declines. Ultimately, beyond repair, it just stops working altogether.

The human body has one capability, however, that no machine can match: the ability to reproduce itself. But this is not an assembly-line operation that turns out an endless succession of identical reproductions. Far from it, for while each new generation has the same basic structure and function as the old, each also has a great many highly individual variations and characteristics of its own. This ability of species reproduction combined with individual variation is not ever likely to be duplicated by a man-made machine.

Reproduction is, in a sense, the body's way of cheating death. The ability to reproduce is not really vital to the life of any individual; it is necessary only to preserve and replenish the species. The mule, a cross between a horse and a donkey, is usually unable to reproduce. Except for such genetic curiosities, however, all living organisms reproduce themselves in one way or another. A one-celled creature like the ameba accomplishes this simply and directly. It draws the genetic material in its nucleus into two sections, splits it apart and then divides the rest of its protoplasm into two new cells in a process called *mitosis*. Each new ameba is half the size of the parent cell, and after growing to maturity it can itself divide to form two more amebas. Fortunately for us, most of these one-celled creatures meet with violent ends before they have reproduced. Otherwise the Earth's surface would long since have been covered with a wriggling sea of ameboid life.

Most tissues in the human body are also formed by simple cell division or mitosis, in which a complete, mature cell divides to become two complete new cells, each only half the size of the parent cell but each containing a perfect replica of the parent cell's genetic material—including the capacity to divide again into two more cells at some later time. This process is the major form of tissue growth within the body: the tiny liver of an infant, for example, grows to

SIMPLE CELLULAR DIVISION (MITOSIS)

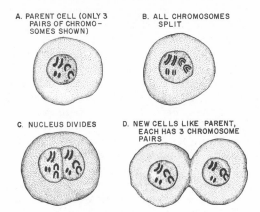

A. PARENT CELL (ONLY 3 PAIRS OF CHROMO- SOMES SHOWN)

B. ALL CHROMOSOMES SPLIT

C. NUCLEUS DIVIDES

D. NEW CELLS LIKE PARENT, EACH HAS 3 CHROMOSOME PAIRS

Figure 10–1.

its full size in the mature adult by simple cell division. Normally a rigid control mechanism, not yet fully understood, carefully regulates the rate of this cellular growth; new cells are provided, so to speak, only when they are needed. Unfortunately, this regulating mechanism occasionally gets out of hand. The reproduction of cells in a cancer, for example, while still occurring by simple mitosis, appears to be utterly unrestrained by natural hazards or normal body controls. In cancer so many cells are found in one stage or another of cellular division that doctors have nicknamed it "the mitotic disease."

There is, however, a big difference between the way in which the one-celled ameba reproduces itself and the reproduction of human life, although it too begins as a single cell, the fertilized egg. The two new amebas that result from the division of the parent cell receive all their characteristics from that cell; in fact, the parent cell ceases to exist. Thus the ameba has remained virtually the same in form and function for millions of years. But the single cell that begins the human reproductive process receives its characteristics from two parents in the union of the sperm cell from the male with the egg cell or ovum of the female. These sperm and egg cells are produced in the body by a very special process called *meiosis,* quite different from the simple cellular division of mitosis. Almost every cell in the human body is capable of mitotic

division, or merely duplicating itself. But certain cells in the male and the female have a special capability. In dividing by meiosis, they do not duplicate themselves, but rather produce the unique male and female sex or "germ" cells which, when united, are responsible for the reproduction of a totally new human organism.

To understand the difference between mitosis and meiosis, we must again look at the basic unit of life, the cell. The structural and functional characteristics of every living organism are determined by a so-called genetic code contained in special structures in the nucleus of each of its cells. In the case of very simple creatures, every living cell is capable not only of duplicating itself but also of reproducing the organism of which it is a part. But in higher, more complex organisms the various cells are coded to perform only very special functions. In the cells of the human body, the genetic code is built into the structure of certain extremely large molecules located in the cell nucleus. These molecules, called deoxyribonucleic acid (or DNA, for short), are composed of double spiraling chains of different amino acids, linked together like the

PRODUCTION OF GERM CELLS (MEIOSIS)

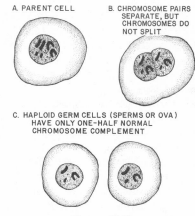

A. PARENT CELL

B. CHROMOSOME PAIRS SEPARATE, BUT CHROMOSOMES DO NOT SPLIT

C. HAPLOID GERM CELLS (SPERMS OR OVA) HAVE ONLY ONE-HALF NORMAL CHROMOSOME COMPLEMENT

Figure 10–2.

steps of a circular staircase. The sequence in which one or another of twenty possible amino acids are joined in these molecules determines the particular information coded into the cell, in much the same way that a punched card in a computer carries specific, transmittable information according to where and in what pattern the holes are punched.

The DNA molecules form packets of information in the cell nucleus which, together with related packets, make up a "node" or *gene*. Genes in turn are strung together in long, chainlike *chromosomes* (so called because they can be identified under the microscope by means of colored stains) that always occur in pairs in each cell nucleus. In mitosis when the cell divides, each chromosome in every pair splits down the middle; thus, as the dividing cell draws apart into two "daughter cells," each of the daughters has a full complement of chromosome pairs. As a consequence, the daughter cells are virtual carbon copies of the parent cell.

But in meiosis there is a difference in the way the cells divide—and a vital difference. In certain cells in the sex glands of both male and female, the individual chromosomes in each pair do *not* split down the middle as in the ordinary cell. Instead, as the cell begins to divide, the two chromosomes of each pair merely draw apart, so that one—and only one—chromosome from each pair goes to each daughter cell. The result of such a "meiotic" division is two new cells of a very specialized nature, each containing only half the genetic material of an ordinary tissue cell. These so-called *haploid cells* ("half-cells") are, of course, the special sex or "germ" cells which alone are capable of creating a new life when a male sperm cell and a female ovum meet and fuse. These germ cells by themselves, however, are literally genetic cripples. Alone, they are unable to divide again and are doomed to die very quickly unless joined by similarly attenuated cells of the opposite sex.

Both the male and the female have special glands or *gonads* specifically designed for the formation of germ cells. In the mature male the sperm cells are formed in the *testicles* or *testes*. In lower animals, sperm production may vary seasonally, but in the human male, sperm cells are manufactured in great quantities—up to millions per day—over a period of five decades or more without any seasonal variation. In the human female, ovum production is far more sparing. Only once every 28 days, on the average, does a rudimentary ovum mature in one of the *ovaries* and descend to the uterus, and the woman's ability to manufacture ova eventually comes to an end, lasting only from puberty to menopause, a period usually of about 35 years.

Obviously the mere development of sperm in the male and ova in the female is not enough. To make reproduction possible there must first be a means of bringing sperm and ova together so that the process known as *fertilization* or *conception* can take place. Second, there must be a means for protecting and nurturing the fertilized ovum through the early stages of embryonic growth, and then for supporting it throughout the nine-month period that must elapse before it can be delivered from the mother's body as a full-term baby capable of sustaining its own life. These goals are accomplished by the closely interrelated yet strikingly different functions of the male and female genital or reproductive organs.

The structure and function of both the male and the female genital organs are discussed in detail in Part XII, "Patterns of Illness: The Urinary and Genital Systems." Here, in summary, it can be said that the male genital organs perform two essentially simple functions: the manufacture of sperm in the testes and the introduction of sperm cells into the vagina of the female in the act of *sexual intercourse* or *coitus*. The female genital organs are much more complicated than the male and perform more complicated functions. The manufacture of ova and the reception of sperm from the male in the act of intercourse are two of their functions. The mature ovum must pass from the ovary to await fertilization in the process known as *ovulation*. If fertilization does not occur the ovum dies and the special uterine lining prepared to receive it in the event of fertilization is discarded in the process of *menstruation*. If fertilization does occur, the fertilized ovum is implanted in the special uterine lining and begins life as an embryo. As it develops it must be protected and nourished within the uterus during the period of *pregnancy* or *gestation*, which normally lasts for nine months and ends with childbirth or *parturition*. Both pregnancy and childbirth are complex physiological processes involving far more than the female genital organs, and are far different from any function of which the male is capable. (*See* p. 811.) So, too, is *menopause*, the gradual decline and eventual cessation of the woman's reproductive functions. But different as these functions are in male and female, they act in wonderful complement. Both are regulated by powerful sex hormones, and equally powerful physical and psychological forces are responsible for the attraction between a man and woman, their desire and ability to mate, to reproduce, and to love and care for the new human life they have created together.

Thus human anatomy, physiology and psychology conspire to make sexual intercourse between man and woman a remarkable means to an important end, reproduction. But the act of intercourse is not only a means of reproduction. Far from being the mindless and compulsive drive of the lower animal species, it can be a unique and wonderful form of human communication, an expression of mutual love, a source of shared pleasure and a means of enriching a human relationship. We are sexual beings, and it is a normal and healthy part of our natures to be drawn by powerful physical and psychological forces to mate. But we are also human beings whose actions and reactions can be controlled by common sense and consideration for others. And we are social beings who have devised laws and customs, for the most part necessary and sound, to regulate the circumstances of mating, to moderate indiscriminate intercourse, to provide women—in the event of conception—with protection and care during pregnancy and childbirth, and to ensure that both parents assume responsibility for the newborn child until it can care for itself.

As complicated as the process of human reproduction may seem, it all begins with the union of a single sperm and a single ovum. The result is the creation of a "supercell," the fertilized ovum, which has a full complement of chromosomes once again, half from the mother, half from the father, and a new human body begins its embryonic development completely equipped with the genetic material that will determine its structural and functional characteristics. But because only half of this material came from each parent, and because it combines in a unique way in the fertilized egg, the embryo will become a unique individual.

Precisely how this combination takes place in the new human being is still far from clear. The first man to try to spell out the ground rules of genetic variation was Gregor Johann Mendel (1822–1884), an Augustinian monk who began studying the hereditary traits of peas in his monastery garden near Brünn in the mid-1800s. A quiet man, Mendel was patiently working out the basic laws of heredity during the same years that Charles Darwin wrote his celebrated *Origin of Species,* without any knowledge whatever of genetic laws, and only a few years after the German pathologist Rudolf Virchow and his followers had discovered the way living cells reproduced by mitosis. Unlike the writings of these famous contemporaries, Mendel's work, which was first published in 1866, remained buried in obscurity until 1900, when Hugo De Vries, a Dutch botanist, repeated the same work independently and then discovered to his chagrin that Mendel had already done it years before. Geneticists today know that the transmission of body characteristics from generation to generation is far more complicated than either Mendel or De Vries suspected, but the lonely work of an unassuming man from an Austrian monastery still remains basic to our understanding of heredity.

For all its complexity, the formation of haploid germ cells by meiosis in the sex glands, and the subsequent pooling of genetic material from both parents within the fertilized egg after conception to create a new individual life both similar to and different from its parents, is far from haphazard and is remarkably free from pathological or disease-producing errors. As with any other physiological process, however, things occasionally can go wrong. Many individuals, quite innocently and unknowingly, may have defects in the genetic makeup of their cells which can be carried on to the germ cells they produce. In most cases the results of such defects, if any, are so minor that they cannot even be recognized as abnormalities at any time during the entire life of the offspring. But occasionally such defects can cause serious health problems. For example, defects causing *astigmatism,* a common disturbance of vision, or an abnormally narrow jaw may result in certain members of one family having impaired eyesight or crooked teeth generation after generation. During the 1800s and early 1900s several members of the royal families in Europe—most notably the young heir to the throne of Russia—were afflicted with a far more deadly hereditary condition, *hemophilia.* In this disease, which afflicts only males, although females are "carriers," the normal blood-clotting mechanism is seriously impaired by the action of a defective "black gene," and the victim may bleed to death from an internal hemorrhage or even the most minor of external injuries.

In other diseases, such as diabetes mellitus, no one has yet been able to pin down the exact role of hereditary defects, but a "family pattern" is so strongly characteristic that heredity must certainly play a major role in its occurrence. Finally, medical researchers in recent years have become aware that so-called inborn metabolic defects due to abnormal hereditary factors are at the root of a number of uncommon but tragic disorders. This knowledge has led to an effective treatment for a once incurable condition known as *phenylketonuria* which, if untreated, produces irreversible feeble-mindedness in its infant victims. It is strongly suspected that *mongolism,* another form of inborn or congenital mental and physical impairment, may be due to a similar hereditary abnormality.

Aside from diseases and disorders that are caused by genetic defects arising from the reproductive process, or are passed on as a result of it, there are, of course, a number of disorders of the reproductive organs themselves. As in any organ system, these afflictions fall into certain now familiar categories. First, congenital defects —outright malformations of both male and female genital organs—may occur. However, once these defects have been diagnosed, modern surgical techniques, in most cases, can correct them. But certain defects may not only be anatomical but hormonal as well, a matter of concern, since the sex hormones have a profound influence over the development of the genital organs and, in fact, the whole human organism. Occasionally, for example, the sex specificity of

the developing fetus becomes muddled, and one of a variety of "mixed sex" abnormalities or *hermaphroditism* occurs. The victim not only may possess functional and nonfunctional genital organs of both sexes, but may also be subjected to a baffling mixture of hormonal influences. In many such cases, however, corrective and reconstructive surgery may enable the victim to assume the most natural sexual role, physically as well as emotionally.

Disorders of the genital organs can also be caused by infections, particularly those venereal diseases almost invariably contracted through sexual intercourse or other sex-related activities, although the infectious organisms that attack other organs and tissues in the body may also afflict the genital system. Finally, cancer and other tumors can develop in both the male and the female genital organs; the female in particular is vulnerable to a number of disorders related to the processes of ovulation, menstruation, pregnancy, childbirth and menopause; and a variety of emotional afflictions, with or without underlying physical causes, can interfere with both male and female sexual function.

The diseases and disorders of the male and female genital organs are discussed in detail in Part XII, "Patterns of Illness: The Urinary and Genital Systems," while those disorders that are specific to pregnancy and childbirth are described in Part XIV, Chapter 57, "Progressing Through Pregnancy." Human reproduction is an incredibly complex process, and any one of many disorders may interfere with it in part or prevent it entirely. Nevertheless, it is in general resoundingly effective in perpetuating the human species and, in addition, serves as the body's only means of cheating death. But once reproduction has been achieved, the newborn infant, no less than the mature adult, is subjected to environmental hazards and to physiological and psychological malfunctions of all sorts. Given the gift of life, every individual must then find the means to preserve and sustain it in good health and comfort. Fortunately, the human body with which man has been equipped is in itself his first—and often the best—line of defense.

The human body has certain built-in mechanisms that aid enormously in protecting and preserving itself. The most obvious of these mechanisms is its almost incredible capacity to heal itself when injured or when attacked by disease processes. Whether the damage involves the most superficial scratching of the skin or a massive destruction of liver cells by the virus of infectious hepatitis, the self-healing capacity of the body immediately goes to work. There is virtually no kind of disease or injury known which the body does not at least *attempt* to heal. In multitudes of cases the attempt is splendidly successful without the slightest intervention. Every doctor knows (and every patient ought to know) that the most powerful medicine in the fight against disease is tincture of time—the patience to allow the body to take care of its own healing if it can.

However, the body's attempts at self-healing may not always succeed, or may succeed only imperfectly. For example, the body may wall off an area of tuberculosis within a lung without actually destroying the organism that is causing the infection, allowing the disease later to break free and become active again when conditions are right. Fractured bones may heal imperfectly, so that full, normal use of a limb is never recovered and permanent crippling results. In certain cases the body's attempt to heal a destructive lesion may even result in dangerous or fatal pathological changes: in acute rheumatic fever, for example, the body's attempt to heal the swollen and inflamed tissue of a heart valve may result in such severe scarring that the valve can no longer work and the victim may ultimately die from resultant heart failure. But, overall, these are the exceptional cases; the real miracle is how often the body's self-healing capacity succeeds where any amount of medical intervention might have failed.

In addition to self-healing, the body has a remarkable series of self-regulating mechanisms to help maintain its internal environment in the delicate balance necessary for life. There is an intricate mechanism that regulates body heat, for example, to help cool us down when the world outside is too warm, or to help us conserve heat when we are cold. Other mechanisms regulate the amount of fluid in our bodies and

control its exact chemical balance within extremely narrow ranges of tolerance. Still others maintain acidity within the parts of the body where acidity is necessary and provide alkalinity where that is needed. Circulation, respiration, the acuity of sense perceptions, the state of sleep or of wakefulness, all are self-regulated, proceeding effectively unless injury or disease interferes.

We are also protected against invaders from the world outside our bodies. The moment dangerous bacteria find entry, the body mobilizes white blood cells to combat infection. Simultaneously a "draft call" is sent out to the bone marrow to start manufacturing more white cells to replace the ones that may be lost in the battle. In a pinch these "ready reserves" of white cells may be poured out into the blood stream before they are even completely matured, much as a nation might throw raw recruits into the field if an invading force threatened in overwhelming numbers.

There are built-in protections against other kinds of invaders as well. The body has an intensely sensitive, unconscious "awareness of self"—a means of assessing and "approving," so to speak, the chemical substances that properly belong within that individual body, and a means of detecting and "disapproving" the presence of foreign or alien substances, especially proteins and certain kinds of complex carbohydrates that may find their way into the body by mistake. Although no one yet fully understands just why such foreign substances constitute a threat, we do know that the body has an elaborate mechanism for confronting and destroying or neutralizing these substances whenever they appear.

It is this mechanism, for example, that accounts for the *immune reactions* that occur when a virus enters the body; special "combat troops," the antibodies, are formed to neutralize and destroy the virus, when possible, and then remain on reserve to counteract that same virus more swiftly if it attempts to gain entry again at some later time. This same mechanism accounts for the *allergic reactions,* sometimes quite violent, that we can suffer when other foreign material—pollens, house dust or insect venoms, to name only a few—get into our bodies. There is no doubt that these allergic reactions play an important role in protecting us from a myriad of potentially dangerous foreign substances in the world around us.

But often it seems that our bodies carry things a bit too far, in effect overreacting to relatively minor threats, like trying to drive a carpet tack with a 20-pound sledge hammer and inadvertently smashing a hole in the floor. It is precisely such overreactions that result in the thoroughly uncomfortable and sometimes dangerous allergies that so many people suffer. And this very same "awareness of self" possessed by each individual's body accounts for the so-called rejection reaction that hinders or, more often, completely blocks the successful transplantation of new tissues or organs from one human body to another even when such a transplant may be the only possible means of saving an individual's life.

The human body's built-in capacity for self-preservation is perhaps the most fascinating and ironic aspect of the many problems associated with proper health care. Although we must assume that there is some deeply entrenched, vital reason for them to exist, the body's unconscious or "mindless" self-preserving reactions *are not always rational,* even though they are regulated by the brain and nervous system as well as by other body tissues. Sometimes they unquestionably act to protect and preserve the body; but at other times they may do just the opposite. In the case of organ transplants, for example, the body's rejection reaction is nothing more or less than a living time bomb, and for such truly lifesaving procedures to become widely usable, we must yet find some reliable means literally to trick the body into "believing" that a transplanted organ is really "a part of itself" and not an "outside invader."

But whether the body's natural defenses are rational or not, whether in a given case they are actually *useful* or not, they often require some conscious, rational, deliberate help from the person most concerned—the individual possessing the body—in order to be truly effective. Such help may include, among other things, the commonsense wisdom to slow down and take it easy in some circumstances, to avoid obvious physical abuses, to eat properly or to seek medical help

when necessary. Here the element of teamwork between the mind and the body is of incalculable benefit in prolonging life and preserving health. If the average man of fifty, for example, were to attempt to maintain the eating and sleeping habits, the physical exertions and the living pace of a fifteen-year-old boy, he would soon be in trouble. In such matters, in a subtle way, our bodies help protect us. As we grow older we are naturally prevented from such excesses of exuberance. Our energy level declines, we require more sleep, we feel the effects of exhaustion more quickly, and we are generally satisfied to do things more slowly and sedately. Even if we are not satisfied, we are nevertheless restrained by joints that become less agile and hearts and lungs that become less resilient and adaptable. As if in compensation, we have the rich depths of years of experience, of lessons well learned, all stored and available in the memory vaults of our mature minds, to enable us to find better answers with less effort and energy than a youngster would have to expend. The capacity to age gracefully is only one of the quiet mechanisms built into our bodies to help preserve and protect us.

Taken together, our built-in physical protective mechanisms and our rational mental capacities—our physiological "awareness of self" combined with our psychological "awareness of self"—are an almost unbeatable combination in our body's conspiracy against death. But the human mind, however ingenious, has not yet found a way either to create life or to prevent death, even though we have been able to figure out why and how each occurs. Perhaps one day we will, but until then it is the body alone that first achieves life and ultimately succumbs to death. In between, body and mind must work together to achieve continuing health, well-being and long life.

The normal human body is truly marvelous in all its complexity—complexity of structure, function, and capacity not only to reproduce new life but to protect itself against untimely death. When things go wrong (as they inevitably do, sooner or later), the body is superbly equipped to handle the trouble itself in the vast majority of cases.

But not always. There are many times when medical intervention is absolutely essential to help heal injury and disease and to preserve optimum good health. Even more often, medical intervention, if not absolutely necessary, is at least highly desirable to anticipate and avoid trouble before it begins, to relieve distressing symptoms when they occur, and to facilitate the healing processes. Once this kind of intervention was considered exclusively the doctor's province. Today we know better. More and more we have come to recognize the obvious: that the most fruitful intervention possible for continuing good health or speedy recovery must be a joint venture in which doctor and patient work together in mutual cooperation and confidence, each contributing in a vital—and knowledgeable—way.

Knowledge is the key that makes such a cooperative venture work. Doctors and medical personnel are carefully trained and highly skilled professionals. But every individual, whether he happens to be a patient or not, should share in at least a part of that professional knowledge: knowledge of the normal, and abnormal, structures and functions of the human body; knowledge of the sudden emergencies that can strike and what can be done about them; knowledge of the patterns of illness as they can affect all the organ systems of the body; knowledge of the particularly trying or stressful times of life when vulnerability to certain types of illness may be especially great; and finally, knowledge of the remarkable wealth of medical facilities that are available today to help make the maintenance of optimum good health a realistic and realizable dream for everyone in our society. It is knowledge of this sort, in the hands of the patient as well as his doctor, that can revolutionize our concepts of health care and make happier and healthier lives possible for all of us.

EMERGENCIES, FIRST AID AND HOME HEALTH CARE

11. When Seconds May Save Lives: The Serious Emergencies   103

12. Minor Injuries and Other Emergencies   124

13. Temperature, Fever and Febrile Illnesses   148

14. Home Health Care   157

Many human illnesses take hours, days or even months to evolve, with ample time to consult a doctor and begin treatment. But in an emergency, trouble can strike with alarming suddenness, and someone—a member of the family, a friend or even a passer-by—must be prepared to take appropriate first-aid measures before medical help arrives. In a minor emergency, first aid may require little more than quick thinking and common sense. But in urgent emergencies the swift, effective application of certain special first-aid procedures can spell the difference between life and death. Everyone should have a practical knowledge of these vital procedures and be able to use them any time the need arises. Further, even nonemergencies may require immediate and knowledgeable action. The appearance of a fever, for example, is perhaps the most commonplace and familiar of all early warnings of illness. It is important to know what a fever means, why it occurs, and in some cases—as with a sudden feverish illness in a child—what to do until a doctor can be reached. Finally, there is the problem of providing home health care for the sick. Modern medical techniques have made it possible to treat many illnesses at home, and even when hospital care is necessary, convalescence at home is often desirable, especially in the case of a child or an elderly patient. Just as a knowledge of first-aid procedures is vital in an emergency, knowledge of certain commonsense principles of home nursing care during an illness or convalescence is an essential adjunct to the maintenance of optimum good health for the entire family.

11

When Seconds May Save Lives: The Serious Emergencies

All sorts of medical emergencies can arise in the course of everyday life. Many are relatively minor and require little more than common sense in the way of first-aid treatment. At the other extreme, there are certain crashing emergencies for which no conceivable first-aid treatment is possible; the victim's life may be saved only if he can be taken to a doctor, or a doctor to him, in time to help. *Diabetic coma* is one such emergency, especially when it occurs for the first time in a child. There is nothing anyone but a doctor can do in such a case. Treatment of this condition requires immediately available laboratory facilities, experienced hospital nursing care and expert medical direction, and the difference between life and death may hang on the few minutes it takes to rush the child to the hospital. *Insulin shock* is also an emergency situation, but there *is* a first-aid measure in this case—rubbing honey on the inside of the patient's cheeks and under his tongue—which can materially aid recovery even before the patient arrives at the hospital. (*See* p. 700.)

An *acute myocardial infarction* or *coronary attack* is another crashing medical emergency. Again, the only thing to do is get the victim to a hospital as quickly as possible, or call a Medic I or other mobile emergency care unit if the community has such facilities available. Much the same can be said for the kind of head injury that causes *intracranial hemorrhage* and increased intracranial pressure. One neurosurgeon at a famous eastern medical school used to delight in telling his students that any one of them

might some day save a life by using a rock to drive a ten-penny nail through a patient's skull. His point was valid enough: this is one emergency means of relieving a possible fatal increase in intracranial pressure. But of course no untrained layman should undertake such a measure as a means of first aid.

Apart from situations like these, however, there are certain other kinds of extremely serious emergencies for which highly effective first-aid measures not only can, but often *must,* be taken before medical help arrives. What a parent or anyone else at the scene of such an emergency does in the way of first aid may determine whether the victim survives or not, or, in less serious cases, how long it will take for his recovery. These are emergencies everyone should be able to recognize and for which everyone should have certain clear-cut principles of action in mind as part of his "emergency equipment." Doing the right thing at the right time may not be merely helpful to the victim; it may save his life.

Among these overwhelming emergencies there are four in particular which require swift and knowledgeable action: *massive bleeding or hemorrhage; respiratory failure from suffocation, choking, drowning or some other cause; abrupt and often inexplicable collapse,* usually due to sudden *circulatory failure;* and the complex group of symptoms known as *shock.* Each of these will be discussed separately and in detail below, but very commonly *more than one may be present at the same time.* That means a

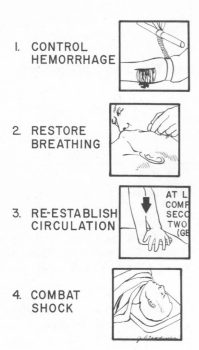

1. CONTROL HEMORRHAGE

2. RESTORE BREATHING

3. RE-ESTABLISH CIRCULATION

4. COMBAT SHOCK

Figure 11–1.
The order of priority in administering first aid.

As a basic rule, massive hemorrhage—especially bleeding from a major artery—must be controlled first. Second most important, breathing must be restored in some way, even by means of prolonged artificial respiration if necessary. Third, circulatory failure must be dealt with, insofar as possible, until medical help arrives. Finally, but by no means to be ignored or overlooked, steps must be taken to prevent, minimize or counteract shock. *This order of priority is the Bible of emergency first aid.*

Arterial Hemorrhages

Arterial hemorrhages are infinitely more serious than the sort of bleeding that occurs from minor lacerations, abrasions and flesh wounds, or even the copious steady bleeding from scalp lacerations or the blood loss from persistent nosebleeds (which is rarely as great as it may

seem). An arterial hemorrhage is the massive, spurting bleeding that occurs when a major artery has been torn or severed. So much blood can be lost so quickly in such an emergency that the victim may exsanguinate if the bleeding is not effectively stopped within minutes at the most, and preferably within seconds, from the time it begins. It takes, for example, approximately two minutes—120 seconds—for a person to exsanguinate from the rupture of a femoral artery, the great artery that carries the main blood supply through the groin into the leg. This is the sort of accident that can occur when a leg is crushed or when a fracture of the femur causes one of the fragments of bone to cut the femoral artery and tear through muscle and skin to the outside. An injury to the neck or head can cause tearing of the carotid artery which carries blood to the head, or to the temporal artery which supplies the front upper portion of the face and scalp or the mandibular artery which

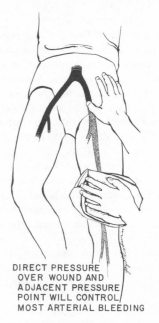

DIRECT PRESSURE
OVER WOUND AND
ADJACENT PRESSURE
POINT WILL CONTROL
MOST ARTERIAL BLEEDING

Figure 11–2.

supplies the jaw, both of which are branches of the carotid artery. Injuries such as these are often caused by automobile accidents and the like, but they occur far more frequently in accidents in the home. Serious lacerations involving broken windows, broken bottles or mishandled carving knives are commonplace, and surgeons can testify how very often life-threatening lacerations of carotid or femoral arteries are sustained from walking through sliding glass doors.

In any case involving hemorrhagic bleeding, it is urgently important to try to stop, or at least control, the excessive bleeding before doing anything else. It may save the victim's life. The best way to do this is to *apply direct pressure to the wound.* Use a clean handkerchief, bandage or

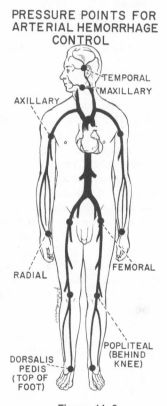

PRESSURE POINTS FOR ARTERIAL HEMORRHAGE CONTROL

TEMPORAL
MAXILLARY
AXILLARY
RADIAL
FEMORAL
POPLITEAL
(BEHIND KNEE)
DORSALIS
PEDIS
(TOP OF FOOT)

Figure 11–3.

any firmly rolled cloth pad as a compress and hold it tightly to the wound for four or five minutes. If you see rhythmic spurts of bright red blood coming from the wound, an artery has been damaged and you should apply additional pressure with the other hand on the side of the wound *toward* the heart, or on the familiar pres-

sure points where a strong pulse is normally felt: the underside of the wrist for wounds of the hand, in the armpit for wounds of the arm, directly in front of the ears for wounds of the scalp, or on either side of the groin for wounds of the leg. You will know that arterial bleeding is under control when the spurting stops. If it continues, readjust the pressure over the wound and on the "pressure point" toward the heart from the wound. Once the bleeding is controlled, maintain the pressure for at least five minutes before relaxing it, and be prepared to reinstate the pressure immediately if the spurting starts again.

If the wound is bleeding in a steady flow of rather dark-colored purplish blood, it probably comes from a vein rather than an artery, and additional pressure should be applied on the side of the wound *away* from the heart. Bleeding from a vein is generally under much less pressure than from an artery, and consequently is less copious and more easily controlled in a shorter period of time.

Control of any kind of bleeding from an extremity, and especially arterial bleeding, will be greatly simplified by *elevating the extremity* while other control measures are being taken. Obviously the heart has a harder time pumping blood uphill than if the limb is level or hanging down. A bleeding limb can be raised or propped up above body level, or it can be held in an elevated position by an assistant, and bleeding will be easier to stop.

What about using a tourniquet? This age-old device—any kind of constrictive band tightened around a limb—has fallen into disrepute as a first-aid measure in recent years. Many first-aid teachers instruct their students never to use them, on the grounds that they can do more harm than good. And indeed they can, when used improperly or in the wrong situations, but such a blanket rejection of the tourniquet is a mistake. There *are* occasions when tourniquets should *not* be used; but there are also occasions when *nothing but* a tourniquet, properly applied, can effectively stop dangerous arterial bleeding and, perhaps, save a life.

What are the real dangers of a tourniquet? First, most laymen *do not apply a tourniquet tightly enough.* Arterial bleeding may be slowed, but it is not stopped; at the same time the tourniquet blocks the return of venous blood, so that venous bleeding becomes steadily worse. In such cases a point may even be reached when venous bleeding cannot be stopped by any means until the tourniquet is taken *off*. Second, if the tourniquet *is* applied tightly enough to stop arterial bleeding, it may also be applied so excessively tightly that it crushes tissue, especially nerve tissue, and long-term or even permanent nerve damage can result. In either case, the use of a tourniquet may result in more harm than if it had not been used at all. Oddly enough, the concern that use of a tourniquet may cut off all blood supply to the limb and thus cause oxygen starvation of the tissues is not a serious worry, at least for the length of time necessary to control bleeding and obtain medical help. Surgeons use tourniquets freely and routinely to stop all blood flow to a limb for as long as an hour or more during surgical procedures without fear of tissue starvation. But they always take careful measures to see that the tourniquet is not crushing tissue.

TOURNIQUET

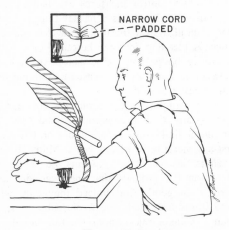

NARROW CORD
---PADDED

Figure 11–4.

These safe rules should be followed in using a tourniquet for emergency control of bleeding:

1. First, *direct pressure over a wound should always be applied if possible.* It will be enough to stop any arterial bleeding in an extremity except when the limb has been mangled, crushed, shredded or amputated. *Use of a tourniquet should be limited specifically to these conditions, and only these conditions.*

2. If you must use a tourniquet, fashion it from some *inelastic* material—a necktie, a piece of rope, or a twisted piece of clothing. An elastic tourniquet may shut off only venous bleeding. If the tourniquet is very narrow, it should be padded to prevent cutting or crushing tissue. The bleeding extremity should be elevated and the tourniquet immediately applied between the wound and the heart. A piece of stick or a similar lever should be twisted into the tourniquet so that pressure can easily be increased or decreased.

3. Tighten the tourniquet gradually just to the point where the arterial bleeding stops *completely.* If you know where to feel for a pulse on the opposite side of the wound, tighten the tourniquet until the pulse is lost. If the limb beyond the tourniquet is mangled or missing, cessation of blood flow alone must be your guide.

4. Maintain the tourniquet at this pressure—but no tighter—until medical aid can be obtained. If this takes longer than an hour, release the tourniquet at that time to see if bleeding has stopped, but be prepared to reapply it if the bleeding starts again.

In short, never use a tourniquet except under the conditions stated above; direct pressure over the wound will control bleeding in other cases. But when you must use a tourniquet, don't be afraid to use it properly and adequately. With the above rules in mind you will not go wrong.

Since hemorrhagic bleeding from a major artery can lead to exsanguination and death within as little as two minutes, control of excessive bleeding should always take *first* priority in any emergency. Someone else should be sent to summon a physician and/or ambulance without delay, while the person providing first aid stays with the victim at least until excessive bleeding is controlled. Remember that most people tend to overestimate the actual amount of blood that is lost from a wound. Also remember that, in case of an accident, other things may also require attention as well as bleeding. Once excessive bleeding is controlled, for example, a moment should be taken to make certain that the victim is breathing freely.

Respiratory Failure (Asphyxia)

Asphyxia is another potentially disastrous emergency. Lack of oxygen for more than four minutes at a stretch can cause permanent damage to body tissues, especially to the delicate nerve cells in the brain, and death may occur if oxygen is cut off for as long as 6½ to 7 minutes. Thus after any accident it is vital to make sure that the victim is breathing through a free and unobstructed airway. An auto accident, a fall downstairs or a blow to the throat during a fight may partially collapse the trachea or the larynx, causing breathing obstruction. Or a person may accidentally suck in or *aspirate* a chunk of food that can lodge in the trachea and completely block any movement of air. In a child an aspirated peanut or cough drop could do the same thing; so could the aspiration of stomach contents during vomiting. If a child is choking, he can be turned completely upside down so that the force of gravity will help dislodge any obstruction. In the case of an adult, placing his head lower than the rest of this body may accomplish the same purpose. A sharp slap on the back also may jar an obstruction loose. Even the victim's tongue can obstruct his airway; pull the tongue forward in his mouth to make sure it does not prevent free breathing.

If these measures fail, or if a person is not breathing at all as a result of drowning, heart attack, electric shock or some other accident, breathing must be restarted artificially by using an effective method of resuscitation. By far the most effective, and the most often recommended, of all methods of artificial respiration is *mouth-to-mouth,* or alternatively, *mouth-to-nose resuscitation,* which depends upon the fact that the air you normally exhale from your lungs contains quite enough oxygen to resuscitate someone who has ceased breathing, even though there is more carbon dioxide in exhaled air than in fresh air. Mouth-to-mouth resuscitation is

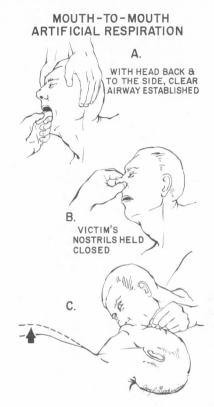

MOUTH-TO-MOUTH ARTIFICIAL RESPIRATION

A. WITH HEAD BACK & TO THE SIDE, CLEAR AIRWAY ESTABLISHED

B. VICTIM'S NOSTRILS HELD CLOSED

C.

Figure 11–5.

both easy and safe to undertake by means of the following step-by-step procedure:

1. Clear the victim's mouth and airway. Remove any visible foreign matter with your fingers. Then turn the victim on his side and slap his back sharply several times to dislodge obstructions. Remove dentures. Pull the tongue forward, since it may also obstruct breathing. *Do not proceed with resuscitation if you suspect there is still an obstruction in the way.* You could inadvertently lodge it even more firmly in place.

2. With the victim lying on his side, tilt his head backward so that his chin is pointing upward. (*See* Fig. 11–5.) Open his mouth, pulling his jaw forward to straighten the airway. Then pinch the victim's nostrils shut with your thumb and forefinger. No air must escape through his nose when you begin breathing into his mouth.

3. Take a normal breath through your mouth, place your lips against the victim's with firm pressure, and exhale with gentle, steady force. You should see his chest rise and expand moderately when you do this. If it does not, there is still something obstructing the free flow of air into his lungs. Repeat Step 1, recheck the position of the head, make sure no air can escape through the victim's nose, and then breathe into his mouth again.

4. When you succeed in inflating the victim's lungs, take your mouth away to allow that air to be exhaled. This will occur naturally, even though the victim is not inhaling for himself. Continue breathing into the victim's mouth with a steady rhythm, about one breath every four seconds. *If the victim is a child, remember he has less lung capacity than you do.* Use only half-breaths to avoid overdistending his lungs. Also remember that an accident victim or drowning victim may regurgitate at any time. If he does, keep his head turned to one side and use a finger to help empty his mouth of emesis (vomited material) before continuing resuscitation.

5. Continue the above procedure until the victim begins taking regular breaths for himself, or until medical aid arrives.

Some people, are reluctant about breathing into an accident victim's mouth. An emergency of this sort is no time for squeamishness, but mouth-to-nose resuscitation can often be used as an alternative method. The procedure is exactly the same as above, except that you seal the victim's mouth tightly with your hand and breathe gently with a steady rhythm into his nose. In accidents in which the mouth has been injured or the jaw broken, this alternative method may be the best choice.

Certain simple mechanical devices can be helpful in administering mouth-to-mouth resuscitation if they happen to be handy, although no time should be wasted trying to find them if they are not immediately available. For example, an ordinary kitchen basting syringe with a rubber suction bulb can be used to suck secretions or vomitus from the victim's mouth. Any modern first-aid kit should contain a small curved plastic airway device (*see* Fig. 11–6), obtainable at your local drugstore. Once the victim's mouth has

been cleared of debris, anyone can safely insert the curved end of this plastic tube to the back of the victim's throat, pulling the tongue forward at the same time. The mouth guard will prevent inserting it too far. Such a device will help hold

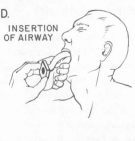

D. INSERTION OF AIRWAY

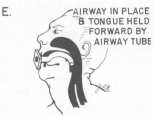

E. AIRWAY IN PLACE & TONGUE HELD FORWARD BY AIRWAY TUBE

Figure 11–6.

the tongue forward, keep more debris out of the airway, and permit more effective movement of air in mouth-to-mouth resuscitation.

There are other methods of artificial respiration, but none is anywhere near as effective as mouth-to-mouth or mouth-to-nose resuscitation, and they should not be used unless the infinitely superior mouth-to-mouth procedure is impossible for some reason—in cases of severe head injury, for example, or when bones of the face or jaw are broken. Most familiar of these alternative procedures is the old-fashioned *prone-pressure method* of artificial respiration, which involves a rhythmic pressing and releasing of the victim's lower rib cage some fifteen or sixteen times a minute. Place the victim face down on a solid surface with his head turned to one side. Be sure his mouth is open, his tongue drawn forward and his airway free of obstructions. Then straddle his hips, placing your hands at the lower edge of his rib cage on either side. By leaning forward for two seconds, applying pressure on the ribs, and then relaxing the pressure for three seconds, rhythmically, you will force exhausted air out of the victim's lungs and allow fresh air to be drawn

PRONE-PRESSURE ARTIFICIAL RESPIRATION

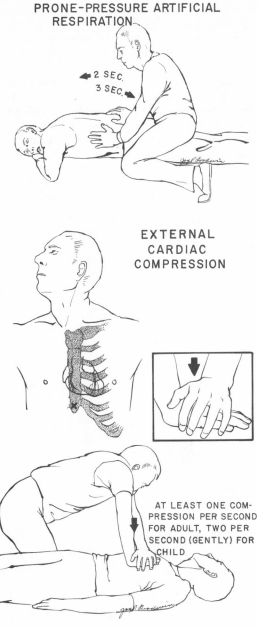

EXTERNAL CARDIAC COMPRESSION

AT LEAST ONE COM-
PRESSION PER SECOND
FOR ADULT, TWO PER
SECOND (GENTLY) FOR
CHILD

Figure 11–7.

before the victim begins breathing for himself or until medical help arrives.

Less familiar, but somewhat more effective, is the *supine arm-lift* or *Sylvester method*. Again, this procedure should be used only when mouth-to-mouth or mouth-to-nose resuscitation is impossible. Place the victim flat on his back with his head turned to one side, his mouth and nose well above the ground. Remove all obstructions from his mouth and draw his tongue forward. Then kneeling over him, draw his arms rhythmically up above his head and return them to his sides about fifteen times a minute, thus mechanically expanding his rib cage and forcing at least some air exchange. Again, you may have to continue this procedure for a prolonged period of time until the victim begins breathing for himself or until medical help arrives.

ARM-RAISING ARTIFICIAL RESPIRATION

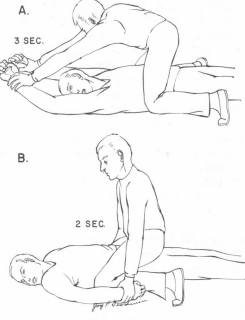

Figure 11–8.

in each time the lungs expand after the pressure is released. This method will allow some fresh air exchange from the moment you begin, but it may have to be continued steadily for an hour or more

Whatever method of artificial respiration is used, however, it is imperative to remember that it must be begun at once and continued until medical help arrives. If necessary, have someone relieve you from time to time without any break in the rhythm of the artificial respiration. There have been cases in which normal breathing was restored after several *hours* of apparently fruitless work. Certainly as long as the victim's heart is still beating there is hope that he will begin breathing again.

Restoring the heartbeat and circulation is third, after hemorrhage control and artificial respiration, in the order of first-aid priorities. While the first two conditions are most often present in victims of serious accidents, circulatory failure may first be discovered, quite without warning, when a person suddenly collapses, or is found unconscious, for no apparent reason. There may be no sign of injury or external hemorrhage, and the victim may be breathing well enough on his own that no artificial respiration is necessary. In cases such as these, some form of circulatory failure, usually due to *cardiac arrest* or spontaneous heart stoppage, must be suspected, and can be quickly confirmed by checking the heartbeat and pulse, either at the victim's wrist or the pulse in the large carotid artery at the base of the neck or the femoral artery in the groin. A wide dilation of the pupils of the eyes upon exposure to light is also an indication of some kind of circulatory failure.

If circulation has stopped—specifically, if you can feel no heartbeat or pulse—swift action must be taken to start the victim's blood flowing again until he can be taken to a hospital. *Sometimes a sharp blow with your fist to the left side of the victim's chest over his heart may succeed in restoring heartbeat.* If it does, the victim should be kept completely at rest until medical aid arrives, even though the attack seems to have passed. But if it does not succeed, a form of "artificial circulation" can be maintained by means of a technique known as *external cardiac compression,* a first-aid measure that can be performed safely and easily by anyone on the scene, and which may well save the life of a victim of cardiac arrest.

The heart normally lies almost midline in the chest, under the breastbone, with just the lower tip projecting to the left. To achieve effective artificial circulation of the blood by using external cardiac compression, put the victim on the floor on his back and kneel beside him. Place the heel of one hand firmly on the lower third of the breastbone overlying his heart (*not* in the notch of the rib cage at the lower end of the breastbone) and place your other hand on top of the first. (*See* Fig. 11–9.) Then roll forward with your arms kept stiff until the weight of your upper body is exerting some 60 to 90 pounds of pressure straight down on the victim's breastbone. This will compress the heart enough to make it expel blood from the ventricles into the aorta. When you relax the pressure, the victim's

CLEARING THE AIRWAY

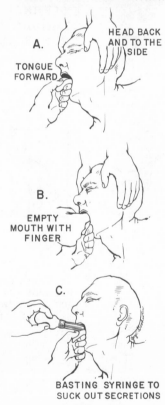

A. HEAD BACK AND TO THE SIDE
TONGUE FORWARD

B. EMPTY MOUTH WITH FINGER

C. BASTING SYRINGE TO SUCK OUT SECRETIONS

Figure 11–9.

heart will refill with the same amount of blood from the veins that is expelled into the arteries. By rapidly and rhythmically compressing for a half second and then removing pressure for a half second, keeping your hands in place all the time, you can establish a certain amount of regular blood flow to and from the heart—not as much circulation as a healthy heart would maintain on its own, but enough to restore a palpable pulse and maintain circulation with a blood pressure sufficiently high to keep the brain and other vital parts of the body at least minimally supplied with blood at an "artificial circulation rate" of at least 60 heart compressions a minute. *A rate of less than 60 compressions a minute will accomplish nothing in an adult, and for small children a rate of 100 to 120 compressions a minute is required.*

If a victim's breathing has stopped as well as his circulation, a far more difficult situation exists, but there is no need for confusion or panic. Simply remember your first-aid priorities. Respiration must be restored first, or simultaneously with restoration of heartbeat. If there are two people on the scene, one may perform mouth-to-mouth resuscitation while the other performs external cardiac compression. If you are the only person present, you can in fact do both yourself, if necessary. Maintaining both artificial respiration and artificial circulation at the same time is known as *heart-lung resuscitation,* and is safe for anyone to perform in any emergency. The necessary procedure is easy to remember with the help of a simple mnemonic device: the A-B-C-D of heart-lung resuscitation.

A—*Airway must be opened.* As with any form of artificial respiration, the victim's breathing passage must be cleared of all foreign bodies and obstructions. Pull the tongue forward. Remove dentures. If a foreign body is lodged in the throat, try to remove it with the fingers or jar it loose with a sharp blow on the back.

B—*Breathing must be restored.* When the airway is cleared, one rescuer should immediately begin mouth-to-mouth or mouth-to-nose resuscitation exactly as described on p. 107 of this chapter.

C—*Circulation must be restored.* Another person, if present, should immediately begin external cardiac compression in the way and at the rate described on p. 110 of this chapter.

D—*Definitive medical treatment.* Summon medical assistance as quickly as possible. Preferably a third party should do this. The victim *should not be left alone,* nor should the rhythm of either artificial respiration or external cardiac compression be interrupted.

If only one person is present at the scene, the procedure of heart-lung resuscitation is obviously more difficult. It may seem like a great deal for one person to undertake on his own in a time of stress, but it can be done successfully, and often must be. Again, simply remember your first-aid priorities: respiration first and then circulation. In addition, the so-called Rule of Five can be applied. Heart-lung resuscitation must be started within *five* minutes from the beginning of respiratory or cardiac arrest. Clear the victim's airway, then give him *five* good breaths by mouth-to mouth resuscitation at the required rate, once every *five* seconds. Then start external cardiac compression at the required rate, pausing only long enough to give the victim one resuscitating breath after every *five* heart compressions. Try not to interrupt the compression procedure for more than *five* seconds at any one time, and do not stop either procedure as long as there is even the faintest hope for restoring respiration and circulation. If you can help maintain just a flicker of life until medical help arrives, the battle may be all but won. Heart-lung resuscitation has been known to sustain life for as long as an hour with complete recovery.

The Specter of Physical Shock

One of the most baffling, misunderstood and truly dangerous conditions that can silently accompany almost any emergency is the complex of symptoms and physical changes known as *shock.* We are not speaking here of electrical shock, a totally different condition which is discussed later in detail, but of physical shock, the massive, total-body response to injury, pain, hemorrhage, asphyxia, circulatory arrest, exposure to the elements or any other grave physical or emotional trauma to the body—even fear, which can, in itself, actually cause death if it is not effectively combated. Any of these emergencies is serious enough in itself, but in each case the shadowy specter of physical shock inevitably threatens the life of the victim still further, although in much more subtle ways. Indeed, shock alone can kill just as surely as massive hemorrhage, asphyxia or cardiac arrest. Anyone attempting to deal with any emergency must also be prepared to face this additional threat and to take the necessary first-aid measures, limited as they are, to combat it at the same time he is dealing with the more apparent and urgent hazards.

Shock is difficult to describe, and even more difficult for the layman to recognize. In fact, it is only since World War II that medical personnel have learned enough about it to be able to combat it effectively. Before then, no one knows how many millions of lives were lost owing to the complication of shock in both battlefield and civilian injuries. To understand the condition of shock, imagine a prize fighter who has just been struck a foul blow to the solar plexus by a vicious opponent and is curled in on himself, breathless, hurting, jolted and temporarily helpless. He knows the blow was treacherous, and if he can somehow fend off other blows until his breath returns and the pain subsides, he may be able to come back slugging. But if the foul blow was hard enough, or if his opponent connects with other crippling blows, he may not be able to recover in time and the fight will be over.

Shock is precisely such a state of physical drain and imminent collapse caused by some "foul blow" of nature—a serious accident, a painful injury, a fractured leg, a coronary attack, a truly jolting emotional blow, or virtually

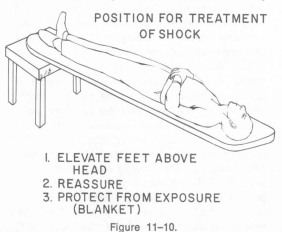

POSITION FOR TREATMENT
OF SHOCK

1. ELEVATE FEET ABOVE
    HEAD
2. REASSURE
3. PROTECT FROM EXPOSURE
    (BLANKET)

Figure 11–10.

any other kind of severe insult to the body. The state of shock that results is the body's "low ebb" in the interval following such an insult before various built-in survival mechanisms can be called upon—a period of time that is necessary for the body to rally or *adapt* to the effects of the trauma. Both the depth of this state of shock and the difficulty the body has in recovering sufficiently to "come back slugging" depend upon the nature of the trauma. It may be mild and short-lived, or it may be exaggerated by hemorrhage, severe pain, or a serious crushing type of injury, but the shock that results is still shock.

How does shock manifest itself? The victim begins to look gray and apprehensive. His pulse is rapid and thready, indicating a diminishment of blood circulation. His mouth feels dry, as if he were spitting cotton, and he finds himself short of breath. Blood vessels in his skin constrict, leading to a sense of chill, compounded by a wave of excessive perspiration. But even as the surface blood vessels constrict, larger and deeper veins tend to dilate, causing a pooling of blood in such areas as the lower back, the thighs, and the intestinal tract. Blood pressure drops, sometimes precipitously, robbing such organ systems as the brain and the kidneys of vitally needed fresh oxygenated blood. Unless the shock is exceptionally severe, the victim remains conscious, but lack of oxygen to the brain may cause him to become confused, muddled, apprehensive and often irrational, while his kidneys, if robbed of sufficient blood supply for a prolonged period, may virtually stop functioning altogether.

The definitive treatment of shock is best handled by a physician in a well-equipped hospital, or in a medically staffed emergency car or ambulance. Details of this treatment are discussed elsewhere. (*See* p. 538.) But obviously any help the victim of an emergency can receive in terms of combating shock, before medical help arrives or before he can reach a hospital, may save his life. Unfortunately, there is relatively little that a rescuer can do on a first-aid basis to combat a profound level of shock, or prevent it from developing, but what little can be done is very important. *The first step is to keep the victim at rest, stretched out on the ground or floor, with pillows, rolled-up bedding or garments, or anything else immediately at hand placed under his buttocks and legs so that his head is lower than the rest of his body.* (Hospitals keep "shock blocks" handy for such emergencies, actual blocks of wood six inches across and a foot high that can quickly be placed under the foot of a patient's bed, thus tilting the lower part of his body up into a suitable "shock position.") *The second most important step is to reassure the victim.* The rescuer should remain as calm, encouraging and reassuring as possible, regardless of how frightened he may actually feel. He must tell the victim that things are under control, that he does not need to worry, that if pain is present it will soon be taken care of, and that help is on the way, even if he is not sure this is entirely true. Remember, the victim's own fear of what is happening to him, his own sense of impending death, and his own emotional response to pain all may work together to create a state of shock far more profound than would otherwise develop. *Finally, keep the victim reasonably warm and protected from the elements, with the use of blankets, overcoats or other warm wraps.* Do not use electric blankets or heaters for artificial warming, however. Never give any injury victim fluids by mouth; he may vomit and then breathe in the vomitus. Solid food should also be withheld if the injury is serious enough to require hospital care. None of these measures can compare with the definitive treatment of shock possible only in a hospital, but they may provide the margin of time and control that will make the difference.

Because first-aid measures to combat shock are so essentially simple, they can easily be applied even when the rescuer is dealing with other life-threatening emergencies. Hemorrhage control, artificial respiration, and artificial circulation must take first, second, and third priorities, of course; but even while these procedures are being followed, the victim can be kept at rest with his feet elevated, he can be reassured, and he can be kept warm. Whatever the circumstances, vigorous treatment of shock must not be forgotten or ignored. And shock can be extremely deceptive. Remember that the victim

may never lose consciousness, yet still be in profound shock. Remember also that you may not be able to tell, from appearances, whether someone is in shock or not, whether he is conscious or unconscious. Do not look for any clues. *You must assume that shock is always present in case of injury or trauma to the body, assume that it is severe and dangerous and work to combat it.* You may well feel you are making a fool of yourself overdoing things. And you may be right. But it is far better to risk looking foolish by doing too much than to risk the victim's life by not doing enough.

Other Cases of Unconsciousness or Sudden Collapse

Many of the gravest emergencies are first discovered when someone who appeared to be functioning quite normally a moment earlier suddenly collapses, or when someone is found lying unconscious, with or without any apparent reason. Any such occurrence must always be considered serious until proven otherwise. Unfortunately, the underlying cause of the collapse or unconsciousness may be impossible to determine, and sometimes apparent "clues" can be dangerously deceptive. But it is not imperative to know for certain what has happened; diagnosis can be left to a doctor when he arrives. It *is* imperative to recognize that a life-threatening situation may exist and that something must be done about it immediately. With unconsciousness or sudden collapse, whatever the cause, the four basic priorities of emergency care still apply: control any hemorrhagic bleeding, restore respiration and circulation if they have been arrested, and treat for shock.

If someone suddenly collapses, or if you discover someone unconscious, the first thing to do is to be sure that he is not actively hemorrhaging from some source that you can see. The second thing to do is check to make sure that he is breathing and that his heart is still beating. If he is hemorrhaging, control the bleeding if you can. If he is not breathing, commence some form of artificial respiration—preferably mouth-to-mouth or mouth-to-nose resuscitation—after making certain that his airway is unobstructed. If circulation has stopped, begin artificial cardiac compression. And in any event, take measures to combat shock.

Always bear in mind that the acute needs of the victim, determined by looking at him critically and checking the items mentioned above, must *always* take precedence over worry about what is causing the trouble, as far as immediate lifesaving emergency care is concerned. But then it is fair to ask: What sorts of things can bring about sudden collapse or unconsciousness? Many things can, some common enough and easily recognizable, others less so. One of the most frequent reasons for a sudden collapse, which usually occurs at the dinner table, is that the victim has inadvertently aspirated a piece of food into his trachea and is literally choking to death. When this happens the victim often starts up from his seat, clutching his throat; his face rapidly turns purple, and he is unable to speak as he struggles to take in a breath of air before he loses consciousness. In some cases the asphyxiating chunk of food can be felt with the fingers in the back of the victim's throat and carefully dislodged. If this does not work, lower the victim's head and raise the rest of his body (preferably with help, if it is available) and strike him sharply on the back. A jarring blow and the aid of gravity may help dislodge the obstruction enough to reach in and remove it with a finger.

Once an aspirated object is removed, the victim will usually resume breathing spontaneously; if he does not, mouth-to-mouth resuscitation may succeed in restoring natural breathing within a very short time. Obviously, artificial respiration must *not* be attempted if the asphyxiating object cannot be removed. When that is the case, the victim is in grave trouble and a doctor must be found immediately. The victim's life may depend upon making a surgical opening—a so-called *tracheostomy*—in his windpipe, below the level of the obstructing object, to provide an airway until it can be surgically removed.

There are a number of cases on record, in fact, in which a layman has performed this emergency operation, using a sharp-pointed knife to pierce a hole in the victim's windpipe in the midline of the throat just above the collar-bone but below the widened cartilage of the larynx (the "Adam's apple") and then thrusting some open tube, such as a pipestem or the cap of a fountain pen with the closed end broken off, through the wound into the windpipe to provide a temporary airway. Few surgeons would recommend this as an acceptable first-aid measure for a layman to undertake. Yet it *has been done successfully* by laymen in cases in which the choking victim was obviously dying and there was no other alternative. Moreover, it has saved lives, whereas there have been few if any cases reported in which such a heroic effort has *cost* the victim his life.

There are, of course, other quite different causes for sudden collapse. The victim may be suffering a *coronary occlusion*—a serious form of "heart attack"—which cannot be helped significantly by any first-aid measures. On the other hand, cardiac arrest with circulatory failure may present much the same sort of collapse, and there may be no way for a person on the scene to distinguish between the two. One can only assume that emergency measures may help, and start them. If the unconscious victim is apparently breathing all right but there is no pulse, cardiac arrest should be suspected. Administer a sharp blow with your fist to the left side of the victim's chest over his heart. If this simple maneuver fails to restore a palpable pulse, begin external cardiac compression immediately and summon medical aid. Even if a blow to the chest *does* restore the heartbeat, a doctor should still be summoned, since cardiac arrest might reoccur at any time.

Other causes of collapse or unconsciousness may have nothing to do with respiratory or circulatory failure. And here again, some of these situations can be dangerously deceptive. For example, an individual suffering from diabetic coma might be found unconscious, breathing stertorously, with a sweetish odor on his breath that can all too easily be mistaken for alcohol. Victims of diabetic coma have been known to die simply because onlookers hurried by, or because the police assumed they were drunk and ignored them, or even took them in to jail for the night to "sober up." Most known diabetics today carry some sort of identification indicating their condition, and an unconscious and apparently intoxicated individual should be checked for such a clue. But in all humanity, *no* unconscious person should be ignored. He may well be in an alcoholic stupor, but even then he could be dying from exposure or some other abuse or illness. Or he could just as well be a victim of diabetes, a heart attack, an overdose of narcotics or some other accident or illness. Notify the police if nothing else. At least then he will not die of total neglect.

There was a time when fainting was considered fashionable. Today it occurs only rarely, and always deserves medical investigation, even though the cause is usually benign. The young acolyte who faints while assisting at a long church service on an empty stomach, or an onlooker who grows faint at the sight of blood at the scene of an accident, can easily be restored if he sits down and places his head between his knees for a few moments. If necessary, make him lie down flat on the floor or ground and raise his feet up a foot above his head, using any convenient block of wood or pile of clothing. The problem will quickly disappear. Other causes for apparent "fainting" may be more serious. A broken blood vessel in the brain ("apoplexy") or a blood clot in a cerebral blood vessel may cause collapse, unconsciousness or *coma,* a more profound form of unconsciousness in which respiration and heartbeat continue but the victim cannot be aroused at all, even by severely painful stimuli. Such individuals may not be in acute danger, from an emergency standpoint, but medical aid should be called or they should be taken to a hospital as quickly as possible.

In addition to these problems, sudden collapse or unconsciousness may result from heat exhaustion, a fainting type of collapse due to excessive exposure to heat, with resulting loss of body salt and water from excess perspiration. It may also be caused by heat stroke or "sunstroke," a more serious condition due to prolonged exposure to excessively high temperatures or the direct rays of the sun, resulting in a sudden dangerous elevation of body temperature. (*See* p. 136.) Finally, collapse or unconsciousness may result from convulsive seizures.

(*See* p. 342.) In any of these situations, a person at the scene of the accident or illness should assess the potential danger to the extent that he is able, begin the appropriate first-aid procedures immediately, and call for medical assistance.

Carbon Monoxide Intoxication

Any sudden accident or illness may involve hemorrhage, cessation of breathing, heart stoppage or shock necessitating use of one or more of the four emergency first-aid priorities. But there are, in addition, certain specific emergencies that may present special problems and require special kinds of emergency aid. Among these are such disasters as carbon monoxide poisoning, a wide variety of chemical poisonings, electrical shock and serious or severe burns.

Most people are well aware of the danger of death from carbon monoxide poisoning, particularly as a result of inhaling the exhaust gases from a running automobile engine. Yet people still go into closed garages to warm up their cars on cold mornings, and some die each year for just that reason. Inhaling exhaust fumes is also a common (and often successful) means of attempting suicide. But other accidental sources of carbon monoxide should not be forgotten: a leaking muffler or exhaust system can allow engine gases to filter into the car from underneath, even when the car is on the road, causing drowsiness and the possibility of a serious accident. Driving in heavy traffic with the windows open can cause similar drowsiness. *Any time exhaust fumes are smelled in the car, a careful check of the exhaust system should be made.* In addition, drivers of station wagons should never drive with the rear window open while all other windows are closed; exhaust gases can be sucked into the rear window by the force of air pressure. Carbon monoxide may also be given off as furnace gas from a badly constructed coal furnace, from a poorly drawing fireplace fire, or from any other fire in which fumes from the partial combustion of wood, coal or oil can collect in a closed space. In recent years, for example, many accidental deaths have resulted from portable gasoline heaters used in poorly ventilated house trailers and hunting cabins.

Carbon monoxide combines more readily than oxygen with the hemoglobin in the red cells of the blood stream. When a sufficient concentration of carbon monoxide piles up in the blood, little or no oxygen is carried to the body tissues and asphyxia and death can follow quickly. Anyone found unconscious in an enclosed place with a fire going, or in an automobile with the engine running either inside or outside a garage, should immediately be suspected of carbon monoxide poisoning. Carry him to the open air as quickly as possible. If breathing has stopped, give artificial respiration, preferably by means of mouth-to-mouth resuscitation, until spontaneous breathing begins. If the victim is without a pulse as well, external cardiac compression may also be necessary to help restore circulation. Finally, shock may also be a complication and must be counteracted. And, of course, medical aid should be sought.

Carbon monoxide poisoning must be considered one of the most serious of all emergencies because it can kill swiftly, without warning. It is, however, one of the most preventable. Its danger is so widely known that only the most foolhardy will risk any situation in which the gas might reasonably be present. Fortunately, quick thinking and quick action on the part of the rescuer can frequently save the victim's life.

Poisoning

Accidental poisoning can be a serious emergency to which small children are especially vulnerable. Their natural curiosity and ignorance of possible danger can lead them to explore pantries, bathroom medicine cabinets and cleaning closets, often sampling various substances as they go. Ironically, most accidental poisonings are not caused by those substances with prominent skull-and-crossbones labels that are usually locked up out of children's reach, or at least should be. By far the greatest majority, particularly among small children, occur from the ingestion of familiar household products often considered "harmless." Number One among them is ordinary aspirin when taken in overdose. Also posing particular danger are tinc-

ture of iodine; petroleum products such as kerosene, gasoline and turpentine; ammonia and other powerful cleaning compounds; bathroom antiseptics such as Lysol, Sani-Flush and Drano, all containing high concentrations of lye (caustic soda or sodium hydroxide); and—perhaps most treacherous of all—various automatic dishwashing compounds, which are capable of inflicting horrible chemical burns of the mouth, esophagus or stomach.

In a case of poisoning, or suspected poisoning, it is imperative to act swiftly, calmly and knowledgeably. The following emergency measures, taken in the order listed, may save a life:

1. Call a doctor, a hospital or the nearest Poison Control Center on the telephone without delay, or have someone else at the scene do it. *It is of the utmost importance to be able to describe, over the phone, exactly what the poison was.* Keep the bottle or box containing any of the substance that is left immediately at hand when you call, so that you can read off the label. (Also take it with you to the hospital later, if that step is required.) With this information, the doctor or hospital or Poison Control Center may be able to give you specific instructions regarding what to do *right then,* thus saving precious time that might be lost trying to track down the nature of the poison later.

2. If a swallowed poison is a *noncaustic substance* such as aspirin, Clorox or sleeping pills, the victim should be induced to vomit by tickling his throat or even using the fingers to stimulate gagging and vomiting. Once the poison has been expelled by vomiting, or even if vomiting cannot be induced, the victim should be encouraged to drink milk, water, a cream soup or even a thin gravy to help dilute whatever poison remains in the stomach. This is one of the few cases in which an accident victim should be given fluids, but you should be especially alert to the danger of his choking or aspirating the vomitus. Unless specifically directed otherwise, this effort to induce vomiting should be made *before* medical help arrives, or *before* or *while* the victim is rushed to the hospital. Although it may work more slowly than mechanical gagging, *syrup of ipecac* is a safe and inexpensive emetic to use to induce vomiting, and a supply should be kept in

every medicine cabinet, especially in homes with small children. One teaspoonful of this pleasant-tasting syrup given every five minutes for three or four doses will usually stimulate vomiting. *Save any material thrown up,* if possible, in some sort of emesis basin or bowl for later laboratory analysis.

3. If the poison is a *caustic substance* such as lye or an automatic dishwashing compound, or an *oily substance* such as kerosene, gasoline or turpentine, *do not induce vomiting;* it could do more harm than good. You can often spot poisoning from such substances by looking for evidence of burns inside the mouth, or sniffing for the odor of a petroleum product on the victim's breath. In such poisonings the best first step is dilution of the poison in the stomach, using the bland fluids mentioned above, unless specifically directed otherwise by a doctor, hospital or Poison Control Center.

4. Finally, a physician should always see a victim of poisoning as promptly as possible. When you first call a doctor, the hospital or the Poison Control Center, you will be advised that an ambulance is on the way, or asked to drive the victim yourself to the nearest hospital emergency room. If for some reason neither is possible, call the police or your local emergency ambulance service.

Today more and more communities have special Poison Control Centers staffed by doctors and nurses around the clock. Keep the telephone number of the nearest center close at hand and call immediately, even if it is long distance, for advice any time you suspect a poisoning. Poison Control Centers have access to information about thousands of potentially poisonous household substances, cross-indexed by brand name as well as generic or chemical name, and can give you quick, responsible advice about antidotes.

In recent years practicing physicians all over the country have joined forces with local pharmacists and Poison Control Center personnel to spread the word to householders everywhere about a few simple measures which can help avert serious poisoning, or provide possibly lifesaving aid when poisoning occurs. These measures include the following:

1. Every home should have a supply of syrup of ipecac *on hand* at all times, to be replaced any time it is used. As a reliable (and usually rapid) means of inducing vomiting, this medicine is unparalleled.

2. Every home should have a can of one of the so-called all-purpose antidotes obtainable inexpensively from any drugstore. The main ingredient in these antidotes is powdered activated charcoal, a substance with a strong capacity to absorb many chemicals, together with a weak buffering alkali such as magnesium hydroxide to help neutralize an acid poison, and a weak buffering acid such as tannic acid to help neutralize any alkali present. This type of antidote is particularly useful in cases of poisoning in which it is best not to induce vomiting. Antidotes are often listed on the labels of many potentially poisonous products, but finding the ingredients and mixing them takes up valuable time. It is far better to have an all-purpose antidote already at hand.

3. Child-resistant containers—that is, bottles with "safety caps" that can be opened only with difficulty or only if you know how—should be used wherever possible for drugs kept in the home. These containers are common now for children's aspirin and *ought* to be used for any other potentially dangerous substances. Poison Control Centers also urge manufacturers to "strip package" all drugs which are not enclosed in child-resistant containers; that is, to seal pills or capsules individually in a plastic strip which is rolled up in a box much as postage stamps are rolled up in a dispenser, to be pulled out and torn off one at a time as needed. Simple as it may seem, this one measure, when used, has noticeably reduced the incidence of accidental poisoning.

Electrical Shock

Perhaps the least familiar of all serious emergencies, yet the most swift and potentially dangerous of all, is the electrical shock that can be caused by an electrical appliance in the home, contact with a live wire or, in the extreme case, being struck by lightning. There is no way to predict the gravity of the injury that may be sustained; the results may be trivial or extremely serious. On one hand, an individual may endure the passage of a high-voltage current through his body and suffer from nothing more serious than deep, blackened burns where the current entered and left. Such burns—on the hands, for example, and at the point of grounding on the soles of the feet if the victim was standing on the ground—can be very severe, but contrary to widespread belief, this is not the major danger of electrical shock. The chief danger is that even a low-voltage current may cause death by respiratory paralysis, cardiac arrest, or both. In fact, the low-voltage currents (110 to 120 volts) commonly found in household circuits are among the most dangerous, since muscle spasm tends to "freeze" the individual in continuing contact with the live wire or appliance, and such low-voltage current, if sustained for more than two or three seconds, may produce a frequently fatal disturbance of the heartbeat known as *ventricular fibrillation*. When electrical shock causes the cessation of breathing or heartbeat, two steps must be taken immediately.

1. *Remove the victim from continuing electrical contact.* If possible, shut off the power at its source or cut the wire with an insulated instrument—an ax with a wooden handle, for example. If this is not possible swiftly, the victim should be forcibly separated from the wire by means of a quick blow or a pull accomplished with some nonconductive material like a wooden pole, a piece of rubber hose, a belt, or a rope. If you must resort to actually touching the victim to separate him from the live contact, you must first protect yourself by wrapping your hands and arms in several thicknesses of dry woolen cloth—a blanket or a thick overcoat. Without this protection you yourself may become involved in the live contact, which can be quite as deadly to you as to the first victim.

2. *Once contact is broken, determine immediately if the victim's breathing or heartbeat has stopped. If one or both have occurred, follow the A-B-C-D procedure for heart-lung resuscitation and summon a doctor as quickly as possible.* Remember, A is for *Airway must be opened;* B is for *Breathing must be restored* using mouth-to-mouth resuscitation; C is for *Circulation must be restored* by means of exter-nal cardiac compression, used either separately or combined with mouth-to-mouth resuscitation; and D is for *Definitive medical treatment.* The victim should be taken to a hospital as quickly as possible. Precautions should also be taken to combat physical shock.

It is, of course, equally important to avoid or prevent situations that might lead to tragic electrical shock. See that your household wiring is in good condition, that circuits are adequate to carry the load demanded of them, and that any electrical appliance which is malfunctioning in any way is either repaired by a competent electrician or discarded. Beware of frayed electric cords, or extension cords and plugs that have to be jiggled to make them work. Avoid overloading *any* single household electrical outlet with multiple sockets. The all too familiar "ball of snakes" surrounding a particularly handy outlet is an open invitation to disaster; it may not only electrocute you, it may also start your house on fire. Teach small children *never* to touch electrical outlets, cords, plugs or appliances, whether they are in good repair or not.

Other precautions also depend upon common sense. *Never* remove the third or grounding wire from such devices as electric drills, saws or hedge clippers. Always use a three-wire extension cord for such appliances if an extension is necessary, and if you cannot plug them into a three-hole outlet, be certain that the grounding wire is well connected to some known ground-source in the house—a steam radiator, for example, or a copper plumbing pipe. *Never* use *any* electrical appliance outdoors when it is raining or when the ground or your clothing is wet. No matter how much you may pride yourself as a handyman, leave all but the most minor electrical repairs to an electrician, particularly repairs involving high-voltage devices such as electric ranges and television sets. If you *must* engage in home electrical repairs, throw *all* the circuit breakers in the house, not just the ones you think affect your repair job, or even better, pull the main switch, before you begin; the legends on household fuse boxes are notoriously inaccurate. And in any questionable situation, remember the wise man's rule of thumb: *When in doubt, don't go near it.*

High-tension wires are less frequently encountered, but are an even greater potential danger. Do not climb an electric pole for any reason, not even to rescue a cat. Call the Fire Department. Never touch or even go near a wire hanging down from an electric pole, and remember that such "recreation" as shooting at insulators on top of power poles is fraught with hazard; people have been electrocuted by flailing high-tension wires severed by a rifle bullet.

What about lightning? The very profusion of bizarre ideas that people have about lightning discharges merely reflects how little we actually know about protecting ourselves from this hazard, and it is small comfort to realize that if you are ever struck by lightning you will probably never know it. If you are caught out in an electrical storm, get indoors if possible; a building will both dissipate and ground a direct strike. If this is not possible, get to the lowest ground in the vicinity and sit or lie down until the storm passes. Trees are excellent natural lightning rods, but the intensely high voltage of a lightning bolt is such that you do not want to be anywhere near anything it is likely to strike if you can help it. Rubber shoes are advisable for golfers, and if you are caught out in a boat, get to land—*any* land—as quickly as possible. Perhaps the safest place of all during a lightning storm is inside an automobile, which is splendidly insulated against grounding a lightning bolt by virtue of its rubber tires and their air cushion. If someone has been struck by lightning, you should follow precisely the A-B-C-D procedure described for the emergency treatment of any kind of electrical shock. However, in this case, there is also the possibility of lightning burns, which require the same special emergency care necessary for any kind of serious burn.

Emergency Care of a Serious Burn

A serious burn represents a unique emergency situation. In a true emergency, one or more of the four first-aid priorities almost invariably apply. Someone skilled in their use can make the difference between life and death; even someone who is awkward or inefficient seldom does the victim any real harm and may, in fact, succeed in providing that extra margin of time and aid that will save a life. But in a burn emergency, the four first-aid priorities do *not* apply. With a severe or extensive burn—the sort which may well ultimately be fatal—death is not likely to occur immediately if the victim has survived the accident. Usually, even in severe burns, there is time to get the victim to a hospital and skilled medical care. But the aftereffects of a serious burn often depend heavily upon what is done when it first occurs, and here *too vigorous or misdirected first aid can indeed do harm, complicate the injury and quite possibly increase the threat to the victim's life.* For this reason, aside from a few simple steps, an inexperienced person dealing with the victim of a serious burn should be very cautious. In this particular case, it is better to risk doing too little than take the possibly greater risk of doing too much.

The seriousness of a burn can easily be underestimated, and in dealing with any but the most obviously minor burn it is always wise to assume the worst. First aid depends to some degree on the nature of the burn—a *chemical burn,* for example, should be washed off immediately with copious amounts of water in order to dilute the substance causing the burn and help prevent further damage. *But the most helpful thing that can be done for any burn, large or small, is immediate immersion or soaking of the burned area in ice water, or in the coldest water available if no ice is at hand.* Complete saturation is necessary. In addition to immediately cooling down hot, scorched tissue, soaking the burned area in ice water will also halt any continuing damage due to smoldering clothing in contact with the surface. After the burned areas have been thoroughly doused, clean blankets or sheets may be wrapped loosely around the victim to keep him warm, combat shock and help prevent contamination of the burn until he can be transported to a hospital or doctor's office. But once ice water has been applied copiously, *leave the burn itself alone. Never* try to strip clothing away from a burned area if it does not loosen and come away quite freely. If the burn beneath the clothing is deep, the cloth is better left adhered until the physician can remove and debride it, probably with the aid of an anesthetic. *Never* smear grease, butter, oil, burn ointments or any other medication on a burn more serious than a mild sunburn or a scorched finger. Contrary to popular notions, such greasy or oily applications do no good whatever, and may make the injury many times more difficult for the doctor to treat later. In addition, various chemicals contained in many burn ointments can all too easily reach toxic levels within the body due to absorption and may even endanger life.

It may seem downright sadistic to soak a burn victim with ice water, but recent experience in burn treatment has shown that this procedure actually limits the severity of burns and increases chances of survival very materially. All other considerations—even first-aid treatment of shock—take second place. Keep the burn victim at rest, his head lower than his feet. If he expresses thirst, moisten his tongue with cool water but give nothing to drink. Anesthesia may be necessary for the treatment of his burn once he reaches the hospital, and if he has any significant quantity of fluid in his stomach, the surgeon may have to postpone treatment for several hours or else risk subjecting the burn victim to the additional threat of vomiting and aspirating the emesis. All too often the death of a burn victim results from some additional physical insult, such as aspiration pneumonia, rather than from the burn itself. As for the problem of pain, protecting the burned area from movement of air around it will help reduce pain; so will the administration of aspirin in about the same amount you would use for a serious headache, swallowed if possible with only a small amount of water. Anything else may interfere with definitive hospital treatment later.

As soon as these simple steps have been taken, get the victim to a hospital as quickly as possible, if he can be moved, preferably calling ahead to alert the doctor. If he cannot be moved, call for medical help and an ambulance. The victim of a serious burn has a long and agonizing road to recovery lying ahead of him, and every minute saved in getting him started on active treatment may reduce that recovery time by weeks.

Definitive Hospital Treatment of Serious Emergencies

All first-aid measures used to combat serious emergencies are predicated on the assumption that medical help is on the way or that, if the victim can survive long enough to reach a hospital, the definitive treatment of the emergency will be taken care of there. In recent years, giant strides have been made in the science of medicine that enable doctors in a hospital setting to deal effectively with these emergency situations. There is nothing magic about what they do, but definitive hospital treatment is naturally far more successful than first aid in establishing control of an emergency simply because of the availability of trained personnel and the most modern medical equipment. Today, in fact, trained personnel and portable medical apparatus are usually part of an emergency ambulance service. Thus definitive treatment can often begin at the scene of the accident or while the victim is being transported to the hospital. Once he reaches the hospital he is usually taken to a special emergency station, staffed on a 24-hour basis by medical personnel, with all the necessary equipment at hand, ready to swing into immediate action.

Hospital emergency care follows exactly the same order of priorities as first-aid care, except that with ample personnel and equipment several procedures may be undertaken simultaneously. But even the most highly trained medical personnel will resort to first-aid measures in an emergency until their equipment can be brought in. Doctors have no reluctance about using mouth-to-mouth resuscitation, for instance, and nurses will slap chests to try to restore heartbeat or commence external cardiac compression.

But as soon as more definitive means of dealing with an emergency are at hand, they will be put to work. If the victim is still hemorrhaging, for example, it can be definitively controlled with pressure, tourniquets, surgical clamps or ligatures to tie off the bleeding vessels. Simultaneously a hypodermic needle will be inserted in a vein, by means of a surgical incision if necessary, so that intravenous fluids can instantly be administered to replace lost blood or support falling blood pressure. Medication can be given by the same intravenous route if swift effect is desirable. In cases of respiratory failure the victim can be resuscitated and his breathing sustained by using one of a variety of *positive pressure breathing devices,* machines which are triggered by the force of the victim's exhalation to supply oxygen-enriched air under pressure sufficient to inflate his lungs. If the victim's airway is obstructed, a tracheostomy can be performed and a breathing tube inserted directly into the windpipe below the obstructing foreign body until it can be removed. If the obstruction is still lower, a long, slender lighted instrument called a *bronchoscope* can be inserted into the trachea or even into the major bronchi, and the obstructing item can be located and withdrawn. When it is necessary to perform major surgery because of an urgent emergency, an anesthesiologist can maintain the victim's respirations with the use of an oxygen bag and an anesthesia machine until such time as he can resume breathing normally again.

Hospital emergency rooms are also equipped to deal with circulatory failure and dangerous heart rhythm abnormalities such as *ventricular fibrillation,* the major cause of cardiac arrest. Most hospitals now have some form of electrical instrument known as a *defibrillator* (sometimes called a "shock box") with which a brief, low-voltage electrical shock can be administered in order to stop the abnormal twitching or "fibrillating" of the heart muscle and trigger the resumption of a normal rhythmic heartbeat. In critical emergencies, open chest surgery can be performed to provide for direct cardiac massage by the surgeon to restore circulation. And in many medical centers, the use of an operating room heart-lung machine can by-pass both normal respiratory and cardiac functions of the patient for a period of time—at least long enough to intervene surgically when necessary.

Hospitals also have facilities for the immediate administration of plasma-expanding medications intravenously, or they may draw on a supply of stored freeze-dried plasma to use in fighting blood loss or shock until whole blood can be cross-matched and administered. A wide variety of "pressor" medications to support fall-ing blood pressure are available as well, and laboratory facilities help the physician judge such things as dehydration of the patient, excessive concentration or dilution of the whole blood, and the balance of dissolved serum electrolytes—sodium ion, chloride ion, potassium ion, etc.—so that the proper balance can be restored if it has been upset.

In poisoning cases hospitals have equipment such as stomach pumps which can be used to empty the victim's stomach thoroughly, massively dilute any residual poison with water and then pump it out with a minimum risk of the victim's aspirating stomach contents into his lungs. Poisoning with caustic substances may require extremely watchful and continuing medical care because of the risk of perforation of the stomach or the esophagus, or such severe scarring of the esophagus that the injury must be treated by prolonged artificial dilatation of the scarred area or even surgical intervention. In cases in which severe burn damage has been done to the gastrointestinal tract, it is even possible to make a direct surgical opening into the stomach (a so-called gastrostomy), by-passing the damaged esophagus altogether until the healing process can begin.

Definitive hospital care of severe burn cases is far too complex for detailed discussion here, yet it is one of the greatest triumphs of modern hospital medicine. A burn involving 10 percent or more of the surface area of the body is considered a gravely serious burn, and as recently as 30 years ago a second-degree (blistering) burn involving as much as one-third of the surface area of the body was considered almost certain to be fatal. Today, thanks to multitudes of new drugs, including the antibiotics, and vastly improved hospital techniques, victims with as much as 90 percent of the surface area of their bodies involved in the burn have, on occasion, been saved. This is still most uncommon; even the 70 percent burn victim has only the slenderest of chances, but the record is infinitely better today than a few decades ago.

Any burn, however, can be painful, destroy tissue and require long and careful treatment. The pattern of recovery is often set in the first few hours or days of hospital care. The main dangers to the patient at this time are: (1) the threat of shock, which must be combated vigorously; (2) the threat of fluid and protein loss due to the steady "weeping" of serum from the denuded burn areas, with the additional threat of kidney failure if protein and fluids cannot be replaced and circulation sustained; (3) infection of the burn, which must be combated with the use of antibiotics and meticulous "operating room" sterile techniques, together with a vigilant alertness for the development of tetanus from a contaminated burn wound; and (4) the general toxicity of the body as a result of the tissue destruction occasioned by the burn. All of these dangers are faced and combated as quickly as possible by an emergency medical team much like the team that comes together in cases of diabetic coma. Debridement of dead skin and tissue together with adherent clothing must be performed swiftly and completely by a surgeon. Dressings must be applied, and then removed and reapplied at regular intervals, which often requires prolonged soaks of the burn victim in a warm bath prior to redressing, and administration of general anesthesia while it is being done.

As the patient passes the crisis and moves at least temporarily out of danger from immediate post-burn threats, the long process of taking skin grafts from unburned areas to cover denuded areas must begin, a procedure that may consume months before it is completed. And even when the patient is finally restored to physical wholeness, still more time may pass before he recovers from the staggering emotional trauma of living in pain and fear for a period of weeks, months or even years. Fortunately burn treatment techniques are improving constantly, and new forms of dressings are being developed to eliminate much of the pain of dressing changes, so that the outlook for ultimate survival of severe burn cases is becoming better year by year.

Emergency situations, whatever their cause, occur all too frequently, and almost invariably some time is lost before the victim can receive definitive medical treatment. For that reason, it is essential to have a working knowledge of the first-aid measures that can be used to combat them: how to stop hemorrhagic bleeding by the direct pressure method; how to apply artificial respiration by mouth-to-mouth resuscitation, how to restore circulation by external cardiac compression, or the use of both methods in heart-lung resuscitation; how to combat physical shock; and the immediate care of an unconscious victim or a person who suddenly collapses, as well as victims of carbon monoxide or other forms of poison, electrical shock and serious burns. It is heartening to know that such first-aid measures, taken during the first few minutes of an emergency, can save lives. But it is even more heartening to know that in most cases, in most parts of our country, medical help is only a telephone call away. Often a hospital, a private ambulance or a police department emergency unit can arrive at the scene within a matter of minutes with personnel trained to deal with every emergency. The recent development of helicopter rescue services in population centers all over the country has further increased the speed with which emergency victims can be taken to well-equipped hospitals for care, and has made speedy help available even in the most remote or inaccessible areas. These emergency services can always be improved and expanded, however, and individuals, as well as civic and professional groups, should be informed about the services available and press for the very best emergency facilities in their community.

Knowing whom to call for help in your community is, of course, vitally important. In many cases your own family doctor is your best and most reliable port in a storm; he can swiftly mobilize the help that is needed whether he himself is able to come or not. In addition, you should have readily at hand, not only by your telephone at home but also in your wallet or purse, the phone number of the nearest hospital emergency service and of a reliable local ambulance service. The local police, the local sheriff's office, the local fire department and the nearest state police or highway patrol office—even the Mountain Rescue Services established in many of our western states—are prepared in almost any locality either to come to your aid themselves or to mobilize medical help for you. If phone numbers are not immediately available, dial "O" for operator and ask her to contact help for you—but make sure to give her *your name, the address* and *phone number,* and then if possible have someone stand by the phone for contact. Many communities today have instituted the "Dial 911" emergency call system to speed help on its way; the front pages of your telephone book will indicate whether you should dial 911 or the operator. If you cannot leave the victim long enough to telephone, or if yourself are the victim, send an onlooker or a passerby to get help for you. If you live alone, particularly in the case of an elderly person, make arrangements to have friends telephone or look in on you at regular intervals; and if they live alone, do the same thing for them. Serious emergencies are everybody's business—each of us knows that he may one day need help himself—and in spite of a few tragic and widely publicized incidents involving fear-induced public indifference to an emergency, the fact remains that very few people will fail, when the chips are down, to come to the aid of a fellow human being when he is in desperate trouble.

12

Minor Injuries and Other Emergencies

In addition to the extreme emergencies that pose an immediate threat to life, we encounter other accidents and injuries almost daily, some of minor importance, some of major importance, but all capable of causing varying degrees of discomfort or concern. Many of these "lesser" emergencies arise from the simple fact that we are highly mobile beings but, unlike many other creatures, relatively awkward and unprotected. We live in a world of sharp-pointed objects and blunt, unyielding surfaces, and our bodies can easily be cut, punctured or crushed. As warm-blooded creatures we are also vulnerable to extremes of heat and cold, and compared to many animals, we are heavy, clumsy and extremely susceptible to injuries like fractured bones which occur only rarely in other species. We have no natural predators (except other men), but occasionally we are subject to attack from stinging or biting insects, irritable dogs and poisonous snakes. There are plant substances, too, that can cause us pain and discomfort. And finally, there are the hazards devised and often inflicted by the hand of man himself—gunshot and stab wounds, for example, or radiation poisoning, to name but a few.

Man's best protection against injuries and accidents of this sort is his intelligence—the intelligence to avoid them in the first place if possible, and the intelligence to know how to handle them if and when they do occur. Minor injuries and lesser emergencies differ chiefly from major injuries and more serious emergencies in that they do not ordinarily pose the threat of imminent death; there is usually sufficient time to use common sense and the proper first-aid procedures to counteract them. But it is well to remember that even a minor injury can lead to serious consequences if it is ignored or treated improperly.

Lacerations, Abrasions and Contusions

Any break in the normal integrity of the skin, or any crushing injury to the skin and underlying soft tissue, carries two main hazards: the threat of introducing infection into the body and the threat of later disfigurement or even interference with function as a result of improper healing and scarring. Ordinarily we do not worry too much about a minor *laceration* (or cut), a small *abrasion* (a scraping wound which scratches, scrapes or denudes a small area of skin), or a minor *contusion* (a crushing blow which may not break the skin but squashes it and the underlying connective tissue). For such minor injuries we need do little other than wash the wound with soap and water, press it with a sterile dressing until any minor degree of bleeding stops, and then cover it with a small gauze dressing to keep it clean until it heals. But obviously all such injuries are not minor. The victim of an automobile accident, for example, may have a deep laceration of the scalp and forehead from one side of his head to the other down to the bone. In such a case, the laceration must be painstakingly sutured by the surgeon to bring the edges of the wound together in correct approximation and to avoid any more scarring in the healing process than is necessary. The motorcyclist who "spins out" and slides across fifty yards of gravel road on his face and shoulder may have abrasions with so much gravel, dirt and other foreign bodies ground deeply into the skin and subcutaneous tissue that it takes a doctor ten hours in the operating room to do an admittedly imperfect job of cleaning the wound. And a crushing injury of the thighs can cause not only contusion of the skin and subcutaneous tissue but deep damage to muscle as well. There is also the real threat of such dangerous complications as a kidney shutdown when breakdown products from the torn muscle are released into the blood stream and obstruct normal kidney function.

Obviously major injuries of this sort require immediate medical attention and hospital care. In fact, almost all cuts, scrapes and bruises, with the exception of obviously minor or superficial ones, should be brought to a doctor's attention and his orders followed. He will close lacerations, if necessary, clean and dress abrasions, and check the extent of damage caused by contusions. He may also prescribe antibiotics to combat infection. There is almost invariably swelling and congestion of these injuries, and during the first 12 to 24 hours following the accident, the doctor may recommend that the injured area be treated with an ice bag or simply crushed ice wrapped in a towel to minimize swelling. Thereafter healing can be speeded by hot water soaks (if the skin has not been broken) or the application of dry heat by means of a heating pad for 20 minutes four times a day. In particular, a doctor should see anyone with the following kinds of lacerations or abrasions:

Lacerations of the Fingers, Hand or Wrist. The tendons which permit extension (pointing out straight) or flexion (bending double) of the fingers can very easily be injured or even severed in what might appear to be a minor laceration of a finger. This kind of injury requires immediate care, since the movement of a finger may be saved by prompt repair of the severed tendon. The same is true for injuries of the hand, through which these tendons pass, or of the wrist, which has a fibrous tunnel through which

extensor and flexor tendons to all of the fingers pass after leaving the muscles of the upper arm. We depend too heavily upon the fine and unhandicapped use of our remarkably sensitive hands and fingers to risk any long-term disruption of function because of an overlooked tendon injury or improper treatment of a hand or wrist wound.

Lacerations of the Face. Almost any laceration of the skin or soft tissue of the face is going to involve some of the facial muscles as well— the thin layer of muscles responsible for the incredibly subtle nuances of facial expression which we use to communicate with others, whether we realize it or not. Thus, quite aside from the cosmetic concern, any laceration of the face should be treated as soon as possible by a physician. In the case of serious facial lacerations, a plastic and reconstructive surgeon may also be called in consultation.

Lacerations of the Scalp. Because all parts of the scalp are abundantly supplied with blood vessels, even a small, superficial scalp laceration may cause bleeding of hemorrhagic proportions. In addition, because the scalp and the hair itself are normally covered with a wide variety of bacteria, scalp wounds tend to be particularly vulnerable to contamination and require special attention to cleansing and debridement before the laceration is closed in order to avoid infection. Bleeding from a scalp wound is relatively easy to control simply by applying firm pressure with a gauze pad or other clean cloth directly over the wound, but once the bleeding is under control the victim should be brought to a doctor as quickly as possible for more definitive treatment.

Lacerations of the Lip. Even the most minor scar or functional defect in the lips is usually quite noticeable. Surgical repair of any laceration about the mouth or on the lips is therefore very important and should not be delayed, ideally, more than an hour or so after the injury.

Penetrating Chest Wounds. Any wound penetrating the chest from the outside, whether inflicted as a stab or gunshot wound, acquired by falling on a sharply pointed object, or even occurring as a result of an open fracture of a rib, poses a particular threat. (*See* p. 138 *and* p.

297.) Such a wound may allow air to enter the chest cavity and cause a lung to collapse, thus severely impairing respiration even if the wound is comparatively small. Any wound that appears to penetrate the chest, whether accompanied by respiratory distress or not, should be sealed off airtight with adhesive tape, or with a compress held against the wound by hand, and the victim then taken to the nearest doctor or hospital for careful medical examination and whatever definitive treatment is required.

Puncture Wounds. Wounds such as those caused by stepping on a nail, being jabbed by a dry branch or deeply pricked with a thorn or a large splinter, should at least be called to a doctor's attention even if no repair of the injury is required. As is commonly known, this kind of injury can often introduce tetanus bacilli into the body and permit them to grow under sealed "oxygen-free" conditions, thus leading to serious, and possibly fatal, infection. (*See* p. 219.) During recent years it has been demonstrated repeatedly that immunization against tetanus, once completed either in childhood (as is usual now) or later in adolescence, has a surprisingly long period of effectiveness. Ordinarily no booster to a complete tetanus immunization series is needed for five or more years after the original vaccination; and even twenty years later, a booster shot will quickly bring immunity up to the high level which immediately follows the initial series. Thus, the administration of tetanus toxoid boosters following puncture wounds or dirty lacerations may well be overdone. Indeed, it is often the patient or the patient's parents who insist upon the tetanus booster, and the doctor complies even though he is perfectly aware that it is not really necessary. In any case, he should examine a potentially serious puncture wound or contaminated laceration, and then he will decide whether or not a tetanus booster is called for. But certainly it is not necessary to give one booster after another to a child who may turn up with a new puncture wound every few weeks.

One of the most common of all puncture wounds occurs when fishermen, both young and old, embed fish hooks in their skin. If the hook is barbed, it may not be possible to withdraw it without causing further damage. However, the barbed point of the hook can usually be pushed forward and upward, following the natural curve of the hook, until it comes through the surface of the skin a short distance from where it went in. Then the barb can be clipped off with a wire cutter and the shank of the hook withdrawn the way it entered. The victim should call a doctor within a day or so about such an injury if he has not had a tetanus booster for more than a year.

Commonsense care of these surface wounds to keep them clean usually ensures healing without infection. Swelling, redness and increasing pain about such a wound, sometimes accompanied by a spiking general fever, are indications that infection has started, and a doctor should be consulted so that antibiotic drugs can be prescribed. Occasionally an infected laceration that has been closed may have to be reopened in order to drain the infection. More commonly an overlooked foreign body embedded in the wound —perhaps nothing more than a virtually invisible shred of clothing or a tiny bit of wood—will be the source of the infection. Often, if the circumstances seem to warrant, a physician may order an X-ray examination of an injured limb before treating a laceration to make certain that there is no radio-opaque foreign body that can be discerned, and no fracture. If a fracture is present, the risk of possible bone infection is great enough that the physician may wish to use antibiotic drugs prophylactically to prevent osteomyelitis, as well as to close the wound.

Usually infections in wounds will tend to drain through the broken surface of the skin. If drainage does not occur that way, an abscess may form deep in the tissue. Abscesses can generally be detected, surgically opened and drained without difficulty. But some of them can be particularly troublesome. Bacteria introduced into the tissue of the tip of the finger by means of a minor laceration, for example, can develop into an exquisitely tender and painful abscess of the fingertip, known as a *felon*, which requires a surgeon's attention to open and drain. (*See* p. 207.) Infection in the nailbed, similarly, is particularly troublesome because it may damage the plate of cells from which the fingernails grow and cause permanent abnormalities of nail growth.

First-aid care of minor lacerations or abrasions is first directed to control of bleeding, then cleaning the wound of as much dirt and debris as possible, and finally treatment for shock if it occurs. As with major wounds, bleeding control is best accomplished by applying pressure over the wound, but sometimes a minor laceration can most easily be cleaned by *permitting* bleeding briefly while the injured part is held under running water. Minor lacerations can often be held in good position after cleaning by using a Band-Aid or "butterfly bandage" to push the edges of the wound together.

TREATMENT OF LACERATIONS

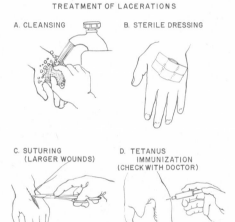

A. CLEANSING   B. STERILE DRESSING

C. SUTURING (LARGER WOUNDS)   D. TETANUS IMMUNIZATION (CHECK WITH DOCTOR)

Figure 12–1.

If the laceration is serious, or if there is the possibility of infection or other complications, a doctor should be consulted. But most minor cuts and scrapes can be handled by the accident victim, or the parent of an injured child, without much difficulty or unnecessary alarm. In the case of a child, soap and water, sympathy and a prominent bandage are usually the only first-aid measures required. After that, the wound and the bandage should, of course, be kept as clean as possible to prevent infection and facilitate healing.

Contusions. In many injuries the skin may not be broken, yet crushing damage is done to the underlying connective tissue or muscle, with tearing of small blood vessels and resulting bleeding into the injured tissue. Such injuries, known as contusions, may be so minor that nothing need be done; the injured area remains sore and sensitive for a day or two, and a bruise appears under the skin as an *ecchymosis* or "black-and-blue mark" which persists for a few days and then gradually fades. When larger blood vessels are torn, there may be marked pain and swelling in the injured tissue, with more persistent and extensive bruising. Extravasation of blood in the tissue can be slowed, following such an injury, by applying an ice pack to the injured area and preventing motion that may stimulate further bleeding. Once any active bleeding has stopped and the injured area has been rested for 24 hours, application of hot moist packs, or soaking in a hot tub for 20 minutes at a time three or four times a day, will speed the breakdown and absorption of the extravasated blood. It is well, however, to have a doctor check any but the more minor contusions, because occasionally such injuries can result in quite extensive bleeding deep into the body of a muscle, with the blood forming a large clotted mass or *hematoma* in the injured tissue. In such an event, the doctor may think it advisable to incise the injured area with the aid of an anesthetic and remove the hematoma to permit speedy healing. Even when surgical incision and drainage are not necessary, the blood that leaks into the tissues from a severe contusion may spread through the tissues along natural planes of cleavage and appear as ecchymoses in areas quite distant from the injury. A contusion of the calf, for example, may lead to the appearance of black-and-blue marks around the heel or at the side of the foot several days later, and it is not at all uncommon, when a blow to the cheek has caused a "black eye," for the skin beneath the *opposite* eye to turn purple a day or more after the injury. Although this in itself is no cause for alarm, extensive ecchymosis is often a reflection of the severity of the injury, and a doctor should be consulted to make sure no potentially long-term damage has been done.

Fractured Bones

Although a fracture may not constitute a life-threatening emergency, it does in most cases represent a more serious injury to the body than a minor laceration, abrasion or contusion, and should always be examined and treated by a physician in order to ensure optimum healing of the broken bone in the briefest possible time. The definitive medical treatment of fractures is discussed in detail elsewhere (see p. 300), but in many cases the ultimate overall success of treatment can depend heavily on the first-aid measures used by a layman on the scene at the time of the injury. Fractures occur commonly enough that everyone should know how to tell—or at least suspect—when a bone has been broken, what special dangers certain kinds of fractures can present, and what basic first-aid measures should be taken when a fracture is encountered.

Identifying a Fracture. Most fractures occur as a result of a fall, a blow, or a sudden and unexpected twisting motion of the body, and the following cardinal signs are usually present when a bone is broken:

1. Severe or persisting pain in an injured area, usually aggravated by motion.

2. Abrupt, dramatic swelling of a painful area of injury.

3. Limitation of motion of a body part, usually because attempted motion causes a sharp increase in pain.

4. Shortening or distortion of a limb, or some other change in the normal contour of an injured area.

Other less serious injuries may also produce such signs, but if one or more is present it is necessary to assume the worst and apply first aid as if a bone were broken until X-ray examination proves otherwise.

Special Hazards of Fractures. Certain kinds of fractures present special dangers which must be recognized and guarded against by anyone applying first-aid treatment:

Skull Fractures. Any blow severe enough to cause a fracture of the hard vault of the skull is also severe enough to cause either injury to the brain or intracranial hemorrhage, or both. If a portion of fractured skull is actually pressed in against the brain, there is even greater probability of brain damage. Further, fractures involving bones of the face, the nose, the rim of the eye or the jaw may lead to permanent distortion of the facial features unless they are expertly treated. First-aid measures should be confined to controlling external bleeding by means of gentle pressure over any bleeding area, and supporting the victim's breathing by means of mouth-to-mouth resuscitation if necessary. Then transport him to the nearest hospital emergency room or summon an ambulance. Remember that the victim of a head injury may be dazed or confused; someone should remain with him at all times to keep him at rest and reassured until medical help is obtained.

Neck and Spine Fractures. The overriding danger of a fractured vertebra is that sharp bone fragments may pierce or cut the spinal cord, leading to irreparable nervous system damage and possible permanent paralysis. (See p. 298.) Whenever a fracture of the neck or spine is even a remote possibility, the victim must be kept reclining and completely motionless until medical help is obtained. If he *must* be moved, he should be lifted flat (*not* rolled) by two or more people working together and transferred to a stretcher, a flat door or some other rigid support so that there is no motion of the injured area.

Fractures of the Extremities. The broken fragments of the long, hard bones of the arms or legs can be sharp as knives and can easily sever arteries, veins or nerve trunks, or lacerate muscle tissue, in the region of the fracture. Thus fractures of the upper or lower arms or legs must be *immobilized* insofar as possible by means of splinting (see below) before the victim is transported to a hospital or doctor's office. When a wrist, elbow, knee or ankle joint is involved in the injury, the entire affected limb should be splinted to prevent motion of the joint as well as any bone fragments that may be present.

Fractured Ribs. The major hazard of rib fractures is that a sharp bone fragment may puncture and even collapse a lung as a result of breathing motion, causing severe respiratory distress. Pain can often be controlled and motion of a broken rib minimized by applying a snug cloth binder around the lower half of the chest, with the binder holding the upper arm on the injured side firmly against the chest until the victim can be moved to a hospital or doctor's office. As long as the ribs on one side are uninjured, the victim will usually get enough air with his own respirations, but if ribs are fractured on both sides, the blue-gray skin color of cyanosis due to oxygen lack may appear, and respiration must then be supported by mouth-to-mouth resuscitation until medical help can be summoned.

Fractured Pelvis. The kind of massive trauma necessary to fracture the heavy bones of the pelvis can also cause serious internal injury as well. In particular, the urethra may be severed by displacement of bone fragments. Thus anyone suspected of a possible fracture of the pelvis should be kept reclining until he can be lifted flat onto a stretcher or other firm support for transportation to a hospital. Any evidence of bleeding from the urethra, or of blood in the urine, should be reported to a doctor as soon as medical help is obtained.

First Aid for Fractures. Bearing in mind that certain kinds of fractures require particular attention to avoid special hazards, the first-aid treatment of any fracture is largely a matter of common sense. First, of course, the four first-aid priorities must be undertaken where necessary: control of external hemorrhage, support of respiration, maintenance of circulation, and steps to combat the physical shock which almost invariably accompanies a fracture injury. Next, certain basic first-aid measures and precautions applicable to any suspected fracture should be undertaken:

1. Avoid use of the injured region unless it is absolutely essential. There is no way, of course, to avoid "use" of a fractured rib; the best that can be done is to strap or splint the injured side of the chest in order to minimize the movement of the fractured rib during respiration. In general, however, the victim of a fracture or even a suspected fracture should be kept immobile until medical help arrives. If he must be moved, it should be done in such a way that the fractured

limb or the area of injury remains as immobile as possible.

2. Whenever possible, use a soft bulky material for supportive splinting to prevent movement and the possibility of further injury from broken

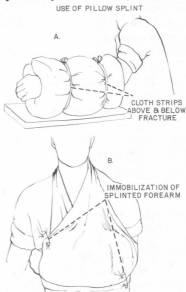

USE OF PILLOW SPLINT

A.

CLOTH STRIPS
ABOVE & BELOW
FRACTURE

B.

IMMOBILIZATION OF
SPLINTED FOREARM

Figure 12–2.

bones or bone fragments. A folded pillow, for example, is excellent for splinting a fractured arm or leg. Well-padded splints of wood may also be used, but in any case the ligatures used to tie the splint in place should not be so tight that they impair circulation.

3. Do not try to "reduce" a fracture (return the bones to their normal position) by means of traction or traction devices unless you are fully prepared to continue applying that traction continuously until the victim reaches a hospital for treatment. Traction on a fractured limb can be exquisitely painful, and if a major blood vessel in the area has escaped injury from the original fracture, it may well be severed by sharp bone fragments if traction is applied and then later released. In most cases immobilizing the victim or simple splinting of the fractured limb and then rapid conveyance of the victim to a doctor or a hospital is the best way to deal with a fracture.

4. *Never* attempt to reduce or set an open fracture; that is, a fracture in which a fragment of bone has penetrated the overlying skin. It will merely compound the doctor's problem in treating the fracture later by possibly introducing bacteria from the skin surface deep into the wound, with the obvious risk of infection. Any significant amount of bleeding should be controlled and the wound covered closely with a clean cloth or sterile bandage.

5. Take protective measures against shock. The victim should be reassured and kept quiet and warm with his head slightly lower than the rest of his body. Mild analgesics such as aspirin and *small* amounts of hot coffee or tea can be given if the victim is conscious.

Dislocations, Sprains and Strains

In addition to fractures, a number of other injuries to bone, joint or muscle may arise from falls, blows, and excessive use or sudden wrenching of various parts of the body. A *dislocation* occurs when the bones of an articulating joint are forced out of the normal joint position, usually with an associated tear or rupture of the joint capsule. (*See* p. 303.) In a *sprain*, the bones of a joint are not dislodged, but the injury tears supporting ligaments and fibrous connective tissue adjacent to the joint. (*See* p. 304.) A *strain* is an injury involving excessive stretching or tearing of muscle tissue. (*See* p. 283.) All three kinds of injury are usually accompanied by pain, swelling and bleeding into the injured area, and X-ray examination may be necessary to be sure that no fracture is involved. If medical help is not immediately available, first-aid measures must be taken to prevent additional harm until a doctor's examination is possible.

Dislocations. Virtually any articulating joint in the body may be dislocated: the shoulder, the hip, the ankle, the wrist, the elbow, one or more joints of a finger, the jaw—even the spine can be dislocated as a result of a massive trauma such as an automobile accident. Dislocations can usually be recognized by marked distortion of the normal body contours in the injured area, by severe pain and swelling of the joint area and by the inability of the victim to use the joint

normally. Frequently dislocations are complicated by fractures of the dislocated bone ends, and in many cases the blood supply to the joint can be severely impaired, or adjacent nerve trunks can be damaged by stretching or tearing unless the dislocated bones are quickly and expertly *reduced* or returned to their normal anatomical position. Although many older first-aid manuals contain instructions for reducing dislocations, most authorities today agree that inexpert attempts to manipulate a dislocated joint are likely to fail, and may well do more harm than good. First-aid treatment should be confined to immobilizing the injured joint with padded splints or cloth bindings so that no movement of the joint is possible, keeping the victim warm and at rest to help combat shock, and then transporting him to medical aid as quickly as possible. Time is of the essence, however, because the longer the joint remains dislocated, the greater the risk of permanent damage to nerves or dangerous impairment of circulation to the joint. Once the physician has reduced a dislocation he will immobilize the joint with a plaster cast or with firm cloth bindings to allow the torn joint capsule to heal before normal use of the joint is resumed.

Sprains. Hard-working, weight-bearing joints are the ones most commonly sprained, particularly the ankle, the knee, the wrist or the thumb. Sprains, by definition, are less serious injuries than fractures or dislocations; bone is not fractured and the normal functioning position of the joint has not been disrupted. Despite this, ligaments supporting the injured joint have been torn, so that the joint is rendered weak and unstable until healing occurs. In addition, there may be bleeding into the joint or adjacent soft tissue, swelling of the tissues surrounding the joint and considerable pain. First-aid treatment is first directed to supporting and immobilizing the injured joint and to minimizing soft tissue swelling. This is most safely accomplished by the use of adhesive plaster or an elastic roller bandage to provide both pressure and supportive protection to the joint. *Care must be taken not to cut off circulation by tight circular strapping around a limb.* This can best be avoided by using a figure-of-eight type of strapping above and below the injured joint in the case of a knee, wrist or thumb sprain, or a basket-weave strapping to support an ankle. (*See* Fig. 12–3.) Ice packs applied to the joint during the first 24

STRAPPING SPRAINED JOINTS
(ELASTIC OR ADHESIVE BANDAGE)

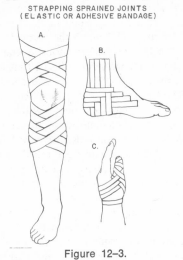

Figure 12–3.

hours following the injury will help control swelling. Thereafter hot soaks or hot moist packs applied for 20 minutes at a time three or four times a day will promote healing. The joint should be rested until the acute pain subsides; then motion and weight-bearing can be cautiously resumed *with the strapping still in place*. A doctor should be consulted and X-rays taken to rule out possible fractures in the case of any severe sprain, or even in the case of an apparently minor sprain if pain and swelling do not subside within two or three days.

Strains. Muscle strains are perhaps the most familiar of all injuries involving the musculoskeletal system. Sometimes acute strains occur because of sudden pulling or muscle-wrenching accidents, but more commonly they result from plain overuse of muscles that are out of condition, leading to a form of muscle stiffness and soreness known as *overuse myositis*. (*See* p. 284.) Acute muscle strains can be recognized by the sudden onset of pain in the injured muscle, often accompanied by cramping—the typical "charley horse"—and followed by such familiar inflammatory symptoms as swelling and hotness in the injured area. Often a bruise will appear in

the vicinity as the pain subsides, indicating that small blood vessels within the muscle, or muscle fibers themselves, have been torn. First-aid treatment of an acute muscle strain includes application of an ice pack to the injured area during the first few hours after the injury to slow down bleeding and counteract swelling, together with rest of the affected muscles. After 24 hours hot moist packs or hot tub soaks will reduce pain markedly and promote healing. Aspirin in adult dosages of 10 grains every four to six hours is usually sufficient to relieve pain. A doctor should be consulted if the pain and swelling fail to subside within 24 to 48 hours, or if there is any suspicion that an associated sprain or fracture may be present.

Muscle strain resulting from overuse of unconditioned muscles is manifested more slowly than acute muscle strain, with the pain and soreness of overuse myositis usually first appearing several hours after the injury. When pain and stiffness are severe, the same first-aid measures recommended for acute muscle strain may be necessary, but in less severe cases a hot tub soak followed by gentle exercise of the stiff, sore muscles will help relieve the condition. Again, aspirin is helpful in relieving the pain; in fact, if overuse can be anticipated in advance, the amount and duration of the discomfort can be greatly reduced by taking 10 grains of aspirin prophylactically before the muscle stiffness and soreness appear and repeating the dosage every four to six hours until the myositis has subsided, usually a matter of a day or two. Ideally, however, the best treatment of overuse myositis is to anticipate in advance the kind of muscle use that may lead to it, and then gradually prepare the muscles to handle the load by a program of daily exercise and muscle conditioning. (*See* p. 931.)

Foreign Bodies

Various kinds of foreign bodies may become embedded in the skin or soft tissues of the body, accidentally or purposely thrust into various body orifices, or swallowed or aspirated. In most cases foreign material that gains entrance anywhere in the body sooner or later becomes painful or irritating, and often introduces infective bacteria into unprotected tissues. Frequently the removal of a foreign body can be accomplished easily without medical help providing the proper techniques are used, but certain kinds of foreign bodies pose special threats and do require a doctor's attention. Thus everyone should have some knowledge of potential dangers that foreign bodies may present, and recognize when a doctor's help is advisable.

Foreign Bodies in the Skin or Soft Tissues. These include such things as wood splinters, cinders, bits of broken glass, fragments of wire or metal shrapnel that may become lodged in the skin or driven into the deeper soft tissues. Such foreign bodies are usually painful, and will almost always produce infection if they are not speedily removed. Such superficial objects as cinders ground into the skin or large wood splinters can often be removed easily with a pair of tweezers; the injured skin area should then be washed with soap and water and dressed with a sterile gauze dressing until healing is under way. Surface antiseptics such as tincture of iodine or tincture of Merthiolate may be applied safely, but soap-and-water cleansing of the wound is the best guard against infection. Deeper splinters can often be removed either with the aid of a needle sterilized in a match flame or by making a small incision in the skin adjacent to the protruding end of the splinter and then working it out with a needle or knife point. The injured area again should be cleansed after the removal and covered with a sterile dressing until healing begins. Continuing pain, irritation or swelling usually indicates that all the foreign body has not been removed. Any foreign body that is not easily removed, or that has been deeply imbedded in subcutaneous tissue or muscle, should be treated by a physician as soon as possible so that it can be removed and the wound cleaned and dressed.

Foreign Bodies in the Eye. Small cinders, broken eyelashes, large dust particles or bits of wood or metal sawdust may become lodged in the eye, usually under a lower lid but occasionally on the clear corneal surface of the eyeball itself. Even the tiniest particle in the eye is extremely irritating, and the temptation to rub the eye may be all but irresistible; but it must be resisted just the same, for rubbing can embed an easily removable particle so deeply into the tissue surrounding the eye that surgical removal becomes necessary, or may cause the particle to scratch the cornea and possibly create a serious eye injury. If a foreign body in the eye can be seen under the eyelid or on the corneal surface, it can often be wiped away by using the corner of a clean handkerchief or the cotton-wrapped end of a moistened Q-Tip. *Never attempt to dig an embedded foreign body from the eye, and never use any sharp or pointed instrument;* if the foreign body cannot be gently and easily wiped away, cover the closed eye with an eye patch—a 2-by-2-inch gauze pad taped across the eye will do—and then have a doctor remove the foreign body as soon as possible. If the surface of the eye has not been scratched or injured, pain and watering of the eye should stop immediately after the object has been removed. If there is persistent irritation or pain, let the doctor know, and keep the eye closed with an eye patch. This will minimize the pain and permit speedy healing of a corneal scratch or early infection.

Foreign Bodies in the Ear or Nose. Any small object—a pea, a small pebble, a plug of hardened wax, even an insect—may become accidentally lodged in the ear canal and cause the most intense annoyance imaginable. If the object is an insect, it can often be "flooded out" by turning the head with the affected ear up and dropping warm water into the ear canal until the insect can be wiped away with a Q-Tip. If the object is vegetable matter such as a pea or a grain of wheat, water should not be used, since it may cause the lodged object to swell. If the object can be seen, an attempt can be made to lift it *gently* from the ear canal using the rounded end of a hairpin, but under no circumstances should one dig deeply into the ear canal with any instrument. Poking and prodding may drive the object deeper into the canal or even rupture the eardrum. If the object cannot be easily and gently removed, let it remain where it is until a doctor's help can be obtained.

The same principles hold true for a foreign body lodged in a nostril. If the victim is an adult, he may be able to blow the object out while holding the opposite nostril closed. If the object can be seen, try to dislodge it *gently* with the rounded end of a hairpin. In the face of any resistance, let it be and consult a doctor. In the case of a child no attempt should be made to dislodge a foreign body in a nostril without a doctor's help, and parents should be especially watchful that the object is not snuffed back into the throat and aspirated into an air passage. Take the child to a doctor's offce or a hospital emergency room at once to have the object removed.

Foreign Bodies in the Rectum or Vagina. Occasionally children, following their natural desire to explore their bodies, will insert and "lose" small foreign objects in the rectal canal or the vagina. Less frequently an adolescent girl or woman may forget to remove a tampon or diaphragm from the vagina. A foreign body in the rectum can do little harm unless it has sharp edges or points, and will usually be expelled with the next bowel movement with no need for medical attention. Objects inserted or left in the vagina, however, may not become dislodged naturally and, if retained for a period of time, will usually cause a *vaginitis* or inflammation of the vagina which will manifest itself as a progressively copious and malodorous vaginal discharge. In the case of a female child, *any* vaginal discharge should arouse suspicion of a foreign body in the vagina, and should be investigated at once by a physician. A mature woman may be able to dislodge a foreign body from the vagina by means of a gentle douche using a tablespoonful of white vinegar mixed in a quart of lukewarm water. Should this be unsuccessful, or should a vaginal discharge persist for more than a few hours following removal of the foreign body, a doctor should be consulted and a pelvic examination performed.

Foreign Bodies in the Throat or Air Passages. The most common foreign bodies to become lodged in the throat are bones or bulky masses of food. If the foreign body becomes lodged in the esophagus it may be possible to grasp a portion protruding into the throat with the fingers and extract it or, alternatively, to carry the object down with a swallow of water or by swallowing a piece of dry bread. If the object is too firmly lodged to be freed in this fashion, a doctor's attention should be sought as soon as possible; the object will remain painful until it is removed, but unless it obstructs breathing it does not pose an imminent threat to life. If the foreign object is large enough to completely block the throat and cause choking, however, or if it enters the air passages to obstruct the trachea or one of the bronchi, a life-threatening emergency may be present, and the victim may die of suffocation if medical aid cannot be obtained swiftly. Emergency first-aid procedures in such a case are discussed in detail elsewhere. (*See* p. 114.)

Swallowing a Foreign Body. This is probably far more common an occurrence than is generally recognized, and perhaps it is best that parents are mercifully spared knowledge of the multitudes of small objects their small children may swallow from one day to the next. For the most part these objects—bits of plastic, marbles, coins, small pebbles, pieces of crayon and so forth—are passed on down the gastrointestinal tract and ultimately expelled unnoticed in the stool. As a general rule any object small enough to be swallowed will do no harm, and require no medical attention, unless it is pointed (like a thumbtack or a pin), sharply angular (a bit of broken glass) or poisonous. If there is any question that the swallowed object might be harmful, however, a doctor should be consulted and his advice followed. Even sharp or pointed objects may pass harmlessly through the intestinal tract and out if the victim is fed substances that leave considerable residue to cover and protect the sharp points—potatoes, bananas or bread, for example. Laxatives should be avoided, since they tend to liquefy the stool, leaving sharp points exposed, and also increase the risk of intestinal injury by increasing intestinal motility. Occasionally X-rays may be needed to trace the progress of a swallowed foreign body, but only rarely is surgical intervention necessary to remove such an object.

Other Minor Emergencies

A variety of other minor but distressing problems may require first-aid measures before a doctor can be seen, or may be resolved without the need for medical attention as long as certain basic precautions are taken.

Blisters. The most common blisters are water blisters that occur as a result of continuing friction on some relatively unprotected part of the skin. Blisters may form on the heels or feet, for example, as a result of wearing tight or ill-fitting shoes; or they may form on the hand while gardening, playing golf or making home repairs. Obviously the first thing to do when a water blister is discovered is to put an end to the friction that caused it. A blister on the heel, for example, can be prevented from enlarging or breaking by changing shoes or protecting the blistered area from further friction with a patch of adhesive tape. If a blister is unbroken, it should in most cases be left that way to subside. If breaking is inevitable, one edge of the blister can be punctured with a pin or needle sterilized in a match flame. Water can then be gently squeezed out and the area dressed with a sterile gauze pad without peeling the dead skin. Since the only real risk from a water blister is the possibility of infection, keeping the area clean and protected until the new underlying skin can toughen is usually the only treatment necessary. Hemorrhagic blisters, commonly called "blood blisters," are less common than water blisters, and usually arise when an area of skin is pinched or traumatized so that there is bleeding from broken skin capillaries into the outer layers of the skin. Treatment is exactly the same as for water blisters, except that healing may also be speeded up by applying moist heat to the injured area for 20 to 30 minutes three or four times a day until the dead skin overlying the blister sloughs off.

Nosebleed. Most nosebleeds occur when tiny capillaries in the mucous membrane lining the nostrils are ruptured, usually as a result of excessively hard nose blowing. Nosebleeds can be stopped in the vast majority of cases simply by grasping the nose between the thumb and forefinger and squeezing the nostrils tightly shut for a period of five minutes measured by the clock. If the nosebleed resumes when the pressure is released, the procedure should be repeated. Once a nosebleed has stopped, care should be taken not to blow or pick at the nose for at least 24 hours to permit the ruptured capillaries to heal. Packing the nose with gauze or other absorbent material is not advisable because it tends to stretch the torn capillaries open, thus defeating efforts to stop the bleeding, and subsequent removal of the pack will also often dislodge the clot and permit the nosebleed to resume. Persistent or recurring nosebleeds may be an indication of underlying blood clotting disorders or other abnormal conditions, and should be investigated by a physician. (*See* p. 534.)

Toothache. The aching of a tooth may arise when an area of enamel and dentine has decayed away, exposing the pain-sensitive pulp cavity, or it may arise from infection or abscess formation at the root of the tooth. In any case, a toothache is a warning of more trouble to come, and a dentist's attention should be sought without delay. Often, however, a toothache caused by tooth decay can be temporarily soothed by touching the decayed area with a drop of oil of cloves, obtainable at any drugstore and applied with a cotton swab. If the toothache arises from infection or abscess formation at the root of the tooth, pain can be temporarily eased by an adult dosage of aspirin (10 grains every four to six hours) and the application of an ice bag to the painful area of the jaw. Relief of the pain should not, however, encourage the victim to postpone a visit to the dentist; the conditions that cause a painful toothache do not ordinarily take care of themselves, and delay in seeking dental care may result in needless pain and permanent damage to the teeth.

Earache. Like a toothache, an earache is usually a warning of underlying trouble that requires medical care—a middle ear infection, for example, or an unsuspected bacterial or fungal infection of the ear canal. In an emergency pain can be controlled with aspirin and application of an ice bag to the affected ear, but medical attention should be sought as soon as possible. Many children have earaches due to infections that have spread from the throat up the Eustachian tube to the middle ear; frequently dramatic pain relief can be obtained by dripping ice water into the ear canal, three or four drops every five minutes until the pain subsides. But in such a case it is important that the ears be examined by a doctor as soon as possible, and definitive treatment of the infection started. (*See* p. 436.)

Stomach Ache. This is a vague term that may refer to virtually any form of abdominal discomfort, and it may arise from a multitude of sources. (*See* p. 612.) When it is cyclical, coming in waves and then subsiding, it usually indicates gaseous distention in the small intestine or colon and can often be relieved completely by a bowel movement. If need be, a laxative suppository or small chemical enema such as the squeeze-bottle Fleet Enema available at most drugstores may help the victim pass a stool and relieve distention and pain. Laxatives by mouth should *never* be taken in the presence of undiagnosed abdominal pain, since the increased intestinal motility stimulated by oral laxatives could be harmful if such conditions as acute appendicitis or intestinal obstruction are causing the pain. Another common cause of stomach ache is simple indigestion from overindulgence in food or alcoholic beverages. In this case the abdominal pain may be more steady, with some associated nausea, and can often be at least partially relieved by taking an antacid preparation such as Tums, Rolaids or Alka-Seltzer. Any abdominal pain that persists for more than an hour, or grows progressively worse, may indicate more serious trouble; first-aid measures should be abandoned in such a case, and a doctor consulted without delay. Even if the pain proves to be a result of a viral "stomach flu" or a bacterial intestinal infection (*see* p. 253), treatment with antibiotics or other prescription medications may be indicated, and close medical observation for any change in the condition is necessary.

Motion Sickness. The onset of nausea, abdominal discomfort and a feeling of faintness that overcomes many people riding in buses, automobiles, airplanes or boats is often interpreted as a "stomach ache," but arises from totally different causes. Motion sickness usually occurs as a result of a disturbance in the balancing mechanism of the inner ear, usually associated with continuing irregular motion of the body. Motion of the eyes such as may occur when a person spends time reading on a moving bus or airplane may also trigger the condition.

Finally, there seems to be a strong psychological element to motion sickness in many cases, although no one has ever clearly identified how or why this works.

Motion sickness is more of a temporary annoyance than a health threat; it usually disappears as soon as the motion stops, and can be prevented completely by avoiding the kinds of motion that trigger it in each individual case. For those subject to this problem who must expose themselves, motion sickness can usually be prevented by taking doses of Dramamine or other over-the-counter, antivertigo medications according to label instructions. Unfortunately, most of these medications tend to induce drowsiness, and should not be used by anyone who must drive a car or operate machinery.

Surviving the Elements

Because the human body is warm-blooded, and unprotected by any significant amount of hair or fur, human beings are vulnerable to certain disorders related to sunlight, temperature or climate. Among the most notable of these conditions are sunburn, heat exhaustion, sunstroke, frostbite, immersion foot (or trench foot), and exposure. Each requires special first-aid attention when it occurs, and each can be prevented if the causes and predisposing circumstances are clearly understood.

Sunburn. The causes and treatment of this disorder are discussed in more detail elsewhere. (*See* p. 382.) For those with fair skin who are especially vulnerable, sunburn can be extremely uncomfortable and even dangerous. Avoidance of prolonged exposure to the sun, or extreme care in the use of indoor sunlamps, is the best of all preventive measures. So-called sun-screen lotions may be effective, but should be used cautiously until their value can be assessed in each individual case. Severe, blistering sunburns can be as dangerous as any thermal burn, and should be treated in the same fashion. (*See* p. 119.)

Heat Exhaustion. A relatively minor but sometimes alarming disorder, heat exhaustion or "heat prostration" arises from exposure to direct sunlight or excessive heat usually during some form of physical labor or exercise, which causes a loss of fluid and salt from the body through excessive sweating. Dizziness, weakness, headache, nausea, sometimes muscular cramps, and a sudden feeling of faintness are the usual early warning symptoms of this condition and should be the signal to stop activity, get into the shade, and lie down with the head slightly lower than the feet. Water and salt loss should be replenished a little at a time by drinking small amounts of water for a half hour to an hour, together with a small amount of salt in the form of salt tablets or some other source of easily ingested salt. One should avoid gulping down great quantities of cold water, which can irritate the stomach and trigger vomiting. If the early warning signs are ignored and heat exhaustion actually occurs, the victim may faint. The pulse rate is usually low, but there is no significant elevation of body temperature, and the skin is blanched, cool and moist. The condition is usually transient, and only rarely profound enough that medical treatment is necessary. What is necessary, however, is rest in the shade, replenishing the body's salt and water supply, and greater caution in the future.

Sunstroke (Heat Hyperpyrexia). Although sunstroke can be caused by the same circumstances that result in heat exhaustion, it is a much more serious condition. Sunstroke arises from a profound breakdown in the body's mechanism for heat regulation, with the development of a dangerously high body temperature, a raging fever and collapse. Generally this condition occurs during more prolonged exposure to heat or direct sunlight than is the case with heat exhaustion, and strikes older people more often than the younger age groups. Sunstroke is also preceded by headache, dizziness and nausea, but the victim tends to sweat very little, and collapses with skin that is markedly flushed and hot but dry, a racing pulse (up to 160 beats per minute) and a temperature rising rapidly to the level of 105° or 106° or even higher. Collapse may be followed by fever convulsions, coma and even death if body temperature cannot be swiftly reduced.

Unlike heat exhaustion, sunstroke is a serious threat to life, and heroic measures must be taken to reduce the victim's body temperature as quickly as possible. If possible, the victim should be placed in a tub of cold water; then the skin should be rubbed vigorously until the temperature begins to drop. Temperature should be checked with a rectal thermometer as frequently as every ten minutes, until it falls to 102°. Artificial cooling mechanisms should be discontinued at that point, and if the temperature continues to drop, the victim may even have to be kept warm. Massage of the skin should be continued even after the cooling bath because cold water tends to constrict the blood vessels in the skin and thus defeats its own purpose after a while. Once temperature has fallen to manageable proportions, the victim should be placed at rest in a cool, well-ventilated room, preferably with an electric fan to keep air moving around his body, and close check should be kept to see that his temperature does not rise again. Remember that a rectal temperature of 106° is dangerously high, and at 107° or 108° the fever can cause irreversible destruction of brain cells. First-aid measures should be started immediately, since the condition may cause death in as much as 20 percent of cases unless vigorously treated as soon as it occurs. Medical help should also be summoned and the victim transported to a hospital as quickly as possible.

Frostbite. When body tissues are chilled to the point that the skin and subcutaneous tissue actually become frozen, the condition is known as frostbite. It is particularly common in parts of the body that are covered with tight clothing, and occurs as a result of moist cold rather than dry cold. Although it may "creep up" on the victim because cold tends to have an anesthetic effect on the skin, it is usually easily recognized because of slight swelling, a dead gray-white color to the skin, and increasing pain as rewarming begins.

In treating frostbite, it is important to remember that any kind of mechanical manipulation of the frostbitten area can further damage skin and underlying tissue. In very mild cases—a part of an ear or a spot on the cheek, for example—slow rewarming of the area by exposure to cool room air or cool to lukewarm moist packs, together with gentle massage of the skin *sur-*

rounding the frostbitten area, will usually be sufficient to rewarm the tissue and restore circulation. There may well be peeling of the skin thereafter, but mild cases of frostbite usually recover without incident. More profound frostbite, however, may require careful medical attention, since thrombosis of the veins in the affected tissue can cause tissue death, sloughing of tissue or even gangrene. Medical treatment depends upon slow rewarming of the area, with the surrounding environmental temperature kept low in order to reduce metabolism in the surface areas of the body and ensure adequate circulation. Medications are given to counteract spasm of the blood vessels and induce dilatation, while in extreme cases, anticoagulating medications may be given to prevent clotting of blood in the vessels as normal circulation returns to the injured areas. Tobacco, which induces spasm of blood vessels in the skin, should be avoided completely until recovery. If pain is severe during the recovery period, analgesic medicines are also given.

Trench Foot (Immersion Foot). Trench foot is a cold injury quite similar to frostbite, except that it can occur in the absence of freezing temperatures. The condition is brought on by prolonged contact of the extremities, particularly those in constrictive clothing, with moderately cool or cold temperatures under conditions of continuing moisture. The feet are usually the most vulnerable, and when they are continuously cold and wet, blood vessels, particularly in the toes, constrict, followed by thrombosis of the veins and then, soon thereafter, a sort of anesthetic gangrene that can destroy all the tissues in the toes, or even the entire foot, and necessitate amputation.

By far the best treatment is, of course, prevention. Cold, wet feet should be completely warmed and dried and full circulation restored at least every six to eight hours, and one or even two pairs of thick wool socks with relatively loose-fitting boots should be used, since wool can absorb a great deal of moisture and yet keep the feet warm even when it is wet. Treatment of mild cases of trench foot is the same as treatment for frostbite. In more profound cases or cases of longer duration, expert medical care is necessary in order to reduce the amount of gangrene.

Exposure (Hypothermia). Oddly enough, the most commonplace, and truly life-threatening, disorder that can arise from man's struggle with the elements is not caused by excessive heat or freezing cold, but occurs under relatively mild climatic conditions—for example outside temperatures not much less than 45° or 50°. Known simply as "exposure," it is all too often a tragic cause of death which results from nothing more than a gradual cooling of the entire body due to environmental conditions to the point where the metabolism can no longer sustain life. Death by exposure typically results from a combination of circumstances; often the victim is lost in a wilderness area without food or the proper protective clothing. He may become physically exhausted trying to find his way out; chilled, damp and hungry, he may have to spend the night, or even several days and nights, with no way to keep warm. Gradually his physical energies and mental faculties begin to fail from continuous chilling and total exhaustion; he sinks into unconsciousness, and unless he is found and can be revived, death follows.

Clearly, adequate preparations are the best way to combat the danger of exposure. Anyone who ventures into the country on camping, fishing or hunting trips, and even weekend hikers, must take certain commonsense precautions. Everyone, not just one member of a group, should carry a minimal backpack containing a change of woolen clothes, an extra change of woolen socks, a windbreaker-raincoat (a cheap plastic parka-like raincoat will do), a packet of moisture-resistant matches, a small bottle of charcoal fire starter and a small amount of extra food. Then if someone is lost or becomes chilled, he can build a fire, and the fire should be big and hot enough to sustain itself even when fed damp wood. Dead branches found on trees, particularly the lower trunks of firs, will almost invariably be dry enough to start and maintain a fire even if the rest of the area is sodden. Besides keeping warm by the fire, the individual should also engage in physical exercise from time to time, jogging in place, whittling wood chips, or almost anything else to keep his circulation going. Sleep is not terribly important, but protection from physical exhaustion is; it is far better to hole up for the night and stay warm and dry than to wear oneself out attempting to struggle through underbrush in the darkness. One excellent protection against exposure is a so-called space blanket, a thin, light aluminized cloth or plastic sheet which, when folded up, can be held in the flat of one hand and easily carried in a pocket, and which provides excellent insulation from chilling cold when the individual wraps himself up in it. In short, exposure is one disorder that no one need suffer *as long as he recognizes that it is a serious threat and takes simple steps to counteract it.*

When treating someone who is suffering from exposure, the basic principles are both simple and logical. First, *prevent further chilling;* build a fire to help warm the victim, and wrap him in dry clothing or blankets to help him retain his natural body heat. Second, *keep him at rest* to help him conserve his physical energy, with reassurances that help is on the way and that he will be all right. Remember that the victim of exposure may be mentally confused, frightened, perhaps even hostile because of temporarily impaired brain function; *never* leave him unattended, and be watchful that he does not get up and wander off in confusion. Finally, *replenish the victim's energy* with small amounts of warm food accompanied by warm coffee or tea. Avoid alcoholic beverages, which will only compromise the victim's brain function even further. Once the situation is under control, transport the victim to a hospital, or send for someone to either bring a doctor or help transport the victim. Unlike shock, even profound exposure is usually reversible as long as the victim is still alive—but the basic principles noted above can make the difference between life and death.

Gunshot and Stab Wounds

Injuries from guns and knives usually occur as the result of hunting accidents, although they also occur on the battlefield or as the result of a criminal assault. The four first-aid priorities apply here exactly as they do in any other serious accident: any copious bleeding must be stopped by applying direct pressure to the wound or by means of a tourniquet (if the victim is alone and conscious he must accomplish this himself); heartbeat, circulation and respiration must be maintained; and shock must be vigorously combated. However, with wounds of this sort the possibility of injury to internal organs must always be considered. A single rifle shell or a piece of shrapnel can shatter the bone of a leg or leave fragments of lead embedded in the tissue from one end of the limb to another. Gunshot or stab wounds to the chest are particularly dangerous if the liver has been injured, and wounds to the abdomen may tear parts of the gastrointestinal tract, allowing intestinal contents to pour into the peritoneum. All gunshot and stab injuries must be considered "dirty" wounds, since bits of contaminated clothing or other foreign bodies may have been carried into the wound. An injury to the chest may not only pierce the lung but also may cause it to collapse, either suddenly or slowly due to sucking of air into the chest cavity from the outside through the wound during breathing motions. Such a "sucking wound" of the chest should be sealed as tightly as possible, using adhesive tape, a rolled-up bandage, the hand, or almost any other means of preventing air from leaking in. Other than this, there is little that the layman can do to combat internal injuries. External bleeding must be stopped, however, and the wound covered loosely with a sterile bandage or a clean cloth to prevent further contamination. Shock is the deadly and almost inevitable accompaniment of wounds of this sort; the victim must be reassured, kept warm and, if possible, immobile, until medical help arrives. If necessary, and if the wounds are relatively minor, the victim may be able to move of his own volition, but if the wounds are more serious and complicated by internal injuries, he must be kept immobile and moved carefully on an improvised stretcher. Summoning medical aid, or transporting the victim to a location where medical aid is available, is also among the first priorities with injuries of this sort, since definitive diagnosis and treatment are possible only in a hospital.

Animal and Insect Bites and Stings

In almost every part of the world men are vulnerable to a variety of biting or stinging flies, mosquitoes, lice, ants, bees, wasps, hornets, spiders and scorpions. Most insects are not much more than a nuisance, with the notable exception of those that are carriers of infectious disease: the mosquitoes that carry malaria or yellow fever, for example, the body lice that transmit epidemic typhus, or the wood ticks that transmit Rocky Mountain spotted fever. *Insect infestation,* however, is a much more serious matter and requires vigilant preventive measures as well as active medical treatment. (*See* p. 268.) Purely nuisance insect bites can be very effectively prevented by application of such familiar insect repellents as 6-12 or Off to the skin prior to exposure, or spraying living quarters with Black Flag or other insecticides. When stinging or itching bites occur, the discomfort can often be relieved by applying a paste of baking soda and water to the bitten areas of the skin. Even more effective relief is possible with the use of calamine lotion preparations containing a small amount of phenol as a skin application, or with the use of ointments containing small quantities of one of the Novocaine-like drugs. Certain individuals, however, develop allergic sensitivity to the bites of even such common nuisance insects as mosquitoes and develop large itching welts whenever bitten. Such individuals should take particular care to avoid the kinds of insect bites that so affect them, and may require the use of small doses of Benadryl or other antihistamine drugs for relief when they are bitten.

Bees, Wasps and Hornets. The venoms of this group of insects contain toxins or chemicals which tend to hemolize or break down red blood cells in the body, but the pain they cause is largely due to the fact that they contain histamine, and their main danger lies in the possible shock that may result from multiple stings, or in the severe allergic reactions which sometimes occur. For the person who is not allergic to beestings, a single sting may require no treatment other than an ice pack for a few moments until the pain subsides. Some stinging insects, however, notably the honeybee, leave the stinger behind in the wound, and this should be carefully removed. In addition, an antihistamine such as a cold tablet may help to relieve the discomfort by counteracting the histamine in the bee's venom. Multiple stings can be much more serious and can result in massive edema all over the body, severe systemic illness and even shock as a result of the large amount of venom injected by the stings. In such a case emergency first-aid measures must include steps to combat shock—keeping the victim wrapped in a blanket for warmth and lying at rest with his head slightly lower than his feet—until he can be transported to a doctor's office or hospital emergency room for care.

In certain persons, however, even a single beesting can bring about a far more profound kind of trouble. Bee venom is one of the most powerful allergens or "allergy stimulators" known, and in people who have developed an allergy to the sting of certain bees, a single sting may cause the appearance of giant hives all over the body, obstruction of the breathing due to swelling of the mucous membrane lining the larynx or voice box, an asthmatic attack or even a profound degree of allergic shock characterized by rapid pulse, collapse and a sudden precipitous fall in blood pressure—all of which may occur within a few minutes of a single beesting once the individual has been sensitized. This kind of allergic shock, known as *anaphylaxis,* is precisely the same as the dangerous reaction that can occur in a person sensitized to horse serum or to penicillin. When it occurs, no time must be lost getting the victim to a doctor or a doctor to the victim, since anaphylactic reactions can prove to be fatal, sometimes in as little as a few minutes.

Unfortunately there are no emergency first-aid measures that can help combat anaphylactic shock unless one has certain indispensable medicines on hand, and knows how to use them, before medical help can be contacted. This means that the person allergic to beestings must always be *prepared in advance* for a possible emergency. Anyone who has ever had anything more than a very mild reaction of transitory pain and localized swelling following a beesting should be carefully examined by a physician and skin-tested to determine hypersensitivity. Further, the family of a person who is hypersensitive to beestings should keep a "beesting kit" on hand; it contains potent antihistamines that can be taken by mouth and some injectable medication such as adrenalin to counteract shock, both of which can be used to start treatment the moment symptoms of allergic shock first appear. It is wise to have a similar kit in the automobile, and in the hiker's pack, since tragedies from this condition usually occur on distant travels or camping trips where medical aid is not readily available.

Spiders. There is only one commonly encountered spider in North America whose bite is sufficiently venomous to cause trouble—the black widow. It is a small, shiny-black spider, easy to identify if one wants to turn it over and look for the bright orange-red "hourglass" spot on its underside. Most people do not. Thus any sharply painful bite from a rather small black spider should be regarded with suspicion. Black widow venom is a toxin to the nervous system which may produce severe rigidity of the abdominal muscles and abdominal cramps, followed by weakness, tremor and excruciating pain in the limbs. Convulsions may also occur, especially in small children. There is no effective first-aid treatment other than reassuring the victim and keeping him warm and at rest until medical help arrives. A doctor's care is imperative as quickly as possible to manage treatment using antivenin and to provide supportive treatment by regulating body fluids and controlling muscle spasm. In general the virulence of the black widow spider has been exaggerated, but children or the elderly can become extremely ill or even die from the bite of this creature.

Scorpions. There are at least two species of scorpions in the southwestern United States which can produce dangerous stings, and a multitude of other species scattered throughout desert and coastal regions of Mexico and Central America. The toxin in the scorpion venom causes severe pain, numbness and weakness of the area (usually a limb) that has been stung, with swelling in the region of the wound. Scorpion stings may be fatal to children or infants,

but adults usually recover. Local pain can be relieved with an ice bag, or with the use of a local anesthetic such as one of the Novocaine family.

Snakes. Anyone who lives in a rural area in the United States, or who goes on hiking or camping trips, should familiarize himself with the species of poisonous snakes he may encounter, and should be prepared to render first-aid treatment to himself or someone else who is bitten. There are two principal varieties of poisonous snakes in this country: the *coral snakes* and the so-called *pit vipers*. The coral snakes are found throughout the southwestern United States and into Sonora State in Mexico, as well as in southern Texas and Louisiana eastward to the Carolinas, Georgia and Florida. These snakes are by far the more dangerous, since their venom, like that of the Asian cobra, contains a powerful nerve poison which can very quickly reach and affect the cells of the spinal cord, respiratory center and brain. Death can result within a few hours because of respiratory failure or widespread paralysis, and therefore any first-aid measures other than keeping the victim at rest and incising and sucking the bite wound itself should take second place to getting him to a hospital and a doctor as swiftly as possible. Fortunately coral snakes are relatively retiring creatures and rarely bite humans, accounting for only perhaps 1 or 2 percent of all venomous snakebites that occur in the United States.

The same cannot be said for the other principal group of poisonous snakes: the pit vipers, so called because they have a noticeable sensory "pit" located on either side of the head adjacent to the eye. Among the pit vipers in the United States are the copperhead snake found in the eastern, southern and central states, the water moccasin or "cottonmouth" found throughout the south from Virginia to the Rio Grande, and a variety of rattlesnakes, most notably the timber rattler found in hills and woods of the eastern United States and the western diamond-backed rattler found in many areas of the west.

All these snakes are both dangerous and aggressive, often striking promiscuously without any provocation. Their "bites" are actually a combination of stab wounds and hypodermic injections; when they open their mouths to strike, a pair of retractable fangs in the upper jaw drop down and are actually stabbed into the flesh for a distance varying from a millimeter to a centimeter or more. Venom carried in venom sacs is then injected into the stab wound through hollow channels running down the fangs. Since most pit viper strikes hit the victim's leg or perhaps lower arm, anyone who is out in the woods or brush where snakes might be found is wise to wear high-topped rubber or leather boots and dungarees or trousers made of a thick, heavy, closely woven material which can provide at least partial protection from snakebites. It is also wise to avoid places frequented by these snakes: rock ledges, stone walls, wood piles or rocky desert land in particular.

When a person receives a snakebite, there is immediate excruciating pain in the area of the wound, followed by swelling of the area, generalized weakness, tingling or numbness of the extremities, a feeling of suffocation and often prostration. Unlike coral snake venom, however, the venom of pit vipers is composed primarily of a group of substances which weaken blood capillary walls and dissolve red blood cells, so that frequently internal hemorrhages occur throughout the body, sometimes with frank bleeding around the lips or mucous membranes of the eyes or mouth. Death can result from extensive internal bleeding and circulatory collapse.

In recent years there has been considerable controversy about first-aid treatment for snakebites. No one argues with the first principle of keeping the snakebite victim at rest and sending for medical aid as quickly as possible, or transporting the victim if a doctor or hospital is nearby. Most authorities also still agree that incising the skin and subcutaneous tissue over the bite wounds and applying suction by means of a rubber suction cup (never by mouth if any other device is available) can be of help in eliminating some of the venom before it gets into the circulation, but this is effective only if it is done within the first half hour after the snakebite. A light tourniquet above the wound should be applied with enough pressure to prevent venous drainage from the area but not enough pressure to prevent

arterial circulation. If possible, it is advisable to keep the affected limb cool, with the use of dry towels containing ice to help control pain and to slow circulation. Once the victim is hospitalized, it is possible to support circulation with intravenous infusions and to prepare blood for transfusion to help make up for the hemolysis (red blood cell destruction) caused by the venom. In addition, a polyvalent antivenin which effectively neutralizes all North and South American pit viper venoms can be administered to counteract any of the venom which remains. In fact, anyone who has a summer cabin or spends much time camping or hiking in wilderness areas during the warm summer months should have a snakebite kit on hand or in his pack, including antivenin, the distilled water necessary to reconstitute it and the syringe necessary to administer it. Even with the use of a snakebite kit, however, medical aid should be sought promptly. With competent first aid and speedy medical care, the great majority of snakebite victims in the United States can be saved, although the bite may cause thoroughly unpleasant illness and disability.

Dog Bites. Any animal scratch or bite must be considered a "dirty" or bacterially contaminated wound; dog bites in particular may cause deep, contaminated contused lacerations, and any but the most superficial should be cleaned, debrided and dressed by a physician. Aside from the threat of superficial bacterial infection, however, dog bites are associated with two extremely dangerous possible threats: tetanus infection from deep puncture wounds, and the possibility of rabies. The threat of tetanus can be minimized by administration of a tetanus immunization booster, if such a booster shot has not been received within a period of one year prior to the injury, or by the administration of tetanus antitoxin if the individual has never had a series of tetanus immunization shots before.

Rabies is an even greater threat. In most parts of the country rabies is well controlled and only rarely appears in domestic pets, but there is always the possibility that a dog may have contracted rabies from contact with some infected wild animal. Thus any victim of a dog bite should report the incident not only to his physician but to the local police or public health authorities, so that the animal can be isolated and observed for any signs of developing rabies. In cases in which the dog has been destroyed, or cannot be found or identified, the doctor must decide on the basis of rabies statistics in the area whether antirabies immunizations must be started or not. Immunization against rabies and the nature of the disease itself are discussed in detail elsewhere. (*See* p. 239.)

Wild Animal Bites. The bites of wild animals carry the same threat of superficial infection or tetanus infection as dog bites, but in this case the threat of possible rabies is even more alarming. In this country there is a natural reservoir of rabies infection among wild creatures, so any bite must be suspect. In addition, most wild creatures are sufficiently wary of man that a healthy wild animal will more likely turn and run than bite a human that comes near; only sick ones are inclined to bite. Animals particularly associated with rabies in the United States include wild bats, skunks, rodents (especially chipmunks, squirrels, marmots, rats and field mice), foxes and coyotes.

Any wild animal bite should be examined and treated at once by a doctor. The creature should, if possible, be captured alive for examination, though not at the risk of further bites. Above all, however, adults and children alike should be taught *never to go near or touch an apparently dead, sick or strangely behaving wild animal.* The best possible way to guard against rabies is to avoid any possible contact with it.

Poison Ivy and Other Plant Pests

A variety of wild plants common in the United States are capable of causing extremely uncomfortable skin reactions upon contact because of irritating oils or other chemicals contained in their leaves. Most familiar of these is, of course, *poison ivy,* a deciduous plant easily identified by leaves that grow in groups of three with serrated edges and a shiny or oily surface appearance. Poison ivy is found in most wooded areas of the United States and southern Canada. The most common species tend to grow as twining vines, but some species grow as a low bush with leaves more oval or oakleaf shaped than

the more common variety and are sometimes locally known as *poison oak*. Either species contains an irritating oily chemical, similar to carbolic acid, in the leaves, and mere contact with this oil causes a severe itching of the affected skin area several hours after contact, followed by blistering of the skin and—if the blisters are broken—the threat of secondary bacterial infection. The best treatment for poison ivy, by far, is recognition of the plant and careful avoidance of contact. Irritation can be caused even by touching some object, such as a shoe, that has contacted the plant and carried off some of the irritating oil; and oil droplets can be carried for miles in smoke from brush fires when poison ivy is burned. The soft skin of the eyelids, forearms or legs is most readily affected, and the oil can be transferred from one person to another.

In case of a known contact with poison ivy or poison oak, the irritating skin reaction can often be prevented by repeated gentle washing of the exposed area with warm water and mild soap, taking care not to scarify the skin by scrubbing. Once the itching reaction begins, it can be treated with such surface ameliorants as calamine lotion or a paste made of baking soda or Epsom salt in a small amount of water. Care should also be taken not to spread the irritating oil by scratching and then touching other parts of the skin with the fingers. So treated, the irritation will resolve and go away without further treatment in a matter of a few days. In areas where contact with poison ivy can be expected frequently, a vaccine exists which can be given *prior* to contact either by injection or by mouth. This, however, is useful only if the vaccine is administered long enough prior to contact to permit an immune condition to develop—a matter of two to three weeks—and the immunization is relatively short-lived and may have to be readministered annually.

Poison sumac is similar to poison ivy, and can cause similar skin irritation upon contact, but it is more difficult to identify. Most varieties of sumac, poisonous and nonpoisonous, grow as small trees bearing long spikes of paired leaves with a single leaf at the tip, and produce clusters of red-orange berries. Since both varieties look much the same, all wild sumac should be avoided when encountered. Treatment of contact irritation from poison sumac is the same as for poison ivy or oak. However, if irritation persists or spreads, or if a secondary bacterial infection occurs, from contact with any of these plants, a physician should be consulted.

Another plant pest common in northern latitudes is the so-called *stinging nettle,* a low-growing weed with fronds of four leaves that appear covered by a soft, velvety coat. This "velvet" is made up of multitudes of tiny bristles that release an extremely irritating chemical upon contact with the skin. The reaction is so instantaneous that the victim may feel as if he had suddenly been stung by a bee, and the stinging persists for several minutes, giving way to itching of the affected skin area for an hour or more. No treatment is required, nor is any effective, but anyone living in a region where nettles are common should learn to recognize the plant and avoid contact with it.

A number of berries, leaves and roots are also extremely poisonous if eaten. It would be impossible here to list all the poisonous plants or fungi that grow in the various parts of the country, but everyone should at least be familiar with those indigenous to his own area. Some of those plants may cause no more than a transitory gastric upset if taken internally, while others—berries from the deadly nightshade, for example, or various of the *Amanita* mushrooms—can actually cause death. Parts of certain highly prized garden shrubs can also be poisonous—the rhododendron, for example—and many plants or herbs produce chemicals which, when used in the proper dosage, can be beneficial, but can be dangerous in overdosage. Leaves of the common foxglove weed, for example, were the original source of the poisonous glycoside *digitalis,* useful in treating congestive heart failure when used in small doses, but capable of producing severe interference with heart function when taken in large quantities.

Most people, of course, have sufficient common sense to avoid eating berries, leaves or roots of unknown plants. Obviously, no wild herbs or mushrooms should *ever* be used for food unless the individual is absolutely certain of the plant's identity. Unfortunately, children are the most frequent victims of plant poisoning, and they should be taught never to eat any wild berry or plant without first bringing it home for identification. If a child becomes ill and plant poisoning is suspected, try to determine what the plant might have been, and if possible obtain a sample for identification after calling a doctor or Poison Control Center for emergency instructions.

Radiation Reactions and Injuries

Radiation sickness as a result of overexposure to high-energy therapeutic X-rays or to the radiation of nuclear reactors, cyclotrons or radioactive medical supplies is a highly dangerous but still quite rare disorder. Nevertheless, it is very much in the public mind, not only as a result of the dreadful plight of victims of the atom bombs dropped on Japan, but also because of the well-publicized dangers of radioactive fallout from testing nuclear weapons. Indeed, a great many people have become so apprehensive about exposure to excessive radiation that they often respond irrationally to what they regard as any possible threat of radiation injury. Thus in recent years the use of diagnostic X-rays in medical treatment has been attacked as dangerous because of the possibility of overirradiation, and many people react heatedly in opposition to the construction of nuclear reactors to generate electric power proposed for their communities.

In considering the danger of radiation, however, it is essential to separate fact from falsehood. X-ray radiation, for example, can indeed cause radiation burns or radiation sickness when it is used at high energies and in really massive doses for treatment of such diseases as cancer. However, this threat is clearly recognized, and techniques for its prevention are universally used by highly skilled therapeutic X-ray technicians. (*See* p. 975.) Equally stringent precautions are taken in the use of diagnostic X-rays. (*See* p. 975.) In fact, the benefits of diagnostic X-rays so far outweigh any conceivable harm they could do that most fears about excessive radiation are totally groundless. In short, there is probably no other area in medicine in which more fastidious care is taken than in the use of X-rays.

The dangers of a nuclear generator are also largely exaggerated. The major problem such installations present to the environment lies not in radioactive pollution but rather in the disposal of the heated water that results from the cooling process. However, all the procedures used in nuclear generation of electric power, including the disposal of radioactive wastes, are rigidly controlled by federal standards, and there is little reason to believe that they pose any serious threat. Today nuclear weapons tests are also rigidly controlled, at least in this country. Nevertheless, they are universally recognized as a major potential threat to all forms of life on Earth because of the danger that long-lasting radioactive materials may be released into the atmosphere. Thus any tests—even those conducted far underground—present a risk of accidental environmental contamination that cannot be ignored.

In spite of precautions to avoid exposure to radiation, rare cases of "radiation sickness" do occur, either following overexposure to therapeutic radiation or accidental exposure to radioactive materials. In an acute case there is an immediate effect which appears within 24 hours of exposure, including pain, nausea, vomiting, diarrhea, loss of appetite, rapid heartbeat and shock. This acute reaction is followed by a so-called latent period during which the body degenerates with internal hemorrhages, high vulnerability to infection, delirium, coma and ultimately death within a week or so. Cases of this sort occur only when the victim has received a sudden, lethal dose of radiation, and death is inevitable; the best that treatment can accomplish is to make the victim as comfortable as possible as the symptoms progress.

Far more commonly radiation sickness follows a less rapid course as a result of prolonged or repeated sublethal doses, particularly when the exposure is due to localized radiation of a small part of the body for therapeutic reasons. In such cases symptoms appear more slowly; there is a loss of hair from the skin surface in the exposed area, followed by atrophy or shrinking of the skin and ulceration of the affected region. Generalized symptoms may also appear: cessation of menses in the female, for example, or depression of the activity of the blood-forming elements in the bone marrow, resulting in a marked diminishment of circulating white and red blood cells. When exposure has been widespread there may be an alteration in the genetic "information system" in the body cells or germ cells, which can lead to the development of leukemia or other cancers, and an increase in the likelihood of mutations or other genetic defects. As long as the radiation exposure has not exceeded the lethal level, however, the chances for survival are good if the victim is in good general health and has the benefit of the necessary supportive medical care.

There has been a great deal of experimentation to find some means of counteracting the dangerous effects of radiation and increasing the survival rate of its victims. A number of drugs and chemicals have been discovered which help in this regard in experimental animals, but so far none has been found to be of practical value in humans. This is not, however, a closed issue, and we may well see marked advances in prevention or control of radiation sickness within the next few years.

Handling Emergencies, Large or Small

Nobody deliberately seeks out emergency situations, and months or years may pass between the sort of accidents that require prompt first-aid attention. Under these circumstances it may be hard to keep a mass of detail about emergency treatment constantly in mind, but the basic and really important principles are few enough and can be summarized as follows:

1. Stop any copious bleeding.
2. Restore breathing.
3. Restore circulation.
4. Treat for shock.

These are the four first-aid priorities, and the techniques necessary to perform them should be part of everyone's knowledge. In addition, there are a few do's and don'ts that almost always apply in an emergency situation:

Do summon medical aid as quickly as possible.
Don't give an accident victim anything to eat

or drink, except in the case of poisoning with a caustic or oily substance.

Don't move an accident victim unless absolutely necessary.

Don't leave an accident victim alone.

The special techniques necessary to give first aid to severe burn and poisoning victims should also be learned and remembered, along with the commonsense precautions that can prevent many minor accidents and injuries from occurring in the first place, and the first-aid measures necessary to treat them if and when they do occur. But perhaps the two most important general rules of first aid are: be prepared for the common emergencies in advance; and use your head in an emergency.

Be Prepared for the Common Emergencies in Advance

The best insurance that anyone can have in coping with an emergency, large or small, is advance knowledge and training. Everyone from the age of twelve on up should have the benefit of a comprehensive course in first-aid techniques. Those provided by many public schools, the Boy Scouts or Girl Scouts, the Red Cross and a number of other agencies, including many hospitals, are excellent, and it is a good idea to have a refresher course at five-year intervals to keep up to date with changes. First-aid training can also be obtained in a Health Mobilization Medical Self-Help program. Inquire about this or similar programs by writing to your state health department or Civil Defense office, or directly to the program offices, c/o Medical Self-Help, Public Health Service, Washington, D.C. 20201.

Such training programs deal with all the basic first-aid principles and precautions in far greater detail than is possible here. In addition, they provide an indispensable opportunity to practice those principles in simulated emergencies. Special techniques for bandaging or supportive strapping are taught, and the techniques for moving a victim safely are practiced under experienced guidance. Many first-aid courses, to be complete, include information and practice training in such important special subjects as water rescue techniques. Indeed, swimming is such a widespread activity in this country, and swimming and boating accidents are so common, that everyone should first learn *how* to swim proficiently, ideally in a Red Cross training program, and then learn and practice water safety and lifesaving techniques. Information about such training programs in your own community can be obtained by inquiring of the nearest Red Cross field office, or from local fire, police or public health departments.

In addition to adequate first-aid training, everyone should own a good first-aid manual for handy reference, and a copy should be carried in the car, on camping trips, or in the backpack on hiking trips. An excellent first-aid instruction manual can be obtained for a small fee by writing to the American Medical Association, 535 N. Dearborn, Chicago, Illinois. An equally fine manual can be obtained from the American Red Cross, and the Boy Scout Handbook available in most bookstores contains a brief but comprehensive section of first-aid instructions.

Finally, a small but basic first-aid kit should be readily available in your home, with another kept at all times in the car or carried in a hiking pack. They should be kept out of the hands of children and, of course, checked periodically to see that they are complete and in usable condition. Kits bearing the approval of the American Red Cross can be obtained quite inexpensively from your local drugstore. Alternatively, an excellent first-aid kit can be made up from materials available at the drugstore and at home. The basic materials that should be included in a good first-aid kit are as follows:

Sterile Dressing Materials

Adhesive (Band-Aid) dressings—assorted sizes
2 × 2″ sterile gauze pads—1 dozen, individually wrapped
4 × 4″ sterile gauze pads—½ dozen, individually wrapped
2 × 4″ "nonstick" sterile pads (Telfa)—½ dozen, individually wrapped

Bandaging Materials

2″ gauze roller bandage—one 6-yard roll
4″ gauze roller bandage—one 6-yard roll

1″ adhesive tape—one 1-yard roll
2″ adhesive tape—one 1-yard roll

Supporting Materials

2″ elastic (Ace) bandage
4″ elastic (Ace) bandage
One triangular bandage (1 square yard clean sheeting or muslin, folded diagonally, for use as sling or wrapper)

Additional Items

1 pair bandage scissors
1 pair tweezers (surgical quality)
1 snakebite kit with rubber suction device and light elastic tourniquet
Sunburn ointment
Small bottle germicidal soap (Phisohex or Septisol)
Small vial tincture of Merthiolate (optional)
First-aid manual

Since an important part of being prepared for emergencies is knowing whom to call for help and how, every home should have an up-to-date list of emergency names and telephone numbers. Among these should be the numbers for your doctor, the nearest hospital emergency room, a nearby ambulance service, the local police department, the local fire department and the telephone number of the closest Poison Control Center. Keep a copy stapled to the front inside cover of each telephone book, or posted near the telephone, with a carbon copy taped to the back of the medicine cabinet door. Then be sure that everyone in the family, including children, knows where these numbers are listed and why. In addition, all baby-sitters should be carefully instructed where these numbers are posted, as well as where parents can be reached in an emergency.

Use Your Head in an Emergency

Accidents and injuries always occur without warning, but it is imperative that you *use* your head—and *keep* your head—in an emergency. With a minor accident that is not a matter of life or death, you will have plenty of time to call for medical help and take the necessary first-aid measures, and it is important to remember that how you behave can markedly affect the victim's reactions. There is no need to create an emergency situation where none exists. But in a true emergency, you must act quickly, calmly and knowledgeably no matter how frightened you may feel. *Do not panic.* In calling for help in particular be certain to say *who you are, where you live, exactly where the emergency has arisen, what the problem is* or appears to be, and *what you have already done about it.* Never be ashamed to telephone for help, but don't deliberately exaggerate circumstances just to get a quicker response. *Stay on the telephone* until some decision has been reached, until you are certain that medical help is on the way, or until you understand clearly what you should do in regard to transporting the victim elsewhere. Many doctors feel strongly that precious time can be wasted in going to the victim's home and then proceeding to the hospital, and they often recommend that the patient be taken to a hospital immediately. This does not necessarily mean that the emergency is grave, but in any case, the doctor's telephone instructions should be followed to the letter.

It is always harder to find doctors in the evening or on weekends than at other times. Thus you should know which hospital in your community has around-the-clock emergency outpatient clinics to handle problems that arise when your own doctor cannot be immediately reached. These clinics can also help in the event of relatively minor emergencies which may not need the immediate attention of your personal physician but which should be seen by some medical attendant: minor lacerations and abrasions, for example, or minor eye injuries, annoying allergic reactions, earaches, nosebleeds, toothaches and similar disorders. In such cases a nearby outpatient service can provide prompt and competent interim care and save you time, discomfort and worry.

Perhaps the most frightening emergency is one that arises when you are in some remote area where no help of any sort is nearby—on a camping or hunting trip, on a deserted beach, or on a hike in the mountains. Indeed, you may be the only one around to help prevent an emergency from turning into a disaster. In such a situation your own common sense is your greatest asset and panic your greatest threat.

Obviously, you must first administer whatever first-aid measures are necessary. Then you must think of the best way to get help quickly. Do not leave the victim alone if there is any possible alternative; rather, always try to find some way to *bring help to you*—light a signal fire or use light-colored clothing or a metal or mirror flasher to draw the attention of passing aircraft, and then give help time enough to arrive. If for some reason you *must* leave to get help, be sure that the victim is covered warmly and protected from the elements, and at least conscious and moderately able to take care of himself unless the circumstances are truly extreme. Finally, insist that he remain precisely where he is until you return.

Of course, no amount of training and advance preparation will make an emergency situation pleasant to deal with, but if you are armed with a basic knowledge of the important first-aid procedures, if you keep your head and use good sense and judgment, you can be confident of doing your best if and when you are the man on the spot in an emergency.

Temperature, Fever and Febrile Illnesses

A three-year-old child, normally active all day long, becomes strangely subdued in the evening, and by bedtime has developed a fever of 104°. The man of the house, aware of a slight headache on going to bed one night, wakes up next morning with aching muscles, a tight chest and a temperature of 101.6°. A housewife, bothered by a scratchy throat all day, takes her temperature and then treats herself with a couple of aspirin when the thermometer reads only 99.2°.

These are, of course, familiar situations. Since childhood we have learned to recognize a fever as abnormal, and the common clinical thermometer is the most familiar diagnostic instrument in the home. It is also the most useful household guide to the severity and urgency of certain kinds of illness. We may sometimes make the mistake of assuming—incorrectly—that if no fever is present, no illness can be present either; but more commonly it is the presence of fever that first alerts us that an illness exists.

Indeed, fever is probably the most widely recognized of all early-warning signs that something is going wrong in the body. For this reason we can properly consider it an "emergency," not necessarily a serious one, of course, but always a warning of trouble which *might* be serious and should never be ignored. Certain diseases and disorders—infections, for example—are so commonly characterized by elevated temperature that they are called *febrile* ("feverish") *illnesses*. But fever is an early symptom of so many other diseases as well that everyone should know exactly what it is, where it comes from, what it may mean and what should be done about it when it occurs.

The Origins of Fever

What is a fever; where does it come from? All the basic physiological processes of life—digestion, respiration, muscle contraction, metabolism, circulation, excretion—are a result of multitudes of biochemical reactions taking place in cells and tissues throughout the body. Many of these reactions involve oxidation—the consumption or involvement of oxygen in the reaction—and oxidation characteristically results in the production of heat. If the body produces too much or too little heat, it is logical to assume that these reactions are not taking place at their usual rate. And when this happens, there is almost invariably a reason for it.

In the healthy human body, the internal temperature usually varies only slightly within the so-called normal range, no matter how hot or cold it is outside or how strenuous the activity. Slight variations are regulated very carefully, not only for comfort, but because many of the chemical reactions in our cells, especially certain very important ones involving the enzymes, can proceed only within a narrow temperature range. To maintain this "normal" temperature our bodies have a number of complex regulating reactions all working at once. Most familiar, of course, is the tendency to perspire when the temperature outside or inside the body begins to rise, so that the evaporation of perspiration on the surface of the skin will help cool us off. By the same token, when the body is literally "overheated" the tiny capillary blood vessels in the skin tend to dilate, bringing more blood closer to the cool surface of the body and causing the familiar flush we see during strenuous exercise or when a fever is present.

By means of these regulating devices—built-in thermostats, so to speak—our body temperature is maintained within a surprisingly narrow range. Ordinarily the internal temperature of the body varies only a few tenths of a degree above or below 98.6° F. as measured under the tongue by an oral fever thermometer, or 99.6° F. if the temperature is measured rectally. (Rectal temperatures always run about one degree higher than oral measurements.) Every person has his own "normal" temperature very close to these averages. However, normal body temperature does vary slightly from one hour to the next, depending upon the day's activities; it may be a trifle lower than "normal" the first thing in the morning, and then may rise to perhaps half a degree above "normal" by late afternoon or evening. Many women also experience a slight change in temperature (two-tenths to four-tenths of a degree) for a few days right at the time of ovulation—the basis for the so-called rhythm method of birth control. But for all practical purposes any temperature a degree or more higher than these averages is abnormal, and is therefore considered a "fever."

When a fever is present, there is more going on than just a rise in body temperature. For some reason, the cells are consuming fuel at a faster rate. The heart beats faster, breathing is more rapid, and the whole tempo of internal body activity increases. These changes often provide the first clue that a fever is present, especially in children, where they are more marked and dramatic. A feverish child will often look flushed and heavy-lidded. He may seem more thirsty, more cranky and less active than usual. In some children, sudden vomiting is the first sign that a

fever is developing. An adult may complain of nagging headaches, sensitivity to light or pain behind the eyes, dryness of the mouth or aching muscles. An accurate temperature should be taken when any of these signs appear.

Two other signs often associated with a high fever are chills and fever crisis. Neither is dangerous in itself, but either may provide a clue that fever is present and may even suggest the cause of it. A *chill* is a sudden uncontrollable attack of shivering, accompanied by a feeling of coldness and a marked skin pallor; a child's teeth may actually begin to chatter. Chilling occurs when a fever is rising very rapidly, usually due to some septic or toxic condition in the body—a fast-moving bacterial or viral infection, for example.

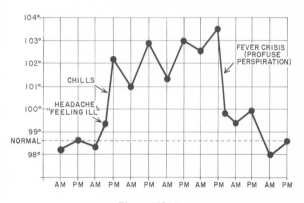

A FEVER CHART

Figure 13–1.

A *fever crisis* occurs when a high fever suddenly breaks and temperature drops to normal, whether from treatment of the fever or from natural causes. This may happen quite dramatically and be accompanied by profuse sweating—sometimes enough to soak pajamas and bedclothes. Some kinds of infections are characterized by fever crises followed by recurrent bouts of fever. In case of either chills or fever crisis, how the person *feels* may not be a safe indication of what his temperature is. Remember that how warm or cool a person feels to the touch is *never* a reliable gauge of body temperature. The temperature should be carefully *measured* and a doctor notified.

Measuring a Fever

Obviously a good fever thermometer is required to measure a temperature accurately. Always keep one handy (two, if there are children in the house, since one will inevitably get broken before an illness is over), preferably in a solid protective case out of the reach of children. Be sure to store it in a cool place; if it is left near a heat source (a hot water pipe, for example) it may be ruined when the mercury is driven up beyond the thermometer's maximum range, and a broken thermometer in a crisis is no help. A druggist can supply either the oral variety or a rectal thermometer with the mercury in a rounded bulb. Since the mercury in a fever thermometer does not fall back to normal spontaneously after a temperature has been taken, it must be shaken down before each use. Hold the end of the thermometer opposite the mercury bulb tightly in the fingers and snap the wrist until the mercury level is below 97° on the scale. Always cleanse the thermometer both before and after use with soap and cool (*not* hot) water, and then disinfect it with rubbing alcohol on a piece of cotton.

The most accurate temperature reading is taken with a lubricated rectal thermometer inserted approximately two inches into the rectum. This provides the truest possible measurement of the internal body temperature. In the case of infants, a rectal measurement is a necessity; babies just cannot hold a thermometer in their mouths. Turn the baby over on your lap, insert the thermometer and hold it loosely between two fingers, like a cigarette, to keep it gently in place. Three minutes is enough time for an accurate reading with a rectal thermometer.

If older children or adults find rectal thermometers uncomfortable, an oral thermometer can be used. It should be held as far under the tongue as possible for five minutes with the mouth kept closed. Remember that everyone has to breathe; be sure the nose is unplugged before taking an oral temperature, or else take the measurement rectally. Also bear in mind that oral temperatures can be affected by recent smoking or by drinking of hot or cold fluids. It is best to take the temperature before a meal, or wait at least half an hour after smoking.

Temperature readings *can* be taken with the thermometer held under the arm, but this method, however much more comfortable it may be, is too inaccurate to be relied upon. And the fact that someone has a hot forehead or "feels warm" has no significance at all. *The only way to judge a temperature is by actually measuring it.*

Don't feel foolish if you have trouble reading a fever thermometer. It does not look like the familiar alcohol thermometer hanging on the front porch, and it can be hard to read until you learn how. Your doctor can show you in a minute how to do it. The best way is to hold the thermometer between your thumb and forefinger with the scale side up. Then roll it back and forth slightly until the light catches the silver-colored mercury column. Each full degree on the scale is usually about a quarter of an inch long, and is marked in fractions of two-tenths of a degree so you can easily tell degrees and tenths. Most fever thermometers, in addition, have an arrow pointing at the 98.6° mark so that any variation from normal can easily be noted.

Foreign travelers should remember that in most countries other than the United States and Great Britain temperatures are normally measured on the Centigrade scale, instead of the Fahrenheit scale that we use, so fever thermometers purchased abroad may bear degree markings ranging from 35° to 40° Centigrade. Our familiar 98.6° Fahrenheit is exactly equivalent to 37° Centigrade, usually marked by an arrow or a change in color in the numbered scale.

Contending with a Fever

When a fever is present, several questions should come to your mind immediately. What does the fever mean? Why is it there and what does it signify? Should you call a doctor about it? If so, when? And what, if anything, should you be doing about it right away, whether you call a doctor or not? Obviously none of these questions has a simple, categorical answer that always applies, but each one is worth special consideration.

What does the fever mean? It may mean something entirely trivial and benign, or it could be a warning of serious trouble. It might mean one thing if a child has the fever and something quite different in an adult. Knowing something about fever in general will help you judge.

First of all a fever—*any* fever—means that *something* in the body has gone awry. Our built-in temperature-regulating reactions are far too efficient to allow temperature to rise more than momentarily as a result of "overheating" or some other nonspecific cause, except under extreme conditions like heat stroke or heat exhaustion.

Most often a fever means that infection of some kind is present in the body, whether it is an ear infection, an abscessed tooth or a case of measles. Sometimes noninfectious illnesses may also raise the body temperature, but this is far less common, and a concern that should be left to the physician. In general it is safe to assume that when someone develops a fever an infection is probably brewing somewhere and take it from there. You can often even judge the kind of infection just by observing the way the fever behaves. The body temperature may increase mildly, say to 100° or 101°, accompanying a head cold or flu. A child coming down with tonsillitis, an earache or one of the "childhood rash" illnesses may push up a temperature to 102° or more, early in the illness. In conditions such as meningitis, pneumonia or rubeola (the "red" or "hard" measles), fever can climb to 105° or above. A child is more likely to spike a high fever faster, with less apparent cause, than an adult—but whatever the fever, there is always a cause.

Should you call your doctor about a fever? If so, when? There is no cut-and-dried answer; it depends on the fever and the circumstances. Some people consider *any* fever a crisis and call the doctor whenever someone registers a temperature above 99°. This is overdoing it, perhaps, but it is certainly preferable to waiting until a child has had a raging 105° fever for

three days before deciding the time has come to call for medical help.

Aside from the threat of infection or whatever else is causing the temperature, is the fever *in itself* ever a danger? Sometimes yes. A mild fever does little harm even over a prolonged period of time, but a very high fever (106° or above) can actually damage nerve cells in the brain. In a child especially, a sudden high fever of 104° or more may cause sufficient nervous irritation to bring about delirium or even convulsions. *Any time a child with a fever begins to show twitchy or jerky movements of the arms, legs or fingers, you should take steps to get the temperature down without delay.* Even if a child has already begun convulsing, it is essential that someone in charge keep his wits about him and begin working to bring the temperature down. (*See* p. 154 below.)

A *febrile convulsion* in a child can be a dramatic and frightening thing to observe. Usually it is simply a response to a very rapidly rising fever, although some children may have seizures without fever later. Children with a high "convulsion threshold" may show no sign of convulsing even at temperatures of 105° or higher; other children can begin to show signs of nervous irritability as temperatures rise to 102° or 103° and may convulse any time a temperature rises much higher than that. Pediatricians believe that, as with chills, it is the rapid rise of a temperature that causes a seizure rather than the actual height of the temperature.

In some children subject to febrile convulsions, a sudden seizure may be the first clue that a feverish illness is present. But more often a child will show some evidence that a fever convulsion is imminent. Typically, his arm and hand motions become jerky, his fingers may twitch, and his body movements become uncoordinated. During the convulsion itself (which may last from a few seconds to half a minute) the child will apparently lose consciousness, clench his teeth, stiffen his arms and legs and then show characteristic jerking or convulsive body movements until the seizure passes. At such a time the child may hurt himself by striking his head, biting his tongue, hurling himself off the bed or other such uncontrolled movements. Protect him by placing him—and keeping him—on a bed or mattress, and insert something soft (such as a rolled-up handkerchief) between his teeth if you have an opportunity. Once the convulsion is over the child may be confused or disoriented for a period of up to an hour or more, and if the fever is not controlled, repeated convulsions may occur.

Frightening as febrile convulsions may seem, there is no need to panic. Recognize them as the reaction of a body and nervous system that have temporarily become too warm because of the fever, and take steps to reduce the fever as quickly as possible. Call your doctor, but see that fever control has been undertaken first.

Often a child who has once convulsed with a high fever will do so again any time a fever turns up, even a comparatively low fever, unless it is carefully controlled. No one knows why one child suffers this kind of sensitivity to fevers while another does not, but it should be emphasized that sensitivity to a fever does not necessarily mean that the child is, or will ever become, epileptic. Fever convulsions are generally outgrown eventually, but as long as the sensitivity exists there should be close cooperation among parent, child and doctor to spot incipient convulsions before they occur and, whenever possible, to prevent them by combating the child's fever—*any* fever—the moment it appears. In such a case the doctor may well prescribe a standby supply of a mild sedative such as elixir of phenobarbital which can be given to the child in a prearranged dose the moment fever is discovered, along with aspirin for fever control. Or he may prescribe small daily doses of a sedative for a longer period of time as a protection against febrile convulsions. Above all, you should carefully observe the individual "fever patterns" demonstrated by your children, since each child may display his own consistent and distinctive reactions.

Aside from the threat of febrile convulsions, when should you call your doctor about a fever? Many people hesitate, especially if they have been rebuked for "bothering" a doctor some time in the past about a fever that he considered unimportant. If your own doctor has certain special procedures he wants you to follow when someone in your family develops a fever, by all means follow his advice. Otherwise you must rely on your own good judgment and common sense. Obviously there will be times when an immediate call is not necessary; at other times a doctor should be notified without delay. Following are some useful guidelines that doctors often recommend.

When a person has a mild fever of a degree or two and neither feels nor looks particularly sick, there is usually no cause for alarm. Minor upper respiratory infections, simple "flu-like" gastrointestinal upsets, etc., can cause a slight temperature and may disappear by morning. In such cases you can safely postpone calling the doctor and wait to see what happens.

With a child, you may be able to guess from other indications whether a mild fever is likely to climb higher during the night. Does he have a sore throat? An earache? A harsh or croupy cough? Any sign of stiffness of the neck? In such cases, your doctor will probably want to know (and the earlier the better) about any fever higher than a degree or two. A doctor would rather be alerted at eight in the evening about a child with a fever of 101° which may get worse than to be called at 2 A.M. when the fever has reached 105° and the child is convulsing. He may simply recommend fever control at first, but at least he will know something is up, and will be prepared if you have to call him again later on. Doctors know full well that small children in particular can become very ill very quickly, and that fever is often the first warning.

In an adult, most infections do not move so rapidly, and fevers seldom climb so high. Here, you can often safely temporize with simple things such as aspirin and fluids, at least for the night. If the temperature is normal again by morning, it should be checked periodically the next day to see if it goes back up. If it does, call the doctor regardless of how high it is.

Any temperature of 102° or more in either an adult or a child should at least be reported to your doctor as soon as it is detected. He will decide whether he thinks a formal visit is necessary. But when you *do* call the doctor, be sure you have actually *taken* the temperature, because that will be the first question he asks. It is no help at all if your answer is, "Well, I don't have a thermometer, but his forehead feels awfully hot."

Often a doctor will want to see a patient who has just begun developing a temperature, and may ask the patient to come to his office, or to meet him at the hospital. Many people have the mistaken idea that some grave harm may result from taking a person with a fever outdoors, or from driving him to the doctor's office in a car. Usually these fears are unfounded. If the person is warmly clothed, a short trip will do no harm whatever, and it may help the doctor immensely in coping with the situation quickly under ideal medical conditions. Again, once the doctor has been called, follow his instructions scrupulously in taking repeated temperature measurements. In any feverish illness, the *pattern* of the fever may be a vital clue to the diagnosis, and your doctor will rely on you to keep a close and accurate record if he considers it necessary.

In most serious infectious illnesses, fever is usually high enough to serve as a good warning. But perhaps most dangerous of all, especially in adults, is the fever which appears consistently day after day in the afternoon or evening—perhaps only a degree or two, never quite high enough to call a doctor, but either persisting or recurring for a prolonged period of time. Such a persisting or recurrent *low-grade fever* may have a perfectly benign explanation, but it *could* be a subtle early signal of a dangerous illness—of tuberculosis, for example, or chronic urinary tract infection, or cancer. In such cases, early diagnosis might well mean the difference between life and death. *Never ignore a persistent or recurring fever, no matter how mild or insignificant it may appear.*

Fever of Unknown Origin (FUO)

The cause of most fevers is clear-cut and readily apparent. But occasionally, particularly with a low-grade, persisting or recurring fever, the cause may be much more subtle, and both patient and doctor are faced with one of the most difficult of diagnostic problems—the dilemma of an FUO.

A fever always means something, and the reason for it must be found. But an FUO cannot be accounted for by any indication, sign or symptom that either patient or doctor can discover, at least immediately. Sometimes an FUO is not even recognized at first. Fortunately, many people can tell quite accurately when they have even a slight fever because of accompanying signs and symptoms they have learned to recognize—a so-called fever headache, an odd feeling about the eyes, a sense of thirstiness, a characteristic kind of stiff neck, muscle aching or other suggestive symptoms. Such "recognition patterns" are not at all uncommon, and usually they are followed by other symptoms and reactions that clearly indicate their cause. But when no further symptoms appear and the fever persists, apparently without cause, a thorough diagnostic search must be undertaken. Such a study may seem a troublesome bother; a person with an FUO generally does not feel very good in the first place, his energy (and patience) are at low ebb, his appetite poor, his sleep disturbed. Why should he have to put up with a doctor's examination and a lot of costly lab tests? The answer is that an FUO may be an early sign of very serious trouble. The sooner its cause is identified the better.

Usually an FUO is caused by some kind of hidden or *occult infection.* If a careful history and physical examination fail to provide clues, laboratory studies may help pin down the cause. These will usually include a complete blood count, a urine examination, a bacterial culture from the nose and throat, and an X-ray film of the chest. A high white blood cell count may provide a clue to an acute or chronic bacterial infection somewhere in the body, whereas an unusually low white cell count often indicates virus infections. A common site for hidden infections, especially in girls and young women, is the urinary tract; such infections may be identified by the presence of white blood cells in the urine. A chest X-ray may reveal an unsuspected lung infection—perhaps a viral pneumonia, or even early tuberculosis—and a nose and throat culture may disclose an active streptococcus or staphylococcus infection before other signs and symptoms begin to appear.

Failing to find the source of the fever from

these screening examinations, the doctor must dig deeper to rule out the most likely or most dangerous causes of FUO's for each age group. In babies the doctor will think of bacterial infections of the respiratory tract, especially pneumonia or meningitis. A baby, of course, cannot tell a doctor that he has a headache and a stiff neck, two common symptoms of meningitis, so most pediatricians will perform a "spinal tap" or lumbar puncture on a baby if no other reason for an undiagnosed fever can be found.

In children of preschool age, persisting upper respiratory infections continue to be the most likely cause of fevers of unknown origin—especially tonsillitis, middle-ear infection (otitis media) or pneumonia. In this age group certain kinds of childhood cancers, particularly leukemia, may first manifest themselves with an otherwise unaccountable fever. Congenital malformation of the kidneys, ureters, or bladder may also be discovered at this age through the appearance of occult urinary tract infections. Repeated urine examinations may prove diagnostic in these cases.

Children from six to fifteen years old are generally quite resistant to infection, but hidden respiratory infections may still cause FUO's in this age group. So can chronically infected tonsils, kidney infection or virus diseases such as infectious hepatitis or infectious mononucleosis ("glandular fever"). Later symptoms and further tests and X-rays usually pin down the diagnosis, but the FUO is often the first indication that such an examination is necessary.

When an older child or an adult develops an FUO, the doctor must worry about other possible causes as well as occult infection. Pulmonary tuberculosis may first appear in young adulthood and reveal itself only by a low-grade evening fever and night sweats. The so-called *collagen diseases* (connective tissue diseases) such as rheumatic fever, lupus erythematosus, or cancers such as Hodgkin's disease (cancer of the lymph glands) may also first appear as puzzling fevers with no apparent cause. Finally, the possibility of bacterial infection of the inner lining of the heart or the heart valves (known as *subacute bacterial endocarditis* or "SBE") must

be considered in any patient with a persisting fever, especially if a heart murmur is present.

It should be emphasized, however, that an occasional, sudden fever—even a high one—by no means implies some grave underlying cause. Everyone develops a fever now and then, and it should be no reason for panic. But a truly worrisome FUO is something clearly and recognizably different. It is *always* persistent and *always* recurrent. And when it is present, diagnosis may require time, patience, and the utmost cooperation with your doctor. The tip-off may lie in some relatively minor change the doctor notices from one visit to the next, and therefore repeated examinations and laboratory studies may be necessary.

Usually diligent and patient observation will at last reveal the cause of an occult fever—but not always. Sometimes an FUO is *never* satisfactorily diagnosed. Occasionally it will just disappear spontaneously, and not return. More often, your doctor, even in the absence of a diagnosis, will finally prescribe some antibiotic. If he does this, it will be only after he has carefully weighed the possible risk of "flying blind" against the risk of delaying treatment while a hidden infection becomes more deeply entrenched. Often there is no "right" or "wrong" answer to this dilemma; each doctor must resolve it on the basis of his impression of the individual case and his experience in dealing with occult infections, and then, perhaps, only after securing expert consultation. No one knows better than he that a fever of unknown origin is not to be trifled with.

Controlling a Fever

The simple fact that a low-grade fever is present does not necessarily mean that the fever itself must be treated. Indeed, treating a low fever too actively before the cause of the fever has been determined may simply mask the fact that it is there, and possibly cover up other signs and symptoms that might help with the diagnosis. Thus you should not attempt to fight down a fever of a degree or so too militantly before notifying a doctor and obtaining some idea of the cause, unless the temperature is rising rapidly or the victim is subject to febrile convulsions.

Once a diagnosis is made and treatment begun, it is generally *desirable* to reduce a mild fever by conservative means, and *necessary* to do so when the fever is high—103.5° or above. Several effective steps can be taken. First, especially in the case of children, keep the house comfortably warm (72° to 75°) but *cover the child with only a minimum of clothing or bedclothes*. The first thing mothers tend to do with a feverish child, especially if he is chilling, is to bundle him up with blankets—and nothing can be more foolish. A hot child cannot be cold at the same time, and piling on blankets can only *increase* the fever. Dress a feverish child lightly —underclothing or light pajamas are plenty— and use no more than a sheet or light cotton blanket on the bed. This alone will help control fever, or at the least will not make it worse.

The safest and most effective medicine for reducing fever is ordinary garden-variety aspirin. Adults or children over age ten may safely use two five-grain tablets every four hours. For smaller children, a rule-of-thumb dose is one grain for each year of age given at four-hour intervals. But dosage should not be continued for longer than 24 hours at a time without a doctor's permission, since children of that age may develop aspirin toxicity. Children's aspirin comes in 1¼-grain tablets, pleasantly flavored and chewable. For very small children use *aspirin suppositories*—aspirin prepared in small waxy pellets for insertion in the rectum. These can be very helpful in the middle of the night, especially if the child is vomiting, as so many do when fever is spiking up. Liquid aspirin (trade name Tempra) is also excellent for infants and small children, and is even more reliable than suppositories. One warning: because most forms of children's aspirin are flavored, they can easily be mistaken by the child for candy and eaten in a dangerous, and possibly fatal, overdose. In fact, aspirin is the number one killer of children who ingest a poison. Incredibly enough, some children will even eat unflavored aspirin. *Keep any aspirin, flavored or not, locked up in a cupboard.*

Another way to bring down a high fever is by sponging the patient with either lukewarm water or a half-and-half mixture of water and rubbing alcohol. (*Never* use ice-cold water except on a doctor's specific orders; an ice-water sponge bath can reduce the patient's temperature so abruptly that he goes into shock.) Get the patient sloppy wet on his neck, back, chest, arms and legs and then fan the skin dry with a magazine or an electric fan. Children may object violently— after all, it feels cold. But it will almost always bring a dangerously high fever under control. At the same time, keep the patient *in bed* and urge him to drink fluids. Any fever that fails to respond to these measures, or that spikes up again, may require special medication for control. In any case, let your doctor know what is happening.

With some kinds of illnesses, particularly those lasting a long time, fever may present a problem in long-term care. Prolonged fever in itself is debilitating, often accompanied by a decrease in appetite and a resultant loss of weight. In addition, with faster metabolism, faster breathing and heavier perspiration, more body fluid is lost than usual, so the patient may become dehydrated. The amount of urination is an excellent measure of dehydration; if a child is just not urinating very much, he is dry and needs fluids. In febrile illnesses of any duration, encourage the patient to drink extra fluids to combat dehydration. It is usually better to urge a feverish patient to drink two or three ounces of fluid at hourly intervals rather than a pint or two twice a day. Under these conditions he is unlikely to drink too much fluid, so don't worry about exceeding any maximum amount per day. Bear in mind that a patient with a fever will not feel particularly well, so try to choose fluids he especially likes. Water and other liquids (short of wine or any alcoholic beverage, which tends to increase dehydration) are fine, but fruit juices and noncarbonated soft drinks are even better. Kool-Aid, Hawaiian Punch and Gatorade are outstanding. Remember that in a young child or infant a combination of high temperature and vomiting (with or without concomitant diarrhea) can result in extreme dehydration within a very short time. Any time a child has a fever associated with either vomiting or diarrhea, even in small amounts, a doctor should be notified without delay. In addition to supplying extra fluids, nutrition should be maintained with a high-vitamin, high-protein diet, perhaps broken up into several small feedings instead of three large meals a day.

Special Causes for Fever

Most fevers are related to infectious illnesses, but some of the highest and most dangerous fevers may result from actual damage to the heat-regulating mechanism in the brain, either as a result of a head injury of some sort or because of a hemorrhage or *vascular accident* (often called a "stroke") that has taken place inside the skull. Often such accidents occur suddenly, accompanied by an excruciating headache; in many cases the patient will become unconscious or comatose. *Any* fever over 103° in an unconscious person, or a high fever that does not respond to the normal, conservative temperature control methods discussed above, should be called to a doctor's attention without delay.

Finally, the body may become feverish in extremely hot weather, particularly if the individual engages in heavy physical exercise. This is *heat stroke* or *sunstroke,* and it should be suspected whenever a person, exposed to high outside temperatures, spikes a fever without any other apparent cause. He feels warm to the touch, has a flushed face and rapid pulse, becomes prostrated and has difficulty breathing. Temperatures as high as 105° or 106° are common, and convulsions or coma may ensue. The condition is a serious threat to life and carries a mortality as high as 20 percent.

Sunstroke should not, however, be confused with *heat exhaustion,* a far less dangerous response to extreme outside temperatures. The victim of heat exhaustion will have a near-normal temperature, but his skin will be ashen, cold and damp, with profuse sweating, much as if he were going to faint. He will usually respond quickly to rest in the shade, cool water and good ventilation, but the sunstroke victim's life may depend on prompt first-aid treatment to reduce his temperature. (*See* p. 136.)

14

Home Health Care

When illness strikes, whether it is acute or chronic, one of the decisions that must be made is just where and how the patient can be most effectively treated. Often, of course, no such decision is necessary. If the illness is comparatively minor or usually quickly curable, the patient simply consults the doctor in his office, perhaps undergoes certain diagnostic laboratory or X-ray studies there, and then returns home for the duration of treatment, with follow-up visits to the doctor if necessary. In the case of sick children, in particular, most doctors are reluctant to put their young patients in the hospital unless it is absolutely essential, and try instead to treat the illness at home whenever possible. At the other extreme there are certain kinds of acute illnesses in which at least some period of hospitalization may be imperative, since a hospital offers certain advantages in the treatment of the seriously ill which simply cannot be duplicated anywhere else.

Aside from these extremes, however, there are many instances in which a real choice exists between treating the patient in a hospital, in some intermediate facility such as a nursing home or an extended-care unit of a hospital, or caring for him at home. Even in cases of serious or prolonged illness in which hospital care is mandatory at first, the time usually comes when full-scale hospitalization is no longer necessary and convalescence can be safely undertaken either at a nursing home or in the patient's own home. In such cases the decision for or against home care is an important one, and should be made only with a full awareness of all the factors involved.

In the long run it is the doctor who carries the major responsibility for a patient's speedy recovery, and it is he who is best able to judge when the patient's condition is such that hospitalization is no longer necessary. Until the doctor himself feels that a patient can be treated as effectively at home as in the hospital, no attempt should be made to force the issue. It is true, of course, that a hospitalized patient is not a prisoner, and that an adult patient or the parent of a sick child has, in most cases, the legal right to terminate hospitalization even against medical advice. But in the vast majority of cases this is a foolish step and is rarely in the patient's best interests. Doctors have no reason to keep a patient in the hospital any longer than necessary, and they are as aware of the burgeoning cost of hospital care as their patients. But when the time comes that a patient can be safely released, or treated just as effectively at home as in the hospital, there should be a frank discussion between the patient, his family and the doctor regarding all of the factors that must be considered in a given case.

Expense is often a major consideration; hospital care is costly, and few medical insurance plans cover *all* the expenses of hospitalization. But other factors must also be considered. Are conditions at home suitable for home nursing care of the patient, or can they be adapted to this purpose? Just who will do the nursing, and how much time will it take? What psychological effects will home nursing care have on the patient and on other family members? How closely and effectively will the doctor be able to follow the patient's further progress? What special nursing procedures may be necessary on account of the nature of the patient's illness, and how can provision be made for taking care of them? What help is available to the family of the patient in terms of home nursing services, preparation of special diets, the assistance of housekeepers or the administration of medication?

In many cases, these questions can be satisfactorily answered, and it may be entirely possible, far less costly and generally better for the sick patient to be treated at home as soon as it is medically plausible. And while home nursing care can be time-consuming and requires patience and diligence, with the application of common sense and knowledge of a few basic skills, it need not be as difficult as it may seem.

Caring for Sick Children

Just as the important considerations related to home health care vary greatly depending upon the nature of the illness, they also vary according to the age and special needs of the patient. Children's illnesses are most often of the kind that do not require hospitalization. The vast majority of them are infectious diseases, sometimes serious, but more often comparatively mild and self-limited. Either they are quickly curable with antibiotic treatment or else, as in the case of virus-caused childhood rash diseases, they tend to clear up by themselves after a few days of moderately acute illness. But even with more serious or prolonged illnesses—acute rheumatic fever, for example, or infectious hepatitis or acute glomerulonephritis—most doctors encourage treatment of the child at home rather than in the hospital, or, when hospitalization is necessary, they try to get the child home for convalescence as quickly as possible. This is because children do not ordinarily have much experience with illness, and when sickness strikes they are often confused, frightened and very unhappy. At such times they require the comfort, reassurance

and sympathy of parents and other family members, and friendly faces and the familiar environment of their own homes are more conducive to speedy recovery than the strange and often impersonal environment of a hospital.

Home nursing care of most relatively minor childhood illnesses is simple and easily managed. A generation ago it was widely believed that a sick child had to be rigidly restricted to bed, isolated from other members of the family, and forced by one means or another to "rest" continuously until the illness was over. Modern pediatricians regard many of these restrictions as ridiculous. They have come to recognize that an acutely ill child will generally remain in bed simply because he *is* ill, will show little interest in activity or play and will naturally get as much rest as the requirements of the illness demand without any special effort on the part of his parents. Further, when the acute phase of an illness subsides, there is no point in forcing a child to stay in bed; he can be treated quite as well, and will usually recover quite as fast, if he is allowed to be up and about, dressed warmly in a bathrobe and slippers, kept indoors, and encouraged to content himself with quiet forms of play. He should also be encouraged to sleep as late in the morning as he can, and to take an afternoon rest or nap, and then gradually be allowed to resume normal activities as the illness subsides.

Since fever is a surprisingly reliable measure of the activity of an infectious illness in children, the temperature should be taken and recorded at three regular times during the day: when the child first awakens in the morning before he is up and about or has eaten breakfast, again in the late afternoon and a third time just prior to going to bed. Typically fevers are lower in the morning and rise steadily throughout the day, and many pediatricians feel that a childhood infectious illness should not be considered over until the temperature remains normal throughout the day for two consecutive days. At the time the temperature is taken the parent can also check closely for the appearance, or disappearance, of any unusual conditions—coughing, the progress of a skin rash, swelling of lymph glands in the neck, axillae or groin, difficulty in breathing, or any other symptoms of interest to the doctor. He will tell the home nurse just what to look for, and obviously his orders for medication, including aspirin for fever control, diet and additional liquids throughout the day, or the administration of antibiotics, should be carefully followed. It is also important that any medications, including aspirin, be kept out of the child's reach to avert the possibility of accidental overdosage.

Most doctors today do not attempt to separate a sick child from other children in the family, recognizing that most infectious diseases that can be spread by contact will spread within the home anyway, whether or not the child is isolated, and isolation is likely to be more discouraging to the youngster than it is helpful in preventing the spread of an infection. When the disease is infectious, however, it is advisable to use a special set of dishes and utensils for the sick child, washing them separately from the rest of the family dishes and, if the doctor recommends it, sterilizing them in water at a rolling boil for a period of 20 minutes after each washing. In the case of some illnesses it is also advisable that bed linens, towels and washcloths be boiled before returning them to general use. With some particularly dangerous infectious diseases—infectious hepatitis, for example—particular attention to rigid procedures of toilet hygiene may also be necessary, making certain that both the patient and others in the family are especially fastidious about hand washing following the use of the toilet and, where necessary, disinfecting the toilet after each use. The doctor's advice should be sought with regard to any special sanitary procedures required for a specific illness, and his recommendations should be followed closely.

Finally, while the sick child requires sympathy, understanding, comfort, and perhaps a special effort to keep foods and beverages varied and interesting, he should also be allowed to do as much for himself as he can, and he should not receive so much attention that he feels being sick is more pleasant than being well. His care should be primarily directed toward encouraging him to get well as quickly as possible.

Home Care of the Handicapped or Chronically Ill Patient

Most childhood illnesses are fairly brief and do not require any basic changes in the organization or management of the household. When the illness involves a physical handicap which may be long-term or permanent, however, or the kind of disorder which may cause prolonged disability either in a child or in an adult, certain special home nursing techniques are usually necessary, and prolonged home nursing care may require some basic adjustments in the family's way of life, not only to make home care of the patient possible, but also to take into account the everyday needs of the other members of the family. If a child contracts such comparatively long-term disabilities as acute rheumatic fever, fibrocystic disease, or chronic nephrosis, for example, actual confinement at rest in bed for prolonged periods may be necessary, and certain specialized kinds of care may be required. It may be advisable to provide for tutoring and home study so that he does not fall too far behind in his school work. It may also be advisable to arrange his room so that toys, books, games and television are easily available without requiring too much physical activity. In short, a great deal of imagination and ingenuity may be necessary to help the child keep up with his lessons or find things to do for amusement, including arranging for company and allowing the child to participate in normal household activities at least as much as his illness will permit.

If the patient is an adult who is physically handicapped—a person recovering from a stroke with residual paralysis, for example, an automobile accident victim with paraplegia as a result of a spinal cord injury, or a person seriously handicapped by Parkinson's disease—long-term care must be integrated with other household activities so that the needs of both the patient and the rest of the family can be met. In such cases, too, home care may involve the skills of physical therapy or rehabilitation, carefully graduated and supervised periods of exercise, and other nursing techniques that require special instruction and practice to perform. For example, the paraplegic patient who has lost the normal neurological control of his bladder may have to use an "in-dwelling" or permanently placed catheter to drain his bladder, and when a catheter must remain for prolonged periods, the doctor may order that it be irrigated once or twice daily with special sterile solutions to prevent the catheter from becoming clogged with sediment and to reduce the chances of bladder infection. These and other special nursing techniques must, of course, be learned by the individual in the family responsible for the care of the patient, or by the patient himself, but in many cases mastering such procedures can make home nursing care possible in situations that would otherwise require hospitalization.

Special home care requirements must also be met if the patient is chronically ill or a long-term convalescent, but again they usually vary widely according to the illness. For example, the patient convalescing at home from pulmonary tuberculosis must have medication at regularly specified times, his temperature must be measured and recorded at regular intervals, and sputum specimens must be collected periodically for examination. The patient convalescing from an acute coronary attack must have daily exercise as specified by the doctor, with adequate periods of bed rest and a steady but graduated resumption of everyday activities, all designed to rebuild the strength and capability of a damaged heart as quickly as possible without subjecting it to an intolerable overload. Other chronic illnesses also require special nursing techniques or precautions which must be spelled out by the doctor and then checked periodically by him, a visiting nurse or some other qualified professional to assure that they are being performed effectively and that no unexpected problems have been encountered.

Obviously in providing home health care for such patients it is imperative that the person undertaking the primary responsibility be as fully informed about the nature of the illness as possible, in order to be able to recognize problems when and if they arise and to provide knowledgeable contact with the attending physician. But when the patient is suffering from a long-term disability, emotional support may be at least as important as the physical necessities

of nursing care, if not more so. It is critical that the patient be helped to adjust to his illness or disability as fully and as quickly as possible, and he must be encouraged to do as much as he can for himself, so that he does not come to feel that he is a total burden. Efforts must be made to vary his daily routines to some degree in order to help counteract boredom and depression, and above all, the patient (whose illness may seem literally interminable to him) must not be allowed to become a "forgotten man" in the household, left out of family councils and isolated from family activities. The more chronic his illness or the more long-term his convalescence, the more important it is that he feel that he is still wanted, useful and cherished by the other members of the family. This kind of emotional support can make an important difference in helping the patient resume his normal, healthy place in life with a minimum of struggle or trauma when his convalescence at last is over, or if the illness is permanent, and destined ultimately to be terminal, it will help immensely in enabling him to maintain his dignity and to draw as much active enjoyment from life as possible.

The Elderly Patient

Home nursing care of the elderly patient can present many of the same problems as the care of the handicapped or chronically ill, depending upon the nature of the illness, but there may be certain other problems as well. Whatever the particular disabilities of the elderly patient, he may also be physically weak and handicapped or partially crippled. An illness that has required a long period of bed rest may have completely sapped his strength, he may be limited in helping himself by failing sight or failing hearing, and not infrequently he may be exceptionally slow, because of his various disabilities, in such normal activities as getting in and out of bed, dressing, using the bath or toilet and feeding himself. Finally, the elderly patient may also suffer a degree of senility and be confused or disoriented, exceptionally irritable, querulous or demanding, or otherwise difficult to care for. For such a patient the ordinary routines of waking up and getting out of bed in the morning, going to the toilet, getting dressed, and eating breakfast may, in themselves, constitute an exhausting day's work; many are unable to accomplish some or all of these procedures and, indeed, many may be permanently bedridden.

If the patient is bedridden a number of special nursing procedures may be necessary. For example, he must be turned from side to side, propped up in bed or placed flat at regular intervals throughout the day, not only to ensure proper aeration of the lungs and prevention of stasis pneumonia, but also to relieve too much continuing pressure on certain parts of the body which can impair circulation, break down the skin and ultimately lead to the formation of pressure sores. (*See* p. 386.) Such areas as the shoulder blades, the skin of the low back overlying the sacrum, and even the heels are particularly vulnerable to pressure sores. Other problems in the care of a bedridden patient include such procedures as bathing in bed, feeding him and assisting him with the use of a bedpan or the toilet. (*See* below.) Obviously home nursing care of an elderly patient can require considerably more time than the care of younger or more able patients, but with the elderly as with anyone else it is important to provide reassurance and emotional support in addition to physical comfort. Again, the patient should be encouraged to do as much as possible for himself, even when some of the simplest everyday procedures could be done for him much more quickly. Great patience and understanding are essential, allowances must be made to accommodate the patient's specialized needs and interests, and family and friends alike should do everything possible to make the patient feel wanted and useful. In the long run this kind of emotional support will do much to speed recovery or convalescence when this is possible, and may greatly reduce the nursing care burden even in those cases in which full recovery is not expected.

General Pointers for the Home Nurse

It is impossible here to discuss in detail all the nursing procedures that might be necessary to provide home health care for a sick patient. More specific information is available in a number of excellent manuals or textbooks of bedside nursing, and anyone about to undertake home nursing care should ask the attending physician, the visiting nurse service or even the head of the nursing department of the local hospital to recommend the books that will be most helpful. In addition, the special nursing techniques related to the individual patient's illness should be discussed thoroughly with the physician and, if necessary, instruction obtained under professional guidance. There are, however, a few basic general pointers that everyone should know with regard to home nursing care, whether nursing duties are to be brief or prolonged.

The Home Nurse's Attitude. Perhaps the most important consideration in approaching the very real problems of providing home nursing care is the attitude of the individual upon whom the bulk of the responsibility will fall. Home nursing care is often hard work, it can consume surprising amounts of time, and it may require considerable planning in order to make it practicable. But if the home nurse looks upon it as an unpleasant "duty" or a burden, it should probably not be undertaken at all. Not only will such an attitude make the necessary work even more difficult; it will also inevitably be communicated to the patient, affecting his progress or causing him additional distress. Home nursing care must not be regarded as a burden, but rather it must be undertaken willingly and cheerfully if it is to be truly effective. If the amount of time consumed is such that it detracts from other household duties, plans should be made either to delegate household chores to other members of the family during the critical period or to obtain temporary outside help. It is of equal importance that someone else take over the nursing care from time to time so that the home nurse can be relieved at regular intervals.

In addition, the individual primarily responsible for home nursing care must be capable of close observation of the patient and clear communication with the doctor about the patient's condition. The doctor depends upon the home nurse to keep him informed about the patient's progress, to recognize and report any significant changes and to follow his instructions meticulously. Thus the home nurse must keep the necessary health records, be alert for symptoms of decline or improvement, accept responsibility for giving the necessary medications in the right amounts at the right times in addition to providing the all-important physical and emotional support the patient needs.

The Patient's Room. Careful attention must be paid to the selection of a room that will lend itself most satisfactorily to the patient's, as well as the home nurse's, needs. Because rest and quiet are essential, the room should be, if possible, secluded and out of the main traffic pattern of the house. It should be close to a bathroom—certainly on the same floor—and inasmuch as possible close to cooking and eating facilities as well. Remember that stair climbing may be impossible for the patient, and an additional burden on the home nurse, so that everything necessary to the patient's care should be located on the same floor. When stair climbing is a must, it may be of value to investigate rental or purchase of a mechanical lift device. Finally, the sickroom should be clean and easy to keep clean, quiet, attractive, well ventilated, properly heated and provided with ample light.

The Patient's Bed. The bed in the sickroom should be chosen both for maximum comfort for the patient and for maximum convenience for the home nurse. If the patient's regular bed is to be used, a bed board should be placed underneath the mattress to prevent it from sagging—a piece of quarter-inch plywood slightly smaller than the mattress is ideal. A triangular backrest for use when the patient is sitting up in bed is preferable to the use of two or three pillows, and will minimize the tendency of the patient to slide down in the bed. Such a backrest can be purchased in a hospital supply store or can be constructed out of a large cardboard carton padded with foam rubber or sheeting. In addition, a footboard should be installed at the end of the bed to prevent the patient from sliding down in the bed and to provide support for his feet. If a long illness is anticipated, it may be wise to rent or purchase a hospital-type bed, with cranks that tilt the mattress in various ways. A hospital bed is higher than a normal bed, and thus a stool will be necessary for the patient to get in and out of it, but it is an ideal height for nursing care and

lends itself splendidly to shifting and changing the patient's position.

The bed should be placed in the room so the home nurse can move around it easily, and light, clean bedding should be used and changed frequently—as often as twice or three times a week if the patient is in the bed continuously. Use of a natural lambskin sheet against the skin will help prevent pressure ulcers. When treating a child or an elderly patient who may suffer from urinary incontinence, it is well to use a protective rubber or plastic undersheet over the mattress beneath the regular sheet. Care should be taken, however, that the undersheet is kept tight and as wrinkle-free as possible. The doctor should be consulted about the advisability of an overhead frame for the bed to enable the patient to help move himself about. In cases in which exercise and physical therapy are important adjuncts to care, such a frame, which can be rented or purchased from a hospital supply company for fitting to a hospital bed, can be invaluable.

In making a patient's bed, one must tuck the lower sheet in tightly or miter it in order to avoid any creases or wrinkles which may be irritating to the patient's skin. The upper sheet and blanket should be arranged to leave the patient as much freedom of motion as possible. If the patient can be out of bed for intervals, it is, of course, easy to make the bed. But even if he cannot get up, the bedmaking procedure is not difficult. The patient should simply be moved or rolled to one side of the bed while the unoccupied side is made, and then rolled back to the newly made side while the other side is made. With care and practice, this can be done with even the sickest patient.

Bathing the Patient. In the vast majority of cases the patient will be far more comfortable and contented if he is allowed to bathe himself, either in a bathtub or, if possible, in a shower. If the patient is weak or debilitated, of course, someone should stay in attendance to help him while he bathes. If bathing in the bed is required, the patient may still be able to do most of it himself with the use of a pan of warm wash water, a pan of warm rinse water and a washcloth and towel within easy reach on a bedside stand. In order to avoid getting the bed wet, it is wise to dry each part of the body as soon as it has been washed and rinsed before going on to the next part. When bed bathing is necessary, either by the patient himself or by the home nurse, the home nurse will have to assist in washing the back, shoulders, and buttocks. Bear in mind that bathing in bed is a slow and inconvenient process and may be quite exhausting for the seriously debilitated patient. Thus it should be planned for early in the day, and the patient should have a period of rest afterward.

Feeding the Patient. In most cases the patient will be able to feed himself from a bedside tray of convenient height or from a hospital-type bed table that slips over the bed. Eating is easiest with the patient sitting upright, and care should be taken to keep the food warm and make it as varied, appetizing and attractive as possible; a sick patient often has little enough appetite as it is, and every effort should be made to encourage him to take the nourishment he needs. If for some reason the patient must be fed by the home nurse, instructions from the doctor or from a hospital or visiting nurse acquainted with the procedure will greatly simplify the process. Since the patient may be extremely slow about chewing or swallowing food, he must be given plenty of time, and mealtimes should be unhurried and cheerful.

Helping the Patient Go to the Toilet. The use of regular toilet facilities in a nearby bathroom is by far the most satisfactory if the patient is able to get to it with or without aid. For patients who cannot get out of bed, a hospital urinal, a bedpan or both may be necessary. Again, the techniques for using these devices can most easily be learned with instructions from the hospital or visiting nurse. The use of both a urinal and a bedpan is much easier if the patient can be propped up in a sitting position. Be sure the bedpan is properly placed for reasonable comfort and an even distribution of the patient's weight. After use of the bedpan for a bowel movement, cleansing of the patient may best be accomplished by having him roll off the bedpan onto one side. A urinal or a bedpan should be promptly emptied, washed with hot water and

disinfectant and then thoroughly rinsed and dried.

Other Nursing Techniques. Other common nursing care procedures may or may not be necessary according to the nature of the illness, and the age and the capabilities of the patient. Temperature should be measured and recorded morning, midafternoon and evening, and the patient's pulse rate (the number of pulses per minute, usually measured at the wrist) and respiration rate (the number of inhalations or exhalations per minute) should also be recorded. If blood pressure measurements are necessary, the doctor can give instructions for the use of a blood pressure cuff and stethoscope. He will also spell out any other special nursing requirements: exercise, massage, applications of heat or cold, enemas or like procedures. One of the most important aspects of home nursing care is, of course, seeing that the patient receives prescribed medications in the dosage and at the time ordered by the doctor. Anyone responsible for home nursing care should have no hesitation about consulting the doctor as soon as any problem arises. Most problems can be easily resolved and can spare both the home nurse and the patient a great deal of needless worry or inconvenience.

Help for the Home Nurse

There was a time as little as a generation ago when anyone responsible for home nursing care of a family member was largely on her own, with no one but the doctor to turn to for help when problems arose. And the doctor, although competent in prescribing treatment and following the patient's progress from the medical point of view, was often as inexperienced as the home nurse about the details and specific techniques of nursing care. Today the home nurse has a wealth of professional services available to her, and home health care is frequently more effective with the help and guidance of a professional nursing facility.

Among the most important adjuncts to home health care that have appeared in recent years are the so-called extended care programs developed by many major hospitals to help meet the needs of the patient who does not really require intensive nursing care in the hospital, yet does require professional nursing supervision of his care at home. More than 250 hospitals in the United States have already instituted these programs to provide continuing and regular nursing supervision of the patient after he has returned home, with professional guidance and instruction for the member of the family who is responsible for the patient. In many cases these extended care programs permit the patient to return home from the hospital far earlier than would otherwise be possible. They are flexible enough to meet the needs of each individual patient, and their cost is usually a mere fraction of the cost of full hospital care. They also cost a great deal less than a nursing home facility, and in the case of prolonged illness, they can provide the means for a smooth, safe and gradual transfer from full-time hospital nursing facilities to home nursing care.

Other resources that the family may call upon at reasonable cost are the public health nursing services or the visiting nursing services available in most large communities. These services provide fully trained professional nurses who make regularly scheduled home visits, often frequently enough to take care of more difficult nursing procedures and special medication regimens; they also can help train the individual responsible for home health care and supervise its effectiveness. Information about the availability of these services in a community can be found by checking the telephone book under "Visiting Nurse Service" or inquiring of the County Health Department.

In cases involving the care of someone who is seriously ill or who requires particularly difficult or specialized nursing procedures, the problems of home care may be greatly simplified by calling on the services of a private duty nurse. Information about the availability of private duty nurses and their fees in your locality can be obtained by calling the Nurses' Professional Registry listed in the telephone book of most major cities. Private duty nurses ordinarily work eight-hour shifts, and around-the-clock private nursing can be very expensive. In many difficult

cases, however, a single eight-hour shift each day may be sufficient to take care of major nursing care problems at a reasonable cost, at least through the critical portion of an illness, and provide a workable alternative to full-scale hospitalization. If professional nursing supervision or services are not required, but the home nurse does need skilled help in caring for the patient, the services of a nurse's aide or a licensed practical nurse may be obtained. Registries of completely trained personnel in this field can be found in most major cities by checking the yellow pages of the telephone book under "Nursing" or "Nurses' Registries."

Finally, in a great many cases home nursing care is not in itself beyond the capability of a responsible family member but consumes so much time that many other household duties cannot be handled simultaneously. Hiring a part-time or full-time housekeeper may help solve this problem, and other members of the family can also contribute by helping the home nurse in any way they can. Home nursing can be difficult and time-consuming, even on a short-term basis, particularly when the home nurse must divide her time between the patient and the equally important needs of other members of the family. But with the many kinds of assistance available, it can be both practical and effective.

Home Medical Supplies

Home nursing care often requires a certain amount of special equipment to meet the specific needs of an individual patient. The doctor or other home nursing adviser can provide information about such special equipment and where to obtain it. Other than this, however, there are certain items of medical equipment and a variety of nonprescription medications that ought to be kept on hand under any circumstances in every home. The following is a representative list of the items which should be available for use at any time in the average home.

Nursing and Hygienic Equipment
Fever thermometers—one oral, one rectal
Cotton swabs (Q-Tips or similar)
Wooden tongue blades
Elastic bandages (Ace or similar)—2" and 4" widths

Band-Aids—assorted sizes
Ice bag
Vaporizer—preferably the "cold vapor" type, high
  output
Enema bag
Chemical enema units with lubricated tip—Fleet or
  similar in plastic squeeze bottle
Douche bag or other douching equipment
Electric heating pad

Medications and Hygienic Solutions

Milk of magnesia—tablet or liquid
Antacid tablets (Tums, Rolaids, Gelusil or similar)
Aspirin
Antinausea medication (Dramamine or per doctor's
  prescription)
Antihistamine tablets
Antidiarrhea medication (Kaopectate suspension or
  per doctor's prescription)
Hydrogen peroxide (3 percent solution)
Insect repellent
Calamine lotion
Surface anesthetic ointment (Nupercainal, Benzo-
  caine or similar)
Vaseline
Alcohol ("rubbing" type)
Syrup of ipecac

Wherever these items are stored, they should obviously be kept out of the reach of children, and replenished for immediate use whenever needed. With such items as a vaporizer, electric heating pad or enema bag, which may be used only infrequently, it is wise to keep the instructions stored with the item to be sure that it will be used properly each time.

Finally, a word of warning about the use, storage and disposal of prescription drugs. Most drugs that are available only on a doctor's prescription are restricted in this fashion because they are potent medications to be used only for specific illnesses in specific dosages. Not only may they be dangerous if taken in overdosage, but virtually all prescription medications can bring about undesired side effects, even in the treatment of the illness for which they are intended. Thus nothing can be more foolish than to keep unused supplies of prescription medications on hand to be "used next time" if someone thinks (rightly or wrongly) that a given disorder has recurred. Also, many prescription medica-

tions tend to lose their potency or effectiveness over a period of time, so even if the same medication is required for a similar condition at a later date, a fresh supply of the drug should be obtained.

In the case of most such drugs the doctor prescribes precisely the amount of medication he thinks a given illness or disorder will require, and intends that the entire prescription be used according to his directions until the supply is exhausted. Unfortunately, many patients with a misguided sense of economy stop taking a prescription medicine as soon as the symptoms of the illness begin to subside, thus taking the risk that the medication will not have done the job it was intended to do. *No* prescription medication should be stopped without first checking with the doctor. When the doctor anticipates that more prolonged use of the medication will be necessary, he may for the sake of convenience authorize one or more refills of a prescription. However, the patient should understand clearly under what circumstances a prescription is to be refilled and should, ideally, check with the doctor by telephone before refilling it.

All prescription drugs should be kept stored in a closed—and preferably locked—medicine cabinet so that they do not fall into the hands of children or anyone else for whom they are not intended. All prescription medications are designed for a specific patient with a specific illness and for no one else. It is not only foolish but downright dangerous to "lend" a prescription medication to a friend who seems to be having "similar" symptoms.

In any case in which an illness is over before a prescription has been completely used up, any remaining medication should be disposed of, preferably by flushing it down the toilet. If the doctor wishes a patient to have a continuing supply of a prescription medication, the name of the medication together with the proper dosage and the date of the original prescription should be written legibly on the label of the container. This will make it possible for patient, doctor and pharmacist all to communicate knowledgeably about a given medication without any unnecessary problems of identification.

PART

IV

PATTERNS OF ILLNESS: THE INFECTIOUS DISEASES

15. The Causes of Infection 169

16. The "Childhood Rash" Diseases 178

17. The Preventable Killers of Childhood 185

18. A Rogues' Gallery of Other Childhood Infections 191

19. "Strep" and "Staph"—The Omnipresent Invaders 204

20. Tuberculosis, Pneumonia and Other Bacterial Infections 211

21. The Variable Viral and Rickettsial Infections 224

22. The Venereal Diseases—Ancient Plague, Modern Threat 243

23. Intestinal Infections and Parasites 253

24. Malaria and Other Parasitic Infections 262

25. Leprosy, Bubonic Plague and Other Uncommon Infections and Parasitic Diseases 271

The infectious diseases are the largest and perhaps the most dangerous of all classes of health disorder. They are among the most ancient of all recorded human afflictions, and even today they remain a constant threat. Some 40 percent of all human illness is caused by infectious organisms, and while many of us may escape other common illnesses such as heart disease or cancer, no one from infancy to old age can escape an infection of one kind or another. The medical conquest of many of these infections in the 20th century will surely be remembered as one of the greatest and most far-reaching of human accomplishments. But that conquest is by no means complete. It may well never be. For that reason, a basic knowledge of the patterns of infection and the means we have to prevent, detect and treat infectious diseases is still a vital first step in the maintenance of optimum good health.

15

The Causes of Infection

Of all the diverse illnesses to which human beings are vulnerable, certain infectious diseases were among the earliest recognized. Ancient medical writings contain surprisingly accurate descriptions of such infectious diseases as boils, pneumonia, leprosy and tuberculosis. Today we know that these and a multitude of other disorders arise as a result of invasion of parts of the body by a variety of dangerous microorganisms —bacteria, viruses, one-celled protozoan parasites, and so on. In fact, the "germ theory" of disease, once a highly radical idea, is so much a part of our everyday thinking that when we feel sick we frequently tell our doctors, "I think I have a strep throat" (i.e., a streptococcus infection of the throat) or "It must be this virus that's going around." But it was only within the last 100 years that the direct relationship between infectious diseases and specific causative organisms was established. Before then no one had any clear idea where these diseases came from.

That certain diseases *were* infectious was, of course, recognized many centuries ago, even if their causes were unknown. People who came into close physical contact with lepers knew they could develop leprosy themselves. So lepers were forced to live as outcasts from society, warning others of their approach by calling out their affliction and ringing hand bells. The meticulous food rituals and proscriptions dating from Old Testament times and still practiced by Orthodox Jewish families today actually had practical as well as religious significance. Parasite-infested

pork and quick-spoiling shellfish were proscribed as "unclean," for good reason in those days, and dairy foods and meats were handled in separate utensils, thus avoiding cross-contamination. Centuries later, during the Middle Ages, bubonic plague was recognized as a communicable disease; its victims were "avoided like the plague" and everyone who was able tried to flee from the disease, usually to no avail. But for all that, no one understood *how* an infectious disease could be spread from one person to another, or what caused the disease in the first place.

With the invention of the microscope, scientists of the 1600s and 1700s discovered a whole new world of organisms never previously suspected, a world of bacteria and one-celled protozoa so small they could not be seen with the naked eye. Many of these tiny organisms were found to be normal—or at least very common—inhabitants of the human body, and a great controversy raged for decades about where they came from. Some very sound and highly respected scientists of the time maintained doggedly that they were generated spontaneously from dead or dying matter; certainly they seemed to be closely related to the decay of dead creatures. Then barely a hundred years ago, Louis Pasteur (1822–1895) proved beyond doubt that "spontaneous generation" of bacteria and other microorganisms was impossible, and further demonstrated that certain kinds of these organisms were responsible for the fermentation of grape juice into wine, for example, and for the souring of milk. It remained for the German bacteriologist Robert Koch (1843–1910) to prove beyond question that infection with certain specific microorganisms brought about specific and characteristic diseases, and that the transmission of such diseases from one human being to another depended upon transmission of the specific causative microorganism.

In the decades immediately following Koch's work, medical scientists identified a wide variety of infection-causing organisms and the diseases associated with them. In those days infectious diseases were far and away the leading cause of death, and giant strides were made in combating them by knowing what the causative organisms were, how they behaved, and what might, conceivably, hinder their invasion and growth in the body. Today we have many different weapons to protect ourselves against infections, or to eradicate the infection before it does grave harm. But many infectious diseases remain dangerous threats, even with all our modern antibiotics and immunization techniques.

To understand these infectious diseases better, we must first take a look at the characteristics of the various microorganisms that most commonly cause them. What are these organisms, and how do they differ from one another? How do they live and propagate, and what do they do, once inside the body, to cause the dramatic symptoms of infection and sometimes even death? There is no single answer to these questions, for different kinds of organisms behave in quite different ways. But all share the ability to invade human tissues, to multiply there, and in doing so to set off the chain of events which we recognize as infection.

The Families of Bacteria

The earliest recognized group of infectious microorganisms was the bacteria—a wide variety of tiny, one-celled creatures, more plantlike than animal-like in their characteristics. Early bacteriologists found that our world is teeming with these organisms, too small to be seen except under a microscope, yet varying in size and shape from comparatively large, fat, rodlike bodies detectable under a low-power microscope, down to small round organisms clustered in chains or bunches so tiny that they can be seen only under high magnification.

All bacteria, however, have certain characteristics in common. All are single-celled organisms, but they are very simple life forms and differ from other one-celled creatures in that most have no cell nucleus. Even so, they are able to grow as well in nutrient broths or on plates of agar gel in the laboratory as inside the human body. (An exception is the family of spirochetes which causes such diseases as syphilis and yaws; they are too delicate and sensitive to be grown on any artificial medium yet developed.) All but a few will not only grow but reproduce in the laboratory, dividing by mitosis just as more complex one-celled creatures do. Although most of these bacteria are colorless, they can usually be stained with various kinds of dye, thus making them much more easily detectable under the microscope. In some cases the staining is difficult—for example, the bacilli which cause tuberculosis and leprosy. A few cannot effectively be stained at all—bacteria such as the spirochete of syphilis, which is best seen in a living preparation viewed by means of a special indirect lighting method known as a "dark field." Most bacteria, however, can be easily identified and differentiated when stained by a special method developed by the Danish physician Hans Christian Gram (1853–1938). By Gram's method, a dried slide preparation of bacteria is first stained with a blue or violet stain, then washed with an alcohol solution and stained again with a contrasting bright red stain. Certain bacteria absorb and retain the first stain, appearing blue-violet on the slide, and are called "gram-positive." Other bacteria take on only the scarlet stain, appear bright red under the microscope, and are said to be "gram-negative." Among the most well-known gram-positive bacteria are organisms of the streptococcus, staphylococcus and pneumococcus families, as well as the bacteria that cause tetanus and gas gangrene. Gram-negative bacteria include the organisms that cause typhoid and paratyphoid infections, gonorrhea, bacterial dysentery and cholera.

Decades of study of the shape, growth characteristics and staining qualities of multitudes of bacteria have resulted in a system of classification so extremely complicated that even bacteriologists cannot agree upon it. Here, however, we need only mention a few broad families or categories.

The Bacilli. These are long or short rod-shaped bacteria, comparatively large in size, which grow either singly or in chains. Some bacilli, such as the members of the salmonella family which cause typhoid fever, salmonella food poisoning and other intestinal infections, are equipped with hairlike tails or *flagellae* which enable them to move about from place to place. Others, such as *Pasteurella pestis,* which causes bubonic plague (the Black Death), or the anthrax bacillus, are nonmotile and tend to grow in chains. Bacilli in the *Clostridium* family succeed in weathering hard times by forming a protective capsule or spore around themselves, and thus can lie dormant in the soil for indefinite periods until they are by chance introduced into a wound and "come to life" to cause tetanus or gas gangrene. Many bacilli are look-alikes under the microscope, especially the many varieties of intestinal bacilli that are gram-negative; but the individual organisms can be differentiated by the way they grow in special culture mediums. One, for example, may have the ability to ferment a certain kind of sugar in the medium, whereas others closely related cannot; thus, identification may require both examination of stained slides and culturing of the bacilli to observe their growth patterns and habits. And although many bacilli are pathogenic or disease-causing in man, certain kinds that take up residence in the human body are not only harmless but actually beneficial. For example, certain bacilli that normally live in the colon serve a useful purpose in the end stages of the breakdown of waste materials, and also produce vitamin K, a substance that is vitally important to the proper function of our blood's clotting mechanism.

The Cocci. This second great family of bacteria is markedly different from the bacilli. The cocci are extremely small and spherical in shape, sometimes growing in long chains (typical of the streptococci) or in grapelike clusters (a characteristic of staphylococci). In some of the cocci family the spherical shape gives way to a double-oval form, the so-called *diplococci* or "double cocci." The pneumococcus, for example, is often found in oblong pairs as though two oval or bullet-shaped cocci were laid end to end. The gonococci and the meningococci, in contrast, grow in pairs with the ovals side by side, looking much like coffee beans. Most of the cocci are pathogens—that is, they cause disease—even though some may inhabit the body for years without causing trouble. Thus, *Staphylococcus aureus* is a normal inhabitant of the skin and usually will only cause infection if introduced into a wound or other incision, or otherwise breaks through the skin's defenses. But the cocci include some of the most dangerous pathogens known to man, responsible for such dread diseases as bacterial meningitis, scarlet fever, blood poisoning and osteomyelitis (bone infection).

A few of the cocci family—the pneumococcus, for example—can form spores in order to survive in a dormant state when conditions for growth are unfavorable. Others, such as the gonococcus, are very sensitive to hostile environments and are extremely difficult to grow in the laboratory. For the most part, however, the cocci are hardy organisms, and they posed a continuing threat to human life until the discovery of sulfonomides and antibiotics in the 1930s and 1940s.

Some bacteria have the odd characteristic of appearing at one time like rod-shaped bacilli and at other times more like cocci. This characteristic is known to bacteriologists as *pleomorphism* (literally, "many shapes"). The most common example of such a pleomorphic organism is the *Corynebacterium diphtheriae,* the dangerous customer that causes diphtheria.

The Spirochetes. Still a third family of bacteria is a group of comparatively large spiral-shaped organisms, the best-known of which is the *Treponema pallidum* that causes syphilis. Characteristically, spirochetes do not stain particularly well and must be detected in live preparations with "dark-field" indirect lighting. One notable exception is a spiral bacterium which appears to live in close partnership with a rod-shaped bacterium, working together to cause the nasty infection of the gums, tongue and mouth known as Vincent's infection or "trench mouth."

Whatever their forms, disease-causing bacteria live, grow and multiply vigorously at body temperature in various human tissues. In many infectious diseases the bacteria invade some localized area, and the symptoms we notice are a result of the body's attempts to destroy them. Thus infected areas become inflamed and swollen, and the blood vessels in the area become enlarged. We feel this swelling and tumescence, together with irritation of nerve endings, as the characteristic "sore throat" of tonsillitis or the painful irritation of a boil. In most bacterial infections, white blood cells are mustered and come swarming to engulf the invaders and destroy them. This leads to an exudate of body fluid, dead white cells and destroyed bacteria which we call *pus*. Most commonly a discharge of pus, while it always indicates infection and often contains bacteria which could contaminate others, is not in itself terribly dangerous; it is merely the body's way of eliminating infectious debris. But sometimes the exudate is thick and sticky, forming a firmly adhering gelatinous membrane in the area of the infection—a real threat in diphtheria, for example, when such a fibrinous membrane can obstruct breathing and suffocate the victim.

Bacteria may also spread from the original invasion site and escape into the blood stream, triggering a more generalized body reaction characterized by chills and spiking fever, symptoms typical of septicemia (blood poisoning). Some bacteria may lodge in capillaries in various organs throughout the body and begin growth there, thus causing a localized infection to become generalized. In some cases the infecting organism spreads directly through the tissues from its local entrance, a condition known as cellulitis (inflammation of the cells).

In many instances the body's natural defenses can successfully fight down such a bacterial invasion, and the infection gradually reaches a peak and then subsides. When resistance is low, however, or when the individual is a victim of poor nutrition or repeated infections, the bacterial invasion can become overwhelming and lead to widespread bacteremia, delirium and death. Some bacteria have an even more unpleasant characteristic: the ability to form violently poisonous substances known as *toxins* which can then seep into the tissues and the blood stream. Thus even a relatively small localized streptococcus infection can create a toxic or "poisoned" condition in the body and render the victim far sicker than would be expected from the area of infection. Some bacterial toxins become attached to specific tissues with devastating effect. A toxin formed by tetanus organisms growing in the body, for example, causes the extreme sensitivity and irritability of the nervous system that leads to the convulsive muscle spasm and jaw tightening of tetanus. The toxin formed by the diphtheria organism can also attack the nervous system, sometimes even obliterating the brain center that regulates breathing.

Fortunately, most bacterial infections today can be cured—or at least effectively controlled—by means of various chemotherapeutic drugs and antibiotics. But with another great class of disease-causing microorganisms, no antibiotics are effective. In fact, it is only within the last two or three decades that we have learned very much about them at all. This group of infectious agents are the ones known as viruses.

The Strange Nature of Viruses

Scientists, as a general rule, like nothing better than a good, solid working theory that seems to hold water. Thus, when the "germ theory" of infectious disease became well established in the late 1800s, it was almost inevitable that they would assume that *all* infectious diseases were the result of different bacteria-like microorganisms and begin diligently searching for the specific organisms that caused them. And they were eminently successful. Between 1849 and 1906 medical bacteriologists and microbiologists identified the organisms that cause some 28 different major and minor infectious diseases, including such traditional killers as typhoid fever, tuberculosis, pneumonia, cholera, diphtheria and tetanus. It was indeed a splendid achievement, a giant step forward in the understanding of human disease rarely matched in the entire history of medicine.

But the "germ theory" could not adequately explain a number of the most widespread and dangerous of all infectious diseases—among them rabies, smallpox, red measles and yellow fever. There was no serious doubt that specific microorganisms of some sort *did* cause them; in the case of rabies and smallpox, for example, highly successful immunization techniques had been discovered which always involved the inoculation of some kind of infectious material from one patient into the body of another. But no one had ever been able actually to observe the causative microorganisms in these diseases and a number of others, or to cultivate them in any type of laboratory culture medium.

Then in 1892 the Russian botanist Dmitri Iosifovich Ivanovski (1864–1920) made a remarkable discovery. The agent causing the spread of a certain destructive disease of tobacco plants could pass right through special porcelain filters with pores so small that all known bacteria were unable to pass. Soon other scientists demonstrated that the previously unobserved causes of other infectious diseases could also pass through these fine bacteriological filters. Early investigators spoke of such a mysterious filterable disease-producing agent as a *contagium vivum fluidum*—a "contagious living fluid." Later these "fluids" came to be called "filterable viruses."

At first bacteriologists assumed that viruses were, in actuality, nothing other than extremely tiny bacteria, so small that existing microscopes could not reveal them. Indeed, with one or two exceptions (such as the vaccinia virus causing cowpox or the virus of psittacosis or "parrot fever" that affects birds, both of which could be seen as vague, fuzzy images under the microscope), most viruses were so exceedingly tiny that the wavelength of ordinary light in a conventional microscope moved right past them. It was not until the late 1930s, with the invention of the electron microscope that used beams of electrons instead of ordinary light waves, that the first clear shadow images of these elusive virus particles could be seen, at magnifications from 40,000 to 100,000 times. It was then discovered that the largest viruses are only about one-third the diameter of streptococci, and the smallest are some 35 times smaller—less than

one-millionth of an inch across, smaller even than some individual protein molecules.

During these years of early virus investigation, scientists began seriously questioning the hypothesis that viruses were merely "tiny bacteria." In fact, they began questioning whether viruses could really be called "living organisms" at all, for they demonstrated some very perplexing characteristics that the more familiar bacteria did not possess. For one thing, viruses did not seem to reproduce until they had entered the cells of a living host. Unlike bacteria, which grow and reproduce exuberantly in simple solutions of beef broth, sugar or nutrient gelatin, viruses seemed to "come to life" only when they found lodging in living tissue cells. On the other hand, although viruses can be destroyed by the intense heat of sterilizing ovens known as autoclaves, or with various chemical germicides, they do not "die" the way bacteria do when deprived of nutriment but merely become inert. To add to the puzzle, in 1935 Dr. Wendell M. Stanley actually succeeded in crystallizing the virus causing mosaic disease of tobacco plants in a pure form as a dry, inert powder. Certainly this did not seem to be characteristic of a "living" organism. It was later discovered that viruses are completely unaffected by any of the sulfa or antibiotic drugs which destroy disease-causing bacteria so readily. In fact, it was finally concluded, viruses are not really "cells" at all, by any normal definition. They contain none of the life substance of cells known as protoplasm. They are not surrounded by a cell membrane, as bacteria are. They cannot even use simple sugars or amino acids to obtain energy or build protein for themselves, and thus they cannot grow. And in an inert state they can survive indefinitely, perhaps even in outer space.

But "living" or not, viruses have one unique characteristic: although they cannot perform any of the basic life functions for themselves that even the lowliest bacteria perform, they have the frightening capacity *to make the living cells of their hosts do their work for them.* And herein lies the deadly danger of virus infections.

Today we know that viruses are really little

more than small bundles of a kind of chemical substance known as *nucleic acid,* surrounded by protective coatings of protein. And it is this nucleic acid—similar to the remarkable genetic material found in the chromosomes of all living cells—that makes viruses so threatening and potentially deadly to human beings.

Within the chromosomes of all living cells the special kind of nucleic acid known as DNA acts as a sort of "master molecule" of the life processes, controlling the cells' biochemical activities, making certain that faithful duplicates of the cell result when it reproduces, and directing a similar nucleic acid called RNA in the manufacture of energy-building proteins and enzymes. (*See* p. 93.)

When an infectious virus enters the body (through the mucous membrane of the nose and throat in the case of respiratory viruses, or by contamination of food by virus-infected waste materials), the virus particles attach themselves to susceptible cells and literally *inject* their own virus DNA or RNA into the cell. These virus chemicals thereupon set up a control system all their own, making use of the cell's vital capacities for totally alien purposes. Instead of manufacturing chemicals and substances useful to the invaded cell, the virus nucleic acid takes over the cell's entire chemical system—much as a dictator might take over a country's armed forces, news media and production capabilities—and forces the cell to manufacture more virus nucleic acid molecules and protein coatings, enough to form hundreds or even thousands of new virus particles. In a matter of hours—in some cases in a matter of minutes—a single virus particle attached to a cell can create 200 new particles, using the cell's manufacturing capacity. These newly formed viruses then burst through the cell's walls and go on to parasitize other cells, leaving the host cell behind, often permanently damaged or even destroyed. Other kinds of viruses follow an alternative battle plan, attaching their nucleic acid to the DNA molecules in the host cell and then "hiding out" within the host cell for prolonged periods, while their nucleic acid is being reproduced each time the cell reproduces its own. Thus several generations of a cell can be infected from the invasion of a

single virus particle so that an overwhelming number of new particles are ready to be released long before even the first signs or symptoms of illness appear.

Obviously viruses can do enormous and rapid damage to cells in the body once they have made their attack. Certain kinds of viruses prefer special tissues: several varieties, for example, grow best in cells of lung tissue, and viral pneumonia may develop within a few days after the deadly invasion. Other viruses prefer nerve cells, causing paralysis or even death as these delicate cells are destroyed in the course of their slavish effort to make more virus particles. Still others can attack cells in the liver or in the lining of the intestinal tract. In recent years, researchers have become increasingly suspicious that viruses may have an even deadlier long-term effect, that they may cause insignificant symptoms or undetectable damage at first, yet may still trigger vast changes in the normal reproductive mechanisms of living cells. No one is yet certain, but it may well be that many kinds of wild and uncontrolled cell growth that we know as cancer are triggered in just such a fashion by apparently innocent and innocuous viruses.

Innocuous or not, no virus can be regarded as benign, for unlike bacteria, which include certain strains that are of real benefit to the human body, all viruses are totally parasitic and no one has yet found a single virus that does anything beneficial for its victim. Fortunately, we are not entirely without defenses against these destroyers. The protective protein coatings on viruses, foreign to the normal biochemistry of the body, tend to stimulate the formation of special protective substances in the blood stream called *antibodies,* which are capable of blocking the entrance of newly formed viruses into the cells. Thus normal bodily defense mechanisms gradually slow down and prevent further virus reproduction. But the production of defending antibodies takes time, and medical researchers are still looking for ways to help speed up body defenses after a virus infection has started, or better yet, to develop antibodies to fight deadly viruses before they ever have a chance to cause infection. There have been some signal successes in this latter approach, as in the case of vaccination against smallpox, or the use of immunizing doses of killed or crippled polio viruses to help the body build up defenses before outright infection with polio begins.

Rickettsiae and Pleural Pneumonia-like Organisms (PPLO)

Although the vast majority of infectious diseases are caused by bacteria or viruses, a small but significant number are caused by members of two other families of microorganisms, each family distinctively different in certain ways from either bacteria or viruses. They are the rickettsiae and the so-called pleural pneumonia-like organisms, or PPLO, which have been recognized as a significant factor in infectious disease only in the past two or three decades.

Infections Due to Rickettsiae. About midway in size between the average bacteria and the average virus is a family of infectious organisms known as rickettsiae, named after Howard Taylor Ricketts, one of a small group of investigators who first studied these organisms at the turn of the century and who died of typhus fever, a rickettsial infection, in 1910. Together with the microbiologist Stanislov von Prowazek (who also died of typhus fever during his investigations in 1915) and Simeon Volvak (who finally first discovered a rickettsial organism under the microscope in 1916, and named it after the deceased Ricketts), he spent several decades studying rickettsial infections without really knowing what the nature of the causative organism was. With the discovery that these organisms could be detected with a conventional microscope and could be prepared for observation with a special stain usually used to stain blood cells, it became obvious that these rickettsiae were not viruses—but then, neither were they conventional bacteria. Rickettsiae are roughly half the size of a streptococcus or staphylococcus organism (among the smaller of the bacteria) and, like other bacteria, are held back by most bacteriological filters which allow even the larger viruses to pass. On the other hand, rickettsiae resemble viruses in that they can reproduce themselves only within the living cells of the infected organism, and cannot be cultured on any ordinary media used for bacteria. But unlike viruses, they are sensitive to various of the modern broad-spectrum antibiotics, particularly Aureomycin, and thus rickettsial infections, which once were extremely dangerous with a high mortality rate, today can often be treated successfully.

Finally, there is one other curious fact about rickettsial infections of man: without exception the causative organism is insect-borne and transmitted to man by the bites of various insect vermin. For example, among the more familiar rickettsial infections, epidemic typhus fever and other forms of typhus are transmitted to man by the bites of human body lice or rat fleas, while Rocky Mountain spotted fever is passed on by the bite of ticks. Less familiar infections such as trench fever, tsutsugamushi disease and Q fever are passed on by the bites of itch mites or ticks. Thus, control of these infections today depends as much upon control of the vermin carriers as it does upon effective antibiotic treatment.

Infections Due to Pleural Pneumonia-like Organisms (PPLO). In 1898 bacteriologists first isolated yet another kind of infectious organism apparently in a class apart from bacteria, rickettsiae or viruses. These agents appeared smaller than rickettsiae or even some of the larger viruses, yet resembled bacteria in that they could grow and reproduce on artificial culture mediums. Since the first organisms discovered seemed to be associated with an infectious disease of cattle known as pleuropneumonia, they were called "pleuropneumonia-like organisms" or PPLO for short. We know now that they produce neither pneumonia nor pleurisy, but the name has stuck. In fact, we are still not entirely sure *what* diseases they produce, if any, at least in human beings. They are often found in women with chronic pelvic infections and in men with urethritis (inflammation of the urethra), but there is no definite proof that they cause these conditions. They have also been indicted, at various times, as a possible causative agent for rheumatoid arthritis or for conjunctivitis (an inflammation of the inner lining of the eyelids), but again proof has not been established. These organisms are impervious to treatment with penicillin or sulfa drugs, but seem sensitive to certain broad-spectrum antibiotics, notably streptomycin. At present they are not considered a serious disease threat to man.

Disease-Producing Fungi

Among the other organisms capable of producing diseases in the human body, there is quite a variety of different fungi—members of a class of plants somewhat more complex than bacteria. Many of these fungus infections are superficial, more nuisance and annoyance than threat, yet often difficult to eradicate. Other more deep-seated fungus infections, however, can be downright nasty, difficult to diagnose and treat, and sometimes fatal.

The fungus group called the *Tinea* causes a variety of familiar skin infections including ordinary ringworm (caused by *Tinea corporis*), ringworm of the scalp (*Tinea capitis*) and athlete's foot (*Tinea pedis*). In addition, certain of the *Tinea* can become lodged under the fingernails and cause a prolonged and unsightly fungus infection of the nailbed known as onychomycosis which can be very difficult to eradicate.

Another commonplace fungus infection, called moniliasis or thrush, caused by a fungus known as *Candida albicans,* thrives on warm moist mucous membrane surfaces such as the inside of the cheeks, the gums, the intestine or the vaginal canal. Once comparatively rare, *Candida* infections now frequently occur as an "overgrowth" in cases in which broad-spectrum antibiotics have been used (perhaps too effectively) to treat bacterial infections. In the absence of the harmless bacteria that normally inhabit various mucous membranes of the body, which are destroyed along with pathogenic bacteria by the antibiotic, *Candida albicans* seems to thrive.

In addition to these relatively harmless but annoying superficial infections, other types of fungus can invade the body and cause far more dangerous, prolonged and deep-seated disease. Most of these organisms are normal inhabitants of soil, and most infections occur as a result of inhalation of the spores, particularly among farm laborers, causing a variety of lung or upper respiratory tract infections. These infections may be difficult to diagnose; they are often mistaken for bacterial or viral respiratory infections, or even pneumonias or tuberculosis. Our bodies develop resistance to these invading fungi with the formation of antibodies, and therefore most such infections are self-limited and may often be completely eradicated without treatment. In some cases, however, the organism can escape from the primary infection in the blood stream and spread to a wide variety of places in the body: the liver or kidneys, the bone, the nervous system or the skin, for example. There are a number of antifungal antibiotic drugs available today which speed the treatment of these infections, once they are diagnosed, and help eradicate even the more dangerous ones.

Infectious Protozoa and Other Parasites

Although most infectious diseases are caused by organisms that are generally considered members of the plant family (bacteria, viruses, rickettsiae, fungi, etc.), certain of the most prevalent diseases of man, and a number of the very obscure and mysterious ones, are caused by single-celled organisms of the animal kingdom, the protozoan parasites, or even by animal parasites of higher orders. In many cases these organisms gain entry to the human body indirectly; they spend part of their life cycle in the bodies of other animals or insects and are then transmitted to humans either by means of insect bites or by ingestion of contaminated food. Thus, the secret of controlling these diseases has been in great part a matter of tracking down the intermediary host—that is, the organism that transmits the disease to man.

A great many protozoan and higher parasitic diseases (or more correctly, *infestations*) are rarely encountered in northern latitudes and are more characteristically tropical diseases. However, many of them can and do occur in this country, or among travelers returning from those parts of the world where the diseases are endemic. Amebiasis or amebic dysentery is one, an infestation by a pathogenic ameba. Malaria is another, caused by one of a group of protozoa called plasmodia which must spend part of their life cycle in the body of the anopheles mosquito.

The tsetse fly plays host to another protozoan parasite, the trypanosome, which when transmitted to the human body causes trypanosomiasis, more commonly known as African sleeping sickness. An oval, one-celled parasite with a long whiplike tail called *Leishmania donovani,* transmitted from human to human by the bite of a small sand fly, causes an infection of the liver or spleen. And the *Trichomonas vaginalis,* another parasite, can cause a minor but persistently annoying vaginal inflammation and discharge.

The animal parasites of man are not limited to single-celled protozoa. Certain more complex organisms, most notably roundworms and flatworms of one variety or another, can infest parts of the human body and cause symptoms ranging from the very minor to the very serious. Trichinosis, caused by the round *Trichinella* worm and contracted by eating infested and improperly cooked pork, is perhaps the most serious. Less serious but much more common are pinworm infections and hookworm disease, both caused by small roundworm parasites. The most familiar of the flatworms that infest human victims are the *Cestoda* or tapeworms.

Thus the kinds of microorganisms that can cause infectious diseases in man—bacteria, viruses, rickettsiae, fungi, protozoa or more complex parasites—are many and varied, a constant threat to health from birth to death. Some result in only minor illness or superficial discomfort; others can be vicious killers. But no matter how various, peculiar or dangerous these "bugs" and the diseases they cause may be, modern medicine has found ways to identify and combat most of them.

16

The "Childhood Rash" Diseases

Among the most familiar of all infectious diseases are a group of "children's diseases," so called because they are usually contracted during childhood and characterized by various forms of skin eruptions or rashes called *exanthems*. These illnesses are so commonplace a part of childhood that it is more often the mother who makes the diagnosis than the doctor. Indeed, they are sometimes regarded as so benign that a doctor may not be consulted at all.

Unfortunately, this viewpoint is not always correct. Today doctors realize that all these "benign" childhood illnesses can be hazardous under certain circumstances. All but one are caused by potentially dangerous viruses, and all can have troublesome, even tragic, side effects or complications. Nor are they necessarily restricted to children. Adults can contract these infections if they missed them during childhood, sometimes with an extra measure of discomfort, inconvenience or even tragedy, as in the case of rubella (German measles).

The "Measles-Type" Exanthems

The three main diseases in this group—rubeola (measles), rubella (German measles) and roseola—appear at first to be closely similar "rash diseases," but they are actually quite distinct infections. Each has a feverish onset, each exhibits a characteristic red skin rash, and each is a highly communicable virus infection spread

by upper respiratory contact. But here the resemblance ends.

Measles (Rubeola). Often called red measles, hard measles, ten-day measles and occasionally black measles, this most long-lasting and severe of the measles-type illnesses has been known to mankind for thousands of years. Historians speculate that the "great plague" that crippled ancient Athens in the war with Sparta might have been a particularly virulent epidemic of measles. Today the disease commonly appears in springtime epidemics among schoolchildren between the ages of five and twelve, but isolated cases can occur at any age from six months on and at any time.

Measles is caused by a very specific virus (that is, a virus that causes this one disease and no other) which is believed to enter the body through the moist mucous membranes of the upper respiratory tract, but which then is spread in the blood stream—a so-called *viremia* reflected by a high fever—to attack virtually all the tissues and organs in the body. The *incubation period*—the interval between the time a person contracts an infection and the time the first symptoms appear; in short, the time it takes the invading organism to become entrenched in the body—is from seven to fourteen days, but a child at school may actually be spreading the measles virus to other people for several days before he himself comes down with the characteristic symptoms, so a source of contact is hard to pin down. Almost any child who seems to have a bad cold *could* have early measles. What is more, it is the one childhood disease that can be spread by an uninfected third person—say, the immune brother or sister of an infected child—who is wearing clothing, for example, contaminated by the virus.

The illness begins with a high fever, a runny nose and a very typical harsh, irritable cough. At the onset, fever may suddenly spike to 104° or more and is hard to bring down; in fact, the sudden onset of a high, stubborn fever from no apparent cause may be the first clue that measles is under way. On the second or third day of fever, the child's eyes become bloodshot and sensitive to light, and the inside of his mouth takes on an angry orange-red color. Small, white cottony-looking spots (the so-called *Koplik's spots*) also frequently form inside the cheeks, a sure diagnostic sign. Finally, between three and five days after onset of symptoms the characteristic rash appears, first on the face and neck, then spreading over the trunk and limbs. The rash has a mottled, brownish-pink aspect, with spots the size of a match head running into each other, and is slightly raised so that the skin feels rough. The beginning of the rash coincides with the highest fever and the most discomfort from coughing and runny nose. After four or five days it begins to fade, with some flaking of the skin, but the last traces may not disappear for another week or more. When the rash is especially severe, tiny capillary hemorrhages may appear in the spots, which will later turn an unattractive black-and-blue—hence the common name "black measles." But this occurrence is nothing to worry about. It just means the child will be extraordinarily unpleasant to look at during his convalescence.

What should you do when you suspect a child is coming down with measles? The steps that follow below apply to all the "childhood rash" diseases discussed in this chapter, and indeed to most infectious illnesses in general, particularly when children are involved.

1. First, take the temperature, and if it is 102° F. or above (or if you see any signs of the "twitchiness" that might warn of impending febrile convulsions) start fever control with aspirin and sponging (*see* p. 154). At the same time, look for other significant symptoms: a rash if one is present, for example, or the presence of a cough, noting how it sounds (i.e., whether it seems to be loose or dry, harsh, "barking" or croupy). The cough of measles is usually harsh-sounding, with very little sign of coughing anything up.

2. Notify your doctor, describe what is going on, and follow any advice he may give.

3. If you are quite sure measles (or some other "childhood rash" disease) is afoot, notify the school as well as the parents of any children that have been in close contact with yours during the past few days. They may not be terribly pleased by the news, but they will be grateful that you have warned them. In the case of measles, if an unimmunized child has been exposed to the disease, there may be time to give him special protective shots of gamma globulin that may modify his infection so that it will not last as long or be as serious. *Don't* take your child to your doctor's office or the hospital emergency room unless you are specifically directed to do so—no one wants this infection spread any more than necessary. But if your child's cough seems to be getting worse instead of better after the rash appears, or if his temperature begins spiking up again after it seems to be controlled, be sure your doctor knows about it without delay.

4. During the illness, keep the child in bed (insofar as possible); check his temperature at least morning and evening and use aspirin to control it as necessary; and encourage him to drink plenty of fluids while the fever lasts. Darken the room for a day or two if light seems to hurt the child's eyes, but do not make a big fuss about it. This step is mostly for comfort—nothing terrible will happen to a child's eyes on account of exposure to light. Fortunately, the rash of measles is usually only slightly itchy, and then only toward the end of the illness, when the skin may flake slightly. It is advisable to limit activity while the fever is high and the patient is acutely ill, but later increases in the activity allowed are a matter of common sense. Many mothers worry unnecessarily because they "can't

keep the child down" during convalescence from measles or other children's diseases. But as a rule of thumb, the child who is too sick to be up will not feel like being up, and when he becomes irrepressibly determined to be out of bed, it is unlikely to hurt him. As long as the fever is up, insist on at least an hour's nap morning and afternoon, but except in certain specific illnesses such as rheumatic fever (*see* p. 560) or infectious hepatitis (*see* p. 200) a certain amount of physical activity is harmless enough.

5. Today formal quarantine is not required for measles or other "childhood rash" diseases, but it is common sense not to invite guests into the home during these illnesses.

Measles at best is an uncomfortable disease. For the first few days the victim will feel miserable and will not want to be up and around much. By the third or fourth day after the rash appears he will begin feeling better, and by ten days or so from the beginning of the symptoms he will be feeling quite well in most cases, although the rash may not completely fade for several days more, especially if black-and-blue spots have appeared. The cough may also persist. If so, let your doctor know and follow his advice about returning the patient to school or other normal activities.

Recovery from measles is usually spontaneous without the use of any specific medicine. Antibiotics, for example, have no effect whatever against the measles virus, but your doctor may decide to prescribe them to guard against a secondary bronchitis or pneumonia caused by bacteria after the measles virus has weakened the patient's resistance. Aside from the threat of these secondary bacterial infections, the most dreaded complication of measles is *encephalitis* (brain fever), which can occur when the measles virus mounts an especially severe attack on the cells in the patient's brain and spinal cord. Measles encephalitis occurs only about once in every 1,500 cases of measles, but in those few cases it can result in extensive and permanent brain damage or even in death. Rare as it is, post-measles encephalitis can take such a grim toll that most pediatricians today urge measles vaccination for *all* children, beginning as early as nine months of age, in hope of preventing measles altogether.

A safe, effective vaccine against measles has been available since 1962 and has been administered to many children without charge in community-wide "Measles Must Go!" campaigns. The vaccine is made from live measles virus in *attenuated* or weakened form. In effect, it gives the vaccinated child a very mild, almost symptom-free case of measles. The immunity conferred by this vaccination is now believed to last for many years, possibly for life. (Infection with measles itself confers lifetime immunity after recovery.) Because some children may have a slight reaction to the vaccine, with a low-grade fever and even a mild rash appearing a week or so after vaccination, most doctors give an injection of *gamma globulin* at the same time the vaccine is given to prevent even this minor discomfort. Gamma globulin is a protein substance in the blood believed to have a powerful antibody effect against many viruses, including the one causing measles. To date no record has appeared of serious post-measles complications from the vaccine, and in future generations measles may become as much a "forgotten disease" as smallpox or poliomyelitis, thanks to modern immunization techniques.

Rubella. Often called German measles or three-day measles, this virus infection also starts with a fever and a runny nose, but the fever is not as high as with measles and the hacky cough is usually absent. Like measles, however, rubella is very contagious and often occurs in epidemics among schoolchildren during the spring months. Like the rubeola or "red measles" virus, the virus of rubella attacks all tissues of the body, but seems to affect the mucous membrane of the nose, throat and bronchial tubes most seriously in most cases. It is also spread by "droplet infection" from upper respiratory secretions, and has a longer incubation period than measles—about sixteen days, on the average. Adults who have not had the disease may contract rubella almost as commonly as children, and will usually first complain of a headache, muscle stiffness and general discomfort.

The rash of rubella appears within a day or

so of the onset of symptoms. Unlike the coarse measles rash, it is fine and pink, slightly rough to the fingertips, and persists only two or three days before fading away completely. Along with the rash, there may be a characteristic swelling of the lymph nodes behind the ears—a sure sign of rubella. In most cases the whole illness is over in three to four days. During that time the same home treatment program should be followed as outlined above. Again, fortunately, the rash does not usually itch, and no specific medicines change the course of the disease much, although antibiotic treatment may be ordered by the doctor to guard against secondary bacterial invaders if the case is severe. In addition, any girl or young woman who has been in close contact with a rubella victim during the three or four days before symptoms begin should be notified.

The reason for this is now widely understood. For many years rubella was considered a completely innocuous disease which did not even make the victim particularly ill. To all appearances, no serious complications ever seemed to occur. But since the early 1940s we have learned that the rubella virus is far more treacherous than anyone suspected. Although its effects on children or adults may be mild, it can wreak havoc on the embryo of an unborn baby if the mother becomes infected during her pregnancy, especially in the first three months. Attacking the embryonic baby in a singularly vicious way, the rubella virus can cause crippling malformations of the heart, congenital cataracts or permanent deafness. So frequently does this virus attack the fetus during the first trimester of pregnancy that the occurrence of a rubella infection in a newly pregnant woman is considered by many obstetricians to be grounds for terminating the pregnancy.

Because of this singular danger, a great effort was made to perfect a vaccine against rubella, and late in 1968 that effort was rewarded. Extensive tests proved a new rubella vaccine to be safe and effective for protection against the disease. In 1970, massive immunization programs were carried out among grade school children all over the country. It is hoped that such mass vaccinations will eradicate the threat of rubella damage to unborn babies within a few years. It is particularly important, however, that young girls be vaccinated before they reach childbearing age if they have not already had the disease (which would confer lifelong immunity). Today one combined vaccine can be used to provide protection against both rubella and rubeola in a single injection.

Roseola Infantum (Exanthem Subitum). Many parents are unacquainted with this illness of babies, probably the least familiar of all the common "measles-type" rash diseases. Even doctors do not know very much about it. It is believed to be caused by a virus, but so far the virus has never been identified.

Roseola occurs most commonly in children under the age of two. The first sign is the abrupt onset of an uncommonly high fever—often 105° or 106°—with no other signs or symptoms to account for it. The fever may remain high and difficult to control for three or four days before breaking spontaneously, followed by the fleeting appearance of a very fine, paprika-like red rash spread diffusely over the body. This rash usually disappears completely within 24 hours, or may even come and go in the course of the night and never be seen at all. The doctor should, of course, be notified in the event of any high fever, but the diagnosis of roseola is often made only by hindsight, based on the age of the child and the abrupt onset of an unexplained three- or four-day fever. Once the fever breaks and the rash comes and goes, the illness is virtually over and there are no grave complications to be feared. Like the other "measles-type" diseases, one attack of roseola is believed to confer lifelong immunity.

The only real threat posed by this rather dramatic but benign illness of infancy is the danger of febrile convulsions from the high fever. If aspirin in the proper dosage (one grain per year of age every 3 to 4 hours for three or four doses) and frequent sponging with alcohol and water do not hold the fever down to 102° or so, call a doctor. He may want to prescribe a mild sedative to help protect against convulsions. If convulsions do occur, take the necessary steps immediately (*see* p. 151), notify a doctor, and follow his instructions.

Other "Measles-type" Diseases. Measles, rubella and roseola are the most commonly recognized of the virus-caused "measles-type" infections, but they are not the only ones. Many people who insist they have had one of these diseases "more than once" have in reality had one of a group of similar but distinctly different infections commonly known as "fourth disease," "fifth disease," or even, recently, "sixth disease."

Not much is known about these odd infections except that they are caused by viruses and are associated with fever, cough and runny nose, and often mimic measles or rubella with a red skin rash. Perhaps they are caused by new, mutated strains of the measles or rubella virus, or by long-existing viruses which ordinarily produce nothing but head-cold symptoms and only rarely cause rashes. No one knows for sure. None of these infections yet stands out clearly enough to become established as a recognized medical entity. Perhaps they never will. Whatever their source, however, they are generally not serious or long-lasting, and have no known complications. The same principles of care discussed above apply to these infections.

Chicken Pox (Varicella)

This benign but highly unpleasant disease enjoys several dubious distinctions in the roster of "childhood rash" diseases. First of all, it is one of the most highly communicable diseases known to man, occurring in the same locale in epidemics every three or four years, an interval just about long enough for a new batch of susceptible children to appear. In addition, it is one of the most uncomfortable of all children's diseases, and certainly about the most unattractive. Finally, chicken pox is probably the most widely self-diagnosed of all infections. The appearance of the rash is so typical and characteristic that it is almost impossible to miss, and in mild cases with little or no fever the doctor may not be called at all.

Chicken pox is caused by a virus, very similar or perhaps identical to the virus that causes the adult disease of skin nerve endings known as *herpes zoster* or "shingles." It is spread by droplets from the nose and throat of an infected person and invades the new victim through the mucous membrane of the nose and throat, with the virus spreading quickly to all the tissues and organs of the body. But in spite of its messiness and discomfort, chicken pox remains a mild disease, more annoyance than threat to the children and occasional adults whom it attacks. The incubation period is from two to three weeks after exposure, and the first symptoms—low-grade fever, headache and general discomfort—are often so minor they are overlooked until the rash appears some 24 hours later.

The typical rash occurs suddenly as a crop of small water-filled blisters about the size and appearance of teardrops, first on the face, then on the upper trunk and then all over. These lesions appear in recurring crops at one-day intervals for three or four days. In mild cases they may be confined mainly to the trunk and upper extremities, but in severe cases the ears, the soles of the feet and even the inside of the mouth may be affected. Gradually the blisters become filled with pus; then in a few days they begin to crust and dry up. In the meantime, unfortunately, they itch. *If left alone and unbroken, chicken pox lesions will heal leaving no scar,* but if scratched so that secondary bacterial infection can get started, permanent scarring may result.

The home care of chicken pox should follow the principles already discussed for other "childhood rash" diseases. Notify the doctor if the victim's temperature climbs to 102° or higher, and use aspirin and gentle sponging, when necessary, for fever control. Notify the school and parents of other children who may have been exposed, as a courtesy. Bed rest and extra fluids are indicated during the early, acute phase of the illness. No special diet is indicated unless chicken pox lesions appear on the inside of the mouth; in that case soft or liquid foods should be used to avoid abrasion. The major care problem centers on the itching of the rash. Older children should be urged vigorously not to scratch. Trim younger children's fingernails down to the quick and, if necessary, bundle their hands up in fluffy gauze bandages to make scratching more difficult. Finally, steel yourself for a dreadful-looking sight as the disease progresses. Nothing is more forlorn-looking than a three-year-old, covered from head to foot with pus-filled, itching lesions, sitting sadly in a crib with gauze mittens taped to both hands.

The main illness of chicken pox is mild. Recovery largely involves waiting the 10 to 14 days needed for the skin lesions to dry up and heal. Calamine lotion offers some relief from the itching, and in severe cases your doctor can prescribe additional medicines that will help. Don't be afraid to bathe the child; a daily sponge bath with warm soap and water, followed by gentle fluff-drying with a Turkish towel, will help prevent staphylococcus infection in the lesions. If the pustules break and ooze, no harm is done, nor is there need to apply any antiseptic or dressing. They will heal faster undisturbed in open air. If infection does begin in the vesicles, call your doctor so that appropriate antibiotic therapy can be started.

Once the last of the lesions have become crusted the child is no longer infectious and can go back to ordinary activities. As with the "measles-type" illnesses, one attack of chicken pox confers permanent immunity.

Scarlet Fever (Scarlatina)

Unlike the "measles-type" diseases and chicken pox, scarlet fever (sometimes called scarlatina) is caused not by a virus but by a member of the singularly dangerous streptococcus family of bacteria, and consequently is quite a different kind of illness. In fact, it is included here chiefly because it is another common children's disease and is accompanied by a rash that is easily confused with the "measles-type" rashes.

Essentially scarlet fever is nothing more than a streptococcus throat infection caused by a particular type of strep bacteria (known as Group A beta-hemolytic strep) which produces a severe body-wide illness and a characteristic generalized red skin rash. Both the symptoms and the rash are caused by a bacterial poison or toxin produced by this particular strep organism. It is another "upper respiratory droplet" infection which may strike at any age, but is by far most common among school-age children. Before the widespread use of penicillin and other antibiotics

in treatment of upper respiratory infections, scarlet fever often occurred in epidemics, but today it occurs more sporadically.

Typically, scarlet fever begins quite suddenly three or four days after exposure with a severe sore throat, a sudden fever which may spike as high as 103° or 104° and other symptoms of severe illness: headache, general discomfort, vomiting, sometimes even prostration. The sore throat gets rapidly worse and becomes red and raw-looking, with a yellowish-gray patchy membrane forming over the inflamed surface. Within 24 hours red patches can be seen on the inside of the cheeks, and the tongue takes on the sore, inflamed, red-spotty "strawberry tongue" appearance typical of the disease. Then, between 24 and 48 hours after onset, the rash begins to appear on the inside of the arms, the neck and the chest, later spreading to the abdomen and legs. It often appears more as a diffuse scarlet flush than as a discrete rash and, once established, is best seen in the skin folds of the neck, under the arms and on the insides of the elbows and wrists. Here the rash may even appear as dark red lines in the skin creases. The victim's face will appear flushed as with a high fever, except for a pale circle around the lips. He will remain infectious from the first appearance of symptoms until the illness is completely over, and until the strep organisms can no longer be found growing in cultures of exudate taken from his nose and throat.

Potentially scarlet fever is a much more dangerous infection than the other "childhood rash" diseases. Not only can the strep organism be a killer during the acute illness, but aftereffects due to the body's attempts to fight off the disease can result in long-term illness. What is more, it is a very toxic infection which makes the victim feel thoroughly miserable. Nevertheless, it is best treated at home if possible rather than in a hospital because of its very infectious nature. The doctor should be called as soon as the disease is suspected, because in this case specific antibiotic treatment can greatly affect the duration and ferocity of the infection. Fever control is important; so is bed rest during the acute phase. A soft or even liquid diet may be necessary because the patient's throat may be so raw and sore that coarse foods would be painful, and often nausea and vomiting are present early in the disease. If necessary, fluids should be given only in small amounts—1½ to 2 ounces at a time every hour. Keep other children away from the patient, and use either paper plates and cups (which can then be burned) for his meals, or sterilize his dishes and silverware separately from family utensils at a *rolling boil* for twenty minutes after use to avoid spreading the bacteria.

As soon as the diagnosis can be established, the doctor will start vigorous antibiotic treatment to knock out the germ as quickly as possible. Penicillin is still the medicine of choice, but other drugs can be used if the patient is allergic to penicillin. Before he starts treatment the doctor may wish to take a bacterial culture from the patient's nose and throat, and perhaps even a blood culture; but the response to treatment may be so dramatic that improvement is often seen within 24 hours.

Even with early treatment, however, the general body effects of the infection may linger for ten days to two weeks before the patient's strength and appetite are fully recovered; strep infections can be fast-moving and debilitating. During convalescence, follow your doctor's instructions for bed rest and other convalescent measures. He may well want to perform a urine examination at weekly intervals for a month or more after convalescence seems complete, and will want to be alerted to *any* evidence of recurring fever. Although the rash of scarlet fever is not usually itchy, the skin may desquamate, or flake slightly, as the rash fades.

In the days before antibiotics scarlet fever was far more dangerous than it is today under active treatment. The acute phase of the disease lasted from seven to ten days and complete recovery might take three weeks or more. Death from the disease was not uncommon, especially among young babies, who could suffocate with their inflamed throats clogged with sticky exudate. Among those who recovered, a certain number continued to harbor strep organisms in their throats for months or years, becoming "carriers" even after their own active illness was over. But even more dangerous than the effects of the acute illness were the serious secondary effects of strep infection and the body's reaction to it, leading to such conditions as acute glomerulonephritis (a dangerous kidney inflammation) or acute rheumatic fever.

Penicillin and other modern antibiotics are extremely effective in destroying strep bacteria, so a typical untreated case of scarlet fever is rarely seen anymore. Today there are only about 6 or 8 deaths per 1,000 cases, and most cases heal without continuing complications. But the subsequent appearance of acute rheumatic fever or acute glomerulonephritis still remains a hazard to anyone who has had such an infection. Thus even today scarlet fever is a threat, and it deserves the patient's respect as well as swift medical attention.

17

The Preventable Killers of Childhood

The whole pattern of childhood diseases today is far different from what it was as little as 30 or 40 years ago. Infections such as measles, rubella and chicken pox are still with us, but the more dangerous full-blown scarlet fever is rarely seen, thanks to vigorous early treatment with antibiotics. Ordinary tonsillitis and bronchitis are still familiar enough, but such notorious killers as diphtheria and whooping cough, once major threats to the lives of children, have faded from the scene—at least for the moment—and the most dreaded child killer of them all, poliomyelitis, seems to be vanishing like a bad memory.

Why such a great change in the space of only a few decades? For one thing, more babies today are hospital-delivered under medical supervision, and are seen by doctors at regular intervals through infancy and childhood, than ever before. In addition, great advances have been made in the diagnosis and treatment of dangerous childhood illnesses, especially in the use of antibiotic drugs to stop certain primary infections and to prevent secondary infections from starting. Above all, safe modern immunizations are widely available today to protect both children and adults from childhood illnesses that once took a frightening toll.

As a result we tend to think of many former killers as "conquered diseases," no longer a matter for concern. But this is a dangerous illusion. Far from being conquered, they are merely held at bay by modern medical techniques, ready to burst forth again, as dangerous as ever, the moment we relax our vigilance. Thus, uncommon as they may be today, certain of these infections deserve more than passing attention.

Diphtheria: The Forgotten Killer

Diphtheria is a fast-moving, debilitating infection caused by a distinctive form of bacteria known as *Corynebacterium diphtheriae*. It is spread from person to person by means of infected nose and throat secretions from one who has the disease, or from an apparently healthy "carrier" who harbors the organism in his nose and throat. The initial throat infection may seem relatively minor, with only a degree or two of fever and a slightly sore throat. Small children may show no sign at all until the bacteria are well entrenched.

Within 24 hours, however, the infection becomes extremely dangerous in two exceptional ways. First, the bacteria invading the tissues in the nose and throat begin killing cells, which then form a thick, sticky, false membrane adhering to the entire back of the throat and even extending down into the larynx and trachea. As the infected tissues swell, this tenacious membrane of dead cells and mucus can obstruct breathing, and may even cause death from suffocation, especially in small children. As if this were not dangerous enough in itself, the invading bacteria also produce a powerful poison called an *exotoxin* which not only destroys tissues in the nose and throat but is carried in the blood stream to distant parts of the body, causing a prostrating generalized illness.

This poison can attack the heart muscle, leading to severe damage and heart failure, or it may damage the kidneys. In severe cases it may even destroy spinal nerve cells, sometimes causing permanent paralysis of the extremities if the victim recovers at all.

CORYNEBACTERIUM
DIPHTHERIAE

Figure 17–1.

Anyone with a sore throat and any sign of difficult breathing, especially a child, should be seen by a doctor at once. Often diphtheria can be diagnosed just from the appearance of the membrane forming in the throat. If he even suspects it, the doctor will first take a throat culture to confirm the diagnosis, and then immediately begin treatment with antibiotics to destroy the bacteria and with diphtheria antitoxin to neutralize the exotoxin that has already been formed. Even with vigorous treatment, recovery is slow, often requiring weeks before full strength is regained. During the acute phase, special care must be taken to keep an airway open for breathing; in severe cases a *tracheostomy* (an opening into the trachea) must be performed and a breathing tube inserted to aid respiration. Sometimes there is no choice but to treat such cases in the hospital. Complications from pneumonia and heart failure must be watched for, and even after the acute illness has subsided, middle ear infections or abscesses in the tonsils may occur. A victim is not considered fully recovered until all symptoms have passed and at least two negative throat cultures have been obtained.

Early diagnosis and vigorous treatment have sharply reduced the death rate from diphtheria in this country. But if the disease has, in fact, become a "forgotten killer" it is due to the highly effective immunization most individuals receive in childhood—the basic DPT "baby shots" or so-called triple vaccine that protects children from diphtheria, pertussis (whooping cough) and tetanus (lockjaw) all at the same time. Immunization is given during a baby's first six months with three successive doses at monthly intervals of the DPT vaccine. These shots are available from your family doctor, or free of charge at Public Health Service clinics everywhere in the country. Six months after the three-shot series a booster shot is necessary; thereafter boosters should be given at three-year intervals until the child is twelve years old. If there is any question whether or not a full series of DPT vaccine was obtained, children of six years and older can be given a special "DT" preparation containing just diphtheria and tetanus vaccines. In addition, a simple skin test known as the Schick test can be performed to determine whether a child is immune or susceptible to diphtheria at any given time. In this test a tiny amount of diluted diphtheria exotoxin is injected between the layers of the skin on the forearm. If a person is immune, antibodies in his blood stream will neutralize the injected toxin, and no reaction will be seen. In a susceptible person the area around the injection site becomes inflamed and swollen in reaction to the injected toxin. *A high level of immunity should be maintained into young adulthood to protect against diphtheria.*

In spite of ready availability of the DPT vaccine, a surprising number of children have never received the complete series. Families move to a new community and forget to resume basic immunizations where they left off. Sometimes financial difficulties arise, and families neglect to take children to the nearest Public Health Service office where the DPT vaccine can be obtained without charge. But failure to provide a child with full protection against such diseases as diphtheria can be a tragic oversight. There are still some 50 deaths out of about 7,000 reported cases of diphtheria each year in this country alone. Parents should keep a permanent Immunization Record (*see* p. 873) for each of their children. If a child has somehow missed a basic shot or booster, consult your family doctor or the nearest Public Health Service office to bring his immunizations up to date. No disease can ever be truly "forgotten," but today there is no reason why *anyone* should contract diphtheria.

Whooping Cough (Pertussis)

While diphtheria is no respecter of age, striking children and adults alike, whooping cough most commonly attacks babies. Fifty percent of all cases occur before the age of two. One attack of the disease confers lifelong immunity, but among unimmunized victims under a year old, the death rate is still high enough even today for whooping cough to be considered a dangerous threat.

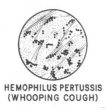

HEMOPHILUS PERTUSSIS
(WHOOPING COUGH)

Figure 17–2.

The disease, which got its common name from the "whooping" sound of the cough associated with it, is caused by the bacterial organism *Hemophilus pertussis*. It is highly communicable, occurring in epidemics among young children at intervals of two to four years, and typically lasts for six to eight *weeks* from onset. The bacteria attack tissues of the upper respiratory tract, trachea and bronchial tubes, forming a sticky mucus which is easily coughed up at first but later becomes very tenacious and irritating. The first symptoms, beginning from one to three weeks after exposure, are like those of a common cold: runny nose, sneezing and coughing. There is usually no fever, but the child's appetite falls off and the cough becomes increasingly severe, especially at night. As sticky mucus forms in the victim's respiratory tract the coughing becomes paroxysmal; the child will cough 10 or 15 times in rapid succession, all in one breath, followed by a deep inspiration or "whoop." Great quantities of mucus may be coughed up during these paroxysms, but the irritation continues and the combination of coughing and gagging on the secretion often leads to vomiting.

This whooping type of cough is at its worst between two and three weeks after onset of symptoms. From then on, the disease goes into a convalescent stage, and the coughing becomes progressively less frequent and severe. At the height of the disease the child may die from suffocation, from complicating pneumonia due to other bacteria, or from aspiration of vomitus during a paroxysm of coughing. Most children ultimately recover, but many are excessively sensitive to other respiratory infections for months to come, with recurrence of the paroxysmal cough even with minor infections. Others suffer enough permanent lung damage to be vulnerable to chronic, recurring bronchitis or to the injury to lung tissue known as *emphysema*.

Whooping cough can be treated effectively today with such broad-spectrum antibiotics as tetracycline, thus markedly shortening the course and severity of the disease. Even so, it remains a real danger to children under the age of four, and in babies younger than six months old the death rate may be as high as 20 percent—still a major cause of infant mortality. In older children and adults the infection is more annoyance than threat, but long-term lung damage may still prove disabling years later.

When a child has whooping cough, other children should be kept away from him, chiefly to protect him from other complicating infections. Your doctor may prescribe an *expectorant,* a medicine designed to loosen sticky bronchial secretions so that they can be expelled. Later in the illness a cough *suppressant* may be indicated, but this decision should be made by a doctor. It is often the long convalescence, with continuing coughing, that worries parents especially. About all that can be advised is patience, and special care not to expose the patient to other upper respiratory infections. Presently the coughing will subside—but final recovery may take months.

The best "treatment" for whooping cough is obviously prevention. A baby can be immunized against the disease beginning at age three months by means of the same DPT vaccine used against diphtheria. Some degree of protection is attained within ten days after the first shot of the series, but in an emergency a child can even be given temporary protection by administering immune blood serum from people who have a high level of immunity themselves. However, this so-called passive immunity (which is transferred, so to speak, from an immune individual to a child with no immunity) will last only a few weeks at best. It can help an unprotected child known to have been exposed to whooping cough, but the DPT vaccine should be given concurrently so that the child can begin developing his own long-term "active" immunity.

Poliomyelitis (Infantile Paralysis)

If the DPT vaccine has been highly effective in controlling diphtheria and whooping cough, recent mass immunization programs have had an even more dramatic effect against one of the most vicious virus diseases known to man. In 1952 in the United States, during a nationwide epidemic, some 57,000 children and young adults were stricken with poliomyelitis, resulting in permanently crippling paralysis or death in more than half the cases. In 1964, just twelve years later, only *91* cases of paralytic polio were reported, with just 17 deaths. This almost incredible turnabout will surely go down in history as a major medical triumph of the 20th century.

Poliomyelitis, known for years as "infantile paralysis" because it so commonly struck children under the age of five, has one of the strangest histories of any major disease. Caused by any one of three very closely related viruses which are now known to be primarily gastrointestinal invaders, paralytic polio was a relatively uncommon affliction throughout the world until the late 1800s. Then, for no apparent reason, epidemics of the disease began to appear, usually during the summer and fall, first in Sweden and Norway, then in the United States and western Europe. Sporadic at first, these epidemics gradually became so widespread and severe that by the early 1950s polio was one of the most dreaded of all diseases, killing or crippling tens of thousands of young people every year.

Finally in 1955, after years of intensive research and testing, Dr. Jonas Salk and his associates at the University of Pittsburgh introduced an injectable vaccine made from killed viruses of the three deadly polio strains and capable of preventing paralytic poliomyelitis. Massive vaccination programs were begun at once in both the United States and Europe. Seven years later a quite different "live virus" vaccine developed by Dr. Albert Sabin of Cincinnati was licensed for use—a more convenient vaccine because it is taken by mouth and is capable of preventing polio infections in the gastrointestinal tract as well as the paralytic infections. The widespread use of these two vaccines brought the incidence of poliomyelitis to a virtual standstill in the United States in just a few short years.

Why this strange historic pattern of polio epidemics? And how could newly developed vaccines work so swiftly to turn the tide of this rampaging disease? The answers, in part, lie in the nature of the disease itself. Today it is believed that in unvaccinated populations poliomyelitis may be one of the mildest and most commonplace of all virus infections known, usually appearing unrecognized in early childhood and causing no symptoms other than mild fever, headache and sore throat for two or three days. It is only in the rare case, perhaps one out of a hundred, that the dreaded symptoms of stiff neck, muscle spasm and paralysis occur at all. What is more, because polio viruses are most commonly transmitted by intestinal contamination of food and water, the mild or "silent" form of the disease is most widespread in parts of the world where crowded living conditions are combined with poor hygiene and primitive sanitation. Thus the polio viruses are widely disseminated, and most children in those areas contract unrecognized infections before the age of two or three and then develop lasting natural immunity.

This pattern of polio infection also prevailed in the United States and western Europe, until the end of the 19th century brought vast improvements in sanitary facilities. Then the pattern began to change. More and more children missed contact with polio viruses during early childhood and reached adolescence or young adulthood completely unprotected by naturally acquired immunity. Thus when virulent strains of polio virus appeared, vast populations in these countries were susceptible, and great epidemics of paralytic polio began to occur. This strange infection pattern still prevails today where polio immunization is not widely available. In under-developed countries with poor sanitation, full-blown paralytic polio appears only in isolated cases, never in epidemics, but in countries with rapidly improving sanitation, it strikes more and more older children and young adults in annual epidemic waves.

When polio infection attacks an unprotected child today, the first or mild stage of the disease may still go unrecognized, mistaken even by doctors for a mild case of three-day flu. In most cases a low-grade fever, a sore throat and aching muscles are all there is to the disease. But on rare occasions a second and far more severe stage of the illness begins several days later with the onset of high fever, severe headache and stiff neck, painful muscle spasms and—all too often—increasing muscle weakness and then paralysis of various groups of muscles as the virus begins permanent destruction of nerve cells in the spinal cord or the base of the brain. It is the motor nerve cells controlling the motion of voluntary muscles that are attacked, and the extent of the paralysis depends upon which of these cells are destroyed, and how many. If enough are damaged in the lower spinal cord, paralysis will affect the legs and feet; higher up it may affect the diaphragm, the accessory breath-ing muscles, one or both arms or the muscles of the shoulder girdle. Most dangerous of all is *bulbar polio,* in which the virus attacks nerve cells at the base of the brain, causing paralysis of the throat muscles, the larynx, the facial muscles or the tongue. Bulbar polio accounts for the great majority of deaths from the disease.

So far there is no effective treatment for the acute polio infection itself once the disease has struck. Hospital care, however, is imperative as soon as diagnosis is made, both to protect the patient against respiratory failure and to limit the damage done by the disease insofar as pos-sible. The patient must be watched closely and constantly for evidence of paralysis, especially of the diaphragm and other breathing muscles. Painful muscle spasms during the paralytic stage of the illness can be relieved somewhat by hot moist packs to the affected areas several times a day. Mechanical support of respiration may be

necessary, either with a tank respirator ("iron lung") or by means of a positive-pressure breathing apparatus. Death from polio in this stage usually results either from respiratory fail-ure or from the inability to cough up secretions which pool in the lungs and can literally suffo-cate the patient. Life itself may depend upon vigorous, experienced hospital nursing care, especially when the respiratory failure proves temporary, and recovery is possible as long as the victim survives the crisis.

Once the acute illness is over, a long period of convalescence may be necessary before it can be known for certain if the paralysis is to be tempo-rary or permanent. If *all* the motor nerve cells controlling a group of muscles have been de-stroyed, no recovery is ever possible; but if only a scattering of nerve cells has been knocked out, those remaining can take over and gradual re-turn of muscle strength is possible. During this phase physical therapy is vital to help retain good muscle tone and to ensure the full range of joint motion. We know today that much of the tragic crippling from polio that occurred earlier in this century could have been prevented if more had been known about proper convales-cent care. Most recovery of lost muscle function occurs within the first six months, but further improvement may continue for a year or more. Above all, the patient with persisting paralysis will need moral and psychological support. Too often the victims of this disease are teen-agers or young adults, totally unprepared for the perma-nent physical impairment that can result.

What are the real dangers of poliomyelitis? Among those victims with paralytic symptoms, more than half will recover with *no* residual paralysis, although certain of their muscles may tire easily. Others are less fortunate: about 25 percent with paralytic symptoms will have some degree of residual paralysis, and another 20 per-cent may be severely crippled for life with per-manent paralysis of the breathing muscles, legs, arms, facial muscles or the muscles controlling eye movements. Between 1 and 10 percent will die, depending upon how virulent the virus hap-pens to be and upon the victim's age; older children and young adults are the most vulner-able to fatal affliction. In some cases death can result in a matter of days; in others the acute disease and its effects may linger for months.

Poliomyelitis today is a wholly preventable disease. There are two different types of vaccine available for protection, each with advantages and disadvantages. The Salk vaccine, developed from polio viruses killed with formalin, was first given by injection in a series of three shots beginning as early as two months of age, with four to six weeks between the first and second doses and the third given some seven months later. It soon became evident, however, that the Salk vaccine did not always provide lasting immunity. Today the American Academy of Pediatrics recommends a fourth or booster shot a year after the basic three, and subsequent boosters every two years until adulthood. Furthermore, the Salk vaccine did nothing to prevent immune "carriers" from harboring the living polio viruses in their intestinal tract and spreading them far and wide.

The newer Sabin vaccine seems to solve these problems. Taken by mouth, not by injection, it contains living polio viruses which have been weakened or attenuated in order to cause a mild, symptom-free polio infection in the intestine. This vaccine produces more permanent immunity and also makes later intestinal reinfection with the polio virus difficult, thus preventing its spread in the community as long as enough people have been immunized. Today the Sabin vaccine has largely displaced the injectable Salk vaccine, especially for use in community-wide mass immunization programs. But for all of this, some virologists still regard this "live virus" vaccine with considerable uneasiness. They point out that rare cases of polio occur in people who have received the Sabin vaccine, possibly brought on by the vaccine itself. They also point out that we still do not know just how long the attenuated virus from the vaccine may stay in the intestinal tract—possibly for years—nor can we be absolutely certain that those viruses might not some time "change back" to a more virulent form.

It may be years before we know for certain which vaccine offers the most protection at the least possible risk. For now, some cautious doctors recommend a full course of the Salk vaccine first, *followed* by a course of the Sabin vaccine, to be as sure as possible that the "live virus" vaccine has no chance to cause an active case of paralytic polio. But whichever vaccine is recommended, one thing is certain: *all* preschool children should have at least one or the other immunization against polio, either as part of a community-wide program or at the family doctor's office. In less than a dozen years polio epidemics in this country have been brought to a halt, saving thousands of lives and sparing tens of thousands who might otherwise have been permanently crippled. The challenge today is to keep up the immunity levels of whole populations so that some day poliomyelitis can truly be conquered throughout the world.

A Rogues' Gallery of Other Childhood Infections

Fortunately, a great number of relatively familiar infections that occur most commonly during childhood and youth are not marked by the kind of virulence that characterizes such preventable killers as diphtheria, whooping cough and poliomyelitis. Even so, many of them are acute illnesses that can cause serious danger and discomfort and often lead to prolonged convalescence. Naturally, some are more dangerous than others, but all of them should be a matter of concern to families with children or young people.

Mumps (*Acute Parotitis*)

One of the most common and readily identifiable of these infections, ordinarily occurring among children or adolescents, is mumps, or more accurately, acute parotitis, a virus infection which characteristically causes painful inflammation and swelling of the parotid salivary glands that lie in the cheeks just in front of the ear, as well as the salivary glands under the chin. When mumps occurs during childhood, the infection is most commonly confined to these glands, although the virus may in some cases also attack the pancreas, the liver, or the meningeal lining of the brain or spinal cord. Often the disease starts with a day or two of high fever, lassitude, loss of appetite and generalized illness before the salivary gland swelling appears to cinch the diagnosis. But at that age the virus rarely attacks other parts of the body. If the infection is contracted after puberty, however, it may also involve either the testicles in the male or the ovaries in the female, as well as other glandular organs such as the pancreas or the breasts. The infection is quite contagious and may occur in epidemics in crowded city areas in the late winter and early spring. But it is not at all uncommon for some children in a family to develop severe cases of mumps while others are apparently untouched. In fact, mumps is typical of many virus infections in that it may attack some more dramatically than others, and it is not unusual for an individual to have a so-called subclinical case—that is, an infection that is so mild that no real symptoms ever appear.

How can you tell if a child in the family is getting mumps? The traditional technique of feeding the child a pickle may be painful, but it is also diagnostic. When a child complains of pain in the cheeks and there is some puffy swelling, any acid food such as vinegar or orange juice which stimulates salivation will help differentiate mumps from swellings that might occur as a result of an infected tooth, a tumor of the salivary gland or an obstruction of one of the salivary ducts by a stone; salivation is acutely painful in mumps. Once the full-blown glandular swelling occurs, diagnosis is even simpler. There is just no other condition known to man which causes first one side of the face to swell up, then the other, perhaps both at once, and sometimes swelling under the chin as well. The location and amount of swelling, however, can vary greatly from patient to patient. Some children may have swelling on only one side of the face with the other glands unaffected; others may have swelling all around, giving the face the appearance of a pear. Contrary to the popular notion, people probably do not contract mumps a second time after recovering from the infection. "Second cases" of mumps are usually shown to be other infections, since the first attack confers a lasting immunity which can be confirmed by skin tests.

There is no specific antibiotic that will alter the course of mumps in the slightest. Treatment of the illness consists primarily of bed rest, symptomatic treatment to reduce fever and relieve pain, and a light, bland diet to help ameliorate the period of nausea and vomiting that often occurs a few days after onset of the infection. Glandular swelling, at its height, may be quite painful for a period of two or three days—sometimes longer—but applications of cold cloths to the swollen areas and an appropriate dosage of aspirin every four hours will often help with the pain. After two or three days the swelling and pain begin to decline, and recovery is usually complete within another seven to ten days. Mothers often become alarmed, at the height of the infection, because of the grotesque distortion of the child's face. But they need not worry. As the infection subsides, so does the swelling, and there is never any residual disability or deformity. In severe cases, the pancreas gland or the liver may be affected, causing abdominal pain and often nausea and vomiting, but these symptoms too will subside in a few weeks as the infection subsides.

More serious, and more difficult to deal with, is the development of *acute orchitis*—inflammation and swelling of the testes—in adolescent or young adult males. Not only is this complication of mumps extremely painful, it may also result in such long-term damage to the glandular structure of the testes that one or the other of them will cease to be functional and will atrophy. In rare cases in which both testes are severely affected, permanent sterility may result. A doctor should always be consulted when a male at the age of puberty or beyond has developed mumps or is known to have been exposed; administration of the synthetic hormone diethylstilbestrol can often prevent involvement of the testes with mumps, and if orchitis does develop, later atrophy of the testes may be prevented by a simple surgical incision to relieve pressure. Symptomatic treatment is also important. The patient's scrotum should be supported on cotton with an adhesive-tape bridge between the thighs. The doctor will direct other aspects of nursing care as needed and can prescribe medication to control pain if necessary. In any event, the patient should be kept at absolute rest in bed, not only to avoid aggravating the pain and discomfort, but to help shorten the period of disability. In adolescent girls, involvement of the ovaries, a less common complication, is not usually accompanied by any permanent damage or residual impairment of ovarian function and fertility. But complete bed rest is still advisable during the acute phase of the illness.

Because of the length of the illness (anywhere from ten days to two weeks or more) and, more significantly, because of the risk of damage to the testes in older boys, virologists in recent decades have been searching vigorously for an effective vaccine to provide artificial immunity against the infection. A vaccine developed in the early 1960s was effective, but provided such short-lived immunity (six months to a year) that it was not very practical protection. More recently a much better vaccine made from live but attenuated mumps virus has become available. A single dose of the vaccine gives an effective antibody response in about 98 percent of susceptible persons and produces an active immunity that persists for at least two years. This is a considerable improvement over the earlier mumps vaccine; most pediatricians now recommend it for children of any age over twelve months, since by then any immunity passed on to the baby by the mother is gone. A few more conservative doctors, however, are nervous about *any* live-virus vaccine and feel that vaccination against mumps should be performed only when a child has reached puberty without contracting the infection. They argue that younger children might better be allowed to contract the illness if possible. Rely on your own doctor's opinion. Although usually uncomplicated in children, the disease is a distressing nuisance, and—even more important—it *can* be complicated by meningitis or encephalitis in some cases as a result of an attack of the mumps virus on the spinal cord or brain.

Susceptible adolescents and young adults, however, do need protection in the event of exposure to the infection. A skin test can be performed on older children in order to tell if they have already had mumps. If they had subclinical infections during earlier childhood that went unrecognized at the time, they will usually demonstrate an immune reaction to the skin test. If they prove susceptible, however, a special mumps-immune gamma globulin can be administered in case of exposure to provide temporary protection.

Familiar Upper Respiratory Infections (URI's)

No one with children in the family requires an introduction to the commonplace infections of the throat, tonsils, adenoids or middle ear to which young people are so frequently susceptible. Doctors speak of infections in these areas (as well as those of the bronchial tubes) as "URI's"—upper respiratory infections—whether caused by bacteria or viruses, and include among them infections of the sinuses, the nasal passages, the larynx or voice box, and the major air tubes leading to the lungs. URI's are not actually a single disease entity, but can be caused by any one of a number of organisms. Those most commonly at fault are streptococci or staphylococci, but a wide variety of relatively nondescript viruses can also be the culprits.

The site of infection is most frequently a ring of a special glandular tissue, known as *lymphoid tissue,* that forms a sort of circle at the back of the nose and throat. This glandular tissue, which includes the tonsils in the throat behind the base of the tongue, the adenoids located above the soft palate where the nasal passages open into the back of the throat, and patches of tissue coating the base of the tongue, was once thought to serve as a vital protective system, trapping microorganisms that entered the body through the mouth or nasal passages before they could pass into the bronchial tubes and the lungs. Today most doctors tend to doubt that these lymphoid tissues actually play any significant protective role, unless it is in the case of infants,

but we know that the tissues themselves, after repeated bouts of infection and scarring, can become the site of continuing chronic infection, sometimes to such a degree that surgical removal is advisable in a procedure known as a tonsillectomy and adenoidectomy, or T and A.

Tonsillitis. The most familiar of these upper respiratory infections, tonsillitis usually begins abruptly with a fever spiking to 103° or more and the sudden onset of pain and swelling in the back of the throat. When a streptococcus is the causative organism, the whole ring of lymphoid tissue is involved, and the back of the throat looks bright red. After a day or two an exudate begins to form on the tonsils, and a number of yellowish-white spots or streaks of pus can be seen on these swollen structures at the back of the throat. At the same time lymph nodes surrounding the infected area become swollen and tender, and can often be felt on the neck underneath the jaw or at the angle of the jaw and just below the ears. The fever continues for several days, if no treatment is begun, and then gradually subsides as the body conquers the infective organism.

Before antibiotics, a bout of tonsillitis could last from 10 to 14 days and sometimes even longer before all symptoms were relieved. Today vigorous treatment of bacterial tonsillitis with appropriate antibiotics—penicillin, tetracycline, or the like—helps limit the infection to a matter of two or three days and, especially if a streptococcus is at fault, also helps prevent the danger of later strep-related illnesses such as rheumatic fever or acute nephritis. But virus-caused upper respiratory infections, unaffected by antibiotics, will persist somewhat longer. When the patient's throat is extremely sore, pain and swelling can be alleviated by the use of an ice collar around the neck, and by frequent gargling with a warm salt-water solution, a teaspoonful of salt to a cup of warm water. As with any acute infection, bed rest is indicated until the fever subsides, as long as the child feels like staying in bed. (Only rarely is it either wise or worthwhile to try to *force* a sick child to stay in bed if he does not want to. He can rest just as effectively up and about the house in robe and slippers, and may even agree to a truly restful morning and afternoon nap in return for such "privileges." It is only adults who usually welcome bed rest when they are sick.) When the throat is sore, a bland, soft or liquid diet is advisable in order to spare the patient unnecessary throat irritation from coarse or spicy food.

Tonsillitis and related infections of the throat, tonsils and adenoids do not usually confer lasting immunity. New infections can occur at any time, sometimes one right on the heels of another. Many children in fairly robust health can endure an occasional bout of tonsillitis without any ill effect. If such infections are infrequent enough, a child's adenoidal tissue gradually shrinks away and disappears, and his tonsils grow smaller and less prone to infections year by year. Other children have bout after bout of recurrent tonsillitis, often two or three or even more attacks a year, with resulting deleterious effects on their general state of health and normal growth and nutrition. In such cases, the possibility of surgical removal of the tonsils and adenoids should be considered.

The Question of a T and A. Thirty or forty years ago tonsillectomy was much more in vogue among doctors and patients alike than it is today. It was a rare child indeed in those days who made it past the age of five without having his tonsils and adenoids removed. Even now there are experienced and responsible physicians who seem to regard all tonsils as "bad tonsils" and recommend a T and A at the earliest possible age for a child who has had any trouble with tonsillitis at all. On the other hand, many modern practitioners go to the opposite extreme. They regard such surgery as a last-ditch measure to be undertaken only when everything else has been tried, and unfortunately may permit their patients to suffer for years with recurring and debilitating infections before they are finally willing, most reluctantly, to recommend the operation.

Which medical approach is right? The answer probably lies somewhere between these two extremes. And furthermore, the attitude of the child's parents may play an important role in making the decision. If you have a child suffering from recurrent bouts of tonsillitis, and wonder if a T and A may not be beneficial, have enough confidence in your doctor to consider carefully whichever course he recommends. But at the same time, have enough faith in your own common sense to question him about his advice, and do not hesitate to ask for a second opinion if you feel it necessary. There are, after all, several important considerations that both you and your doctor must bear in mind in reaching a decision.

First and foremost, there is the question of medical necessity. No physician today can justify subjecting a child to a surgical procedure for the removal of tonsils and adenoids just because they are there. Nor is a history of one or two bouts of tonsillitis usually an adequate reason for such surgery. On the other hand, when the child suffers from recurring bouts of infection every year, when his tonsils are obviously enlarged, scarred by old infection and chronically infected, and when his general level of health, resistance and growth has been beaten down by these recurrent infections, there is no virtue in postponing or avoiding a T and A without a specific and valid reason. Among other important medical indications for a T and A are recurrent episodes of ear infection along with chronic infection of the tonsils and adenoids, or so much enlargement of the tonsil and adenoid tissue that there is obstruction of the nose and throat, with resultant changes in voice or breathing. True, the surgeon will quite properly insist that such a child be free of active infection at the time the surgery is done, and in many young patients this can mean scheduling and postponing the operation repeatedly, perhaps for as long as a year or more.

Second, there is the age of the patient to consider. Most surgeons prefer not to perform T and A's on children under two years old, partly because of the technical difficulty of operating on such a tiny patient, partly because of the risk involved in the anesthesia techniques necessary, and partly because enough lymphoid tissue may remain after surgery that recurrent infections still continue. (Contrary to popular belief, tonsils never "grow back." But small patches of lymphoid tissue at the back of the throat or in the area of the adenoids can indeed enlarge and become the focus of new recurring infection, giving much the same appearance as the re-moved tonsils and adenoids.) Even when children reach the age of twelve years or so, additional risks, mostly related to the possibility of severe hemorrhage, must be taken into consideration.

With the use of modern anesthetics and surgical techniques, however, a T and A is generally regarded as a relatively safe procedure, even for small children—so much so, in fact, that the real risks of the operation are often underrated even by the surgeon. Yet all too often this "innocuous" procedure can become a true surgical emergency. For one thing, there is a certain risk involved in the administration of any general anesthesia. In the very young, swelling of the larynx and injury to the trachea can result from the tube inserted to give the anesthesia. Recovery from the anesthesia can be complicated by vomiting and—occasionally—aspiration of the emesis with the development of a chemical pneumonia as a result. In older teen-agers and adults the greatest risk is that of severe post-operative hemorrhage from the raw bed of vascular tissue from which tonsils and adenoids have been removed. Such a hemorrhage can sometimes be massive or even fatal before the physician can be summoned to deal with it.

Does this mean that the T and A procedure should be discarded, or undertaken only as a last-ditch measure? Of course not. It simply means that a T and A is *never* an innocuous procedure. It should be undertaken only when medically necessary, and under circumstances in which any risk is reduced to the barest possible minimum. Thus a T and A should be regarded not as a routine operation for every child between the ages of three and ten, but rather as a relatively safe surgical procedure, bearing certain calculated risks, to be used in individual cases only when necessary.

When this kind of selectivity is practiced, what results can be expected? Occasionally they can be dramatic indeed; once in a while a child who has been "held back" in terms of normal growth, resistance and overall physical development owing to chronic and recurring throat infections will show a remarkable improvement after a T and A. In such a case the frequency of upper respiratory infections declines sharply, and when they do occur they are mild and easy to control with modern medications. The appetite often improves, and the child may literally blossom after recovery from the surgery with a rapid weight gain and a marked spurt in growth. Unfortunately, this kind of response is rare, even though many parents tend to expect it, often with the encouragement of their doctors. In most cases changes are far more subtle, and may seem disappointing. This does not mean that a T and A that was medically necessary has been a "failure." It does mean, however, that a child with occasional tonsillitis should not be subjected to surgery unnecessarily, just in the hope that some miraculous change will take place. The T and A question must be examined carefully on all sides by both doctor and parents, and performed only in those individual cases in which the advantages clearly outweigh the possible risks.

The performance of T and A is not a guarantee that a child will no longer suffer from upper respiratory infections. True, he may well be free of infection in the tonsils and adenoids, since they are no longer there; but bacteria or viruses can still cause acute infections of the throat. Without the lumps of poorly vascularized lymphoid tissue in the tonsils and adenoids, these infections are usually less severe and more generalized, involving all parts of the throat and nasopharynx, and sometimes extending to the upper part of the trachea. Referred to medically as pharyngitis, they do not tend to be chronic and recurrent; and those that occur after a T and A has been performed are usually caused by viruses, since there is not so much tissue in which bacteria can lodge and grow. Other infections such as laryngitis (inflammation of the larynx), tracheitis (inflammation of the lining of the trachea) or bronchitis (inflammation and infection in the smaller air tubes within the lungs) may even be somewhat more prevalent than before tonsils and adenoids are removed.

In any case, the occurrence of all these infections deserves attention by a doctor, proper culturing of the nose and throat in order to determine if a bacterial organism is at fault, and then specific treatment with the antibiotics of choice.

Fortunately, as a child grows into adolescence or young adulthood these infections become less and less frequent, possibly because they are often virus-caused and the body develops lasting immunity against them.

Otitis Media

A more aggravating and distressing condition, which may occur either before or after a T and A, is otitis media, an inflammation and infection of the middle ear. This is the familiar and typical "earache" of childhood, and it results either from bacteria in the throat and nasopharynx making their way up the Eustachian tube to invade the middle ear or from viruses which find entry by the same route. The Eustachian tubes are the narrow passages that extend from the middle ears to the back of the throat to permit equalization of air pressure inside and outside the eardrums, especially with changes of altitude. Swallowing or yawning usually opens the throat end of the Eustachan tubes—provided they are not swollen shut by infection—and leads to the familiar "popping" of the ears when riding an elevator or an airplane.

Otitis media may occur in conjunction with other upper respiratory symptoms, or it may occur without the usual warning of fever, malaise or general illness, manifesting itself for the first time through the sudden onset of severe pain in the ear. It also may occur in a child who is apparently recovering from an infection of the nose or throat. The earlier illness appears to be under control, medication has been stopped, and the child is back at his normal activities when suddenly he wakes up in the middle of the night with an extremely painful earache.

Aside from the pain involved, otitis media can cause other problems. In the days before antibiotics, infection of the middle ear commonly spread into the bony air pockets of the mastoid region behind the ear, setting up permanent housekeeping there and leading to chronic recurrent *mastoiditis*. A *mastoidectomy,* the surgical removal of the infected mastoid area of bone, was once considered the treatment of choice when this occurred. But today when both

upper respiratory infections and otitis media are usually treated vigorously with antibiotics—penicillin, ampicillin, or one of the tetracycline family—mastoid infection is rarely seen as a complication.

Any evidence of middle ear infection deserves the prompt attention of a doctor, since both the severity of the infection and its duration can be markedly decreased by proper treatment. To treat the acute pain that arises with this condition, the appropriate dosage of aspirin is often sufficiently effective. An ice bag applied to the ear may also help relieve pain. When these measures fail, another simple technique often works, uncomfortable as it may seem. With the child lying on his side, ice water can be dripped into the affected ear canal, using an eyedropper or even holding an ice cube in the fingers and allowing melted water to drip directly into the ear. Instill three or four drops every five to ten minutes for an hour or so, using a tissue to sponge up water which has been warmed in the ear canal. Although this kind of treatment may sound like a new sort of Chinese water torture, it will often reduce the acute swelling and pain of a midnight earache quite effectively.

In a small percentage of severe infections, however, none of these measures is effective. The pain does not subside and the collection of fluid and swelling of tissue in the middle ear may cause the eardrum to bulge, a condition the doctor can easily observe with his otoscope. In such cases, rupture of the eardrum or *tympanic membrane* is a distinct possibility, and the doctor may decide to open the membrane by means of a small, clean surgical incision called a *myringotomy* which will later heal without scar or other damage to the eardrum. A spontaneous rupture, on the other hand, may cause a long, ragged opening that heals with scarring and possibily some later impairment of hearing. In either case, there may be a copious drainage of pus and lymphatic fluid out of the middle ear for a day or two. The surgical procedure is usually preferred because, like incising and draining a boil, it often leads to a much speedier recovery with less permanent scarring and damage than if the eardrum ruptures, or if the infection is allowed to run its course and subside on antibiotic treatment alone.

Most middle ear infections respond readily to treatment and only rarely result in chronic infections or permanent damage to the anatomy of the middle ear or to the hearing function. But some children (and even some adults) seem far more prone than others to developing otitis media any time they contract an upper respiratory infection. Part of the reason for this may lie in the amount of adenoidal tissue that surrounds the opening of the Eustachian tubes in the nasopharynx. Not infrequently recovery from a T and A is complicated by transient irritation of the middle ear simply as a result of scraping adenoidal tissue away from the Eustachian tube openings. Nevertheless, infections of this tissue often block the Eustachian tubes and move into the middle ear. Thus recurrent otitis media is another valid medical indication that a T and A may be necessary. Infection may also reach the middle ear via the Eustachian tube as a result of blowing the nose too vigorously during a head cold. Children should be taught to blow their noses only gently, if at all, and if possible to sniff up mucus and spit it out rather than to blow. Finally, *any* drainage from an ear is ample reason to see a doctor whether there is pain present or not. Many people tend to neglect this because they feel all right, but permanent damage to an ear can result from a painless chronic ear infection.

Infectious Mononucleosis (Glandular Fever)

One of the most peculiar and variable of all the illnesses afflicting human beings is infectious mononucleosis, a disease which often presents the doctor with a diagnostic challenge because of the many different ways it can affect its victims. But generally it proves to be more nuisance than threat because of the length of time (from a couple of weeks to several months) that is needed to throw it off. A comparative newcomer among infectious diseases, mononucleosis was first recognized as a clinical entity by Emil Pfeiffer in 1889, who described an epidemic among schoolchildren of a disease which he

called "glandular fever" because of the swelling and tenderness of lymph glands that was consistently present among victims of the infection. Later investigators found that the disease was characterized by a marked increase of lymphocytes in the blood stream of infected persons, the kind of white blood cell formed in the lymph glands and lymph tissues. Because these cells were commonly called *mononuclear leucocytes* (literally "one-nucleus white cells") to distinguish them from polymorphonuclear leucocytes ("many-shaped-nucleus white cells") formed in bone marrow, the disease was later given the name "infectious mononucleosis." Since the early 1900s the disease has been recognized throughout the world, often in epidemic form among younger children but today more common in adolescents of high school and college age or even, more rarely, in adults. No one has yet isolated or identified the microorganism which causes the disease, but it is commonly believed to be a virus infection that is spread by close upper respiratory contact, thus accounting for its wry nickname, "the kissing disease." On the other hand, oddly enough, two cases are rarely seen in the same household, and some authorities doubt that kissing has anything to do with it.

The most perplexing thing about infectious mononucleosis is the wide variety of ways it can affect its victim, and the multitudes of differing symptoms it can cause. No two people ever seem to have *exactly* the same symptoms. Sometimes the disease appears abruptly as an acute upper respiratory infection, with cough, fever, chills, headache and general malaise. When this occurs it makes things easier for both the doctor and the patient; at least they know something is wrong. More commonly, however, the onset of the infection is vague and insidious, characterized by increasing fatigue, listlessness, loss of appetite, recurrent daily headaches and perhaps daily low-grade fevers. Also quite frequently there is an apparent inability to get sufficient rest, so that when the victim finally, perhaps after several weeks, consults a doctor, he complains mostly of just being constantly tired. He may also complain of a mild and persistent sore throat, nothing very serious, just an annoying scratchiness that seems to come and go from day to day but never entirely clears up. In these cases, except for the unusual fatigue, the doctor has little or nothing to go on.

Further investigation, however, may help pin down the diagnosis. Characteristically the virus affects the lymph tissue in the body. There may be swelling of the glands in the neck, under the arms or in the groin, and this is often an important clue. In other individuals an intermittent high spiking fever, which appears recurrently without any apparent cause, may be the tip-off. With perhaps 10 percent of the victims, a transitory reddish skin rash, much the same as the rash of German measles, will appear at some point early in the infection, persist for a day or longer, and sometimes recur again and again accompanied by severe itching. In about half the cases of mononucleosis the patient's spleen will be so swollen that the doctor can actually feel it protruding down under the edge of the ribs on the left-hand side of the abdomen. More rarely, the patient's liver becomes so filled with lymphocytes which have been trapped there that the function of that organ is impaired and a transitory jaundice (yellow coloring of the skin and whites of the eyes) appears.

In the absence of specific symptoms like these, however, diagnosis can be very difficult. Fortunately, most physicians have had enough experience with the disease to be highly suspicious of vague complaints and nondescript symptoms, and two laboratory tests will often confirm the doctor's suspicions. First, he checks for changes in the patient's white blood count. Lymphocytes normally make up only about 30 to 35 percent of all the white cells present, but in mononucleosis lymphocytes may make up as much as 70 or 80 percent of the white cells, many of them showing certain characteristic changes in their form when they are stained and examined under the microscope. Second, he checks the antibody content of the patient's blood. Whatever microorganism causes the infection, the body responds by forming special immune antibodies which are pathognomonic of infectious mononucleosis; that is, these special antibodies appear in vastly increased quantity in the blood stream in re-

sponse to this one type of infection and no other. These so-called *heterophile antibodies* begin to appear anywhere from a few days to three or four weeks after the onset of the disease; they can be detected quite readily in the laboratory and the concentration or *titer* accurately measured. Thus when heterophile antibodies are found in a patient's blood stream in high titer, the doctor can be quite certain that infectious mononucleosis is present.

Ironically, once a doctor has accurately diagnosed the disease, there is little else he can do. There is no specific cure other than bed rest during its acute stages and symptomatic treatment of the various discomforts that may occur, such as headache, fever, abdominal pain or itching of the skin. No antibiotic seems to affect the organism causing the disease or shorten the course of the illness, which is almost always benign, yet it may seem to the patient that it lasts forever. The acute stage usually spends itself within three or four weeks, but the side effects—lassitude, fatigue and a sense of just "not feeling well"—may persist for two to six months or even more. But once recovered, the patient will usually have no residual problems to worry about except the risk of recurrence, which is common. Recovery is marked by a return of blood tests to normal, and—more significant to the patient—a gradual return of a feeling of health and well-being.

The only real danger of infectious mononucleosis lies in certain very rare complications. When a patient's spleen has become swollen and engorged with lymphocytes during the acute stage, that organ may rupture spontaneously, or may be ruptured by a very slight accidental blow to the abdomen, leading to internal bleeding that must be treated by emergency surgery to prevent exsanguination. Occasionally the virus may cause inflammation of the pericardium (the outer lining of the heart), leading to acute pericarditis. Even more rarely, a viral meningitis (inflammation of the protective outer lining of the brain and spinal cord) or encephalitis (brain fever) may be caused by the mononucleosis virus. The likelihood of any of these uncommon complications can be markedly reduced by an adequate period of bed rest during the acute stage of the disease. When the body has been invaded by the mononucleosis virus, it has adequate work without any other demands upon its supply of energy.

So far no kind of vaccination or immunization is possible against infectious mononucleosis, and considering the benign nature of the illness, it seems unlikely that immunization would ever be widely used, except in the case of epidemics, even if the virus could be isolated and a vaccine prepared. Like any virus disease, mononucleosis strikes most often when the victim's natural resistance is low as a result of some other infection (such as an acute URI) or due to exhaustion, exposure or malnutrition. Thus the best way to prevent the illness is adequate rest and care in the event of *any* infection, and the avoidance of excessive or chronic physical or mental strain.

Meningococcal Meningitis (Epidemic Spinal Meningitis)

If mononucleosis is a benign infectious disease even though no specific treatment is known, certain meningeal infections are just the opposite, fulminating and viciously dangerous diseases which even today take many lives and leave numerous other victims crippled in spite of the number of effective antibiotics that can be used to treat them. One form of meningitis in particular can move so swiftly that there is often barely enough time for treatment to be started before the patient is dead. Other forms, less fulminating, still represent a serious threat, especially to children, and may cause permanent neurological damage before the infection can be stopped.

People tend to think of "spinal meningitis" as a single disease caused by a single microorganism. In truth, one or another kind of meningitis may arise when any of a dozen different bacteria or viruses cause inflammation and infection of the *meninges,* the delicate membranes that enclose the spinal cord and the brain itself in a protective sheath. Any of these organisms can cause the group of symptoms characteristic of irritation of the meninges which doctors call *meningismus:* severe headache, pain on movement of the head or neck, marked stiffness of the

neck, the appearance of certain abnormal reflexes, and other changes in the normal nervous system responses of the victim that may vary all the way from marked excessive nervous irritability to coma. Any of these organisms may also

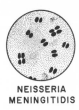

NEISSERIA
MENINGITIDIS

Figure 18–1.

bring about permanent damage, particularly to the higher nerve centers in the cerebral cortex, leading to impaired mentality or even feeblemindedness, and to the cranial nerves which make vision and hearing possible.

But of the many kinds of meningitis, the most common and dangerous is the so-called epidemic spinal meningitis or "spotted fever" caused by one of the most virulent of all the bacteria, the *meningococcus.* It is most commonly spread by upper respiratory contact and can become epidemic among schoolchildren, for instance, or in crowded living conditions such as military barracks. The organism first enters the body by means of a mild infection in the nose, throat or middle ear, then gains access to the blood stream, multiplying constantly and causing a meningococcemia, or meningococcus blood poisoning. Soon after it converges in the meninges covering the spinal cord and brain and causes an incredibly swift and devastating infection there.

The first sign of the disease is usually a severe headache, a sudden high, spiking fever, vomiting, and the rapid onset of mental confusion, delirium, or even coma. The victim's neck and back become rigid, sometimes to such a degree that the whole body seems to be bowed outward, and presently muscle twitching or even convulsions begin. In severe cases these meningeal symptoms may be preceded or accompanied by an odd rash of pinhead-sized spots, hence the name "spotted fever." These spots are really tiny capillary hemorrhages under the skin, and microscopic examination of a drop of blood taken from one of them will often show the meningococci present. In addition to the characteristic symptoms, diagnosis is made certain when meningococci are discovered in these blood samples, or when large numbers of the bacteria and pus cells are discovered in a spinal fluid sample taken by means of a lumbar puncture (LP).

If the infection becomes overwhelming before it can be diagnosed and treated, death may ensue in convulsions or coma, or the bacteria may cause hemorrhages in the cortex of the adrenal glands, leading to abrupt circulatory collapse and death. Among those who survive a severe attack, sometimes even when treated promptly and heroically, the disease may leave grim permanent scars: partial or complete blindness, deafness, partial paralysis, permanent convulsive disorders or sufficient brain damage to cause irreversible mental retardation. The organism causing meningococcal meningitis is very sensitive to both penicillin and the sulfa drugs, as well as other antibiotics. Massive doses of these drugs must be given swiftly, and expert nursing care must be available in the hospital during the critical few hours while the antibiotic is beginning to take effect. But quick diagnosis is the single most vital factor to successful treatment. It is for this reason that *any sudden high fever in a child, any evidence of tiny pinpoint hemorrhages under the skin or any sign of stiffness of the neck and severe headache should be called to a doctor's attention immediately*. Meningococcal meningitis is not seen nearly as often today as it

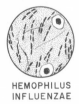

HEMOPHILUS
INFLUENZAE

Figure 18–2.

was 20 or 30 years ago, thanks to the widespread use of antibiotics in treatment of all kinds of upper respiratory infections, but outbreaks still occur, and the danger of death or permanent

disability is still so great that no chances should be taken.

Other organisms may also cause meningeal infections, most notably the tuberculosis organism, a bacterium known as *Hemophilus influenzae* (*not* the influenza virus), the pneumococcus, the streptococcus or even the staphylococcus. In addition, numerous virus infections may cause meningeal irritation or inflammation. Any of these organisms may cause symptoms such as those described above, but rarely with the devastating swiftness of the meningococcus. Meningitis caused by these other organisms at least offers the physician some leeway and time in which to make the diagnosis and institute treatment. Meningococcal meningitis, on the contrary, is literally a race against death. But with acute diagnostic acumen and swift treatment more and more victims today than ever before are saved and returned to normal health without any devastating residual effects.

Infectious Hepatitis (Acute Infectious Jaundice)

Infectious hepatitis is often only a mild to moderately severe illness, but in some instances it can follow an extremely serious course. Out of every hundred people who contract the infection in recognizable form, most at worst suffer a two- or three-week acute illness, followed by a prolonged convalescence; but some 10 percent suffer irreparable damage to the liver which permanently cripples them and shortens their lives, and some 2 to 4 percent die, either during the acute infection or within a year or two after chronic illness as a result of liver damage.

The disease ordinarily strikes children and adolescents, but adults are by no means passed by. And as with many other virus infections, there is no way to tell in advance who will be severely stricken and who will have only a mild case. The infection is caused by a tiny and elusive virus, even yet never definitely isolated or cultured, which is excreted in the stools of infected persons, so the disease is transmitted through contamination of water, milk or food and can be passed from person to person by close physical contact. It often attacks in epidemics, particularly in areas with poor sewage disposal or other sanitary facilities (seafood from sewage-contaminated water is a notoriously dangerous source) or in crowded cities, most commonly in the heat of midsummer and early fall. Like many other virus infections, authorities suspect that a great many people may contract the disease in such a mild form that telltale symptoms never appear and the disease is shrugged off as a mild case of intestinal flu. It is also suspected that many people who do have such unrecognized cases of hepatitis may nevertheless carry the virus in their bodies for prolonged periods, thus acting as carriers of the disease—one reason why careful attention to isolation of an infected patient and meticulous sanitary precautions are so vital when someone in the family is afflicted.

Typically, the disease starts with intestinal flu-like symptoms—a spiking fever, a severe headache, aching muscles and nausea, vomiting and loss of appetite—as the virus enters the body and travels through the blood stream to find lodging in the liver. Here it multiplies rapidly, causing widespread destruction of cells. In response to the infection the liver becomes swollen and very tender, causing a deep-seated aching in the right upper abdomen and acute pain on pressure just below the ribs.

At this point, the victim may still believe he only has a case of flu and postpone seeing a doctor. But in fact, he is acutely ill and highly infectious. In a few days, his skin and particularly the whites of his eyes take on the yellowish-orange color of jaundice, caused by the backing up of bile formed by the liver into his blood stream. He develops a sickly sweet fetid odor on his breath, his urine turns dark brown owing to excretion of abnormal amounts of bile through his kidneys, and his stools lose their normal color and become a characteristic grayish-white. His fever and loss of appetite continue, and he feels exhausted with even the slightest physical effort. Incredibly enough, some victims ignore even these obvious symptoms. When they finally do seek medical help, the doctor has every reason to be alarmed and begin immediate and vigorous treatment.

Treatment of the disease, under ordinary circumstances, consists of strictly enforced bed rest, careful attention to diet and a great deal of patience. Little else can be done. There is no medicine or antibiotic that has any effect on the virus, although the doctor may prescribe one or another antibiotic to forestall secondary infection by bacteria. The very sick patient is usually best treated in a hospital where he can be kept in strict isolation and where intravenous feedings are sometimes necessary while nausea and vomiting are prominent symptoms. Less serious cases can often be treated at home, but there, too, the doctor's directions must be followed to the letter, including isolating the patient from the rest of the family, reserving one set of dishes for his use alone, keeping all but the one person responsible for nursing care out of his room, strict attention to personal hygiene, hand washing, etc., and close adherence to dietary instructions. A bland liquid diet is best during the acute stages of the infection, later followed by a diet rich in protein and with restricted amounts of fat.

After a week to ten days of bed rest, the disease will usually subside. The patient's body has time to form antibodies to counteract the virus, the jaundice in most cases recedes, fever drops, appetite returns, and the patient once again feels like getting up and moving around. Indeed, he may feel *too* much like normal and try to return to his usual activities too soon, with a subsequent relapse and return of the jaundice. Even in relatively mild cases, the infection saps the energy of the body tremendously, and a convalescence of weeks or even months may be necessary. Depending on the severity of the disease and the extent of damage to the liver, the doctor may prescribe continuing dietary restrictions, decreased physical activity and often, for adults, total abstinence from any form of alcohol for several months.

In most cases the patient regains his strength gradually and there is no evidence of residual or long-term damage from the illness. But not all cases have such a happy ending. Sometimes the infection is so severe and so much of the liver is damaged that the victim can go swiftly and steadily downhill. The jaundice deepens as he lapses into a stupor or coma characteristic of liver failure, and ultimately he dies during the acute phase of the infection. This kind of devastating course is rare, however; more often there may be sufficient damage to liver cells that regeneration and return of normal liver function is impossible. Healing progresses with massive scarring and distortion of the liver's normal structure so that a *post-hepatitis cirrhosis* or hardening of the liver occurs. When this happens the victim may appear to recover completely from the acute virus infection, but laboratory studies will reveal continuing and permanent impairment of liver function, and the victim may remain forever vulnerable to acute liver failure any time a later infection or disability places a demand on his liver function. If the cirrhosis is severe, the circulation of blood through the liver may be permanently impaired. Veins in the abdomen, or around the stomach and esophagus, which normally carry blood into the liver become tremendously distended or *varicosed,* ultimately leading to severe bleeding into the stomach or intestine.

No one knows definitely to what extent improper rest and care during the acute stages of the infection may lead to permanent damage and threat to life, but most physicians agree that the danger of impairment, however seldom it may occur, is sufficient to warrant the most cautious approach to care any time the acute infection strikes. Some recent studies suggest that such caution may be unwarranted, but until we know for certain, a few weeks or even months of enforced bed rest and convalescence are a small price to pay for complete recovery from an infection which can result in chronic illness, disability and even untimely death.

The early detection and diagnosis of infectious hepatitis is obviously of critical importance. Often the first clue is the appearance of jaundice in the midst of an acute flulike illness. Jaundice, of course, can occur as a result of many conditions other than infectious hepatitis, but this is one symptom which is *always* abnormal and should always be called to a doctor's attention immediately. The patient's medical history, a careful physical examination and a variety of laboratory tests measuring liver function will help the doctor pin down the diagnosis. Labora-

tory studies, which may be repeated several times during the course of the illness, will also help him follow the progress of the disease so that he can better judge when it is safe for the patient to resume normal activity.

Once infectious hepatitis is diagnosed and treatment is started, it is important to protect other members of the family, or friends who have been in close contact with the victim, against infection insofar as possible. Although no vaccine has yet been developed to confer long-term immunity, individuals who have been in contact with the infection can receive short-term protection lasting as long as six weeks to two months by means of gamma globulin injections. But the success of the injection depends upon the swiftness with which it is administered after exposure. Certainly when one member of a family comes down with hepatitis, other members who have not had the disease should receive gamma globulin shots. When the disease occurs in epidemic form in military installations, in schools or in crowded city areas, widespread use of gamma globulin can materially decrease the incidence of new infections and help bring the epidemic to a halt. A person who has previously had hepatitis and recovered, however, will carry a lasting acquired immunity to reinfection, so that gamma globulin need be used only as an added precaution if the individual is elderly or otherwise in ill health.

Serum Hepatitis. Infectious hepatitis is the most common virus liver infection, but there is, oddly enough, another type called serum hepatitis which produces virtually the same symptoms but is believed to be caused by a different virus agent, and is transmitted in an entirely different way. Unlike the virus of infectious hepatitis, the serum hepatitis virus is not excreted through the intestine, and thus is not transmitted by means of contaminated water or food or close physical contact. Rather, it is spread from person to person only by the use of contaminated hypodermic needles, lancets, or other medical or surgical instruments, or by the administration of blood or plasma taken from a donor who is a carrier of the virus. Serum hepatitis is virtually identical with infectious hepatitis except that its incubation period is much longer

—symptoms may not occur until five or six *months* after inoculation—and its course is usually much more severe, with a markedly higher incidence of acute fulminating illness leading to death and a higher incidence of post-hepatitis cirrhosis.

Until recently serum hepatitis was a relatively unusual infection, occurring primarily among doctors or medical researchers who came in contact with contaminated needles and syringes, or occasionally spread by contaminated equipment used in mass vaccinations. Recently, however, there has been a sharp increase in this particularly deadly form of hepatitis as a result of the use of contaminated syringes and needles for the self-administration of narcotics and other drugs. The virus of serum hepatitis is extremely hardy, impervious to ordinary antiseptics such as a 70 percent alcohol solution or even to a few minutes of boiling. Indeed, the only procedure that can guarantee its destruction is the sterilization of instruments in an autoclave which uses live steam under pressure for periods of 20 to 30 minutes. Obviously, young people experimenting with drugs do not have autoclaves; often they do not want to be bothered even with such elementary precautions as prolonged boiling of their needles and syringes. As a result, much of the increase in serum hepatitis in recent years has been among teen-agers and young adults who are using drugs for "kicks" and sharing their hypodermic equipment. To make matters even worse, individuals who survive an attack of serum hepatitis may carry the live virus in their blood streams for prolonged periods, acting as "healthy carriers" of this dangerous disease. Thus, quite apart from the perils of drugs and narcotics, anyone experimenting with their use is exposing himself to the additional, and possibly fatal, danger of serum hepatitis.

"Strep" and "Staph"—The Omnipresent Invaders

Many of the infectious illnesses, particularly those associated with childhood and youth, are type-specific; that is, they are individual diseases with specific symptoms caused by specific micro-organisms. Mumps, for example, is an easily discernible disease caused by one particular virus and no other, while diphtheria is a discrete disease easily distinguishable from other diseases and caused by a particular species of bacteria. However, this pattern does not hold true for all infectious illnesses. Two groups of the most common of all disease-producing organisms known—various *streptococcus* bacteria and two or three varieties of *staphylococcus* bacteria— can be responsible for several different forms of infection without necessarily being invariably identified with any one illness. (Scarlet fever, which is caused by a specific strain of strepto-coccus bacteria, is an exception to this rule.) And to make matters even more complicated, many of the forms of infection most commonly caused by either strep or staph organisms can, occasionally, be caused by other bacteria as well. But here we will consider those various forms of infection most often caused by strep and staph organisms, including some of the most familiar and annoying diseases that a family, both chil-dren and adults, can encounter.

These infections are so commonplace for the simple reason that strep and staph organisms themselves are so commonplace and in such omnipresent contact with the human body. Staph organisms are normal and usually per-fectly benign inhabitants of the skin of the face, neck, trunk, arms and scalp. Two predominant strains, in fact, the *Staphylococcus albus* and the *Staphylococcus aureus,* are under normal cir-cumstances not disease-producing organisms at all. It is only when they are introduced inside the body through a break in the skin or an abrasion of a mucous membrane that they become infec-tion producers. Strep organisms, while less com-monly found as benign inhabitants of the human skin, often exist in the nasal passages, throat or other areas of the body, again without causing infection. But many people who are completely free of active infection themselves nevertheless "carry" these strep organisms and can spread them to more susceptible individuals. Once these organisms invade an individual with low resis-tance to infection, they may become very dan-gerous indeed. At best they can cause relatively mild infections, but at their worst, they can be responsible for serious and sometimes life-threatening illness.

Superficial Skin and Eye Infections

Impetigo. Many people have had personal experience with a disease commonly known as impetigo—an itching, slowly spreading infection of the surface layers of the skin, especially on the face, scalp or arms. It is characterized by shallow weeping lesions that start as tiny fluid-filled blebs or blisters which subsequently burst and become covered with a dirty-looking grayish scab or crust of dried exudate. The first lesion of a case of impetigo can begin with an abrasion, a scrape or a cut, but sometimes it appears, often in the ears, even though no break in the skin has been noted. Once begun, however, the urge to scratch becomes almost irresistible, and the infection can then be spread further or even transferred to others in close contact.

Characteristically, impetigo, which is generally caused either by a strep or a staph organism, afflicts schoolchildren, and sometimes appears almost epidemic in form, spreading quickly from one child to the next. Untreated, it tends to involve more and more skin area, and also to invade deeper tissues, becoming a more deep-seated cellulitis. It may even enter the blood stream to become a blood-borne infection or bacteremia. In general the disease represents a real threat only to newborn babies in hospital nurseries, and when a nursery is involved in an epidemic of impetigo resulting from antibiotic-resistant strains of staphylococci, the disease can constitute a very serious health hazard. The spread of the infection is particularly facilitated any time some other skin rash associated with itching is present—a diaper rash in an infant, for example, or an allergic rash in an individual of any age.

Most cases of impetigo respond very promptly to proper treatment with local applications of antibiotic drugs in the form of salves, or water-soluble creams or lotions, which are usually more satisfactory. It does little good, however, merely to smear an antibiotic salve or lotion over the surface of the crusted lesions, since the infecting organisms are living and multiplying in the moist tissue *underneath* the crusts. For most effective treatment, the crusts over the lesions should be cleansed away with warm soap and water, applied gently with a washcloth. If the lesions are particularly tender, they can be soaked with a solution of a teaspoonful of salt in a quart of warm water, applied with warm compresses. Once the crusts have been removed, the antibiotic medication can be rubbed directly into the denuded surface of the lesions. Carried out faithfully two or three times a day, this sort of treatment will produce quite dramatic results in most cases, with the itching relieved in a matter of a few hours, and the lesions diminishing in size and drying up in two or three days. Treatment should not be abandoned too soon, however; as long as any open raw area is still present, the infection can easily recur as soon as treatment is suspended. Your doctor may also prescribe injectable or oral antibiotics to speed recovery.

In families with numerous children it is particularly important to realize that impetigo is highly contagious, and vigorous efforts should be made to prevent its spread. The easiest way to do this is to see that *all* members of the family use a bactericidal soap, such as Phisohex, and make sure that washbowls or tubs used by an infected individual are scrubbed thoroughly with a chlorine-containing scouring powder or with a Phisohex-type soap. All washcloths, hand towels and bath towels used by the infected individual should be kept separate from the regular household supply, and should be disinfected by boiling for 20 minutes or more at a rolling boil in a large pan before being returned to general use.

If treated early and effectively, impetigo will heal quickly without scarring. It is only when it has been neglected and allowed to invade deeper tissues or form boils that scars or pockmarks may remain after healing.

Acute Conjunctivitis ("Pinkeye"). Another annoying superficial infection, usually caused by a staph organism but sometimes by pneumococci or other bacteria, is an acute infection of the *conjunctiva*—the mucous membrane inside the eyelids—in a highly contagious condition known as acute conjunctivitis or, more commonly, pinkeye. The first warning a victim has is usually a period of intense itching and excessive tearing, often in only one eye but sometimes occurring simultaneously in both. The lining and even the white of the eye redden as tiny capillaries become engorged, and sometimes there can even be edema or swelling of the eyelids. After a few hours, a discharge of pus begins to form which may tend to "glue" the eye shut during sleep; this is accompanied by even more intense itching and irritation. Again, pinkeye is an infection which is readily spread among children, so it is well to warn children to avoid close contact with an infected individual as well as his clothing and other personal effects.

Treatment of acute bacterial conjunctivitis is best accomplished with either an ophthalmic salve or eyedrops containing one of the broad-spectrum antibiotics, sometimes combined with one of the cortisone-type medications to help quiet the inflammation and itching quickly. Self-medication with nonprescription medicines can be hazardous. A doctor should always be consulted and his prescriptions used in treatment. Over-the-counter medications may not contain suitably effective drugs to treat the condition or may not carry the drugs in high enough dosage to be effective. More important, however, is the fact that the symptoms of pinkeye are sometimes mimicked by the comparatively uncommon virus infection herpes zoster, or shingles, which may afflict the eye and actually cause ulceration of the cornea. The cortisone-like drugs tend to aggravate this kind of herpes infection, sometimes increasing the risk of permanent impairment of vision if they are used mistakenly. Such a herpes infection can easily be distinguished by a doctor in a simple office examination and appropriate medication prescribed to avoid this hazard.

Bacterial conjunctivitis will usually respond to antibiotic treatment within a day or two, but medication should be continued for 48 to 72 hours after symptoms have disappeared in order to avoid recurrences. If the medication prescribed is an ophthalmic salve, the easiest way to apply it is to pull down the lower eyelid and lay a line of the salve direct from the applicator tip across the moist mucous membrane. Then the patient should close his eye and roll his eyeball around to distribute the salve. Many doctors, however, prefer to use a water or saline solution of an antibiotic in the form of eyedrops, which can be applied every two hours during the day, and during the night if the patient wakes up. In either case, pinkeye should heal promptly and is unlikely to have any complications or residual ill effects. During recovery it is well to avoid irritation of the eye from wind, dust, smoke or intense light. The infected individual should avoid close personal contacts, and the towels and washcloths he uses should be disinfected by boiling to prevent spread of the infection.

Sepsis and Septicemia (Blood Poisoning)

Far more grave than impetigo and pinkeye is a different form of strep or staph infection that involves deeper soft tissues in a cellulitis, frequently causes a generalized bacterial poisoning of the body spoken of as sepsis, and sometimes leads to the invasion of the blood stream by the infecting organisms, resulting in a condition known as septicemia or, more commonly, blood poisoning. These are dangerous conditions indeed, and they must be recognized and treated early in order to avoid serious or even fatal consequences. *Cellulitis* arises from a superficial strep or staph infection which, owing to the breakdown of the body's defense barriers against it, is able to invade and spread in the soft tissues beneath the skin.

One common and dangerous form of cellulitis is a strep infection called *erysipelas*, in which the bacteria spread from a local wound or infection into surrounding tissues. The infection follows the lymph channels and often first appears as angry-looking red streaks visible on the skin extending toward the trunk from a formerly minor infected area on the neck, face or a limb. This type of cellulitis is accompanied by acute pain, tenderness, and some swelling in the lymph nodes and affected areas. The toxins manufactured by the streptococci cause a high spiking fever with chills, severe headache, sometimes delirium from the fever, nausea and vomiting, and other general symptoms arising as a result of the body's being literally poisoned by the spreading infection. A cellulitis and septic condition resulting from a staph infection, however, usually spreads more slowly and less dramatically, and more often forms a localized pocket of infection, spoken of as an abscess, which ultimately becomes filled with pus, swollen, tense and extremely painful. The abscess will finally "point" or work its way toward the surface by means of pressure stretching the layers of tissue. Then it will either break and drain spontaneously or can be incised and drained by a physician. Adolescent pimples are nothing more than small abscesses formed by staph organisms trapped in plugged-up pores in the skin. Larger staph abscesses frequently form on the back of the neck.

Various forms of cellulitis and sepsis are known by different names. In the days before antiseptic methods were recognized as necessary in childbirth, streptococci were often introduced into a mother's womb in the process of delivering a baby, causing a singularly vicious strep infection involving the entire uterus that often led to fatal blood poisoning, a condition that is known as *puerperal sepsis* or "childbed fever." It was the Hungarian obstetrician Ignatz Semmelweiss who demonstrated in 1847 that doctors and midwives themselves were responsible for transmitting childbed fever from one innocent victim to another. He proved that the incidence of this dread plague could be sharply reduced by the simple expedient of having the attendants wash their hands thoroughly in a solution of calcium chloride before deliveries and change and boil the garments they wore after each delivery. This was the first consistent application of the principle of antisepsis in medical history, and the mortality rate in Semmelweiss' clinic fell from 12½ percent in May to 2 percent in June and 1 percent in July of the same year; in March and April of the following year there was not a single death from puerperal fever in the wards of his obstetrical clinic. Sad to say, Semmelweiss himself finally died of streptococcal blood poisoning.

Today the appearance of childbed fever is a medical rarity, but it still remains a threat, especially in a case of prolonged labor which requires repeated vaginal examinations. The first sign, much the same as erysipelas, is the sudden onset of spiking fever and chills. Because childbed fever, as well as other forms of streptococcal cellulitis, is quite sensitive to treatment with either penicillin or other of the broad-spectrum antibiotics, mortality from these infections today is extremely rare except in cases that simply do not come to the doctor's attention until the sepsis has become overwhelming.

A common form of staph cellulitis (and one of the most painful types of infection known) is the *felon*—an infection of the soft tissue in the pad of a finger or thumb. Felons often arise as a result of minor skin breaks on the fingers, splinters, or torn hangnails. The initial infection seems to have healed completely when days or even weeks later a new, exceedingly painful, throbbing infection develops in the ball of the finger. The infection causes an abscess and swelling in an area that has little elasticity, and thus the pain nerves in the fingertip involved are literally crushed. If neglected even for a short time, it can lead to early bone infection of the finger. Conservative treatment of a felon is rarely successful; quite radical surgical incision of the fingertip, followed by drainage of the abscessed area, is necessary to permit healing. The pain can be so severe that even morphine does not help, yet it can be relieved within an hour simply by adequate incision under local anesthesia and release of the tension.

Any form of cellulitis, accompanied by the generalized sepsis or "poisoning" that such infections cause, can evolve into septicemia—a condition in which bacteria gain access to the blood stream and travel throughout the body, setting up secondary infections in capillary areas and posing the most severe threat when the site of these infections is the kidney, for example, or the brain. Septicemia is the classical picture of a dangerous infection gone wildly out of control, with bacteria in large numbers literally overwhelming the body's natural capacity to counteract them by means of the white blood cells. Before antibiotics, blood poisoning was a serious complication of any kind of infection, and it led to innumerable deaths, often as high as 25 or 30 percent when the infecting organism was a virulent one such as the streptococcus. Today, thanks to early antibiotic treatment of almost any diagnosed infection, blood poisoning is rarely seen because the bacterial infection can be stemmed before it reaches this stage. Even in cases in which it has already begun, it still can often be stopped by heroic antibiotic therapy, unless it is so far advanced that death ensues before the antibiotic has time to work.

Thus, from a very practical standpoint, infected wounds, no matter how minor they may seem, require the attention of a doctor. In addition to the antibiotics prescribed by the physician, the home treatment of such infections should include soaking with hot water or hot, moist compresses to help increase the blood flow to the infected area, thus carrying more white blood cells to the body's defense there. Substances dissolved in the water—salt, Epsom salt, powdered mustard or other popular "home remedies"—do no good. Plain hot water, at a temperature that can be comfortably tolerated, applied three or four times a day for fifteen or twenty minutes at a time will help the body fight infections, and in the case of pus-forming infections will help the lesion to "point" or come to a head so that it will rupture spontaneously or it can be incised and drained by a physician, if necessary.

Furuncles (Boils), Carbuncles and Other Staph Infections

Strep infections causing cellulitis or blood poisoning can be virulent, swift-moving and highly toxic, striking down an apparently healthy person with the blitzkrieg swiftness of an invading army. But staph infections are generally "borers from within," a sort of dogged, entrenched fifth column always present and always ready to take advantage of a lapse in physical resistance. They, too, can get out of control and overwhelm the victim with severe toxic illness, but they are more likely to grow quietly, spread and fester rather than fulminate. For that reason, it might be assumed that staph infections pose little threat to the body, and this assumption would be correct except for two facts: staph infections, by their very indolence and relative lack of symptoms, can sometimes advance to a highly dangerous state before they are recognized; and second, the staph organisms themselves have a most diabolical ability to change their genetic nature readily and very quickly develop new strains or families that are resistant or immune to the protective antibiotics that are being used to combat them. As a result, they all too often can cause prolonged and dogged battles for health before they are finally eradicated.

Staph infections are among the most commonplace that a person is likely to encounter. Everyone has suffered, usually in adolescence, from an outbreak of unsightly pimples or acne on the face, almost invariably caused by staph infections of the pores of the skin. (*See* p. 393.) This affliction is nothing more or less than a form of staphylococcal furuncles or, to use the more common name, "boils." Almost everyone has also suffered from a more serious form of furuncle, the deep-seated boil in which pus ultimately collects, and which is extremely painful owing to the swelling and tension caused by the infection.

If left untreated, a boil may eventually be conquered by the body's resistant forces, gradually resolving, with absorption of the purulent material, but leaving an indurated area of scarring in the soft tissue. However, proper treatment by a doctor can significantly reduce the duration of the infection. The first step in treatment consists of medication for pain (often simple aspirin will suffice, or in more severe cases aspirin combined with a mild prescribed tranquilizer), and the application of frequent hot moist packs to the boil—or hot tub soaks—for the purpose of bringing the lesion to a head. This type of conservative treatment is usually combined with the prescription of appropriate antibiotics, more for the purpose of preventing spread of the infection than for the effect the medicine may have on the active lesion. Once a boil has come to a head, surgical incision and drainage is usually indicated. Evacuation of the pus material will promote more rapid healing, and a portion of the material extruded can be cultured in the laboratory to determine the sensitivity of the causative organism to various antibiotics. If the boil is large or extensive, the surgeon may leave a sterile gauze drain or rubber wick in the incision for a day or two to promote further drainage. Characteristically the pain of the boil disappears quite abruptly once the incision has been made and the pressure of pus within the wound has been released.

The terms "furuncle" and "boil" are used to describe an infection involving the skin or the subcutaneous tissue just beneath the skin. Typically a boil contains a collection of pus and destroyed tissue, and often a "core" of cheesy material that is extruded during drainage. The term "abscess" is used to describe both superficial furuncles and deep-seated infections, accompanied by destruction of tissue and formation of pus, that can form in almost any part of the body, often by means of transmission of the infecting organism through the blood stream. A brain abscess, for example, is a large lesion within a portion of the brain caused when bacteria from some apparently benign superficial lesion are transmitted through the blood stream and lodge in the brain. Other deep abscesses can form in the liver, usually as a result of infection by the protozoan ameba which causes amebic dysentery, and at the site of a removed appendix when some of the bacteria-laden content of the intestine is inadvertently spilled into the abdominal cavity during an appendectomy.

Typically the body attempts to wall off or seal an abscess so that it may be held in a capsule and does not spread widely. However, a hidden deep abscess can produce a mysterious recurrent fever and other symptoms of generalized bacterial poisoning. Although relatively uncommon, such deep abscesses sometimes prove excessively difficult to diagnose. Diagnosis may become even more difficult if the bacteria in the abscess have been successfully destroyed by the body's defenses, leaving a so-called cold abscess or sterile abscess which indicates its presence only by the pressure it exerts on adjacent organs or parts of the body. Any brain abscess, for example, whether actively infectious or sterile, will usually cause recurrent or continuous headaches as well as other neurological symptoms as a result of pressure.

In addition to hot soaks to help bring furuncles or abscesses to a head, followed by surgical incision and drainage, broad-spectrum antibiotics help limit the infection and speed healing. Laboratory identification of the offending organism and its sensitivity to a variety of antibiotics is wise, since it may be a staph strain that is impervious to the more commonly used antibacterial drugs. These infections do not ordinarily spread through the tissue. However, if the infection is deep-seated in connective tissue beneath the skin and is left untreated, or is inadequately treated, spreading can occur. The result is a comparatively large area of tissue afflicted by multiple localized pockets of infection, often connected to each other by scarred channels of fibrous tissue known as *fistulas.* When a staph infection evolves in this manner, an area of multiple boils several inches across may form, with some parts actively breaking the skin and draining while other parts remain tense, swollen and actively infectious. Such a multiple boil is spoken of as a *carbuncle,* and is usually associated with severe pain in the area, spiking fever and general toxicity or bacterial poisoning of the body. Often there is open oozing of pus, blood or serum from the lesion, and sometimes extensive sloughing of dead tissue from the wound.

A carbuncle is one type of infection that should emphatically *not* be treated by home remedies and self-medication. The attention of a physician, and probably a surgeon, is vital to speedy healing of the lesion with a minimum of scarring and permanent tissue damage. Even with surgical incision and drainage, debridement of dead tissue and opening of channels connecting different areas of infection, the healing of a carbuncle may require weeks. The doctor or surgeon will probably combine his treatment with antibiotic medication and will take antibiotic sensitivity studies as soon as purulent material from the lesion is available for culture. In some cases extensive surgical excision of a carbuncle followed by skin grafting may be the ideal method of treatment. But every case of this sort is different; the important thing is to seek professional help early and follow the medical or surgical regimen indicated, even if it means a prolonged period of treatment.

All staph infections may be complicated by the fact that the causative organism is "immune" to many commonly used antibiotics. There is the further danger of superficial infections of this sort finding their way into the blood stream and seeding infections far distant from the primary source. One of the most serious complications of a staph infection results when the bacteria are transmitted via the blood stream into areas of bone, a tissue which has a poor blood supply, poor defense mechanisms, and thus a vulnerability to extensive infection.

Osteomyelitis, the generic term for any bone infection, often begins this way. Although it can be caused by numerous other organisms and not infrequently arises as a result of an open or compound fracture of a long bone, it is one of the most serious sequelae of staph infections. (*See* p. 304.) Nor is it the only one, of course; any part of the body *can* be affected. Because of their insidious nature and their antibiotic resistance, staph infections are a matter of serious medical concern. Unfortunately, they can actually be spread in modern hospitals as a result of unsuspected contamination of wards, instruments and other care facilities. Any infection of the skin, eyes or other parts of the body which appears shortly after a period of hospitalization should be reported without delay to a doctor for diagnosis; if it is a staph infection, the hospital should be notified, so that steps can be taken to prevent any further spread of the infection there.

No discussion of strep and staph infections would be complete without at least brief mention of the so-called strep-sensitivity diseases. It is true that strep infections, as a general rule, are quite responsive to penicillin or other antibiotic drugs—even to sulfa drugs—and once correctly diagnosed can usually be swiftly stopped. Even so, these infections can sometimes be followed by a form of late complication or side effect that has nothing to do with the streptococcus organism itself. Among these late side-effect diseases, perhaps the most dangerous are rheumatic fever and acute glomerulonephritis, an inflammation of the kidney that is more often called acute nephritis.

Both of these conditions were medical mysteries for many centuries. Even today much remains to be discovered about their nature. But within recent decades it has become increasingly clear that both result not from any direct infection with strep organisms, but rather as a result of an odd sort of overreaction of the body to the presence of certain particular strains of strep organisms or to substances they produce. In other words, they begin as a hypersensitivity or exaggerated body defense reaction which itself becomes a serious illness. Both diseases occur most commonly in children and young adults and can follow strep infections that were so mild that they went virtually unnoticed. Both are heralded by similar symptoms—a high spiking fever, nausea and vomiting. Here, however, the diseases begin to differentiate, for rheumatic fever particularly attacks the heart and acute nephritis the kidney; but both, without prompt diagnosis and vigorous treatment, can cause crippling disability and permanent damage. (*See* p. 560 *and* p. 723.)

Thus, strep and staph infections, as common as they are, should never be taken for granted. Even though they may begin as superficial infections, there is always the danger that they may evolve into more deep-seated and generalized illness. Strep organisms pose a particular threat because of the virulence of their original attack and the possibility of later side effects, while staph organisms can also cause serious complications and may prove to be resistant to antibiotic treatment.

Tuberculosis, Pneumonia and Other Bacterial Infections

Type-specific diseases like mumps or diphtheria are each caused by one particular microorganism and no other, while other infectious organisms like strep or staph may each cause a wide variety of different infections. This by no means exhausts all the possible varieties of infection, however. Certain diseases, such as tuberculosis, are always caused by a single specific bacterial organism but may involve a multitude of organ systems in the infection, even though one organ system (the lungs, in this case) is more commonly invaded than the others. Conversely, certain forms or classes of infectious illnesses may involve only one organ system but may be caused by any one of a wide variety of different bacteria, even though one particular agent is the most common cause. The most familiar examples of infections of this class are the bacterial pneumonias. Other infections, such as Vincent's infection (trench mouth), are caused by two or more bacteria working together as a sort of infectious team. Still others, including tetanus and gas gangrene, are type-specific diseases but have certain unique and remarkable characteristics, owing either to the nature of the causative bacteria or to the singular ꞌ way in which they affect the body. All these infections are fairly common, and all are equally impartial in their selection of victims.

Tuberculosis: Modern Plague-in-Waiting

There is probably no other major affliction of mankind that has undergone a more staggering revolution in medical management or a more dramatic decline in incidence and death rate in the Western world in the past twenty years than the infectious disease tuberculosis. Once called the Great White Plague, it has possibly taken more human lives, in total, than any other infection in all the history of medicine.

For many of us today, tuberculosis has become almost a forgotten disease. Since 1945 we have heard less and less about it; the incidence of newly discovered cases and the death rate have both tumbled sharply. One by one the special hospitals and sanatoriums for treatment —as many as 100,000 such institutions operating in the United States alone in 1950—have been closing their doors. Community-wide campaigns for early diagnosis of the disease have faltered. The programs of tuberculin tests for schoolchildren have fallen off. Surgical treatment of the disease, once commonplace, is now performed only rarely. Yet for all this, tuberculosis is by no means a "conquered" disease. It remains an ever present threat, a plague-in-waiting, ready to strike once again any time we drop our guard or relax our hard-won control over this killer infection.

Tuberculosis is caused by an odd organism known as the *Mycobacterium tuberculosis* or tubercle bacillus. It can attack virtually any organ system in the body, but the most common form in man is *pulmonary tuberculosis,* a chronic infection of the lungs, once known as pthisis or, more commonly, consumption. Studies made of human mummies have shown that it was active in the earliest Egyptian civilizations, surely one of the most ancient of all known diseases; it was also commonplace in the societies of ancient Greece and Rome, and throughout the Middle Ages. With the Industrial Revolution in England and America, tuberculosis became an increasing threat; by the year 1900 it was the most frequent cause of death in all Temperate Zone countries where health records were kept. Yet by 1960 it was only sixteenth among causes of death in the United States, and the death rate has continued to fall every year since.

MYCOBACTERIUM TUBERCULOSIS

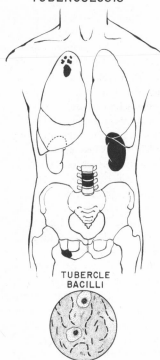

TUBERCLE BACILLI

Figure 20–1.

What is the nature of this disease, and what has caused the sudden decrease in its incidence? Many theories about the cause of "consumption" flourished during the Middle Ages; everything from evil spells to the malign influence of night air was blamed for the disease. It was not until the early 1800s that the great French physician René Laënnec (1781–1826) first accurately described its pattern and suggested that it was an infectious disease passed from one person to another. Robert Koch finally identified the causative organism in 1892: a slender, rod-shaped bacillus with an odd, waxy coating that made staining and microscopic detection very difficult. Koch finally found a crimson dye that would penetrate the organism and color it for observation even after the stained specimen had been rinsed with a mild acid solution. Doctors still sometimes refer to tuberculosis as "red-bug" or "acid-fast infection."

But discovery of the tubercle bacillus did not help much with control of the disease. Typically, the infection would begin silently and insidiously, with no early symptoms to help identify it. Bacteria invading the lung would involve small patches of lung tissue with infection; often the body's resistance would work to wall off these infected areas, and months and even years would pass as the germ multiplied and spread, destroying tissue and forming infected nodules filled with a cheesy material that was often teeming with the bacteria. Eventually these "tubercles" would form cavities in the lung tissue, and the bacteria would spread to adjacent areas. Sometimes they would enter the blood stream and travel to the kidneys or bone and begin destroying tissue there. Finally great segments of lung tissue would be destroyed, but it all happened so slowly that symptoms, when they appeared, were often vague and only very slowly progressive.

Among the earliest symptoms were chronic fatigue and gradual weight loss, accompanied by a mild progressive cough. As the infection became entrenched, the victim would begin having afternoon fevers, not very high but occurring daily, and a pattern of night sweats. The coughing would become persistent, and when small blood vessels in the lung were involved in the infection, the victim might begin coughing up blood. Sometimes massive hemorrhages would occur, causing death from suffocation or even exsanguination. Appetite would depart and the victim would become skeletally thin and almost too weak to move, literally "consumed" by the disease until death finally ensued. The course of illness was often prolonged for years, with intermittent periods of improvement and relapse. Indeed, we now know that the body's fight against the invading bacteria is valiant, and some areas of infection may be trying to heal spontaneously at the same time that others are being invaded.

With the discovery of X-rays in 1896, medicine at last had a splendid new means for early diagnosis: a chest X-ray could often reveal the presence of the infection in the lung before any symptoms had begun. The bacteria could also be identified in the sputum of victims. It was recognized that fatigue and poor nutrition increased the body's susceptibility to the disease and that crowded housing and poor hygiene contributed to its spread, particularly in the heavily populated English industrial cities and in American tenements and slums, although the disease was by no means limited to these areas. It is contracted, it was learned, by contact with the infectious discharges from a victim's lungs, and special hospitals and sanatoriums were built where patients could be isolated from their uninfected families and treated with total rest and nutritious diets. Cure was possible in the less advanced cases, but the course of treatment took months and sometimes years. Even then, the infection was merely arrested, the damage already done to the lungs could not be repaired, and the patient, if not careful, was susceptible to a relapse and the continual threat of other respiratory infections. In advanced cases, nothing could be done. Often the patient was merely sent away to die.

Slowly, however, more and more was learned about the disease. For example, it was found that virtually everyone, at one time or another, comes in contact with the bacillus. In most cases no active infection gets started. When it does, the body's natural resistance rises to the challenge with the formation of antibodies, and usually the disease is aborted before it gets well started. When this occurs, the individual remains extra sensitive to reinvasion by the bacillus, often for many years, an important natural defense against later recurrent infection. In order to help distinguish between those who had had such early contact with tuberculosis and those

who had not, scientists devised a special skin test in which a protein extract known as tuberculin derived from the bacillus was injected or placed in contact with the skin. Anyone who had once had, or who still had, the bacillus living in his body, even though with no sign of active infection, would develop an angry red spot on the skin at the site of the tuberculin test. This test was particularly useful in detecting early tuberculosis in schoolchildren, or in helping to rule out hidden tuberculosis when trying to diagnose upper respiratory or lung infections.

In the 1920s and 1930s public health authorities began mass screening programs to try to detect victims of tuberculosis and reduce the high incidence of the disease. People with positive reactions to tuberculin tests received chest X-rays to help identify the disease early, when it might respond more quickly to treatment, but thousands still died every year. Even with drastic treatment techniques such as *artificial pneumothorax,* in which a diseased lung was temporarily collapsed to allow it to "rest" completely and promote healing, or *thoracoplasty,* in which a lung was permanently collapsed by removal of ribs, or *pneumonectomy,* the surgical removal of a diseased lung, and with increased public awareness and a gradual improvement in living conditions and nutrition, progress was slow. As late as 1940 public health officials thought gloomily in terms of a centuries-long struggle to control this devastating disease.

Then in 1943, Dr. Selman Waksman discovered a substance formed by certain earth-mold bacteria which seemed to have the power to kill tubercle bacilli, or at least slow down their growth. Later he received a Nobel prize for his discovery; streptomycin proved to be the first antibiotic effective against this disease. The drug had its drawbacks; when used in sufficiently large doses to affect active tuberculosis, it could also damage the auditory nerve, causing permanent hearing impairment or even deafness. But in 1952 another drug known as isoniazid was discovered; it was even more effective than streptomycin, and for the first time doctors had a choice of weapons with which to fight the active infection. By using streptomycin and isoniazid alternately, together with a third mildly effective drug known as para-amino salicylic acid (PAS), it was possible to turn the tide against tuberculosis, to arrest the progress of the disease in advanced cases and to bring about permanent cures in earlier or milder infections.

What is the state of things today? Experts universally agree that the eventual disappearance of tuberculosis as a major cause of disability and death is possible, but this millennium has not yet been achieved. There are still deaths from pulmonary tuberculosis, and also from infection of the kidneys by the bacillus. Tuberculous infection of the spine, now known as Pott's disease, once a common cause of hunchback deformities, still occurs, as does tuberculosis of the larynx and tuberculous destruction of hip and shoulder joints or other bones. People still reach advanced stages of tuberculosis without ever seeing a doctor or taking the precaution of a chest X-ray. The disease still occurs among the poor and malnourished who live in crowded slums, and among American Indians and Eskimos who seem inherently more susceptible to the infection than others. And among the ill-fed and ill-housed populations of other parts of the world, scarcely a dent has been made in controlling the disease.

Today the discovery of early tuberculosis is not the social and economic disaster that it was 20 or 30 years ago. Often the disease can be effectively and quickly treated with modern antibiotics without necessitating a long layoff from work or prolonged hospitalization. Long-term follow-up is absolutely necessary whenever the disease has been discovered, for it is difficult to be absolutely sure that it has been destroyed or that reinfection has not occurred. Surgical treatment, rare today and generally applied only after the active disease has been halted with medicines, may be used to remove a portion of lung permanently scarred and possibly still harboring the bacteria, or to excise a kidney or segment of bone badly damaged by the infection. But until tuberculosis has been completely eradicated as a major destroyer in all parts of the world, it remains a potential pestilence, just waiting its chance to attack.

The best possible protection against tuberculosis today lies in a few everyday commonsense precautions combined with simple periodic medical checkups designed to detect the disease in its earliest stages. An adequate and nutritious diet, warm dry living quarters and sufficient daily rest are all essential to keep the body in fighting trim against the infection. Children should have tuberculin skin tests at the time of entering school and at two- or three-year intervals thereafter—more often if someone in the family has had tuberculosis. These tests can be given by a doctor or obtained free of charge at Public Health Service offices; some school systems also provide them. Screening chest X-rays or mobile unit X-rays are no longer recommended unless specifically ordered by your physician, but a doctor should be consulted about any recurring fever, night sweats, unexplained weight loss, persistent coughing, or any prolonged respiratory trouble. Raw milk was once a dangerous source of tuberculosis; today most dairy herds are regularly inspected, but a doctor or the Public Health Service should be consulted before buying unpasteurized milk. Again, extra vigilance is necessary for individuals in close contact with someone who has or has had active tuberculosis, although with modern antibiotic treatment isolation of these people is rarely considered necessary. Above all, no one should allow fear to deter him from regular health examinations. Symptoms may be few until the infection is well under way, but modern treatment can stop even advanced cases, and the social stigma and economic burden once connected with the disease are a thing of the past. What *is* to be feared is that complacency, individual negligence and the deterioration of health facilities, especially among overcrowded, malnourished city populations, may once again allow tuberculosis to move in, out of control. The tiger is waiting at the door; only vigilance and strong public health controls can prevent a modern-day resurgence of this ancient plague.

The Bacterial Pneumonias

The respiratory tract, which extends from the back of the throat and larynx to the great air tube or trachea, and then divides into the smaller air tubes or bronchi and then into the smaller bronchioles, is completely lined with a moist membrane abundantly equipped with special mucus-forming cells. It leads finally to the air sacs or alveoli in the lungs, which are also moist and are endowed with a rich capillary blood supply. It is, in short, a perfect breeding ground for bacteria, and considering the incredible number of bacteria and other potentially infectious organisms that we draw in every time we breathe, it seems a small miracle that we are not constantly afflicted with recurring infections throughout the entire respiratory system. Fortunately, the protective devices of the body work so well that we are surprisingly free of such infections. Nevertheless, they can and do occur quite often, in a spectrum ranging from the mildest case of laryngitis or bronchitis to the gravely dangerous pneumonias.

Pneumonia, an inflammation of the lung, is a type of infection which can be caused by a wide variety of bacteria and/or viruses. But the disease that we think of when we hear the word—the disease that took so many lives prior to 1936 that it was considered the number one killer of them all—is the so-called lobar pneumonia. It is caused by a distinctive bullet-shaped bacterium which usually occurs in pairs in a gelatinous capsule and is known as *Diplococcus pneumoniae,* or more commonly *pneumococcus.*

These bacteria (of which there are some 20 or more known strains, all appearing alike under the microscope but revealing their differences in certain kinds of laboratory tests) usually reach the lung tissue by means of infected water droplets inhaled from the air. If the natural resistance of the victim is low on account of another recent infection, poor nutrition, exhaustion from overwork or other afflictions or debilities, the bacteria can successfully invade the lung tissue, multiply rapidly and destroy cells in the tiny air sacs or alveoli. When the infection is caused by the pneumococcus, it is characteristically centered in one lobe of the lung, and often will progress to involve almost all of the lung tissue in a lobe before diagnosis can be made and treatment started. In attempting to fight off the disease, the body mobilizes hundreds of thousands of white blood cells at the site of the infection, and the exudate formed there can

literally fill up the air sacs in the portion of lobe affected. Thus it becomes virtually solidified and completely unable to maintain the oxygen exchange necessary to life.

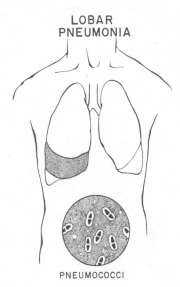

LOBAR PNEUMONIA

PNEUMOCOCCI

Figure 20–2.

Typically, lobar pneumonia reveals itself first with a high fever, nausea, vomiting and general malaise. Soon after the onset of infection, coughing begins, accompanied by a sense of pain or tightness in the part of the chest where the infection is located. As it progresses, the fever continues to climb, sometimes to 103° or higher, and the victim begins coughing up quantities of phlegm, often mixed with blood, thus giving the sputum a rusty appearance. At the same time there will be a marked increase in pulse rate owing to the increased metabolism of the body caused by the fever, and also to the difficulty of circulating blood through the damaged and infected portion of lung. Finally, the victim becomes noticeably short of breath and has difficulty getting enough air; when an entire lobe or even two lobes of lung tissue are affected, the remaining lung may not be able to supply adequate oxygen to the body, and the victim's face and trunk take on a dusky purplish hue known as *cyanosis.* At this point, the victim becomes prostrated and unable to manage any physical activity, using all his energy literally just to breathe.

In the days before antibiotics a high percentage of victims died in the eighth or ninth day of the disease from suffocation or heart failure or both. Those who survived endured a prolonged disability lasting from two to three weeks, with a continued high fever and a general wasting away due to the effort of breathing and a disinterest in food. Then, in a dramatic change, a "fever crisis" occurred during which their temperature spiked up to 105° or 106° and their difficulty in breathing increased for a few hours. After that their fever suddenly broke, returning abruptly to normal, with profuse sweating and a dramatic reversal of symptoms. Their bodies had licked the infection and there was gradual improvement of their overall physical condition through another two or three weeks of convalescence.

Today we seldom see pneumococcal or lobar pneumonia follow this once typical course, since virtually anyone so gravely ill seeks medical attention, and since antibiotic treatment usually destroys the bacteria and helps terminate the illness far more quickly. Before the first effective drugs were discovered, bacteriologists had learned how to "type" the kind of pneumococcus causing a given infection, and had moderate success treating the disease with immune serum from patients who had recovered from a pneumonia caused by the same type of organism. However, the laboratory work required often took so long that the battle was lost before the proper antiserum could be determined. Then, in 1936, a new chemical drug discovered in Germany in 1932 and known as sulfanilamide was introduced in this country and was found to kill the pneumococcus organism effectively in a matter of three or four days' treatment, thus reversing the progress of the disease. Within a year of the introduction of sulfanilamide, the death rate from pneumococcal pneumonia dropped dramatically from some 50 percent of infected cases to fewer than 5 percent, and the heyday of lobar pneumonia as the number one killer was over. A few years later penicillin was discovered and found to be equally or even more effective against this infection than the sulfa drugs, and

today any number of broad-spectrum antibiotics can also be used.

This does not mean, however, that lobar pneumonia is no longer a threat. Early diagnosis and immediate treatment are still essential. Diagnostic clues are the onset of fever, chest pain, the coughing up of rusty sputum and, most important, evidence of the infection appearing on a chest X-ray. After diagnosis the doctor will take a sample of sputum for culture to determine the type of organism causing the disease, and will then begin vigorous antibiotic treatment. In advanced cases it may be necessary to use an oxygen tent or nasal tube to provide extra oxygen to the part of the lungs that is still able to function, but the infection will usually subside in a matter of a few days after treatment has been started. With this form of early treatment, there are no residual ill effects, although the patient may remain surprisingly weak and shaky for several weeks after recovery from the infection—an indication of the enormous drain on the body's energy this disease makes even when it is treated with wonder drugs.

What should you look for to avoid an active pneumonia infection? For one thing, any upper respiratory infection which persists or develops into a prolonged irritative coughing disease should be regarded with suspicion. Simple laryngitis can often progress to tracheitis or bronchitis, all less serious bacterial or viral infections of the respiratory tract, and all characterized by irritating, persistent coughing, the bringing up of quantities of sputum, and sometimes a low-grade fever. These conditions often resolve themselves fairly quickly even without treatment, but there is also the possibility that they may lead to pneumonia. A high fever, chills, a feeling of tightness in the chest, an increase in pulse rate and in frequency of respiration (sometimes up to 45 respirations per minute) and acutely painful coughing are the danger signals that pneumonia is under way, and no time should be lost in calling a doctor.

Pneumococcal pneumonia is a highly contagious disease, particularly during long winter months when whole families may be especially vulnerable owing to the debilitating effects of a long series of head colds or other mild URI's before the pneumonia appears. Once diagnosed, the disease is usually best treated in a hospital until the active infection is stopped and the patient is free of respiratory difficulty. However, convalescence may take place at home. The convalescing patient will be very weak and may have a persisting cough. A disposable sputum cup (available at any hospital or pharmacy) should be placed by the bedside, replaced each day and disposed of with the garbage or by incineration. Bed rest, plenty of fluids and tasteful high-protein meals will all speed recovery.

BRONCHIAL PNEUMONIA

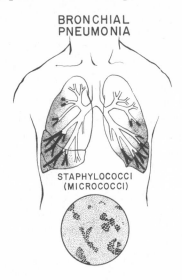

STAPHYLOCOCCI
(MICROCOCCI)

Figure 20–3.

Statistically, in cases of lobar or pneumococcal pneumonia, 95 percent of those who are treated with modern antibiotics survive. But patients who are treated during the first day or two are far more likely to recover than those treated later. Age also plays a part: the disease is more dangerous in older persons, in those afflicted by some other chronic disease, and in those whose bodies have been weakened by chronic alcoholism or by some earlier debilitating disease such as viral influenza. Indeed, pneumonia deaths today, whether arising from pneumococcal pneumonia or other varieties, are most common among elderly people who have

first been hard hit by influenza and then contract the pneumonia as a complicating infection at a time when their bodies are too weak and debilitated to fight the infection effectively even with the aid of antibiotics.

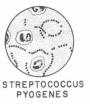

STREPTOCOCCUS
PYOGENES

Figure 20–4.

All pneumonia is not caused by pneumococcal organisms; the staphylococcus and streptococcus can also cause infections very similar to lobar pneumonia. Further, not all pneumonias are of the "lobar" type, which involves large sections of individual lobes of the lung. Pneumonia that arises from acute bronchitis may frequently involve patchy areas of both lungs and present a mottled or "moth-eaten" appearance of the lungs on X-ray examination. Such a condition, whether caused by pneumococcus or by a staph or strep organism is sometimes called bronchial pneumonia or bronchiolar pneumonia because only the areas immediately adjacent to the small bronchiolar air tubes in the lung are affected. A similar condition results from a form of pneumonia caused by an uncommon organism known as Friedländer's bacillus. In this infection, thick, sticky mucus is formed and tends to plug up the bronchioles so that the victim can become gravely ill and have great difficulty breathing even while antibiotic treatment is going on. This form of pneumonia and another, caused by the plague bacillus and known as pneumonic plague or plague pneumonia, move rapidly, involve such large areas of lung tissue, and are often so far advanced before the victim reaches a doctor that mortality rates are very high.

Equally dangerous is a form of pneumonia caused by a bacterium called *Hemophilus influenzae* which is sensitive to sulfa drugs but may be resistant to or unaffected by other antibiotics.

Pneumonias caused by these other bacteria also may affect patchy areas throughout both lungs rather than a single lobe, so that more of the breathing apparatus of the lung is compromised and the victim is in serious trouble very early in the course of the infection. Rare as they are, diagnosis and treatment of these forms of pneumonia are in the nature of true medical emergencies. Even the loss of an hour or two in making the diagnosis and beginning heroic treatment can prove fatal.

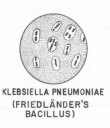

KLEBSIELLA PNEUMONIAE
(FRIEDLÄNDER'S
BACILLUS)

Figure 20–5.

Still other forms of infectious pneumonia are caused by viruses (*see* p. 228), and in addition, certain pneumonia-like inflammations of the lungs may occur which have nothing to do with infectious microorganisms at all. These conditions include *chemical pneumonia,* resulting from inhalation of irritating gases, industrial vapors or sprays; *aspiration pneumonia,* which may arise when acidic gastric material is regurgitated from the stomach and then inadvertently aspirated or inhaled into the lung; *oil pneumonia,* owing to the aspiration of nonabsorbable oily substances into the trachea and bronchi; and the so-called *hypostatic* or *stasis pneumonia,* which may occur as a result of excessively shallow respiration due to prolonged bed rest or other forced inactivity, especially among aged and debilitated patients. All these conditions, as well as some of the serious complications that can follow infections or inflammations of the lungs, are considered in detail in Part VIII, "Patterns of Illness: The Respiratory Tract."

Vincent's Infection (Trench Mouth)

For many years, this rather odd form of mouth infection, also known as Vincent's angina, suffered a bad reputation for a high degree of contagion, but today most authorities agree that the underlying causes, such as poor mouth hygiene, nutritional deficiencies, other prolonged and debilitating diseases, or heavy smoking, play as large a part in causing Vincent's infection as the contagion of the causative organisms. It has probably never been fatal, but even so, it is an extremely unpleasant, painful and embarrassing infection. First described by the French physician J. Henri Vincent (1862–1950), the disease as well as its causative organisms were given his name. It acquired the more familiar name "trench mouth" from its frequent occurrence among soldiers in World War I.

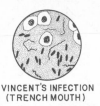

VINCENT'S INFECTION
(TRENCH MOUTH)

Figure 20–6.

In most cases Vincent's infection is caused by a pair of quite different bacterial organisms working together—a small cigar-shaped bacillus and a nonvenereal spirochete. Usually the infection is confined to the gums and appears as painful, punched-out red ulcers which form at the rim of the gum or gingiva and gradually accumulate a foul-smelling membrane of dead tissue. Often the disease occurs after a prolonged bout with some other type of nose or throat infection, and on occasion it can extend to involve the inside of the lips, the inside of the cheeks, the roof of the mouth or even the pharynx. It is usually easily diagnosed by the physician from its appearance and the malodorous breath of the patient. But before treatment he will make a smear of the pus material from the lesions for staining and microscopic examination of the causative organisms in order to cinch the diagnosis, since there are other conditions (such as very grave blood diseases) which can account for lesions of similar appearance.

Treatment of Vincent's infection varies with the degree of severity. When there is a minor degree of involvement centered in the gums alone, a simple program of home treatment will often be effective. First the infected areas should be cleansed and debrided gently with a cotton swab dipped in a full-strength hydrogen peroxide solution. Then a quarter of a cup of hydrogen peroxide diluted with a quarter of a cup of water should be used as a thorough mouthwash, followed by rinsing the mouth with a saline solution of a teaspoonful of salt in a cup of warm water. In many cases this procedure, repeated at least three times a day, will quickly quiet the infection to the point where gentle brushing of the teeth with a soft-bristle toothbrush is possible, and the maintenance of good dental care with tooth brushing after each meal will prevent recurrence. In more severe cases, a doctor or dentist may administer penicillin by injection or one of the broad-spectrum antibiotics such as tetracycline by mouth for the first few days, in combination with the hygienic care program mentioned above. When the infection is advanced and widespread, even this more vigorous program of treatment may have to be continued for days before the infection quiets down. Some refractory cases continue to plague the victim for weeks, apparently simmering down and then flaring up again the moment treatment is relaxed. Ultimately, however, it can be quelled and—unless there is an underlying infection of the gums such as pyorrhea—will heal with no long-term damage or complications.

Even though it is believed that contagion is of less importance than it was once thought to be, it is well to have the victim of Vincent's infection use his own eating utensils and dishes. Keep them carefully separate from the household supply, especially if there are many children in the family, and sterilize them by immersion in boiling water for 20 minutes or more before they are returned to general use. Alternatively, disposable paper dishes and plastic utensils may be used.

Tetanus (Lockjaw)

Of the many kinds of pathogenic organisms, there is probably none more thoroughly vicious and dangerous than the *Clostridium* family of soil bacteria, spore-forming organisms which live practically everywhere in dirt and manure, are able to survive extremes of both heat and cold, and are responsible for such afflictions as tetanus (lockjaw), gas gangrene and botulism, the most deadly form of food poisoning. All three deserve a special place in the rogues' gallery of infectious diseases, but of the three tetanus is perhaps the most frightening.

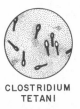

CLOSTRIDIUM
TETANI

Figure 20–7.

Even in the days before there was any immunization against tetanus, this infection was comparatively rare except during wartime when many soldiers received mutilating wounds. At first this seems strange considering that the bacillus that causes tetanus, *Clostridium tetani,* is extremely widespread, particularly around farms, manure-fertilized gardens, and even in dusty, dry desert areas. But the low incidence of tetanus can be explained by the peculiar nature of the bacteria that causes it. The tetanus bacillus, like others in the *Clostridium* family, is anaerobic; that is, it cannot grow well except under conditions in which no atmospheric oxygen is available. Indeed, the presence of oxygen prevents the organism from forming the deadly toxin that accounts for the severity of the disease. Thus tetanus arises only when the organism is introduced into the tissues of the body in such a way that atmospheric oxygen cannot get to it: carried into the foot, for example, by a puncture wound from a rusty nail on the ground, or introduced deep into the tissues when a compound or open fracture occurs, or when a penetrating shrapnel wound is sustained. On the other hand, the wound does not necessarily have to be deep or serious if anaerobic conditions are present. Tetanus has been known to result from a superficial puncture wound in a finger inflicted by the thorn of a rose, and it is a special hazard in the wake of any third-degree burn when dead tissue has not been thoroughly debrided.

Curiously enough, it is not the growth of the tetanus bacillus in the local area where it enters the body that does the harm. The danger lies in the powerful protein poison or toxin, one of the most violently poisonous substances known to man, that the organism produces. This toxin, which travels through the blood stream, quietly becomes fixed in the nerve tissue of the spinal cord and brain, and it is this that brings about the terrible symptoms of tetanus.

Typically, an incubation period ranging from three or four days to as long as three weeks will pass from the time the bacillus enters the body to the time the first symptoms of tetanus appear: a headache and a low-grade fever, followed by irritability, stiffness of the neck, difficulty in swallowing and a characteristic stiffness of the jaw caused by tightening of the powerful masseter muscles normally used for chewing. As poisoning by the toxin continues, the jaw stiffening may increase so severely that the teeth remain clamped together (hence the common name of the disease, "lockjaw"), and the slightest physical stimulation, such as tapping the jaw muscle with a finger, causes an agonizing spasm of muscle tightening that may last as long as ten or fifteen minutes. Gradually other muscles also become involved, owing to excessive irritability of the central nervous system. Then the severely afflicted victim will respond to virtually any stimulus—a touch, a sound, a change in the lighting of the room—by stiffening his whole body and arching his back. Swallowing becomes impossible, and the victim must be fed by means of a gastric tube. As the disease progresses into a second and third day of symptoms, the victim may actually convulse from the stimulus of a draft of cold air, a noise or a slight jarring of the bed. And throughout all this, until death comes or recovery begins, he remains perfectly clear of mind, fully aware of everything going on as his body is racked by agonizing spasms. If he dies, the immediate cause of death often cannot be determined; and in the victim lucky enough to recover, the muscle spasms may subside only slowly over a period of weeks.

Before the days when immunization was available or tetanus antitoxin had been discovered, the death rate from the disease varied from 20 percent in relatively mild infections to as much as 85 percent in massive infections with swift onset of symptoms. Treatment in those days depended upon surgical opening and debriding of the wound, if it could be found, good nursing care in a hospital, and hope. Even today when antibiotics are used to attack the tetanus organism itself, and when tetanus antitoxin capable of neutralizing the poison being produced by the growing organism is also used, the death rate ranges from 20 to 50 percent of those cases in which symptoms of the illness appear before treatment is started. The trouble is that the tetanus toxin that has already become "fixed" in the cells of the spinal cord and brain cannot be neutralized in any way. The best that can be done is to administer the antitoxin (which is made from the blood serum of tetanus-infected horses) in order to destroy the toxin still being formed but not yet fixed in nervous tissue. When a wound from an open fracture, or a war wound, is the source of the infection, surgical removal or debridement of all dirt and dead tissue is still important. Penicillin given by injection helps destroy the tetanus organism, and tetracycline can be used in persons who are penicillin-sensitive.

Since 1936, no one from earliest infancy on need contract a tetanus infection, for it was in that year that a highly effective vaccine for the prevention of this disease was introduced in this country. The vaccine is made from tetanus toxin which has been neutralized or detoxified with a weak solution of formaldehyde to form *tetanus toxoid*. When injected into the body, this substance stimulates the formation of extremely long-lived antibodies, just as an actual infection with the tetanus organism would do. Once formed, these antitetanus antibodies remain in the circulating blood for years to prevent growth or toxin formation by any tetanus bacteria that might later gain entry.

This immunization has proven remarkably effective and reliable in preventing tetanus. Since the beginning of World War II, pediatricians have routinely provided an initial immunization against tetanus for all babies with the triple DPT vaccine, the so-called baby shots, which contain diphtheria toxoid, pertussis (whooping cough) vaccine and tetanus toxoid all in one mixture and are usually given in three shots spaced a month apart beginning at three months of age. Further, at the beginning of World War II the entire military personnel of the American armed forces were actively immunized against tetanus with tetanus toxoid. When soldiers on the battlefield were subsequently injured, they were given an immediate booster dose of toxoid. The almost miraculous effectiveness of this immunization was shown by statistics gathered at the end of the war. During World War I more than 10,000 American soldiers contracted tetanus as a result of contaminated war wounds; but after immunization with tetanus toxoid, only *12* cases of tetanus developed in soldiers between 1942 and 1945, and in each of those cases some irregularity in the administration of the basic immunization series was found.

The use of this immunization against tetanus has, in fact, proved far more successful than originally predicted. At first booster shots were recommended every four years, and physicians always gave additional booster doses to any patient who suffered a penetrating wound even if he had been given a tetanus booster as little as a year before. But today we know that a single booster dose of the toxoid will push the level of immunity up to the maximum within a matter of a few days, even if the basic immunization or subsequent booster immunizations were given many years before. Doctors now often refrain from using tetanus boosters in case of injury as long as an earlier immunization was completed within the previous five or so years. It is better, however, in dealing with such a serious infection, to be safe than sorry. The important thing is to be absolutely sure that everyone in the family has been given the basic immunization series. It is also important to consult the doctor any time someone in the family sustains a potentially dangerous wound. He will decide, based on the nature of the wound and the immunization record of the victim, whether or not a tetanus booster shot is indicated.

Gas Gangrene

Like the tetanus organism, the most common bacterium that causes gas gangrene, *Clostridium perfringens,* is an anaerobic bacillus, growing well and producing toxin only when introduced deep into the tissues by a penetrating wound or open fracture. Once the organism gains such entry into the body, however, it tends to grow rapidly and spread in a fast-moving cellulitis or tissue infection. And like the danger of tetanus infection, the danger from this member of the *Clostridium* family lies not so much in multiplication and widespread invasion of the bacteria as it does in the potent toxins that the growing organism produces.

Technically, gangrene is not a bacteriologic disease at all, but rather a condition which can arise in any number of ways in different parts of the body, often with no relationship whatever to any particular bacteria. The term "gangrenous" describes any area of the body in which living tissue has been destroyed, often in large quantities, usually as a result of loss of blood supply to the area. Only then is it often followed by bacterial invasion and subsequent putrefaction. An inflamed appendix, for example, can have its blood supply diminished by swelling and edema and become gangrenous, just as a loop of intestine trapped in an inguinal hernia may become gangrenous because of the loss of its blood supply, not necessarily associated with infection. In other cases gangrene may develop at the center of a cancerous tumor which has enlarged so swiftly that it has outgrown its blood supply, and severe diabetics may develop an "aseptic" or noninfectious gangrene in their extremities because advancing arteriosclerosis has blocked the arterial blood supply to the area. Gangrene can also result from frostbite.

Further, not all tissue infections caused by the gas gangrene organism necessarily become "true" gangrene with widespread tissue destruction. In some cases the organism may grow in the body, invading the connective tissue between the muscles in a slowly spreading, relatively painless infection characterized by the formation of a putrid-smelling gas. In such cases the afflicted individual may run a low-grade fever and become generally ill or "toxic," but the process is slow enough that it can be arrested by the use of antibiotics, and treatment with these drugs together with surgical incision and drainage of the wound can save the affected area.

This sort of cellulitis or general tissue infection by the gas gangrene bacilli is generally far milder and slower than the true gas gangrene that arises when they grow in the absence of oxygen in a deep, dirty flesh wound. In this case the infective process is swift, beginning as little as six hours after the injury has been sustained, and is associated with pain that rapidly increases in severity. The toxin produced by the organism invades muscle in the area, destroying muscle tissue swiftly, and causing *hemolysis,* the destruction of red blood cells reaching the area. Again foul-smelling gas and pus are formed in the area of infection, and the physician can sometimes feel or even *hear* the movement of gas in the tissue as he rubs it with his finger. Widespread death of muscle and other tissue follows in the wake of this infection; the tissue literally rots away in a rapidly spreading area, and the victim becomes generally ill, with prostration, stupor and even delirium or coma.

In civilian life the most common site of this kind of swift-moving gangrenous infection is probably the uterus, as a result of an abortion with the use of contaminated instruments. It may move very swiftly in these cases, with massive hemolysis of blood reaching the uterus. The patient rapidly goes into shock and often dies before a doctor is ever called—particularly when the patient is trying to conceal the fact of the abortion.

True gas gangrene can also result from the massive injuries often sustained in automobile accidents and on the battlefield, or even from less serious punctures and lacerations. When it occurs, treatment is primarily the province of the surgeon. If the infection is still in its early stages, the infected area must be opened for drainage, with the destroyed or necrotic tissues debrided and excised, together with any dirt or foreign material from the initial wound. If the gangrene is well advanced in an extremity such as an arm or a leg, a swift decision for amputation may be necessary to prevent spread of the infection and toxic death of the patient in shock. When the uterus is the affected organ, curettage must be performed and sometimes even hysterectomy (surgical removal of the uterus) if the condition is not too far advanced. In any case, surgical intervention must be accompanied by the use of massive doses of penicillin or one of the broad-spectrum antibiotics. At the same time supportive measures such as the administration of blood, plasma, intravenous glucose or electrolytes must be taken in an effort to alleviate shock.

The main organism involved in gas gangrene was first discovered by William Henry Welch in 1892 at Johns Hopkins University in Baltimore. As soon as medical researchers realized that the chief damage resulted from a tissue-destroying toxin, the search was on to identify the toxin and find out how it acted. It was soon discovered that a number of different toxins could be involved, and subsequently a so-called *polyvalent antitoxin* was developed from the serum of infected horses in the hope that its use would slow down the wildfire activity of the disease. Although effective, these antitoxins are by no means the final answer in the fight against the infection. Many experts today question their value, but most will still administer them in severely ill patients. Although a toxoid to be used for active immunization against gas gangrene is possible, it is still in the theoretical stage. Unlike tetanus, there is as yet no way to prevent the infection, and once it is contracted treatment still depends upon prompt surgical attention and the use of antibiotics to save lives and limbs.

The most important thing to remember is that *any* puncture or penetrating wound (particularly wounds such as cuts with broken glass or sharp beer can tabs), any wound contaminated with dirt, foreign bodies or torn clothing, or any crushing or macerating injury in which the skin is broken can lead to infection by either tetanus or gas gangrene or both. Such injuries should be seen by a doctor as quickly as possible, preferably within six hours. Even then a correct diagnosis cannot always be made, and any sign of increasing pain, swelling or redness around a wound even after it has been treated and debrided should again be called to a doctor's attention. It may only be some minor infection, but the possibility of major infection is too great to be ignored.

The Variable Viral and Rickettsial Infections

Everyone is familiar with the symptoms of the common cold—a stuffy nose, a scratchy throat, a dry, hacking cough, aching muscles, a low-grade fever and that "tired feeling." But a doctor, after making a thorough check of his patient's nose, throat, ears and lungs, may very well shrug apologetically and say, "Afraid I don't see much wrong. It's probably some kind of virus." Is the doctor being intentionally vague? Of course not. Once he has determined that the cold is caused by some kind of virus, there is not much more he can say. For virus infections are among the most vague and mysterious, as well as the most frequent, of all the infectious illnesses.

Like bacterial infections, many virus diseases are type-specific. The measles diseases, mumps, and infectious hepatitis, for example, which were discussed in earlier chapters, are each caused by particular viruses. But many virus infections are not nearly as specific. The common head cold, for example, may be caused by any one of dozens of viruses. In fact, the various "cold vaccines" have proved to be largely ineffective simply because so many different and unidentifiable viruses are responsible for coldlike symptoms. Influenza, or flu, as it is commonly called—a disease which is distinctly different from the common cold despite the fact that many people erroneously use the terms "cold" and "flu" more or less interchangeably—is caused by specific groups of viruses, many of which can be identified in the laboratory; but even so, these organisms may cause influenza

infections of widely varying severity. Usually influenza is a relatively mild affliction, requiring nothing more than a few days of rest in bed to ensure complete recovery. But occasionally a virus mutation may appear that brings about a massive epidemic of severe influenza such as the one that killed millions of people in 1918–1919, or the "Asian flu" that swept across the world in the early 1960s, or the "Hong Kong flu" that reached epidemic proportions in the United States in 1968 and 1969.

Apart from causing the most common of infectious illnesses, viruses are also responsible for a large number of much more serious or even dangerous infections, often transmitted to man by insect or animal carriers. Some of these virus diseases, such as yellow fever and rabies, are fortunately quite rare today, at least in most advanced countries. Others, like dengue fever, are still all too common, and one of them—smallpox—deserves special attention not only as an ancient scourge but as another modern plague-in-waiting which, like tuberculosis, is by no means the "conquered disease" many people assume that it is. Finally, a number of infections caused not by viruses but by rickettsiae—the curious organisms that lie halfway between viruses and bacteria in size, but which have many virus-like characteristics—are both prevalent in the world today and decidedly dangerous. Especially notable among these are Rocky Mountain spotted fever and various forms of typhus fever. And although doctors may appear to be vague and casual when it comes to the common cold, they have a very healthy respect for the damage that viruses and rickettsiae can do. Through the heroic efforts of medical science

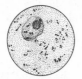

RICKETTSIAE

Figure 21–1.

many of the more serious of these viral and rickettsial infections have been brought under control, but there is still much to be learned about these organisms and how they work, and in particular the challenging science of virology is providing us with important new information every year.

The Common Cold

The common garden-variety head cold is not a single disease entity caused by a single virus, but any of a group of very similar infections which may be caused by a wide variety of viruses, some resulting in mild illnesses, others in quite severe ones. Often the dividing line between a simple head cold, virus-caused infections of the pharynx, the larynx, the trachea or the bronchi, viral pneumonia and influenza itself can be extremely narrow, with one condition shading into another and all displaying similar symptoms. Indeed, an illness which begins as a simple head cold may easily progress into a more serious upper respiratory infection or even, occasionally, into pneumonia. Strictly speaking, however, the common cold is an upper respiratory infection that primarily involves inflammation of the mucous membranes lining the nose, throat and larynx, with symptoms including the sudden onset of a scratchy throat and an acute rhinitis (inflammation of the nasal mucous membrane) with the formation of a watery discharge which later becomes filled with mucus and pus. Other symptoms sometimes include swelling of the eyelids, swelling shut of the Eustachian tubes so that the ears feel "plugged," and hoarseness owing to inflammation of the larynx. Frequently

the mucous lining of the nasal sinuses is also involved, leading to additional mucus drainage, a sense of pressure under the eyes and, often, severe pain or "sinus headache." There is often a bronchial element to the common cold, too, either due to direct involvement of the bronchial membranes in the infection or due to an irritative trickle of nasal discharge down into the air tubes, so that the symptom complex includes a persistent hacking cough which may or may not produce any sputum. Sneezing resulting from nasal irritation is a common early symptom. Occasionally the common cold will be accompanied by a low-grade fever, and the overall result is a general feeling of discomfort along with nasal stuffiness and coughing.

Where do the viruses of the common cold come from? We probably come in contact with some any time we come within three feet of another human being; they are literally all around us, and are constantly being spread by droplets from people's upper respiratory tracts. Ordinarily the body fights off this continual invasion quite well, although we are not entirely sure how. Usually the cold strikes when natural resistance is low—when we are overtired, for example, or have got overchilled or thoroughly soaked in winter weather, or are recovering from some other infection. Contrary to popular myth, however, these conditions do not in themselves bring on a cold, nor will open bedroom windows at night or sitting in a draft. At worst they may *predispose* a person to catching a cold when he is exhausted or has not been eating an adequate, balanced diet. On the other hand, nasal allergies are believed to help facilitate a cold infection, a notion supported by the well-recognized fact that dosage with one of the antihistamine medications at the very beginning of symptoms will frequently relieve nasal swelling and dripping quite dramatically and sometimes even abort a cold altogether. So far as we know now, immunity to reinfection does not necessarily follow the common cold. Further investigations are still trying to unravel whether this apparent lack of immunity is due to some failure of the body's normal immune response to viruses, or whether successive common colds are simply caused by different viruses each time. *All* cold viruses, however, temporarily injure the mucous membranes of the nose and throat, so that secondary bacterial infections of the throat, ears, sinuses and bronchi are extremely common—some doctors say inevitable—complications of common colds. What is more, with the myriads of cold viruses in circulation at the same time, reinfection is the rule rather than the exception; many people who acquire colds tend to keep them, or rather suffer a long succession of new cold infections, for weeks or even months. In such "protracted colds" secondary bacterial infection is virtually inescapable, and complete recovery is likely to be delayed unless antibiotic therapy of some sort or another is begun.

Treatment of a common, relatively uncomplicated cold is aimed primarily at relieving symptoms. By far the greatest majority of common colds never come to the doctor's attention; victims simply treat themselves at home. And as long as there is no evidence of any marked interference with respiration (that is, tightness of the chest, persistent nonproductive coughing, chest pain, etc.) home treatment is perfectly safe. Many age-old home remedies are just plain silly—mustard plasters on the chest serve no more real purpose than do hot water bottles on the feet—but other measures can do much to make the victim of a cold more comfortable and shorten his illness. Beyond question the best home remedy of all is *an excess of rest*. If you *must* continue to work with a head cold and cannot afford a day or two of rest in bed, at least go to bed as soon as you get home from work and stay there until you have to go back to work again; 12 to 14 hours of sleep and bed rest a day will do more than anything else to knock out a severe cold. Aspirin can be taken, up to 10 grains every three to four hours, and will do as much to relieve fever and general discomfort as any of the "compound cold tablets" which claim all sorts of miraculous benefits and cost ten times as much.

The use of astringent nose drops at regular intervals helps greatly in controlling the amount of nasal discharge. Best and safest are nose drops in a weak saline solution containing Neo-Synephrine (phenylephrine) or ephedrine—adrenalin-like medicines capable of shrinking the congested capillaries in the nasal mucosa and thus "unplugging" the nose and reducing drainage. These can be used effectively every four hours or so during the day. It does little good, however, to instill nose drops in the nostrils while standing or sitting upright; 95 percent of the effect will be lost because the medicated solution will immediately run down the floor of the nose into the throat and be swallowed. To get the full effect from nose drops, lie on your back on a bed with your head hanging over the edge and your nostrils pointing straight to the ceiling; then have someone instill about five drops in each nostril while you remain in this position. This way the nose drops pool at the back of the nose in continuing contact with the swollen mucous membrane—the place where they are needed the most. Maintain this position through a slow count to 15 and then, rather than sit upright, simply roll over so that the excess nose drops can run out the nose again and be caught in a tissue. This procedure will not only provide the most effect from the nose drops but will also prevent swallowing the excess. These nose drops should, however, be avoided in the evening because the medications they contain, even in weak saline solution, can cause such undesirable side effects as pounding of the heart, headache or wakefulness at night.

If you buy nose drops without a prescription, check the label to make certain that they are saline or water-based solutions. Many widely advertised preparations are nose drops containing menthol or other aromatic chemicals dissolved in oil. These medicines are not dangerous, but the oil is. Any oil-based nose drops should be avoided, particularly if they are to be used several times a day. The danger of these solutions is that some of the oil may get into the trachea and run down into the bronchi without stimulating a cough reflex to get it up again. If oil trickles down into the air pockets in the lungs, there is no way for it to be absorbed, and a so-called *oil pneumonia* can result. (*See* p. 488.) Water- or saline-based nose drops do not pose this threat.

Coughing due to bronchial irritation is a common feature of most head colds, and any number of cough preparations are available. Cough syrups containing cough *suppressants* such as codeine, dihydrocodeinone or dextromethorphan, some of which are purchasable without prescription, should be avoided unless specifically recommended by a doctor in a given case. Coughing is, in fact, the best way for the body to empty the bronchi of infected mucous secretions, and it should not ordinarily be suppressed. But a cough syrup containing an *expectorant*—a drug such as ammonium chloride or glyceryl guaiacolate which helps to moisten and loosen mucus—may offer considerable relief from dry and apparently fruitless coughing. If the coughing is continuous or severe enough to disrupt sleep, the doctor may prescribe a suppressant cough preparation for limited use, but in general it is better to allow the coughing to do its job. A safe and beneficial homemade cough syrup, especially for children, can be made by mixing a teaspoon each of honey and lemon juice in 1½ ounces of whiskey. Half-teaspoon doses given every one to two hours can help soothe the irritation of a cough and also act as a gentle soporific to help the uncomfortable child relax and sleep. Whiskey and lemon juice in larger doses, an ancient "home remedy" for colds, is nice for those who like whiskey but has no real medicinal value whatever, and certainly should not be given to children.

Many widely advertised cold pills contain various antihistamine medications. For those whose head colds are commonly complicated by an allergic factor, these drugs can be extremely beneficial both in relieving symptoms and in helping to speed recovery; they are available either by prescription or over the counter, usually in half-strength dosage. But be sure to check the labels on such preparations to be certain that you reduce the amount of plain aspirin you are taking if the cold pills also contain aspirin, as most do. As for antibiotics, these should never be taken except on specific doctor's orders in a given case, even if you have a supply left over from treatment of a previous cold. Medical opinion still varies regarding the use of antibiotics in the treatment of mild upper respiratory infections; for many years they were often prescribed in "shotgun" fashion anytime a cold began. Today most doctors prefer to take bacterial cultures of the nose and throat before starting any antibiotic, so that the specific drug, if one is needed, can be geared to the particular infection. In cases involving very small children or aged and debilitated patients, or in cases in which the doctor feels that a secondary bacterial infection can be particularly dangerous, he may order penicillin or other broad-spectrum antibiotics at once, even though he knows they will do no good against the cold virus itself. In still other situations he may temporize, confining treatment to symptomatic remedies at least until a throat culture can be grown. In any case, however, it is wise to abide by his decision and *never* urge him to use antibiotics against his better judgment.

What about "cold shots" to prevent colds? A few years ago virologists, believing that most common colds were caused by two or three "major offenders" among the many cold viruses, developed vaccines to block these organisms. In actual practice, however, use of such cold vaccines has proved disappointing. They are still available, and some doctors feel that they provide at least some protection against common colds when given to a debilitated elderly patient, but for the most part they do not seem particularly effective. Not only are there far too many viruses that can be responsible for colds to make a single vaccine effective, but many of these viruses mutate or change so rapidly that even if vaccines could be provided against them all today, there would be whole new families of slightly different cold viruses to contend with tomorrow.

The best preventive measures known include plenty of rest, good nutrition, avoidance of chilling and dampness through use of sensible bad-weather clothing, avoidance of people actively suffering from colds, and maintenance of adequate exercise during the fall, winter and spring months. In addition, if you live in a dry winter climate, adequate humidity should be provided in the air of your home. Dry air tends to parch and irritate the nasal and bronchial mucous membrane, a threat that can be prevented by maintaining humidifiers or even open pans of water over radiators and heaters during the dry winter months. Finally, avoid the various fad preventatives or remedies that you hear about until you have discussed their value with a doctor. For example, no one yet has scientifically demonstrated the value of massive doses of vitamin C (ascorbic acid) in preventing colds despite periodic widespread claims, and while this substance in large amounts does no known harm, it can be a totally useless and needless expense. In the long run, the best home remedy for head colds, and also the cheapest, is tincture of time. Most colds will subside within a matter of two or three days to a week providing you get adequate rest, plenty of fluids and a nourishing diet. If complications occur—persistent coughing, chest pain or rising fever, for example—see your doctor without delay; specific therapy, including antibiotics, may be indicated.

Virus Bronchitis and Pneumonia

These are more serious viral infections, and although some of the symptoms of a head cold may also be present, these infections are clearly centered in the lower respiratory tract. The victim runs a higher fever, with more coughing, often pain in the chest accompanying the cough, and frequently a feeling of tightness in the chest or shortness of breath. Usually these virus-caused bronchial or lung infections can be distinguished from the lobar pneumonia caused by the pneumococcus bacteria because the areas of infection are widely disseminated throughout both lungs, rather than localized in one section. Thus an X-ray film of the chest will often show a mottled or patchy appearance of swelling and fluid collection centered in the lung tissue immediately surrounding the smaller bronchial tubes. Along with these specific symptoms, the viral pneumonia patient in particular is likely to suffer acute fatigue, loss of appetite, sometimes vomiting and an overall feeling of generalized discomfort.

Any "bad cold" that persists, affects the chest, or seems to be more deep-seated or severe than usual should *always* be brought to the attention of a physician early in its onset. One of the most foolish things a victim can do is attempt to continue his normal activities, for the body is literally expending all its available energy to fight off an invasion of viruses which, if allowed to

become overwhelming, can be fatal. The doctor will do certain laboratory studies to rule out the possibility of a bacterial pneumonia; but he will usually administer a broad-spectrum antibiotic even when he is quite sure the disease is viral, since secondary bacterial infection immediately following a viral infection is most commonplace —and indeed, can prove the dangerous straw that breaks the camel's back. In less serious cases, hospital treatment is usually not necessary, but the doctor's recommendations for strict bed rest at home, ample fluids and a nourishing diet should be followed to the letter. This type of virus infection is notorious for recurring if the patient, eager to be up and back to work as soon as acute symptoms disappear, overtaxes his energy too soon. Again, aspirin will help relieve fever and aching muscles, and nose drops should be used as needed. In addition, an expectorant cough syrup, either prescribed or purchased over the counter at a drugstore, will relieve coughing and help bring up sputum. As in the case of common colds, cough syrups containing cough *suppressants* should be avoided unless specifically recommended by your doctor.

If small children or elderly people in particular are infected, or in the case of a severe infection, the doctor may decide that treatment can best be handled in a hospital. He will never make this decision lightly, but if he advises it, do not hesitate to do it. Sometimes virus pneumonia can move very swiftly, even in previously young and healthy adults, and all the facilities of expert nursing care and careful hospital surveillance may be necessary to check the infection and prevent complications.

Influenza

Influenza, also often called flu, grippe or cat fever, is not a single disease entity but rather a group of similar diseases. It differs from the common cold and other viral URI's in that it is caused by certain specific adenoviruses and para-influenza viruses, most of which have been isolated, cultured and studied, thanks to the great amount of medical research in virology in the last ten or fifteen years. Three major families of viruses, known as types A, B and C, cause the majority of cases of influenza that occur sporadically throughout the year in widely scattered areas, and infection with any of these organisms confers at least a short-lived immunity against reinfection. But influenza viruses appear to have a singularly unpleasant capability. From time to time "mutant" strains appear, apparently spontaneously, which are just different enough in their genetic makeup and disease-producing capability that they can cause brand-new types of influenza, often virulent infections, against which none of the antibodies already built up in the blood stream as a result of previous influenza infections seems to be effective. It is believed, for example, that the great world-wide pandemic of influenza in 1918–1919, in which more than 20 million people died of the disease and millions more died as a result of secondary infections, was a result of such a virus mutation. Another pandemic of influenza in 1957 and 1958 was due to a type A virus, but the particular strain apparently had not recently been involved in any epidemic, so much of the world population was not immune to it. Both the Asian flu virus that caused epidemic infection in 1960–1961 and the Hong Kong flu virus of 1968–1969 were probably mutant forms of ordinary flu viruses. Unfortunately, such mutant forms very often cause much more severe and widespread infection than the ones which normally exist in the population all the time. For that reason, epidemics of influenza caused by a virus strain that is demonstrably new and different from previously known strains are a matter of serious concern and often require special medical and public health emergency measures to check their spread.

Influenza is more than just an upper respiratory disease; although the virus is spread by upper respiratory droplets or secretions, it is a "whole-body" infection with wide-ranging symptoms. The ordinary case is a severe but relatively short-lived disease which usually begins quite suddenly, with a fever spiking up to 101° or 102°, and very prominent physical symptoms such as excessive fatigue, generalized headache, weakness, nausea, loss of appetite and a characteristic ache in the joints and muscles of the back and legs which is sometimes quite painful.

Respiratory symptoms are usually mild: a slightly sore throat, a dry, hacking cough, and sometimes a runny nose. In mild cases the temperature may rise to 102° and persist for two to three days, with rapid recovery from the acute symptoms as soon as the fever breaks. In more severe cases the temperature may go as high as 104° or 105° and persist for as long as six or seven days before it finally subsides. When nausea, vomiting and diarrhea are the predominant symptoms, the disease may be called intestinal flu or stomach flu, although this term is also often applied inaccurately to virtually any gastrointestinal upset and is thus not very scientifically accurate. But perhaps the most consistent and striking symptom of *any* form of influenza is the massive fatigue the victim feels for days or even weeks after the other symptoms have subsided. Patients who try to go back to their normal activities as soon as their fever is gone often find that they are literally exhausted after being out of bed for only two or three hours.

The most potent and useful treatments known for influenza are a light but nourishing diet, plenty of fluids, rest in bed and sufficient patience to stay there until the characteristic fatigue begins to lessen. In severe cases it is wise to seek the advice of a doctor. Diagnosis is usually made from the whole clinical picture and the history of the infection, although it is possible with modern sophisticated techniques of virology to isolate the virus from the back of the throat in the early stages of the disease or to have serum tests for antibodies run during the acute phase and convalescence. Generally, however, these examinations are not considered necessary, and the doctor is far more concerned about the possibility of a secondary bacterial infection occurring on the heels of the influenza. Anyone who has a persistent cough, fever and other respiratory symptoms for more than five or six days following the onset of a case of flu should see a doctor without delay, for the threat of a dangerous and swift-moving bacterial pneumonia is very real. Many people who think they are merely suffering a "relapse" a few days after the influenza seems to have subsided are actually suffering from a secondary bacterial infection which should be treated promptly with antibiotics.

Most sporadic cases of common influenza are not dangerous in themselves, but epidemic influenza caused by a new or mutant virus strain is quite another story. In some cases a fulminating pneumonia may accompany the infection, resulting from either the influenza virus itself or secondary bacterial invasion, and may occasionally lead to shortness of breath, spitting of blood, gathering of fluid in the lungs and death in as short a period as 48 hours. The threat of such a virulent attack is particularly great in small children, who may have had upper respiratory infections prior to the onset of influenza, and in aged and debilitated persons with relatively low natural resistance.

For some years vaccines to create temporary immunity against types A, B and C of the influenza viruses have been available and are remarkably effective in blocking active infection by those specific types. Furthermore, various virology laboratories throughout this country, working in cooperation with the U.S. Public Health Service, are armed and equipped to analyze the nature of any new mutant virus that may be causing widespread infection. In most cases, they are then able to create new vaccines to immunize potential victims and prevent a large-scale epidemic. In terms of commonsense prevention, elderly persons, especially those with chronic lung diseases or other debilitating illnesses, are well advised to have the polyvalent (that is, types A, B and C) influenza vaccine every year in a two-shot initial vaccination with a booster shot in the early fall. When a mutant epidemic strain makes its appearance, these same people, as well as children, should be protected by the new vaccine as soon as it becomes available. In addition, most doctors recommend vaccination for the breadwinners of families, since a pandemic of a new type of influenza can knock out a great many family providers for a period of days or even weeks. Most doctors, office nurses and hospital personnel take protective immunization shots themselves under these circumstances. This at least assures a full complement of medical and hospital workers to help handle the great influx of patients that appears with the onset of an epidemic wave of influenza.

Can we expect that some day a single vaccine will be developed to give lasting protection against all forms of influenza? Probably not. Immunity to one influenza virus does not "cross over" to provide immunity to another, and even natural immunity to one virus acquired as a result of an active infection does not persist much more than a year or two. The best protection available is therefore the use of such vaccines as we have or as become available against the more common influenza viruses, with special attention given to small children and aged people. Commonsense preventive measures—avoidance of chilling, dampness or exposure, and attention to adequate rest and nutrition—will help guard against flu. When it is contracted, the best treatment is alertness to the symptoms, early medical attention and, most particularly, complete bed rest for long enough to permit the body's own defenses to fight the infection effectively. This will reduce not only the severity and duration of the disease but also the risk of secondary infection.

Viral Infections of the Skin and Eyes

A "cold sore" or a "fever blister" on the lip or adjacent to the mouth is a relatively familiar affliction that often appears in the wake of an upper respiratory infection involving a high fever. The cause of this type of lesion, known by the medical name of *herpes simplex,* is a comparatively large virus which may live within the skin on the face, around the lips or around mucous membranes anywhere in the body. Most authorities believe that the initial herpes simplex infection is actually a generalized virus infection that occurs in infancy or childhood and is mistaken for a cold or a mild case of influenza. Thereafter, however, the dormant virus can be "awakened," so to speak, and cause the localized fluid-filled blisters and clusters of small vesicles to appear as a result of overexposure to sunlight, fever illnesses of any kind, upper respiratory infections or severe physical or emotional stress.

In most cases herpes simplex is a minor irritation. Usually after a few days it begins to dry, forms a thin yellowish crust and ultimately heals —or appears to. However, the lesions may recur in the same location again and again, with gradual evidence of scar formation after repeated infection. When the infection is active, it is contagious. Oddly enough, in many cases there seems to be a strong emotional or psychological factor involved in recurrences of this infection, and on occasion psychotherapy has been recommended as an aid in treatment. Similarly, smallpox vaccinations repeated at weekly intervals for a period of several weeks also seem to help heal the lesion and prevent its recurrence, although this treatment may have more psychological than physical value. In most cases, however, the best treatment is simply to leave the lesion alone. Whatever the cause, no antibiotics or local antibiotic salves have any effect, and the lesion should not be covered with anything, for fear of introducing a bacterial infection in the area and compounding the damage.

Herpes simplex may on rare occasions occur on the mucous membranes of the genitals, causing a highly irritating and embarrassing infection; but it responds to patience and the same treatment outlined above, although more slowly. Occasionally the disease may also flare into a generalized body infection, which must be treated much the same as influenza, with systemic antibiotics given as an extra protection measure. The main danger from this disease, however, is that the virus can sometimes cause a painful affliction of the transparent corneal surface of the eye, which the victim often mistakes for a foreign body in the eye. A careful office examination by a doctor involving the use of a droplet of fluorescent stain will usually make a herpes eye infection clearly apparent. In such cases the expert advice of an ophthalmologist may well be indicated, since herpetic lesions recurring in this area can form tiny ulcers that may subsequently impair vision.

Herpes zoster or "shingles" is an odd disease affecting the nerve endings in the skin caused by a virus similar to the herpes simplex but also closely related (some say virtually identical) to the virus of chicken pox. Actually, herpes zoster is a virus infection of the central nervous system which primarily involves the nerve cells that extend from the spinal cord but makes itself known by an eruption of blisters on the area of skin served by the affected nerve cells. First symptoms may include a mild fever and chills, malaise or gastrointestinal disturbances for a day or so, similar to the symptoms of mild influenza, but within four or five days a crop of exceedingly painful blisters or vesicles appears on the skin, often on the chest, back, neck or thigh, and usually only on one side. The most characteristic feature is the nature of the pain; it is felt right in the skin and is often described as "sharp," "searing" or "burning." It may be so severe, in fact, that codeine or even morphine is necessary to control it. Often any motion, touch or stretching of the skin stimulates the pain, and some patients cannot even bear to have clothing come in contact with the infected area.

To date there is no specific treatment that is consistently effective against herpes zoster. Fortunately, in most cases the vesicles begin to dry up and heal some five days after their occurrence, the pain subsides, and one attack apparently confers a lasting immunity. Some physicians feel that the pain is markedly reduced and healing of the lesions speeded up by the use of intramuscular injections of certain proteolytic (protein-destroying) enzymes, but the results of this treatment do not seem to be consistent, and no one can explain why it helps, if it does. Thus, most treatment is conservative and expectant, simply a matter of waiting for the body to overcome the infection and for the lesions to go away. In a few cases a persistent neuralgia may result, with the continuation of some degree of pain, either constant or sporadic, for a matter of months or years. In most cases, however, this complication (which occurs most frequently in elderly people) may be readily controlled with mild analgesics such as aspirin; but when it is severe, more radical treatment with X-ray irradiation of the nerve roots of the spinal cord or even surgical intervention to cut the pain-transmitting nerve channels may be necessary. If morphine or other habit-forming drugs are prescribed for the pain, there is a very real danger that the victim may become addicted. The doctor should, of course, be told that pain is there, but if he insists on the use of mild and harmless analgesics rather than prescribing potent narcotics, he is not being indifferent. He is simply protecting the patient against a long-term disability more dangerous than the neuralgia.

While both herpes simplex and herpes zoster can involve the eye, another virus infection of the eye known as *trachoma* is far more severe. It is uncommon in the United States except in southern mountainous regions, but it is extremely prevalent in the Arabian desert countries of the Middle East, central and southern Europe and parts of the Far East, perhaps due to the desiccating, dust-filled winds of those regions. Essentially trachoma begins as an inflammation of the conjunctiva, the mucous membrane lining the eyelids, and it usually occurs in both eyes. The disease tends to get progressively better and then worse as periods of inflammation lead to the formation of small, yellowish granulations of the eyelids and conjunctiva. Over an up-and-down course lasting from several months to a year or more, blood vessels may grow in the inflamed tissue to form a veil over part of the cornea; or the cornea itself, the vital "clear-viewing screen" that covers the front of the eye and makes vision possible, may become involved with the infection. The tear ducts may also be afflicted, so that the formation of tears is reduced and the corneal covering of the eye becomes chronically dried and thickened. If left untreated, the end result is progressive loss of sight and eventually blindness.

Fortunately, trachoma is one type of virus infection which can be aided by specific drug therapy. The sulfa drugs taken by mouth and used as eyedrops often speed healing, and even certain of the broad-spectrum antibiotics appear helpful. Work is under way today to prepare an effective vaccine against the virus of trachoma, but to date no preventive is available for the disease. Although trachoma is rare in this country, other eye infections are not. The eye is a delicate mechanism and *any* continuing or progressive irritation or inflammation should be brought to the attention of a doctor as quickly as possible.

The Scourge of Smallpox

Many of the virus infections are relatively benign and commonplace, often dreadful nuisances but not ordinarily terribly grave illnesses. Even the deaths ascribed to severe influenza are far more often due to secondary bacterial or viral infections than to influenza itself. But not all virus infections are so innocuous, by any means; some are truly dangerous killers. This fact is illustrated dramatically in the case of smallpox (variola), an epidemic virus-caused disease which resembles chicken pox—at least on the surface. But unlike its benign cousin, smallpox is a vicious infection which can take the lives of from 20 to 40 percent of its victims in an epidemic and subject the survivors to prolonged, severe illness and lifelong disfigurement.

Smallpox is one of the oldest afflictions in human history; it was known in the early centuries A.D. in China, India and Africa, and numerous epidemics occurred in Europe and the Middle East during Greek and Roman times. Later the disease was disseminated widely by the Crusaders, and was brought to America very soon after Columbus' first voyage. In the early days, the disease was called simply "the pox," referring to the pustular skin lesions so commonly associated with it. But during the Renaissance it became known as "the small pox" to distinguish it from "the great pox," the common name then given to syphilis.

Throughout its history, smallpox has been notorious as a highly contagious disease, and it still occurs in epidemics in India and southeast Asia and in occasional outbreaks elsewhere in the world. It is particularly virulent when it attacks populations that have never before been exposed to it. Thus, when American Indians were infected by white settlers and soldiers, whole tribes fell to the disease in vicious epidemics. The Mandan Indians of the Dakotas, for example, were virtually wiped out by it.

Smallpox can be contracted by virtually any kind of contact with an infected person, or even by contact with contaminated clothing, household articles or bedclothes, for the virus is present in all the victim's secretions or excreta. It is even present—and infectious—in the dried scales from the pustular skin lesions it typically causes. Initial symptoms of the infection resemble severe influenza: chills, high fever and prostration, headaches, aching muscles, sometimes vomiting. Then after two or three days a skin rash appears, round red spots about the size of a match head which soon enlarge and become fluid-filled blisters. After another day or two, these blisters become purulent and presently rupture and crust as they begin to heal gradually by the eighth or ninth day. Unlike chicken pox, the lesions of smallpox all appear at the same time in a single crop, and thus heal at approximately the same time, but the healing is slow, and death may occur at the height of the eruption. Among those who recover, the larger and deeper skin lesions leave permanent pockmark scars when they finally heal.

There is no effective treatment for smallpox once it has been contracted. Penicillin or other antibiotics help protect against secondary infection in the skin lesions, and extremely sick and prostrated victims may need supportive treatment with intravenous fluids. Typically, the acute illness lasts about three weeks, with an additional two or three weeks of convalescence necessary before the victim can return to normal activities.

Fortunately, smallpox *can* be prevented, and in most of the Western world mass vaccination has made the disease a rarity today. The English physician Edward Jenner (1749–1823) is often credited with performing the first successful vaccination against smallpox in 1796 on a farm near the country village where he practiced. The truth is that a crude form of vaccination was known in China and India as early as the 11th century A.D., but this method used infected serum from active smallpox lesions as the vaccine and often produced a full-blown case of the disease it was supposed to prevent. Jenner's great discovery was that people who had been infected with cowpox, a mild disease common among English milkmaids, rarely if ever became victims of smallpox, even during epidemics. Jenner used serum from a cowpox lesion to vaccinate young James Phipps, a healthy boy of eight; a single

pustule formed on the boy's skin at the site of the vaccination, but it healed quickly and the boy thereafter remained immune to smallpox. Today we know that the "vaccinia" virus of cowpox so closely resembles the virus causing smallpox that the antibodies we form in reaction to a mild induced cowpox infection can also effectively block any later invasion of smallpox viruses. The level of immunity, however, diminishes with time, so revaccination is recommended at intervals of three years for people who expect to be traveling in smallpox-stricken areas.

Today most children in the United States are vaccinated in infancy. A small amount of the vaccine is gently scratched into the baby's skin. Within 48 hours a small, raised red pimple appears at the site of the vaccination; a few days later it becomes a blister filled with clear fluid, and within two weeks turns into a crusted pustule. This is considered a full primary vaccination reaction or "full take." About three weeks later the crust falls off, leaving a reddish scar which then gradually turns white—the typical "vaccination mark." When a child is first vaccinated, the vaccination itches and he usually tries to scratch it. This can introduce skin bacteria into the vaccination site and cause an angry, swollen secondary infection. If this happens, a doctor should be notified because the child may begin to run a fever and may then require treatment with antibiotics. The cowpox virus in the vaccination can also be spread to other breaks in the skin by scratching, bathing, etc. Generally it is best to postpone vaccination if the child has any kind of skin rash or other skin outbreak; in fact, many pediatricians by-pass smallpox vaccination altogether for children with skin allergies. They feel the hazard of spreading the vaccine to other areas outweighs the risk of contact with smallpox—at least until the child has outgrown his skin allergies or is going to be taken to smallpox areas.

If an individual of any age is revaccinated more than four or five years after his primary vaccination, one of two things will ordinarily happen. If his level of immunity has fallen low, he may have a reaction similar to a primary vaccination, except with a much smaller lesion on the skin and much more rapid healing and peeling of the scab. If his primary vaccination is still in good effect, however, he will merely have a so-called immune reaction. A very small, reddish pimple will develop within 24 hours, often with quite vigorous itching, but will disappear again without forming a scab in a matter of two or three days. Even with this mild "immune reaction," however, the revaccination boosts the level of immunity.

If a primary vaccination or revaccination does not "take," a number of things may be responsible. The vaccine may be outdated, for example, or may have lost its potency because of improper refrigeration. And unless the skin is actually broken and scratched with the needle point, the vaccine may not reach the cells under the skin to cause the vaccination infection. In the case of a primary vaccination, it is very important to be sure that a rather nasty-looking sore forms at the site of the vaccination within ten days to two weeks. If it does not, the doctor should be notified that the vaccination did not "take" and arrangements should be made to have it redone.

Up until the last decade, smallpox vaccination in this country was considered a must for everyone, and there is no doubt that mass immunization has kept the United States completely free of epidemic smallpox for many years. Recently, however, a number of doctors (particularly pediatricians) have begun to question whether routine vaccination for smallpox is such a good idea in a country or community where little or no smallpox exists. The reason for this sudden caution is simple: it is now suspected that vaccination is not the completely benign procedure it was once assumed to be. Secondary infections in the vaccination site are quite common, and can sometimes lead to extensive and severe bacterial infection. Even worse, an occasional individual may develop a generalized skin eruption as a result of the cowpox virus in the vaccine—a condition which can be particularly dangerous to infants. This complication is rare, granted, but some pediatricians still feel it is wrong to take even that slight risk when smallpox is so seldom

seen, and so easy to identify when a case does appear that protective immunization can be quickly provided where it is needed. The question is by no means settled even today, as statistics about vaccination reactions are still being gathered, but it is quite possible that within the next few years routine vaccination of small children, at least, will no longer be recommended unless the child is going to be taken abroad. Probably adult vaccination will still be urged, most particularly if any kind of foreign travel is contemplated. If you travel abroad frequently or expect to be going to any area where epidemic smallpox still occurs—to India or Southeast Asia, for example—you must be sure that you maintain a high level of protective immunity against this still-deadly disease. Indeed, for years the U.S. Public Health Service required a certified smallpox vaccination within three years, before traveling citizens were allowed to reenter this country. This rule has been relaxed recently, but still applies in many countries and may be reinstated here at any time. Thus it is wise to check current rules with a Public Health Service office before embarking on foreign travel.

Yellow Fever

Yellow fever is not a serious threat to health in the United States today, for it is mainly a disease of the moist tropics of Africa and the jungles and swamps of South and Central America. However, epidemics of this dangerous virus-caused disease have occurred from time to time in the last few centuries in heavily populated urban areas. In 1793, long before anyone understood the nature of the disease and how it was spread, there was an epidemic of yellow fever in Philadelphia, and an epidemic in New Orleans occurred as recently as 1905. The disease is caused by a virus acting in deadly partnership with certain kinds of mosquitoes. The chief villain is the *Aedes aegypti,* a mosquito which transmits the virus by feeding on the blood of an infected person during the first few days of his attack and then biting an uninfected person within ten days to two weeks later. In the deep tropical jungles, yellow fever can also be transmitted by certain kinds of forest mosquitoes; and in some areas where the disease is prevalent, various monkeys can act as a natural reservoir of the virus. Indeed, in the mid-1960s a yellow fever epidemic virtually wiped out the monkey population in the jungle areas of southern Mexico and Guatemala, although few human beings were affected.

The disease itself, a generalized infection, is swift, severe, dangerous and often fatal when an unprotected person is attacked. The victim suddenly spikes a fever to 102° or 103°, often accompanied by chills, within three to six days after being bitten by an infected mosquito. Nausea, vomiting and constipation are characteristic symptoms, as are generalized muscular aches in the thighs and legs, and the victim becomes prostrated with a severe headache and irritability. Within a week of the onset of symptoms, his temperature rises even higher and a marked jaundice appears, for the virus attacks and destroys liver cells. In addition, kidney cells are affected, so that albumin appears in the urine, and the victim often begins to vomit quantities of black stuff which is blood that has leaked through the mucous membranes into the stomach. Finally, in severe cases, delirium and convulsions occur, and ultimately the victim may die in coma. In areas of epidemic the fatality rate can climb as high as 85 percent, but in areas where the disease appears sporadically it seems milder, with a fatality rate of only about 10 percent.

There is no specific treatment known for yellow fever, other than bed rest, good nursing care and, if necessary, intravenous feeding. By far the best treatment is prevention, which is so simple that it is surprising that few people in this country, other than world travelers, seek immunization. A single shot with a yellow fever vaccine will confer an active immunity against infection for a period of at least six years, and frequently as long as ten, and boosters are not required except during epidemics. Yellow fever shots are given free of charge by the U.S. Public Health Service. A telephone call to the nearest Health Service office will provide you with information about where and when they can be obtained. Certainly anyone who travels extensively in the southern United States, Mexico or other tropical and subtropical areas should have this painless and effective protection against a dangerous disease.

The history of the conquest of yellow fever, or yellow jack as it is sometimes called, is one of the most fascinating in the annals of medicine. The disease has been known for hundreds of years. According to medical historian Charles Singer, the legend of the Flying Dutchman arose from the story of a ship on which a murder was committed, followed by an epidemic of yellow fever. No port would give sanctuary to the unfortunate crew, and all of them finally died of the disease. The legend has many variations, but in one of them the deserted "phantom" ship was believed to sail the seas around the Cape of Good Hope, bringing misfortune to all sailors who saw it. Wagner's opera *The Flying Dutchman* was based on another variation of the legend, and Coleridge's famous poem "The Rime of the Ancient Mariner" also deals with a ship stricken by yellow fever. Although the disease is tropical, it extended from time to time as far north as Boston, and there were repeated plagues of yellow fever in Spain, Portugal, Italy and the islands of the West Indies. Many different things were blamed for its spread, including a "miasma" supposed to emanate from the earth when the soil was turned over. Benjamin Rush, the early American physician who worked during the great outbreak in Philadelphia in 1793, thought the disease was contagious, but the true cause was not proposed until 1881 when Dr. Carlos Juan Finlay of Havana, the son of a Scottish physician who had emigrated to Cuba, deduced that the *Aedes aegypti* must be the transmitter. Unfortunately, Finlay's work was ignored until the year 1900, when the United States government appointed a commission headed by Walter Reed of the Army Medical Corps to investigate the high mortality rate in American soldiers from yellow jack in Cuba. Reed confirmed Finlay's experiments and further proved that the disease was not transmitted in any other way. The next step was obvious; all infected persons must be treated in screened enclosures to prevent mosquitoes from biting them and transmitting the disease to others, uninfected persons must take precautions against being bitten and, finally, the mosquitoes themselves must be eliminated by destroying their breeding grounds. These measures were instituted in Havana and then in Panama, at the time the Americans had taken over construction of the canal from the French, under the direction of William Gorgas, the American sanitation expert and later United States Surgeon General. They were so successful that Gorgas was instrumental in reducing the number of deaths in Panama from the three to four thousand a year suffered by the French workers who earlier attempted to dig the canal to literally no fatal cases in 1906.

Finding a means of immunization was a more difficult and time-consuming process. For many years researchers assumed that a bacteria caused the disease. There were bacteria, in particular a spirochete known as *Leptospira icteroides,* which caused a similar sort of disease in experimental animals and in man, but it was not until 1927 that an Irish physician, Adrian Stokes, and his collaborators showed conclusively that yellow fever was caused by a filterable virus. Stokes himself died in 1927 of yellow fever while doing post-mortem work on infected monkeys, but in 1928 the first vaccine was prepared for preventive purposes by weakening or attenuating the virus with phenol or formaldehyde. Viruses thus treated lost their power to produce the disease, but nevertheless could stimulate formation of antibodies in the blood of susceptible people who were inoculated. Finally the virus was grown in tissue culture in 1932, and by 1935 a vaccine conferring a prolonged active immunization was perfected.

Yellow fever is not by any means a "conquered" disease today. Although it has been largely eradicated from urban centers in the tropics by vaccination and control of mosquito breeding, great areas of jungle continue to harbor mosquitoes capable of transmitting the infection. Even so, no one need die from yellow fever if the simple precaution of immunization is taken, particularly before travel in tropical areas.

Dengue Fever

Although dengue fever (pronounced den'-gee) has been recognized as a distinct disease syndrome since an epidemic occurred in the Dutch East Indies in 1779, it was not until World War II when large numbers of American soldiers fighting in the South Pacific encountered the disease that medical researchers were able to demonstrate that it was caused by a virus and transmitted by an insect—interestingly enough, the same *Aedes aegypti* and other related mosquitoes that spread yellow fever. There is little similarity between the two diseases, however, and dengue is not nearly as dangerous as yellow fever in terms of mortality rates, although it too is a generalized disease affecting all tissues of the body, and its symptoms can be almost as severe. Essentially it is never fatal, but victims commonly complain of being so sick they wish they could die during the characteristic seven-day course of the fever. A typical case, which begins with a day or two of rapidly rising fever to the level of 103° to 105°, is characterized by a very intense headache, severe pain in back of the eyes, especially on eye movements, and excruciating pain in the back, muscles and joints. This pain, which accounts for the common nickname of the disease, "breakbone fever," may be so severe that codeine is required to relieve it, and it persists from four to seven days after onset. Finally, on about the third or fourth day of the infection, a conspicuous red rash, sometimes so fine that it looks like a blush or the red flushing rash of scarlet fever, appears on the trunk, face and extremities. Again, typically, when the fever and pain resolve, the victim is left with a feeling of complete physical exhaustion and often an extreme emotional depression, both of which may persist for two weeks or more before he is able to resume his regular activities. There is no treatment for the disease other than bed rest and administration of aspirin or codeine analgesics during its acute phase.

Dengue fever usually occurs in epidemic outbreaks, and although it appears in temperate as well as tropical zones, the insect that spreads it is not active in winter, so the disease occurs only in a "summer-like" climate. Once it appears, the cycle of infection and reinfection is insidious. The infected human being has enough virus in his blood stream during the first three to five days of his illness to infect a mosquito that bites him. After biting an infected man, the mosquito requires an incubation period of eight to twelve days at summer temperatures before it too becomes infectious. Then it is capable of initiating a new infection by biting a susceptible victim, who after a five- to six-day incubation period comes down with symptoms and can pass the infection on to another mosquito. The infected mosquito remains infectious as long as it lives.

As with yellow fever, control of the disease rests with preventing both infected and uninfected individuals from being bitten by the carrier mosquito, and with eliminating the mosquitoes by destroying their breeding grounds. Thus far no effective vaccine is available to provide immunization. Researchers continue to work on the problem, but experimental vaccines have caused such severe dengue-like symptoms themselves that they are not practical for general use. Luckily, the disease is rare in the United States, but it continues to be a threat to servicemen in Southeast Asia and on tropical islands, and to travelers in the southern Orient, India and Ceylon.

Rocky Mountain Spotted Fever and Typhus

The infectious microorganisms known as rickettsiae are quite distinct from either viruses or bacteria, yet seem to occupy a position halfway between them. They are smaller in size than the smallest known bacteria, but larger than large viruses; and although they behave much as bacteria do, they resemble viruses in that they must invade living cells in order to grow and multiply. The most serious diseases caused by these microorganisms are Rocky Mountain spotted fever and various forms of typhus fever, and like the viruses that cause yellow fever and dengue, the rickettsiae must depend upon an insect carrier to reach their human victims.

Rocky Mountain spotted fever has been recognized as a separate disease only since the beginning of this century, although medical historians now believe that it probably existed in Idaho and Montana at the time white men first settled there, and it may have been known to the Indians long before then. The disease is limited to the Western Hemisphere, but the name is now somewhat misleading, for today it also occurs in the mountainous and wooded areas of the East as well as in the Rocky Mountains.

Rocky Mountain spotted fever is primarily a disease of wild rodents—squirrels, chipmunks, field mice or rats—which human beings largely acquire by accident. Certainly the wild rodents serve as the natural reservoir of the disease. The rickettsia that causes the disease is transmitted to man by various species of wood ticks which first bite the infected animals and then later bite human victims. These wood tick "carriers" can be picked up on the clothes during forest camping trips, mountain hikes or any other wilderness activity during the three-month summer tick season. When the rickettsia is introduced into the human body by means of a tick bite, the organisms first invade the tissue at the site of the bite, but then quickly enter the blood stream and cause a generalized infection.

Two to five days following the tick bite there is a gradual onset of an almost influenza-like illness with a low-grade fever, malaise and loss of appetite. Then, after two or three more days, the victim begins to develop a severe headache and his temperature climbs to 103° or 104°. Often the first skin lesion to appear is a small sore or ulcer at the site of the tick bite, a raised and reddened pimple which later becomes an open sore with a black crust over the top. Then, on approximately the third day of the fever, a generalized mottled red rash appears on the skin of the face, neck, chest and legs. The rash spreads quite rapidly, and in severe cases the mottled splotches tend to coalesce. At the same time tiny hemorrhages under the skin in the rash areas occur, so that the color of the rash changes from a pale pink to a deep red or purple after a day or two. In areas where the splotchy rash does not occur, tiny pinpoint hemorrhages called *petechiae* often appear. When the fever of the disease subsides, the rash also begins to disappear, often with peeling or desquamation of the skin overlying the areas where the rash was present.

Before the availability of antibiotic drugs, Rocky Mountain spotted fever was a very dangerous disease, with an overall death rate of about 20 percent. In certain parts of the country it was even more serious. The Bitterroot Valley of Montana, still today one of the most dangerous reservoirs of the disease, once reported a death rate as high as 80 percent for infected adults and almost 40 percent for children. Fortunately, the rickettsia causing the disease is quite sensitive to broad-spectrum antibiotics such as members of the tetracycline family or chloramphenicol. Thus early diagnosis and vigorous early treatment save the lives of most victims today. Even so, individuals in whom treatment is started late are still in danger of death, and prevention is by far more sensible than having to fight the disease once it has been contracted.

Since there is no practical way to eliminate either the tick "carriers" or the rodents that harbor the disease, the major means of prevention is, of course, to avoid tick bites. In any area of the United States where ticks are commonly found, and especially in the western mountains of Montana, Idaho and Wyoming and the eastern mountains of Virginia, North Carolina and Tennessee, everyone should be carefully examined for ticks in the clothes or on the skin at least daily, and children twice daily. Any ticks that are discovered should be removed with care. It appears that they do not transmit the disease until after having been attached to the skin for some hours, so early detection and removal can be effective protection. Applying a drop of ether or kerosene to the tick, or holding a lighted cigarette near it, will often cause it to disengage and back off. If this fails, use a pair of tweezers, grasping the tick as close to the skin as possible and tugging gently to release it without leaving its mouth parts embedded in the skin. *Do not crush the tick on the skin or between the fingers.* That will contaminate the area with the tick's body fluids. It should be destroyed, but only after it has been completely removed from the skin. Once the tick has been removed, disinfect the area by washing with soap and water, and treat the tick bite site proper with a drop of silver

nitrate, iodine or phenol applied with a toothpick or cotton swab. Remember that dogs or other house pets may also pick up ticks. Use the same precautions in removing them; there is no way you can tell if a tick is infected or not.

Even better, avoid tick bites in the first place by using a good insect repellent when you are out in the woods or fields where ticks may be present. Commercial insect repellents containing diethyltoluamide which can be applied directly to the skin are very effective. One company markets this repellent in either concentrated liquid form or aerosol spray under the trade name Off. Finally, vaccines containing chemically killed spotted fever rickettsiae are of value for immunizing those who spend time or work in tick-infected areas—forest rangers, loggers, campers, etc. The immunization is carried out in a course of three injections given in the spring before ticks become prevalent. Repeated injections are necessary each year, however, to maintain a high immunization level.

Typhus fever exists in several forms throughout the world, caused by various strains of rickettsiae and all transmitted by the bite of body lice, itch mites (chiggers) or rat fleas. One form, epidemic louse-borne typhus fever, was probably prevalent in antiquity and has played a major role in modern history for at least four centuries. It has always been associated with famine, poverty, overcrowding and other human misfortunes, but it has been particularly prevalent in time of war, among both military and civilian populations, with body lice transmitting the disease from one person to the next. Epidemics of typhus in eastern Europe and Russia immediately following World War I are believed to have caused as many as 3 million deaths. Even today with effective immunization techniques, the disease is a constant threat in poverty-stricken and war-torn areas of the world, and in the city slums and isolated rural areas of the most advanced countries.

The disease is characterized by an abrupt onset of a severe headache and generalized aching throughout the body, with a rise of temperature to 104° over a period of three or four days. On the fifth day a rash appears, pinkish-red in color and spreading from the back and chest to the abdomen and extremities, but usually absent on the face, palms and soles. Although similar in color to the rash of Rocky Mountain spotted fever, the red splotches do not usually coalesce, nor do pinpoint lesions appear except in severe cases. The fever remains elevated in untreated cases for two to three weeks, and the patient develops bouts of active delirium and may presently go into a profound stupor or coma. The invading organisms cause the formation of thrombi or clots in the small blood vessels and capillaries, with the result that the victim's toes, fingers, genitals, ear lobes or the tip of his nose may not receive enough oxygenated blood and may become gangrenous. Death from typhus, in approximately 20 percent of all untreated cases, occurs as the patient progresses from stupor to coma and then dies in an episode of vascular collapse.

Treatment of louse-borne epidemic typhus with broad-spectrum antibiotic drugs is highly successful providing it is begun early in the disease. Often diagnosis cannot specifically be made until the appearance of the typical rash, and today, when broad-spectrum antibiotics may be prescribed for any highly febrile disease without waiting for a specific diagnosis, the rash may well *not* appear in those cases in which treatment and healing are begun before the disease becomes full-blown. However, apparent recovery from the acute infection must be followed by a period of convalescence of two to three weeks because the patient is constantly tired and weak, and requires fairly prolonged bed rest for a complete recovery. Active immunization against typhus is now possible on a wide scale, using a vaccine containing killed rickettsiae, in an initial course of two inoculations ten days to two weeks apart, followed by booster doses at intervals of a few months if exposure is likely. Even when complete immunization is not achieved, the individual who has been partially immunized has less chance of acquiring typhus fever, and if it is acquired has a far less severe illness with little or no risk of death. Again, since the disease is transmitted by body lice, treatment with a 10 percent DDT powder will help kill the insect vector and reduce the incidence of the disease sharply. Today scientists are also searching for equally effective and less dangerous insect killers.

Other types of typhus include so-called *murine typhus fever,* a disease occurring in urban slums, particularly in the southern United States and Mexico, which is transmitted by rat fleas; and *scrub typhus* (also called tsutsugamushi disease or tropical typhus), which is transmitted by itch mites or "chiggers." Both types, while similar in symptoms to louse-borne typhus, are milder infections and shorter-lived illnesses with much lower death rates. Murine typhus, even when untreated, lasts only between six to twelve days, with a less extensive rash and fatalities only in the very young or very old. It responds to broad-spectrum antibiotics much as epidemic typhus does, and although vaccines are available for medical personnel likely to be exposed to the disease, mass immunizations of the general population are rarely considered necessary.

Scrub typhus, while known for centuries, emerged from obscurity during World War II as a major infection of Allied armies in the South Pacific. This disease again brings symptoms similar to epidemic typhus—headache, fever and a generalized rash—and, like epidemic typhus, is treated with chloramphenicol or the tetracycline antibiotics with a high degree of success. No effective vaccine is yet available to prevent infection, so the best prophylaxis against acquiring scrub typhus is the use of insect repellents to remain free of the chiggers that spread the disease.

Rabies (Hydrophobia)

The fear of a "mad dog" is well founded, for the bite of such an animal can result in one of the most horrible and universally fatal illnesses known to man. Rabies is an acute infectious disease caused by a rather large virus which attacks virtually all warm-blooded animals, including man. Although it does cause a generalized illness at first, the virus primarily attacks the brain and other parts of the central nervous system. It also finds its way into the salivary glands of the infected host, so that it is transmitted from animals to man by means of animal bites, and once symptoms of the infection have begun it is almost invariably fatal. Rabies is primarily an infection of wild animals—wolves and coyotes in the Arctic regions, mongooses and bats in tropical Africa and Central and South America, foxes, coyotes, skunks and wild rodents in the United States—but it is most commonly transmitted to man by dogs which have been infected by contact with infected wildlife. Even in areas of the world such as the United States, where control of the disease has been at least partly accomplished by vaccination and licensing of dogs and collection and disposal of strays, the disease maintains a widespread "natural reservoir" among wild animals throughout the country, most particularly among bats.

In domestic dogs rabies can appear in two different forms. In the "agitated" form, the animal becomes excitable and then irritable owing to the infection of brain tissue, often ferocious, tending to snap or bite at anything that comes near it, and finally goes into convulsions and dies after a period of about ten days. Alternatively, the disease may manifest itself in a "mute" form in which the dog becomes sluggish, with violent spasms of the throat muscles, excessive salivation and a creeping paralysis first of the hind limbs and then of the trunk, finally ending in coma and death. In either case the virus is present in the saliva of the animal and can be transmitted to man by means of a bite or contact of any open sore, cut or scratch with the animal's saliva.

When a human is infected in either manner, the disease may have an incubation period anywhere from ten days to as much as several months (some say a year) before symptoms begin. The first signs of the disease are the onset of fever, headache, nausea, sore throat and loss of appetite—symptoms so common to other less dangerous virus infections that the diagnosis is often missed at this point unless there is a clear-cut history of a fairly recent animal bite. As the infection progresses to involve the nervous system, there is a general hypersensitivity, particularly of touch, sound and sight. Evidences of

muscle spasm and paralysis soon make their appearance, with extremely painful spasms of the muscles of the mouth and pharynx and the muscles controlling swallowing. Because swallowing is so painful, these spasms can be triggered at the mere sight of water, the explanation for the common name of the disease, hydrophobia ("fear of water"). Ultimately, after a period of eight or ten days of progressive debilitation, the victim may have episodes of delirium, widespread muscle spasms or convulsions, finally giving way to coma, general paralysis and death. When the infection has been contracted as a result of the bite of certain kinds of bats, it may have a "mute" course of progressive paralysis without any evidence of the "agitated" form of the disease. But whatever the form, there has, to date, been only one medically verified case in which a victim has recovered once symptoms began. To all intents and purposes the infection, once entrenched, is invariably fatal.

There is, however, a course of crash treatment that can be used after the infection has been contracted but before symptoms have begun. But, obviously, protection against the infection and possible infective contact is the best way to control the disease. For that reason, everyone should be certain that house pets, particularly dogs and cats, receive rabies shots from a veterinarian, and that those shots are adequately "boosted" at prescribed intervals. When rabies makes an appearance in a community, local public health offices usually publicize the fact and make arrangements for free inoculation of house pets. Many communities require such protective vaccination as a prerequisite to licensing pets—perhaps the best protection of all.

Vaccinating domestic animals is a simple and effective procedure, but, of course, there is no practical way of vaccinating wild animals which may infect each other and transmit the infection to domestic animals or humans. Nor is there any completely safe human immunization procedure. This means that the only sure-fire method to prevent the disease is to avoid being bitten. *No one should attempt to feed or come in close contact with any wild animal anywhere,* particularly one which appears sick or dead, or is behaving strangely. This includes chipmunks, squirrels, rabbits, skunks or woodchucks. *Contact should also be avoided with any domestic animal that is behaving strangely.* Children in particular should be discouraged from approaching or teasing unknown and possibly unfriendly pets.

In spite of every precaution, animal bites do happen. In that case, there is only one thing to do. *A bite from any animal, wild or domestic, in which the skin is broken should be reported to a doctor.* If the animal that inflicted the wound is known, it should also be reported to the police and local health authorities who will keep it under observation until absolutely certain that it is not infected. If the animal is a pet in your own household, it too should be confined for observation, preferably under the guidance of local health authorities. If the animal is infected, clearcut symptoms will appear within a ten-day period and it must be destroyed. *Never destroy the animal prior to the expiration of this observation period.* If for some reason it dies or is destroyed, its head should be preserved for examination by public health officials for pathological evidence of the infection in the brain. Further, if a pet shows any signs of odd behavior or an abrupt "change of personality," or if it has been in a fight with another domestic or wild animal, it is a sensible precaution to take it to a veterinarian, even if it has not bitten anyone.

Most bites from known domestic animals are relatively harmless, thanks to the prevalence of vaccination. The doctor will simply disinfect and dress it. But if the animal that inflicted the wound is wild, like a fox, squirrel or chipmunk encountered on a camping trip, or a domestic animal that cannot be found for observation, then additional precautions must be taken. World health authorities have worked out a guide for physicians to follow when a patient has been bitten by a possibly rabid animal. The guide is complex, seeking to cover all possible circumstances, but the basic idea behind it is simple. First, *no* animal bite should be ignored, even if the animal inflicting the bite is a family pet. Second, if the animal at fault proves, after observation, to be free of infection, the patient requires no further treatment. But if the animal does display symptoms of rabies, protective anti-

rabies treatment of the patient should begin immediately. Third, if the patient has been bitten by an animal whose condition cannot be observed and determined, treatment should begin at once. And fourth, when the patient has received multiple bites, or bites on the face, head, fingers or neck, treatment should also be started immediately. In cases of a minor wound, treatment when necessary consists of disinfecting and dressing the wound, followed by a course of inoculation with a vaccine containing the rabies virus in attenuated form which builds up the body's resistance to the infection. In cases of severe or multiple wounds, doses of rabies-immune serum taken from previously vaccinated animals are given to provide immediate protection, followed by the course of vaccination.

Why not give rabies vaccinations to anyone who has been bitten by an animal, or for that matter, to everyone to provide immunity even before he is bitten? There are, after all, effective vaccinations against other dangerous virus infections like smallpox and yellow fever. The main reason is that simple vaccinations, such as are given to house pets, are just not safe enough for widespread human use. There is always the risk that such vaccination might, on rare occasions, actually cause an active rabies infection, and nobody can afford such a risk with a disease like this. As for giving full-scale antirabies treatment to anyone who has been bitten by an animal or as general protection, this is by no means as simple a matter as a one-dose smallpox vaccination or the three-dose influenza series. Modern antirabies treatment, which is essentially the same procedure that Louis Pasteur pioneered fifty years before viruses had even been discovered, involves a series of fourteen daily and often quite painful shots, followed by additional booster doses at intervals thereafter. Few people care to go through such a program on the off chance that they might one day be bitten by a rabid animal, and of those who *must* have the treatment a small percentage (about one out of every 2,500 patients) may suffer nervous system complications, conceivably even with fatal results. Even in the milder and less dangerous vaccines recently developed from strains of rabies virus grown in duck eggs rather than in animal brain tissue (which Pasteur used), the course of treatment is long and tedious—certainly impractical for mass immunization. Work is under way to develop a completely safe live-virus vaccine which might make a one-shot vaccination possible, but many health authorities feel that far too little is known about the long-term effects of any live-virus vaccine once it is introduced into the body, particularly one involving such a deadly virus, to be enthusiastic about the prospects.

For the time being, then, vaccination against rabies is reserved for those who may have been exposed to infection from animal bites, and the advice of your doctor should be sought in any such accident. He, in turn, is kept advised by local public health authorities about the frequency of rabies known to exist in various animal species in the area. Many parts of our country have been relatively rabies-free for decades, and in certain localities health authorities do not feel that any antirabies treatment is necessary under these circumstances. Many authorities believe, however, that the natural wildlife "reservoir" of rabies is increasing both in open country and in heavily populated urban areas. In any case, rabies can be a serious threat, and it may well be that a new, safe and uncomplicated type of vaccine will be developed within the next few years and prove to be the best possible protection against this disease.

22

The Venereal Diseases—Ancient Plague, Modern Threat

Considering the enormous advances in medical science in the last few decades, it is easy to persuade ourselves that we have "conquered" many of the infectious diseases. After all, the discovery of sulfonamides and antibiotics has completely altered our approach to their treatment, and several former killers are no longer any more than a minor concern. Even with infections that do *not* respond to antibiotics we have found ways to protect our health by means of immunization. But for all of this, there are still a great many dangerous infections which have not been "conquered" by any means. A handful of these enduring afflictions have been tormenting human beings for centuries and continue to do so today. Among these ancient plagues is a group of infections commonly known as VD or venereal disease—infections most commonly transmitted by sexual contact. Although these infections at least nominally attack the genital organs—the penis or urethra in the male, the urethra, vagina, uterus or Fallopian tubes in the female—they can often, if undetected or untreated, spread throughout the body to play havoc with organs and tissues far distant from the point of contact. In times past social taboos limited frank and open discussion of these diseases, but today they represent such a serious and burgeoning health hazard, particularly among young people, that it is foolhardy to ignore them or pretend they do not exist.

Syphilis

Of all the infectious diseases that plagued mankind in ancient times, there is little doubt that the one which continues to present the most active and insidious threat is syphilis—in spite of the fact that many medical authorities as little as ten or fifteen years ago seriously believed that the disease was totally under control. More recent statistics indicate quite the opposite. Although the incidence of syphilis indeed fell off sharply immediately after World War II, thanks to the great effectiveness of penicillin in combating it, the disease is now again sharply on the rise in our society. But perhaps even more alarming, by far the greatest number of its victims today are teen-agers between fourteen and eighteen years old, young people who all too often fail to seek medical help through ignorance of the serious nature of the disease, or through fear of their parents' anger, or both. With early diagnosis and treatment, the disease can be completely cured, but there is no medical cure for ignorance and fear. Only knowledge can do that, and everyone today should be armed with facts about this vicious killer, particularly the parents of teen-agers and—above all—teen-agers themselves.

No one knows when syphilis first made its appearance on the historical scene. It was recognized as a distinct disease entity in Europe in the late 1400s, but may have been widely confused with leprosy. Very possibly the disease was in existence in some parts of the ancient world as many as a thousand or more years earlier and was simply mistaken for something else. In the 1490s, however, an epidemic of an extremely virulent form of syphilis spread all over Europe, and it was recognized even then that whatever caused it, the infection was spread primarily by means of sexual contact. Because of the characteristic skin rash that often appears in the moderately advanced stage of the disease, it was commonly known as "the pox" (later called "the great pox" to distinguish it from smallpox). It was also, typically, known as "the French disease" in Spain and Italy and as "the Spanish disease" in France. Because of its venereal nature, it was widely considered to be a sort of divine punishment for sexual sins and regarded with grave social approbation, an attitude which unfortunately persists to the present day. In 1530 the Italian physician Girolamo Fracastoro coined the modern name "syphilis," drawn from a legend about a Greek shepherd, Syphilus, who insulted Apollo and for punishment was afflicted with a loathsome disease. In modern medicine the infection is also referred to as "lues," or in medical shorthand simply by the capital Greek letter sigma (Σ).

In the days before any really effective cure was known, syphilis was a dangerous killer, as well as one of the most complex and baffling of all diseases. Indeed, it was known as "the great imitator" because of the many different forms it could take in its natural history, and huge textbooks were written by specialists who devoted their entire medical careers to the study of this single disease. Today many of the mysteries have been solved, and we know a great deal about the natural history of syphilis. Oddly enough, this hardy and perennial infection is caused by one of the most sensitive and vulnerable of all infectious microorganisms—a comparatively large spirochete known as *Treponema pallidum*. Removed from a moist, warm environment such as the mucous membranes or internal organs of the body, the organism will die within a matter of five minutes or so, and contentions that the infection can be acquired from unsanitary toilet facilities are largely nonsense. It is this sensitive vulnerability of the syphilitic spirochete that accounts for the fact that far more cases of gonorrhea, which is caused by a hardier organism, are contracted than of syphilis, even when the contact has both diseases in highly infectious form at the same time. In many cases ordinary washing or douching with soapy water immediately following sexual intercourse with an infected individual will destroy the *Treponema pallidum* before it can become entrenched, while the gonorrhea organism may be unaffected by this procedure. Syphilis *can* be acquired nonvenereally on rare occasions by kissing an individual who happens to have an open, infective lesion on his lip or in his mouth, but such an event is so unlikely as to approach the ridiculous. Syphilis is by far most commonly contracted by genital contact with an individual who has an infectious stage of the disease. Both men and women may be infected, and the disease may be spread just as readily by homosexual contact as by heterosexual, and by way of oral and anal intercourse as well as by the more usual sexual contact.

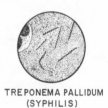

TREPONEMA PALLIDUM
(SYPHILIS)

Figure 22–1.

At first the natural history of syphilis is fairly simple and straightforward. Lodged on the warm, moist mucous membrane of the penis, vulva, vagina, anus or mouth, the organism penetrates the surface and begins multiplying rapidly, forming a small, painless lesion at the site of the contact. It may occasionally attack the external skin surface of the penis (or, more rarely, any skin surface), finding entrance through a tiny scratch or abrasion. Within a period of from four to eight days after exposure, this primary infection usually becomes a shallow, painless ulcer—the so-called hard or primary chancre—teeming with the spirochete.

The lesion may persist for a matter of three or four weeks before healing itself spontaneously, and it is during this interval that the newly infected person is himself most actively infectious. In some cases the lesion may become sore and swollen as a result of secondary infection with other bacteria, occasionally accompanied by swelling of lymph glands in the groin; but far more frequently it is small and apparently innocuous, often so nondescript that it escapes notice altogether, or in the female it may be concealed internally. Occasionally no actual ulcer appears at all, and the primary lesion is nothing more than a small pimple which forms for a few days and then disappears spontaneously. If the primary lesion goes unnoticed until it has healed, further symptoms may not appear for as long as 90 days or more.

During this "primary stage" of the infection, however, the spirochete multiplies rapidly, finding access to small blood vessels and spreading widely throughout the body, where it can set up a multitude of foci and begin growing actively. The disease then enters its "secondary stage," and in most cases after a period of one to three months, but sometimes as late as eight or nine months after the primary infection, a widespread skin rash appears briefly. Often this rash is not very impressive: an outbreak of flat, plaquelike, dusky red splotches on the back, abdomen, arms, face, genitals and in the mouth. This "secondary rash" also disappears spontaneously within a brief time, but scrapings taken from an area of rash reveal the presence of myriads of spirochetes, and at this time the infected person again can transmit the disease, particularly by sexual contact. The "secondary rash" phase is probably a manifestation of the body's natural and vigorous attempt to eradicate the spirochete, for we know that in some 25 to 30 percent of victims the manifestations of the disease disappear at this point, never to recur. In the great majority of cases, however, spirochetes in one or another part of the body *do* survive. Even though not present in large numbers anywhere, they begin a long process of tissue destruction which may continue for years unsuspected and undetected and ultimately may result in the death of the victim.

Exactly what form this "tertiary stage" of syphilis takes depends upon what particular area of the body the organism invades. Virtually any part or organ can be affected, but certain sites are by far the most common. For reasons no one understands, the arch of the aorta—the point at which the great artery leading from the heart curves down into the lower chest and abdomen—is particularly vulnerable to the spirochete. The organism lodges in the aorta walls and, over a period of months or years, creates an area of inflammation in which the strong fibrous connective tissue of this great artery is broken down and destroyed. As a result, a so-called *aneurysm* or "bulging out" of the aorta wall develops, much as a damaged tire will form a swelling or bubble when the cords in its walls have been weakened or broken. Once started, this process may continue over a period of eight or ten or even as many as twenty years, and if undiscovered and untreated the aneurysm will inevitably rupture and cause death by uncontrollable hemorrhage.

Another favorite focus for attack in advanced syphilis is the nervous system, either the spinal cord or the brain itself. In the spinal cord the spirochetes invade and destroy the *dorsal horn cells,* the neurons that regulate sensation and muscular coordination of the hips and lower limbs. As the infection progresses in this area, many of the vital reflex arcs that help control the balance and function of the legs without direct orders from the brain are broken down; the "knee jerk" reflex disappears, and in typical *tabes dorsalis,* as this form of syphilis is known, the victim ultimately becomes a shuffling wreck unable to coordinate such functions as walking, dependent upon support in order to walk at all and, eventually, confined to a wheelchair for locomotion. If the organism attacks the brain itself an even worse form of nervous system degeneration known as *general paresis* occurs. Vital nerve cell centers and connecting links within the brain are gradually destroyed; various of the cranial nerves controlling facial expression, use of the tongue, and so on, are impaired; the victim's memory and intellectual capacity begin to disintegrate slowly until life terminates in a sort of moronic premature senility. Like other aspects of tertiary syphilis, these changes may occur over a period of years or may be delayed for decades before any sign of the damage occurs.

Other less common late sites of infection and damage can involve almost any part of the body. Draining sores appear on the skin, and typically the organism will cause swollen, thickened and indurated areas of inflammation known as *gummas* which may occur on the tongue, in the bone of an elbow joint, in the wall of the stomach, or practically anywhere else. But perhaps saddest of all the unpleasant aspects of this disease is the capacity of the spirochete in an expectant mother's blood stream to penetrate the placenta and infect her developing unborn child, who will not only have active syphilis at the time of birth, but may bear for the rest of his life certain stigmata of *congenital syphilis:* destruction of cartilage of the baby's nose, leaving a flattened, saddle-shaped deformity of the nose and forehead; misformed, peglike teeth; and a variety of other tragic physical defects.

Considering the grisly natural history of syphilis, it is hardly surprising that medical research for centuries was directed at finding some means of early diagnosis and treatment. This research was impeded by the peculiar nature of the spirochete itself, which could not be readily stained for observation and has never successfully been grown on artificial culture mediums. In fact, it was not discovered and identified with the disease until 1905 when Fritz Schaudinn succeeded in spotting the organism in a fresh specimen under the microscope by means of dark-field lighting techniques. Today diagnosis of early syphilis depends heavily on two laboratory procedures, each complicated in its own way. Most ideally, dark-field examination of serum freshly removed from a suspicious ulcer or other lesion found on the mucous membrane of the genitalia or elsewhere on the skin may reveal the spirochete itself—diagnostic of the disease in its earliest stage when treatment is most likely to be successful and when control of its spread can best be managed.

The disease can be diagnosed at a later stage by means of identifying the footsteps, so to speak, left behind by the organism. Natural body defenses swing promptly into action to fight off an invasion of the spirochete of syphilis; therefore, within two or three months of the initial infection a victim of the disease will have in his blood stream a high titer of antibodies formed to fight off the organism. A variety of extremely sensitive laboratory examinations have been devised to detect the presence of these antibodies in the victim's blood, and the most familiar of them, the so-called Wasserman test, or others similar to it, will almost invariably spot the infection if it has been present for more than a few weeks. Such a *serological test for syphilis* (STS) is now usually done routinely at the same time as a blood count examination, so that anyone who has a routine physical at regular intervals will be protected against the unsuspected development of the disease. Furthermore, because of the dreadful threat of congenital syphilis in newborn babies, most advanced nations and most of the states in the United States require that blood tests be given the prospective husband and wife before a marriage license is issued, and as an added precaution an STS is routinely performed on expectant mothers at the time they first come to a doctor's office or clinic for care of a pregnancy.

Finally, both before effective means of treatment were discovered and today as well, spread of the infection is combated by the diligent and relentless efforts of the venereal control division of the U.S. Public Health Service, working in cooperation with local health departments and other social agencies. Not only do these agencies provide free treatment for the disease, but each time a new case of syphilis is discovered, a skillful team of investigators swings into action. The infected person is encouraged to reveal the possible contacts from whom he might have acquired the disease as well as any later contacts to whom he might have spread it. Then each contact is painstakingly tracked down and examined in order to break, if possible, an insidious chain of infection. There is no social stigma or embarrassment connected with the investigation. It is done with extreme diplomacy, and care is taken to conceal the names and protect the privacy of every individual involved. In fact, the only shame and guilt connected with the disease lie in *not* reporting it, both to public health officials who are well equipped to handle it and to any known contacts who may have been infected and require immediate treatment. Because doctors are required by law to report cases of venereal disease to the public health authorities, even patients consulting their private doctors may have to undergo questioning. This should not be regarded as a threat, but rather as a responsibility. Syphilis is a terribly dangerous and often tragic disease which can, and does, literally ruin lives. It is only by cooperation of victim, private doctor and public health authorities that this scourge can ever be checked.

Of course, such cooperative efforts would be of only limited value if there were no effective means of treating syphilis. Over the centuries, many treatment methods were tried. Most failed, but certain chemicals and drugs were found to have at least some effect in slowing the progress of the infection. Mercury preparations, for example, were widely used and helped retard the infection, but such treatment was limited by the toxicity of the medicine itself. In the Renaissance decoctions of guiac wood also seemed to be effective. But it was not until the early 1900s that Paul Ehrlich, a German physician and bacteriologist, discovered his "Magic Bullet"—the first time a specific chemical substance was found that could cure a specific infection without having intolerable deleterious effects on the body at the same time. Convinced that preparations of arsenic and bismuth might be used to attack the syphilis organism alone, Ehrlich tried literally hundreds of combinations of these chemicals in organic forms on infected rabbits before he found one called Salversan 606, which had the effect he was seeking. For the first time physicians had a relatively safe and nontoxic drug that could be used not merely to curb but to cure syphilis, and Ehrlich in his work gave birth and substance to the electrifying concept of specific chemotherapy for the treatment of infection.

Unfortunately, treatment with these new arsenic and bismuth compounds often took months or even years, and although they were effective in many cases, there were also disappointing and inexplicable failures. Then in the early 1940s the newly discovered penicillin, first of the true antibiotic drugs to be used against infection, was found to be deadly to the syphilis organism. At last there was a simple, safe and effective means of eradicating this age-old killer. Early penicillin treatment required low-dosage injections every four hours around the clock for several days to be effective, but today penicillin given in doses of one million units or more in a single shot will often destroy an infection completely. Particularly when treatment is started early in the infection, penicillin is truly a "wonder drug" against syphilis; not only are detected cases effectively treated, but with the widespread use of penicillin for other kinds of infections following World War II, hundreds of thousands of undiscovered cases of syphilis were undoubtedly treated and cured along with coughs, colds and tonsillitis without the victim's ever knowing he had the infection. The growing incidence of new cases of syphilis dropped precipitously, and medical authorities were optimistic that the disease was on its way out as a serious threat to society.

Today we know that this optimism was premature. Although the *Treponema pallidum* does not seem to form penicillin-resistant strains as readily as other bacteria—notably the staphylococci—do, recent cases of syphilis have been found to be considerably more refractory to penicillin treatment than when the drug was first used. Widespread "shotgun" use of penicillin for multiple minor ailments has also come to an end, as more and more people have developed sensitivity to the drug and as better and more convenient antibiotic preparations have been discovered. Also, inevitably, physicians became lax in reporting syphilis to public health authorities, and the search for contacts became less diligent. Even many of its victims came to feel that the disease was not much worse than a head cold. Finally, the relaxation of many traditional restraints on sexual activities—or the rebellion of youth against those restraints as "old-fashioned" and "square"—has exposed a whole new generation to the recurring specter of syphilitic infection. With little or no knowledge or training about the nature of the disease, and without the mature common sense to recognize the dangers of exposure or to take the simple prophylactic measures that could help prevent infection, many young people simply ignore syphilis, to their later regret. Perhaps even worse, the social and moral stigma too long connected with the disease, and aggravated today by the generation gap, still encourages concealment. The result is that syphilis, one of the ugliest of the ancient plagues, is sharply on the increase among both young and old in our society.

The first step in avoiding infection is simply to avoid sexual contact with anyone known to be promiscuous. It is well to recognize, however, that *any* sexual partner may be infected; syphilis is no respecter of social classes, and the infection can be acquired from any kind of sexual contact, even oral or anal contact, with an infected person. The second step is to take the simple prophylactic measures that can help prevent infection after intercourse. The use of a condom or "safety" during intercourse is no insurance against infectious contact for either partner. In the male the best possible prophylaxis is a thorough washing of the penis, scrotum and surrounding skin areas with warm water and soap as soon after intercourse as possible—preferably within five to ten minutes. In the female, careful and complete washing of the external genitalia with soap and water should be supplemented by use of a thorough douche with warm soapy water, again as soon as possible after intercourse. Thereafter a careful inspection of the external genitalia should be made daily for a week to ten days to detect the development of any suspicious pimple or open sore, whether it is painful or not. Any such lesion should be called immediately to the attention of a private doctor or public health personnel, and even if no such physical change appears, a blood test should be taken approximately two months after exposure as an additional precaution. It is also essential, both for the victim of the disease and for anyone who may have unknowingly come in contact with it, to cooperate fully with a public health investigation. Guilty secrets and mistaken loyalties have no place in dealing with this disease. Any friends who may have been exposed *must* be informed about it, either by the contact or through public health channels, so they may be given tests and treatment if necessary. In its

primary stage syphilis is easy to combat and cure. It is only when fear or ignorance allow it to progress to its secondary and tertiary stages that the disease becomes a serious threat. In these later stages, it is more difficult to treat—repeated courses of medication may be necessary—and the damage it has already caused can never be repaired. In addition, no reliable immunity is developed as a result of infection; the disease can be contracted again and again, even though it can be successfully treated each time.

By its very nature, syphilis may never be eradicated from our society. But aided by the common sense, knowledge and prompt action of its victims and potential victims, modern medicine may again be able to bring this ancient plague under tight control.

Gonorrhea

Although syphilis is the oldest known and by far the most dangerous of the venereal infections, gonorrhea is certainly the most common, occurring in a ratio varying from 100 to 200 cases of gonorrhea to each case of syphilis in heavily populated areas. Really accurate information about the incidence of this infection is very hard to obtain, since reporting of the disease is poor and since so many people with characteristic symptoms obtain penicillin or other antibiotics for self-treatment. Gonococci, red-staining, coffee-bean-shaped bacteria which are usually found in pairs, cause the infection. Once one of the most sensitive of all organisms to penicillin, gonococci were easily destroyed by

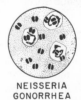

NEISSERIA
GONORRHEA

Figure 22–2.

relatively low doses of penicillin shortly after its discovery and widespread use in the early 1940s. For some five years thereafter, there was a very sharp decline in the total number of gonorrhea infections reported, and many optimists assumed that it was soon to become a vanishing disease. But within the last ten years, incidence of cases has once again been climbing sharply, partly owing to the ignorance or carelessness of its victims and their failure to obtain treatment under the false impression that the disease is not particularly dangerous anymore. Even worse, the disease is also on the rise because a growing number of strains of gonococci have become increasingly resistant to penicillin. The disease goes hand in hand with prostitution and promiscuity and is also widespread among poorly educated, low-income populations. As with syphilis, much of the recent increase in the incidence of gonorrhea has been among teen-agers, and since infection with the organism leads to no immunity, the same individual may have repeated attacks of the disease as a result of new exposures, even though each attack is properly treated. The public health problem is further aggravated by the nature of the infection itself. Whereas the symptoms are quite straightforward and recognizable in the male, gonorrhea is very often difficult to detect in women, particularly in its early stages, so that they can become essentially symptom-free carriers of the infection for prolonged periods of time.

The earliest symptoms of the infection, which may appear any time from two to seven days after sexual contact, are an itching or burning sensation in the urethra, particularly when urinating, accompanied by a whitish watery discharge, most commonly noted when first awakening in the morning. Within a day or so the discharge becomes frankly purulent. In either male or female these symptoms, if overlooked or ignored, will tend to recede after a few days, but the infecting organism itself may persist for weeks or months, continuing steady and progressive damage to tissues in the urogenital tract and elsewhere. In the male the infection may travel up the urethra to affect the prostate gland, or it may do so much damage to the urethra itself that healing and scarring cause a stricture or partial obstruction of the urinary outlet. In the female, local infection of the Bartholin glands at the entry to the vagina can lead to abscess formation; the bacteria can also remain in the vagina and gain entry to the uterus, passing upward and ultimately lodging in the Fallopian tubes extending from the ovaries to the uterus. Infection in this region, known as *gonorrheal salpingitis,* may lead to large collections of infected pus in the tubes and, ultimately, to total obstruction with resultant sterility which can only occasionally be corrected by later surgery. In other cases in the female, the disease may involve vagina, uterus, tubes and all in a painful type of widespread infection, accompanied by fever and chills, commonly known as *pelvic inflammatory disease* or PID, usually readily diagnosed, but sometimes mimicking the symptoms of an acute surgical disease in the abdomen such as appendicitis. In either male or female the bacteria also enter the blood stream and, as a late complication, can attack the glossy synovial membranes that line the joint capsules in the body, most particularly the knees, and cause *gonorrheal arthritis,* which can be permanently crippling. Finally, a baby born to a mother afflicted with gonorrhea may suffer a swift and frightful infection of the lining of the eyes, acquired at the time of childbirth, which can lead to permanent blindness in a matter of a few days. In modern delivery rooms silver nitrate or penicillin drops are routinely instilled in the eyes of newborn babies within minutes after birth to protect against the possibility of this disaster.

Both acute destruction and late complications resulting from gonorrhea can readily be prevented if the disease receives adequate treatment as soon as symptoms appear. Various means of prophylaxis against infection are the first step in prevention. Here, for example, use of a rubber or fiber condom may help protect either the male or the female from contact. As in the case of syphilis, thorough washing of the external genitalia with soap and warm water immediately after contact is an additional protection, and, in the female, so is a warm douche with soapy water. (*Never* use an irritative or corrosive chemical in a douche, since this may simply excoriate the vaginal mucous membrane and make invasion by the organisms of gonorrhea or syphilis all the easier.) At one time special "prophylactic kits" were recommended by medical authorities for use by people who had been exposed to gonorrhea. Most such kits, still available in drugstores, contain solutions of various bacteriocidal silver compounds which can be used externally, at least by males, or introduced into the outer end of the urethra by means of an eye dropper. This prophylactic technique tends to be more irritating than beneficial; in most cases it is better to rely on thorough external cleansing and then to seek immediate medical attention in the event that a discharge appears.

Obviously the best prophylaxis of all is to avoid sexual contact with any individual who might be carrying the infection. Amateur or professional prostitutes are so commonly and repeatedly infected that any contact should always be assumed to have been infectious. Teenagers should be equipped with full knowledge of the nature of gonorrhea as soon as they begin dating and should fully realize that the disease can be transmitted just as readily by "heavy petting" with superficial or incomplete sexual contact as by completion of the sex act. It can also be passed from one person to another by means of oral-genital or anal intercourse, both heterosexual and homosexual. Contrary to popular myth, the gonorrheal organism is so extremely delicate and so easily destroyed by cooling or drying that blame cannot possibly be cast upon contact with contaminated toilet seats or the like; for all practical purposes the infection is contracted *only* by intimate physical contact.

Fortunately early gonorrhea is often still quite effectively treated by large doses of injectable penicillin, even though more and more strains of the organism are becoming increasingly resistant to this drug. Recent rumors of the appearance of "new" or "incurable" types of gonorrhea or syphilis among servicemen in Vietnam are unfortunate and dangerous exaggerations. What actually has happened is that many of the prostitutes in contact with military personnel in the Far East have taken small or sporadic doses of penicillin over prolonged periods in a misguided attempt to keep themselves free of transmittable infection, and have consequently become infected with virulent penicillin-resistant strains of both gonococci and *Treponema pallidum*. These organisms do, however, respond quite well to treatment with other antibiotics and are by no means "incurable." If an individual with the symptoms of gonorrhea does not respond to penicillin therapy, or is allergic to that drug, a variety of alternative antibiotics may be prescribed by a doctor. However, such treatment (or even penicillin treatment) must be carried on for a prolonged period in the case of advanced or complicated gonorrhea. Again, as in the case of syphilis, gonorrhea is a legally reportable disease and the best way to help prevent its continuing increase is by cooperating with public health officials in tracking down the sources of infection. Finally, most doctors treating gonorrhea will take blood tests for syphilis before treatment is begun and at monthly intervals for three to six months thereafter, since a syphilis infection contracted at the same time as gonorrhea may be masked by antibiotic therapy but not eradicated.

Chancroid and Other Venereal Infections

Although syphilis and gonorrhea are by far the most common venereal diseases, several other types of infection may also occur, or may complicate the "big two." *Chancroid* is a localized infection of the external genitalia caused by a bacillus. It begins, within three to five days of sexual contact, with the formation of a tender ulcer on the external genitalia. Unlike the primary lesion of syphilis, the ulcer of chancroid is usually painful and does not tend to heal spontaneously. Progressive ulceration may erode deeply into the tissues of the penis or labia, or may spread to involve various parts of the groin and thigh. Often a markedly swollen lymph gland or bubo appears in the groin. Chancroid is treatable with sulfonamides or tetracycline, but simultaneous infection with syphilis must be ruled out before treatment is commenced.

Lymphogranuloma venereum is caused by a very large virus, one of the few that can be observed with a light microscope, and is characterized primarily by the appearance of large swollen lymph glands in the groin or around the rectum which appear from ten to thirty days after exposure. These buboes may erode to the surface of the skin and drain, or the infection may be complicated by the formation of rectal abscesses. Syphilis should be ruled out before treatment with sulfonamides or broad-spectrum antibiotics is begun. Such treatment may have to be prolonged up to thirty days, but it is usually effective.

Granuloma inguinale is an indolent, chronic and progressive viral infection usually confined to the genitals, anus or surrounding areas, considered a venereal infection although it may be impossible to trace the precise infective contact because of the long period (eight to twelve weeks) usually required for the infection to begin. Early symptoms are the appearance of raised, beefy-red, usually painless ulcers on the external genitals which often bleed readily when traumatized—for example, during sexual intercourse. Since the early lesions are not painful, the victim rarely seeks medical care until the disease is well advanced, with the ulcerated area extending widely in the genital region. After other venereal diseases have been ruled out, treatment can be accomplished with broad-spectrum antibiotics.

Compared to syphilis and gonorrhea, these venereal infections are relatively uncommon in the United States, and no special prophylactic measures are helpful other than those already described. Thorough soap-and-water cleansing of the external genitalia after possible infectious contact is nothing more than obvious common sense. It is equally obvious common sense to call *any* unusual discharge, sore or other lesion of the genitals to the attention of a doctor without delay. Left untreated, all these infections are progressively damaging to the body and, in the case of syphilis, ultimately fatal. Yet all can effectively be cured. Procrastination in seeking medical aid when an infection is suspected is a tragic foolishness which can harm not only the infected individual but anyone with whom he or she may have sexual contact.

The Role of Education in VD Control

Most mature adults today have at least some rudimentary knowledge about the various venereal diseases, their cause and the availability of treatment. Judging from current statistics, many

of today's young people do not. All too often they are either totally ignorant of the danger or even the possibility of venereal infections, or else they are thoroughly confused by locker-room misinformation. This potentially tragic situation is bound to get worse instead of better unless both parents and school authorities can muster the courage and common sense to teach young people the truth about sex and the threat of venereal disease early enough for the information to do them some good.

Many parents object strongly to the institution of sex education programs in the schools, which would naturally include teaching the facts about venereal disease. Many contend that sex education is their responsibility and theirs alone. In some cases their opposition is based on moral grounds. They regard any sexual experimentation outside of marriage to be morally wrong and fear that "impersonal" classroom discussions of sex may be interpreted by young people as some sort of social sanction or licence for promiscuous sexual activity.

No one can argue that teaching moral values and personal standards of behavior is not a parental responsibility and prerogative. Yet when it comes to teaching the facts about sex and venereal disease, the sad truth is that far too many parents do *not* fulfill their responsibility, either because they themselves are misinformed or because they find it difficult or embarrassing to talk about such topics. Adolescents, too, seldom feel completely free to talk to their parents about sex until some unexpected event forces them to do it. Parents who assume that sexual knowledge is "instinctive" or that "setting a good example" is all there is to sex education are no less mistaken than the adolescent who thinks he knows it all or assumes that his parents could not possibly "understand." Parents in particular must come to realize that in matters of sex and venereal disease ignorance is never bliss.

Wise parents today, knowing that the upsurge of venereal disease in our society is a very real threat and that their children are vulnerable no matter how careful and proper their upbringing, recognize their responsibility to teach their children the facts about these diseases. Many have also recognized that their local schools can, and should, contribute to this aspect of their children's education by instituting sex education programs, ideally commencing in the early elementary grades before children reach puberty. With cooperation among parents, teachers and school boards to determine subject matter and teaching methods that will be acceptable to the majority of families in the community, these sex education programs have proved to be resoundingly successful. There is no reason for any parent to fear that such programs will pervert the minds or morals of their children. Excellent factual but tasteful teaching materials have been developed which satisfy the standards of the most critical and conservative of professional educators, and widespread experience has shown that the teachers charged with presenting even the most sensitive material have almost invariably approached their task with a high degree of respect and understanding and, above all, with the deepest sense of the responsibility that has been placed in their hands.

Parents and—most especially—their children have everything to gain and nothing to lose from these programs. This does not mean that parents can or should abdicate their own responsibility in the sex education of their children, but sex education in the schools, organized and presented with parental cooperation, can be a valuable adjunct and can help protect the children of this generation, and of generations to come, from needless tragedy.

Intestinal Infections and Parasites

Whenever something is wrong, our bodies almost always react with a variety of striking, sometimes even alarming, signs and symptoms. In the case of infectious diseases, fever is one of the earliest and most universal signs. Perhaps second most common is the appearance of some form of gastrointestinal (GI) upset: nausea, vomiting, abdominal cramps or diarrhea, sometimes all together. People often speak of these symptoms as "stomach flu," a sort of wastebasket term that is used, quite inaccurately, when virtually any illness stirs up some kind of abdominal discomfort. Such disturbances may occur even when the infection is far removed from the intestine itself; but in certain infections that have their origin there, these GI symptoms may be the most striking characteristic of the illness.

Gastrointestinal infections, often lumped together under the generic name *gastroenteritis,* occur in many forms, some relatively minor, some more severe, some even life-threatening. But all share certain features in common. All are caused by bacterial organisms or various other parasites which can flourish in the gastrointestinal tract, particularly in the small intestine or the colon. All are most often transmitted by fecal contamination of food, milk or water. And all are most common in areas where poor sanitation and poor hygienic practices prevail. This does not mean, however, that these infections are confined to underdeveloped foreign countries. The mild ones, like bacterial food poison-

ing and "traveler's dysentery," can happen to anyone; and even the dangerous ones, like typhoid fever, dysentery and cholera, can occur anywhere, often in epidemic form, any time a lapse in sanitary control occurs.

The Mild Intestinal Infections

Staphylococcal Food Poisoning. This benign but singularly nasty illness often turns up at the most inopportune times—following wedding receptions, for example, or large summer picnics or banquets—and may dramatically afflict large numbers of people all at the same time. Literally hundreds have been hit simultaneously with the short-lived but violent symptoms of this infection if they have eaten the same food, and in spite of our knowledge of how to avoid it, it still remains the most common of all easily identifiable gastrointestinal afflictions.

Strictly speaking, staph food poisoning is not just an "infection." The violent symptoms arise from ingestion of an *enterotoxin*—a poisonous substance exuded by certain kinds of staph bacteria growing in contaminated food. Milk, cream sauces, meat and fish are the most frequent offenders, after first being contaminated by staph organisms from the skin of food handlers and then allowed to sit without proper refrigeration for a period of time before serving. Chicken salad is a notorious source of this trouble; so also are cream-filled pastries and tuna fish salad.

The most striking feature of the illness is the

swift onset of symptoms some two to four hours after eating the infected food. Victims are suddenly doubled up with cramps, nausea, vomiting and diarrhea. Headache and fever may occur, and in some the symptoms are violent enough to cause prostration. Then, after about three to six hours, the attack clears up with complete recovery the rule. There is no effective treatment except in cases in which fluid loss from vomiting and diarrhea is extreme. Then the patient may require intravenous fluids.

Diagnosis is usually obvious: no other gastroenteritis strikes so fast or affects so many people from the same table. If you suffer an attack, you probably will not be alone, and staph organisms cultured from the offending food will remove all doubt. The best possible treatment is, of course, prevention. If you are preparing food ahead of time for any occasion, be sure all ingredients are absolutely fresh and then kept either piping hot or well refrigerated until served, especially in warm weather. Also be sure when preparing food that your hands, as well as all utensils and surfaces, are clean. Make sure, too, that all cream-filled pastries and prepared meat or fish salads bought in a store are absolutely fresh; it is a good idea to avoid such foods in restaurants and at large public dinners. In your own home, use up leftovers as quickly as possible, and keep them well refrigerated in the meantime. If there is even the slightest question in your mind that some food may have "gone bad," throw it out. Staph food poisoning is not a threat to life, but it is quite unpleasant enough to warrant taking no chances.

Paratyphoid (Salmonella) Infections. Almost as commonplace as staph food poisoning is the type of acute gastroenteritis popularly, if not quite accurately, called salmonella, or paratyphoid infection. It is also commonly but incorrectly called stomach flu. The terminology is admittedly confusing, for these infections are caused by intestinal bacteria closely related (but *not* identical) to the salmonella bacteria that cause typhoid fever. They are true intestinal infections arising from eating virtually any food contaminated by these fecal bacteria, usually by way of unsanitary food handling. The offending bacteria are usually from the *Salmonella* family,

but various other colon bacteria—sometimes even the supposedly "friendly" ones—may occasionally be at fault.

Symptoms are quite similar to those of staph food poisoning: abrupt onset of cramping, nausea, vomiting and diarrhea, often with chills and fever thrown in. Salmonella infections may also strike large numbers of people at once if they have inadvertently eaten the same contaminated food at a dinner or in a restaurant. Widespread outbreaks are not uncommon, and when reported are often a problem to the public health authorities who try to track them down. It can be all the more difficult because infected food is not invariably the source of trouble; one of the worst salmonella outbreaks in recent years, in Riverside, California, was traced to contaminated wells.

Unlike staph food poisoning, salmonella infections require from 6 to 48 hours to "hatch" before symptoms appear, and the misery of the illness may last two to three days or more. In most cases it then clears up spontaneously, but recovery can often be speeded by treatment with antibiotic drugs (especially neomycin or tetracycline) or with sulfonamides. Many commonly prescribed remedies also contain kaolin and pectin, which are added to help stem the diarrhea. In a severe case, a doctor may prescribe tincture of paregoric for the diarrhea, or one of the belladonna preparations to reduce the cramping.

The main danger of salmonella infection is dehydration from recurrent vomiting and diarrhea, and the upsetting of the biochemical balance of the body that may result. Thus extra fluids should be taken during recovery, together with a balanced diet of bland foods. In many victims the illness is so mild that regular activities may be continued; in others it may be extremely severe, prolonged and prostrating, and occasionally even fatal. In some cases the infecting bacteria may form abscesses in the appendix or gall bladder, or enter the blood stream to cause localized abscesses in the lung or even in the bone. Some people remain "carriers" for weeks or months after recovery from the active illness, adding to the difficulty of public health control.

Even though they are relatively mild, salmonella or paratyphoid infections constitute a growing public health hazard in countries such as our own, where the many public restaurants may have substandard sanitary facilities. Any suspected salmonella infection, however mild, should at least be reported to your doctor so that an attempt can be made to isolate the source. The increasing threat of these infections can be controlled only by awareness of the danger, and close cooperation among patients, doctors and public health authorities.

"Traveler's Dysentery." From the number of derogatory nicknames for this common bane of tourists and travelers—the "Mexican two-step," "Montezuma's revenge," "La Turista"—one might imagine that it is an affliction specially reserved for visitors to Mexico. That is, of course, grossly unfair. Since time immemorial travelers in *all* parts of the world have periodically been attacked and their holidays interrupted by the sudden onset of abdominal cramps and frequent, urgent watery stools. For that reason, the infection is generally, and more appropriately called "tourist diarrhea" or "traveler's dysentery."

Oddly enough, given its universal frequency, no one knows a great deal about this annoying illness, nor is any single treatment reliably effective. Tourists who travel through foreign countries subsisting solely on canned foods and bottled water can still come down with the disease. Others can travel the length and breadth of the world, eating native fare and drinking local water, yet never suffer for a moment. But beyond doubt, many cases of "traveler's dysentery" are in fact salmonella infections or the more severe bacillary dysentery that arises from ingesting contaminated food or water. Other cases have been blamed on various strains of colon bacteria which are perfectly harmless to the people who are in constant contact with them but can be infectious to a tourist. Many cases result, however, not from infection so much as from chemical irritation of the bowel caused by plain overindulgence in unfamiliar foods and alcohol. And that can happen anywhere in the world, even in your own hometown.

"Traveler's dysentery" is seldom severe or dangerous. If it strikes, the best cure is to slow down, rest and let it pass without excessive concern. If it does cause prolonged and miserable discomfort, treatment with sulfa drugs or antibiotics supplemented by kaolin and pectin preparations will often afford speedy relief. However, treatment may fail to help; the symptoms may persist for days before subsiding and may even recur. But this happens only in rare cases. Most experienced travelers in any part of the world expect to come down with at least a mild case from time to time on their journeys and they do not worry about it. For that reason, inexperienced travelers should not let the prospect of a mild case frighten them off, even if they want to visit strange and exotic places. Nor should they allow worry about it to hang like a cloud over their whole trip, and render themselves and their companions foolish and uncomfortable by taking unnecessary precautions.

Naturally, the best preventive measures are caution and common sense, but the degree of caution necessary depends on where you are. Travelers to Canada, Hawaii, Europe, Japan, Australia or other areas with modern sanitary facilities need not be seriously concerned about getting into trouble; to avoid buying an Italian ice in Rome or an orange from a peddler in Valencia for fear of dreadful gastrointestinal reprisals would be a pity. Elsewhere in the world the food and water served at most of the major hotels and restaurants frequented by tourists are usually perfectly safe. In less-traveled small towns and out-of-the-way places, where sanitary standards may not be quite so high, the tourist is well advised to avoid local water, even for brushing teeth, in favor of bottled water or boiled drinks, and to sample unfamiliar and highly spiced local dishes with care. Milk and other native dairy products should also be avoided in such areas, and uncooked fruit and vegetables should be both washed and peeled. Finally, the tourist who plans to travel in Central or South America, Africa, the Middle East, India, Southeast Asia or the Orient should be sure that his typhoid and paratyphoid immunizations are up to date, and check with an office of the U.S. Public Health Service before any given trip to see what other immunizations (against cholera, plague or yellow fever, for example) may be recommended or required. Those who travel anywhere *frequently* would be wise at least to keep typhoid and paratyphoid immunizations current, even when there seems to be little threat. These shots are harmless, inexpensive and readily available in any medical or Public Health Service office; and they offer a measure of protection that may be as useful in New York as in Bangkok.

Nonspecific Gastroenteritis. The mild intestinal afflictions described so far are clearly recognizable clinical illnesses, arising from identifiable causes, with predictably benign courses. But in addition, there are multitudes of vague minor GI infections that can never be clearly identified. Some are mild bacterial infections, while many may be caused by intestinal viruses, including even the polio viruses. They are collectively called nonspecific gastroenteritis, and for the most part, symptoms are minor: a little nausea, perhaps one or two episodes of vomiting, abdominal cramps and transitory mild diarrhea. These infections are rarely disabling and rarely require a doctor's attention. Symptomatic home treatment (as outlined below) will afford some relief, and you need worry only if the illness persists more than a day or so, or recurs. Of course, *any intestinal distress that persists or recurs should be reported to your doctor,* just as a matter of common sense. So should any symptoms that seem to become progressively worse in the course of a few hours. It is pointless to get excited about a mild episode of GI distress, but it is downright dangerous to ignore a progressive pattern of symptoms that might prove to be acute appendicitis, a severe dysentery or a gall bladder attack.

Treatment of GI Symptoms. Whether caused by a mild infection or something more serious, the symptoms of gastrointestinal illness can make you miserable, and a few simple remedies will often help without aggravating a more serious disorder if it exists. Small doses of Dramamine (dimenhydrinate), now available without prescription, can relieve nausea and vomiting, and antacid tablets may also be helpful. Simple aspirin helps with cramping, and a kaolin-pectin

suspension, taken according to dosage directions on the bottle, will help firm up loose stools. *Never* take a laxative, not even milk of magnesia, in the face of these symptoms except on doctor's orders.

Prescription drugs can offer more specific relief, if your doctor considers them necessary. Paregoric (technically, camphorated tincture of opium), in combination with a bismuth suspension, sharply reduces intestinal motility and can provide effective relief from diarrhea. A variety of so-called tranquilizing drugs also relieve nausea, while drugs of the belladonna family, as well as various new synthetic drugs such as Lomotil, can relieve painful abdominal cramping. Any of these medicines, however, can get you in trouble if you assume that a double dose will be twice as helpful as a single dose. Follow your doctor's instructions to the letter and *never* increase the dosage of prescription drugs without his permission.

The Dangerous Intestinal Infections

Typhoid Fever. Until quite recently, this severe and treacherous intestinal infection occurred not only in individual cases but in periodic plaguelike epidemics in almost every corner of the world, including the United States. And while it is caused by bacteria of the *Salmonella* family similar to those causing the milder "paratyphoid" infections, typhoid is far more dangerous, not only because of the intestinal infection, but because of the severe systemic illness that accompanies it.

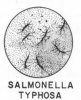

SALMONELLA
TYPHOSA

Figure 23–1.

Typhoid fever is an acute generalized infection which may affect all parts of the body. The offending organism, usually spread by fecal contamination of food and water supplies, first invades the gastrointestinal tract, but then makes its way to the blood stream through the lymph channels and can lead to involvement of the throat, the respiratory tract, the kidneys or the nervous system. Unlike milder salmonella infections, typhoid is a prolonged illness which starts with gradual onset of fever, chills, malaise and headache. In one victim out of five, abdominal cramps and diarrhea may appear early in the disease, but more often there are no specific GI symptoms at first, so the diagnosis may be missed for several days.

Typical of typhoid, however, is a continuing, spiking fever that increases in stepwise fashion for the first seven to ten days as the illness grows steadily worse. The victim's appetite disappears, and he feels progressively more debilitated. After the eighth day or so, the high fever levels off and remains at its peak for another week or more; febrile delirium or even a stuporous state may appear during this stage. In many cases a characteristic pink "rose spot" rash appears on the abdomen and chest at this time, persisting for two or three days before it begins to fade.

Subsequently cramping and diarrhea appear, sometimes minimal, sometimes severe. The bacteria cause inflammation and ulceration of the lower end of the small intestine, which in untreated cases often leads to such dangerous complications as intestinal hemorrhage or intestinal perforation. Before antibiotics, such complications occurred in some 25 percent of all typhoid victims, with an overall death rate ranging from 6 to 15 percent during epidemics. In those who did not die, the fever would fall quite suddenly about the beginning of the fourth week of illness and a prolonged convalescence would begin. Among those who seemed completely recovered, about one out of twenty would become chronic carriers of the deadly bacteria, unknowingly contaminating food or water everywhere they went.

In the early days no one understood how typhoid was spread. Epidemics would sweep whole countrysides, armies in the field and huge segments of urban populations, particularly in slum areas. Once the offending organism was discovered, and once the threat of healthy carriers was recognized, control of the disease be-

came possible by improving methods of sewage disposal, purification of drinking water, and teaching such hygienic measures as washing the hands before handling food and after using the toilet. By the early 1900s such control measures in the United States had so greatly reduced the incidence of typhoid that it was confined to sporadic outbreaks in communities where lapses in sanitary precautions had occurred. The carrier's role in spreading typhoid received wide publicity in the famous case of Mary Mallon ("Typhoid Mary"), an Irish-American housemaid who carried the infection into many homes in the late 1800s. A careful study of her case made it clear for the first time that typhoid could be harbored and spread by apparently healthy people.

Typhoid is uncommon in America today, occurring only sporadically in single cases or in small groups. Diagnosis is confirmed by culturing the typhoid bacteria from the victim's stool or blood stream. Most cases are traceable to food contaminated by typhoid carriers or are contracted abroad by unimmunized travelers. When the disease occurs, active treatment with antibiotics—particularly chloramphenicol—reduces the fever and toxicity within four to five days and prevents most of the serious or fatal complications, although a long convalescence is still the rule. Unfortunately, the indiscriminate short-term use of antibiotics for "shotgun therapy" against all kinds of intestinal infections before diagnosis is made has undoubtedly "masked" many unrecognized cases of typhoid and helped to perpetuate the carrier state in many who have no idea they have ever had the disease. Thus the threat of recurrent outbreaks remains—partly as a result of misuse of modern treatment methods.

The best protection today is immunization with modern vaccines that guard against attacks of both typhoid and paratyphoid organisms. Anyone who has been exposed to typhoid, or who works in medicine or in contact with sick people, should have full vaccination—usually a series of three typhoid- paratyphoid shots given at intervals of one week. None of the available vaccines affords complete protection, but a full immunization will usually be effective for a year or more, and at least will markedly reduce the severity of the infection if it is contracted.

Cholera: Plague of the Orient. If typhoid is an indolent, slow-developing intestinal infection, Asiatic or epidemic cholera is a veritable bombshell—one of the most acute and violent infections known to man. Even today cholera is a devastating disease, sweeping whole subcontinents in India, Pakistan and Southeast Asia in huge epidemics. Untreated, it has a staggering 50 percent death rate. Yet the infecting organism, a strange comma-shaped bacillus known as a *vibrio,* is thrown off by the body in a matter of two weeks or so if the victim can somehow survive the massive dehydration and depletion of body salts that occur in the first few days of the disease.

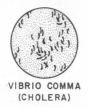

VIBRIO COMMA
(CHOLERA)

Figure 23–2.

Like most other intestinal infections, cholera is spread by fecal contamination of water and food. After two or three days of incubation, the disease strikes abruptly with fever, abdominal cramps, nausea, vomiting and finally an almost unbelievable, fulminating diarrhea which may result in the loss of as much as 15 or 20 *quarts* of body water in a single day. The diarrhea is caused by a poison, produced by the cholera vibrio, which alters the intestine's normal ability to reabsorb water; in fact, it reverses the process, so that water is actively drawn into the intestine from the rest of the body. So much water is lost so swiftly in this way that severe dehydration occurs in a matter of hours. The victim becomes intensely thirsty, then prostrated. Without treatment he may die from circulatory collapse when there is insufficient fluid left in his blood to permit circulation.

Treatment of cholera is aimed more at vigorously replacing lost fluids and electrolytes than at destroying the bacteria, which are conquered

by the body anyway in a matter of a few days. Under such treatment, full recovery is the rule. Because the infection burns itself out so fast, antibiotic therapy is of limited value. Antibiotics may better be used prophylactically by travelers coming out of endemic cholera areas.

Infection with cholera confers only a short-lived immunity (up to one year), so the disease can be contracted repeatedly. Control depends upon widespread public health measures to purify water and safely dispose of sewage, combined with effective quarantine at points of entry to a country. Vaccination is possible, involving two shots of cholera vaccine given a month apart, and will protect against the disease for a short while. But boosters are required at intervals of six months to maintain lasting immunity, and really effective mass immunization in endemic areas is virtually impossible. The use of boiled water and careful attention to hygiene and sanitation offer the best promise for control in areas where the disease is common. Cholera is now rare in the United States and western Europe, but it remains a very real threat any time war or natural disasters upset normal sanitary facilities, as was the case when a violent typhoon and flood ravaged the coastal areas of East Pakistan in 1970. Waves of both cholera and typhoid followed that disaster, and it was only prompt and heroic medical teamwork that prevented these diseases from taking even more lives than they did.

Bacillary Dysentery (Shigellosis). Similar in some ways to the milder salmonella infections, yet quite different in its clinical course and its threat to life, this dysentery caused by bacteria of the *Shigella* family is a constant health hazard in any overcrowded area where sanitation facilities are inadequate, particularly big-city slums and areas with open sewage systems or public outhouses. Extremely dangerous and often fatal, the disease is spread by fecal contamination of water, food, clothing or household objects by infected individuals. Common house flies are also active agents in its spread.

Bacillary dysentery strikes quite abruptly, first with fever, loss of appetite, and vomiting, then with severe abdominal cramps and the onset of massive diarrhea; stools may be as frequent as

20 times a day or more. The bacteria attack and ulcerate the inner lining of the large intestine or colon, so that stools soon begin to contain blood, pus and mucus. With so much diarrhea, dehydration is a threat, especially among young children, in whom it may become severe before it is even recognized. Most deaths occur among young victims who cannot tolerate the loss of water and other body chemicals as well as adults can.

Before antibiotics were available, bacillary dysentery killed as much as 25 percent of infected infants and some 5 percent of older children who contracted it. Among untreated survivors the illness may last from four to five days to as long as six weeks. Then it gradually subsides without any residual problems, except that relapses may occur. The infection does not confer immunity, so recurrent infections are also possible. No protective immunization is available, but after repeated attacks, adults seem to develop a certain natural resistance to the bacteria, and reinfections become less severe.

The *Shigella* bacteria have proved to be highly sensitive to sulfa drugs, as well as to broad-spectrum antibiotics such as tetracycline. Modern treatment often combines sulfas and antibiotics to reduce the length and severity of the attack quite significantly. In addition, the victim requires adequate replacement of lost fluids and sufficient bland food to maintain his strength until recovery is complete. Infected children are still best treated in the hospital to combat the threat of dehydration and to supervise replacement of lost body salts and minerals.

Control of the disease obviously depends upon good public sanitation and personal hygiene. Exclusion of flies from toilets, latrines and outhouses and protection of food from contamination are major steps toward control. Washing hands before eating or handling food also helps break the chain of contamination and new infection. But in spite of modern public health programs, bacillary dysentery is still commonplace in our country in crowded slum areas, especially among infants and children during the hot summer months. During wartime it is an even greater threat among military personnel in the field. It was this kind of dysentery that took so many American lives in filthy prison camps during World War II and—especially—the Korean War. Even in peacetime the disease remains a constant hazard in underdeveloped countries and in overcrowded poverty areas throughout the world.

Amebiasis: The Pandemic Dysentery. Of all the really dangerous intestinal infections, amebiasis or amebic dysentery is by far the most common in the United States, where as much as 35 to 40 percent of the population in some southern communities is either actively infected or has been at some time. In tropical countries infection rates are even higher, and 55 to 60 percent of the population in some areas may be symptom-free carriers of the offending organism.

Amebic dysentery is caused not by bacteria but by a rather large one-celled organism named *Endamoeba histolytica*—a cousin to the familiar ameba often studied in high-school biology classes. Infection is almost always acquired from food or water contaminated by sewage containing the ameba, either in active form or in a quiescent "encysted" state. Transmission by healthy carriers is by far the most common, but epidemics of the disease have swept through whole communities as a result of a breakdown in the plumbing of a single hotel or factory.

The disease itself is tricky, appearing as a mild, benign, intermittent diarrhea, yet it is actually the most insidiously destructive of all the intestinal infections. Once taken in, the ameba may live quietly in the intestine for weeks or months, or it may begin dividing and multiplying rapidly. Symptoms are often very vague—occasional mild diarrhea, occasional bouts of constipation, recurring unexplained fevers, chronic fatigue and intermittent episodes of abdominal pain. Once entrenched in the intestine, the ameba penetrates the mucous membrane and forms small abscesses, causing mucus and pus to begin to appear in the stool. As the organism propagates, many such lesions are formed, but the victim may ultimately consult a doctor more on account of chronic fatigue and weight loss than because of gastrointestinal symptoms. Diagnosis is often exceedingly difficult, since repeated stool examinations do not always reveal the ameba, and the disease is frequently misdiagnosed as anything from thyroiditis to malingering. Once identified, however, it must be treated by prolonged courses of various noxious drugs, some of which have quite toxic side-effects and can be thoroughly unpleasant.

Unpleasant or not, treatment is essential, for amebiasis is a deadly threat to life if it is not eradicated. The danger is not from the dysentery, but from the fact that the ameba can find its way through the intestinal wall into the blood stream and may set up housekeeping and form huge abscesses in other parts of the body, especially in the liver. Amebic abscesses of the liver have been known to grow as large as baseballs, destroying vital liver tissue and even eroding through the diaphragm to involve the lung, or the outer or pericardial lining of the heart. Nor is the liver the only target; amebic abscesses have occasionally been found in virtually every organ in the body, from the kidneys to the brain. During treatment, certain drugs are most effective against the ameba in the liver and other organs, while different medicines hit the organism best in the colon. It is very difficult, however, to be completely certain that the infection has been eradicated. Repeated stool examinations over a period of years may be necessary, together with observation for any sign of recurring symptoms.

No immunization is possible against amebiasis. The only way the disease can be controlled and eradicated is through personal cleanliness and hygiene, sanitary sewage disposal, discouraging the use of raw human sewage for fertilization of soil (a common practice in many areas of the world), and the institution of other well-established sanitary practices. Of all the intestinal infections, amebiasis will probably be the last to be completely controlled; but each family's attention to personal hygiene will go a long way to help. In addition, both patients and doctors should be highly suspicious of any vague illness characterized by unexplained fatigue, low-grade fevers and mild, recurrent diarrhea.

Botulism. Technically, this dangerous disease is not an infection at all, but rather a poisoning which arises from ingestion of food containing a toxin produced by a bacillus known as *Clostridium botulinum,* close cousin to the organisms that cause tetanus (lockjaw) and gas gangrene. The disease almost invariably results from eating improperly preserved food, especially home-canned products, which have not been adequately heated before serving. Home-canned vegetables, mushrooms, olives or seafoods are frequent offenders. The affliction is quite common throughout the United States in spite of well-publicized warnings, and the death rate among victims is appalling, averaging as high as 65 percent.

One reason for such a death toll is the difficulty in diagnosing the disease early. Although vomiting and diarrhea are sometimes present, in most cases there is no clear connection between onset of symptoms and the eating of spoiled food. The poison attacks the nervous system, not the gastrointestinal tract, and symptoms typically begin, some 18 to 36 hours after the food is eaten, with visual disturbances, double vision, difficulty in swallowing and sudden weakness in the muscles of the extremities and trunk. Thus even expert diagnosticians can confuse botulism with bulbar poliomyelitis, viral encephalitis or a variety of possible drug poisonings unless the vital clue of an offending food product is brought to light.

Death from the disease may occur at any time in the first ten days from respiratory paralysis or from aspiration of vomitus and resulting pneumonia. Antitoxin can be administered to neutralize any of the poison not yet "fixed" in the nervous system, but often the damage is already done by the time of diagnosis. Successful treatment depends upon expert nursing care in a hospital, with intravenous feedings, suctioning of saliva and other secretions the victim cannot swallow, even mechanical breathing support if respiratory failure threatens. The effects of the poison on the nervous system wear off after the first ten days of illness and leave no permanent paralysis, although a recovered victim may have residual weakness of the eye muscles for several months before recovery is complete.

Obviously, the best approach to this frightful disease lies in prevention. Take extreme care that proper techniques are used in home canning, and swiftly discard any foods, home-canned or otherwise, that show evidence of spoilage. Occasionally cans of commercially prepared foods show a telltale bulging at the ends of the can. Report any such discovery to both your grocer and your doctor and *don't* use the contents of the can. In addition, it is wise to discard home-canned foods prepared by someone else if you are not sure they are perfectly safe. Botulism is far too dangerous and too tricky to take any chances.

Malaria and Other Parasitic Infections

Most of the infectious diseases are caused by small and primitive bacterial or viral parasites that invade the body. There are others, however, caused by larger and more complex parasitic organisms. The ameba responsible for amebic dysentery is one, but there are several more, ranging from single-celled protozoa all the way to multicelled and highly specialized creatures. Not all of the tiny bacterial parasites that live on or in the human body are pathogenic; a few of them, in fact, even do some good. But very little can be said in favor of the larger parasites, for among them are the organisms that cause malaria and the nasty worm and insect infestations that are still common in this country in spite of modern methods of prevention, treatment and control.

Malaria

Malaria must certainly be ranked along with smallpox, typhoid fever, cholera and yellow fever as one of the most ancient and deadly of the human plagues. This debilitating and often fatal disease was accurately described by the great Roman physician Celsus during the reign of Tiberius Caesar in the first century A.D., but it quite possibly had played a tragic role in human history for thousands of years before that date. It is a strange disease in that it is caused by an invasion of the blood stream by a protozoan organism—a one-celled animal—which in order to grow and multiply must spend part of its life cycle within the body of a certain species of

tropical or subtropical mosquito. Thus in any warm climate where both man and the anopheles mosquito live, malaria is usually found, and although today we have the knowledge and drugs with which to wipe the disease off the face of the Earth within 14 days flat, it still remains just as much a threat in many parts of the world as it was centuries ago.

Why this paradox? The reason is simply that the major areas of the world where malaria occurs—India, Southeast Asia, China, Indonesia and parts of central and equatorial South America—are heavily populated and underdeveloped, and it has thus far been impossible to organize and carry out the intensive medical campaign necessary to destroy the disease. Interestingly enough, there is a zone in the central and south Pacific, including the Marshall Islands, the Carolines, Fiji, New Caledonia, New Zealand and Guam, that is free of anopheles mosquitoes and hence malaria-free. In other areas where massive mosquito control measures combined with widespread availability of drug therapy have been effectively utilized, the disease has been virtually eradicated. For example, 25 years ago malaria was prevalent in the subtropical parts of the United States; today it is rare, and has also been eradicated in such places as Puerto Rico, Taiwan, parts of Venezuela and other areas. Even so, travelers and servicemen returning from malarious areas of the world continue to bring the disease back home, so that malaria control requires constant vigilance.

We tend to think of malaria as a single disease, but actually there are four or more types of malarial parasites, each with a somewhat different biologic pattern and thus causing a different form of the disease. In all cases, however, the disease begins when an anopheles mosquito carrying undeveloped parasites in its salivary glands bites a human victim, releasing them into the human blood stream. The immature parasites, called sporozoites, then migrate through the blood stream to the liver, where they may remain from a week to up to five years or more in a sort of hibernation, the length of time depending to some degree on the particular species of parasite. After hibernation, however, the mature parasites, known now as plasmodia, reenter the blood stream in force and take up residence within human red blood cells. The disease can also be spread, of course, by transfusions of blood containing the parasite or by reuse of unsterilized syringes used by individuals infected by the parasite.

In the red blood cells the plasmodia begin reproducing by cell division, rupturing the cells and releasing the newly formed parasites to enter other cells. It is in this stage of the infection that the characteristic symptoms of intermittent high spiking fevers and chills occur, often the first hint that the individual has been infected. All but one of the varieties of malarial parasite send successive waves of the organism out of hibernation to invade red cells in a cyclical pattern, and thus the fever and chills of the acute disease seem to follow cycles that can vary from every 48 hours to every three or four days depending on the species of parasite. But to complete the life cycle, certain of the parasites in the red cells reproduce not by ordinary cell division or mitosis, but by meiosis, forming special cells called gametocytes or "seeds" which circulate in the blood serum until the individual is again bitten by an anopheles mosquito. The blood containing the gametocytes sucked in by the mosquito then goes to the mosquito's stomach, where the "seeds" are transformed into the sporozoite or "larval" stage of the parasite, and migrate to the mosquito's salivary glands, thus completing a perfect life cycle and preparing the mosquito to infect the next human being he bites.

The characteristic acute symptoms of malaria are the sudden and unheralded appearance of a high fever, usually accompanied by severe chills and sweating, which last only a few hours and then subside so that the victim may feel entirely well again until the next wave of fever and chills. During these paroxysms the temperature may rise as high as 104° or 105°, sometimes accompanied by delirium. Incredibly, there was a time in the late 1800s and early 1900s when individuals were deliberately infected with malaria as a cure for syphilis, since the delicate syphilis organism could not survive the repeated high fevers brought on by the malaria. The trouble with this approach, of course, was that while malaria was doubtless a more socially acceptable disease than syphilis, people could still die from it, and in most cases the "cure" was at least as bad as the condition it was "curing."

Untreated, the course of malaria can vary widely. It is not necessarily fatal, nor usually swiftly so, but the chills and fever may continue intermittently for months. Even when acute symptoms subside, the body remains infected with the parasites, the disease may recur at any time, and the victim is still capable of transmitting the infection. Traditionally, quinine, a chemical originally extracted from the bark of the cinchona tree, was used to reduce the fever and treat the infection. It certainly had the effect of slowing down the growth and development of the parasites in the blood stream, but it was not curative. Often after the discontinuance of quinine as a suppressive therapy, the malaria would recur as many as ten or twelve times in a row, or victims seemed to develop a partial immunity so that the disease would be held in check, so to speak, for months or even years between recurrences. But once infected, the body was unable to destroy the disease completely without treatment. The parasite continued to live either in the blood stream or in various tissues, particularly the liver and spleen. Gradually both spleen and liver would become enlarged, packed full of parasites, malarial pigments and destroyed red cells. Victims of chronic malaria would often show jaundice, a yellowish coloring of the skin and whites of the eyes, in this case caused by the pigments from destroyed red blood cells. In victims who died from certain kinds of malaria, the brain was found on autopsy to be a slate gray in color, with many tiny hemorrhages scattered throughout and the capillary blood vessels packed tight with parasite-infested red blood cells. In some chronic cases "black water fever" would occur, in which hemoglobin from the red cells was passed out in the urine in such quantities that it turned a dark brown or blackish color.

Although the symptoms of malaria are highly characteristic, and the victim usually has a history of travel or residence in a tropical or subtropical malarial zone at some time in his life, there are other infections which display similar symptoms, and therefore absolute diagnosis of the disease depends on actually observing under a microscope the parasites in a blood sample taken from the victim. Quinine is no longer in wide usage as a form of treatment, but a variety of drugs have been discovered which can be used either to treat an acute attack or to prevent it from occurring. American troops sent to the South Pacific during World War II were given regular daily doses of quinacrine hydrochloride, more familiarly known as Atabrine, which successfully protected them against malaria but unfortunately stained the skin and whites of the eyes an unpleasant yellow color and often caused chronic nausea, vomiting and diarrhea at the dosages necessary to suppress the infection. Today less toxic drugs are available which can be taken only once a week by individuals going into a malarial region; and in case of an acute attack, combinations of drugs can be used to destroy both the mature parasite in the blood stream and its gametocyte or "seed" forms. A course of treatment extending for fourteen days will not only cure most malarial infections but will also destroy the form of the parasite taken in again by the biting mosquito, thus breaking the life cycle completely. Widespread treatment of the active disease in this fashion, combined with drainage of swampy areas, spraying of jungles and other extensive mosquito control measures, if accomplished all over the world at once, could conceivably eradicate the disease competely.

Is this kind of world control likely to happen in the foreseeable future? Probably not. Too many mosquito breeding grounds are inaccessible, and adequate medical facilities have not yet been made available to the many populous areas of the world where the disease is still prevalent. Such a program would require the utmost in peaceful cooperation between nations, which is, unfortunately, seldom possible in today's world, even under the leadership of the World Health Organization (WHO) of the United Nations. Malaria can be effectively attacked on a national basis, however, and there is hope that gradually more and more areas of the world will become malaria-free. Meanwhile, when it does occur, the disease can be cured, as long as treatment is persistent, at least in the forms that we now know it. But there is always the danger of new and different forms of the parasite evolving. When large numbers of American troops were sent to South Vietnam in the middle 1960s, a particularly fast-moving and virulent form of malaria was found to attack them, requiring increased doses of suppressive drugs to check the infections. But even this form of malaria does yield to persistent drug therapy as long as the active disease is recognized and treated quickly enough. One day, it is hoped, this ancient disease will be eradicated in larger and larger areas of the world and treatment in any form will no longer be necessary.

Parasitic Worms

The parasitic worms that cause human disease are of various kinds and sizes, but they are generally divided into two categories—roundworms and flatworms—and infestations can range all the way from the mild and almost symptomless to the massively debilitating and even fatal. The most common of these parasites have strange and complicated life cycles which unfortunately include infesting the intestines of human victims.

Hookworm disease is one of the most prevalent of the really dangerous roundworm infestations that occur in the United States. It is commonplace in most of the southern states bordering on the Atlantic and Gulf coasts, and in the southern Appalachian region extending into North Carolina. Adult hookworms are not very large, perhaps half an inch in length, but one female attached to the human intestine can produce from 5,000 to 20,000 eggs per day. The eggs hatch into larvae in the intestine, pass out in the stool and contaminate the ground in areas where sanitary facilities are nonexistent or unused, or in other areas of the world where human feces are highly prized as fertilizer.

The disease is contracted by coming into contact with the contaminated matter. The hookworm in its larval form invades the body through the skin, usually the skin of the feet when the victim is barefoot, so that prevalence is high particularly among children in climates where barefootedness is commonplace. Some six weeks are required from the initial invasion for the larva to make its way to the intestine and become an adult worm. It then literally hooks itself to the lining partway down the small intestine and begins feeding on blood and producing eggs.

Most of the symptoms of hookworm disease come as a result of a progressive anemia, increasing malnutrition and possibly heart failure. A single hookworm may ingest as much as one-fifth of a cubic centimeter of blood each day; if, as is often the case, a victim is infested with dozens or even hundreds of hookworms, the daily blood loss can easily exceed the body's capacity to generate new blood cells. The victim usually develops a pallor and then anemia, first moderate and later severe, together with muscle weakness and a sharp increase in appetite. In heavily infested victims the same symptoms appear in exaggerated proportions, with a very severe anemia, marked weakness and fatigue, and evidence of heart enlargement due to its frantic work to circulate enough of the impoverished blood to provide for the body's needs. The victim develops shortness of breath even on minimal exertion, and in the case of a child there is a marked depression of both physical and mental development. Ultimately, in the absence of treatment, the disease can produce all the symptoms of chronic starvation, although the victim may be voraciously eating whatever food is available, as well as earth, minerals, bits

of wood or other unusual substances—the odd symptom complex known as pica. A mild untreated infection may last for as long as 15 to 20 years, but in more severe cases the parasite will destroy the victim, usually with death resulting from heart failure and such marked anemia that the blood may contain less than 10 percent of the normal amount of hemoglobin for carrying oxygen.

Treatment for hookworm disease (when it is sought, and when the drugs are available) can be completely curative. Tetrachloroethylene, a drug which destroys the adult worms attached to the intestinal wall, has been used in millions of cases with only minor toxic side effects. Another drug, hexylresorcinol, seems about equally effective without as much toxicity and will also kill simultaneous infections with larger roundworms such as the *Ascaris*. Part of the treatment, of course, should include a high-protein diet and supplementary iron to help the body produce more red cells and reduce the anemia.

In the long run, however, hookworm disease can be reduced in incidence only by two major control measures: rigid sanitary disposal of human feces in areas where the disease is commonplace, using pit toilets or trench latrines when enclosed plumbing is unavailable; and wearing shoes to protect against infestation from contaminated earth. Both these measures are all too often ignored in many parts of the southern United States and other areas of the world where sanitary and bathing facilities are limited or seldom used, shoes are often not economically possible, and protein and iron in the diet are practically nonexistent. The belief that the impoverished peoples of the South of whatever race and the native populations of other areas of the world are naturally "slow-witted," "lazy" and "underdeveloped mentally and physically" is erroneous. Where these conditions exist, they are almost invariably the direct result of poverty, ignorance, malnutrition and widespread hookworm disease in populations where both social and economic conditions make it difficult if not impossible to carry through adequate preventive programs. Public health officials in the South and all over the world, however, have recognized this vicious cycle and are working hard to provide the education and the funds necessary to establish control of the disease.

Ascaris infection, like hookworm disease, is also commonplace in the warm, moist areas of the world, including the southern United States. But it is not limited to that region; children in the midwestern or northern parts of the country can also contract the disease from close association with an afflicted pet dog. The *Ascaris lumbricoides* or giant roundworm is one of the largest of man's intestinal parasites, often measuring from 8 to 15 inches in length. Unlike the hookworm, the *Ascaris* larva cannot enter the body through unbroken skin; it is usually ingested in fecally contaminated matter. Once in the intestine the larva becomes an adult worm and lays multitudes of eggs, subsisting in the meantime on food materials present in that region. Larvae, eggs and even whole worms can be identified in the stool. The first clue that a child has an *Ascaris* infection may be the discovery of the adult worms in his bed, passed through the rectum during the night.

Often the disease is without symptoms or is accompanied by only vague intestinal discomfort. Undoubtedly the worm impoverishes the nutrition of the victim to some degree, although the anemia of hookworm infection does not occur. But unfortunately the *Ascaris,* when they have become adult worms, tend to migrate to various parts of the body and cause all manner of mischief. They can, for example, invade the bile ducts, the gall bladder, the liver or the appendix, carrying intestinal bacteria to these areas so that acute infections or even abscess formations may result.

Once diagnosed, treatment is relatively easy, safe and simple, using the inexpensive vermicide piperazine (trade name Antepar) for two consecutive weeks, followed by repeated treatment in two weeks. Like hookworm disease, the spread of this infection can be reduced by proper sanitary facilities, careful attention to personal health habits and avoiding the use of human feces as fertilizer. It is easy to think of both these infestations as the products of poverty and improper sanitation, but even in families that observe the most fastidious health habits,

Ascaris infection can be transmitted to children, for example, from an infected house pet. *Ascaris* is one of the most common of all worm infections suffered by dogs, which can contract it and transmit it the same way that a human carrier does. Any evidence of worms passed in a dog's stool should be reported to a veterinarian so that the dog can be examined and wormed. If such a problem occurs in your family, it is wise to consult your family doctor immediately so that he can check the various members of the family for infection.

Pinworm infection is by far the most pervasive and annoying of the roundworm infections in man, and the most difficult to permanently eliminate. Caused by a worm that is only approximately one-sixteenth of an inch long, the *Enterobius vermicularis,* it is found in virtually all geographical areas of the world, particularly in cities, and in all economic classes, even where the most modern sanitary facilities are used.

The adult worms inhabit the lower part of the small intestine and the upper part of the colon, often in overwhelming numbers, where they feed on the intestinal contents or even, possibly, on tissue fluids from the intestinal wall. A single mature female pinworm may store as many as 10,000 eggs in her body, then migrate down the colon and out the rectum. There the eggs are expelled and develop infectious larvae within a few hours. The presence of worms and eggs in the region around the anus is highly irritating, causing the victim to scratch and—particularly among children—to carry the larvae under their fingernails or on their fingers to later contaminate their food. Then the worm's simple life cycle is completed when the eggs are swallowed, hatch and go to the lower end of the small intestine. Thus a victim can continually reinfect himself as well as others. Often the most fastidious attention to personal hygiene does not break this life cycle, for the pinworm eggs can be released in such numbers that they permeate the victim's clothing and bedding, escape into house dust, and may even be carried by air currents and spread through whole families or groups living in the same environment. Most physicians treating this disease assume that if one member of the family is infected, all members are infected, and treatment is likely to be recommended for everyone.

A great many symptoms and complaints have been ascribed to or "explained" by pinworm infection, especially in children: poor appetite, failure to gain weight, bed-wetting, grinding of the teeth during sleep, pain in the abdomen, nausea and vomiting, and even appendicitis, among others. The fact is that there is no real scientific proof that these symptoms are the result of pinworms; even so, their presence in a child's stool is often accepted by parents (or even the doctor) as the explanation for numerous vague symptoms that cannot be explained any other way. Even the experts cannot agree about whether or not pinworm infection causes appendicitis. Some surgeons feel that it definitely can while others reject the idea, and no real proof exists. Nor is there actual proof that pinworm infection necessarily has any ill effects on the victim's nutrition or growth. Many pediatricians are convinced that it does, and feel that eradication of the infection is often followed by a striking improvement in the child's overall well-being.

There is no question, however, that pinworms cause a severely annoying itching in the anal region, particularly at night, and mothers often make the diagnosis themselves by observing the worms in a child's stool or around the anus when he has been awakened from sleep by itching. Laboratory examination of the stool may fail to reveal any of the parasites, but the eggs can often be detected by using a length of Scotch tape folded sticky side out over a tongue depressor which is then pressed against the region around the anus. When the tape is placed on a microscope slide and examined, the typical eggs containing immature larvae can often be observed, clinching the diagnosis.

Pinworm infection can be effectively treated with piperazine, or Antepar, taken in divided doses over seven consecutive days according to the weight of the victim. Because all the parasites are not always killed in one course of medication, the same course is usually recommended throughout a second week following a

week without medicine. Since effective treatment of one member of the family really requires treatment of everyone in the family at the same time, this program can be both inconvenient and expensive. But another chemical sold under the trade name Povan is equally effective and has the advantage that only a single dose is required for each member of the family, followed by a second dose one week after the first treatment. Whether this medicine is taken in tablet or liquid form, it contains a chemical dye which will color the stools bright scarlet, and if the liquid is spilled it will stain. The color, however, leaves the stool a day or two after the dose has been taken and causes no problem other than the annoying possibility of staining underclothes, bedclothes, etc.

Once contracted, pinworm infection can be very insidious. Even with treatment victims tend to become reinfected unless the strictest preventive measures are taken. Extreme care in personal hygiene by everyone in the family is essential, including hand washing after use of the toilet and before meals, the use of diapers or close-fitting cotton underpants when the infection is present, boiling diapers, underpants, pajamas and bed sheets two or three times a week, and taking pains to keep the house as dust-free as possible. Even then reinfection is possible.

Considering this, and the lack of proof that pinworm infection actually causes any dangerous pathology, many victims—and even their doctors—become discouraged by having to treat and re-treat the infection and maintain such a demanding program of prevention in the household. Is it really worth it? Many doctors are inclined to say no, as long as the infection is not so overwhelming that real distress and symptoms occur. Probably the best guide to follow is the denominator of common sense. If one or more members of the family are obviously suffering from nighttime itching, irritability, poor appetite or general failure to grow and gain weight as expected, and pinworms are present, all the family should undertake a course of treatment and tighten up on family sanitary precautions. On the other hand, if pinworm infections recur repeatedly and there is no evidence that the children are really suffering any debility or symptoms as a result, a period of calm watchful waiting may be the wisest course rather than entering a frantic cycle of treatment and retreatment. Pinworms can certainly be an annoyance, but probably even at their worst they rarely pose a serious health threat.

In addition to these various roundworm infections, certain flatworms, commonly called *tapeworms*, can infest the human body, taking up residence in the intestine and feeding both on digested food materials there and—more importantly—on blood from the intestinal lining. Tapeworms are primarily animal parasites living in cattle, swine or fish; most cosmopolitan in the world is the beef tapeworm. Human infections occur when the eggs or larvae of these worms are ingested either from poorly cooked infested meat or from food that has been fecally contaminated by an infected person. The eggs or larvae mature in the upper part of the large intestine, hooking into the lining and then growing into a series of short, flat segments. In mature worms the end segments, called *proglottids*, contain tiny larvae of new worms. These may break off and be passed out in the stool, where they can often be detected by careful microscopic examination. The worms also lay eggs which are passed in the stool and can sometimes be discovered microscopically.

Symptoms of tapeworm infection are often vague, including abdominal cramps, diarrhea and a general mild toxemia marked by physical exhaustion, loss of appetite and sometimes a low-grade fever. Contrary to the popular myth, tapeworm sufferers do not ordinarily have voracious appetites, but certain varieties of the worm can grow to be many yards long and require considerable sustenance, so weight loss and anemia frequently develop. Once infestation is diagnosed, tapeworms can be destroyed by treatment with quinacrine hydrochloride (Atabrine), one of the drugs also used to prevent malaria, or with other drugs, depending upon the particular variety of worm. The fish tapeworm, in particular, can cause pernicious anemia (*see* p. 516), and treatment includes dosage with vitamin B_{12}.

Scabies and Other Insect Parasites

We live in a world vastly more overpopulated with insects than with people, and while many insects are beneficial to man's existence on earth in one way or another, others constitute very real health hazards. These hazards can vary widely. Biting or stinging insects are usually more nuisance than threat, except in rare cases (*see* p. 139). Other insects spread infectious diseases by mechanically carrying the causative bacteria from one place to another—for example, the common house fly. Still others play a more direct role in spreading infection. Anopheles mosquitoes spread malaria from victim to victim by biting, while wood ticks transmit the rickettsiae of Rocky Mountain spotted fever in much the same way. In the case of malaria, however, the causative parasite depends upon residence in the mosquito to complete a vital part of its life cycle, while with rickettsial diseases, the insects merely carry the organism from one infected creature to the next. Finally, there are a host of insect pests which themselves live on or beneath the surface of the body as parasites, often burrowing into the skin to feed. Some of these also carry infectious microorganisms into the body, but many that do not are nevertheless themselves annoying or even dangerous health hazards, and cause specific parasitic diseases.

A prime example of the latter is a skin disease known as *scabies*, caused by an itch mite so tiny it can hardly be seen by the naked eye. Infestation becomes apparent when the female insect burrows into the superficial layers of the skin to lay her eggs and deposit excreta, leaving a tiny red pinpoint lesion which itches intensely. The eggs hatch, the insects multiply, and the victim may eventually be covered with these lesions, especially where clothing is tight, between the fingers and in the area of the genitals. The itching often becomes continuous and unbearable, and leads to scratching which may introduce a secondary bacterial infection into the lesions. The infestation is transmitted by close body contact—children sleeping together in the same bed, for instance, or by sexual contact—during which the itch mites on the skin may simply change hosts. Scabies occurs world-wide, and is particularly prevalent among people living in crowded dirty quarters with poor bathing facilities.

The infection is often difficult to diagnose, particularly when a secondary infection is present. But once diagnosed it can be treated quickly and effectively under a doctor's supervision with a chemical ointment or lotion applied over the whole body from the neck down, followed by thorough soap-and-water washing. Sometimes two or three treatments are required to completely eradicate the insect. Prevention is the best approach, however, with careful attention paid to personal hygiene and avoiding contact with infected persons. Clothing, towels and bed linen used by an infected person should also be carefully washed to prevent reinfection. House pets such as dogs and cats, particularly those with skin infections of one sort or another, are often blamed for spreading scabies. Although they are usually quite innocent, the mites that cause mange in house pets may infect human beings; and when human scabies infection is found, treatment of house pets can be important to prevention of reinfection.

Chiggers (or "redbugs" or "harvest mites"), while causing an itchy infection similar to that of scabies, are usually picked up during the summertime while walking in grass or shrubs, while baling hay, or by other exposure to the outside habitat of the insects. Chiggers, which are so tiny they can barely be seen, characteristically burrow in warm, tightly bound areas of the body, such as under the belt line, under bra straps or around the ankles where constrictive socks are worn. Like the mite of scabies, chiggers can also cause intense itching, but they may be eradicated by the use of one of several chemical ointments applied to the affected regions. If you live in an area where chigger infestation is common, check with your doctor about an effective repellent to use on the skin and in the clothing before going out where exposure is likely. Once again, prevention is ten times the value of cure.

Pediculosis (infestation with lice) may occur in various forms and in various areas of the body, depending upon the particular insect involved. Certain species of lice infest the hairy region of the head and scalp (head lice), while a variety of the same insect makes its home on the body, often also residing in clothing (body lice). A completely different form of louse, the crab louse, usually lives in the pubic hair and is commonly passed from one person to another during sexual contact. It may also infest the underarms, chest, or even the eyebrows and eyelashes. Head lice and crab lice lay eggs, called nits, attached to the hair of the host, while body lice usually lay eggs in the clothing. All three varieties suck blood for nourishment and cause severe itching.

In many undeveloped areas of the world where bathing facilities are inadequate or nonexistent and where medical care is unavailable, lice are widespread, a "fact of life" that people take for granted. In this country such infestations are usually the result of personal uncleanliness or unsanitary living conditions. However, even the most fastidious person can become infected by either accident or carelessness. Treatment is possible with safe insecticides used in solutions, creams or ointments wherever the lice are found. Reinfection is prevented by thorough daily baths, boiling of bedding and wearing apparel, and avoidance of infected persons.

Domestic animals, especially dogs and cats, are often infested with fleas, which may become especially annoying to humans in homes in which flea-ridden house pets have died or been disposed of, leaving their fleas behind them. Fleas not only jump about in an irritating fashion; they also *bite* people. Today they are chiefly a pest, with the notable exception of certain varieties of rat fleas which transmit the deadly bubonic plague bacillus from infected rats to people. Various chemical insecticides can be used to rid humans and their living quarters of fleas—either your doctor or your druggist can advise you—and many veterinarians now recommend the use of chemically treated collars for house pets to help keep them free of fleas.

Wood ticks of several species are common throughout the United States in wooded or brushy areas at various times throughout the summer season, particularly during July and August. Although these insects are easy enough to see, being about one-eighth of an inch long and brownish or brown-speckled in color, they may attach themselves to clothing while a person is walking through brush or woods and later make their way to the skin—usually to hairy areas—unnoticed. Once they find a likely, protected spot, they attach themselves to the skin by means of a painless bite and begin feeding on the victim's blood and tissue juices, often swelling to as much as one-half inch long if they are unnoticed for several days. Even once fed, they may remain with their heads embedded in the skin and may be the source of secondary bacterial infection at the site of the bite.

The best treatment against wood ticks is prevention (*see* p. 237), including careful inspection of all parts of the body and removal of the insects at least once and preferably twice a day during the season in those areas where ticks are prevalent. Remember that ticks are very flat with a hard protective coating, so that squeezing them may not destroy them. Furthermore, if they happen to be infected with the organism of Rocky Mountain spotted fever, squeezing them could conceivably introduce the organism into the body. If part of a tick is left in the site of the bite, it is wise to have a doctor assist in removing it.

Very rarely an odd form of temporary paralysis can develop as the result of poisons introduced into the body by a biting tick. If there is any sign during the summer season of weakness or poor control of legs, trunk, arms, neck, tongue or swallowing, the victim should consult a doctor without delay. This so-called tick paralysis is transitory, but sometimes supportive respiration with a respirator is necessary until the condition recedes.

Finally, no discussion of insect pests should close without mention of the lowly bedbug, *Cimex lectularius.* Most commonly found in crowded urban ghettos and aging tenement buildings, these small, flat insects hide in bedclothes and mattresses and come out at night to feed on their sleeping victims. The bites itch and are frequently infected with bacteria as a result of scratching. Thorough fumigation of bedding, clothing and rugs may be necessary to rid a house of this pest, but insect repellents may be effectively used to protect the sleeper.

Leprosy, Bubonic Plague and Other Uncommon Infections and Parasitic Diseases

A list of all the infectious diseases and parasitic infestations known to man would seem to be almost endless. In our discussion, some of these infections have been arbitrarily ignored because they are very uncommon or sharply limited geographically; others have been bypassed because they rarely, if ever, occur in the United States, even though they may be common in other countries. Still, some of these rare infections do occur here, often related to specific areas or occupations, and others have played such a significant role in the history of human civilization that they deserve more than passing mention. As every doctor knows, it is possible to contract any infection, no matter how obscure; and the layman should have at least a passing acquaintance with their history and some of their more unique and outstanding characteristics.

Leprosy (Hansen's Disease)

Leprosy is another of mankind's ancient plagues, far more horrifying to those who lived with it than almost any other disease because of its prolonged course and terrible physical effects. Today it has rather euphemistically been renamed Hansen's disease, after the man who first identified the bacteria that cause it, in hope of lessening the dreadful social stigma still attached to its former name. Like tuberculosis, leprosy tends to be a slow-developing and long-chronic infection, pursuing its course over years and decades; but unlike tuberculosis, it produces stigmata in its victims which are easily recognizable. It was once believed that the touch or the very presence of a leper could spread the infection, and it was so deeply dreaded that its victims were cruelly ostracized from society, sent to remote and isolated colonies or locked up in leper houses.

In the ancient world the disease was endemic to the subtropical and tropical countries of the Middle East and Africa; and for a period of time in the Middle Ages it actually became epidemic in southern and western Europe. But then its incidence suddenly declined quite sharply, ironically due to the great epidemics of bubonic plague and the increasing incidence of syphilis which probably wiped out the leper population. Today, although leprosy is not an active, widespread threat, it still occurs in Spain, Portugal, north and central Africa, China, the Gulf Coast states of the United States and Hawaii. It is even more common, however, in Indonesia and Southeast Asia, and there is reason to believe that a number of U.S. servicemen are becoming infected abroad and are bringing the disease back home with them. According to recent Public Health Service estimates, there are approximately 3,500 cases of leprosy in the continental United States today.

Victims of leprosy are, of course, treated much more humanely now that we have discovered the actual pathology of the disease. It is caused by a waxy-coated, crimson-staining bacterium so very closely related to the tubercle bacillus that the two organisms can be differentiated only by special and complicated bacteriological procedures. But unlike the tubercle

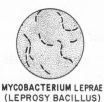

MYCOBACTERIUM LEPRAE
(LEPROSY BACILLUS)

Figure 25-1.

bacillus, which characteristically attacks the deep-seated, warm and highly vascular internal organs such as the lung or the kidney, the *Mycobacterium leprae* of leprosy tends to infect the cooler and more superficial tissues of the body: the subcutaneous tissue just beneath the skin, for example, especially of the hands, eyebrows, cheeks, forehead or ears, and the superficial nerve endings in the skin as well as the nerve trunks lying close to the surface. The bacteria ordinarily grow very slowly, first infecting small patches of tissue and forming indurated lumps and nodules, then spreading locally from there to destroy more tissue as they grow. The spread of infection is not only insidious but usually painless, for the sensory nerve endings are destroyed along with surrounding tissue and the victim develops areas of anesthesia as the disease progresses. When motor nerves to an area such as the fingers are involved, loss of movement occurs gradually and the subsequent shriveling of unused muscle causes contracture and the ultimate formation of the typical "claw hand" of moderately advanced leprosy. When the bacteria attack the subcutaneous tissue of the face, facial nerve endings are destroyed and parts of the face become immobile and expressionless, hair follicles in the scalp are destroyed and the hair falls out, and the cartilage of the ear may eventually be completely eroded away. Ultimately bone destruction follows, and then other parts of the body may be affected bit by bit. Untreated, the course of the disease may extend for 15 or 20 years with the steady destruction and erosion of

tissue, scarring and disfigurement. Death often ensues as a result of some other intercurrent infection rather than from the leprosy infection itself.

Obviously this kind of slow, indolent infection is not one that lends itself to instant contagion. It cannot be contracted by a mere touch, nor is it hereditary as was once believed. It is transmitted only after *prolonged and intimate* contact with an infected person. The bacterium causing the disease was first discovered in 1868 by Gerhardt Henrik Hansen (1841–1912), a Norwegian physician in charge of the leper hospital near Bergen. With that discovery, it was found that commonsense health precautions would prevent the spread of the infection, and although those in the advanced stages of the disease were usually isolated, they were no longer treated as social outcasts. Still there was no effective treatment until many years later. Even streptomycin and isoniazid, so effective against the tubercle bacillus, proved to be of little significant help. But in the early 1940s a group of chemicals known as sulfones (not to be confused with sulfonamides) were found capable of arresting the progress of leprosy. Today the infection can be cured with prolonged sulfone therapy extending over periods of three to eight years, and other drugs are also now known which help control or cure the disease.

Unfortunately, the damage done to nerves and tissues by the infection before it is diagnosed and treated can never be repaired. But it is now possible for a victim of the disease in its early stages to be safely and effectively treated at home and to continue his daily life and work without threat of infecting others. If this is not practical, he may be sent to the U.S. Public Health Service Hospital in Carville, Louisiana, where he will receive expert care and may soon be able to resume his normal life. If the benefits of sulfone treatment could be carried to all parts of the world where the disease still occurs, leprosy could probably be completely eradicated. Thus the only real threat that remains is the age-old fear of the disease and the absurd social opprobrium that still goes along with it, felt by both its victims and those close to them. One day, it is hoped, these too will be completely eradicated.

Bubonic and Pneumonic Plague

Leprosy is one of the ancient destroyers which is rapidly declining in the modern world, but the same cannot be said for bubonic plague. The Black Death which swept repeatedly across Europe like a deadly brush fire during the Middle Ages and the Renaissance, leaving indescribable slaughter in its wake, still remains endemic in many parts of the world today.

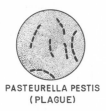

PASTEURELLA PESTIS
(PLAGUE)

Figure 25–2.

Plague, which is certainly among the most violently infectious diseases known to man, is caused by a hardy bacillus known as *Pastuerella pestis,* one of the microorganisms that Louis Pasteur studied and proved to be a dangerous disease vector. Two forms of the disease have long been recognized. Most commonly seen during the murderous epidemics that swept Europe in the Middle Ages was the so-called *bubonic* form, a sweeping infection of the entire body in which the bacteria were carried through the blood stream and the lymphatic channels to virtually every organ system. From the symptoms of this form of plague it is easy to understand how it came to be called the Black Death and the horror in which it was held. The disease began abruptly, usually with repeated chills, and a rapid rise in temperature as high as 103° to 106°. The victim grew deathly ill with vomiting, an unsteady gait and a headache, often becoming stuporous within a matter of a few hours. Convulsions and coma often followed. As the infection increased, the victim's face would become puffy, his spleen swollen, and multitudes of capillary hemorrhages would appear under the skin, at first red, but rapidly turning into coalescing black-and-blue splotches. The lymph glands in the groin and under the arms would become markedly enlarged, painful and tender, forming so-called buboes, and these lumps would often become necrotic and break through the skin, discharging quantities of infectious pus and blood. Death, when it occurred, was the result of massive damage done by the bacteria to tissues in the brain, kidneys, lungs and other organs, all combined, or to toxemia or shock, and it would ordinarily come on the fifth or sixth day of the infection when the ravages of the disease upon the victim's body were the most obvious and the most hideous.

A second form of infection, known as *pneumonic* plague, killed even more swiftly and horribly. In this form the bacteria primarily attacked the lungs, leading to a swiftly moving hemorrhagic pneumonia in which the victim literally suffocated coughing up his own blood. When untreated, the bubonic form of plague was fatal in perhaps 20 to 30 percent of cases, although death rates were clearly much higher in certain of the ancient epidemics. The pneumonic form had a fatality rate closer to 80 or 90 percent, with the victims usually dying within 72 hours of the onset of symptoms.

Although plague in either form could be transmitted directly from human victim to human victim, and pneumonic plague in particular was often spread by coughing, such direct transmission was not the usual pattern, at least at the beginning of epidemics. Plague is primarily an infection of rodents, most notably the black rat and the brown rat, which live in such close proximity to human beings all over the world. The disease is ordinarily transmitted to human beings by rat fleas which infest the diseased animals and then bite human victims. Today broad-spectrum antibiotics such as tetracycline and chloramphenicol are used to attack the disease organism, and the infection can be cured if treatment is started early enough. But once the infection is well along on its violent course, even antibiotics often fail to stop it, especially the pneumonic form.

Treatment and cure have been possible, of course, only quite recently. Before that no other single disease had a more appalling effect on human history. The first recorded plague of mammoth proportions occurred in Egypt in A.D. 542, spreading to Asia and Europe and leaving an estimated 100 million people dead. In the early 1300s it appeared again along caravan and trade routes from central Asia and India to Constantinople. From there it was carried to Sicily and the great Italian city-states of Venice, Genoa and Florence in 1347 and on to France in 1348. There it grew rapidly into the most devastating plague in all history, destroying between 25 and 50 million people in Europe—a quarter of the total population at that time—and wiping out as much as three-quarters of the entire population of France. Equally staggering death rates were recorded in Italy and then in England. The disease struck terror in the minds of rich and poor alike, and they went to incredible lengths to avoid it, even though they had no idea how it was caused. Plague victims were abandoned and left to die at the first sign of infection; and ships from plague ports were forced to dock at some remote distance from the main harbor of a city, first for 30 days, a period known as a "trentina," and then later for 40 days or a "quarantina."

In later centuries the countries of Europe were afflicted by plague only in localized epidemics, but even these were devastating. After a series of lesser outbreaks, London was decimated by the great plague of 1665, finally checked by the equally disastrous fire that destroyed almost the entire city. By the 1800s the disease had virtually disappeared in epidemic form from western Europe, but Africa and the Near and Far East were not quite so fortunate. The last great wave of plague began in 1894 in China and India and, for all our modern knowledge of isolation and antibiosis, still recurs there periodically. It is also a threat in areas of Southeast Asia and Africa where control of the rodent reservoirs of the disease has not yet been achieved. Plague was brought under control in the Western world mainly by destruction of the plague-bearing rats and (after the rat flea vector was finally identified in 1914) by use of insecticides to scour out the infected insects. It will probably never occur in epidemic form again, but with modern transportation and travel to and from all parts of the world, individual infections are still very possible.

The United States has been spared any great epidemic of plague. Between 1908 and 1951 only 91 cases occurred in 15 western states, and since then the occurrence of even a single case is a medical rarity. Even so, wild rodents such as field mice, rats, ground squirrels, chipmunks and marmots provide a continuing reservoir of the disease in the mountains and forests of the West Coast and the Rockies. With the growing popularity of wilderness travel and family camping in these areas, everyone should be aware of the potential danger of contact with small wild rodents, especially if they appear sick or behave strangely. Further, the abrupt onset of any illness with high fever, rapid heartbeat and aching muscles on western vacations, camping or hunting trips should be brought to the immediate attention of a physican, together with full details of the victim's activities and any possible proximity to wild rodents.

There have been numerous attempts to produce a vaccine effective in protecting against plague. The results have not been highly satisfactory, although inoculations today can provide some degree of protection for a limited period of time. Routine inoculations are not recommended in the United States, but travelers should be inoculated prior to travel into known plague areas of the world. Immunizations are available at any U.S. Public Health Service office and the Health Service maintains up-to-date information about areas of the world which must be considered dangerous.

Anthrax. Once called "woolsorters' disease" or "rag pickers' disease," anthrax is primarily an infection of grazing animals, especially sheep, caused by a large gram-positive bacillus which can be transmitted to man if a skin abrasion is brought into contact with infected animals, animal hide, hair or waste. It is most prevalent in Asia, Africa and Europe, but uncommon in the United States, although outbreaks do occasionally occur. The characteristic human infection usually begins with an expanding ulcer on the skin at the site of the infection, with an angry red rim and a bluish-red center which soon turns black. It is curable with penicillin or a broad-spectrum antibiotic, but it can be fatal if untreated or if the bacteria also invade the lungs.

Prevention depends upon commonsense hygiene when working with animals and eradication of the disease in the animals themselves.

Brucellosis. More commonly known as undulant fever or Malta fever, brucellosis is another disease which primarily affects animals, especially cattle, hogs and goats, but which can be transmitted to man by direct contact with the infected animals or by drinking milk products containing the *Brucella* organism. The infection develops slowly, characterized by fatigue, muscle ache and a recurrent or "undulating" fever which may repeatedly spike as high as 104° or 105° in the evening and then drop to normal, with profuse sweating, in the morning. Untreated, brucellosis may remain in a chronic stage for months with recurrent exacerbations of fever. It is rarely fatal, even if untreated, but the use of broad-spectrum antibiotics is moderately effective. The disease, most prevalent in rural areas, is also an occupational disease among meat packers, veterinarians and livestock farmers. In any case of a recurring or undulating fever of unknown origin, brucellosis must be considered in the differential diagnosis and, if possible, ruled out as a cause by means of laboratory tests on blood serum.

Tularemia. An acute and severe infection, tularemia is caused by a small bacillus, *Pasteurella tularensis,* which is distributed widely in nature, most particularly in wild rabbits, hence its common name, "rabbit fever." In fact, as many as 90 percent of reported cases can be traced to contact with infected wild rabbits, although eating inadequately cooked rabbit meat can also lead to infection. The disease is spread among rabbits, squirrels and occasionally other animals by deer flies, ticks and lice, which can also pass the infection directly to human victims. It is characterized by sudden high spiking fever, prostration, extreme weakness and a toxemia similar to that of typhoid fever. A skin ulcer is usually found at the site of the infection. Relapses or even death may occur in inadequately treated cases. Broad-spectrum antibiotics are effective treatment, and the best prevention is, of course, extreme care when coming in contact with rabbits, living or dead. Wild rabbit hunters should use kitchen rubber gloves to handle and clean their bag, and thorough cooking of the meat is advisable.

Glanders. This is a bacterial disease of horses which is communicable to man. It need not concern anyone who is not in close contact with horses. Those who are should consult their veterinarians for information about prevention and detection of the disease in their animals.

Relapsing Fever. This infection, caused by spirochetes, is transmitted by lice or ticks and is characterized by recurrent seizures of fever lasting from three to ten days, separated by periods of apparent recovery. The louse-borne infection occurs mainly in Europe, Asia and Africa, while tick-borne infection is also found in Central and South America and the western states of this country. When untreated, recurrences of the fever may appear at intervals of one to two weeks for months. The spirochetes may be found in the blood stream during febrile relapse, and false-positive blood tests for syphilis are found in 20 percent of cases although the infection has no relationship to the venereal disease. Rarely fatal, the disease gradually recedes as the victim develops immunity, but treatment with penicillin or broad-spectrum antibiotics usually speeds the cure.

Yaws. Another nonvenereal infection caused by a species of spirochete similar to that of syphilis, yaws is a highly contagious disease. It is limited, however, to tropical regions, notably Central Africa and equatorial South America, and is predominantly a disease of children. When contracted by contact with discharges from lesions of an infected person or from infected clothing, a primary ulcerating sore appears on the skin, followed later by a generalized eruption of similar skin ulcers, fever and malaise. In severe cases there may be serious disfigurement, and destructive lesions of the soles of the feet or of the bones and joints may also result in permanent crippling. Infection is rarely fatal, and yaws is treatable with penicillin, often in combination with arsenic or bismuth compounds.

Psittacosis. Also known as parrot fever, psittacosis is a pneumonia-like infection caused by a virus transmitted by infected birds. Spread of the infection is a public health concern because it may be brought into this country by way of birds imported for sale as pets. At first the disease may be confused with influenza, bronchitis or bacterial pneumonia. Frequently fatal in the past, it is one of the few virus infections that responds to antibiotic treatment, especially with tetracycline, and today it is seldom diagnosed before antibiotic treatment has been started on the assumption that a bacterial pneumonia is present. Diagnosis usually depends upon a history of contact with wild or imported pet birds.

Q Fever. This rickettsial infection apparently arises from infected sheep, cattle or goats in which the organism is not particularly pathogenic. Its name comes from the tentative name "query fever" given it when it was first noted. It is a pneumonia-like disease, mild and self-limited with a record of very few fatalities. Antibiotic treatment with tetracycline is usually curative.

Systemic (Internal) Fungus Infections. Although most pathogenic fungi attack only the skin and cause such infections as ringworm and athlete's foot (*see* p. 398), a few relatively uncommon fungi invade the body and cause internal infections just as bacteria can. Usually these are indolent infections which may require months to produce notable symptoms and may continue untreated for years before causing death. Various of these fungi involve different and often characteristic parts of the body. The fungus causing *actinomycosis* can enter the body through infected gums or decayed teeth and cause a lesion in the face or neck composed of many small communicating abscesses. The lungs or abdomen may also be affected. The infection persists for months or years and may respond only slowly to medical treatment with sulfas or penicillin, combined with iodine-containing medications which hamper growth and spread of many systemic fungus infections.

Histoplasmosis is caused by a fungus organism which lives in the soil and is spread by inhalation of dust containing the spores. A mild primary infection in the lung is common, but first evidence of the infection is often the appearance of ulcerated areas on the ear, nose, lips or pharynx. Ingestion of the organism may lead to intestinal ulceration, with involvement of both the spleen and the liver. An insidiously progressive infection, often difficult to diagnose, the disease when untreated can be fatal within a few weeks to several months, but it responds dramatically to treatment with such antifungal antibiotics as Amphotericin B. In this country histoplasmosis is most common in damp, humid rural areas on the western slope of the Appalachians and in an area west of the Mississippi and north of the Ohio rivers.

Coccidioidomycosis, also called valley fever or San Joaquin fever, is a highly infectious fungus disease, often chronically progressive, involving first the lungs and then the bones, joints, skin, viscera or brain. Often fatal, this dust-borne fungus infection was first identified in the United States in the San Joaquin Valley, but it is now generally prevalent in all of the Southwest and the western third of South America. Negroes, Mexican Americans and Filipinos appear more sensitive to the disease than Caucasians. Often difficult to diagnose, the infection may prove the source of a "fever of unknown origin." Amphotericin B is the only effective drug known, and is far more effective in treating infections in the early stage.

Blastomycosis is caused by one of a variety of yeastlike fungi about which little is known. Most cases in this country have appeared in the southeastern states and the Mississippi Valley. The fungus causes ulcerating lesions on the skin, but may also invade the lung (sometimes with such rapid growth as to simulate lung cancer on a chest X-ray), the bone, liver, spleen, kidneys or central nervous system. Although quite rare in the United States, this infection is thoroughly nasty when it occurs, is difficult to diagnose and requires long and painful regimens of treatment with antifungal drugs for its eradication.

Trichiniasis (Trichinosis). Occurring far more commonly than formerly suspected, this disease is an infestation of the skeletal muscle of the body by the larvae of a tiny (¼ to ½ inch long) parasitic roundworm known as *Trichinella.* It is usually contracted by eating infested and undercooked pork. (Game hunters should note that undercooked bear meat can also be a source of trichiniasis, and whale meat has been implicated as a cause of the disease among

Eskimos.) When the parasite is ingested, cysts from the diseased meat, containing larvae of the worm, are broken open by digestion in the gastrointestinal tract. The worms mature quickly and mate, and within a few days the females give birth to living young, which are then carried by the blood stream and lymphatics to take up lodging in skeletal muscle fibers all over the body, particularly in the diaphragm, the tongue, the chest muscles, the shoulders, back and legs. These larvae cause an acute inflammatory reaction in the affected muscles. Symptoms include fever, muscle soreness and muscle swelling as the normal defense mechanisms of the body try unsuccessfully to fight off the parasitic invasion. If the heart muscle itself is infested, heart failure may complicate the picture.

Severity of the symptoms depends upon the number of worms involved. In severe cases the temperature may rise to 104°, with acute pain and muscle spasm that may persist for days or weeks. If fewer parasites have been taken in, the victim may suffer only vague muscle aches that never become serious enough to call to a doctor's attention. In either case the larvae ultimately become encapsulated in the muscles and then continue to live there without further activity for years. Diagnosis is usually made by means of microscopic examination of a biopsy of muscle tissue, which can reveal the presence of the encysted larvae between strands of muscle tissue.

There is no effective treatment or cure for trichiniasis yet known, but aside from occasionally causing a very painful muscular disease, the infestation does not usually result in any permanent damage or disability. A very severe infestation may trigger congestive heart failure, or pain in the chest muscles may impair respiration enough to threaten the victim with stasis pneumonia, but these are exceptional cases. Once considered a rare disorder, pathologists now suspect that as much as 15 percent of the entire population of the United States suffers some degree of *Trichinella* infestation at one time or another. By far the best approach to this disease is to adhere rigidly to the ancient hygienic practice of thoroughly cooking all pork that is eaten, with special attention to pork sausage of any

kind. "Never eat pink pork" is an excellent guideline, since even with modern meat inspection procedures it is believed that up to 5 percent of all pork reaching the market may be infested. Freezing the meat at below-zero temperatures for 24 hours or more is also effective in killing the parasite, but most home freezers cannot be counted on to reach that low a temperature steadily, so cooking the meat after it is thoroughly thawed is still the only safe procedure. Cooking a pork roast before it is thawed will leave the center undercooked, a potential source of a thoroughly unpleasant disease.

Filariasis. An infestation of the tropical and subtropical countries, filariasis is a roundworm infection spread by larvae that are ingested by mosquitoes and then passed on to other victims. The adult worms in man enter the lymph channels and cause progressive lymphatic obstruction, sometimes resulting in massive edema (swelling up with water) of either or both legs, a condition known as elephantiasis. Control of the infection depends upon antimosquito measures; there is no known specific treatment. A singularly unpleasant form of this infestation known as *loa loa* is found in West Africa, where the microscopic larvae of the worm are transmitted to man by the bite of certain flies. Loa loa is characterized by the rapid migration of adult forms of the worm through the subcutaneous tissue of the body. The worms may move as much as six or eight inches a day in this way and may even cross the eyeball just under the mucous membrane or conjunctiva.

Dracunculiasis. Also called guinea worm infection, this roundworm disease is uncommon in the United States but fairly common in tropical Africa, some islands in the West Indies, and the tropical Guianas in South America. The larvae are transmitted to man when infected shellfish are eaten. The adult worm, which is often quite long, makes its way to the subcutaneous tissue, where its head may erode through the skin to form an ulcer and release larvae. The traditional native treatment of this condition involves the slow mechanical extraction of the worm by gently pulling it out of the skin and winding it up on a stick, a procedure that may take from ten to fourteen days. Modern treatment involves injection of the tissues in the vicinity of the worm with a chemical poison in order to kill the parasite before extraction.

Schistosomiasis. Caused by a blood fluke, a microscopic flatworm that spends part of its life cycle in fresh-water snails, this disease is common in virtually all tropical regions of the world and frequently is encountered in Puerto Ricans residing in the United States. Man becomes infected by bathing in contaminated water. The disease causes a feverish illness as the parasite invades the liver, then later may attack the urinary bladder or the intestinal wall, causing symptoms of bladder infection or chronic dysentery. It is difficult to control and difficult to treat, often requiring the use of highly poisonous chemicals which may cause severe toxic reactions. Diagnosis is made by detecting the eggs of the fluke in the stool or urine, or by biopsy of the rectum or urinary bladder.

Trypanosomiasis. More familiarly known as African sleeping sickness, this disease is caused by a protozoan parasite transmitted by the bite of the tsetse fly. The parasite ultimately invades the central nervous system and brain, causing a slow-developing stuporous and then comatose state. Death often comes from starvation. Those who survive may suffer convulsions and/or permanent brain damage. Treatment is long and difficult, but infection can be prevented by prophylactic medication before travel into areas of central Africa where the disease is endemic. Control is best achieved by eradicating the tsetse fly in such endemic areas. A similar trypanosome infection known as Chagas' disease occurs in South America, transmitted by a house fly common to the area. These forms of "sleeping sickness" are never acquired in the United States, and should not be confused with certain forms of virus-caused "sleeping sickness" or encephalitis that do occur here.

Leishmaniasis. Called by a number of names, including Oriental ulcer, tropical ulcer, and Dumdum fever, leishmaniasis is a "family name" for a group of infections caused by a variety of related protozoa transmitted by the bite of sand flies. A severe form called kala-azar is found in India, China, Africa, the Mediterranean basin, Brazil and other South and Central American countries. It is characterized by a generalized feverish illness followed by enlargement of the liver and invasion of other organ systems by the parasite, and is 90 percent fatal when untreated. Milder forms common in China, India, the Near East, the Mediterranean basin, northern Africa and South and Central America cause single or multiple nonhealing ulcers on the skin. Still another form, found in southern Mexico and Central and South America, causes ulcerative lesions of the nose and throat. All forms can be treated with greater or less success, but treatment must be prolonged and often involves the use of highly toxic chemicals. None of these illnesses is commonly encountered in the United States except in the very warmest subtropical areas or among travelers who have become infected in endemic areas.

Toxoplasmosis. A severe disease, involving the central nervous system, lymph nodes and spleen, this infection is caused by a protozoan parasite believed to be transmitted to man by eating undercooked rabbit or pork. The parasite may also be transmitted to an unborn baby through the placenta if a mother is infected just before or during pregnancy, a congenital form of the illness that is usually fatal to the infant. In adults, acute symptoms may mimic the pneumonias or a generalized infection resembling typhus fever, with a rash which covers the body, high fever, chills, and involvement of the spleen, liver, heart and central nervous system, often abruptly fatal before diagnosis is made. If the acute attack is not fatal, the disease becomes subacute and chronic and the patient may survive with low-grade symptoms resembling infectious mononucleosis for months or years. No satisfactory treatment is known, particularly for the subacute or chronic lesions, but the acute infection at the beginning may respond to certain of the sulfa drugs, at least to some degree. The infection occurs all over the world, but incidence is higher among slaughterhouse workers, rabbit trappers and farmers. Thorough cooking of all pork and rabbit meat is the best preventative.

Trichomonas Vaginalis. This benign but often highly irritating vaginal infection caused by a protozoan organism is a stubbornly recurring nuisance to a great many women as well as their sex partners, although it rarely has any serious pathological effect. (*See* p. 752.)

PART

V

PATTERNS OF ILLNESS: THE MUSCULOSKELETAL SYSTEM

26. Muscle and Tendon Diseases   281

27. Fractures and Other Bone Disorders   294

28. Arthritis and Other Joint Diseases   310

The musculoskeletal system is a beautifully structured and marvelously coordinated system of bones, muscles, joints and connective tissues that provides the body with structural support, with special protection for certain of the vital organs, and with the capacity for motion. Important as it is, however, this organ system is not "vital" in the sense that the respiratory, circulatory and nervous systems are vital; life can continue even with marked impairment of many of the bones, muscles or joints. But it is, like the other organ systems of the body, subject to a variety of disfunctions—particularly fractures, sprains and strains—and to the normal processes of wear and tear and aging. It is also vulnerable to certain disorders or dystrophies owing to infection or inflammation, to the breakdown or normal biochemical reactions, to exaggerated immune reactions or, like any living tissue, to abnormal forms of growth. The remarkable thing is that truly devastating afflictions of this organ system are relatively few in kind, and when they do occur the body displays an astonishing ability to compensate for them. Even the few long-term, chronic or recurring disorders are not always necessarily seriously disabling. Modern medical science has perfected a variety of ways to detect and treat these afflictions, as well as the means to reduce or overcome the disabilities they may cause.

Muscle and Tendon Diseases

For years, science fiction writers have speculated about the creation of "mechanical men," robots or so-called androids devised in human form. No such machines yet exist, nor are they likely to in the near future, for as far as adaptability, versatility, elasticity and overall performance are concerned, it is hard to imagine any man-made device that could ever surpass the human "machine," and in particular the ingenious structure and function of the human musculoskeletal system. There is no material yet known that possesses the peculiar combination of strength, lightness, supporting capacity and self-repair exhibited by human bone. There is no material even approaching the elasticity, strength, endurance, adhering quality and capacity for self-repair of human muscle and connective tissue. Nor is there any arrangement of levers, hinges or sockets that can duplicate the smoothness of action, the self-lubricating qualities, the generally trouble-free function, or the strength and endurance of the human joint. A robot might well be stronger than a man, but it could hardly match the variety, the delicacy and the finesse of human movement. The only advantage it might conceivably have is freedom from the diseases and disorders that sometimes afflict the human musculoskeletal system.

In discussing these disorders, we can, for simplicity's sake, separate those affecting muscle tissue, bone, and the joints. Yet it is well to remember that no single part of the musculoskeletal system can ever become diseased or break down without affecting the overall co-operative function of the entire system. Even minor stiffness, pain or cramping of muscle tissue in a given part of the body due to strain or tension may effectively immobilize a whole portion of the body. Muscle tissue is perhaps more free of serious diseases and disorders than any other tissue, yet because there is so much of it, and because we depend on it so heavily to perform so many crucial tasks, even minor muscular aches and pains can, at best, be inconvenient and, at worst, seriously disabling. Many minor muscular afflictions can be treated by the victim himself, but persistent, recurrent or chronic disorders may require a doctor's care.

Skeletal Muscle

Muscle tissue in the human body is found chiefly in two quite different forms. (*See* p. 33.) One form is the "smooth" or *involuntary muscle* that forms the muscular wall of the gastrointestinal tract and lines the arteries and arterioles. Smooth muscle cells fit together in layers and contract in a kind of slow, gentle, wavelike motion under the direction of the involuntary or autonomic nervous system, quite beyond our conscious control. Smooth muscle works by means of a recurring squeezing action, but has comparatively little strength.

The other kind of muscle, commonly called *skeletal, voluntary* or "striated" *muscle,* makes up the vast bulk of muscle tissue in the body. It contracts or relaxes in response to our voluntary desires, or to certain kinds of outside stimuli.

The structure of this muscle tissue is totally different from that of smooth muscle, for voluntary muscle cells are long and thin, lying together in bundles or *fascicles,* and are capable of very powerful, sustained contraction. The cells themselves contain a pigment known as *myoglobin,* which gives them a reddish color and is somewhat similar to the hemoglobin in the blood, and their contractile strength seems to be related to the structure and organization of their cellular protoplasm, which gives the cells an oddly striped or striated appearance.

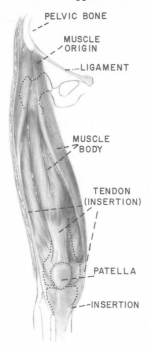

PELVIC BONE

MUSCLE
ORIGIN

LIGAMENT

MUSCLE
BODY

TENDON
(INSERTION)

PATELLA

INSERTION

Figure 26–1.
Skeletal muscle.

Skeletal muscle has a number of interesting characteristics. First, it is usually anchored firmly to bone at either end, with the attachment at one end spoken of as the *origin* of the muscle and the attachment at the other end known as the *insertion.* Sometimes the muscle is attached directly to bone, but more often the muscle ends are gathered together into powerful ropes of a special fibrous connective tissue called *tendon,* which itself is attached to the bone to form the

muscle insertion. In many cases this tendon is comparatively short so that when the muscle contracts it pulls on the bone closely adjacent, but in some cases tendon extends relatively long distances to attach to bone, providing for a sort of "remote control" motion. For example, the motion of our fingers is controlled by tendons connected to muscles in the forearm which extend through a special tunnel in the inner side of the wrist to attach to the bones of each finger. Tendon, however, should not be confused with *ligament,* a similar tough, fibrous connective tissue which has no direct connection with muscle activity but which helps tie the *articular* or *joint* surfaces of bone together and thus works to support the skeletal frame.

The basic difference between tendon and ligament is well illustrated by the way in which many people confuse the two words "strain" and "sprain." A *strain* is an injury that occurs to muscle or tendon owing to severe overuse or stretching. It can occur either when the muscle is unaccustomed to such overuse or when the excessive use happens suddenly or unexpectedly. The actual injury may range from tearing a few muscle fibrils to actually snapping a tendon or tearing it loose from its insertion on the bone. A *sprain,* on the other hand, is a twisting or wrenching injury to a joint which stretches or tears the supporting ligaments. Again, this kind of injury can range from a minor twist with little structural damage to a very severe tearing which may then require surgical intervention and suturing of the torn ligament before the usefulness and stability of the joint can be restored.

Finally, certain characteristics of skeletal muscle set it apart from other kinds of tissue in the body. For one thing, it may range in strength from the incredibly gentle blinking of an eye to the clenching of the masseter or jaw muscle, probably the single most powerful muscle in the body. Second, skeletal muscle tends to *hypertrophy* or increase in mass and weight as a result of exercise and use, and to *atrophy* or shrink in size and weight as a result of disuse. The child who is forced to wear a plaster cast from his navel to his ankle in order to heal a fractured thighbone may be amazed to discover that the large muscles of his thigh on the injured leg will have shrunk to half the size of the muscles of the opposite thigh simply because of disuse while the fractured limb was immobilized. On the other hand, a man with a physically demanding job, or a man who works out with weights, may develop enormously hypertrophied muscles in his arms and shoulders or other parts of his body. In such people certain muscles may hypertrophy to such a degree that their sheer mass actually interferes with delicate muscular movements, and the individual appears surprisingly clumsy or "muscle-bound."

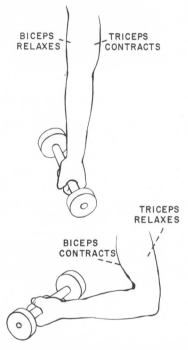

Figure 26–2.

Most skeletal muscles are arranged in teams or pairs, with one muscle bringing about one form of motion and an opposing muscle bringing about the opposite action. For example, the biceps of the upper arm is a *flexor* muscle which acts to flex or bend the elbow. The triceps, on the back of the bone of the upper arm, opposes the action of the biceps and functions as an *extensor* muscle, enabling us to stretch the elbow out straight. These two muscles work in dynamic

balance, the triceps relaxing when the biceps contracts, and the biceps relaxing when the triceps contracts. A similar arrangement is found in the great muscles of the leg; the quadriceps in the front of the thigh acts as extensor of the knee and lower leg, while the hamstring muscles at the back of the thighbone act as flexors or "benders" of the knee. Even the muscles in the back on the right and left sides of the spine work in opposition to each other in a dynamic balance that helps us maintain our upright position.

Normally these muscle pairs perfectly balance each other. But if for some reason one muscle of such a pair ceases to function, the opposing muscle tends to remain in contraction, holding the limb in whatever position is no longer opposed by the other muscle. Thus in cases in which certain muscles have lost their function owing to injury or disease of the muscle itself, or the nerve supplying it, the victim is in danger of developing a kind of crippling deformity known as a *contracture* simply because the healthy muscle, unopposed by the nonfunctioning one, tends to hold the limb motionless in an abnormal position. In any case in which there is likely to be muscle damage or disuse, one of the most important aspects of care is to provide continuing exercise for that muscle in order to guard against the development of contractures. Combating contractures is one of the important jobs of the physical therapist, and forms a vital part of the physical rehabilitation that is so often necessary when an injury or illness affecting the muscles has occurred.

Everyday Disorders of the Musculature

It is one of the contradictions of our everyday lives that we are both too sedentary and, in spurts, too active. Ordinarily we eat too much, sit too much and refuse to walk if we can ride or drive. We take elevators instead of climbing stairs, use the telephone instead of walking across the street to talk to a neighbor and fill our homes with "labor-saving devices" designed to spare us as much physical activity as possible. But then, all of a sudden, we will decide we need some exercise. So after long periods of inactivity, we jog, swim or play tennis to "get back in shape." A week of doing nothing more strenuous than watching television is often followed by a weekend of hard work and play—raking leaves, skiing, hiking, camping or playing touch football in the backyard. And we wonder why we suffer from sprains or strains or just plain sore, aching muscles. But it is this contradictory way of life that accounts, in large part, for many of the most common and annoying disorders of our musculoskeletal system. Frequently these disorders are relatively minor and, while painful and even moderately disabling, they can be treated safely at home with simple remedies if we know what is wrong and what to do about it. Following is a checklist of minor disorders of the skeletal muscles and tendons; their causes and the simple measures that can be taken for their relief are described.

Muscle Fatigue. In our normal, everyday lives our skeletal muscles work hard, and it is not surprising that they grow tired and require rest. A variety of chemical breakdown products, the result of the energy-producing reactions that allow the muscle to contract, build up in the muscle tissue faster than the body can clear them away. If we continue working to the point that certain muscles become somewhat overtired, they begin to ache and need a longer period of rest for recovery. This cannot really be called a disorder—it is a natural, normal, even expectable occurrence. A warm shower or hot bath and a period of physical relaxation with the legs elevated at the end of a day's work goes a long way toward relieving this natural muscle fatigue; a restful night's sleep usually completes the job. This process does not become abnormal unless certain muscles are subjected to either prolonged or severe overuse, or to sudden episodes of extreme overuse for which they have not been prepared or conditioned. It is only then that special measures are necessary to aid recovery.

Cramps or "Charley Horses." Among the most annoying and sometimes alarming of the minor abnormal muscle conditons is the sudden painful cramping of a muscle known as a charley horse. It usually results directly from unexpected and extreme overuse of certain muscles that have not been conditioned to handle the load placed upon them. These cramps

occur very commonly in the large quadriceps muscles in front of the thighbone, often after someone who is unused to running has suddenly raced for a bus or tried for a home run in a sandlot ball game. Such cramps can also occur in the muscles of the upper arms, forearms or shoulders when they have been used far beyond their normal level of activity. Extremely painful cramping spasms may also occur in the muscles of the calf or the hamstring muscles of the thigh just below the buttocks. Often a charley horse appears out of the blue when a person is relaxing, lying in bed or sleeping.

The exact cause of these cramps is not clearly understood. In most cases they are thought to be related to a build-up of biochemical breakdown products that remain in the muscle for a period of time after it has been overused. They are also related to *ischemia* or inadequate flow of blood to the muscle. Not that the circulatory system is necessarily impaired in any way; it may simply not be carrying sufficient blood to the overused muscle at a given time to clear away the lactic acid, calcium compounds and other biochemical breakdown products that remain after exercise. Finally, exceptionally severe and sudden overuse of soft, flabby unconditioned muscles may actually cause the tearing or rupture of some of the fascicles of muscle cells within the tissue. When this happens, the cramping will be accompanied by continuing exquisite tenderness of the involved muscle which may last for days, and *ecchymoses* (black-and-blue marks) may appear in the skin overlying the injured muscle. In all such cases of overuse, from the most minor to the most severe, a certain amount of reactive inflammation will be present, with temporary pain, heat, swelling and a decrease in function of the muscles. Hence this kind of disorder is often known by the general term *overuse myositis.*

Several easy measures will help relieve simple, uncomplicated muscle cramps and help prevent them from recurring. First, immediate moderate exercise of the muscle for a few minutes will increase the blood flow and allow the painful cramp to relax. Leg cramps in particular will usually relax when the victim stands up and walks back and forth, or even does a few deep knee bends to increase blood flow to the leg muscles. Second, a tub soak, with the water as hot as can be tolerated, will further relax the sore, cramping muscle and dilate blood vessels to increase circulation. Aspirin, which is so commonly used as a mild general analgesic for headaches and other minor pains, is also potently specific in relieving aching muscles, bones and joints. Taking up to two 5-grain tablets every three to four hours will relieve the residual pain of a muscle cramp. Various rub-on liniments are widely touted as beneficial for aching muscles. They probably do no harm, but it is doubtful that they do much good, either. At best they act as a counterirritant and cause a pleasant warm feeling when massaged into the skin over the sore muscles. Probably the same amount of massage without any liniment would prove just as beneficial, but if liniments seem to help, by all means use them. Avoid the use of highly irritating chemicals such as mustard plasters, however; the harm they may do to the skin far outweighs any possible benefit to the underlying muscle.

Finally, maintaining moist heat over the affected area for 20 to 30 minutes several times a day will help relieve severe muscle cramping. Probably the best and safest means is to soak a bath towel in very hot water, wring it out, and apply it as a hot moist pack to the sore area. It may be kept warm with a well-insulated electric heating pad so long as it is properly used. Wrap the heating pad in a plastic pillow cover before applying it to the wet pack, even if it is "rubberized" or "waterproof," and never turn the heating pad on higher than the lowest level, since the possibility of a severe burn cannot be overlooked. *Never* go to sleep with a heating pad in place, since the risk of either a thermal burn or an electrical short-circuit fire is always present.

These measures will help relieve the cramps and pain of simple overuse myositis. If severe pain and cramping occur immediately following extreme overuse of a muscle, however, actual tearing or bruising of the muscle may have occurred, and there may even be bleeding into the muscle. In such a case, keep the muscle at rest and apply an ice pack for the first 24 hours. (*See* p. 130.) Then follow with moist heat,

massage and gradually increasing exercise of the muscle.

Lumbago. A rather indefinite term, "lumbago" is often used very loosely to describe any kind of ache or pain in the middle or lower back, but in its medical sense it refers in general to *muscular* aching in the lower curvature of the back, known as the lumbar region, as distinguished from pain owing to injury of the joints or ligaments in that region. (*See* p. 294.) Lumbago often appears insidiously from time to time as a generalized aching in the lower back associated with muscle spasm and usually following some form of physical activity in which a strain has been placed on the back muscles—a form of overuse myositis. Water-skiers, motorcyclists, snowmobilers and other weekend athletes frequently find themselves crippled up with lumbago after a strenuous day's fun. In other cases it may appear quite suddenly and without apparent cause with such painful muscle cramps and spasms in the lower back that the victim is virtually immobilized. This is sometimes—but by no means always—a secondary effect of arthritis in the lower spine. In addition, lumbago is frequently associated with dampness, chilling, drafts or exposure to cold conditions which many fall and winter sportsmen put up with and later learn to regret. The victim of lumbago very often suffers it recurrently, and usually in the same pattern each time.

Since lumbago is primarily due to painful muscle spasm, treatment is aimed at relaxing the cramped muscles, increasing circulation in the region, and relieving the pain with use of analgesics. Hot water tub soaks, hot wet packs and adequate dosage with aspirin will resolve most attacks of lumbago in a day or so without any complications. In more severe cases, rest for a day or two and use of a hard, flat mattress and a bed board (a sheet of plywood under the mattress) will be of great help. If the pain persists or fails to respond to these simple measures, consult a doctor to rule out other possible causes of discomfort in this region—kidney infection, for example, or arthritis in the low back, or the sacroiliac joint syndrome.

Torticollis ("Wry Neck," Stiff Neck). Torticollis is similar in many ways to lumbago, except that it affects the muscles in the upper back, shoulders or neck. Once again, it is a condition of muscle cramping and spasm which may arise from coldness, dampness, chilling or drafts, or even just from prolonged tension of the shoulder and neck muscles. It may occur, for example, after a long day of automobile driving. Like lumbago, torticollis can sometimes be a secondary effect of spinal arthritis. Overuse is less commonly a factor, but tension and anxiety may play a part. Often the cramps are so severe that the victim cannot turn his head without suffering spasms of pain in the neck and shoulder or in the shoulder blade region. If this condition occurs infrequently, hot wet packs or tub soaks, massage, and aspirin to relieve the pain may resolve it without further attention and may help prevent recurrences. But if it is a frequent or recurring condition, a physician should be consulted. As in other muscle spasm conditions, a physician's examination may reveal small nodules or "trigger points" in the cramped muscles, and in many cases marked relief from torticollis can be obtained by injecting a small amount of a local anesthetic or even small amounts of sterile saline solution directly into the trigger area, causing it to relax. In persistent cases, a careful medical examination is also necessary to investigate the possibility of early arthritis in the cervical or dorsal spine which may be contributing to the condition, or to determine other possible underlying causes.

A number of new muscle-relaxant drugs have recently been introduced, some of which seem to help greatly in the treatment of all kinds of muscle-cramping disorders, although none has been universally successful. All are prescription drugs and should be used only on a doctor's order, since there are occasional untoward side effects—temporary muscle weakness, for example, or muscle incoordination or even a degree of drowsiness. In most cases aspirin is still the safest and most effective drug to help relieve the pain of muscle spasm.

Generalized Myositis or Fibrositis. Generalized myositis or inflammation of the skeletal muscle has much in common with such localized forms of myositis as lumbago or torticollis, except that it involves muscles in multiple parts of the body at the same time, and the same elements of treatment apply as with the more localized conditions. The disorder most frequently arises when a normally sedentary person overexercises without getting into condition first. The ensuing stiff muscles stand as mute but painful evidence that the victim should have been more cautious. There is a simple way to relieve much of the discomfort of such muscle stiffness until continuing exercise has adequately conditioned the body. Simply use aspirin prophylactically, ten grains every four to six hours from the start of exercise, and continue during waking hours until the myositis has subsided or until the muscles have become conditioned. This procedure is particularly helpful if an individual who is normally quite inactive knows that he is going to be undertaking a period of unusual exercise.

Even better, however, is to plan a sensible and regular program of exercise to help keep muscles in tone and better prepared for exertion. Any such program, to be effective, must involve the sort of exercise the individual himself enjoys enough to want to continue. The easiest and most underrated form of exercise—to say nothing of the safest—is simple walking. Working out in a gymnasium, playing handball or tennis, jogging and weekend hiking are all excellent ways to maintain a better level of physical fitness. But such programs should be undertaken with some degree of caution, particularly among the middle-aged. Anyone who might be vulnerable to trouble because of age or physical condition should first consult his family doctor before starting a program of exercise.

Finally, a word should be said about the effects of emotion on muscular disease, particularly in the case of such muscle-cramping disorders as torticollis. There is no direct one-to-one relationship between anxiety and emotional tension on one hand and aching muscles on the other. There is, in fact, almost always some physical stimulus that triggers these conditions; but often there is also a strong element of emotional stress and tension involved. This is seen most clearly in people who suffer recurrent episodes of muscle aching or stiff neck while under emotional pressure on the job or at home, and who find that the condition clears up almost miraculously the moment the pressure is eased. For some people, aching muscles appear to be the "target organ" for the release of tension, much as the stomach or duodenum are for individuals who suffer from peptic ulcer.

Rarely do local or generalized muscle aches prove as totally disabling as ulcer disease or other emotion-related illnesses, but they can be a chronic annoyance and often respond remarkably well to a deliberate effort to tone down the degree of emotional tension in the victim's life. Various drugs are also available to help safely decompress emotional strain—the tranquilizers in particular—but use of these drugs should be undertaken only under a doctor's direction. As in so many other cases, tranquilizers alone are not likely to do the job, but used in the proper dosage at the proper time, they can be an enormous help in breaking a vicious cycle of tension and myositis which has become a chronic and recurrent problem.

Tendonitis or Tenosynovitis. Tendons too can suffer from overexertion, trauma or other injury, which may result in a strain, or just in swelling, soreness, stiffness and impaired motion of the extremities the tendons help control. Tendonitis is an inflammation involving the tendons alone; tenosynovitis involves both the tendons themselves and the normally smooth, slippery *synovial membrane* which forms connective tissue sheaths through which the tendons move. Both are very common overuse or overexertion disorders. Tenosynovitis causes swelling of both the tendon and the synovial sheath around it, creating friction in an area that is supposed to be friction-free. Motion of the tendon in its sheath under these circumstances can become very painful. In tenosynovitis of the wrist, for example, friction may become so great that one can sometimes actually hear the moving tendon emit an audible squeaking sound when the fingers are flexed or extended. In extreme cases the pain and swelling in the wrist may be so marked that use of the hand is severely limited.

When the cause of the tendonitis is known, and when the pain and disability are mild, self-treatment with hot water soaks to reduce the swelling and aspirin for pain may be all that is needed. Rest for the injured area is also essential, and if the arm and wrist are affected, they can be held in a sling or immobilized for a few days with a splint. If the inflammation is severe,

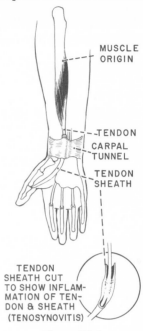

MUSCLE ORIGIN

TENDON
CARPAL TUNNEL

TENDON SHEATH

TENDON SHEATH CUT TO SHOW INFLAMMATION OF TENDON & SHEATH (TENOSYNOVITIS)

Figure 26–3.

however, or fails to respond to these simple measures, a doctor should be consulted. He may administer some form of cortisone to speed healing because of the powerful anti-inflammatory properties of this medicine. It can be very dangerous to ignore a tendonitis or to persist in using the painful limb; enough *fibrin* (a sticky inflammatory exudate) may form in the vicinity of the tendon to anchor it firmly down in its sheath, so that full range of movement becomes impossible. When this happens, surgical intervention may be necessary to free the tendon, a procedure which is far from satisfactory because it can in itself produce still more inflammation in the area. It is far wiser to allow sufficient time for the tendonitis to heal before using the affected tendon further.

Ganglion. Another common disorder of the tendons—or more accurately, of the synovial sheath through which the tendon runs—is the so-called *ganglion,* an outpouching of the tendon sheath which forms a fluid-filled lump, most commonly found at the inner surface of the wrist. (A similar disorder that appears at the back of the knee is spoken of as a *Baker's cyst*.)

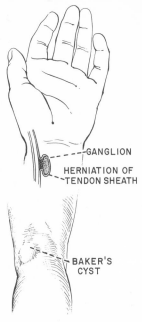

GANGLION

HERNIATION OF TENDON SHEATH

BAKER'S CYST

Figure 26–4.

Although ganglions are more of a nuisance than anything else, and are only rarely painful, people have long been fascinated by them, and an amazing folklore has arisen about their treatment. One favorite old wives' remedy for a ganglion was to hit it hard with the family Bible, thus rupturing the fluid-filled bubble in the hope, seldom realized, that it would heal without recurrence. Today a ganglion can sometimes be reduced in size simply by draining it by means of a needle, injecting a small amount of cortisone to avoid inflammation and then immobilizing the area, with pressure, for a few days to permit healing. This procedure is seldom permanently effective, however, and in most cases when a ganglion is causing symptoms or is in the way, it should be removed surgically, so that the defect in the tendon sheath can be sewed up. This procedure is quite successful in correcting the disorder, with little distress or complication for the patient.

The Major Muscle Disorders

Minor disorders of muscle and tendon may be temporarily painful, and may lead to brief periods of partial physical limitation, but they rarely result in serious or prolonged disability. There are, however, three major diseases of skeletal muscle that are indeed grave afflictions. These disorders—muscular dystrophy, myasthenia gravis and dermatomyositis—are basically very different from one another, but they have certain things in common. All three are long-term, progressive, chronically debilitating diseases which primarily involve skeletal muscle, all three arise from unknown causes, all three are considered incurable, and all three are comparatively rare. But even though no cures are known today, all three can often be controlled to a greater or lesser extent by the use of modern medicines, once the diagnosis is made, so that many victims of these diseases now can lead relatively long and productive lives.

Progressive Muscular Dystrophy. A hereditary disease, muscular dystrophy is somewhat more common in men than in women. It is characterized by a progressive shrinking or wasting of skeletal muscle, with progressive weakness as the diseased muscle deteriorates. In most cases it has its onset at some time during childhood or adolescence, and although only certain groups of muscles seem to be affected in the beginning, ultimately virtually all of the muscles of the body become involved. Sometimes the disease begins so slowly and insidiously that months or even years may elapse before the symptoms are recognized as serious. In other cases, the disability develops much more rapidly, particularly when the onset is during childhood.

When muscular dystrophy manifests itself in early childhood, many skeletal muscles seem to become involved in rapid succession, and the first symptom, which may appear before the age of five, is the child's increasing difficulty in climbing stairs, running, or standing erect from a sitting or lying position. Also at this early age, a degree of apparent hypertrophy or enlargement of certain muscle groups due to edema is often noted, particularly those in the lower legs, and there is a marked discrepancy between the apparently enlarged muscle and its clearly impaired strength. Contractures begin to develop in the leg, owing to degeneration of some muscle fibers while opposing muscle fibers remain relatively unimpaired. At first running and climbing, then walking, become more and more limited. Use of the knees and hips is impaired, and pronounced curvature of the spine may appear due to weakness of some of the back and hip muscles while others remain active. There may also be considerable weakness of muscle in the upper extremities.

This early-appearing form of muscular dystrophy usually runs a rapid course; the child becomes so infirm that he is confined to a wheelchair within a matter of two or three years, and rarely survives through adolescence, with death usually due to respiratory muscle weakness and aspiration pneumonia or other respiratory infection. It is thought that the generalized muscular weakness and the inability to cough effectively account for this kind of terminus to the disease.

Many victims are more fortunate. When the disease does not appear until adolescence or early adulthood, it tends to follow a much less fulminating course. Often in these victims the first symptoms involve weakness of the facial muscles, sometimes only on a single side, so that one eyelid begins to droop. The victim's facial appearance changes gradually; his smile becomes asymmetrical and he may lose the ability to whistle. Presently the muscles of the back, shoulder and upper arm are affected, and ultimately the disease progressively involves more and more muscles. In this later-appearing form of the disorder, however, the patient may remain ambulatory (that is, able to walk about with or without the aid of canes or crutches) for as long as two or three decades before becoming confined to a wheelchair. Still another form of the disease seems to affect first the muscles of the upper arms and shoulder girdle or pelvic girdle, and then progresses even more slowly, but the end result is the same slow wasting and weakness of all muscle groups.

There is no treatment of muscular dystrophy that is particularly effective. With afflicted children physical therapy may help maintain the function of wasting muscles and avoid the twist-ing and crippling effects of contractures for a while, but this has only a limited amount of value. It does not appear to have any long-term influence on the progress of the disease, although it does succeed, in many cases, in postponing the development of contracture deformities and giving the child a few more months or years of ambulation and independence of physical activity before the disease disables him completely. In older patients, physical therapy may be considerably more beneficial, often enabling the victim to continue normal activities for a significantly longer period.

There is no known cause, although heredity is clearly a factor; almost half of all victims of muscular dystrophy have had other members of their families similarly afflicted. Extensive medical research is currently under way in an attempt to discover exactly what happens in the muscle cells that leads to the degeneration, wasting and ultimate destruction of muscle tissue. Many investigators believe that some basic biochemical flaw must be a contributing factor, but so far this theory has not been verified. It is hoped that researchers will ultimately discover the cause or causes of the disease and then find specific drugs or other measures to prevent or limit its effects. In the meantime, society has rallied splendidly to support this research through private donations to such foundations as the Muscular Dystrophy Association of America and other organizations devoted to aiding the tragic victims of this disease.

Myasthenia Gravis. From its name, which literally means "serious weakness or debility of muscle," one might think that myasthenia gravis is similar to muscular dystrophy. Actually, it is quite a different disease, and in many ways more mysterious, even though more is known about its cause and far more hope lies in current treatment. Myasthenia gravis involves little of the deterioration and wasting of muscle fiber seen in muscular dystrophy, but it is characterized by marked fatigability and weakness of various groups of muscles which become progressively worse as the muscles are repeatedly used. There appears to be a breakdown in the chain of biochemical reactions by which the motor nerve impulses are transmitted from the nerve ending in the muscle cell to the muscle itself. Under normal circumstances the nerve impulse is transmitted to the muscle cell by means of an instantaneous chemical change which triggers the muscle response and causes the muscle fiber to contract. Then, in order for the muscle fiber to respond to another stimulus and contract again, there is a split-second resting period in which the chemical reaction carrying the nerve impulse across the bridge from nerve to muscle is reversed by the action of certain enzymes in the muscle cell itself. In myasthenia gravis, this "recovery phase" after muscle contraction is gravely impaired and slowed down, so that the next time the motor impulse comes to the muscle it cannot respond as quickly. Gradually the muscle seems to "run down" much the same as a worn-out automobile battery that is not being properly recharged. The result is that various groups of muscles are unable to carry on repeated activity and seem to "wear out" far more quickly than normal.

The first symptoms of myasthenia gravis usually arise from weakness of muscles powered by the cranial nerves. One of the most common early symptoms is *ptosis*—drooping of the eyelids—which gives the victim a deceptively sleepy appearance. Weakness of the muscles that move the eye in its socket also frequently leads to periods of *strabismus* (turning in or out of one or both of the eyes) and *diplopia* (double vision). Often the muscles of the palate and tongue are affected, causing a marked change in the victim's speech, and a tendency to regurgitate food up into the nose when attempting to swallow it. Actual difficulty in chewing and swallowing food, particularly large pieces, is another common early symptom. Then, gradually, other muscles of the body, especially the respiratory muscles and muscles of the shoulders, neck and trunk, become weaker. The day-to-day pattern of symptoms is often highly variable; one day of marked muscle weakness may be followed by another in which the muscle appears to function perfectly normally—an important clue to diagnosis. The weakness of the muscles often becomes more evident late in the day, but after a spell of severity many or all of the symptoms may disappear spontaneously for days,

weeks or months at a time. Even when they seem to clear up, however, there is usually some residual muscle weakness, and careful testing and measuring of muscle strength with repetitive electrical stimulation often helps seal the diagnosis. Perhaps the most dramatic diagnostic test used in identifying this disease lies in the fact that certain drugs help restore muscle strength quite dramatically for short periods of time. When these drugs are administered to a patient as a therapeutic trial, sudden temporary reversal of the symptoms is an extremely good indication that myasthenia gravis is present.

The same drugs that are used in diagnostic tests can be administered on a regular basis to help control the symptoms and temporarily restore near-normal muscle strength. In fact, three or four different drugs, all with similar actions, may be used, either alone or in combination. None is entirely satisfactory, since the ones that relieve symptoms for the longest period tend to be the most toxic and have undesirable side effects, while the less toxic drugs are also less effective and must be administered more frequently. When the more toxic drugs are used, other medicines must often be taken solely to counteract side effects. In most cases, however, careful observation of the symptoms in relation to the amount of medicine taken makes it possible to obtain good general control of the disease symptoms and allows the victim to live a comparatively normal life.

No one knows exactly why this odd biochemical defect occurs. It does not seem to be related to heredity. Generally it first appears during the young adult years, although occasionally children are affected. There is some reason to think that myasthenia gravis may actually be, basically, a disturbance of endocrine gland function of some sort. For one thing, almost a quarter of its victims are found to have some abnormal enlargement of the thymus, the glandular structure that lies at the base of the throat in babies and seems to have some role in the development of immune responses in the baby's body during the early years of life. The thymus gland usually shrinks away in size and activity almost completely by early adolescence, and the fact that it seems to persist in so many people suffering myasthenia gravis suggests that it may in some way be connected with that disease. In addition, surgical removal of the thymus gland has been found to relieve many victims of myasthenia gravis quite markedly, especially when this little-understood gland is found to be enlarged or affected by benign tumorous growth. But anesthesia is extremely risky in these patients, and such surgery has so high a mortality rate—as many as 4 percent fail to recover—that it cannot be considered an ideal form of treatment. Equally peculiar is the relatively high proportion of victims, some 25 percent, who suffer the onset of the disease during or immediately after an episode of increased or toxic thyroid gland activity. Finally, approximately 25 percent of all its victims seem to undergo complete spontaneous remission of the disease without recurrence, again for reasons unknown.

The main dangers of myasthenia gravis arise from weakness of swallowing function so severe that the victim cannot eat well, or tends to aspirate food into the trachea, and from weakness of respiratory muscles which makes it difficult to cough mucus or other secretions up out of the bronchial tubes. Most fatalities from the disease, in fact, occur from aspiration pneumonia, stasis pneumonia or suffocation due to clogging of the air passages with mucus. Usually, however, treatment with available medicines helps minimize the risk of these complications for prolonged periods, sometimes for years, and with so many clues to follow there is at least reason to hope that one day its cause will be discovered, and means found to prevent or completely cure it.

Dermatomyositis. This disorder, also fortunately quite rare, is one of the family of inflammatory diseases known as collagen diseases because they are characterized by breakdown of collagen or connective tissue throughout the body. (Acute rheumatic fever, lupus erythematosus and rheumatoid arthritis are other diseases in this family.) Connective tissue provides the vital function of binding all the other tissues and organ systems of the body together, including muscles, bones and joints. In this particular disease, inflammation primarily affects connective tissue in the skin and damages voluntary muscles. There is some evidence that dermatomyositis may appear following recovery from an acute streptococcus infection, as is the case with rheumatic fever, but so far no direct one-to-one relationship has been found, and we still must consider the cause of the disease to be unknown.

A prominent feature of dermatomyositis is widespread weakening and degeneration of muscle tissue, but unlike the painless degeneration found in muscular dystrophy or the painless weakness in myasthenia gravis, the onset of dermatomyositis is characterized by very painful and sometimes agonizing swelling and soreness of various muscle groups, combined with redness and swelling of the skin, particularly about the eyes, on the face or over the affected muscles. The disease may start abruptly with fever, painful muscle swelling and even prostration; or it may come on more slowly with vague muscular weakness and a soreness or stiffness similar to the "aching muscles" of simple overuse myositis, except that it doesn't clear up spontaneously after a day or two of rest. Any or all voluntary muscles may be affected, and in severe fulminating cases even the heart muscle may become involved. Indeed, in very acute cases death may ensue within a few weeks or months as a result of severe congestive heart failure that resists all measures to correct it.

Most often, however, the course of the disease is much more chronic and highly variable. As with myasthenia gravis, it seems to wax and wane. But in dermatomyositis permanent damage and scarring in muscle tissue results from each acute recurrence, and this progressive damage leads to continuous permanent weakening of the muscle. In some cases, after a period of time, the disease seems to "give up" and disappear, followed by complete and permanent recovery in which unaffected muscle is able to compensate fully for the damage that has been done. But more commonly the victim suffers recurring waves of acute activity up to a certain level of uncorrectable involvement. Then the disease becomes more or less stationary for years. One of the main problems in this long-term and chronic form of the disease is that weakness in some muscles which does not occur in opposing muscles can cause crippling contractures unless great care is taken to keep the weakened muscles active and as strong as possible by using moist heat and such physical therapy measures as gentle passive exercise. Because the pain of dermatomyositis may be recurrent and agonizing, powerful painkillers are sometimes needed, and there is real danger that the chronic victim may become dependent or addicted to antipain medications.

As soon as the powerful anti-inflammatory action of the cortisone-like hormones was discovered, these and other anti-inflammatory drugs were tried in the treatment of dermatomyositis. Frequently these have proven very helpful in reducing inflammation, pain and swelling in the muscles and skin so that there is less long-term disability due to scarring. But these measures are palliative rather than curative. Once the disease becomes entrenched, it is likely to remain active to some degree or other throughout the life of the victim. Fortunately there is hope that current studies of the body's immune mechanisms in relation to these collagen diseases may eventually result in a cure for dermatomyositis, or at least lead to more effective medications for treating it.

Other Muscle Diseases and Disorders

Certain other muscular disorders are either so minor that they deserve only passing mention or so rare that little need be said about them. Among the former are commonplace muscle *tics* and *tremors,* involuntary twitchings of skeletal muscle which may occur occasionally as a result of overuse of specific groups of muscles, or as a sign of generalized fatigue, but more often stem from nervous causes. (*See* p. 343.) At the other extreme are *muscle cancers,* serious indeed when they occur, but exceptionally rare, since muscle tissue is the least vulnerable of all body tissues to tumor growth. Benign muscle tumors, known as *myomas,* are noncancerous growths of fibrous muscle tissue which may arise anywhere, but occur most commonly in the uterine muscle of middle-aged women and are commonly known as "fibroids." (*See* p. 755.) Malignant tumors or cancers arising in muscle, bone or connective tissue are usually of a special variety known as

sarcomas, and rare as they are, they tend to be exceptionally fast-growing and invasive, often spreading out swiftly into surrounding tissues before their presence is even detected. Those arising from fibrous connective tissue such as tendon or ligament are called *fibrosarcomas;* those beginning in smooth muscle are *myosarcomas,* while rarest of all are the *rhabdomyosarcomas* developing in large skeletal muscles. Almost always these cancers are first suspected because of swelling, soreness and alteration in the normal function of the musculoskeletal tissue at the site of origin, and the best hope for recovery lies in wide or so-called radical surgical excision, not only of the cancer itself but of any surrounding or adjacent tissue that may have been seeded by cancer cells. (*See* p. 938.) Far more common, although less dangerous, is *trichiniasis* (more familiarly known as *trichinosis*), an infestation of skeletal muscle by the *Trichinella* roundworm that is frequently acquired by eating infested, undercooked pork. (*See* p. 276.)

Finally, a number of major diseases causing malfunction of skeletal muscle are actually disorders that are primarily centered in other organ systems, even though symptoms and changes affecting muscle function may be more impressive or debilitating than any others. This is particularly true of certain diseases of the nervous system in which nerves—or portions of the brain—controlling muscle function are damaged or destroyed, so that the muscles they normally control cannot work properly. One familiar condition of this sort is *poliomyelitis,* a virus infection that can permanently destroy certain of the nerve cells in the spinal cord which control the movement of skeletal muscle. The muscle paralysis seen in polio is not primarily due to muscle disease; indeed, if the destroyed nerve cells could somehow be replaced before the muscles they controlled had atrophied and scarred, the affected muscles would soon recover. Unfortunately this does not happen, and this disease can result in permanent and irreparable muscle paralysis when infection has not been prevented by polio shots. (*See* p. 188.)

In another whole group of nervous system diseases, the fatty material that coats the nerve fibers supplying various skeletal muscles can degenerate, causing a sort of "short circuit" that prevents motor nerve impulses from getting through to the muscles. Most prominent of these disorders are *multiple sclerosis* and *amyotrophic lateral sclerosis,* both characterized by loss of skeletal muscle function. (*See* p. 371.) The kind of brain injury resulting in *cerebral palsy* also often causes marked malfunction of skeletal muscle owing to damage to various motor nerve centers in the brain. In many cases muscle function is so disturbed that permanent muscle con-

tractures develop; in other cases the victims are severely disabled due to inability to control the movement of voluntary muscle even though the muscle itself is perfectly healthy. (*See* p. 882.) Thus the physician, faced with any evidence of muscle disfunction in a patient, cannot categorically assume that a primary muscle disease is necessarily at fault. Careful physical examination and assessment of *all* the organ systems of the body may be necessary before the correct diagnosis can be made and appropriate treatment begun.

Fractures and Other Bone Disorders

It is sometimes difficult to think of bone as living tissue. It seems inert, it is obviously very hard, and it does not appear to change much in shape from day to day or year to year. Yet the bone structure of an infant compared to that of an adult is obvious proof that bone grows and changes. When a bone is broken, it is also capable of self-repair and regeneration, another proof that it is a living tissue. And anyone who has suffered from aches and pains in the bones or joints will certainly testify that bone is "alive." It is, in fact, one of the most specialized living tissues of the body. (*See* p. 26.) Like all other tissues, it is composed of living cells nourished by a capillary blood supply, and it is interrelated in structure and function to all the other tissues and organ systems of the body. And like other tissues it is also, unfortunately, subject to traumatic damage from accident or injury, to infection by pathogenic microorganisms, and to the abnormal and uncontrolled growth patterns of cancer. In addition, bone is capable of becoming *necrotic*—literally dying—even when other tissues around it remain living. Even so, the bone composing the human skeletal system is remarkably resistant to physical injury and disease and, given time, is remarkably adept at repairing damage when it does occur.

There are a number of terms, many of them familiar, that are normally used in medicine to describe the skeletal system and its disorders. We speak of the *long bones* of the arms and legs; the *short bones* that are found in the hands, fingers, feet and toes; the *flat bones* of the ribs, the skull or the pelvis; the chunky *vertebrae* that form the backbone or vertebral column; and the small, many-sided bones that form the articulating joints of the wrist and the ankle. Each of these bones is covered at the joint ends by a softer tissue known as *cartilage,* which has a smooth and glistening surface. In normal growth processes cartilage is the precursor tissue of bone, the substance in which new bone cells are formed and in which the growth of bone occurs as calcium is deposited in the cartilage matrix. An X-ray of a newborn baby reveals that a great deal of his skeleton is still cartilage; the full mature development of the bony skeleton is not completed until mid-adolescence. The cartilage at the bone ends also provides the smooth, slippery surface necessary for the movements of the joints which are bound in place by the tough, flexible *ligaments* and the fibrous connective tissue of the *joint capsule*. Bone and joints, powered by the muscles, work together to give the body both support and varying degrees of mobility. Thus a bone injury or infection that also involves a joint may be much more serious than damage to the bone alone.

The most frequent injury to bone is, of course, a break or *fracture*. The term *simple fracture* does not necessarily mean a painless or harmless one, but rather a fracture that has not broken skin and in which bone fragments are not shattered. An *open fracture* (previously called a "compound fracture") is one in which the bone fragments have actually pierced the skin and have thus become contaminated with bacteria. In a *comminuted fracture,* bone fragments are crushed so that there are a number of small pieces of bone at the site of the fracture rather than a clean break. Injuries involving both bone and joint include *dislocations,* in which the bone has been twisted or wrenched out of its normal joint position, and *sprains,* injuries that occur when the ligaments binding a joint (and sometimes special supporting cartilages as well) have been torn or wrenched. Finally, injuries to bone may also lead to *periosteal hemorrhage,* in which the *periosteum,* the thin, tough, fibrous coating of tissue that overlies the bone, rich in sensory nerve endings, has been bruised or scraped in such a fashion that bleeding has taken place. When this occurs, the periosteum may be separated from the bone to which it normally adheres tightly—a condition that can be extremely painful.

Common Fractures

Virtually every bone in the body, even the tiny hyoid bone that lies at the base of the tongue, is vulnerable to fracture, usually in connection with some kind of trauma or accidental injury. Bones are constructed to withstand the stresses and strains of normal movement; they are even surprisingly resilient to many abnormal movements and shocks. But sometimes a fall, a sudden blow or even an apparently minor twist may result in a fracture. Certain kinds of common fractures are, in fact, often associated with specific accidents and injuries.

Fractures of the Long Bones. These fractures may involve one or both of the bones in the forearm, the humerus in the upper arm, the bones of the lower leg, or the femur or thighbone of the upper leg. Fractures of both the forearm and the upper arm occur commonly as the result of a blow or fall. Fractures of the lower leg are particularly common among skiers, who are often victims of a twisting fall at the same time that their weight is borne on the leg. A fracture of the thighbone is much less common; it is an extremely strong and thick bone, and is usually broken only in a very severe highway accident or when a heavy person takes a fall on the stairs. In older people, whose bones have

become brittle with age, fractures of the upper end of the thighbone occur more frequently and are often referred to as a "broken hip." Such an injury can present grave problems to an older

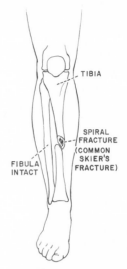

Figure 27–1.

patient not only because of the length of time required to heal the fracture but also because long periods of immobility may leave him vulnerable to pneumonia and other complications. Another danger is the possibility that the thighbone may be fractured in such a way that the blood supply to the ball-shaped femoral head is impaired or cut off, an occurrence which can result in the necrosis or tissue death of the femoral head and lead to permanent crippling of the hip joint. Fortunately, modern orthopedic surgery has developed a variety of means to aid in the quick recovery of elderly patients, as well as to restore by mechanical means at least partial function of hip joints that have been irreparably damaged.

Fractures of the long bones may vary all the way from simple cracks or through-and-through breaks to badly smashed, compacted or multiple fractures. Especially dangerous is *any* long bone fracture in which the break in the bone involves a joint such as the knee, hip or elbow. Such fractures are difficult to set properly; they also heal slowly and always threaten some degree of permanent limitation of function of the involved joint. Of all physicians, the orthopedic surgeon or "orthopedist" is best equipped with the special training and skill needed to treat these complicated fractures successfully, and usually an

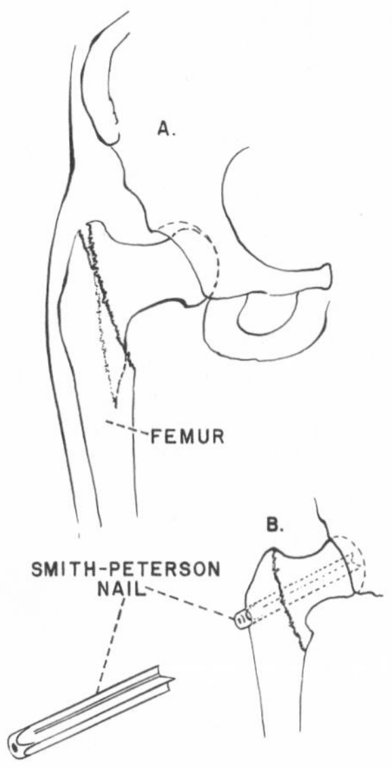

Occasionally one or more of the *carpal bones* —the small bones that make wrist movement possible—may be fractured without any injury to the long bones of the forearm. Such fractures

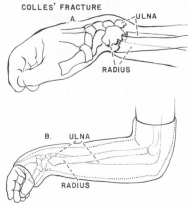

Figure 27–2.
A. Fracture of the femur near ball joint.
B. One means of correcting ball-joint fracture.

orthopedist is at least called in consultation in such cases.

Wrist Fractures. The most common fracture in the wrist is the Colles' fracture, which is usually sustained when a person falls hard on an outstretched hand. The impact breaks the wrist end of one or both of the long bones of the forearm and displaces them in relation to the several small carpal bones of the wrist itself, leaving the hand cocked backward on the wrist to form the so-called silver fork deformity. This particular kind of fracture must be treated with expertise, and the physician must make very sure that the forearm and the wrist bones are returned to their normal position and then held there (often very difficult to accomplish) until healing takes place, so that full functional use of this very important joint may be regained. Even under the most ideal circumstances, a Colles' fracture frequently leaves some degree of permanent limitation of wrist motion.

Figure 27–3.

are just as serious as Colles' fractures and, unless allowed to heal in almost perfect position, may lead to permanent impairment of wrist function. Even after healing, a long period of physical therapy may be necessary in order to recover full wrist motion.

Fractured Fingers. Although relatively uncommon, fractures involving the fingers, or the metacarpal bones of the back of the hand, present special problems because improper healing can often seriously impair the capacity for fine and delicate movement that is so important in the hand. Few people realize how greatly we depend upon the perfect sensory and motor control we have of our hands until some impairment occurs. Aside from actual loss of function, a badly healed finger fracture may also leave the finger stiff or out of proper position so that it is far more vulnerable to future accidents. Fractures of the fingers and the hand usually occur as a result of a direct blow or trauma—hitting a finger with a hammer, for example—or from crushing injuries like catching a hand in a car door. Fractures or dislocations (or both) of fingers also happen so often as a result of catching a baseball without the protection of a mitt that the typical deformity—a finger joint dislocated in the direction of the back of the hand—is commonly spoken of as "baseball finger." It is important that *no* injury of the hand which might have resulted in a fracture be ignored. Have a doctor see it and X-ray it to rule out the possibility of a fracture that could lead to long-term distress if not properly treated.

Skull Fracture. Always dangerous because of the extreme delicacy of the brain structure inside, skull fractures are commonly sustained as a result of unprotected falls, automobile accidents or sharp blows to the head. Special dangers include an undetected *depressed fracture* of the skull, in which a fractured bony plate is dented inward and exerts pressure on a part of the brain; a *comminuted fracture* in which sharp skull fragments actually penetrate brain tissue; and the threat of internal bleeding due to a fracture, in which a gathering of clotted blood or *hematoma* may cause undue pressure on the brain. Any head injury severe enough for the victim to lose consciousness even momentarily should be checked out with a doctor, as should any symptoms occurring a few hours later, such as difficulty with vision, persisting headache, excessive drowsiness or fainting. Often the very same symptoms may result from a *concussion,* a jarring injury to the brain itself which can arise from any sudden blow to the head, whether a fracture is sustained or not. (*See* p. 358.) In either case a doctor's attention is imperative, and only X-rays can rule out the presence of a fracture.

Fracture of the Jaw. Usually the result of a blow, a jaw fracture is often more of a nuisance than a threat, since the jaw is very difficult to immobilize for bone healing without also limiting or preventing two of our most popular activities—talking and eating. It should always be remembered that a blow hard enough to fracture the jaw is also hard enough to cause a concussion injury to the brain. Thus the importance of consulting a doctor about *any* head injury other than the most minor.

Rib Fractures. One or several broken ribs quite commonly result from automobile collisions, falls, crushing injuries, or even from an overexuberant embrace. A rib fracture must always be carefully observed for any evidence of damage to the underlying lung, and fractured ribs are often very painful because there is no effective way to immobilize one side of the rib cage and protect it from the pressure changes and motion of breathing. Ribs also may seem to take an inordinate amount of time to heal. It is not uncommon for the pain of a broken rib to persist for months after the injury, even when the rib itself is healing well, because of irritation of the sensitive pleural membrane that lies beneath the ribs. Fracture of ribs on both sides simultaneously presents an especially threatening situation known as "flail chest" in which the normal pressure dynamics based upon a semi-rigid rib cage that enables us to fill our lungs with air are thrown awry. This kind of injury requires expert medical care as early as possible and in some cases may require mechanical respiratory support until the fractured bones begin to stick and heal. When the fracture has caused actual damage to lung tissue, a much more serious condition exists which also requires expert medical attention, since impairment of breathing or serious respiratory complications may result. (*See* p. 128.)

Broken Collarbone. This is a common injury in all the body-contact sports and may also result from a collision or a fall. Fortunately, this kind of fracture is usually quite easy to treat by means of a simple dressing designed to pull both

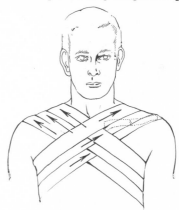

Figure 27–4.
Dressing for fractured collarbone.

shoulders back, thus realigning the collarbone in its normal position, and it heals rather quickly without undue pain or discomfort. (*See* Fig. 27–4.)

Broken Neck or Spine. Always dangerous, sometimes tragically so, any fracture involving the vertebrae in the neck or the back requires expert medical, orthopedic or even neurosurgical attention *from the moment of injury,* if possible, even *before* the victim is moved. Neck fractures all too commonly occur as a result of diving accidents in swimming pools, lakes or streams when the diver strikes his head on the bottom or against some submerged object. And in recent years, with the increasing use of the trampoline as a piece of gymnastic equipment, many tragic neck fractures have been sustained by untrained, or even trained, performers who lose control. Fractures of the lower vertebrae occur as a result of automobile accidents, falls or any massive body trauma. Any vertebral fracture is serious in itself because it damages the body's major up-

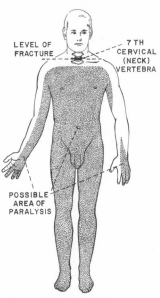

FRACTURED VERTEBRA = DANGER OF PARALYSIS BELOW FRACTURE LINE

LEVEL OF FRACTURE

7 TH CERVICAL (NECK) VERTEBRA

POSSIBLE AREA OF PARALYSIS

Figure 27–5A.

right supporting member. But the overriding danger of such fractures is possible injury to the spinal cord and/or spinal nerves which are encased in the vertebral column. A shattered or cracked vertebra may pinch or even sever the

delicate tissues of these vital nerves, causing partial or almost complete paralysis and in some cases even death. All too often this additional injury occurs *after* the accident that caused the

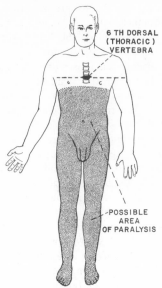

6 TH DORSAL (THORACIC) VERTEBRA

POSSIBLE AREA OF PARALYSIS

Figure 27–5B.

fracture, usually as a result of well-meaning but clumsy attempts to move the victim. If a neck or back fracture is even remotely suspected, medical aid should be summoned immediately and the victim should be moved *only* under medical supervision. These two simple measures may very well prevent serious neurological complications. (*See* p. 356.) If the victim *must* be moved before medical help arrives, it is imperative that it be done in such a way that the neck and spine are kept as motionless as possible. (*See* p. 128.)

Fractured Pelvis. This is a relatively uncommon injury because of the great thickness and strength of the bones that form the pelvic girdle—the "saddle bone" of the skeleton. Usually such fractures occur only in cases of a fall from a considerable height, or some gross trauma such as an automobile accident or a gunshot wound. When they do occur, the victim should not attempt to stand or walk, although the pain is usually great enough to discourage movement. The main danger is the possibility that abnormal movement of the fracture fragments may tear or transect the urethra, the tube through which urine is emptied from the bladder. Thus one of the first concerns of the physician is to obtain a urine specimen to check for evidence of blood. If the urethra has been damaged, surgery to repair it may be necessary as soon after the injury as possible.

Ankle and Foot Fractures. Simple fractures of the ankle or foot bones often fall in the "nuisance" category and are difficult to treat largely because it is hard to immobilize an active person long enough for these thick, tough, weight-bearing bones to heal properly. The ankle and foot are not as delicate as the wrist and fingers, but they are essential for mobility and balance, and not even a broken toe should be ignored or treated lightly. Improper healing of the ankle, in particular, can seriously impede its function. However, time, patience and proper immobilization and care are usually all it takes to heal even a serious break.

Recognizing Fractures

Any broken bone represents a potential threat to the body unless it is promptly diagnosed and properly treated. A broken bone impairs both the structural support and the normal motion of the body, and any movement of fractured bone fragments before the bone has knit may slow down the healing process significantly or even prevent it altogether. This is a special danger if the fracture involves a joint surface in any way. Thus it is foolish to ignore a possible fracture or to delay obtaining accurate diagnosis and treatment. Almost any kind of twisting or wrenching injury, fall or blow to the body may cause a fracture, but even apparently minor accidents can result in broken bones. Any time you encounter one or more of the following symptoms, a fracture may be present.

Pain and swelling in the injured area. The periosteum, the sensitive layer of fibrous tissue overlying bone, causes very severe pain when it is torn or even bruised. Thus most fractured bones are painful, especially upon motion of the injured area, and even if the fracture is only a crack, some bleeding underneath the periosteum will stretch this sensitive tissue and make it hurt. Furthermore, an accident sufficient to break bone will usually cause injury to adjacent muscle, tendon or ligament in the same area, with bleeding into the tissue, often with marked swelling and the appearance of massive bruises. Less serious injuries like sprains and strains may also cause pain and swelling, but a fracture should always be suspected until X-rays can be taken to rule it out.

Limitation of motion. Any injury which makes even minor motions of the body difficult or painful should be speedily checked out for a possible fracture. Difficulty in breathing, for example, may indicate a broken rib, since the muscles of the chest contract to guard or "splint" the fracture from painful motion.

"I felt something snap." Very frequently an accident victim will feel something "snap" or "give." Some even insist they hear a noise—and in the case of a fracture of a large bone, this is entirely possible. Occasionally a sprain or dislocation will create a similar sensation, but again X-rays should be taken to rule out a fracture.

Shortening or distortion of a limb. This is perhaps the most convincing clue of all. When a long bone in the arm or leg, for example, is broken, muscles in the area tend to cramp or contract, often resulting in a shortening of the limb, or an obviously abnormal angulation. Any limb that shows signs of distortion in its length or shape should immediately be protected from movement or weight-bearing, and it should be assumed that a fracture has occurred until proven otherwise. In addition, any motion of an extremity *except* the normal motion of a joint signals trouble. Such "false motion" will usually be extremely painful, and the victim may even be aware of a grating sensation. Moving broken bones even slightly can cause severe damage to muscles, blood vessels or nerves in the area, compounding the injury and slowing up the healing process. Thus it is important in any case of suspected fracture to guard the injured member from any motion at all, if possible, until it can be immobilized by adequate splinting or a plaster cast.

Diagnosing Fractures

Today we depend heavily on the use of X-rays to help identify fractures and plan appropriate treatment. But even the X-ray is not infallible; a crack-fracture of a bone, for example, may not show up at all on an X-ray film immediately after the injury. In such cases, it is sometimes necessary to wait long enough—perhaps a week to ten days—for the first steps in the process of bone healing to begin before a distinct fracture line can be seen on X-ray. But even when a fracture line cannot be seen at first, continuing pain in the region should suggest that a fracture may indeed be present even though as yet invisible. Your doctor will use his best judgment, and may well treat an injury "expectantly"—as if a fracture were present—until he can X-ray again some days later and satisfy himself that no bone injury exists.

How Fractures Are Treated

Since most fractures are the result of sudden and unexpected accidents, the initial steps in treatment are usually the first-aid measures taken at the scene. These measures are discussed in detail elsewhere. (*See* p. 128.) Here it is necessary only to review briefly the proper procedures. In cases of minor fractures where the victim can be safely moved, the injured part should be immobilized, by splinting if necessary, and the victim taken to a doctor. In cases of major injuries, the steps necessary to control hemorrhage and to deal with asphyxiation, heart arrest or shock must be taken first, and then the injured part, or the victim himself if necessary, must be immobilized until medical help arrives. *Do not attempt to apply traction or "set" the fractured bone*. Those are jobs for a physician, or for someone specially trained in first-aid procedures.

Doctors plan the treatment of a fracture according to many factors: the extent of the injury, the nature of the fracture (that is, whether it is simple, comminuted or crushed, or open), the position of the bone fragments, the age of the patient, the necessity of early mobilization, and so forth. But the basic principles in treating any fracture, from the most minor to the most massive, arise directly from the slow and curious manner in which damaged bone tissue heals. The process actually begins at the moment of the injury when bleeding at the fracture site forms a clot of blood or hematoma around the broken ends of the bone. During the first week or ten days, a sort of "reverse healing process" goes on in which the calcium salts from the fractured ends of the bone are partially reabsorbed into the blood stream. At the same time, delicate fibrils of connective tissue begin to grow through the hematoma, bridging the fractured edges of the bone, followed by the growth of a large quantity of fibrous tissue across the fracture line. This process continues for some two to three weeks. It is only at the end of that time that the fractured bone ends become even lightly stuck or "glued" together, and any movement of the bone fragments prior to this can easily tear this tenuous, sticky new fibrous tissue, forcing the body

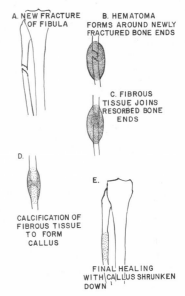

Figure 27–6.

to start producing it all over again. Even at this point the fibrous rejoining of broken bone ends is rubbery and flexible, so that good positioning of the fragments can still be lost by inadvertent movement.

Then some six weeks to two months following

the fracture, depending upon the age of the patient (the speed of this healing process tends to decline as the body grows older), the original fibrous tissue bridge between the broken bone ends is gradually strengthened and hardened by the slow deposit of calcium compounds along the fibrous strands of the bridge. At the end of this time the fracture fragments are usually "glued" quite firmly in place. As the calcium is deposited, it forms a wide area of calcification or *callus* around the fracture. Finally, the callus slowly shrinks into normal new bone bridging the fracture line, often resulting in a union that is slightly thicker and stronger than the original bone itself. If the fragments of bone are in good position when this healing process begins and remain in good position, without motion, until callus forms, full strength will be restored to the broken bone, and after a period of some months or years it may actually be impossible to detect the fracture site with X-rays.

Obviously, then, the most important principle in the doctor's treatment of a fracture is complete immobilization of the fractured area for long enough for this slow healing process to be completed. Any motion of the injured bone will either retard the healing or cause such an overgrowth of fibrous tissue and callus that permanent distortion of the fractured limb may result. In extreme cases of motion at the fracture site, the fracture may not heal together at all, but may form a fibrous "false joint" which seriously impairs the strength and function of the region and may necessitate repeated surgery and bone grafting before healing takes place.

When the fracture is a simple crack, with no displacement of the fragments, this essential immobilization may be accomplished simply by applying a well-padded plaster cast and then waiting for the bone to heal. When the fractured bone is out of position, it must be "set" or *reduced* into normal anatomical position and then held there by means of a plaster cast. Often muscle spasm tends to draw the bone ends together, forcing them to "override" each other and shorten the limb. In such cases the doctor must use traction to pull the bone ends apart again before fixing them in position. Usually this kind of manipulation is best performed under

anesthesia, not only because of the pain involved, but because the anesthetic also helps relax the muscle spasm. If the fracture is closed (that is, if the skin has not been broken) and the bone has not been crushed, the doctor can often reduce the fracture and immobilize the region in a plaster cast without any surgical incision. Perfect positioning of the fracture fragments is not always possible, and in many fractures it is not even necessary as long as the *length* of the bone is maintained; the healing process will compensate remarkably for minor degrees of imperfection.

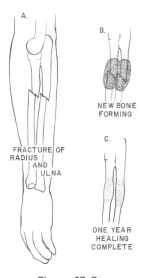

Figure 27–7.

Badly crushed fractures or fractures that have broken the skin pose a more difficult problem. When the skin has been broken, the surgeon must clean and debride the wound thoroughly, removing such debris as dirt and bits of clothing and excising damaged muscle and skin tissue before setting the fracture, in order to minimize the chance of serious bone infection. When the fractured bone has been crushed, an open or surgical reduction is often necessary. Through a surgical incision the surgeon can then apply metal plates, pins, screws or other devices to help hold the bone fragments in position. When the fracture involves a long bone of the thigh or upper arm, a narrow metal rod or "intramedullary nail" may be inserted in the hollow cavity of the bone shaft to accomplish this immobilization. All such surgical hardware is specially manufactured from stainless steel or other alloys which are biologically inert—that is, they undergo no chemical changes or reactions within the body—and thus in most cases can simply be left permanently in place after the fracture has healed.

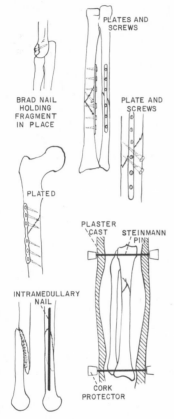

Figure 27–8.
Stainless steel hardware used in setting fractures.

Sometimes bone is so badly crushed or contaminated that part of it must be surgically removed. In such cases the surgeon may take fragments of healthy bone from such places as the upper margin of the pelvic bone, where a natural surplus exists, and use them as "bone grafts" in the injured region. These grafts help fill the gap between fractured bone ends and form a framework on which the bridge of fibrous tissue can form during healing. In most cases such bone grafts work best when taken from the fracture victim himself, but in recent years much experimental work has been done to store bone graft materials in "bone banks" from which they can be drawn for use as needed. Much work has also been done to develop successful artificial joints or so-called *joint prostheses* to partially or completely replace joints that have been irreparably damaged by fracture or disease. (*See* p. 309.) Finally, badly mangled limbs must sometimes be amputated, to be replaced with prosthetic or artificial limbs. But the days of clumsy "peg legs" and the single crude crutch of Long John Silver are gone forever; today the fitting and use of artificial limbs, when necessary, has been developed into a high art through years of research by leading orthopedic surgeons the world over.

Special kinds of fractures require special treatment procedures. Some fractures, for example, cannot be well immobilized and held in place either by means of plaster casts or by surgery; often the victims of such fractures must be kept in bed in the hospital while various external traction arrangements are applied to immobilize their fractures until the fragments have "glued" tightly enough to permit casting. Fractures of the vertebrae may require traction to hold the bones slightly apart and prevent damage to the spinal cord or spinal nerves by the sharp bone fragments. In skull fractures any bone fragments piercing underlying brain tissue, or pressing against it, must be surgically removed and replaced without pressure; sometimes a metal plate is substituted. Occasionally a fractured long bone which has slipped from proper position and then begun to heal must be reset. One hears of "rebreaking" bones in such cases, but this term is a bit overdramatic. Seldom is the misalignment allowed to remain so long that new bone has formed before the situation is corrected.

Because healing of fractures takes so long, medical scientists are constantly searching for new treatment techniques to speed healing and shorten convalescence. One such experimental technique, first reported in 1972, involves the application of low-voltage electric current across the healing fracture site and through adjoining tissues. Early reports indicate that such treatment has, for reasons that remain obscure, apparently brought about a marked increase in the speed of healing in certain fracture cases, and has been helpful in cases where normal fracture healing has failed. At this date it is still too early to evaluate just how useful, overall, such an approach to fracture treatment may be, but if early successes are confirmed during subsequent investigation, this may prove to be an extremely useful adjunct to more conservative methods of fracture treatment.

We think of orthopedic surgeons performing modern-day wonders in their handling of fractured bones, yet the basic principles of bonesetting have not really changed a great deal since ancient times. Archaeologists have unearthed skeletal remains many thousands of years old that show unmistakable evidence of well-healed fractures—fractures that could have healed that well only as a result of proper setting and immobilization at the time they occurred. What is more, recent studies of the techniques used by tribal witch doctors in central Africa today in dealing with many kinds of fractures reveal uncanny similarities to the techniques of our finest present-day orthopedists. These primitive physicians have never heard of plaster casts (they use thick coats of mud baked in the hot African sun) and their bonesetting procedures are very simple, but they obviously understand the basic fundamentals of bone healing.

Probably the single most useful adjunct to fracture treatment, and the hardest to come by, is simple patience. Fractures in general will take from three to six months or longer to heal completely, depending upon the size of the bone and the seriousness of the injury. Nothing is more foolish than to attempt to "speed things up" by using the injured part prematurely. The time devoted to allowing a bone to heal correctly is the best possible investment that can be made, since it will help prevent lasting pain and later disability.

Finally, there is the tedious but extremely important period of time necessary to recover full function of the injured part after bone healing is almost complete. Muscles in the area will have atrophied because of disuse and lost a great deal of their strength. Joints that have been immobilized will have stiffened. Even though the bone may have healed, the surrounding muscles and joints must gradually be brought back into use through a careful program of progressive movement and exercise until normal function has been regained. When this is not done, it is common for a great deal of swelling and pain to recur, signs that too much use may have been attempted too soon. Your doctor will outline a reasonable program for recovery of function, including guarding the injured area from overuse, using hot water soaks to improve circulation and reduce pain and swelling, and performing gradated exercises to help rebuild strength and mobility. All too many victims of fractures, particularly when joint surfaces are involved, never recover full function simply because they have been too impatient or did not recognize the importance of this period of "retraining" and "rebuilding" the injured area.

Of all the questions a physician hears from a fracture patient the most frequent is, "Will I get back full function?" In the majority of cases the answer will be a guarded "Yes—with luck, and if you stick with proper care." Unfortunately, certain fractures are prone to heal with some permanent limitation of function even when they are handled with the greatest of skill. Fractures of the elbow joint, the wrist, the shoulder or the hip, for example, are almost impossible to prognosticate. But these are generally recognized as difficult cases, and the family doctor will probably work with an orthopedic specialist to assure the best possible treatment. It cannot be emphasized too strongly, however, that the outcome of a fracture depends heavily upon the common sense and patience of the victim himself.

Dislocations and Sprains

The same types of injuries that cause fractures can also cause *dislocations,* in which one or more of the bones in a joint are torn or jarred loose from their normal moorings and moved completely out of place. Hip dislocations, for example, frequently occur in head-on automobile collisions when the victim, bracing himself instinctively against the impact, is hurled forward so that his knee jams into the dashboard, causing backward dislocation of the head of the femur from its socket in the hip. Virtually every joint in the body can be dislocated, sometimes by accident or injury, sometimes as the result of weakness in the joint caused by an earlier injury or anatomical defect, but the most common are dislocations of the hip, the shoulder, a finger joint or the knee. The jaw can actually be dislocated, on rare occasions, simply by yawning too widely.

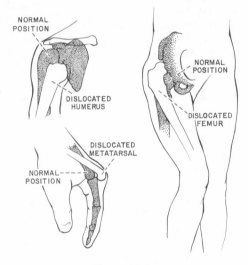

Figure 27–9.

Many people regard a dislocation as far less serious than a fracture because manipulation by the physician to reduce or replace the dislocated bone in its proper position is usually followed by immediate relief from pain and apparently normal function of the joint. However, when a bone is dislocated, the ligaments that hold it in place and the fibrous joint capsule that surrounds the joint and contains the sticky fluid that lubricates it are inevitably stretched and usually torn. Both must be allowed time to heal before the joint is returned to normal use if continuing pain, swelling, arthritic changes or even repeated dislocations are not to occur. Thus a dislocation should always be treated by a

doctor even if it "reduces itself," which occasionally happens, immediately after the accident. Sometimes the ruptured joint capsule must be repaired surgically, but even if this is not necessary, the joint should be immobilized long enough for healing to take place, and then use should be resumed on a gradual basis. There is also the danger that a dislocation may be accompanied by a fracture, and careful X-ray examination should be made both before the dislocation is reduced and afterward to confirm proper replacement of the bone and to rule out the possibility of chips of fractured bone remaining in the joint.

Sprains occur when the ligaments holding the joints together are stretched or torn. These injuries are generally less severe than dislocations, but still cause considerable pain, swelling and disability because they affect the function of a joint. Certain kinds of sprains—a severely sprained ankle, for example—often must be immobilized and treated with as much care as a fracture in order to allow time for adequate healing. X-rays should be taken to make sure that no fracture is present, and the doctor's instructions for treatment should be followed to the letter.

Osteomyelitis: The Scourge of Bone Infection

In this age of antibiotics and sulfa drugs, the vast majority of infections of the body tissues are far easier to control and far less threatening than they used to be. But one type of tissue infection that is still as dreaded as it ever was is infection of bone, known as osteomyelitis.

There are two reasons why this kind of infection is such a grave problem. First, most bone tissue is nourished by a very limited supply of blood, so that when a bone infection has started, it is hard to get sufficient quantities of antibiotic to the infected area, making eradication of the infection extremely difficult. Second, although bone tissue can repair and regenerate itself, the process is extremely slow and damage done to bone by infection may take months or years to heal. This is particularly true if some of the infection remains actively present throughout the period of healing so that there is both destruction and healing of bone going on at the same time. In practical terms, bone infection often means a prolonged illness, with the risk that it may do extensive damage before it can be eradicated completely to permit the bone to heal.

The bacteria causing bone infection are usually either a streptococcus or staphylococcus. More rarely, the infection may be caused by one of the Salmonella coliform organisms or by other bacteria that are present on the skin or in our environment but do not ordinarily succeed in mounting an invasion of the body. A staphylococcus bone infection is usually more dangerous than one caused by a streptococcus because so many of the varieties of staphylococci in existence today have become partially or completely insensitive to such antibiotics as penicillin or tetracycline. One common way in which infectious organisms reach the bone is through open fractures. However, it is also possible for bacteria to travel in the blood stream from some distant focus of infection in the body and become lodged in the marrow of one of the long bones, usually near one end. From there they may infect not only the bone but also the adjacent joint, and destroy the smooth cartilage necessary for joint movement, a serious complication of osteomyelitis.

Most cases of osteomyelitis first manifest themselves with the sudden occurrence of pain in the affected bone and a spiking fever. There may be considerable swelling and tenderness over the infected area, causing movement to be painful or even restricted. This evidence of acute infection is accompanied by a sharp increase in circulating white blood cells, and because of the symptoms a doctor is usually consulted early in the disease. This is fortunate, because successful treatment of osteomyelitis depends heavily upon striking at the invading organism with antibiotics as soon as possible. The danger of delay is easy to see: as the infection attacks bone tissue, the bone itself is killed in progressively greater amounts, and the antibiotic carried to the area by the blood stream cannot reach the dead bone. Ideally, osteomyelitis should be treated even before it can be seen in X-rays, since such evidence may not be visible for several weeks after the onset of infection. Other diagnostic studies are often helpful, however. Cultures of blood samples may contain the offending bacteria and make it possible to test them for sensitivity to various antibiotics. If a joint is involved, it may also be possible to withdraw a small amount of joint fluid for culture and sensitivity studies, and in some cases the infection will cause an abscess to form under the periosteum in the affected region so that incision and drainage are possible and the invading organism can be identified in laboratory tests.

Successful treatment of acute osteomyelitis depends upon finding an antibiotic that will attack the invading bacteria vigorously. But even if the organism is "immune" or not sensitive to the more commonly used antibiotics, certain others are held in reserve specifically for dangerous situations such as osteomyelitis. Thus under ideal circumstances—early symptoms, early diagnosis and effective antibiotic treatment—infection can frequently be stopped before it becomes well entrenched.

In some cases, however, the typical symptoms do not occur, or are overlooked, and the infection is well under way before it is discovered, destroying bone tissue at the same time the normal regenerative processes are trying to lay down new bone to replace it. This odd process may result in the formation of a *sequestrum*—a chunk of infected dead bone covered by thick layers of newly deposited living bone not yet attacked by the infection. This condition can be identified on X-ray films and surgery can be undertaken to remove it. The area of infected bone is laid open and the sequestrum is cut or scraped out to remove all actively infected bone tissue. Then antibiotic therapy is used following the surgery. In most cases even a chronic bone infection can eventually be eradicated in this way, but the illness may still be long and tedious. Many months are required for healing to take place, and frequent checkups are necessary to be sure that no pocket of infection remains.

One kind of osteomyelitis that presents unusual problems is *tuberculosis of the bone,* the invasion of bone by the tubercle bacillus, generally spread from a primary tuberculous infection located somewhere else, such as the lung. The peculiar danger of this kind of infection is that it may start slowly and silently, involving a bone or a joint in a smoldering, painless infection which may then proceed to extensive bone destruction before it is discovered, without the type of bony repair normally seen with other kinds of infection. One of the most frequent places for tuberculosis of the bone is in the vertebrae, and occasionally the first hints that the disease is present are the symptoms of pain and deformity when one or more of the vertebrae are so badly eroded by infection that they collapse. Before the advent of modern antibiotic treatment for tuberculosis, the damage done by this organism in the spine often resulted in a severe "hunchback" deformity known as Pott's disease. But today the disease is usually discovered and treated earlier, particularly if tuberculosis of the lung is present, and many of the grotesque deformities caused by tuberculosis are now seldom seen. Treatment with the anti-tuberculosis drugs, combined when necessary with surgical excision of destroyed bone and followed by fusion of healthy vertebral bone above and below the area, sometimes using bone graft, has proved very successful.

Unfortunately, this infection—like tuberculosis anywhere else in the body—may linger for years or even decades in an inactive state before flaring up. Once a person has suffered tuberculosis of the bone, it is necessary to check with faithful regularity to see that there is no evidence of recurrence, even when drug treatment is continued long after apparent recovery. And since tuberculosis of the bone can also appear without any known tuberculous infection being present elsewhere, it is imperative that a person seek medical attention any time there is some unexplained limitation of motion in a joint, some stiffness or limpness in the lower extremities, or a rigidity of the back that seems to appear for no detectable reason.

Bone Tumors

Although bone is normally a slow-growing tissue, it is, like other tissue, subject to the development of a number of different forms of "new growth" or *tumor,* both benign (noncancerous) and malignant (cancerous). Among the benign tumors, there are simple bone overgrowths called *osteomas* or bone cysts, and overgrowths of unusual cell types such as giant cell tumors that occur within bone but do not have calcium laid down in them, so that they appear as holes in the bone on X-ray. In some of these benign cysts there is no pain and the first clue that something may be wrong is the occurrence of a so-called *pathological fracture,* a fracture that occurs through a weakened area of bone in the absence of any accidental fall or blow. The discovery of any abnormal growth involving bone makes mandatory a thorough examination and surgical biopsy of the affected area, because there is no certain way to tell from X-rays whether the tumor is benign or malignant.

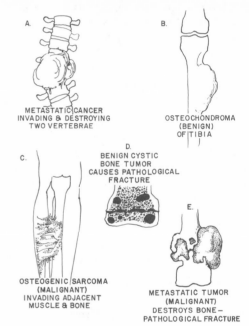

A. METASTATIC CANCER INVADING & DESTROYING TWO VERTEBRAE

B. OSTEOCHONDROMA (BENIGN) OF TIBIA

C. OSTEOGENIC SARCOMA (MALIGNANT) INVADING ADJACENT MUSCLE & BONE

D. BENIGN CYSTIC BONE TUMOR CAUSES PATHOLOGICAL FRACTURE

E. METASTATIC TUMOR (MALIGNANT)—DESTROYS BONE—PATHOLOGICAL FRACTURE

Figure 27–10.

Among the malignant tumors that affect bone, many are *secondary tumors* which develop from cancer cells thrown off by a primary cancer in some distant part of the body. These cells may become lodged in the capillaries of the bone or bone marrow and can then give rise to very painful secondary growths. Cancer of the breast and cancer of the prostate are among the most common offenders, frequently seeding multiple tumors in the bone tissue. Often these growths cause pain before they become evident to X-ray, and in some cases secondary tumors in the bone are discovered before a primary cancer is even suspected.

Among the primary cancers that begin in bone, the most common and serious is the *osteogenic sarcoma* which may occur in bone tissue anywhere, destroying normal bone and replacing it with cancerous cells that form a thick bonelike tissue growth. Usually the growth is very rapid, quickly penetrating beyond the normal confines of the bone and invading the muscle tissue surrounding it. X-ray pictures will often show telltale spicules of bone radiating from the center of such a cancer. Typically these are highly malignant tumors which often have already spread to other parts of the body by the time they are first discovered. The earliest symptom is usually pain, followed by painful swelling over the area of the cancer. Diagnosis is aided both by X-rays and by certain blood tests showing biochemical changes resulting from bone destruction.

The only treatment for osteogenic sarcoma that offers any hope of cure is amputation of the affected limb, usually above or through the joint above the cancer. Radiation treatment has no effect on this kind of cancer, and there has not been much success using powerful anticancer chemicals. Death usually occurs within a year from discovery of the cancer, and statistics indicate that fewer than 5 percent of all cases survive, even when the cancer is discovered early and treated by means of radical surgery.

Among the several other forms of malignant bone growths are *chondrosarcoma,* a cancer that begins in cartilage at the end of bone, and *Ewing's sarcoma,* a highly malignant cancer that develops in the shafts of long bones, particularly in children. One odd form of cancerous growth in bone is the *multiple myeloma,* which usually originates in multiple areas of bone marrow throughout the body and often causes severe anemia because of destruction of the blood-forming elements there. The disease attacks only during or after middle age, and men are affected twice as frequently as women. The lesions are

relatively painless and the illness may not be suspected until it has progressed to such a point that the vertebrae or long bones in the extremities have been weakened and collapse in pathological fractures. Chief symptoms are persistent unexplained pain in the back, the chest or an extremity, and a progressive anemia that cannot be otherwise explained. Diagnosis is aided by X-ray as well as by the study of changes in various chemicals in the blood indicating that some process of bone destruction is going on. There is no cure for multiple myeloma, and death usually terminates the illness within 18 months, although some people survive as long as three or four years. Today there is active investigation of a number of chemical anticancer medicines which show promise of slowing the growth of the myeloma and of relieving the pain that accompanies it.

Other Bone Diseases and Disorders

A few other diseases and disorders affecting bone, mostly fairly rare, deserve mention. One hereditary bone disease known as *osteogenesis imperfecta* involves a general weakness of bone throughout the body, with marked decrease in the amount of calcium laid down, so that pathological fractures occur frequently with relatively minor injuries. A far more common disorder, *osteoporosis,* occurs as a natural degenerative process as people grow older, especially among women. There is a generalized decrease in the amount of calcium in the bones, and the total mass of bone gradually decreases because of a slowing down of the rate at which new bone is formed. This condition explains the "brittleness" of bone in older people and the marked slowing down of bone healing when fractures occur in the aged. In *osteomalacia,* still another condition, there is a marked decrease in the amount of calcium laid down in bone, owing to inadequate concentrations of calcium or phosphorus in the body fluids.

Achondroplasia (sometimes called chondrodystrophy) is a disease of the skeleton which begins while the fetus is developing in the uterus; it is characterized by a marked dwarfism—generalized shortness of the length of all the long bones, together with an enlarged head, short stubby fingers and often a sunken bridge of the nose. (Dwarves should not be confused with *midgets,* individuals who are abnormally small owing to a deficiency of growth hormone from the pituitary gland, but whose skeletons are perfectly proportioned.) There is much that is not yet understood about achondroplasia, but it is clear that the disorder involves a defect of cartilage growth and bone formation. There is a strong hereditary pattern; the child of an achondroplastic parent has a 50 percent chance of showing the disorder. Many achondroplastic babies fail to survive or are stillborn, but achondroplastic dwarves who live, usually growing to a height of from 3 to 3½ feet, often enjoy a normal life span and are able to undertake perfectly normal activities in spite of their size. There is no related mental deficiency, and these individuals have well-developed musculature and relatively greater strength than persons of normal size. Nothing can be done to correct this disorder, nor does anyone understand precisely why a child born to normal parents may be affected by achondroplasia. But statistics indicate that the birth of a second achondroplastic child to such parents is extremely improbable.

Certain disorders occurring in the bones of children are grouped under the name of *osteochondrosis.* It begins as a degeneration of the growth center of the bone, followed by regeneration of bone over the damaged area. A common site of this trouble is the front of the shinbone or tibia just below the knee. Osteochondrosis in this particular area is known as *Osgood-Schlatter disease,* and can cause continuing pain, swelling and disability unless treated by means of rest and inactivity of the affected part—difficult for children, but successful if a period of three months or so of relative inactivity can be achieved. A similar kind of degeneration of bone in the hip is known as *Legg-Calvé-Perthes disease,* in which the head of the femur degenerates, with inadequate or deformed regeneration, leading to progressive disfunction of both hip joints. Although it is difficult to distinguish the joint pain which may be present due to a potentially serious illness such as this from the relatively frequent complaint of joint pain in

children which has no specific cause, it is wise to have a physician examine the child in any case in which this type of complaint is persistent.

One of the most odd and mysterious of all bone diseases is now thought to occur much more frequently than was once believed. It is *osteitis deformans,* more commonly known as *Paget's disease,* first described in 1877 by the English surgeon Sir James Paget (1814–1899). A slowly progressive disorder that seldom appears before the age of thirty, Paget's disease is marked by slow decalcification of certain weight-bearing bones in the body—most notably those of the lower spine, pelvis and legs—and also of the skull. Gradually new bone is generated in the decalcified areas, but with characteristic deformities: the new bone is thicker but softer than normal; the legs become bowed, the spine bent and the skull often grotesquely enlarged. This disorder, which may progress for as long as twenty or thirty years before the victim becomes an invalid, is frequently accompanied by shifting, intermittent bone pain, seldom as severe as it is aggravating; in many cases the victim first suspects that something is wrong when he notices that his hat size is growing progressively larger. No one knows what causes Paget's disease, nor is there yet any known treatment or cure, but most authorities suspect some unidentified metabolic disorder to be at the root of the trouble, and there is continuing research into possible new forms of treatment. Once the disease was considered rare, but researchers today suspect that as many as 3 percent of all males and 1.5 percent of all females develop some degree of Paget's disease, often never detected, at some time in their lives.

Other bone disorders are definitely attributable to disturbances in the body's chemistry or metabolism. Among these are *rickets,* caused by vitamin D deficiency in children (*see* p. 892), and a generalized decalcification of the entire skeleton known as *osteitis fibrosa cystica,* which results from overactivity of the parathyroid glands (*see* p. 893). Other abnormalities of the bones and joints may result not primarily from bone disease, but from disorders of the nervous system or of muscle. Poliomyelitis, for example, may not only permanently paralyze large groups of muscles by irreplaceably destroying the motor nerve cells in the spinal cord that control those muscles, but may also cause shortening and distortion of the bone and joint in an affected leg, if the paralysis occurs before bones are fully grown. When groups of muscles in the back are so affected while the opposing muscles remain strong and healthy, the entire spine may be twisted into a permanent S-curve deformity known as *scoliosis*.

Finally, the musculoskeletal system, just as any other organ system, can be affected by congenital malformations. Such disorders as *congenital hip dislocations* can often be corrected by proper orthopedic treatment soon after birth. Hunchback deformities of the spine due to congenital bone deformation are much more difficult to correct. Indeed, once bone is badly deformed congenitally or damaged by disease or injury, repair and correction may take years of patient work by the orthopedic surgeon, utilizing reconstructive surgery, bone grafts, prosthetic devices, or artificial limbs or joints, and aided by carefully planned programs of physical or occupational therapy. More and more interest in such work has arisen in recent years, and the orthopedic surgeons have been joined in their efforts by physicians working in a comparatively new specialty, *rehabilitative medicine,* to achieve modern miracles in restoring function to victims of bone, muscle and joint diseases who would have been permanently invalided as little as thirty years ago. As a result, there is probably no area of medicine in which the promise of further gains in the future is richer.

28

Arthritis and Other Joint Diseases

The joints in the body are subject to far more physical wear and tear than any other tissue. The bulk of the weight of a 200-pound man, for example, is carried either simultaneously or alternately on his hip joints whenever he stands or walks. The many joints of the spine must act as a semiflexible supporting post which carries far more weight because of man's upright position than does the spine of even a large four-footed animal. The joints of the elbows and shoulders must also support heavy weights in everyday use. In weight-lifting competitions, it has been shown that the bones, muscles and joints of a featherweight 123-pound man, all working together, are capable of lifting 290 pounds or more, and in 1969 the weight-lifting championship of the Amateur Athletic Union in the heavyweight class (competitors weighing 198 pounds or more) was won by Bob Bednarski, who hoisted an astounding 465 pounds dead weight over his head.

Actually the joints are remarkably well fitted for both weight-bearing and motion. The bone ends that meet and articulate in the joints are covered with a layer of smooth, somewhat soft and rubbery cartilage that may vary from one-sixteenth to one-half inch thick. The joint is held together by tough fibrous ligaments, and in such large weight-bearing joints as the knees, there are separate supporting strips of cartilage built into the sides of the joint. All of these structures are enclosed in a joint capsule of fibrous tissue that spans the joint from the shaft of the bone

above to the shaft of the bone below. This capsule is lined with a thin tissue, the *synovia* or synovial membrane, which ordinarily secretes *snyovial fluid,* a viscous and slippery substance, unlike any found elsewhere in the body, that lubricates the cartilage to permit virtually friction-free movement. Finally, certain joints—notably the shoulder and the elbow—are protected from injury by special fluid-filled connective tissue pads called *bursas* which are outside the joint proper but which overlie parts of the joint that are especially vulnerable to trauma.

With this picture of the structure of the joints in mind, it is easy to imagine the kinds of joint disorders that might occur. First, inflammation of any of the tissues surrounding the joint can cause painful swelling which impairs the function of the joint. In fact, the most common of the joint diseases, although differing considerably in detail, all involve inflammation of the joint and thus are called *arthritis.* Some forms of arthritis may occur at any age, but most are particularly common among people at middle age. One type afflicts more elderly people almost exclusively, as a result of the wear and tear and degenerative changes that occur throughout the body with age.

Trauma to a joint is another cause of arthritis, often following such injuries as sprains and dislocations. Infection can also afflict a joint, attacking the soft, vulnerable cartilage surfaces of the bone ends and roughening them so that friction-free function is no longer possible. Finally, biochemical disorders in the body can cause both acute and chronic joint diseases. And in addition to the diseases that affect the joint

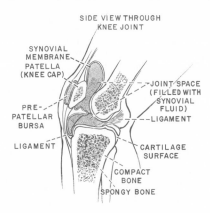

Figure 28–1.

proper, there is a kind of disorder involving inflammation of the joint capsule or bursa that leads to an extremely painful *bursitis*. Minor and temporary afflictions of the joints are all too common, but considering their complex structure and the constant burden of motion and

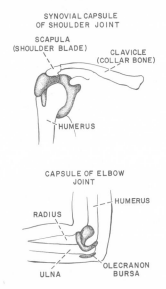

Figure 28–2.

weight-bearing they must withstand, they ordinarily perform their important functions with remarkably little trouble.

Infectious or "Septic" Arthritis

While there is no tissue which is completely immune to invading bacteria, some areas of the body provide these organisms with particularly ideal conditions for growth. Bacteria generally flourish in an area that is moist, warm and rich in protein upon which they can thrive and multiply. If the body's defenses against them—for example, the mobilization of white blood cells carried to the infected area through markedly enlarged blood vessels—are somewhat restricted in a given area, so much the better, as far as the invading organism is concerned. Thus, when bacteria find access to a joint, they are in a highly advantageous situation for growth. The joint fluid provides a splendid culture medium, and because the blood supply to the cartilage surfaces of the joint is relatively limited, it is difficult for white blood cells (or antibiotic drugs) to reach the infected area by way of the blood stream.

Obviously one of the most frequent ways bacteria gain entrance to a joint is by a trauma that breaks the skin over the joint, or by penetrating wounds that deposit bacteria directly into the joint space. Any kind of injury in the vicinity of a joint which is followed by swelling, heat, redness and pain in the joint should be assumed to be contaminated and medical care should be sought immediately. Other joint infections, however, are caused by streptococcus or staphylococcus bacteria which are carried to the joint from some other place in the body by way of the blood stream. Such an infection usually appears suddenly as an acutely sore, painful and swollen joint, often with evidence of *effusion* of an excessive amount of joint fluid into the joint from the irritated and inflamed capsule which lines it. Diagnosis and differentiation of this kind of condition from a noninfective form of arthritis can be made by withdrawing a small amount of fluid from the joint by means of a special needle, a procedure which can be done in the doctor's office quite simply and painlessly with the aid of a local anesthetic. In the presence of an infected joint, the normally crystal-clear joint fluid appears turbid and is found upon microscopic examination to contain pus cells and, frequently, bacteria which can be cultured and tested for sensitivity to various antibiotics.

In any infectious or septic form of arthritis, early diagnosis and vigorous treatment are imperative because invading bacteria can rapidly damage or destroy the cartilage of the articulating surfaces of the joint or surrounding ligament and joint capsule. Most joint infections (other than tuberculosis) reveal their presence early by pain, swelling, stiffness, heat, fever and production of excess fluid in the joint space, often seen as a marked puffiness of the joint. Any combination of these symptoms should be called to a doctor's attention at once.

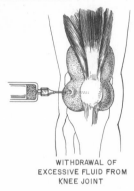

WITHDRAWAL OF
EXCESSIVE FLUID FROM
KNEE JOINT

Figure 28–3.

Certain kinds of joint infections are particularly dangerous. For example, untreated gonorrhea characteristically releases gonococci into the blood stream which lodge and grow in the knees or other joints and cause a particularly fulminating and rapidly destructive septic arthritis. Syphilis may also affect the joints, particularly the knees, during either the secondary or the tertiary stage of the disease, with considerable swelling and fluid formation, but with no particular redness or heat. Arthritis due to tuberculosis tends to be deceptively painless and slower to develop, but it is equally destructive. It is first suspected when a person who has had active tuberculosis of the lung, for example, notices swelling and impairment of joint motion when there has been no history of a blow or injury. Unlike syphilis, tuberculosis occurs most frequently in children. Although almost any joint in the body can be involved, the hip joint

and the joints of the spine are the two most common sites of tuberculous arthritis.

For septic arthritis caused by staphylococcus, streptococcus, gonorrhea or syphilis, the treatment of choice is vigorous administration of an antibiotic that has been found, upon laboratory sensitivity tests, to be particularly effective against the causative organism. Healing may be slower than it is in bacterial infections of tissues with better blood supplies, but adequate antibiotic treatment will usually quiet a septic arthritis within a few days. Arthritis caused by tuberculosis usually responds to the administration of streptomycin, isoniazid and salicylic acid (PAS) just as tuberculosis of the lung does, but often enough damage may have occurred before diagnosis or treatment to require surgical excision of the infected portion of the joint and bone. Sometimes bone excised for this reason may be replaced by bone grafts. In other cases, artificial or prosthetic joints help replace lost joint function.

Finally, septic arthritis can be an occasional complication of other kinds of infections in the body. For example, in approximately one out of every 200 cases of lobar pneumonia due to pneumococcus infection, the pneumococcal organism also affects one or more joints. The bacteria causing typhoid fever and bacillary dysentery also may cause septic arthritis, often quite some time after the acute stage of the infection is over. In these cases, the bacteria can almost always be isolated from a laboratory sample of the joint fluid, and appropriate antibiotic treatment will be effective.

Rheumatoid Arthritis

Not all joint inflammations are infectious, nor do all occur suddenly or follow a rapid course of destruction. One of the most commonplace forms of arthritis, believed to affect as much as 3 percent or more of the general adult population to one degree or another, is a chronic disease known as rheumatoid arthritis, sometimes spoken of as arthritis deformans because of the long-term destruction and deformity of joints that so frequently accompany the disease.

The name of this disorder is misleading, since

it is easily confused with the arthritis of rheumatic fever—a totally different and unrelated disease (*see* p. 560)—or with "rheumatism," a rather vague, old-fashioned term still used in reference to any sort of chronic and recurring aching of muscles or joints common to the middle-aged and elderly. Although the symptoms of rheumatoid arthritis may, at times, be similar to those of rheumatic fever arthritis or "rheumatism," this particular disorder is a very specific, identifiable, chronic disease process marked by progressive and recurrent episodes of inflammation in the joints, accompanied by gradually destructive joint changes. In its earlier stages these changes may be reversible, and rheumatoid arthritis appears primarily as a shifting or "migratory" swelling and stiffness of various joints. In later stages it is characterized by permanent irreversible deformity, destruction or even "freezing" or fixation of certain joints.

Rheumatoid arthritis primarily affects the connective tissues of the joints, and is now considered one of the family of collagen diseases, which also includes rheumatic fever, lupus erythematosus, dermatomyositis and scleroderma, among others. Rheumatoid arthritis appears to be a disease primarily of cool temperate climates, comparatively rare in the tropics but quite common in the relatively cold, wet weather of some of the great northern cities. For some unknown reason it occurs about three times as frequently in females as in males, and although it is often thought of as a "degenerative" or "old-age" disease because of its long chronicity, it actually makes its appearance in the vast majority of cases at around the age of thirty to forty, and may often appear even earlier.

No one knows the cause of rheumatoid arthritis, but there are a number of conditions which seem to "trigger" its onset. Unlike rheumatic fever, which is known to occur in response to a preexisting streptococcus infection, there is no consistent correlation between infections of any kind and rheumatoid arthritis. The things which do seem to trigger the disease are mysteriously varied and interrelated. Sometimes it first appears after a severe physical or emotional shock—a death in the family, some business disaster, a severe surgical illness or a difficult childbirth, for example. Some kind of physical injury is occasionally associated with the beginning of the disease, although it soon clearly involves joints other than those affected by the injury. Physical exhaustion also seems to precipitate the disease, as do sudden or repeated exposures to dampness, rain and cold. Further, there seems to be some familial pattern; very frequently more than one member of a family will have it, but no clear-cut hereditary pattern has yet been determined. Finally, in at least some cases there seems to be a relationship between the onset of rheumatoid arthritis and allergic responses of one sort or another, although just what the relationship may be has not yet been clarified.

The earliest symptoms of this long-term chronic disease are most commonly rather vague, deep-seated aching in one or more of the joints, together with some swelling in the tissue around the joints, and stiffness and limitation of motion. Typically, the joints first affected are the middle joints of the fingers, often involving the same joints on both hands. Indeed, these finger joints are frequently the most seriously affected right from the beginning, but other joints of the extremities may also be involved early in the disease. In a great many cases, at the beginning, the characteristic pain, early-morning stiffness and swelling of the affected joints will be intermittent, growing worse on some days and subsiding on others. Or it may "migrate," becoming worse in one joint even as it appears to improve in another.

The disease has another odd characteristic: the aching and stiffness of the affected joints is far more noticeable upon first arising in the morning than later in the day after the joint has been exercised, and the pain then often recurs later in the day after the victim has been sitting still or resting for a while. Many people in the early stages of rheumatoid arthritis discover for themselves two valid methods of treating the disease: first, they find that the arthritic joint feels much better after it has been "warmed up," either by purposeful exercise or by soaking for a few minutes in hot water; and second, they learn that the pain, which tends to be dull, nagging and persistent, can be relieved almost miraculously by small doses of aspirin.

Not all cases of rheumatoid arthritis begin slowly or insidiously. Occasionally the onset may be marked by some memorable disturbance of the victim's physical equilibrium, such as an acute infection, a period of unusual exposure to cold, a debilitating surgical operation or even fatigue from overwork. In such cases the pain and swelling of the joints may occur rapidly, sometimes associated with chills, fever, prostration and other symptoms of an acute illness. At the other extreme, many individuals trace the onset of the disease to the gradual appearance of pain and stiffness in just one particular joint which continues for weeks or even months without further change. In either case, rheumatoid arthritis eventually assumes a chronic course, usually affecting joints of the fingers, hands, knees or spine, coming and going at first, but then gradually settling down into a chronic and progressive pattern of pain and swelling, followed by gradual deformation of the affected joints.

The deformity occurs because of the basic lesion caused by the disease, an active inflammation that involves various parts of the joint and the surrounding soft tissue, particularly the joint capsule and the synovial membrane that normally exudes the lubricating synovial fluid within the joint. As inflammation continues, this membrane becomes swollen and deep red in color because of the increased dilatation of blood vessels in the area. After a long period of time it begins to form granulation tissue—evidence of the body's attempt to heal the inflammation—which extends into the joint and covers the slippery joint surfaces. Gradually this granulation tissue is converted into a dense fibrous tissue which impedes the natural movement of the joint. In other cases the cartilage on the joint surfaces ulcerates and there is a marked increase in the amount of fluid in the joint cavity, followed by the growth of fibrous tissue. Because the joint becomes stiff and difficult to use with these changes, the muscles around it tend to shrink and atrophy. The bones also shrink as they lose a certain amount of their normal

mineral substance, and the skin over the joint becomes thin, tough and shiny.

Thus, over a period of years, more and more joint destruction occurs as a result of the inflammatory process of rheumatoid arthritis. The fingers become twisted and deformed, the knees knobby and swollen. Other joints, including the ankles, the hinged joint of the mandible, the elbows and even the upper spine may be involved.

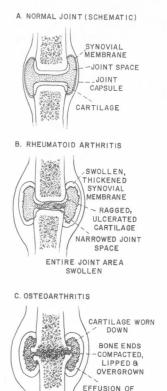

Figure 28–4.

As the disease enters its chronic course, other changes occur. Many people develop odd lumpy nodules beneath the skin over the irritated joint. Some victims feel chronically ill, tend to eat poorly (and look it) and gradually become anemic. In early cases of rheumatoid arthritis the symptoms frequently run a comparatively short course and then disappear for weeks or months, but in most cases the condition returns repeatedly and with each recurrence becomes more severe and chronic.

Diagnosis is usually based on these symptoms and the patient's medical history. Physical examination and X-ray studies of the arthritic joints help determine the progress of the disease. Certain laboratory tests are also helpful: the presence of an anemia, an increased sedimentation rate of the red blood cells, and certain changes in the balance of the blood proteins all may help confirm diagnosis. Fluid withdrawn from an affected joint typically shows no evidence of bacteria but may contain a large number of white blood cells, another diagnostic clue. Finally, doctors today look for a so-called rheumatoid factor in the blood which, when present, is also diagnostic.

Because prompt treatment of rheumatoid arthritis in its beginning stages can markedly influence its course, early diagnosis and differentiation from other kinds of arthritis are extremely important. For that reason, the American Arthritis and Rheumatism Foundation has undertaken a widespread campaign to teach the public the key symptoms of the disease:

1. The tendency of rheumatoid arthritis to occur in young adults as a changing or migratory arthritis.

2. Later changes in the joints which become chronic, persistent and tend to be symmetrical.

3. The characteristic swelling and tenderness of the affected joints.

4. Frequent involvement of joints in the fingers early in the disease, with typical "fusiform" or cigar-shaped swelling around those joints.

5. The tendency for affected joints to become more and more stiff until, gradually, they cannot be used and tend to become fixed or twisted.

6. The characteristic laboratory findings, as noted above.

Everyone at one time or another has sore aching joints as a result of temporary overuse or trauma of some kind, or merely as a side effect of various other illnesses—a case of flu or grippe, for example. But in such cases the aching joints do not appear swollen or inflamed. Any time joint pain involves swelling or the other symptoms listed above, it is time to see a physi-

cian. The earlier rheumatoid arthritis is diagnosed, the better chance there is of controlling or even arresting its course, and in many cases postponing the degenerative changes of the joints for many years.

Once diagnosis is made, the first and most important initial step in treatment of an acute attack is a rational period of *rest*. This does not necessarily mean total bed rest, but ideally it does mean giving up physically active work long enough for the inflammation to subside. Once this has been accomplished, gradual extension of activity is begun—but without heavy work or weight-bearing—to prevent stiffening of the affected joints. Mental and emotional rest is just as important as physical rest; if a rest program in itself creates tension and emotional distress, it may well defeat its purpose.

In addition to rest followed by measured activity, various drugs play an important part in the treatment of rheumatoid arthritis. Of all these drugs, however, there is none that stands up as well month after month as aspirin, which has very specific anti-inflammatory and antipain effects in this disease. Ten grains can be taken three to four times a day, or in even larger doses if they can be tolerated. Individuals who suffer from gastric disturbances due to aspirin may take aspirin combined with antacid materials or aspirin tablets with a so-called enteric coating which prevents them from dissolving until they have passed out of the sensitive stomach into the intestinal tract. Unfortunately, aspirin can be toxic if taken in excessive doses; *any dosage greater than 10 grains four times daily should be taken only under a doctor's supervision.* Occasionally the doctor may prescribe small amounts of stronger drugs for pain if absolutely necessary, but any potentially habituating drugs are usually scrupulously avoided in treating rheumatoid arthritis simply because the disease tends to be chronic and the patient can become excessively vulnerable to addiction.

Various organic compounds containing gold are also used in the treatment of rheumatoid arthritis, and many authorities feel that they frequently help induce a remission of the disease. Nobody understands just why gold compounds have their effect, and in most cases they are used for three to four months and then continued according to the amount of relief they provide. They seem most helpful when administered early in the course of the disease, but many patients using gold compounds sooner or later develop either allergic symptoms or some other form of intoxication, since gold, like other heavy metals, is basically a protoplasmic poison. When this happens, the medicine must be discontinued.

Perhaps the greatest help today in treating the inflammation of rheumatoid arthritis lies in the use of various cortisone-like hormones, particularly hydrocortisone, or the administration of ACTH, the adrenocorticotrophic hormone which stimulates the patient's own adrenals to manufacture cortisone. These substances have an overall tendency to suppress inflammatory reactions anywhere in the body, whether due to infections, injury, wound healing or any other cause. They can therefore prove a great boon in reducing the joint inflammation in rheumatoid arthritis. However, these potent hormones may also have profound side effects. For example, they tend to make the body retain excessive salt and fluid; occasionally they can lead to the development of peptic ulcers; and frequently they can mask the symptoms of infections that may be present in the body and decrease the body's natural defense mechanisms against them. They can also bring about emotional disturbances of varying severity. Because of these untoward side effects, a great deal of research has been done to develop synthetic compounds similar to cortisone and hydrocortisone which have higher anti-inflammatory potential with lower dosage and fewer undesired side effects. Today the doctor has a wide variety from which to choose and can use these compounds for years in controlling rheumatoid arthritis. This kind of medicine may be given in tablet form or by intramuscular injection. In many cases it may even be injected directly into the inflamed joint space, where it can exert a local anti-inflammatory effect precisely where it is most needed with fewer side effects in distant parts of the body. Once a full course of cortisone treatment is started for rheumatoid arthritis, however, arthritis authorities today believe that it should be used continuously for the rest of the patient's life, and therefore initiation of such treatment is usually postponed until all other drugs have failed.

Another drug widely used today is phenylbutasone, a substance completely unrelated to the cortisone hormones, which often produces dramatic relief of symptoms of rheumatoid arthritis and is thought to have a very specific anti-inflammatory effect. Unfortunately, this drug also has a rather high incidence of toxic side effects, including gastrointestinal disturbances, skin rashes and sometimes dangerous bone marrow depression. For this reason the doctor will use it most cautiously, usually only for brief periods at a time and with frequent blood counts to help detect any ill effect on the bone marrow. In early cases of rheumatoid arthritis, however, courses of this medication lasting only two to four weeks can often bring about prolonged relief of all symptoms.

Various forms of physical therapy are useful in treating rheumatoid arthritis in order to increase circulation to the affected joints, and to preserve as far as possible the tone and function of the skeletal muscles, and the range of motion of the joints themselves. Heat, a great help in ameliorating pain and in permitting regular exercise of the affected joints, may be applied either locally to an inflamed joint or to the entire body by soaking in a hot tub. Hydrotherapy with supervised exercises in a warm swimming pool or bathtub is another important aspect of treatment, since the warmth relaxes the muscles and the buoyant water makes movement easier. Skilled physical therapists can also teach the individual patient certain exercises and calisthenics designed to help preserve the function of the affected joints, maintain muscle tone and strength and prevent the progression of deformities. Patients with rheumatoid arthritis are rarely in need of hospital care for this disease alone, but many hospitals provide physical therapy services on an outpatient basis when such specialized therapeutic care is prescribed by the physician. For many years doctors tended to overlook the help that supervised physical therapy could provide patients with this long-chronic affliction, but today more and more physicians are incorporating it in their treatment programs, and any patient with sufficient arthritis to impair joint motion should not hesitate to inquire about the potential of physical therapy in his individual case.

Finally, the question often arises about a change of climate. It was once believed that many rheumatoid patients responded well to the warm dry weather found in such places as the southwestern United States or Mexico, and multitudes of people embarked on such climate changes, expecting overnight miracles. Recent studies, however, have found no correlation between the progress of rheumatoid arthritis and such factors as geography, climate or culture, and most authorities today discredit any change in climate as an aid to rheumatoid victims.

With early diagnosis, treatment and careful follow-up, the course of rheumatoid arthritis can almost always be slowed, and in some 20 to 25 percent of such cases, it will clear up completely for months or years. Generally it does come back, but fully three-quarters of the people afflicted with this condition could be spared much of the pain, distress and misery of the illness by early diagnosis and by faithful pursuit of a rational medical program. The disease rarely, in itself, causes death, and there is considerable evidence that after many years of chronic activity, rheumatoid arthritis tends to "burn itself out" or gradually decrease in severity in later years. Fortunately, it is a disease that can be alleviated greatly by treatment, and research today continues in an effort to find more satisfactory and permanent ways of checking and perhaps even curing it.

Degenerative Joint Disease (Osteoarthritis)

Like rheumatoid arthritis, degenerative joint disease (also called osteoarthritis) most often begins insidiously and runs a long, chronic course. It probably has a far greater incidence than rheumatoid arthritis, especially considering that multitudes of people suffer a mild degree of osteoarthritis for years and just put up with it without consulting a doctor. Unlike rheumatoid arthritis, however, osteoarthritis is not, as far as we know, caused by some internal disorder of the body which results in marked inflammation and swelling of the tissue of the joints. It bears no

mysterious relationship to other vaguely defined physical or emotional problems, nor does it often result in the actual "freezing" of a joint, as rheumatoid arthritis does. Although some women begin to develop early symptoms shortly after menopause, it usually does not begin to afflict individuals severely much earlier than middle age. Rather, osteoarthritis is a joint condition that results largely from wear and tear, from normal life circumstances in which weight-bearing joints have simply carried too much weight for too long or too regularly, and it is one of the numerous quietly progressive degenerative processes that mark the afternoon and twilight of life.

Osteoarthritis affects men and women about equally, and most characteristically it first attacks the major weight-bearing joints: the knees, the hips, the lower spine or the shoulders. It strikes those who have lived hard, physically active lives more frequently than those with sedentary jobs, and is far more common among obese individuals, who carry excess weight around with them, often for years, than among the thin and wiry. Finally, although it does not necessarily progress very rapidly, once started it never goes away. But this is not to say that the disease is hopeless; there are very effective forms of treatment which can markedly prolong normal activity and comfort following the onset of the disease, especially if they are started when the disorder is in its early stages.

Osteoarthritis presents quite a different picture to the physician than rheumatoid or other kinds of arthritis. In the early stages of the disease the overworked weight-bearing joints, responding to wear and tear, develop a slight roughening of the cartilage surfaces where the bones rub together in the joint. At first there is an attempt by the body to heal this roughening; for example, excess amounts of slippery synovial fluid begin to appear in the damaged joint. But inevitably the roughened surfaces tend to grind together, with further weight-bearing, until the cartilage surfaces may be almost completely worn off and raw bone comes in contact with raw bone within the joint. The bone accommodates to unprotected contact as best it can. Its surface becomes very shiny and smooth, and marked compaction or hardening develops at the joint surface. This may be so conspicuous on X-rays that the bone of the joint appears far more dense than elsewhere. At the same time, there is an overgrowth of bone, a sort of "spurring" at the edges of the weight-bearing surfaces, which occurs as a part of the body's natural attempt to regenerate damaged tissue. Often calcium is deposited in these cartilaginous spurs to become true bone; calcium may also be deposited in the tendons and ligaments around the joint, and characteristic nodules of hardened connective tissue, known as Heberden's nodes, appear in the vicinity of the affected joints. Occasionally fragments of cartilage are broken off within the joint to become so-called joint mice. Throughout this process the joint space between the bones becomes narrower and narrower, and in many cases the joint becomes swollen and tense owing to the overproduction of synovial fluid.

It might seem at first that treating this disorder would be like trying to treat old age, but actually there are three characteristics of osteoarthritis which can be helped significantly by treatment: the pain, the limitation of motion and the progressive damage caused by the disease. All three respond well when excessive wear and tear on the joint is either relieved or markedly reduced.

The first step in accomplishing this, as in treating any kind of arthritis, involves *rest*. If the osteoarthritis is acutely painful, it may be necessary for the patient to have complete bed rest until the symptoms subside—perhaps for a few days, perhaps for a week or more. At the same time, if he is markedly obese, as is very often the case, he *must* lose weight to relieve the affected joints of their excessive burden. The best course of action is a rational program of weight loss aimed at changing eating habits so that the weight, once lost, will not immediately be regained. (*See* p. 927.) Often if a significant amount of weight can be lost, especially when the disorder has only begun, that alone can have a remarkable effect in slowing down or halting the degenerative process in the joints and can perhaps provide the patient with months or years of symptom-free life before the process inevitably resumes.

Again, simple physical measures such as hot tub soaks, application of hot wet packs to the joints, mild exercise and massage will help relieve the pain of osteoarthritis and maintain range of motion. If the patient's normal way of life involves physical activity that will inevitably aggravate the disease, serious consideration should be given to making the changes necessary to slow down its progress. It may be possible for such a person, following a careful treatment program, to continue his normal activities for a few months or even years with relatively little pain, but sooner or later he must face the fact that his occupation or mode of living in itself is going to make the condition worse. And if his job depends upon good coordination and agility, the disease may well become hazardous to his very life; no one can count on the proper functioning of joints which have become agonizingly painful. By far the best course, if possible, is to retire from active physical labor or shift to a less physically demanding job.

Among the drugs that are useful in treating osteoarthritis aspirin again is among the most effective and safest in relieving pain and reducing inflammation. Phenylbutasone is also frequently useful, especially when the disease is in its early stages and the patient suffers only occasional episodes of pain and stiffness following spells of extraordinary activity. The cortisone-like hormones may be highly effective if applied cautiously in order to avoid the untoward side effects. If a single joint, such as one knee or one hip, is causing special pain and discomfort, injection of hydrocortisone or a related medicine directly into the afflicted joint will frequently provide dramatic and prolonged improvement. Other measures—periodically removing excess synovial fluid from a painful joint, for example —can also relieve the stiffness and soreness that accompany the disease.

Because osteoarthritis is a long-term, chronic and recurrent disorder that seems largely to be a part of the normal aging process, the prognosis for long-term recovery is poor. But the course may vary greatly from person to person. In most cases marked relief of symptoms and significant slowing of joint degeneration can be accomplished with proper medical care, administration of drugs when needed, and observance of a program of moderation in physical activity combined with weight loss. In older people with osteoarthritis, it is particularly important that their capacity to move about be retained as long as possible so that they do not become vulnerable to stasis pneumonias. It is also important for them to live in an environment where they will not be vulnerable to disastrous falls resulting from arthritic limitation of movement. The use of a cane is a much neglected aid to safe mobility among older people. If everyone over the age of sixty who suffered from degenerative joint disease in the hips or legs would use a cane to provide a wider base for balance, there would be far, far fewer hip fractures and other potentially dangerous accidents as a result of this disease.

Gout or Gouty Arthritis

To many people the mention of gout conjures up a stereotyped picture of a fat old Englishman in a periwig sitting with his flannel-wrapped foot propped up on a stool, crippled because of his chronic indulgence in alcohol and food, particularly beef. This notion, if unscientific, is not altogether inaccurate; the disease is indeed a common affliction of the middle aged and the obese who overindulge, but it is not peculiar to the English, nor is overindulgence always at fault. Gout, or gouty arthritis as it is more accurately called, is surprisingly prevalent in this country, and it may just as well afflict the thin, wiry man or the trim young woman as the individuals who fit the popular picture.

Basically gout is a generalized metabolic disease, the result of a breakdown or defect in the body's ability to handle the normal biochemical reactions involving certain protein food substances—particularly a group of compounds known as purines commonly found in meats and seafoods. Because of this defect, a protein breakdown product called uric acid piles up in the blood stream faster than the kidneys can excrete it, even when the individual does not overindulge. Thus victims of gouty arthritis are often found to have crystals of uric acid in their urine, and may even pass kidney stones composed of agglomerations of precipitated uric acid. In addi-

tion, small concretions of uric acid may be deposited in other tissue, most often in the upper rim or helix of the ear. This condition is pathognomonic of gout; that is, it occurs in gout and in no other disease, and thus the discovery of such nodules is an important clue to diagnosis.

The major symptoms of gout, however, are those of a severe arthritis, a singularly dramatic and painful type of joint inflammation which comes on without warning in acute and recurrent attacks. Ordinarily gout first appears in middle or early old age, but it may sometimes occur in young people as well, and its symptoms are so flagrantly different from other forms of arthritis that the diagnosis is often suspected from the victim's medical history alone. Typically an attack of gout begins very suddenly, often nocturnally, with the onset of excruciating pain in a single joint. Most frequently it involves the joint where the big toe joins the foot, but the ankle, the knee or virtually any other joint may occasionally be the site of the attack.

Unlike the dull, deep-seated ache of rheumatoid arthritis or osteoarthritis, the pain of gout tends to be sharp and agonizing, accompanied by sudden swelling of the affected joint and marked redness of the overlying skin. The pain may be so severe that the victim cannot even bear the touch of light bedclothes on the affected area. Heat does not ease the pain, and aspirin or even stronger analgesics do not help. Untreated, the attack may last for three or more days before it gradually subsides to a completely symptom-free period. During the attack there usually is no question about resting the affected area simply because any movement or weight-bearing is too agonizing to endure. Typically, early in the disease, an attack may occur only once every four or five months or even at longer intervals, usually selecting just one joint. But later the attacks become more frequent and multiple joints may be involved. For reasons that are unclear, the disease occurs almost 20 times more frequently in men than in women, but it cannot be ruled out automatically in women, or overlooked because it does not occur in a "typical" location or at the "usual" age.

In the absence of treatment, gouty arthritis attacks become increasingly frequent, and presently deposits of uric acid in crystal form are laid down in the affected joints, forming large chalky nodules spoken of as *tophi*. Over the years these deposits, combined with degeneration of the chronically inflamed joints, can lead to marked and permanent deformities.

Gout is one of those rare human illnesses in which a therapeutic trial or "test run" with one specific drug will, in most cases, firmly clinch the diagnosis. This drug, known as colchicine, is remarkably effective in relieving the pain of an acute attack of gout, yet it has no significant effect at all in any other disease. Thus, if a trial prescription of colchicine dramatically halts the pain of an attack of an unidentified arthritis, the doctor can be quite certain the arthritis is due to gout.

There is just one problem with colchicine, one of the herbal medicines that has been known to man for centuries. It is highly toxic; even small quantities may cause nausea, vomiting and diarrhea. In order to relieve the pain of gout the patient must take enough of the drug to approach the toxic dosage level. Nevertheless, if colchicine is used at the beginning of an acute attack of gout in small doses on a regular schedule—perhaps one tablet per hour—until either the pain is relieved or gastrointestinal symptoms begin, control of the pain can then usually be maintained with very small and infrequent additional doses until the acute attack has subsided. This makes colchicine a real boon to the doctor diagnosing gout, and to the patient suffering from it, tricky as it may be to use. Indeed, among the relatively high percentage of patients with gout who have some prior warning symptoms that an attack is impending—a tingling in the vulnerable joint, for example, or a sense of stiffness—colchicine taken quickly enough can successfully abort or prevent the attack altogether. Thus many patients subject to frequent attacks choose to take the drug continuously in a low maintenance dosage for prolonged periods of time as a prophylaxis against acute attacks of gout, or keep a supply on hand to use when they feel that an attack is about to start.

Other drugs are also useful. Two of them, probenecid and sulfinpyrazone, stimulate the kidneys to excrete uric acid in the urine and thus lower excessive blood levels of this substance that seem to trigger attacks of the disease. These so-called uricosuric drugs are often prescribed in maintenance dosages for long periods of time, sometimes in combination with colchicine, to help broaden the interval between attacks. Indomethacin helps control the pain of acute attacks. In addition, especially in a patient whose uric acid level seems to be extremely high, the doctor may prescribe a special low-purine diet, eliminating as far as possible many of the foods that permit a build-up of uric acid in the body. In such diets meat, fish and seafood are limited to one serving a day, with necessary protein supplied instead from milk, eggs and cheese. Such high-purine-containing foods as sweetbreads, anchovies, liver, sardines, rich meat extracts and gravies are often eliminated from the diet completely.

These various treatment methods can alter the natural pattern of gout very profoundly; indeed, there are few other diseases in which the patient's understanding and full cooperation are so important. Effective care of this disease may mean the use of certain medications on a daily basis for years; it may mean altering one's eating habits to avoid foods that make the disease worse; it certainly means periodic checkups with a physician to assess progress in combating the disease process; and it means the foresight to have adequate supplies of medicines on hand and the knowledge of how to use them without delay in the event of an acute attack. With this sort of cooperative effort between doctor and patient, a victim of gouty arthritis need not lead the life of intermittent misery that was so characteristic of the disease a century ago.

Other Kinds of Joint Disorders

Rheumatoid arthritis, osteoarthritis and gout account for the vast majority of all serious joint ailments, but a few other disorders of the joints should also be mentioned even though they are either more rare or less debilitating.

Traumatic Arthritis. It is not unusual for a single joint involved in some accidental injury or blow to become extremely painful and swollen. This type of injury, generally known as traumatic arthritis, may range from the most minor annoyance to a severe sprain in which the ligaments and supporting fibrous tissues around the joint are torn. Traumatic arthritis can occur as a result of running, hiking, or any body contact sport or other active physical exercise. It will usually respond to simple measures designed to aid healing. The two main dangers connected with a traumatic arthritis are the possibility that a bone may be fractured and the possibility of doing further damage to an already injured joint by injudicious use before the injury has healed.

For these reasons, any joint injury that involves marked swelling, pain or discomfort that persists for more than a day or so should be examined by a doctor and probably X-rayed to rule out the possibility of fracture. In addition, measures should be taken to reduce the swelling and provide support for the joint while it heals. If the swelling is only in the soft tissue around the joint, this can be accomplished by wrapping it firmly with an elastic bandage extending both above and below the injured joint to help provide additional support. Frequently, however, there is either an effusion of joint fluid or bleeding into the joint space. Thus the normal structure of the joint is altered, and it is both limited in its range of motion and extraordinarily weak and vulnerable to further injury. If the doctor detects fluid within the joint space, or suspects it, he may elect to remove it by means of a hypodermic needle and syringe with the use of a local anesthetic. Often as much as 100 cc.'s or more of clear or bloody synovial fluid may be withdrawn from a knee joint that has been injured, for example, with marked relief of pain and return of normal range of motion. Occasionally this procedure must be repeated over a period of several days, keeping the joint at rest and wrapped with an elastic bandage during the interval. If the injury is such that ligaments, supporting cartilage or the joint capsule have been badly injured, orthopedic surgery may be necessary to repair the damage. For the victim of a painful joint injury, the major rule is to *keep the joint at rest* for as long as necessary for the injury to heal, since premature use can cause prolonged or even permanent additional injury. In extreme cases the doctor may even apply a

plaster cast to immobilize the joint, exactly as if a fractured bone were present. Most traumatic joint injuries, if carefully treated, do not cause lasting defects or recurrent trouble.

Locking Knee. This is a curious joint phenomenon which may occur after a single severe injury to a knee or following repeated knee injuries. The damaged knee becomes unstable and tends to "lock" or become limited in motion in one direction or the other from time to time while behaving perfectly normally other times. In most cases of this kind, one of the *semilunar cartilages* in the knee has been torn and becomes caught in the knee joint periodically, preventing normal function. Any such episode should be called to a doctor's attention. A knee can usually be "unlocked" by simple manipulation, but sometimes surgical removal of the torn cartilage may be the best course to prevent recurrences.

An odd and less common affliction of the knee is the presence of "joint mice," tiny fragments of cartilage that have broken loose from the supporting structure of the knee and simply float more or less freely within the knee joint. In many cases these cause no symptoms, but if they do become symptomatic, as in locking of the knee, surgical removal may be called for. The knee is a complicated and delicate joint whose proper function is essential to the body's mobility. Any disturbance or discomfort in this area should be brought to a doctor's attention.

Neurogenic Joint Disease. The normal function of the musculoskeletal system depends not only upon healthy bone, joint and muscle, but also upon a healthy and intact nervous system. Both the voluntary and involuntary movements of the musculoskeletal system are controlled by the motor nerves that carry impulses from the brain down the spinal cord. Thus, damage to the motor nerve cells in the spinal cord by traumatic injury like a fractured vertebra or by a disease like poliomyelitis can result in complete paralysis of large groups of muscles, bones and joints. Diseases of the musculoskeletal system caused by disfunction of the nervous system are called neurogenic, and both the underlying nerve disorder and the complications it has caused require treatment. Destruction of nerve cells and fibers in the spinal cord due to syphilis, for example, can cause a loss of sensation and position sense in the extremities with the consequent loss of feeling and normal muscular control of a joint such as the knee. In this disorder, known as Charcot joint, the knee joint is repeatedly injured and reinjured without the victim's realizing anything is wrong until the joint becomes permanently damaged, unstable and distorted by the body's continuing attempts to heal it. Although the syphilitic infection can be combated, the damage to the nerve cells cannot be repaired, and it is sometimes necessary to provide support for the knee with a brace, or even to fuse the joint surgically.

Bursitis. This is an acute or chronic disorder in which certain of the *bursas*—the fluid-filled pads or pockets of connective tissue which overlie and protect such vulnerable areas as the bony prominences of the shoulder joint, the elbow or the knee—become inflamed and swollen as a result of trauma, infection or other chronic irritation. The inflammation can be acute and quite painful, sometimes making it almost impossible to move the affected joint because of muscle spasm due to the pain. Bursitis has many colorful and descriptive popular names; "housemaid's knee," for example, is an inflammation of the bursa overlying the kneecap; "tennis elbow" is an acute inflammation of the bursa at the outer side of the elbow. In people who spend a great deal of time sitting on hard surfaces, bursas protecting the sharp bones of the pelvis beneath the buttocks may enlarge; trauma or inflammation of these bursas, once common among tailors or weavers who sat cross-legged on the floor all day, is known by the quaint name "weaver's bottom."

An acute inflammation of a bursa must first be differentiated from some other type of joint disease. Then it can often be treated very effectively by injection of one of the cortisone-like hormones directly into the inflamed area. Recurrent bursitis in the same area is frequently identified on X-rays by chalky calcium deposits in the areas of the bursas, but these are of no particular help in diagnosing new or acute cases, since they stand as "monuments to past bursitis," the result of earlier healing processes. In addition to medication for pain and muscle

spasm, complete rest of the joint and the application of moist heat will help speed recovery. But once a person develops bursitis in one place or another, he should be particularly careful to avoid overuse of the joint, since chronic and recurrent attacks are not at all uncommon.

Flatfoot and Other Common Foot Disorders. Flatfoot is a structural deformity in which the heel is rotated somewhat outward and the natural bony arch of the foot has fallen because the ligaments that support it have given way. It can be caused by an innate weakness, injury, strain, obesity or simply improper walking and standing. The condition frequently causes pain in the arch of the foot, and sometimes in the calf muscles or even the knee and hip as well, with the discomfort increased by prolonged standing or walking. Pain and discomfort can be alleviated by wearing sponge rubber arch supports or even metal or plastic supports in the shoes for walking. Children with flatfeet should be kept *out of tennis shoes,* or footwear such as sandals or thongs, as much as possible, since these provide little or no arch support and encourage exaggeration of the defect. Going barefoot should also be discouraged in such cases, although it does not *create* flatfeet in people with healthy arches. There is no permanent way of correcting the disorder, but in many cases it can be improved. A doctor should be consulted about the use of proper shoes and such other

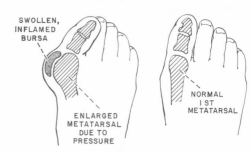

Figure 28–5.
Bunion.

forms of treatment as exercises to strengthen the muscular support of the arches.

Bunion, another common disorder of the foot, is the bony enlargement of the inner and upper sides of the first toe joint with angulation of the big toe away from the midline. Bunions usually occur bilaterally and are a result of prolonged pressure over this section of the foot, with recurrent bursitis which causes calcification and overgrowth of the bone in the area. Almost invariably due to improperly fitted shoes, bunions can become extremely painful, but the pain may be eliminated either by wearing specially fitted shoes or by enlarging or cutting out the portion of a regular shoe that presses on the bunion area. In a very active person in otherwise good health, excellent results can be obtained from surgical removal of the overgrown bone and calcification.

Hammertoe or "clawtoe" is a deformity of one or more of the toes, sometimes due to poorly fitting shoes, rheumatoid arthritis or, more rarely, as an aftereffect of poliomyelitis. In this condition, the toe is pulled upward where it joins the foot and then bent into severe flexion at the tip, often with the formation of a callus or corn at the pressure point at the top of the toe. In many people this deformity causes no discomfort or trouble whatever. Pain due to pressure can be relieved by well-fitting shoes and the use of a protective pad over the corn. In severe cases surgical correction is possible.

Stone bruising is a common injury resulting from a sudden hard blow on the under surface of the heel which leads to either bursitis or actual inflammation of the bony lining of the heel. An injury of this kind often causes alarm far out of proportion to its importance because the pain seems to persist and often appears excessive for the amount of injury. A sponge rubber pad beneath the heel will help relieve the pain due to pressure, and aspirin and hot water soaking, combined with as much rest as possible for a few days, will usually allow healing to proceed quickly.

The Problem of Low Back Pain

A very common complaint, low back pain is also one of the most commonly misunderstood conditions in the body; it is often a result of no discernible physical disease, and yet it can be a very crippling disability. In this condition, pain is centered in the region of the lower lumbar spine, the lumbosacral area where the vertebrae join the bony plate of the sacrum at the base of the spine, or in the sacroiliac region underlying the upper buttocks on either side where the sacrum joins the iliac bone of the pelvis. In some cases pain in these areas may be very sudden and acute and of such agonizing quality that the victim is virtually immobilized; in other cases it may be a very low-grade aching that is never acute but also is seldom relieved. In still other cases the pain may radiate into the legs, sometimes causing more severe discomfort there than in the back

The complaint of low back pain is a trial for everyone, including the physician who is faced with the problem of diagnosing and treating one of the most bewildering symptom complexes known to medicine. The problem is made all the harder by the fact that there may be any number of physical causes for low back pain, or no physical cause at all, and what can be done to help relieve the symptoms depends greatly upon the cause. The doctor's problem is to distinguish low back pain that may be a result of normal or abnormal physiology elsewhere in the body from that which is related to actual disease of some sort centered in the lower spine. In the latter case, he must distinguish muscle fatigue, arthritis, spasm or sprain that is relatively limited in nature and amenable to conservative treatment from the similar pain caused by true nerve damage as a result of a collapsed or "slipped" intervertebral disk. Low back pain may also stem from psychological rather than physical causes, and finally, because of the difficulty of diagnosis, it is frequently a favorite complaint of the malingerer.

Low Back Pain Due to Problems Elsewhere. There are a number of conditions which may cause pain in the back, even though the source of pain is not in the bones and joints of the vertebrae or pelvis. Any muscular disorder of the back—lumbago, myositis and the like—may be the root cause. Many women suffer backache with menstruation, and the disturbance of the body's normal muscular balance during pregnancy frequently results in pain in the low back until after delivery of the baby. Bacterial infections of the kidneys typically cause very severe pain in the lower midback overlying the kidneys; and finally, prostate disease, rectal disorders or even a generalized viral illness such as influenza can cause aching in the low back. In situations such as these, a careful physical examination will usually identify the disorder actually causing the distress, and proper treatment can alleviate the pain.

"Psychosomatic" Backache. All too often an injury or an organic disorder that once caused backache may be followed for a prolonged time by pain in the lower back that is as hard to explain as it is to treat. Details of the history of this sort of back pain are often highly bizarre. Pain may be associated with activities that are not ordinarily unduly strenuous, or with other totally unrelated symptoms in the body, and actual signs of illness—cramping of muscles, identifiable foci of pain and spasm, etc.—tend to migrate from place to place, or be absent altogether. There is no doubt that in many cases psychosomatic back pain is, in fact, painful, even if the cause is only in the patient's mind. There may well be a residual physical cause, but often the real reason lies in the patient's hope for some secondary gain—attention, sympathy or some job-connected benefit. In cases of this sort, the patients, however unconsciously, may actually resist getting well. Like those who complain of other psychosomatic ailments, such patients can be very difficult to deal with—no one is ever sure how much pain they actually suffer—and they present particular problems to the doctor, who must always be wary of some specific organic disease at the root of the trouble. Often the only way he can distinguish between physical and psychosomatic pain is by long observation and careful judgment of the response of the condition to efforts to treat it. Finally, even if the pain is psychosomatic, certain measures can be helpful. Often a patient will be aided just from the knowledge that a physician is taking great care to see that no grave physical illness is being overlooked. In other cases, improvement may result when the patient himself becomes convinced that he has more to gain by getting well than by remaining "ill."

Back Pain Due to Local Mechanical Defect. A variety of conditions can bring about true mechanical defects in the area of the low back. The possibility of lumbago, infections such as tuberculosis or syphilis, various forms of arthritis, congenital defects of the lower spine or vitamin deficiency diseases such as rickets must not be overlooked in a careful diagnostic study. But barring pain that results from fractures of the lumbar vertebrae, the sacrum or the pelvis, which almost invariably are associated with a severe accident, the great majority of cases of acute low back pain are caused by sprains of the joints of the lower lumbar vertebrae or of the lumbosacral joint. These sprains may result from lifting heavy objects, from unexpected twisting, from injury during body contact sports, or, in some people, merely from bending over at an awkward angle. Depending on the actual site of the sprain, such injuries cause pain that is often spoken of as "lumbosacral syndrome" or "sacro-iliac syndrome." In the former case the pain usually begins abruptly in the lumbosacral area, and often then becomes progressively worse, with muscle spasm affecting the whole lower back until the individual is virtually unable to move. In some people there is a regular pattern to these attacks, which can be highly refractory to treatment, and the pattern of pain may recur later as a result of the most minor muscle strain. Usually there is no evidence of nervous system abnormalities, and X-rays rarely reveal anything useful. Occasionally a person subject to such recurrent attacks is found to have some form of minor developmental abnormality in the lower spine, but even in these cases such abnormalities are seldom actually related to the cause of the pain.

These episodes of acute low back pain tend to encourage bed rest simply because the patient is too uncomfortable to do anything but lie still. With rest on a hard, flat mattress, the pain will usually subside without treatment in a matter of a few days to a week. Recovery can be speeded by using hot wet packs on the painful area, aspirin or other analgesics as directed by the doctor, and some of the new medicines which are particularly helpful in relaxing skeletal muscle. Where muscle spasm is present, manipulation of the low back, when performed by someone skilled in such maneuvers, often produces relief by stretching cramped muscle and loosening the spasm. In general, however, there is soft tissue injury involved which has to heal, so that rest and a gradual return to normal activity is advised even if back manipulation is successful.

A variation of acute lumbosacral sprain is a similar type of sudden cramping located not at the midline of the back but on either side of the sacrum in the area of the sacroiliac joint. People speak of "throwing out" their sacroiliacs without quite knowing what they mean. Usually what they are describing is the so-called sacroiliac syndrome—strain or sprain of muscle and ligament binding this long, firm cartilage connection between the sacrum and the iliac bone of the pelvis, with resulting muscle spasm and pain. Typically this injury, which can occur as a result of lifting, twisting, bending in the wrong position or sometimes even sitting too long in a draft, is unilateral, and may well be accompanied by a sensation of pain going down the leg. Treatment is much the same as for the lumbosacral sprain noted above, except that sacroiliac manipulation, a fairly simple maneuver, is often signally successful in bringing speedy relief.

Intervertebral Disk Abnormalities. A great deal of low back pain is casually blamed upon a "disk problem" when, in fact, nothing more is involved than a sprain of the intervertebral joints or strain of the muscles of the low back. However, the thick, padded "disk" of cartilage that lies between the lumbar vertebrae or between the lowest lumbar vertebra and the sacrum is a tissue that takes an enormous amount of strain, and in certain cases can weaken or even degenerate. In some instances the softer cartilaginous material in the center of one of these intervertebral disks will find a weakness in the harder outer lining and will herniate or extrude through the back side of the disk, sometimes merely causing chronic low back pain due to persistent pressure, but occasionally actually pressing or pinching one or more of the roots of the spinal nerves that go to make up the sciatic nerve extending into the leg. This condition is sometimes called a "slipped disk." Typically, pain is felt in one side of the back and radiates down the back of the thigh all the way to the heel and toes, usually on just one side but occasionally on

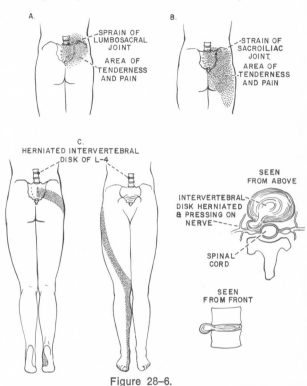

Figure 28–6.

both. Such radiating pain is commonly called "sciatica" because it arises from pressure of the disk on the spinal roots of the sciatic nerve, the great motor and sensory nerve that passes down the leg. (In old-fashioned parlance the word "sciatica" was, and sometimes still is, incorrectly used to refer to virtually *any* pain in the low back and thigh, but true sciatica arises from the very specific causes stated.) The victim's normal motions are sharply restricted by the pain, which is frequently aggravated by coughing, sneezing or straining at defecation. In many respects the symptoms greatly resemble a simple acute low back sprain, but when disk injury is involved, an additional factor is present because of pressure on the nerve: there is marked impairment of certain reflexes in the lower leg and often a loss of touch sensation in parts of the limb, as well as marked weakness of the leg due to loss of muscle tone. Typically the person with a true disk syndrome will be quite unable to lift his weight on tiptoe on the affected side, although still able to do so on the normal side. To confirm the diagnosis special X-rays called myelograms can be taken, in which a radio-opaque dye is injected into the lower vertebral canal where the spinal nerves descend and branch away from the spinal cord. When an intervertebral disk is herniated and pressing on these nerves, a characteristic outline of the defect can often be seen on the X-rays.

Disk syndrome is a difficult disease to manage, and when it is discovered it is usually best treated by a specialist: an orthopedic surgeon, a neurologist or a neurosurgeon. On the first episode of pain, every possible effort should be made to encourage the herniated disk to heal itself without surgical intervention by means of prolonged bed rest, regular use of heat and massage, and moderate medications for pain. Muscle-relaxant drugs may also help, and after an initial period of complete rest, a special series of graduated exercises designed to strengthen the muscular support of the low back can be undertaken. When such conservative treatment is faithfully carried out, the acute symptoms will usually subside in a week or two, but six weeks or more may be necessary before the disk has healed sufficiently for the victim to begin walking more than a few steps. When he is allowed out of bed, he will usually require the support of crutches for a period of time, and will not be considered out of the woods until he has recovered the muscle strength in his leg and his leg reflexes have returned to normal, indicating that all pressure on the nerve roots has been relieved. Sometimes a corset or back brace is helpful in preventing recurrences once the patient is up and about again.

Naturally many patients object to this long and tedious period of rest in bed, but it is by far the best hope for preventing further attacks. If the area is not allowed to heal, there will be recurrent attacks with progressive damage to the disk. This results in continuing chronic pressure and increasing damage to the nerve roots. When this happens, surgical treatment becomes neces-

sary. The operation, done by either an orthopedic surgeon or a neurosurgeon, involves exposing the injured intervertebral disk and removing the disk material from the nerve canal where it has been protruding and causing pressure. In selected cases, when the back is very unstable, the surgeon may also fuse the vertebral body above and below the disk by means of a bone graft in the hope of preventing pain by eliminating motion. Needless to say, recovery from this kind of surgery takes even longer than the bed rest program does, and is usually not undertaken until there is unmistakable evidence of continuing pressure and damage to the nerve roots, including positive X-ray findings, in spite of all conservative measures that have been taken. Nor is surgery by any means always a wholly satisfactory cure; some 25 to 30 percent of surgical patients will have continuing low back pain in spite of surgical treatment of the disk problem.

In summary, low back pain often has very real physical causes, and can be a recurrent and aggravating problem, but in almost all cases significant relief can be achieved by proper treatment, which requires close collaboration between patient and doctor. For the person suffering with a first attack, the goal is complete healing with no recurrences. For the person who has suffered recurrent attacks, the goal is better healing and lengthening of the interval between recurrences, as well as shortening of the disability period when the pain recurs. Meanwhile, as more and more is learned about the nature of low back pain, the symptoms customarily accompanying it and its physical characteristics, it becomes less and less possible for malingerers to use this once vague and uncertain complaint successfully—a boon to those whose very real low back pain requires skilled and sympathetic medical care.

"Whiplash" Injuries of the Neck

Just as muscle and joint disorders of the low back can range from the minor to the serious and often prove difficult to diagnose, so-called whiplash injuries of the neck present both doctor and patient with a bewildering variety of problems. Although everyone has heard of this kind of injury in these days of frequent traffic accidents, there is probably no other disorder of the musculoskeletal system that is more hazily defined in people's minds. Even doctors disagree as to what, precisely, a whiplash injury is and whether or not it really warrants the concern and attention that it so often receives.

Whiplash injuries most commonly arise as a result of the rear-end type of collisions of moving vehicles. The sudden jar of the collision throws the victim's head back before he has enough time or warning to tense the muscles of the neck and shoulders for protection. Any such unexpected jolt can momentarily throw an excessive strain on these muscles and on the tough ligaments that hold the vertebral joints in the neck in place. If the jolt is sharp or severe enough, fibrils of neck and shoulder muscle can be torn, the ligaments can be stretched or sprained, the spinal nerves emerging between the vertebrae from the spinal cord can be bruised or pinched, and, in extreme cases, chiplike or crushing fractures of the bony spurs of the vertebrae themselves may even be sustained. Thus the pathology of a given whiplash injury may range all the way from a minor degree of muscle strain in the neck to actual damage to bone and nerve.

Symptoms vary accordingly. Victims complain of stiffness and pain in the neck and shoulder muscles, sometimes beginning at the time of the injury, but more commonly first noticed some hours later. Considerable muscle spasm may be present, and the pain can be so severe that any motion of the neck is agonizing. Sometimes pain radiates down the arms, accompanied by numbness and tingling in the hands or fingers, and occasionally the victim may complain of some degree of paralysis or inability to coordinate the function of the upper extremities properly. In addition, there may be any number of bizarre symptoms which simply defy explanation, ranging from pounding headaches and disturbed vision to gastrointestinal or even sexual disturbances.

The problem is that in most cases virtually all evidence of real physical injury is subjective—the doctor has the patient's account of his symptoms to go on, and very little else. Of course, in extreme instances chip fractures may be identified on X-rays, or careful physical examination may reveal objective, identifiable evidence of neurological changes—impairment of tendon reflexes in the arms, for example, or distinguishable loss of touch or pain sensation in the fingers. But such findings are extremely rare. And to further complicate things, the circumstances surrounding a great many whiplash injuries are such that the victim is tempted to exaggerate his symptoms, or at least to make the most of any real discomfort he may have. Thus the doctor is often hard-pressed to determine how much, if any, real injury has actually been sustained and how much, if any, treatment and follow-up is really warranted. Some authorities believe that if the question of blame were removed from the automobile accident scene, so that insurance companies indemnified their clients for injuries sustained regardless of who was at fault, the incidence of whiplash injuries requiring extensive treatment would immediately decrease by 90 percent.

This is by no means to say that all instances of whiplash injuries involve malingering. Some people indeed suffer real pain and disability which, on occasion, can be very serious and can even result in injury to bone and nerve. Cases involving no more than strained muscles and sprained ligaments in the neck may cause distress lasting for weeks or months. Certainly anyone suffering pain and stiffness in the neck, back, shoulders or arms following any kind of jarring injury should see a doctor to rule out potentially dangerous physical damage. In most cases a few days of rest, the application of hot moist packs to the aching muscles and the use of a mild analgesic such as aspirin will help resolve symptoms quickly. When severe muscle spasm or sprain is present, a padded supportive collar is often useful to prevent movement of the head and neck, thus forcing rest of the injured area until healing can take place. Follow-up should continue until all symptoms are gone, and—in cases involving nerve injury—until full, normal nerve function has been recovered. Considered in perspective, most whiplash injuries are more annoying than dangerous, and the risk of sustaining such an injury can be substantially reduced by using seat belts and supportive headrests when driving or riding in an automobile.

Scoliosis and Lordosis

Finally, a word must be said about the various forms of "curvature of the spine" which occasionally arise as a result of one or another disorder of the musculoskeletal system. Under normal circumstances the human spine has a perfectly natural S-shaped curvature when regarded from a side view. The vertebrae tend to bow out slightly in the dorsal, or midback, region below the smooth inward curvature of the neck, and then to curve inward again at the small of the back to end in another slight outward curve at the point where the lumbar vertebrae join the sacrum and pelvis. When some pathological condition causes an exaggeration of this smooth, natural curvature, the excessive curvature is called *lordosis*. On the other hand, the spine is normally perfectly straight in the front-to-back view, and even a slight S curvature to the side of

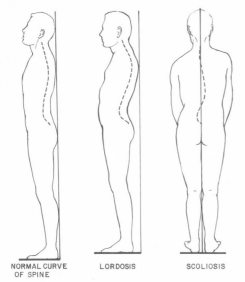

NORMAL CURVE OF SPINE   LORDOSIS   SCOLIOSIS

Figure 28-7.

any part of the spine is known as *scoliosis*.

Either lordosis or scoliosis may result from a variety of disorders. Congenital malformations of the spine account for a small percentage of

cases. Poor posture may contribute. More commonly, pathological spinal curvature results from some disease or disorder which affects the muscles along the spine on one side, so that the normally functioning muscles on the other side tend to pull the vertebral column out of its normal alignment. Any of the muscle-wasting diseases may have this effect; so also may nervous system diseases that impair muscle function. (*See* p. 352.) Arthritis of the spine can lead to varying degrees of spinal curvature, and the destruction of bone in the vertebral column by infection (particularly tuberculosis) or bone tumor can cause marked lordosis, scoliosis or both.

Spinal curvature is often first detected on routine physical examination. Subtle degrees of it may first be noted on X-rays taken for other purposes in which part of the vertebral column appears on the X-ray plate. Treatment in any given case depends upon diagnosis and treatment of any underlying cause; then evaluation by an orthopedic surgeon may be necessary to determine whether conservative treatment measures, including corrective bracing of the spine, may be helpful, or whether surgical treatment is necessary. In a great many cases an individual with a moderate degree of lordosis or scoliosis may have no symptoms whatever, and can go through life perfectly well without treatment, although such activities as heavy lifting or vigorous physical sports may be inadvisable because of additional risk of sprains or strains of the back. Most doctors are not inclined to meddle with such conditions unnecessarily, but cases involving symptoms such as pain, easy tiring, muscle spasm or progressive deformity should never be ignored.

Where to Look for Help

Disorders of muscle, bone and joint are often very closely interrelated, and frequently extremely difficult to diagnose and treat. In addition, many of these disorders, particularly the various forms of arthritis and chronic back problems, tend to cause long-term or recurrent disability for which *no* form of treatment proves wholly satisfactory. It is no wonder, then, that some of the most highly trained and skillful specialists in medicine have devoted their lives to the investigation and treatment of these diseases, using all the auxiliary medical help they can find, ranging from a bewildering array of mechanical and prosthetic devices to the special services of physical and occupational therapists, orthopedic nurses and aides, and many others. Nor is it surprising that this field of medicine has also drawn quacks, faith healers and medical charlatans of the worst sort. For those suffering from musculoskeletal disorders, some guide to whom to consult—and whom *not* to consult—for help will be useful.

Among the fully trained and licensed physicians, the logical first port of call is your regular family doctor, whether he be a general practitioner, an internist or—in the case of children—a pediatrician. No one is better equipped to evaluate symptoms, conduct the necessary physical examination and, in many cases, outline an optimum treatment program. In addition, your family doctor will be able to judge when consultation with a specialist is advisable, or to recommend which kind of specialist, either to provide a helpful second opinion regarding treatment or to take over the care of the disorder if this is indicated.

A variety of specialists have particular experience in dealing with the different musculoskeletal diseases. The *rheumatologist* is a specialist in internal medicine who has subspecialized in the medical treatment of muscle and joint diseases. The *orthopedist* is specially trained in surgical treatment of fractures and other bone and joint disorders. When nervous system disfunction is at the root of musculoskeletal problems, the *neurologist* is skilled at diagnosis and medical treatment, while the *neurosurgeon* is consulted when surgical treatment is necessary. Finally, the specialist in rehabilitative medicine, known as the *physiatrist,* is an internist trained to help patients recover lost function of muscles, joints or nerves—or, if the loss is irrecoverable, to help the victim adapt himself to it and live as normally as possible.

The osteopathic physician, until very recently, dwelt in a strange sort of limbo in the medical hierarchy; many people who have an impression that osteopaths are in some way better equipped to treat bone and joint diseases than regular medical doctors are not entirely clear just what osteopathy is, and hear discouraging stories about osteopathic treatment from their family doctors. Osteopathy began as a variant school of medical thinking and training originated in 1874 by a man named Andrew Taylor Still, and it remains a medical phenomenon unique to the United States and Canada. The first college of osteopathy was organized in 1892, and ultimately six were established, one later to become a regular medical school as a part of the University of California. The osteopath received the same full curriculum of medical training as the allopath (the conventional physician trained to use any and all scientifically effective modes of treatment) but with special emphasis on the structural defects of the musculoskeletal system as the underlying cause of disease. Receiving a D.O. (Doctor of Osteopathy) degree rather than an M.D., the osteopath often took his internship and residency training in special osteopathic hospitals, and proceeded to treat illness primarily by seeking to correct musculoskeletal defects by means of physical manipulation, supplemented by the use of medicines or surgery as he thought necessary.

For many years osteopaths have been regarded as poor relations by most conventionally trained physicians. Educational standards in the colleges of osteopathy have not matched those in regular medical schools, nor have osteopathic hospitals been able to provide the necessary clinical experience for interns and residents in training. Osteopaths have made no significant contributions to our knowledge of musculoskeletal disorders, and are no more skilled in bone-and-joint manipulation than regular M.D.'s or even good physical therapists. Indeed, in recent decades emphasis on "osteopathic methods" of treatment has declined even among practicing osteopaths, and the number of osteopaths in practice in this country—approximately 13,000—is smaller today than it was ten years ago.

Today many osteopathic graduates, encouraged by such medical organizations as the American Medical Association, have accepted the code of ethics of conventionally trained physicians, undertaken their work in regular hospitals, associated more closely with practicing M.D.'s and—in states where it is permitted by law—upgraded their medical training to achieve M.D. degrees. Although this close association has been vigorously opposed by major osteopathic organizations, it probably represents the wave of the future. In the meantime, victims of musculoskeletal diseases should realize that advanced knowledge of the nature and treatment of these disorders always has and still does lie in the province of conventionally trained physicians, specialists in internal medicine and orthopedic surgeons, and should seek out care for their illnesses accordingly.

In addition to physicians, surgeons and osteopaths, two other groups of professional workers are particularly concerned with treatment of diseases of the musculoskeletal system. These are the *physical therapists* and *occupational therapists* who work at the direction of physicians and surgeons to help prevent the physical disabilities these diseases may cause, or to help in the rehabilitation of victims who have lost the function of muscles, joints and nerves. In most cases these people are employed in hospitals, clinics and nursing homes, but some maintain private offices for the care of patients referred to them. They are skilled in the use of such special equipment as whirlpool baths, diathermy machines and ultrasound equipment, muscle-testing devices and machines employing mild electric current to stimulate the contraction of specific muscles. In addition they utilize heat, massage and various forms of exercise to aid the recovery of victims of musculoskeletal diseases. Occupational therapists are also experienced in retraining individuals who have permanently lost muscle, joint or nerve function to do what they still can do, employing the use of specific physical projects as a special kind of incentive or motivation. These workers are not physicians, however, and either physical or occupational therapy should always be carried out to the specific prescription of a doctor and under a doctor's supervision.

Other "physical therapy" measures, including Turkish baths, steam baths, saunas and the services of masseurs, are generally harmless but have little or no true scientific basis or medical value. Many a weary businessman or professional athlete feels rested and reinvigorated after a Turkish bath and rubdown, but these measures should never be considered an adequate substitute for scientific medical treatment in the face of illness or disability.

Finally, a word should be said about chiropractors, naturopaths and various other "healers" who deal in musculoskeletal disorders, some under the imprimatur of state licensure and control and some with no imprimatur at all except a sign on the door. The practice of chiropractic was devised in 1895 as an aberrant theory of the cause of disease by an Iowa grocer and fish peddler named Daniel David Palmer. It has subsequently been taught, in many variations, in a number of "schools of chiropractic" throughout the country. According to Palmer, virtually all human illnesses arose as a result of pinched nerves emerging from the vertebral column, and could be adequately treated by manipulating or "adjusting" the spine by means of a number of curious physical maneuvers. Unlike osteopathy, which has unfortunately been confused with chiropractic, there has never been any demonstrable scientific validity to chiropractic theory; practitioners were (and still are) inadequately trained in even the barest fundamentals of anatomy and physiology. Furthermore, in many areas chiropractic has led to spurious and even dangerous diagnostic techniques such as "whole body X-rays," the use of impressive but useless diagnostic boxes, improper use of electric currents and blatantly fraudulent therapeutic devices. This is not to say that all chiropractors are necessarily charlatans; some can, at least temporarily, relieve the pain of certain low back disorders, and some even acknowledge their limitations and refer patients to physicians when they recognize diseases they are not equipped to treat. But these practitioners are few and far between; most chiropractic patients have little basis upon which to judge whether they are being well treated, victimized or even endangered, and the risk of irreparable harm being done is so great that the practice of chiropractic was roundly condemned across the board in the pages of a major scientific medical journal as recently as 1971. By far the best course to follow, before consulting a chiropractor, is to *ask a licensed physician,* preferably one who knows you and your medical history.

Naturopaths have even less legitimate excuse for their ministrations, employing both the physical manipulations of the chiropractor and the use of "natural medicinal substances," a term so vague that it can include practically anything from simple syrup to cinchona bark. Finally there is a wide, ever present and ever changing variety of self-appointed "faith healers," most of whom are outright charlatans with no interest in anything but cashing in on human misery. None have any real scientific basis for their practices, and all should be scrupulously avoided. The overriding danger of consulting such quacks, many of whom are highly skilled confidence men, is that some truly serious disease or disorder may be ignored or overlooked until it has reached a point where even legitimate medical care can provide little help.

In addition to the many kinds of legitimate physicians and their aides equipped to diagnose and treat disorders of the musculoskeletal system, a large number of public and private agencies may be called upon by the victims of these disorders, or their physicians, for help of various kinds. Among these, the following deserve special mention here:

The American Arthritis and Rheumatism Foundation provides information and physician referrals, supplies physical therapy and loans special therapeutic equipment.

The National Foundation, supported by the March of Dimes, supplies funds for diagnosis, referrals, direct patient care and necessary equipment for victims of congenital defects, arthritis and poliomyelitis.

The United States Public Health Service provides information, nurses, clinics and laboratory facilities, with special services for handicapped children and amputees.

The Society for Crippled Children and Adults makes equipment, prosthetic appliances and transportation available for those who cannot provide their own, helps coordinate medical referrals and operates special summer camps for the handicapped.

The United Cerebral Palsy Association supports sheltered workshops for the handicapped and provides speech and hearing therapy facilities.

Volunteers of America operates summer camps for the handicapped.

The Shriners' Hospitals for Crippled Children provide hospital care, equipment, physical therapy and appliances for the needy.

Physical therapy, loans of equipment and transportation facilities are also provided by the *Elks Therapy Program for Children* and the *American Cancer Society*. In addition, in most states both the public schools and departments of vocational rehabilitation provide personnel and facilities to aid handicapped children and adults recover lost function or find ways to lead relatively normal lives when physical losses are irreparable. Your physician can provide you with further information about these and other agencies and their services.

VI

PATTERNS OF ILLNESS: THE NERVOUS SYSTEM

29. The Symptoms of Nervous System Disease   335

30. Major Nervous System Disorders   352

Most complex of all the organ systems, and often the most poorly understood, the human nervous system performs many crucial functions. It provides us with detailed sensory contact with the external world, and because it is intimately related to all the body's other organ systems, it helps regulate such vital internal functions as respiration, circulation and metabolism. Apart from these purely physical actions and reactions, it also makes possible such higher mental processes as thinking, remembering, judging and decision making, as well as mediating the wide range of emotions that make human beings so distinctively human.

Obviously our overall state of health, and even life itself, depends heavily upon the normal operation of the nervous system. But like any other organ system, it is subject to infection, physical trauma, the growth of benign or malignant tumors and a multitude of distinctive nervous system disorders that can interfere with that operation. Because of the extent and complexity of the system, many of these disfunctions may seem mysterious or frightening; but a clear understanding of the symptoms that may signal nervous system disease, and knowledge of the more frequently occurring diseases themselves, will go a long way to help us keep our nervous systems in peak working order.

29

The Symptoms of Nervous System Disease

The nervous system, like the circulatory system with its vast network of arteries, capillaries and veins, is spread far and wide through every part of the body, a complex organization of cells, tissues and organs that is more intricate and in many ways more immediately essential to life than any other. (*See* p. 42.) The human nervous system, composed of the brain, the spinal cord, the extensive peripheral network of motor and sensory nerves, both cranial and spinal in origin, and the special auxiliary chain of nerve ganglia and plexuses that make up the autonomic or "involuntary" part of the system, works as a whole to motivate and moderate the function of virtually every other tissue and organ in the body. And while certain disorders may primarily strike just one structure or another, the overall effects are likely to be widespread, for no part of the nervous system functions properly by itself.

To most laymen—and, indeed, to many physicians—diseases and disorders of this complex organ system have always seemed more serious and frightening than diseases of any other part of the body. There are several reasons for this very common attitude. For one thing, diseases of other organ systems generally manifest themselves by symptoms and signs that are directly and obviously related to the diseased system. Pneumonia, for example, causes an unmistakable and direct malfunction in the process of breathing. A fractured bone causes immediate and obvious trouble at the site of the fracture. But when a disease affects a part of the nervous system, symptoms may appear most mysteriously in quite another part of the body. Injure the spinal nerves in the lower back, and suddenly the muscles of the lower leg cease to work properly. Damage a certain portion of the brain and vision may be lost, although there is nothing discernibly wrong with the eyes. In all too many nervous system diseases there appears, to the layman, to be a total lack of any direct connection between the site of the active disease and the symptoms it may bring about.

A second reason that nervous system diseases are so deeply dreaded is that more than any other kind of affliction they can cause gross and frightening disturbances in multitudes of body functions that we take utterly for granted. They can suddenly affect our muscle control, interfere with vital sensory perceptions and even alter our state of consciousness. Most alarming of all, perhaps, is the prospect of sudden or gradual impairment of our mental capacities—not in the sense of mental or emotional illness such as the neuroses or psychoses (*see* p. 778), but in terms of outright organic or tissue-damaging disease that can permanently impair or destroy nervous system function. One can live with, and even accommodate to, a damaged liver or lung, but it is far more difficult, for victim and family alike, to live with the consequences of a severely damaged spinal cord or brain. Even lesser nervous system losses can completely alter lives in tragic ways: nerve damage may cause partial or complete paralysis; destruction of the optic nerves or the visual cortex of the brain can plunge the victim into permanent darkness; and loss of the capacity to hear or to articulate words can subject the sufferer to virtual neurological imprisonment.

Finally, when disease affects other organ systems, destroying cells and hindering their function, successful treatment and cure of the disease is, in most cases, followed by healing, regeneration of tissue and the restoration of full normal function. Further, with organs such as the lungs or the kidneys, the body has a wide reserve of functioning tissue so that even total destruction of one of the paired organs may leave the other with quite adequate function to take care of the body's needs. But in the case of nervous system disease there is no such reserve, except in certain unusual situations. And once a nerve cell is destroyed, there is no regeneration—it is irreparably gone and its function lost.

Thus it is that ever since nervous system diseases were first studied as such, about 150 years ago, and certain patterns and symptoms began to be understood, neurology and neurosurgery have always been regarded as among the most challenging and complex of the specialty fields in medicine. They remain so even today, not only because of the difficulty of treating these diseases once they have been diagnosed, but also because diagnosis itself can often be so difficult. Both the general practitioner and the specialist must rely on the patient's oral history and a variety of seemingly mysterious symptoms for their diagnosis. But that is only the first step, for symptoms are only a manifestation of a disease, not the disease itself. Thus the physician must be skilled in interpreting any cause-effect relationship, and in sorting out and tracing those symptoms that may have a direct connection with a possible nervous system disease. The patient, too, in order to aid the physician in his diagnosis, should have at least a general awareness of those symptoms that may signal a nervous system disorder. But perhaps more important, he should lay aside any fear he may have about nervous diseases. Mysterious they may be, but they can be diagnosed and treated, and early diagnosis is a crucial factor in the eventual outcome of treatment.

Common Symptoms of Nervous System Disorders

If injury or disease causes a breakdown in the function of the nervous system in any part of the body, it is logical to assume that there will be certain symptoms which are at least possible clues to what is going on. These symptoms usually fall into three broad categories. Some are *general symptoms* which may or may not be related to nervous system disease, but which suggest that some disorder in the nervous system *may* be present. Others are more *specific symptoms* which suggest at once that something is out of order in the nervous system. A third group of *mixed symptoms* suggests possible nervous system disease but may also suggest disorders of other organ systems as well.

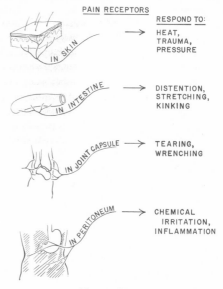

Figure 29–1.

Pain. The most common of all of these symptoms is pain, the general alarm system of the body. It may signal that something has gone wrong in virtually any part of the body, and the alarm is then picked up by pain or other sensory receptors in the area and carried to the brain by way of the sensory nerves. The occurrence of pain does not in itself necessarily mean that something is wrong with the nervous system, but it is often a feature of nervous system disease and requires investigation to determine its source. Sometimes the source is obvious from the *nature* or *quality* of the pain. A sharp, cutting pain is most often associated with injury to the surface of the body—lacerations, tears, abrasions, pinches, etc. A deeper pain which feels dull or diffuse, yet more severe, is often related to fractures or deep tissue infections such as boils, or occurs due to an insufficient blood supply to the heart. So-called visceral pain is related to disease or injury of the abdominal or pelvic organs, and is frequently associated with some degree of nausea.

In most cases pain is centered at the source of the trouble, but in some circumstances it may be "referred" to a distant part of the body. Thus, a pinched or irritated nerve near the lower end of the spinal cord, as in the case of a "slipped" or herniated intervertebral disk, may cause severe pain all the way down the back of the leg into the calf or ankle, along the route of the great sciatic nerve. The pain of angina pectoris due to insufficient blood supply to the heart muscle is often "referred" as an ache extending up the left side of the neck to the jaw and down the left arm as far as the wrist. Some kinds of referred pain are so characteristic of the cause that they immediately alert the doctor to the possible diagnosis.

Pain is probably the most important single symptom that causes an individual to seek medical care. A careful account of when it started, how it started, how it behaved (that is, whether steady or intermittent, throbbing or uniform), and even the words the patient uses to describe the pain, all provide important clues to the doctor in making a diagnosis. When a patient complains of an aching or cramping pain in the abdomen up under the ribs which always seems to be relieved by food or milk but which then recurs a few hours after a meal, the doctor will be concerned about the possibility of a peptic ulcer. A pain described as "stabbing" or "cutting" and felt just in the skin surface around one side of the chest is highly characteristic of herpes zoster or "shingles," a virus infection of the skin nerves.

Minor and transitory pain from known causes —hitting a thumb with a hammer, for example, burning a finger or twisting an ankle—may be safely treated by taking a mild analgesic such as

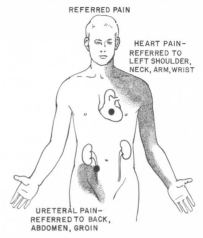

REFERRED PAIN

HEART PAIN—REFERRED TO LEFT SHOULDER, NECK, ARM, WRIST

URETERAL PAIN—REFERRED TO BACK, ABDOMEN, GROIN

Figure 29–2.

aspirin and waiting for the pain to go away. A pain that is more severe or recurrent or a pain whose cause cannot clearly be identified deserves medical attention. Common sense must be exercised in the use of pain medications that may be left over from treatment of some earlier condition. Whereas aspirin will rarely relieve or mask a serious degree of pain, the use of such preparations as codeine, Percodan or other narcotic painkillers without a doctor's advice may well blunt or dull a pain without meeting its source, and may lull the victim into a false sense of security while the real—and perhaps dangerous —cause of the pain gets progressively worse. In judging whether or not to consult a doctor when pain occurs, it is well to remember that *there is always a cause for persisting pain anywhere in the body,* and even when the source of pain is more psychosomatic than organic, it still deserves medical attention.

Finally, everyone has a level at which irritating stimuli become painful, or are interpreted as painful, and this level varies widely from one person to another. This "pain threshold" may be extremely low in certain individuals, so that even a relatively mild irritation is interpreted by them as "painful," and a more severe pain may be agonizing. On the other hand, some individuals with a very high pain threshold may not be bothered by irritable stimuli that would cause extreme discomfort in someone else. An individual cannot influence his pain threshold very much; a low threshold is not a sign of weakness, nor is a high threshold necessarily a particularly favorable sign. It is important, however, for each individual to have some idea where his pain threshold lies in order to help the doctor evaluate the nature of any pain he may be suffering. If a patient knows that he is very sensitive to pain, or relatively insensitive to it, he may well be able to provide the doctor with the critical item of information he needs to make a diagnosis.

Headache. Of the many kinds of pain, headache is one of the most common, and sometimes the most difficult for the average person to evaluate. Headaches may be serious or trivial, but with some knowledge of their cause and the kind of headaches that should be regarded as danger signs, it is possible for anyone to differentiate quite well between a headache that can safely be treated with a couple of aspirin and one for which medical attention should be sought.

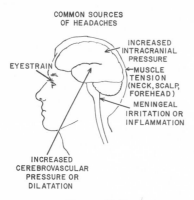

COMMON SOURCES
OF HEADACHES

EYESTRAIN

INCREASED
INTRACRANIAL
PRESSURE

MUSCLE
TENSION
(NECK, SCALP,
FOREHEAD)

MENINGEAL
IRRITATION OR
INFLAMMATION

INCREASED
CEREBROVASCULAR
PRESSURE OR
DILATATION

Figure 29–3.

In general, most headaches are believed to arise as a result of dilatation of arterioles and capillaries supplying the brain or the pain-sensitive meningeal tissues surrounding the brain and the spinal cord. Whether the headache results solely from the dilatation of these blood vessels or from a slight increase in pressure inside the skull as a result of this dilatation, no one knows. Headaches may also be caused by excessive tension of the muscles of the neck where it joins the scalp, or by strain of the muscles that control the eyes, the eyelids or the forehead.

By far the greatest number of common headaches occur only occasionally, are transitory and can usually be attributed to some identifiable cause. For example, headaches accompany most acute infections in the body, and often occur with fever. Sometimes fatigue is the cause, or eyestrain due to excessive reading, long periods of driving, lights that are too bright or too dim, or use of the eyes for too long at a single focal length—watching television, for example, without resting the eyes by intermittent close vision and distance vision. Excessively loud, persistent or irritating noise can also stimulate headaches. Occasionally allergic reactions are accompanied by severe headaches which are relieved by the antihistamine medications used to relieve other symptoms of the allergy. Various toxic substances can be another cause. The "hangover" headache, for example, arises because ingestion of a quantity of alcohol tends to dilate the cerebral blood vessels for a prolonged time, accounting for the throbbing head of the "morning after," often associated with quick movements or position change, and often accompanied by nausea and general dehydration. This kind of headache, which usually persists for anywhere from six to twelve hours, obviously will not be cured by "the hair of the dog," since further consumption of alcohol merely prolongs the state of cerebrovascular dilatation. Even aspirin is inadvisable, since it will only further irritate an already inflamed stomach lining without helping the headache much. The only really useful treatment consists of rest and relative inactivity, and taking fluids such as bouillon to replace salt and water lost by dehydration, and such noncitrus juices as vegetable or tomato juice which are rich in vitamin C.

Any headache which does not clear up quickly, recurs or persists for more than a few hours without any reasonable explanation, or is exceptionally severe should suggest the need for medical attention. Certain disease states which have nothing to do with the nervous system may be characterized by headaches of this sort. Among these, hypertension (high blood pressure) commonly causes a characteristic dull, throbbing headache felt at the base of the skull, especially noticeable upon first arising in the morning, with a tendency to decrease or disappear once the individual is up and about. Similarly, kidney disease which has caused a degree of kidney failure and uremia may also cause a severe generalized pounding headache. In addition, infections of the eyes, the nose, the throat or the ear may account for recurrent headaches. In all of these cases the headache may be repeatedly relieved by a steady diet of some analgesic such as aspirin, but the frequent use of any painkiller should not be undertaken without first discovering the underlying cause of the headaches.

Severe, continuing or recurrent headaches may also arise as a result of some specific disease or injury of the central nervous system. Trauma to the head, for example, may cause a severe headache, sometimes localized at the site of the injury and sometimes generalized. Even in the absence of any other neurological symptoms, such a headache can persist for a prolonged period of time, but a physician should know about the condition and follow it carefully since there is always a possibility of intracranial bleeding resulting from a head injury. Headaches due to meningeal infection or meningeal irritation are usually severe, constant and associated with stiffness of the neck or back, with marked increase of pain on bending the head downward. Any headache that is accompanied by other changes in body function—progressive weakness of one or another set of muscles, visual or speech difficulties, convulsions, vomiting, or persisting drowsiness or unconsciousness—demands immediate attention by a physician in order to establish a diagnosis and institute corrective measures if possible. These symptoms, or combinations of them, may indicate an increase in intracranial pressure from one or another cause: a brain tumor, for example, or other expanding lesion in the brain, an abscess in the brain, a blood clot formed beneath the meningeal layers surrounding the brain due to prior head injury, or active bleeding due to head injury or disease

of the blood vessels in the head. The sudden or abrupt onset of a severe headache for no discernible reason should always be investigated without delay. Such headaches may have perfectly benign causes, but the possibility that the headache arose because of a sudden increase in intracranial pressure due to hemorrhage from one of the blood vessels in the head must be investigated. On the other hand, headaches which persist for weeks or months without any significant change and without the development of any other symptoms or signs suggesting nervous system disease are more often related to psychosomatic or psychological disturbances than to organic disease. But in these cases, also, it is necessary to rule out a possible underlying disease before starting a program of therapy to treat the headache.

One kind of common headache which constitutes a distinct disease syndrome in itself is known as *migraine headache* or "sick headache." It is a severe, generalized headache which characteristically occurs in recurrent attacks, varying in frequency from once or twice a year to once or twice a week. In most cases the victim of migraine headaches is in perfectly good health except for these attacks which, when they occur, may be severe enough to be incapacitating and are frequently associated with nausea and vomiting. They are often heralded by a characteristic *aura* or "warning state" involving light flashes before the eyes, double vision or a feeling of slight nausea; and when not identified and treated early enough, they tend to last for a period of three to four days before they clear up spontaneously.

So far every effort to determine the cause of migraine headaches has failed. This type of headache has been described since the days of antiquity, and before modern treatments were devised it was not uncommon for a victim to be incapacitated for three or four days at a time, two or three times a month or more. For many years migraine headaches were thought to be a purely psychosomatic phenomenon; that is, a manifestation of excessive nervous tension or some other emotional upset. This view seemed to be substantiated by success in treating stubborn cases of migraine by means of hypnosis. But today physicians are not so sure that migraine headaches are entirely emotion-based. Some authorities believe that allergies are involved. There is often a history of people in different generations of the same family having migraine headaches, and there is no question that there is real dilatation of the blood vessels in the meninges and in the scalp during a migraine attack. Furthermore, migraine headaches do respond to certain medications that have little or no effect on any other kind of headache, suggesting a specific physiological cause. Indeed, the response to the administration of drugs of the ergot family, powerful vasoconstrictors, is so dramatic that a therapeutic trial of this kind of drug is often used as a diagnostic test to determine whether a recurrent headache is of the migraine type or not.

Treatment today involves use of drugs of the ergot family, preferably in conjunction with small doses of caffeine, begun as early as possible after the headache has started, if not sooner. In fact, if the individual can recognize an oncoming attack from a familiar aura, he can often abort the headache completely by starting medication before the pain begins. Once the pattern of a given individual's migraine headaches is understood and a successful program of treatment is set up under a doctor's direction, the migraine sufferer can ordinarily keep a supply of the medicine at home and treat himself as necessary. In such a case, however, periodic visits to the doctor are most important to assess changes or progress in the disorder, as some people who experience extremely severe migraines so dread an attack that they tend to overmedicate themselves or use medication even in the absence of any aura or onset of symptoms. On the other hand, migraine headaches characteristically recede in frequency and severity with the use of an appropriate treatment program, or as the individual approaches middle age, so that a review of the situation with the doctor will enable him to judge when medication can be reduced or stopped.

Another type of headache, similar in some ways to migraine but quite different in other ways, is the "cluster" headache, or *histamine headache*. Attacks, which are often severe, will ordinarily involve just one side of the head, temple, neck and face. Frequently they will be associated with pain in the eye on that side, and sometimes with swelling of the soft tissue around the eye and other apparently allergic symptoms such as watering of the eye and running of the nose. Sometimes the headache is so severe that there is actual tenderness to touch on the external forehead, temple and cheek or neck of the involved side, and the conjunctiva of the eye may become reddened. These headaches were once considered a variant of migraine headaches, but the fact that they typically occur on only one side and often do not respond to vasoconstricting drugs suggested some other kind of trouble. Today these headaches are thought to be a result of hypersensitivity to the chemical substance histamine which is released from the cells as part of the body's allergic reaction to some foreign protein. This theory is borne out by the fact that the frequency of these headaches can be sharply reduced and often terminated by the administration of a series of tiny sensitizing doses of histamine given by injection and gradually increased, thus getting the victim's body used to the substance so that a larger and larger amount is required to trigger the headache.

Unconsciousness. This condition is defined as a state of insensibility in which the individual is unaware of any sensory impressions and has no subjective experiences. Under ordinary circumstances every person spends approximately one-third of his life in an unconscious state, since normal physiological sleep is a form of unconsciousness. Indeed, a basic and regular minimum of sleep is an absolute necessity to continued good health and most particularly to normal functioning of the mind. Although we still do not know the exact mechanism that induces sleep, or exactly what it is that happens to the body or mind during sleep that makes it so necessary, we do know that this regular period of obliterating outside conscious impressions seems to be an essential restorative to the vitality of the nervous system, and also permits the overall metabolism of the body to slow down to a certain degree. A person may force himself to remain awake for a period of approximately 36 to 48 hours, sometimes longer, and with the use of certain stimulant drugs can induce sleeplessness up to 72 hours or more, but only at the price of the onset of mental confusion, visual hallucinations, and a tendency to doze off into marginal unconsciousness even while moving around with the eyes open. The disorienting and demoralizing effect of more prolonged periods with inadequate sleep is a familiar technique in "brainwashing" and in the "third-degree" type of interrogations.

Aside from normal sleep, however, unconsciousness is always an abnormal or pathological state and is often a manifestation of severe underlying disease or injury. It may be brief and transitory, as in simple fainting, or it may be prolonged. It may also vary in depth from a semiconscious stupor, from which the individual can be aroused with persistent effort, to the state of coma—unconsciousness so deep that the individual cannot be aroused at all, no matter what stimuli are used.

Fainting is a transitory spell of unconsciousness which may occur as a result of emotional shock, unexpected and sudden physical pain, or undue stress of any sort. Physiologically a person faints when some external stimulus causes a dilatation of the great blood vessels in the lower part of the body; the blood supply to the brain is therefore temporarily diminished, and the faint is a result of a wave of cerebral anoxia or "oxygen hunger." Usually a specific emotional jolt or an injury involving severe physical pain precedes fainting, but it may also occur during times of generalized physical or emotional stress. The main danger from fainting is the risk of a falling injury, since in a true faint there is no reflex action taken to break the fall. In the so-called hysterical faint used either consciously or unconsciously as a means of drawing attention, the "fainting" individual is usually careful to find a comfortable place to land. Other than the possibility of injury from a fall, fainting is self-limiting, since it places the head at a level with the rest of the body, allows the brain to be suffused with blood, and thus leads to speedy recovery of consciousness. An individual recognizing that he is about to faint by a sudden wave of dizziness, chilliness and perspiration can often

prevent it simply by sitting down and putting his head between his knees for a few moments or lying down with his feet elevated. Although some people tend to faint more readily than others, there is no pathological significance to this, and most soon come to recognize the prodromal symptoms and can usually prevent the faint from occurring.

More prolonged unconsciousness, ranging from *stupor* to deep *coma,* virtually always indicates something radically wrong, either some disfunction of the nervous system or some other organic disease or disorder. The most frequently encountered instance of stuporous unconsciousness is probably that of the individual who passes out from drinking. Essentially he falls into a deeper than normal sleep from which he can be partially aroused by painful stimuli, but then drops back asleep as soon as he is left alone again. The characteristic alcohol odor will be on his breath, and his breathing will be deep and noisy, but regular. "Passing out" is not always as harmless as it is often assumed to be. If the person passes out in such a position that his tongue falls back in his throat, it is possible that this, together with secretions from the nose and throat, may obstruct his airway and suffocate him. There is also a very real threat that he may vomit and aspirate material from his stomach into his bronchial tubes, a cause of aspiration pneumonia or lung abscess. Despite its widespread social use, alcohol is very decidedly a poison and a severe depressant to the body's respiratory centers; it is entirely possible for a person to ingest enough alcohol at one sitting to produce a fatal alcohol intoxication. Any individual who passes out from alcohol should at least be observed to see that regular respiration continues, and if there is any indication of irregular breathing or choking, appropriate first-aid measures should be undertaken and medical aid found as quickly as possible.

Passing out from alcohol is seen so commonly, and is so often politely ignored or treated as some kind of joke, that it is easy to overlook a simple fact: a person who has passed out may be unconscious as a result of something else altogether. Innumerable deaths have occurred when an individual who has been drinking heavily terminates his evening by taking a handful of sleeping pills, often in the perfectly innocent but befuddled belief that they will help him get to sleep. His body's respiratory controls are then so massively depressed by the double effect of the alcohol and the barbiturates that he proceeds into deep coma and death. There have also been innumerable deaths in cases in which severe diabetics who have fallen into coma are mistakenly assumed to have passed out from alcohol, partly because the sweetish odor on their breath resembles that of alcohol, and they then expire from diabetic acidosis. Again, individuals who have been drinking are often unsteady on their feet, and not infrequently take falls which could lead to unconsciousness due to head injury and cerebral hemorrhage. In short, it is wise to obtain medical aid for anyone who is found in an unconscious state from which he is difficult to rouse, unless it is a person known to you as an excessive drinker who has passed out from alcohol and who is, to your knowledge, not afflicted with any other illness. Even in that case, he should be kept under observation until the blackout is over.

Other causes of unconsciousness can often be deduced from surrounding circumstances. Evidence of a head injury—laceration of the scalp, distortion of head shape suggesting a fractured skull, or a "goose egg," for example—may indicate that a concussion, brain damage or possible cerebral hemorrhage is at fault. If the unconsciousness occurs in circumstances suggesting a water accident or drowning, with cessation of breathing as well as unconsciousness, artificial respiration by mouth-to-mouth resuscitation may be necessary. (See p. 107.)

Unconsciousness from barbiturate poisoning is very often signaled by the presence of an empty bottle of sleeping pills by the bedside. This method of "suicide" is, in fact, often used by the individual who wants to be sure that he is found in time and consequently leaves the incriminating bottle as glaring evidence. Unfortunately, such people are occasionally more successful in their attempted suicides than they really intend, and although comparatively rare, there are deaths due solely to barbiturate intoxi-

cation. Carbon monoxide poisoning can also cause unconsciousness, but is usually revealed by the surrounding circumstances—a victim found in a closed car, or in a garage, with the car's engine running. Unconsciousness can also occur as a result of a weak blood vessel bursting in the brain or the plugging of a cerebral blood vessel with a clot—both forms of so-called *cerebrovascular accidents.* And finally, an epileptic may have a period of unconsciousness following a convulsion, or unconsciousness may arise due to a tumor or infection in the brain. Speedy medical attention may be lifesaving in all these cases, since a physician can learn a great deal about the possible cause of unconsciousness from a fairly simple and expeditious neurologic examination. Whatever the cause, known or unknown, unconsciousness can be serious. Calling for medical help, and then standing by until it arrives, may well prevent an untimely and unnecessary death.

Convulsions. Convulsive seizures or "fits" are highly dramatic and frightening episodes, and are among the symptoms or manifestations that are almost invariably directly related to some disease or abnormality of the nervous system, specifically in the brain. *Grand mal seizures,* the major form of convulsions, cause the whole body to contort, stiffen and then shake in repeated rhythmic jerks for a period lasting from a few seconds to a minute or so. Less striking but equally symptomatic of some type of disturbance in the brain are the *petit mal seizures,* in which there is a brief, sometimes even split-second, loss of consciousness with immediate recovery. Other types of convulsive disorder include *psychomotor seizures,* in which the victim undergoes a change of consciousness, forgets where he is and what he is doing and wanders off, often recovering at some place nearby without knowing how he got there. And finally, one of the oddest of seizures, virtually always a sign of some destructive lesion in the brain, is the so-called *Jacksonian seizure,* a recurrent convulsive episode which begins with the twitching of an extremity—one thumb, for instance—and then in a matter of a few moments progresses to involve other fingers, the hand and wrist, and finally the whole arm in uncontrollable jerking movements which finally cease spontaneously as abruptly as they began.

Grand mal seizures in infants and young children frequently occur solely as a result of excessive nervous system irritability brought about by fever; frightening as they may be to a parent, they rarely signal serious nervous system disease or imply that the child necessarily will continue to have seizures or become epileptic. Such convulsions can usually be controlled or averted by being alert to the onset of fever and using a combination of antifever measures and a mild sedative until the fever subsides. (*See* p. 154.) Among older children, adolescents and adults who have convulsions, some clearly arise as a result of a specific and identifiable nervous system lesion of some sort. They can appear in brain or meningeal infections, in certain metabolic diseases such as hypoglycemia (low blood sugar) or underactive parathyroid gland function, as the result of poisoning with toxic agents such as lead or from acute alcohol intoxication, as a result of a brain tumor, a hemorrhage within the brain or in the meningeal layers with pressure on the brain, or following severe injury to the head. They may also occur as withdrawal symptoms in individuals who have been taking narcotic drugs, or as a result of withdrawal from heavy doses of barbiturates, certain tranquilizing drugs or large amounts of alcohol. But as many and various as these causes can be, in some 75 percent of cases of individuals beyond the age of three years who have convulsions, no obvious reason for the attacks can be found. It is believed, however, that even those that suffer from so-called idiopathic epilepsy (that is, epilepsy with no apparent cause) actually do have some focus of damage or scarring in the brain, even if it is microscopic in size, which has resulted from the bursting of a blood vessel, a degree of trauma in the process of birth, or some other injury.

The characteristics and treatment of convulsive disorders are discussed elsewhere. (*See* p. 883.) Here it is important to emphasize that convulsions are never "normal" and never "benign." Especially in individuals who have been completely free of any sign of convulsive disorders and then suddenly begin having them, the convulsions strongly suggest the possibility that some new focal lesion has developed in the brain. Anyone with any kind of convulsion should seek medical attention, and a concerted effort should be made to determine any remediable cause. In the case of a nervous system disorder that can be treated if diagnosed, convulsions can be an important clue to the cause of trouble. It is only when all possible causes of convulsions have been ruled out that the doctor will accept the diagnosis of idiopathic epilepsy and start the patient on a long-term program of treatment.

Whether convulsions are idiopathic or due to some identifiable nervous system lesion, the seizures themselves involve certain real dangers. In grand mal seizures especially, the victim may lose consciousness and fall quite abruptly, risking head injuries or broken bones. A clenched jaw is often a feature, and victims can bite their tongues severely if someone does not insert some padding, such as a rolled-up handkerchief, between their teeth. Occasionally the convulsive jerking of the body can involve such intense muscle contractions that compression fractures of the lower vertebrae have been known to occur. Perhaps even more alarming, seizures which occur repeatedly in some adolescents or adults sometimes appear to be related to progressive brain deterioration as a result of the seizures themselves. Thus, in most cases, treatment of convulsive disorders not only involves a search for possibly remediable causes, but is also directed toward preventing further seizures from occurring when this is at all possible.

Tics and Tremors. Both tics and tremors are neuromuscular manifestations which may or may not indicate that something is wrong with the nervous system. *Nervous tics* (sometimes called "habit spasms") are sudden, purposeless movements, often localized in a single area or group of muscles, that occur apparently beyond the conscious awareness or control of the individual. In most cases tics are more often a curiosity, and sometimes an embarrassment, than an indication of nervous system disorder.

The region of the head and neck is usually involved, and tics occur most frequently in children between the ages of six and twelve, although they can appear in any age group. The tic may be such a minor thing as frequent blinking of the eyes, or a facial twitch which involves a whole group of muscles. Other tics may involve grimacing, clearing the throat, inappropriate smiling, swallowing, coughing, shrugging the shoulders, or any "nervous habit" which is seemingly beyond the individual's control.

Tics of this sort may have psychological roots and in some cases can be corrected or controlled. There is rarely a specific physical cause, particularly for minor tics and twitches, but they are seldom related to any serious nervous system disease. But all tics or sudden, involuntary movements do not arise from innocuous sources. Occasionally a tic will develop in a person who has recovered from encephalitis (brain fever) and may represent a minor degree of cerebral palsy which can persist indefinitely. Of even more concern is a kind of tic which develops as a major symptom in acute rheumatic fever (*see* p. 560), appearing in some 50 percent of children suffering an attack of that disease. Known as *Sydenham's chorea,* this condition involves involuntary, purposeless movements of the extremities or trunk, sometimes so infrequent and subtle that only an experienced observer will notice them, sometimes so marked that the child is constantly making odd athetoid ("wormlike") movements of the hands, arms or shoulders. In this severe form the condition has been known for centuries as St. Vitus' dance. The chorea of rheumatic fever is a self-limited condition which clears up spontaneously after six to eight weeks without any sign of residual brain damage, although it tends to recur from time to time in about one-third of its victims. Its chief significance is that it provides an important diagnostic clue to the presence of acute rheumatic fever.

Painless tics of this sort should not be confused with another sort of condition bearing the same name: painful spasms of muscles that result from irritation of a nerve or nerve root. *Tic douloureux,* for example, is a pathological spasm or cramping of muscles on one side of the face or jaw, often agonizingly painful, that results from irritation of a branch of the trigeminal nerve, one of the cranial nerves that arise at the base of the brain. This very distressing condition requires medical attention and sometimes even surgical intervention before relief can be effected. Nor should ordinary tics be confused with another condition known as *Bell's palsy,* a transitory paralysis of the facial nerve, another of the twelve cranial nerves, which supplies the muscles in the cheek and upper face. This affliction, which is totally painless and which comes on without warning for reasons that are not clear, causes the affected side of the face to sag. The victim loses control of his lips on that side and has difficulty chewing or talking. Whatever the cause of Bell's palsy, it is benign, and in most cases the paralysis eventually disappears, although it may take several weeks.

Tremors may be much more serious matters. They are gross, persisting, involuntary movements of one or more parts of the body, usually an extremity, which, while often controllable by an effort of will, tend to recur as soon as the attention is turned elsewhere. In fact, tremors are alternating contractions of opposing muscle groups, and may be either quite fast, as many as eight to ten times per second, or slow, perhaps two to three times per second. Those known as *tremors at rest* occur only when the involved part of the body is relaxed and disappear as soon as motion is started. Those known as *intention tremors* work just the opposite: the tremor disappears when the arm, for example, is at rest but begins as soon as it is put into motion. Some kinds of tremors are highly characteristic of certain specific diseases or disease conditions: the individual suffering from severe liver failure, for example, may frequently develop a coarse, rapid, flapping tremor of the hands or arms much like the flapping of the wings of a bird; in Parkinson's disease there is a characteristic tremor of both hands and forearms in a slow rhythmic motion, with the thumbs brushing the tips of the curved fingers in a characteristic "pill-rolling" motion.

Unlike tics, most tremors have a basis in some kind of organic illness. They appear commonly in toxic states: the person addicted to morphine or cocaine may show a fine tremor of the face and hands which becomes particularly noticeable upon withdrawal; toxicity from an overactive thyroid gland causes a fine and rapid tremor of the fingers together with an elevated pulse; chronic poisoning with mercury compounds can cause tremors, and so can the toxic state that occurs in alcoholism. Finally, tremors may occur as a result of tertiary syphilis affecting the brain, or other nervous system diseases such as multiple sclerosis or a cerebrovascular accident. In old age a generalized arteriosclerosis of the cerebral vessels may bring about a tremor; but a tremor may also be a fairly common symptom in the presence of acute anxiety states. When a tremor appears, a physician should be consulted in order to find the underlying cause, if possible, and begin treatment.

Vertigo (Dizziness). True vertigo is a disturbance in which the individual has the impression of his body moving in space, or of the rest of the world moving around him, as distinguished from a feeling of faintness or lightheadedness. It is always a result of some disturbance of the function of the body's balancing mechanism; that is, of the inner ear, the cranial nerve that controls the balancing mechanism, the eyes or the muscles and joints involved in balance. It is usually associated with a tendency to lose equilibrium and lurch or stagger, and also frequently with a quite disabling and refractory nausea, sometimes accompanied by vomiting. The onset of such a condition after an automobile or bus ride, an airplane ride, or a ride in a boat may mean nothing more than a degree of motion sickness, which tends to disappear as soon as the motion ceases and can be much relieved by such simple nonprescription medicines as Dramamine. Sudden attacks of vertigo, combined with nausea and vomiting, which occur in the absence of motion are always abnormal, and a complete physical examination is necessary to root out the cause. The condition can be brought about by a middle or inner ear infection, by toxic states due to overuse of alcohol, salicylates or various sedatives, or by eyestrain, hypertension or a variety of other things. When no physical cause for the vertigo can be found and when it recurs without warning and lasts for periods of from a half-

hour to a day or more, the symptom complex, given the name *Ménière's syndrome,* can usually be controlled symptomatically until presently it goes away. But vertigo is unusual enough that every possible physical cause should be ruled out before the diagnosis of Ménière's syndrome is made.

Singultus (Hiccups). The common hiccup is another familiar neurological manifestation which, on rare occasions, can become much more than a minor annoyance. Hiccups, the result of spasmodic contractions of the diaphragm, often occur at regular and rhythmic intervals, causing short involuntary inhalations before the glottis in the throat can shut off the airway and permit swallowing. Hiccups may be triggered by a variety of conditions, usually by something which irritates either the diaphragmatic muscle itself or the phrenic nerve which passes from the base of the brain down to the chest to activate the diaphragm. Some people invariably get hiccups, for example, when they drink cold carbonated beverages. Sometimes hiccups are triggered by acid indigestion and heartburn, by pressure on the diaphragm caused by sitting or standing in a certain position (different for different individuals) or other minor irritants. Often there is no apparent reason for their occurrence, and in the vast majority of cases they cease within a matter of a few minutes whatever the cause. When they persist, a number of different maneuvers may help terminate them: holding the breath, for example, for 30 seconds; deep breathing for a few moments; drinking a cup of warm water; or rebreathing air in a paper bag for four or five breaths, thus increasing the carbon dioxide concentration in the blood stream. There is no reason to worry about the occurrence of hiccups unless they persist for several hours in spite of eating, drinking or normal activities, or unless they are disturbing sleep. *Persisting* hiccups, however, could conceivably be a clue to some underlying nervous system disorder that requires medical attention, and a doctor should be consulted if they continue for more than ten or twelve hours or in prolonged recurrences. Extremely rare cases of truly intractable hiccups do occur from time to time, and they deserve thorough medical investigation even though the cause can very seldom be found.

Specific Sensory Disturbances. Irregularities in taste, touch, smell, sight or hearing often provide direct clues to nervous system disorders—sometimes the earliest clues of all to appear. But like so many other symptoms, abnormalities in sensory reception do not by any means *always* indicate nervous system disease; it becomes the doctor's job to differentiate, for example, between sensory disturbances resulting from trouble in the nervous system and similar or identical disturbances arising from some disorder of the sense organs themselves. Numbness and tingling of the fingers and hands is a common early symptom of the kind of neuritis or nerve inflammation that can arise from deficiencies of certain of the B vitamins, or which may occur in diabetes or as a result of severe alcoholism. But the same symptoms may also occur because of impaired circulation in the extremities, perhaps as a result of progressive arteriosclerosis. Any visual disturbance, however minor or fleeting it may be, deserves a doctor's attention without delay, particularly such things as blurring of vision, temporary visual loss, or diplopia (double vision). Transitory hearing impairment is much less common, but recurrent curious noises in the ear—humming, buzzing or ringing—may be an early sign of some neurological disease. Even more suggestive are such sensory changes as an awareness of steady or recurrent abnormal odors, particularly when others notice nothing unusual, or the appearance of a persisting and unpleasant taste in the mouth. Although such abnormalities do not necessarily indicate the presence of some grave neurological disease, and thus need not be a cause for fear or panic, they should at least be adequately checked out by a physician.

The Neurological Examination

With such a bewildering variety of signs and symptoms which may or may not be related to some nervous system disease, how does a physician, whether a family doctor or even a specialist in neurology, manage to sift through them all to arrive at an accurate diagnosis? Nervous system disorders are certainly one of the most complicated and challenging areas of medicine, but no matter how complex such disorders may be, they almost invariably present characteristic warning signs or symptoms to alert the physician. And once he is alerted, there is a specific kind of physical examination which, in conjunction with a careful medical history, will assist him in his diagnosis.

Most of the major procedures in this so-called neurological examination are part and parcel of the ordinary general physical examination. But when something in the medical history or some particular physical symptom suggests the possibility of nervous system disease, there is a more detailed examination procedure the doctor can follow to gain additional information. The purpose of the neurological examination is to make a swift but thorough survey of the nervous system and its functions, and it involves the five major steps outlined below.

The mental state of the patient. This hardly requires any special examination procedures other than the doctor's visual observations and the normal exchange of questions and answers. Any oddity in the patient's general behavior and responses under any circumstances will alert the doctor to the possibility of nervous system disease. Certainly the patient who seems disoriented in time and space, for example, or who has a speech disorder or exhibits an abnormally poor memory for recent events will draw the doctor's attention. The patient who is unconscious when the doctor first sees him is obviously a special case. Even so, with the fact of the unconsciousness uppermost in his mind, the doctor can evaluate the patient's condition on the basis of other characteristic signs and symptoms.

The patient's gait, balance and posture. The alert physician can often note an abnormality in the patient's normal walking gait without any special examination. Oddities may be subtle but still noticeable to an experienced eye: the "duckwaddle" gait typical of the individual who has muscle loss in the pelvis supporting the hip, for example, or the diminished arm swing on one side that may be the clue to the so-called little stroke due to a transitory spasm of cerebral arteries. A person with a disorder of balance may tend to lurch from side to side, common enough in cases of alcohol intoxication but also suggestive of some kind of inner ear infection or acoustic nerve affliction when alcohol is not part of the picture. Balance may be further examined by means of the Romberg test, in which a patient, standing erect, closes his eyes and the doctor notes any consistent tendency to shift weight in one direction or the other.

A review of the cranial nerves. An assessment of the function of the cranial nerves is extremely important in any search for nervous system disorders. These twelve pairs of nerves which arise from the brain stem can very easily be checked for proper function and often provide the doctor with a clue to otherwise obscure neurological disorders. In addition, the cranial nerves account for much of the healthy person's perception of the world around him, and damage or loss of function of any one of them can be a serious handicap. Among others, the cranial nerves include the *olfactory nerves,* which provide our sense of smell; the *optic nerves,* by means of which we see; the *oculomotor nerves,* which permit us to move our eyes in their sockets; the *trigeminal* and *facial nerves,* which control most of the muscles of expression in our faces, lips and jaws; the *acoustic nerves,* which mediate our sense of hearing; the *glossopharyngeal* and *hypoglossal nerves,* which enable us to swallow and control the movement of our tongues; and the *vagus nerve,* which extends from the brain stem to the stomach and helps control the amount of acid secretion present there. All the cranial nerves are easy to check because their functions are so immediate and noticeable; a thorough review of these functions can be managed in a matter of approximately three minutes or less.

The patient's motor and sensory nerve systems. A few simple exercises will help the doctor in his assessment of the relative strength and range of motion of the muscles of the patient's legs and arms—the so-called motor responses that permit us to move about at will. Deficiency or weakness in a muscle or group of muscles does not necessarily imply that something is wrong with the muscle; it may mean that something has happened to the part of the nervous system that sends the motor nerves to that muscle, and the distinction is important in tracking down a possible neurological disorder.

The same is true for the sensory nerves. In this case, rather than testing muscle strength and function, the doctor will test such things as pain, heat or cold sensations in various parts of the body, as well as the patient's position sense. Ordinarily, for example, an individual lying relaxed with his eyes closed has no difficulty feeling the doctor touch his big toe, and then distinguishing whether the toe is being moved down or up. In the presence of certain kinds of neurological disorders, however, this position sense may be lost, and that loss is a vital clue in making the diagnosis.

The patient's reflex systems. In this part of the neurological examination, the doctor watches for two things: the depression or absence of certain normal reflexes and the appearance of others which are not normal and may signal the presence of certain neurological disorders. In the first group, all patients are familiar with the *deep tendon reflexes:* the knee jerk reflex, for example, or the Achilles' tendon reflex in the heel. In addition, most people will demonstrate "arm jerks" when deep arm tendons are tapped with the reflex hammer, and also will normally exhibit a "withdrawing" or "pulling away" type of reflex when the upper or lower abdominal muscles are stimulated by an unexpected gentle touch. Absence of any of these normal reflex actions is a clear indication that something is wrong and will flag the doctor's attention. The presence of abnormal reflexes is equally significant. For example, increased pressure within the cranium and hyperirritability of parts of the brain may cause an abnormal reflex known as *ankle clonus,* which may be elicited by placing the patient on his back and pushing his foot back sharply on his ankle. The ankle jerks rhythmically as long as the pressure is maintained. A similar regular jerking of the tendon across the front of the knee, the abnormal reflex known as *patellar clonus,* can be elicited by pushing the patella or kneecap back sharply. Other abnormal reflexes suggestive of disorder can also be elicited: for example, irritation of the sole of the foot ordinarily causes the individual to curl his toes down, but in the presence of certain kinds of disorders of nerve cells high in the central nervous system, stimulation of the sole of the foot will cause the toes to curl up, the so-called *Babinski sign*.

No part of the neurological examination in itself is necessarily diagnostic; however, a careful assessment of physical signs or abnormal reflexes can be very revealing. Complex as it may sound, a very thorough neurological examination can be conducted in the course of 15 or 20 minutes and often is a source of information which, combined with the history of the patient, will help the doctor pinpoint the diagnosis of neurological disease.

Finally, when nervous system diseases are suspected, the physician has at his command a variety of special diagnostic techniques to help him pinpoint the source and site of the trouble. Among the most common of these are simple X-rays of the skull and vertebral column. Quite frequently careful examination of such diagnostic films can reveal abnormalities that would

otherwise be exceedingly difficult to identify. They are particularly valuable in detecting tumors growing within the skull or in the spinal cord, or revealing such things as arthritic changes in the vertebrae that may be causing pressure or irritation of nerve roots. When impairment of the blood circulation to the brain is suspected, cranial arteriograms can be taken: special X-rays in which radio-opaque dyes are injected into the carotid arteries and then may reveal, in a series of films taken in rapid succession, areas of the cerebral vasculature through which normal blood circulation is blocked, markedly reduced, or abnormally increased.

Additional invaluable information can be obtained by performance of a *lumbar puncture* (often called an LP or spinal tap). After a drop of a local anesthetic has been injected into the skin of the lower back in the midline, a narrow, hollow needle is inserted between two of the lower lumbar vertebrae until it enters the fluid-filled space well below the end of the spinal cord itself. Spinal fluid pressure can then be measured

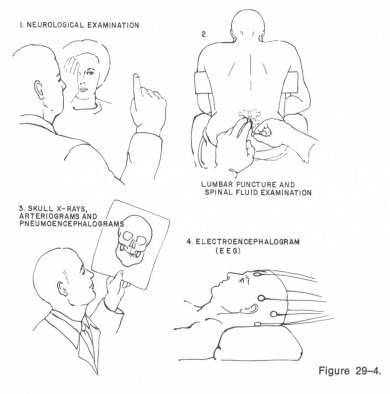

I. NEUROLOGICAL EXAMINATION

2.

LUMBAR PUNCTURE AND
SPINAL FLUID EXAMINATION

3. SKULL X-RAYS,
ARTERIOGRAMS AND
PNEUMOENCEPHALOGRAMS

4. ELECTROENCEPHALOGRAM
(EEG)

Figure 29–4.

directly to detect any increase above normal, sometimes a vital clue that a brain tumor is present or that a blood clot is causing increased pressure within the skull, to mention just two possible causes. In addition, a sample of spinal fluid can be removed or "tapped" for laboratory examination. Ordinarily spinal fluid is crystal clear, colorless, and free from any sign of blood cells or bacteria. If these are found to be present, or if the chemical makeup of the fluid is discovered to be abnormal, such changes may not only indicate nervous system disease but also help the doctor identify its nature.

The lumbar puncture may also provide a means of performing an even more specialized examination of the interior structure of the brain itself, a procedure known as a *pneumoencephalogram,* in which spinal fluid is drained a bit at a time from the spinal column and ventricles of the brain and allowed to be replaced with air. X-rays taken during such a procedure reveal the interior contours of the cerebral ventricles far more clearly than they can be seen by any other means, and dreadful as it sounds, the procedure is actually both safe and painless.

An *electroencephalogram* is a procedure performed by attaching electrodes to the patient's scalp by means of a simple adhesive and then making a graph of the tiny, rhythmic electrical discharges generated by the brain during its normal activity. These so-called brain waves occur in characteristic patterns during normal waking and sleeping periods, but are often markedly altered in the presence of various convulsive disorders or other nervous system diseases. Although electroencephalogram records are complex enough to require expert interpretation, they are so simple to record with ordinary office or hospital equipment that they are often performed whenever any question of neurological disease arises, especially brain disease of any kind. Finally, under certain circumstances, it is possible for the neurosurgeon to determine the extent and nature of brain damage at surgery by means of gentle electrical stimulation of various portions of the brain, with close observation of the response that occurs when one or another area is stimulated.

Thus, by means of diagnostic techniques that range from the most simple and routine to the most highly complex, it is possible today for general physicians or neurologists to identify, diagnose and plan treatment of an immense variety of nervous system ailments, some so obscure or mysterious that they were hardly recognized to exist as little as a few decades ago. Medical progress in this field has done much to reassure the victims of nervous disorders and their families, and it is even more reassuring to know that neurological research continues at a rapid rate, with the promise of many more significant breakthroughs in the future.

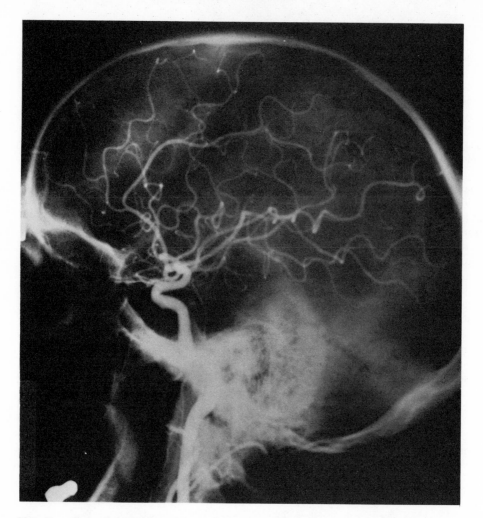

Plate 7a   Normal cerebral angiogram (side view). The cerebral arteries are outlined by a harmless radio-opaque dye injected into the carotid artery just prior to X-ray exposure.

Plate 7c   In another special examining technique, the ventriculogram, radiotranslucent air is introduced directly into the cerebral ventricles by the neurosurgeon in the operating room. Side view.

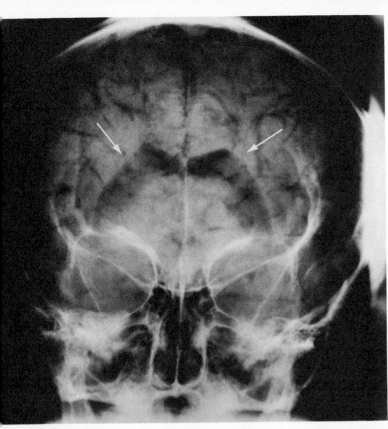

Plate 7b
Normal pneumoencephalogram
(front view) showing radiotranslucent air in spaces within the
brain that are normally filled
with cerebrospinal fluid.

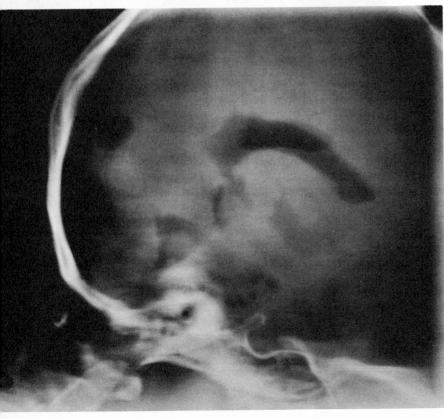

30

Major Nervous System Disorders

Any attempt to catalog human illness according to specific organ systems must inevitably suffer one drawback: the fact that virtually all diseases affect more than one organ system at a time. Although a given disorder may have its root cause in damage or destruction of tissue in one particular organ system, the effects of that disorder, more often than not, may be felt in some completely different part of the body. This is particularly true of diseases and disorders of the nervous system. Because the nervous system is a major "controlling" organ system of the body, almost any nervous disease will have widespread effects elsewhere. The reverse is also true; diseases and disorders centered primarily in other tissues and organs may have a devastating effect on the nervous system.

A great many infectious diseases affect the nervous system, for example. Some, such as poliomyelitis, viral encephalitis (brain fever) and rabies, are caused by viruses. Syphilis, a bacterial infection, can cause permanent destruction of nerve cells in the spinal cord or in the brain itself in its later stages. African sleeping sickness may also cause brain damage as a result of infestation of the body by a parasitic protozoan organism transmitted to man by the bite of the infected tsetse fly. Tetanus is primarily a bacterial infection of soft tissues of the body, but the infective organism releases a deadly toxin that travels in the blood stream and becomes lodged or "fixed" in nerve cells in the spinal cord or brain stem, leading to violent muscle spasms. The diphtheria organism may

also threaten life by its production of a similar deadly "neurotoxin." Finally, many of the disorders of the musculoskeletal system also deeply involve the nervous system because of the close relationship between the function of nerve and muscle. Fractures of the skull, neck or spine, for example, obviously endanger nerve tissue and can cause severe nervous system disfunction. Herniated intervertebral disks, spinal arthritis or whiplash injuries of the neck may also involve irritation or injury to spinal nerves, and the interrelation between nerve and muscle in such conditions as myasthenia gravis is so close that this illness is sometimes classified as a "neuromuscular disease."

In considering diseases and disorders that are primarily centered in the nervous system, it is often convenient to divide the system into its component parts: the brain and spinal cord of the central system; the motor and sensory networks of the cranial and spinal nerves; and the autonomic nerve networks of the peripheral system. But it is well to remember that just as a nervous disorder may impair the function of some completely different organ system, so a disorder in a specific part of the vast network of the body's nerve tissue may very well have a profound effect on any or all of the other parts of the system.

Diseases of the Peripheral Nerves

If nerve cells are the most delicate of all tissues in the body, and the most vulnerable to injury, they are also the best protected, up to a point. The brain and most of the cranial nerves are contained in the solid, bony vault of the skull; the spinal cord is encased within the closely fitted, semiflexible vertebral column. Even the spinal nerves of the peripheral system which arise from the spinal cord and travel to the extremities are bound together in nerve trunks that are generally located as deeply as possible, lying close to the bone in the legs and arms and protected by muscle and connective tissue. Even so, these peripheral nerves are more vulnerable to injury than other parts of the nervous system, and one of the first things a physician checks when he is examining a victim of a serious accident is to see that no injury to nerve has taken place. Even a simple cut finger may become a major injury if the nerve carrying sensory or motor fibers has been severed.

Injuries to nerves can be recognized either by the loss of motion of some part of the body due to tearing or crushing of a motor nerve or by the loss of sensation—pain, touch or heat—due to injury to a sensory nerve. If the nerve is severed, sensory or motor loss will be permanent unless the nerve can be repaired. Severing a nerve in an extremity does not destroy the nerve cell, since its cell body and nucleus are located within the spinal cord; the fibrils in the nerve trunks are merely long extensions of the nerve cell. When a nerve trunk is severed, the part beyond the site of injury atrophies and dies, but if the nerve trunk is carefully repaired by suturing the severed ends together, the living nerve cell can grow a new fibril along the nerve trunk and loss of function may ultimately be restored. Regrowth of a nerve fibril is a very slow process, but in the case of injury to the nerve of a finger, recovery of the loss may be achieved within a few weeks. If the injury occurs in the upper arm, however, recovery may be delayed for months or more because of the longer distance the nerve fiber has to grow. Many accidental injuries merely crush the nerve rather than actually severing it, and in this case the chances of full recovery through regrowth are much better.

Palsy or paralysis, either temporary or permanent, may also result from injury or disease of the peripheral nerve. Bell's palsy is a temporary paralysis of the facial nerve which occurs for unknown reasons, but most probably as a result of nerve irritation due to inflammation, as with a virus infection. Other nerve palsies may arise from chronic inflammation or trauma to a nerve somewhere in the body. For example, the ulnar nerve carrying motor nerve fibers to the ring finger and little finger of each hand passes down the arm very close to the skin overlying the outer surface of the elbow. Hitting the so-called funny bone results in an "electric" tingle felt in the ring finger and little finger, a familiar experience which, in fact, has nothing to do with bone at all; it is a minor trauma to the ulnar nerve. Occasionally a more severe injury in this area may result in inflammation and scarring of the nerve fibers traveling in the ulnar nerve trunk, causing an *ulnar nerve palsy*. This can usually be alleviated by protecting the nerve from further trauma, or in some cases by actually shifting the nerve trunk, by means of surgery, from its normal course across the bone of the elbow to an adjacent area of muscle where it is better padded and protected.

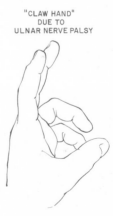

"CLAW HAND"
DUE TO
ULNAR NERVE PALSY

Figure 30–1.

Neuritis and Neuralgia. These two terms, often incorrectly used interchangeably, actually represent two quite different conditions. *Neuritis* is a general term meaning "inflammation of nerve cells or nervous tissue" and is a disease process that may stem from a multitude of causes. *Neuralgia,* strictly speaking, is a symptom rather than a disease and refers specifically

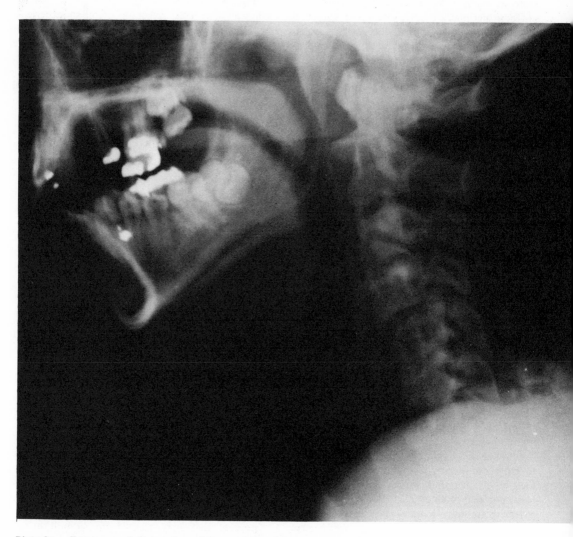

Plate 8a   Fracture and dislocation of the neck involving the 4th and 5th cervical vertebrae.
Side view.

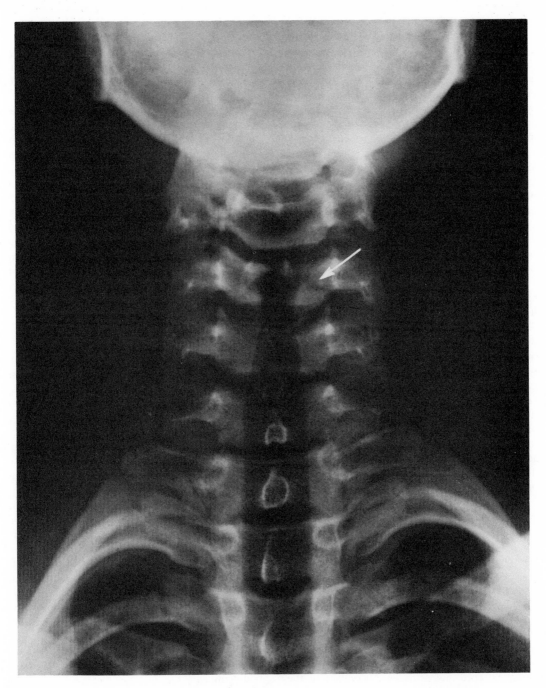

Plate 8b   Same injury, front view, showing the fracture line. This patient was initially paralyzed
by the injury but eventually made full recovery.

to paroxysms of acute pain which occur along the distribution of a single sensory nerve, often for unknown causes but usually related to some kind of irritation of the nerve or nerve root. *Tic douloureux,* a severe spasmodic pain in the jaw and cheek due to irritation of the trigeminal nerve, is a form of neuralgia. Another true neuralgia is characterized by recurrent attacks of acute pain in the back of the throat, tongue and middle ear. Known as *glossopharyngeal neuralgia,* it is an extremely rare condition of unknown origin which, when severe, has to be treated by surgical severance of the glossopharyngeal nerve. Most references to "neuralgia," however, that are found on the labels of aspirin bottles and other nonprescription medications actually refer to vague, generalized pain or discomfort which may have nothing at all to do with nervous system disorders.

Neuritis as a specific disease process can be caused by infection, injury or trauma, chemical irritation such as poisoning by lead or arsenic, alcohol toxicity, and even pressure on a nerve during sound sleep or while under anesthesia. It may involve nervous tissue in the brain, the spinal cord or the nerve trunks, in which case it is often called peripheral neuritis. Neuritis involving several nerves in different areas at once frequently accompanies nutritional deficiency, particularly the lack of vitamin B_1, as is often seen in the alcoholic who fails to eat properly, or as part of the disease process in uncontrolled diabetes mellitus. It is also a typical symptom of pernicious anemia.

Neuritis is characterized by such uncomfortable sensations as tingling, burning, "pins and needles," or even more severe pain. Both sensory and motor nerves can be affected, and the painful sensations are often accompanied by muscular weakness and tenderness; if the neuritis is prolonged, gradual atrophy of the muscles served by the affected nerves may occur.

Certain types of neuritis occur commonly enough to be recognized as separate clinical entities. For example, the *sciatic nerve,* which is made up of nerve fibrils from the lower end of the spinal cord and provides innervation to the entire leg, is quite commonly involved in neuritis because of either disease or trauma to the nerve proper, as when an intervertebral disk degenerates and presses against the sciatic nerve roots in the low back. This causes the syndrome known as *sciatica,* characterized by pain in the buttocks and down the back of the thigh and leg to the ankle, sometimes numbness along the outside edge of the foot, perhaps other disturbances in sensation in the leg, weakness of the calf muscles as evidenced by the inability to raise up on the toes on the affected side, and diminution or absence of such deep tendon reflexes as the knee jerk or the ankle jerk. Neuritis of the sciatic nerve—or any other nerve—will usually be called to a doctor's attention because of pain or discomfort, and a careful examination is necessary to determine the underlying injury or disorder that is causing it. In most cases, neuritis can be successfully treated if the underlying cause is found and corrected, but the condition may recede slowly, and may require extended bed rest and particular care to keep affected muscles in tone until the neuritis is improved.

Spinal Cord Disorders

The spinal cord connects the control centers of the brain with the multitudes of nerves extending to all parts of the body, and obviously any injury or disease that affects the spinal cord will have far-reaching effects on the body's function. The most common and tragic spinal cord injury occurs when one or more of the vertebrae are fractured or displaced and crush, tear or even transect the vertical nerve pathways at the site of the injury. Such injuries may result in the loss of all function, both motor and sensory, in all parts of the body served by the nerves arising from the spinal cord below the injured area. When the injury occurs at the level of the middle of the back, it leads to *paraplegia*—paralysis of both lower limbs from the hips down. Paraplegia is also usually accompanied by pain above the level of paralysis radiating up into the back, and both bladder and bowel function are commonly lost. This is an all too frequent result of automobile accidents, severe falls or other massive bodily injury.

When the injury is higher up, with damage to the spinal cord at the neck level, the result may be *quadriplegia*—paralysis of all four extremities, often including the accessory breathing muscles, in which case the victim's respiration must be supported by an iron lung or positive

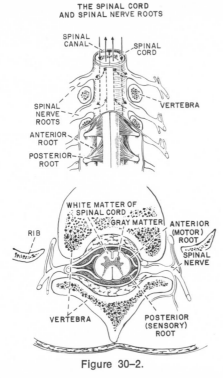

THE SPINAL CORD
AND SPINAL NERVE ROOTS

Figure 30–2.

pressure breathing apparatus. Although fractures of the vertebrae of the neck occur fairly frequently, this dreadful complication is fortunately quite rare, and in most cases can actually be prevented by moving the accident victim with extreme care, under medical supervision if possible. (*See* p. 298.)

Neck fractures with resulting paraplegia are most frequently the result of diving accidents, but recently they have become increasingly associated with the use of the trampoline by untrained amateur gymnasts, both young and old. The trampoline appears deceptively easy to use, harmless and fun; but it is, in fact, an exceptionally dangerous piece of equipment and should be used only by expertly trained, physically mature individuals in superb condition. Many physicians feel strongly that the trampoline is so potentially dangerous that it has no place whatever in any

mandatory physical education program in our public schools, and that parents should be fully aware of the danger before giving consent for their children to engage even in voluntary trampoline practice. Even special precautions, instruction or assistance cannot fully remove the risk of tragic accidents in the event that a trampoline performer loses control.

Although any injury which tears, cuts, compresses or even bruises the spinal cord may cause the symptoms of paraplegia or quadriplegia, the outcome of such an injury can depend heavily upon obtaining excellent and specialized medical care as swiftly as possible. There is no way to determine the exact nature of the injury upon initial or superficial examination; if the spinal cord has actually been torn or transected, recovery may never occur no matter what is done. But when the injury involves only, for example, pressure on the spinal cord caused by bone fragments or by formation of a blood clot or hematoma in the injured area, early neurosurgical intervention can often relieve the pressure quickly enough to permit recovery of motor and sensory loss. If the cord has been injured only by bruising, prognosis for eventual recovery is very good. In general, however, unless the necessary surgery is done very quickly—usually within 24 hours of the injury—potential for recovery diminishes sharply. With any further delay it may be lost completely even though the damage might have been correctable earlier. Once the victim of such an injury is in the hospital, careful X-ray examination of the spine from a variety of angles, examination of spinal fluid from a lumbar puncture, and a detailed neurological examination will aid the neurosurgeon in judging what, if anything, can be done. But in some instances, even during and after surgery itself, the doctor cannot be certain how extensive the injury actually is and what the chances of recovery are. In such cases, one can only wait, provide excellent nursing care to avoid such threatening complications as bladder infections or bedsores, provide physical therapy in order to keep the muscles and joints of the paralyzed extremities in healthy tone, and otherwise prepare expectantly for recovery. Even when that recovery comes, it may not be complete, but *any*

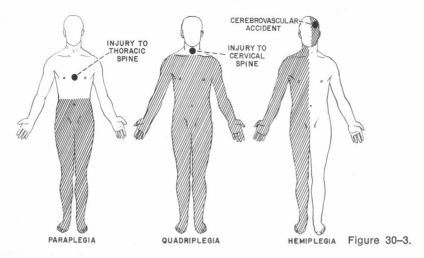

SPINAL CORD INJURIES

INJURY TO THORACIC SPINE

CEREBROVASCULAR ACCIDENT

INJURY TO CERVICAL SPINE

PARAPLEGIA   QUADRIPLEGIA   HEMIPLEGIA   Figure 30–3.

degree of recovery, however slight, is worth the struggle necessary to achieve it.

All paraplegia or quadriplegia is not necessarily a result of injury to the spinal cord. A tumor of the cord, whether a primary growth or a metastatic tumor seeded into the bone of the vertebral column from a distant primary cancer, may gradually exert pressure on the cord and even invade the nerve tissue to cause a gradually developing paralysis. In most cases of this sort, pain in the area is a prominent feature of the illness, and a general physical examination and laboratory tests will reveal the site and nature of the lesion. Surgical removal of as much of the tumor as possible will often permit recovery of lost sensory or motor functions, particularly if the tumor is merely a benign but space-taking growth. But ultimately the prognosis for recovery depends on how much damage had already occurred to the cord and whether or not regrowth of the tumor occurs.

Syringomyelia, another progressive disease of the spinal cord, can lead to destruction of a portion of nerve tissue with consequent sensory loss and muscular atrophy of the extremities. The condition leaves localized holes or cavitations in nerve tissue, permanently destroying the nerve cell bodies in the damaged area. The cause is unknown, although some physicians believe it may be due to some developmental abnormality

in the fetus, and it often occurs in the presence of other developmental defects such as webbed fingers, clubfeet or extra ribs. There is no cure for this slowly progressive condition, but it may be arrested for years at a time so that the victim may live to be as old as thirty-five or forty, much of that time spent in relative comfort.

Finally, the spinal cord or spinal nerve cells may also be involved in various kinds of infection or inflammatory processes. Most familiar and serious of these is meningitis—infection of the meningeal membranes enclosing the brain and spinal cord, and especially the swift-moving and often fatal variety caused by the meningococcus organism. (*See* p. 199.) Meningitis usually occurs when bacteria invade the meninges from within the body, but it can also arise as a serious infectious complication of such injuries as open fractures of the vertebrae. Other infections involving the spinal cord and spinal nerve cells include poliomyelitis and herpes zoster, or shingles.

Head Injuries, Concussions and Amnesia

Blows to the head are among the most serious of all physical injuries, and rightly so, for they are potentially the most dangerous. A fractured leg may cripple the victim temporarily, and a blow rupturing the spleen can cause serious internal hemorrhage, but at least something can be done to relieve such problems when they are discovered. A head injury, however, can lead to permanent—even fatal—destruction of brain tissue, and all too often the damage that is done cannot readily be repaired or corrected. Perhaps it is not coincidence that our most perceptive sensory organs—the eyes and the ears—are located in the head, standing guard against such injuries as well as keeping us posted about other events in our environment.

When they do occur, injuries to the head can cause many different kinds of damage. A skull fracture may exert pressure on the brain, damage brain tissue with fragments of bone, or cause internal bleeding that leads to increased pressure within the cranium which in itself can squash and destroy brain tissue. (*See* p. 128.) An open skull fracture in which the skin is broken poses the additional threat of infection of the meningeal membranes or the brain itself. Even in the absence of a fracture or intracranial bleeding, a mere physical jolt to the head may cause brain damage or disturbance of mental function.

Whenever a head injury has been sustained, even a seemingly minor blow, the victim should be seen by a physician at the earliest possible moment. The severity of the injury, of course, determines the procedures that should be followed. If the injury appears to be minor and the victim can be safely moved, he should be taken to a hospital immediately, *always* in the company of another person, as the victim of even a minor jolt may be mentally confused, perhaps agitated and unable to follow instructions or take care of himself. If the injury is more serious, the victim should *not* be moved until medical help arrives, and appropriate first-aid measures should be taken to combat external hemorrhage, cessation of breathing, cardiac arrest and shock, all of which may complicate a severe head injury. (*See* p. 103.) Again, the victim should never be left alone.

Whatever other damage may result from a head injury, virtually any moderate to severe blow will be accompanied by a *concussion,* a jarring injury to the brain. Even a mild concussion can cause at least momentary unconsciousness—witness the prize fighter who is "knocked out" for seconds or minutes during a boxing match. More severe concussions may result in prolonged unconsciousness, and if there is also intracranial bleeding, it may progress into coma. It is not particularly useful for the layman to try to distinguish between temporary unconsciousness and coma when dealing with the victim of a head injury, nor is the victim helped significantly by first-aid efforts to "bring him around." Any measures beyond the four first-aid priorities are distinctly the physician's responsibility, not the layman's.

Medical or surgical treatment of head injuries is guided by the doctor's diagnosis of the damage that has been done and by observation of any neurological symptoms that may subsequently appear. In many cases nothing but observation is indicated; in other instances neurosurgery may be necessary to stem intracranial hemorrhage, evacuate blood clots or hematomas, or debride bone fragments or destroyed brain tissue. Often the full extent of the injury cannot be determined for weeks or months as lost neurological function gradually returns. Infection can complicate treatment severely; later complications may include convulsive disorders triggered by scar tissue forming in the brain or disturbances in mental function, including episodes of severe depression or agitation. Early and expert treatment and prolonged post-injury observation are always essential. Thus any such injury, no matter how minor it may seem, deserves a high degree of enlightened respect.

A remarkable folklore has grown up around another possible complication of head injuries: *amnesia* or some degree of memory loss, either temporary or permanent. Who has not read novels or seen movies in which the hero recovers consciousness following a blow to the head, unable to remember who he is, where he lives or what he is doing? According to the familiar scenario, memory is later dramatically restored —usually by another blow to the head. While such bizarre occurrences have indeed been reported on rare occasions in medical literature, this picture of amnesia is for the most part utter nonsense in real life. There are, however, certain quite common circumstances in which some form of amnesia does occur. The victim of a head injury and concussion, for example, may well be confused and at least partially amnesic for a short while—perhaps even a few hours—following his injury. Temporary mental confusion misinterpreted as amnesia may also occur due to clinical shock, in a diabetic suffering from insulin shock (*see* p. 700), following the administration of electroshock therapy for certain forms of mental illness (*see* p. 803), following a grand mal seizure (*see* p. 883), or as a symptom in certain emotional or mental disturbances. When true amnesic memory loss is present in such cases, however, it is usually only partial and clears up quickly and spontaneously, once the underlying cause is identified and treatment, when appropriate, is begun.

Amnesia should not be confused with a quite different phenomenon. The mind has a remarkable capacity to "forget" particularly painful, frightening or unpleasant experiences, a familiar phenomenon which psychologists know as *blocking* and which is seldom related to any physical illness or injury. In most such cases the blocked experience can be recalled in perfect detail as soon as the individual is confronted with it, but sometimes blocked memories resist all efforts to call them to mind. Most authorities regard this as a mechanism used by the mind to protect itself from the possible ill effects of memories that might be emotionally harmful.

Perhaps closest to the popular picture of amnesia is the *retrograde amnesia* which is commonly seen in an individual who has suffered some experience that was both physically dangerous and emotionally frightening—following a serious automobile accident, for example. Often the victim of such an accident is later quite honestly unable to remember events that occurred for some period of time *prior* to the accident. For example, the man injured in a collision while driving to work may later be unable to remember anything that occurred from the time he finished shaving that morning. Frequently the accident itself is also blotted out. No one knows for certain why retrograde amnesia occurs; it is not necessarily related to any brain injury. Possibly it is a mind-protecting mechanism very similar to blocking, and usually no treatment is particularly helpful. In most cases the "lost"

memory will return in bits and pieces, more or less slowly, over a period of days or weeks following the incident, but sometimes the memory of the accident itself remains permanently expunged.

Cerebrovascular Accidents

While severe head injuries are certainly a threat, they are by no means as common as another class of disorder that can affect the brain. In fact, *cerebrovascular accidents* (CVA's) are the most frequent of all causes of brain damage, and despite the term used to describe them, they are not usually associated with external injuries. Rather, they are internal "accidents," arising from a variety of different causes, which impair circulation of blood to the brain.

More than any other organ of the body, the brain depends heavily upon a rich and continuing supply of oxygen from the blood stream. It is estimated that the brain ordinarily receives 25 percent of the heart's total output of oxygen-rich arterial blood, even though brain tissue represents less than one-tenth of total body weight. Other organs—even the heart—have at least some degree of reserve, so that temporary interruption of circulation may impair function but will not stop it. The brain does not, and any limitation of oxygen supply due to circulatory distress of any kind will lead to actual death of nerve cells within a matter of a minute or two.

Stroke. The most common cerebrovascular accident is the stroke, commonly spoken of as "apoplexy," the destruction of brain tissue due to hemorrhage or rupture of a blood vessel within the brain. It may also be caused by *thrombosis* or formation of a clot within the brain, usually as a result of severe *arteriosclerosis* or thickening of the cerebral blood vessels. In either case, brain tissue is suddenly deprived of its vital oxygen supply. As the name "stroke" suggests, this kind of cerebrovascular accident usually occurs without warning, and it may cause a degree of neurological loss ranging from a very slight weakness of a few muscle groups on one side of the body to almost complete *hemiplegia* or paralysis of one side of the body. The degree of the damage depends upon which particular vessel suffers the accident, how big it is, where it is located in the brain, and how much of the brain tissue is actually destroyed. This kind of CVA most commonly occurs after the age of fifty; when a stroke occurs in young people or children it is usually the result of an *embolism* associated with heart disease or the rupture of an *aneurysm* or weak spot in a cerebral blood vessel. In the former case, a floating blood clot or embolus is released from the heart into the blood stream and finally lodges in a branch of the cerebral arterial tree. An embolism can also result from rheumatic heart disease or bacterial endocarditis when a vegetative growth from the lining of the heart breaks loose and is carried to the brain. An aneurysm is usually the result of some developmental defect.

When a stroke is impending, the victim frequently experiences premonitory or warning symptoms—dizziness, vertigo, sometimes nausea and vomiting, and transitory weakness of the muscles or disturbance of sensation on one side of the body. Once the accident occurs, headache is a common symptom, nausea and vomiting frequently occur, and—less frequently—there may be an episode of convulsions. From 25 to 50 percent of the victims of stroke go into a

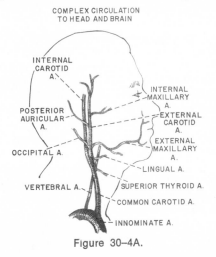

COMPLEX CIRCULATION
TO HEAD AND BRAIN

Figure 30–4A.

deep coma; those who do not may demonstrate weakness or paralysis of muscles of the extremities of one side, a weakness of facial muscles on one side, disturbances of speech (slurring or

inability to control the tongue in order to pronounce words correctly), or even aphasia (inability to speak).

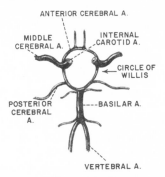

Figure 30–4B.

The outcome of a stroke depends very much on the size of the damaged area of brain and its location, and on the exact nature of the cerebrovascular accident causing it. If there has been a cerebral hemorrhage, it will often be accompanied by prolonged coma, convulsions and various other neurological signs that can be elicited on examination. Blood will usually be found in the spinal fluid, and the spinal fluid pressure is usually increased. Indeed, one of the ways such a patient's day-to-day progress can be judged is by comparing the relative amount of blood present in daily spinal fluid samples. Cerebral thrombosis frequently has less acute signs and symptoms, with the victim remaining awake or recovering from coma in a matter of a few hours, but again the prognosis depends upon how much brain tissue was damaged and where. Fortunately the brain is one of the areas of the body that has excellent collateral circulation; that is, blood can reach most parts of the brain by more than one arterial route, so that when a vessel supplying a portion of the brain is knocked out by hemorrhage or clot, in most cases fresh arterial blood can still reach the damaged area by an alternate route.

Sudden death from a stroke is comparatively rare unless there has been an extensive and massive hemorrhage. If the cause of the stroke is extensive arteriosclerotic disease of the cerebral arteries, there is little that can be done other than to reduce physical and emotional tensions to a minimum and wait for as much recovery as possible. If high blood pressure is a complicating factor, as is frequently the case with a cerebral hemorrhage, vigorous treatment to reduce the hypertension will help reduce the likelihood of a second hemorrhage. In cases of thrombosis of a cerebral vessel, anticoagulant therapy may be useful in reducing the chances of further clots lodging in the cerebral arteries. In addition, cardiovascular surgeons and neurosurgeons in recent years have explored a variety of techniques to restore circulation through occluded vessels supplying the brain with blood, particularly when a major artery such as the carotid is occluded or narrowed. One such procedure is known as *carotid endarterectomy,* in which a carotid artery is surgically opened and the thrombus obstruction is peeled out, together with the inner lining of the artery to which the clot adheres. Sometimes an arterial graft is inserted if a segment of the artery must be removed. Such procedures are considered only in selected cases in which special X-rays known as arteriograms reveal the obstruction in an accessible area. This kind of surgery is still in its earliest stages of development, and surgeons continue to refine techniques to overcome the multiple technical problems involved; but these procedures have saved lives and will certainly become more and more widely used as their value is more clearly established.

In the long run, however, the burden of treatment in this kind of condition today rests in skillful nursing care. Often the victim of a stroke is, at least at first, almost completely incapacitated, and even if he is not, he should be encouraged to rest and let others do things for him. The stroke victim may also be unable to express his needs and desires, or may have periods of irrationality, either of which can complicate the problem of proper nursing care. Since recovery of at least some of the function of limbs paralyzed by a stroke is usually possible, physical therapy is necessary to keep the muscles in good condition and to maintain the range of motion of the joints. Occasionally in cases involving massive and continuing hemorrhage, surgical intervention to ligate or tie off the bleeding vessel may be a necessary life-saving

procedure, providing the victim survives the additional trauma of the surgery. In certain kinds of cases, complete ligation of one of the carotid arteries—the two major arteries carrying blood to the brain—is helpful in controlling hemorrhage. Naturally such surgery is not even considered unless the surgeon is convinced that the risk to the patient of *not* intervening is substantially greater than the risk of the surgery itself.

Many people who have suffered cerebrovascular accidents recover completely with time and patient nursing care; almost all who survive the initial insult of a stroke recover at least some of their loss. Frequently a great deal of work must be directed toward restoring function of paralyzed limbs or retraining the individual in such basic functions as speech. This is possible, in some cases, because of one of the most curious characteristics of the human body, the built-in reserve capacity of the brain, unlike the reserve capacity of any other organ. As far as can be determined, the human body uses the full capacity of the nerve tissue in the spinal cord and in the peripheral nerves, but ordinarily it uses only about half the brain tissue with which it is equipped. A large part of the normal function of the human brain is centered in just one side, the so-called dominant hemisphere; the other hemisphere, while unmistakably tied into the nervous system, appears to have relatively little function under normal circumstances. Because of crisscrossing of nerve pathways in the brain from one side to another, an individual's dominant hemisphere is usually the one on the opposite side from his dominant muscle function; that is, if he is strongly right-handed, the major brain function takes place in the left hemisphere of his brain.

No one has ever discovered quite why we are equipped with a vast mass of brain tissue that generally is not used. We do know, however, that a massive stroke in the dominant side of the brain causes far more motor and sensory loss than a stroke of similar magnitude in the "unused" side. Furthermore, when a stroke has involved the dominant side, there appear to be certain brain functions irreplaceably lost due to cell destruction which can nevertheless be re-learned, apparently by using the equivalent brain centers on the "unused" side. This does not occur in a clear-cut, predictable manner, however, and there is no way to tell in advance the degree to which lost functions may be restored by training the ordinarily "unused" portion of the brain. But *some* improvement is usually possible, and such functions as speech, for example, can often be recovered.

The first ones who have to cope with a stroke, in most cases, are the family or near friends of the victim. Sometimes minor strokes are overlooked or simply ignored by the victim, and may be allowed to pass unnoticed unless a friend or family member calls attention to curiosities of behavior. In a more serious stroke involving massive obstruction or hemorrhage, the victim may be found stricken or comatose in bed, suddenly unable to use certain muscles or to communicate. If the stroke does not cause immediate death, the most imminent threat is that it will affect the vital centers of the brain monitoring respiration, or knock out the respiratory muscles; a secondary concern is that paralysis of the tongue may result, and it may fall back into the victim's throat and choke him. Care to keep the victim at rest, turned on his side if possible with his tongue carefully pulled forward to maintain an open airway, and then the maintenance of respiration by means of mouth-to-mouth resuscitation, if necessary, until medical help can be obtained, may be lifesaving. No effort should be made to encourage the victim to eat or drink anything, even if he is apparently conscious and aware, and of course nothing should ever be given by mouth to an individual who is unconscious or in coma.

Once these emergency measures have been taken, the next critical stage of care depends upon swift and expert medical attention. The victim should be transported in an ambulance to a hospital without delay. But even under hospital care, there may be a period extending from several hours to several days before an accurate diagnosis of the kind of stroke can be made, or before the patient can be considered out of imminent danger.

The third phase of treatment, by far the most prolonged and most likely to involve family or friends of the patient, is the convalescence during which the patient must be maintained with the best nursing care possible for the days, weeks or months that may be necessary for the maximum recovery from paralysis or other neurological losses. Rarely is prolonged hospitalization necessary throughout this convalescent period except in cases of continuing coma, or when nursing care is beyond the capacity of the immediate family. If specialized nursing care is necessary, it can be provided in a nursing home equipped to handle such cases. In the great majority of cases, however, the stroke victim can convalesce at home. A more detailed discussion of home nursing care may be found elsewhere. (*See* p. 157.) But the convalescing stroke victim may pose certain special problems. Obviously, attention to adequate nutrition is important. So is ordinary attention to cleanliness, elimination, and prevention of bedsores. Emotional support is extremely important for the patient who is entirely alert mentally and yet comparatively helpless physically; it is critical that he recognize that his physical limitations are, at least in part, only temporary and that some degree of recovery, perhaps even total recovery, may be expected. Further, a paralyzed limb, which might otherwise recover, can remain permanently crippled if physical therapy measures are not used to help maintain the strength and tone of the affected muscles and to help prevent stiffening of the joints. Thus regular exercise, performed for the patient if necessary, and then in assistance as recovery begins, is essential. This kind of physical therapy can often be accomplished at home by otherwise unskilled individuals as long as a physical therapist can teach them what needs to be done and how to do it, and then supervises their performance and reviews the patient's progress at reasonable intervals. Other forms of physical rehabilitation, under the direction of a physician skilled in this specialty, with the aid of physical and/or occupational therapists, can also gradually speed the victim's recovery and at the same time teach him to adapt to whatever permanent loss may remain. Instruction in the use of a walking frame, for example, may enable the stroke victim to get out of bed by himself and move about far earlier than would otherwise be possible. If recovery permits him to graduate to crutches, he should be carefully taught by an expert in their proper use, essential to both their effectiveness and their safety.

During convalescence a program of medical care should also be instituted to help improve circulation to the brain, to reduce blood pressure if it remains elevated, and to prevent, insofar as possible, any recurrence. Perhaps above all, a stroke should not be interpreted by the victim or his family as the end of life, or the beginning of an invalid existence. This might have been true once, but today, thanks to modern diagnosis, treatment and recovery techniques, it is simply not so in most cases—yet often the hardest one to convince is the stroke victim himself. If medical attendants, family members and friends can help the victim counteract any feelings of helplessness or defeat, there is probably no other service that could do more to speed his recovery.

Once an individual has suffered and recovered from a stroke, what are the chances of recurrent or repeated attacks? If the stroke was due to a cerebral hemorrhage as a result of uncontrolled high blood pressure, the likelihood of a recurrence can be markedly diminished if the hypertension can be brought under control with medications. To the degree that the stroke was due to arteriosclerosis of the cerebral vessels, the likelihood of recurrent strokes sooner or later is very high. However, modification of normal daily activity, provision for adequate rest, and avoidance of sudden physical or emotional stresses all can help prevent or at least postpone recurrent attacks. Not too many years ago it was considered axiomatic that a person who had suffered a major stroke would inevitably suffer another which would terminate his life. Today, with a greater understanding of the mechanism of this kind of disorder and factors that contribute to it, the axiom no longer holds true. A great many people who have had strokes survive for years and ultimately die from other causes as frequently as from recurrence of their cerebrovascular disease.

In recent years we have come to recognize a singular type of "early warning" that future CVA's may be expected unless preventive care is instituted. This warning is in the form of a so-called little stroke, which appears not really to be a stroke at all, but rather a brief episode of circulatory disturbance due to transitory spasm of the muscular wall of the cerebral arteries. In this condition the victim may suffer a very brief spell of fainting, for example, or may find himself suddenly unable to make his words come right for a matter of a few seconds or a minute or two, or may suffer a brief, passing spell of weakness in the use of a limb. In some cases these "little strokes" are so unimpressive that nothing abnormal is noticed at all by the victim, but in others there is just enough disability for just long enough to be unmistakable. These "little strokes" have been recognized as a form of cerebrovascular disease for such a short time that we do not yet know for certain that there is a direct correlation between their occurrence and later more serious CVA's, but it seems likely that they are precursor events in the natural history of disease of the cerebral vessels. And if so, early institution of more rest, less tension, better dietary control, and less smoking may well serve at least to postpone more severe attacks.

Subarachnoid Hemorrhages. A kind of cerebrovascular accident of quite a different sort is the subarachnoid hemorrhage, which results from rupture of one or more blood vessels on the surface of the brain that lie beneath the arachnoid membrane, the middle of the three layers of meningeal tissue that cover the brain. This kind of CVA may occur at any age, usually as a result of a head injury sufficiently severe to tear a meningeal blood vessel, but also occasionally due to the bursting of an aneurysm in one of these vessels. In some people, a developmental defect may cause a number of these aneurysmal swellings of the blood vessels, vulnerable to bursting at any time, but this occurs only rarely. Whether resulting from an aneurysm or from a head injury, a subarachnoid hemorrhage is characterized by sudden severe head pain, nausea and vomiting. Sometimes the victim goes into a deep coma, but more frequently he is semicomatose. The bleeding into the space between the meningeal membranes causes pressure on the brain which can lead to dizziness, convulsions or disturbances of the heart and respiratory rates. The spinal fluid is found to be grossly bloody and under increased pressure, and the hematoma or blood clot that forms at the site of the accident may act very much like a brain tumor, pressing on adjacent brain tissue and even destroying brain cells because of the pressure. In extreme cases death may ensue if bleeding is not stopped.

The kind of headache that accompanies a subarachnoid hemorrhage can hardly be confused with something else; it is characteristically excruciating and is not relieved by any nonprescription analgesic. Once the victim is under medical care, diagnosis is usually established by discovery of blood in a spinal fluid sample. Sometimes the site of the hemorrhage can be pinpointed by *cerebral angiography,* a technique of X-ray examination in which a radio-opaque dye is introduced into an artery leading to the brain so that rapid-sequence X-rays can be taken to determine where the break in the blood vessel occurred.

Once active hemorrhage stops, the broken blood vessel heals and spinal fluid pressure returns to normal over a period of several weeks. A secondary rupture of the vessel may occur, but if no such accident takes place within six months, there is a good chance it will not recur at all. Treatment is directed toward correction of any underlying condition such as high blood pressure which might have caused the hemorrhage, and in some cases surgery may be performed to tie off the weakened blood vessel above and below the area of hemorrhage. In addition, it is sometimes necessary to open "burr holes" in the skull surgically in order to evacuate a large blood clot which may be exerting damaging pressure on underlying brain tissue. If the subarachnoid hemorrhage is due to rupture of an aneurysm, the prognosis for permanent recovery must be very guarded, since a number of such aneurysms may be present, any of which may rupture at any time.

Subdural Hematoma. This condition is also a hemorrhagic disorder involving the meningeal membranes covering the brain—in this case the outer layer or *dura mater*—but it presents a surprisingly different picture from subarachnoid hemorrhages. In this disorder, bleeding occurs between the dural and arachnoid membranes, sometimes in adults as a result of a head injury, but most commonly in infants, due to unusual trauma at birth, and results in formation of a hematoma just beneath the outer meningeal membrane. Often undiagnosed at first, this hematoma tends to form a fibrous membrane and become converted into a fluid-filled sac which grows progressively larger as blood cells within it break down and surrounding tissue fluid is drawn into it by osmosis. Ultimately this sac exerts more and more pressure on the brain as it enlarges. The child may become comatose, abnormal reflexes may appear, and convulsions often become part of the symptom complex. Unless diagnosed in time, permanent brain damage or even death may ensue, but once the diagnosis is made, neurosurgical exploration is possible through burr holes in the skull, and the fluid-filled sac can be drained and removed, with full and permanent recovery the rule.

Other Brain Disorders

All brain diseases and disorders, of course, are not necessarily related to head injuries or cerebrovascular accidents. Certain paralytic diseases or "palsies," tumors, degenerative diseases and toxic conditions or "brain poisonings" also occur commonly enough to merit individual mention.

Parkinson's Disease. Also known as *Parkinsonism* or *paralysis agitans* ("shaking palsy"), this disease is a chronic disorder of the motor control and reflex centers of the brain which involves a progressive weakness and slowing down of purposeful movements of the voluntary muscles of the body, progressive rigidity of muscles of the extremities, and a progressively disabling tremor, most commonly seen as a rhythmic "pill-rolling" motion of the upper extremities and hands which occurs at rest. As the disease progresses it is also characterized by a loss of control of the facial muscles, leading to a typical wide-eyed, unblinking, staring expression. Equally characteristic is a slow shuffling gait with the trunk bent slightly forward and an uncontrollable tendency for the victim to totter ahead more and more quickly until he breaks into a run, exactly as if he were trying to keep from falling forward whenever he walks.

The disease was first described in 1817 by the English physician James Parkinson and has borne his name ever since. Although Parkinson's disease at first seemed to be comparatively rare, it was difficult to overlook because of the very distinctive physical stigmata. Originally it was thought to result from cases of encephalitis (brain fever), from certain kinds of poisoning or from trauma or other injury to the head and cerebrovascular system. In general, it seemed to occur most commonly among middle-aged or elderly people. Then, in the first half of the present century, the incidence of Parkinsonism suddenly and inexplicably began to skyrocket among much younger people; whereas only an occasional individual had developed this condition before, now hundreds and thousands began to appear with the characteristic symptoms. For many years no one could explain this enigmatic increase in the disease. But in the course of just the last decade, investigators have noticed that the incidence of new cases seems to be falling off again quite sharply, and that the average age of new victims of the disease is once again increasing. Today it is believed that Parkinson's disease is, in fact, a delayed or residual effect on the brain of certain generalized virus infections—an effect that strikes only a few of the original victims of these viruses while causing no symptoms at all in the others. According to this theory, the great upsurge of Parkinsonism in the first half of this century resulted as a late residual effect of the devastating influenza epidemic of 1918 and 1919. If this notion ultimately proves true, there is reason to hope that the incidence of Parkinson's disease will revert to its original infrequent pattern as survivors of that epidemic become fewer and fewer.

The exact cause of the disease has not yet been determined, and diagnosis may require time, since the condition is slowly progressive and clear-cut symptoms often appear only gradually. Indeed, they may not become severe enough to be incapacitating for many years. Various drugs have been used to relieve the distressing symptoms, particularly the amphetamines to help combat lethargy and make the patient more active and cheerful, and the belladonna family of drugs to reduce the amount of the tremor and rigidity. But no program of treatment was really successful until experimental work was begun in the early 1960s with a powerful drug known as L-dopa. So far this drug has proved to be extremely useful in controlling both the rigidity and the tremor of Parkinsonism, and helping the patient return to a more normal range of activity. Today it is considered by far the most hopeful medical approach to treatment that has yet been found, despite a number of distressing side effects that may arise from its use. In addition, in recent years techniques of intracranial surgery aimed at destroying certain nerve pathways have permitted at least partial control of tremor and muscle rigidity in many patients. Either the surgical approach or the medical approach may be used, depending on each patient's individual condition, and the next decade or so may see Parkinsonism disappear as a significantly frequent affliction of the nervous system.

Brain Tumors. Among the most serious of all diseases or disorders affecting the brain are *intracranial neoplasms*—so-called brain tumors. Abnormal new growths can begin in virtually any part of the brain and arise from virtually any kind of brain tissue. As with tumors anywhere else, there is an important distinction between *benign tumors,* which may enlarge but do not spread or invade surrounding tissue, and *malignant tumors* with cells that infiltrate surrounding brain tissue or bone and seed cancerous growth in distant parts of the body. In the brain, however, benign tumors within the cranial vault can become just as deadly as malignant tumors as they grow, simply because they take up an increasing amount of space in an area that allows no room for expansion. Thus a *meningioma,* a benign tumor of the meningeal membranes, may grow within the skull to a diameter of several inches, steadily compressing underlying brain tissue and producing gradually progressive symptoms of nervous system loss. A *neuroma,* a benign tumor arising from nerve cells, may begin growing within the skull from one of the cranial nerves such as the acoustic nerve and, without invading surrounding tissue, may still develop to the size of a baseball, first causing loss of hearing and equilibrium and later progressively crushing other cranial nerves and then the whole base of the brain if the tumor cannot be surgically excised. Malignant tumors, on the other hand, can arise either from nerve cells themselves or from the connective tissues which hold those nerve cells in position in the brain, and may invade and destroy surrounding tissue or seed new growths in other parts of the body. In addition, the brain is a likely place for metastatic cells thrown off by cancers arising in other organs of the body to be trapped in a capillary bed and begin to grow. It is particularly characteristic, for example, that the most common form of lung cancer, bronchogenic carcinoma, will seed malignant cells into the brain which then develop in metastatic lesions there. Occasionally the very presence of a lung cancer is discovered in the first place while investigating a sensory or motor malfunction apparently originating in the brain.

Contrary to popular opinion, headache is *not* a common early symptom of a developing brain tumor unless it happens to be pressing on the highly pain-sensitive meningeal tissues. Far more commonly the first signs of trouble are slowly progressive disturbances in balance, vision or sense of smell, or progressive weakening and then paralysis of certain muscles in the extremities for no apparent reason. Often a marked increase in spinal fluid pressure is discovered without evidence of blood in the spinal fluid or any of the other stigmata of a cerebrovascular accident. Naturally as more and more brain tissue is damaged or destroyed by either a benign or a malignant tumor, there is progressive neurological loss, and often the location of the tumor can be deduced from the kind of motor or sensory loss that is present. X-rays of the skull will frequently provide vital information about the location of the tumor; although the tumor itself may not appear on the X-ray, evidence of eroding bone or a location shift of the contents of the cranium may be visible.

Whenever the patient's general level of health permits, a brain tumor, whether benign or malignant, is best treated by surgical excision.

Often the size of the tumor alone, or its duration, will limit the amount of recovery of lost nervous system function that will be possible once the tumor is excised. An acoustic nerve neuroma, for example, may have been growing slowly for years or decades before it becomes large enough and causes great enough pressure on adjacent structures in the brain to become seriously symptomatic. Malignant tumors, of course, generally grow much more rapidly, and surgical removal may be only palliative or even contraindicated if evidence of metastatic spread to other parts of the body can already be detected. As with any other kind of cancer, early diagnosis and surgical treatment remains not only the best but virtually the only hope until we develop a far greater understanding of the nature of cancer, its causes and methods of arrest or treatment.

Senile Dementia. A familiar degenerative condition that is related to impairment of circulation in the brain but which rarely occurs before the age of sixty is the slowly progressive and irreversible impairment or deterioration of brain function known as senile dementia, or just senility. The most common cause of this condition is the presence of long-standing arteriosclerosis of the arteries of the brain, which leads to a progressive shutdown of adequate circulation. The elderly victim of this combination of disease and the aging process begins to suffer lapses of memory, primarily of recent events, while memories of events long past and apparently forgotten come forth with surprising clarity. Often there is periodic disorientation and a progressive change of personality, perhaps better described as a loss of the normal ability to adapt to changing circumstances: the victim becomes more easily angered or irritated, inappropriately amused or moved to weeping without apparent cause, with wide swings of mood from euphoria to depression occurring within a matter of a few hours. At the same time, he tends to become garrulous, talking in a rambling fashion without reaching a point and sometimes repeating himself because he has forgotten what he has just said. There is a progressive deterioration of intellectual power and judgment, and often the victim begins suffering from childish delusions of

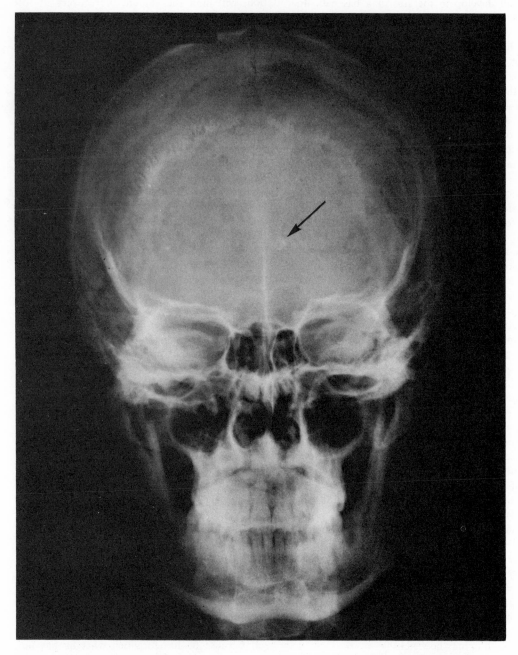

Plate 9a   A large brain tumor, itself invisible in the X-ray, has pushed the calcified pineal gland (see arrow) to the left of its normal midline position within the skull. Detection of such a "pineal shift" aids the radiologist in diagnosing and locating the tumor.

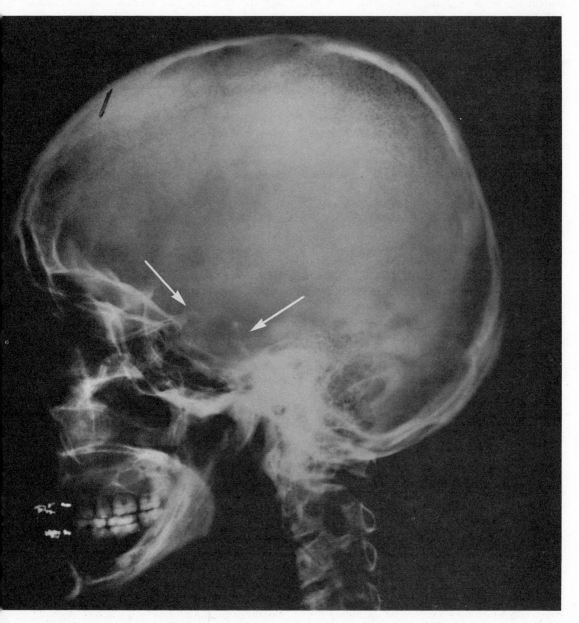

Plate 9b   An intracranial tumor, itself invisible in the X-ray, has eroded the bone at the interior
base of the skull (see arrows) and thus revealed itself to the radiologist.

persecution. In fact, the victim of senile dementia often becomes extremely childlike in overall behavior, as the familiar term "second childhood" suggests. But all too often it is an unhappy, rather than pleasant, childishness; the victim becomes helplessly enraged at minor reverses, suspicious of even the closest friends and relatives, and frequently obsessed with profound guilt feelings about "sins" of the past which may have been only the mildest of transgressions, if not totally imaginary. There may also be a general loss of the sense of propriety; the victim may expose himself, for example, or use profane or obscene language that once would have been unthinkable.

In many cases this gradual breakdown of mental functions progresses over a period of months or even years until finally interrupted by death from a stroke or from some other illness. But occasionally senile dementia occurs quite suddenly and without warning, almost in the form of a mental storm, in which sensory disturbances, confusion and disorientation, incoherence, excitability, delusions of persecution and sometimes even hallucinations all begin at once. In such a form, the disorder is likely to run a much more rapid course of deterioration with death ensuing in a matter of a few weeks.

There is little that can be done to treat senile dementia other than helping the victim maintain good nutrition, personal cleanliness and physical hygiene, preventing him from doing inadvertent harm to himself or others due to impulsiveness or depression, doing whatever possible to quiet and reassure him and providing as much emotional support as possible. Use of medicines should generally be held to a minimum, since elderly people frequently tend to overreact. If sedatives are necessary, it is best to avoid barbiturates or bromides, both of which can accentuate the symptoms of the dementia and induce excitation. Small doses of chloral hydrate are sometimes used instead for their calming or sleep-inducing effects. In general, victims of the disease do better in an atmosphere and environment with which they are familiar, including the presence of family members; but when they are cared for at home, family members should recognize that the anger and suspicion so often

expressed by the victim of senility are a part of the process of mental deterioration and are not really purposefully directed at them. Above all, they should realize that no one is at fault or to blame for the patient's condition; when it occurs, it is something that would have happened regardless of anything that anyone did or did not do. It is particularly important when there are children in a family caring for a senile old person that they be made to recognize the nature of the disorder and not be unduly disturbed by it.

Often the question of institutional or nursing home care for such individuals arises. There is much to be said on both sides of the question, and the decision has to be made purely on an individual basis. A good, well-managed nursing home can provide excellent facilities for care, a comforting and reassuring daily routine for the senile patient, and allow for frequent visits from the family without the disruption of family life or the ill effects of the emotionally charged atmosphere that so often prevails when the patient is cared for at home. On the other hand, good nursing home care is costly; the elderly patient, who already feels desolated by a gradual loss of faculties that he cannot control, may feel abandoned and think, all too often correctly, that he is being sent away to die. Certainly when an individual in senility is massively disruptive to family life, there is an obligation to other members of the family to find a more suitable place to provide care. But, unfortunately, a great many nursing homes are really little more than prisons for the confinement of the elderly ill on a low-protein starvation diet until they give up the struggle. It is important that the concerned family select a nursing home with attention to the quality of care available, the competence and friendliness of the staff and the brightness of the surroundings. Then the effort should be made to visit regularly, to include the old person in family gatherings and celebrations at home whenever possible, and to provide real support, tempered by compassion and concern, so that these already bleak and frightening terminal months or years can be as happy as possible.

Cerebral arteriosclerosis is not the only cause for brain deterioration and dementia, nor is brain deterioration necessarily limited to the elderly. In chronic alcoholism there is often a disintegration of personality which may range all the way from mild impairment of emotional control to outright dementia closely resembling senility. Part of the damage is believed to be a result of long-term deficiency of proteins and B vitamins in the diet, but replacement of these nutriments does not necessarily undo past damage or improve the condition. A common warning of developing brain damage from alcoholism is the occurrence of *delirium tremens* (d.t.'s), an acute alcohol psychosis involving massive confusion, delirium, shaking tremors of the extremities and singularly horrid and frightening visual hallucinations, often of vermin, snakes or insects crawling on the body. An episode of d.t.'s may last from a few hours to several days and often terminates with a period of profound sleep. Occasionally, when the victim is not being cared for, death may occur from exposure, physical accident, trauma or pneumonia. If the alcoholism has been severe for long enough to produce permanent and widespread brain damage, delirium tremens may gradually merge into a more permanent state of disorientation, amnesia, irritability and confabulation (falsification of memory to fill in frightening amnesic gaps). This syndrome of alcoholic brain damage may be reversible to some extent after a period of some weeks if the individual is withdrawn from alcohol, but often the impairment is permanent and merely becomes progressively worse with continuing use of alcohol.

Multiple Sclerosis and Other Nervous System Diseases

In many nervous system disorders the telltale signs and symptoms frequently occur at a distance from the site of the pathology, but may still be specific enough to pinpoint precisely where the breakdown has occurred. There is one disorder of the nervous system, however, which presents such a variety and apparently random shifting of signs and symptoms in so many different areas, either all at once or periodically, that this very symptomatic pattern becomes one of the most important clues to the diagnosis. It is

the strange and baffling disease of unknown origin known as *multiple sclerosis* (MS).

Multiple sclerosis is a mystery in many ways. Basically it is a condition in which scattered areas of nerve tracts within the brain and in the spinal cord somehow become denuded of the waxy coating of myelin which normally ensheaths individual nerve fibrils and, in fact, plays a vital role in the transmission of nerve impulses. There is no apparent reason for why or even where this "demyelinization" of nerve tracts occurs. It seems to be almost entirely random, and, at least early in the disease, it also seems to be a reversible condition in that nerve tracts may be blotted out for prolonged periods and then recover completely and spontaneously. Thus, at first, the disease is characterized by a wide variety of symptoms related to nerve loss which last for a while and then disappear as inexplicably as they arrived.

The pattern of incidence of multiple sclerosis is also mysterious. It occurs primarily in individuals living in the Northern Hemisphere, mostly in Europe and North America, although it does occur in China and India as well. The Japanese, for some reason, appear to enjoy a singular freedom from the disease, as do black Africans, although it occurs as frequently in American Negroes as in whites. Even more baffling, the incidence of multiple sclerosis is some three times higher in the northern United States and Canada than it is in the southern states. So far no one has found any explanation for these curiosities of distribution, nor do they lend themselves to any plausible theory.

The onset of symptoms of multiple sclerosis is usually insidious and sometimes so minor as to be overlooked. The first symptom is very commonly a sudden and inexplicable disturbance of vision—an episode of blindness or blurring of vision in one eye, for example, or double vision —which may last for as little as an hour or two or as long as a week before reverting to normal. Beginning symptoms generally occur in the young or middle adult years, with two-thirds of all cases starting between the ages of twenty and forty. The initial symptom, once it has disappeared, may never again recur, and a period of months or even years may pass before new symptoms begin. Then, gradually, there will be symptoms of transitory weakness of certain muscle groups, unusual tiring of a limb, minor interference with walking, unusual stiffness of muscles, sometimes dizziness, mysterious loss of bladder control and paresthesias (disturbances in the senses of touch, pain and heat) in various parts of the body. At times most or all of these symptoms, or any one of them, will characteristically disappear, only to be followed later by other apparently inexplicable disturbances.

It is not uncommon for the disease to proceed in this on-again, off-again fashion for a period of months or years before a definite diagnosis is possible. But finally the symptoms become unmistakable. The deep tendon reflexes change gradually, tremors appear, and muscles become both weak and spastic—that is, stiff and movable only with difficulty. Urinary retention occurs, and impotence in the male or pelvic anesthesia in the female may cause intermittent disturbance of sexual function. Eventually the victim may become bedridden owing to impairment of motor function of muscles, and there is often a characteristic personality change, at first in the direction of exaggerated cheerfulness and optimism, then later in the direction of irritability and emotional depression as the victim sees his faculties failing him bit by bit, sometimes returning in part but only to be lost again to an even greater degree. Toward the end there may be outright mental deterioration, incapacitation from muscle contractures, partial or complete blindness and difficulty or inability to speak. On the average, victims of the disease live for ten or fifteen years following onset of the first symptoms, with bronchial pneumonia the most common terminal illness. But some victims suffer much more severe attacks and rapid deterioration with death ensuing in less than five years, while others may suffer chronic illness without much change from a certain level of incapacity for decades, ultimately to die of some completely unrelated disease. Occasionally a victim of MS may have a complete or nearly complete remission of all symptoms that can last for as long as 25 years before downhill progress resumes. There has never, however, been any known case

of definitely diagnosed multiple sclerosis in which full and permanent recovery and healing of the nervous system lesions has occurred, and although many approaches have been tried, there is still today no specific treatment for the disease other than general supportive nursing care as needed and efforts to prevent such complications as bedsores or urinary tract infection.

With such a devastating illness occurring as frequently as it does (some 60 cases for every 100,000 people in the northern United States) and with such a uniformly poor prognosis, it is not surprising that great amounts of money and effort have been devoted to the study of multiple sclerosis in the hope of finding its cause and a means of arresting or curing it. In addition, public funds have been directed to the care of victims of the disease which, by its very long-term and chronic nature, can so readily deplete private resources. And in the case of multiple sclerosis this concentration of money, effort, time and research facilities makes remarkably good sense; no one can observe the disease in its various clinical manifestations without the conviction that there must be some basic physiological flaw at fault which, if only the right clue could be found, might yield results as dramatic as those recently achieved with diabetes and poliomyelitis.

In addition to multiple sclerosis there is a wide variety of other comparatively rare degenerative diseases affecting the spinal cord and brain, often similar in their manifestations to MS but with different overall patterns of development. In most cases the characteristics of these diseases are well known only to neurologists, but two have recently come to widespread attention because of having afflicted popular public figures: amyotrophic lateral sclerosis, sometimes described as "Lou Gehrig's disease," and Huntington's chorea, with which the beloved folk singer Woody Guthrie was stricken in his later years.

Amyotrophic lateral sclerosis, a disease of unknown origin, involves a rapidly progressive destruction of the nerve cells in the spinal cord that permit innervation of the muscles in the extremities, as well as the nerve tracts connecting those cells with the brain. Beginning insidiously, there is usually first a loss of such fine movements of the hand as buttoning clothes, writing or handling small objects. There may also be early difficulty in swallowing and speaking, with slurring of speech and hoarseness. In comparatively rapid succession, then, there is a steady destruction of more and more of the cells permitting motion of the extremities and other voluntary muscles, with marked weakness and stiffness of the legs, making walking progressively more difficult, followed by atrophy of the afflicted muscles. There is no consistently useful treatment, and the disease runs a fatal course in from two to five years after the onset of symptoms, except in the rare case in which the disorder seems to level off for a few years before resuming a downward spiral.

Huntington's chorea is also a degenerative disease of nerve cells, in this case primarily affecting the part of the brain involved with the mental functions of thinking and judgment, as well as those parts that help control voluntary muscular activity. This disease, however, is definitely hereditary, transmitted as a Mendelian dominant trait to children, so that those who do not develop the disease rarely transmit it to their children, but approximately half of the children of an individual who ultimately develops the disease will also acquire it. Unfortunately, the disease seldom manifests itself before middle life, long after fathering of children or childbearing is over. The symptoms consist of mental deterioration with forgetfulness, restlessness and childish behavior together with so-called choreiform movements, uncontrollable jerking of the head, arms or legs which progressively interfere with walking or arm movement until the victim is bedridden. There is no known treatment, and the disease is uniformly fatal within ten to twelve years from onset of symptoms.

Congenital and Hereditary Nervous System Disorders

Of the many disorders that can afflict the nervous system, congenital and hereditary defects are among the most tragic because of the age of their victims. These disorders arise at some time during the development of the unborn baby and result in physical deformities, mental retardation or both. Many of these conditions are clearly recognizable at the time of birth, but in other cases their discovery may be delayed for months or even years. Certain of the congenital disorders are purely anatomical deformities— accidents of fetal development, so to speak— that arise for totally unknown reasons. One such anomaly, fortunately very rare, is a condition known as *microcephalus,* in which many of the higher brain centers in the cerebrum fail to develop at all. The afflicted child is born with an abnormally small, deformed skull and is grossly retarded mentally, totally incapable of thought, memory, judgment or the ability to adapt to the world around him. Many of these children are stillborn or die within a few days or weeks of birth; in earlier times those who survived to childhood or adolescence often spent their lives cruelly taunted as "pinheads." There is still nothing that can be done to correct the damage once it has occurred, but today society provides protective institutional care for those who survive. In extreme cases, known as *anencephalus,* virtually none of the brain develops, but almost all these victims are lost by miscarriage of the pregnancy or are stillborn.

A more common, but far less devastating congenital anomaly is *spina bifida,* in which a portion of the developing vertebral column fails to close over the underlying spinal cord, leaving it unprotected except for the meningeal membranes covering it. Frequently the meninges form an outpouching of cerebrospinal fluid in the region of the defect, known as a meningocoele, which may be very small or as large as a football, depending on the size of the defect. The immediate danger of this condition is infection of the meninges and the underlying nerve tissue in the region, but in many cases the development of the spinal cord itself is also flawed in the affected area, so that the child may be partially paralyzed. Neurosurgical correction of a meningocoele is often possible, although this may require a long series of tedious and difficult surgical procedures, and if developmental damage to the nervous tissue involved is not too great, the victim may at least be protected from infection and often restored to a comfortable and productive life, since mentality is seldom

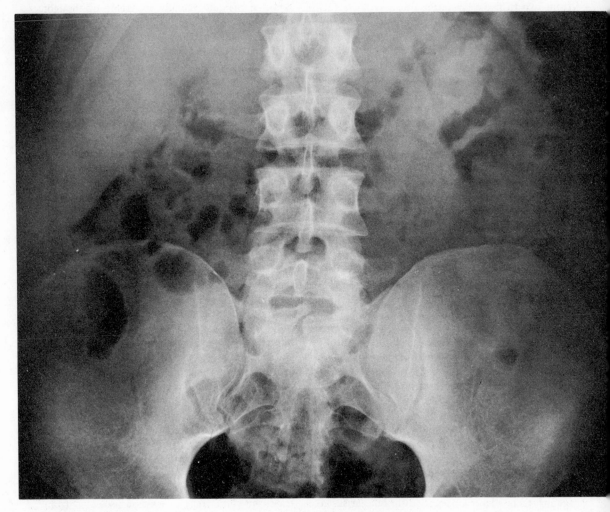

Plate 10   Congenital spina bifida occulta in an adult. This boney defect is seen in the center of the lowest lumbar vertebra, just above the sacrum.

impaired in this condition. In some cases complete restoration to normal is possible.

Hydrocephalus (literally "waterbrain" or "water on the brain") is a condition in which the cerebrospinal fluid which forms in the ventricles deep within the brain is trapped in these cavities because of some mechanical obstruction of the canals or "aqueducts" through which the fluid normally escapes to bathe the meningeal membranes covering the brain and spinal cord. Occasionally this obstruction arises in adolescence or adulthood as a result of scarring or destruction of the canals due to meningitis or syphilis, or due to the growth of brain tumors, but in most cases hydrocephalus is a congenital defect of unknown origin which occurs in unborn babies during the last few weeks before delivery. As increasing amounts of fluid are produced, there is a marked rise in pressure within the brain; the baby's head becomes grotesquely enlarged, with wide spaces appearing between the bones of the skull. Unless this increasing fluid pressure can be relieved, otherwise healthy brain tissue is literally crushed and death ensues within a matter of weeks or months. Once considered a hopeless and incurable condition, hydrocephalus today can sometimes be successfully treated by neurosurgery. In some cases, for instance, polyethylene plastic tubes can be inserted to conduct fluid from the brain ventricles into the spongy mastoid bone behind the ear, where it can be absorbed into the blood stream, or even down the spinal cord to empty into the abdominal cavity. In all such procedures there is still a high risk that infective organisms will find their way into such artificial canals and cause meningitis, but at least some victims of hydrocephalus have been successfully treated by these pioneering procedures, and there is hope that more and more can be saved in the future as the necessary neurosurgical techniques are refined and improved.

Although many congenital deformities of the nervous system arise for no identifiable reason, there is one prominent cause that is well recognized today: infection of the mother with rubella (German measles) during the first six months of her pregnancy. The virus usually causes only the mildest of illnesses in the mother, but the effects on the developing fetus can be devastating. Among the congenital nervous system malformations that can arise as a result of fetal rubella infections are deafness, malformations of the eyes or optic nerves, microcephalus, hydrocephalus and such defects of skull formation as cleft palates and closures of the ducts that normally drain tears from the eyes into the nasal passages. These and other congenital defects (*see* p. 180 *and* p. 823) can be so devastating that a known rubella infection in a pregnant woman today is considered by many authorities to be a valid indication for termination of the pregnancy.

For the most part congenital anomalies are not hereditary, that is, they occur at random and are not generally passed from parents to children as a result of defective genes. Although a few cases of familial or hereditary microcephalus have been reported, most of these conditions occur only once in a family and are not transmitted. But certain other nervous system diseases that first appear at birth or shortly after *are* hereditary. Known by such unfamiliar names as *Friedreich's ataxia, progressive spastic paraplegia* and *familial spastic paralysis,* most of these conditions are exceedingly rare although readily recognizable to the neurologists and pediatricians who must occasionally deal with them. Most involve degeneration of nerve cells in the brain or spinal cord, and are accompanied by progressive paralysis of the so-called *spastic* type in which the paralyzed muscles tend to remain contracted and tense rather than flaccid. Although some pursue a chronic course, virtually all of them are fatal; however, since they appear to be carried by recessive genes, some members of afflicted families remain free of symptoms and survive to mate and produce afflicted offspring.

One of the more prominent of these conditions deserves mention here because a means of prenatal detection has recently been discovered. *Tay-Sachs disease* is an invariably fatal degenerative disorder of the brain which is passed from one generation to the next as a recessive genetic defect; that is, a parent carrying the "black gene" that causes the condition, although not himself afflicted with symptoms, will transmit the active disease to some 25 percent of his children. The primary defect is both tragically simple and totally incorrectable, as far as is known today: the absence of a single enzyme which normally acts to prevent a certain fatty material from building up in the nerve tissue of the brain and the cranial nerves. In its absence, ever increasing deposits of this fatty material lead to progressive blindness, mental deterioration and paralysis in the afflicted baby, beginning long before birth and terminating in death by the age of two to four years.

So far there is no cure for Tay-Sachs disease, and most neurologists doubt that a cure will ever be found. But recently hope has arisen that Tay-Sachs disease and certain other congenital or hereditary disorders may at least be discovered early enough in fetal life that doomed pregnancies may be safely terminated. This hope stems from a revolutionary new examination technique known as *amniocentesis:* when a fetal defect is feared, a small amount of amniotic fluid can be removed from the pregnant woman's uterus during gestation without disturbing the pregnancy. This amniotic fluid contains cells which have been washed away from the baby's skin surface within the uterus, and examination of these cells can often reveal the telltale absence of the critical enzyme which means that the baby will inevitably develop Tay-Sachs disease. Indeed, with further research it may be possible to detect an unsuspecting carrier of the "black gene" of the disease before he or she can conceive a child, thus breaking the hereditary chain.

Amniocentesis also offers hope that still another common and tragic congenital condition—*Down's syndrome,* more commonly known as *mongolism*—may soon be detectable early enough that an afflicted pregnancy can be terminated if the parents so desire. Unlike Tay-Sachs disease, mongolism only rarely occurs in a hereditary pattern; in most cases no one knows why it occurs, although children conceived late in a woman's childbearing years are markedly more vulnerable. A child with mongolism develops with certain characteristic defects in the shape and number of his chromosomes; as a result he is born with a number of physical stigmata—a distinctive "mongoloid" appearance of the eyelids, an enlarged tongue and abnormal creases in the palms of the hands—and is seriously, sometimes profoundly, mentally retarded. Mongoloid children develop much more slowly than normal after birth, and although they may survive to adolescence or even adulthood they seldom achieve a mental age beyond that of a seven-year-old. Although many mongoloid children can be cared for at home, for many others lifelong institutional care is either necessary or strongly desirable. To date there is no cure for mongolism, or even any way to ameliorate it, but it can now be detected long before the baby is born by examining cells in the amniotic fluid, withdrawn from the pregnant woman's uterus by means of amniocentesis, for evidence of the characteristic chromosome abnormalities. This is still a highly specialized technique today, but there is hope that it soon may be performed as a screening test during early pregnancies, especially among older women who have the highest risk of bearing mongoloid children. With foreknowledge that a given pregnancy will result in a mongoloid child, parents can then make a rational, informed decision whether or not to allow the defective pregnancy to proceed to term.

Not all congenital afflictions of the nervous system are necessarily hopeless or incurable. *Cretinism* is a condition, often confused with mongolism because of similar physical stigmata and mental retardation, that sometimes appears in babies born to mothers suffering from extreme underactivity of the thyroid gland. (*See* p. 690.) Untreated, the child with cretinism will be permanently retarded both mentally and physically, but early diagnosis and treatment of the condition immediately after birth will usually restore the baby to normal within a few weeks. Another congenital disease, once thought incurable, is *phenylketonuria (see* p. 878), an inborn metabolic defect which leads to progressive mental degeneration and early death of the child if it remains undetected. Fortunately, within hours of the afflicted child's birth an abnormal chemical can be detected in the infant's urine, and the condition can be cured by the faithful use of special dietary measures during the first few years of life. Today pediatricians routinely perform a simple screening test on the urine of all newborn babies to detect the presence of phenylketonuria so that treatment can be started in time.

Perhaps the most tragic and baffling of all congenital nervous system disorders are those which involve some degree of permanent and irreparable *mental deficiency* or *retardation:* some limitation of intelligence or interference with the child's ability to adapt to the world around him, whether obvious organic disease is present or not. Marked mental retardation is a prominent feature of such conditions as mongolism, hydrocephalus or Tay-Sachs disease, together with either physical stigmata or brain degeneration. In some conditions the mental retardation can be reversed if the underlying affliction can be corrected or effectively treated early enough. But in the vast majority of cases mental retardation is not related to any known organic or physical disorder whatever. Certain children, for reasons unknown, are born lacking the intellectual equipment of the normal child and must live out their lives in the dim half-world of mental retardation—lives which all too often are further scarred by the scorn, ridicule and outright cruelty of others around them. In years past it was customary to classify the mentally retarded according to their relative mental abilities compared to children with "average" IQ (intelligence quotient) measurements between 90 and 110. These classes ranged from slightly retarded *morons* with IQ's between 50 and 75 to the more severely impaired *imbeciles* with IQ measurements from 25 to 50 and the almost totally retarded *idiots* with IQ measurements below 25. Today these terms have largely been abandoned, for authorities recognize that mental retardation can exist in a multitude of different forms and at a multitude of different levels. In some instances mental retardation follows a definite familial or hereditary pattern; in other cases injury of some kind to the baby during the gestation period may be suspected. But universally,

true primary mental retardation tends to be permanent and inalterable.

Any time mental deficiency is suspected, accurate diagnosis is of paramount importance, since many environmental conditions can often create an appearance of retardation in perfectly normal children. Improper diet, for example, especially involving protein starvation, can lead to a slowness of both mental and physical development which can easily be mistaken for mental deficiency. Emotional deprivation in an unstable home, severe infectious illnesses in infancy, or certain early-appearing mental illnesses such as schizophrenia can all have similar effects. Parents should also realize that entirely normal children may have different rates of mental development, even in the same family, so that a slow-developing child may well appear retarded compared to faster-developing brothers and sisters. No conclusions should ever be drawn without consultation and careful examination by a pediatrician and, if necessary, other neurological and psychiatric specialists. Even then a definite conclusion may not be possible without months or even years of periodic follow-up. Many techniques, including charting or graphing both mental and physical development of children, have been devised to help assess the possibility of mental retardation, but all methods have their flaws, and often a final answer must depend upon patience as much as anything else.

Once mental deficiency has been clearly diagnosed, doctor and parents must work closely together to plan a program for the child that will provide the best possible opportunity for him within the limits of his capabilities. In cases of severe retardation institutional care may be necessary or advisable. The effect of such a child upon normal brothers and sisters in the family— and upon the parents—must be carefully weighed. While it may not be possible to improve the mental capacity of the afflicted child, much indeed can be done to protect him from a baffling world with which he is unable to cope and to train him to use both his physical and mental capacities to the fullest extent possible.

VII

PATTERNS OF ILLNESS: THE CUTANEOUS SYSTEM

31. The Skin and Connective Tissue 381

32. Care and Disorders of the Teeth and Gums 415

33. The Special Sensory Organs: Eyes, Ears and Nose 424

34. Diseases of the Breast 444

The very specialized organs of the cutaneous system—the skin, hair, nails, teeth and gums; the eyes, ears and nose; and finally the breasts or mammary glands—may seem to have little in common, but all are derived from cutaneous tissue and all serve the body in extremely important ways. No part of the body is more constantly exposed to view, more vulnerable to the dangers of the external environment, but the skin and the sensory organs provide the body's first line of defense against those dangers, while the breasts play a role in the vital reproductive process. In fact, because all these organs are both visible and accessible, and because they are intimately related to internal as well as external body functions, much can be done in terms of commonsense care and maintenance to protect them, to detect disorders early, and to keep them in peak working order. Thus a knowledge of the normal function of the organs of the cutaneous system, as well as the symptoms that signal disfunction, can pay handsome dividends in preventing illness and ensuring continuing good health.

31

The Skin and Connective Tissue

If the nervous system is the most complex of all organ systems in the body, surely the cutaneous system, made up of the skin and its appendages (*see* p. 55), is the most multipurpose. Not only does it cover and protect all the external organs; it also contains and preserves the "inner sea" of body fluids essential to life. Further, it regulates body temperatures and serves as a major sensory organ by means of its vast network of nerve endings which respond to touch, pressure, heat and cold. And finally, because of its external location, the cutaneous system plays a major role in the overall appearance of the body. Although beauty may be only skin deep, that skin is vitally important.

The skin is the body's first line of defense, and it is therefore understandable, if unfortunate, that it is subject to a wide variety of "nuisance disorders" from the external environment. Cuts, hangnails, bruises, abrasions, lacerations and punctures are all too common afflictions, and because of the danger that infectious organisms may be introduced into the body, even the most minor of such injuries should be cared for properly (*see* p. 124). Burns pose a hazard not only to the skin but to life itself if they are extremely severe (*see* p. 119). Other external causes for skin disorders range all the way from excesses of heat, cold or pressure to inflammation and infection caused by pathogenic bacteria and viruses, as well as plant and animal parasites and pests.

Quite aside from external hazards, the skin is a major "target organ" for various disfunctions of the body's internal environment, including allergic reactions to disorders stemming from glandular disfunctions, malnutrition, metabolic disturbances or even psychosomatic causes. Generalized illnesses of the body or of a particular organ system or tissue may also involve the skin—the "childhood rash" diseases such as chicken pox or measles, for example, or more serious afflictions like smallpox and the venereal diseases. Organic disorders of the skin itself are relatively uncommon, but abnormalities of color, growth or structure are virtually universal, if seldom serious. Like other organ systems, the skin is also subject to malignant or cancerous growths, and last but by no means least, it is certainly the organ system most visibly affected by the normal processes of wear and tear and aging.

It is easy to see why *dermatology*—the medical specialty dealing with the treatment of disorders of the skin, hair and nails—is such a vast and complicated field. The old saying that the dermatologist's patients never die and never get well is not entirely fair; there are indeed fatal skin disorders, just as there are many cutaneous system diseases that can be cured. But even skin specialists themselves may never see or treat certain of the rare or highly regional skin afflictions. Here we can discuss only the relatively familiar and frequent disorders that are specific to the cutaneous system itself. They are surprisingly few considering the large area of the body the skin covers and its continual exposure. But that does not mean that we can take it for granted. Apart from its many important physiological functions, the color, texture and condition of the skin often provide revealing indications not only of a person's age, but of his overall state of physical and emotional health.

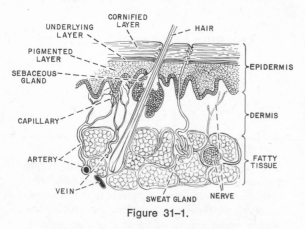

UNDERLYING LAYER

CORNIFIED LAYER

HAIR

PIGMENTED LAYER

SEBACEOUS GLAND

EPIDERMIS

CAPILLARY

DERMIS

ARTERY

FATTY TISSUE

VEIN

SWEAT GLAND   NERVE

Figure 31–1.

Thus "problem skin" deserves a doctor's attention, whatever its cause, and the care of normal, healthy skin should be a part of a sensible and conscientious daily hygienic routine.

Skin Disorders Due to External Factors

Sunburn. This is one of the most common afflictions of the skin, especially among white Caucasians of north European stock who live in areas where a hot, sunny summer follows wet, gray or cold winters. Anyone of any race, complexion or skin color can sunburn with sufficient exposure to the sun at midday, but fair-skinned people burn more easily and severely than dark-skinned people, regardless of race, because they have lesser concentrations of the protective pigment *melanin* in their skins. Exposure to the sun in modest daily doses stimulates the formation of melanin in the tanning process, but the ability to tan may also vary among complexion types.

Other factors involved in sunburning are sometimes overlooked. For example, it is far easier to sunburn—and harder for the fair-skinned to tan—in tropical areas near the equator, where the sun beats down from directly overhead and the burning ultraviolet rays are much more concentrated, than in northern latitudes where the sunlight slants through the atmosphere and more of the burning rays are filtered out. Thus many people in tropical regions tend to burn and reburn rather than tan. In the temperate zones severe sunburns are most commonly acquired during late spring, summer and early fall due to exposure to the sun between the hours of mid-morning and late afternoon. Those who claim to sunburn at night should not be taken seriously. Almost everyone knows that a serious sunburn can be acquired on a cloudy day, if the cloud layer is relatively thin; yet often overlooked is the fact that it is also perfectly possible to sunburn through clothing, particularly the lightweight, open-weave shirts or blouses commonly worn in the summertime. Relatively thick, loose and lightweight clothing, including a wide-brimmed hat, provides the most protection against both heat and sunburn; the white cloth headdress and heavy flowing robe of the desert Arab actually keep him cooler and safer from sunburn than lightweight colored shirts and trousers.

Finally, while air temperature has nothing to do with sunburn, reflection of sunlight most decidedly does. Some of the worst of all sunburns are acquired on the beach, out fishing on a lake, or skiing on snow in bright sunlight, particularly at high altitudes. Reflected sunlight can also cause a painful inflammation of the cornea, the sensitive translucent membrane over the surface of the eye—a condition known as "snow blindness." This condition, much akin to the ultraviolet "flashburns" suffered by welders who do not protect their eyes, is reversible but can cause the sufferer hours of unnecessary agony until the inflammation subsides.

Some people sunburn far more readily and more seriously than others. A mild sunburn affects only the outer layer of living cells in the skin and leads to a mild redness or erythema, itching and very slight pain. In some people a minor sunburn may even raise a multitude of tiny water blisters in the skin. It is probably best to leave a mild burn untreated; even though some peeling may occur, the healing will be conducive to later tanning in those individuals who tan readily. With a more severe sunburn deeper layers of cells are injured. The skin becomes an angry pinkish red soon after exposure and may be followed within a few hours by extensive blistering. The victim may have fever, chills, headache, even nausea and vomiting in the evening following such an exposure. Severe burns are likely to be very painful for as long as a week, finally to be resolved by extensive peeling of the burned skin. Early conservative treatment will help minimize the discomfort and speed healing. Skin emollients, such as suntan lotion, applied copiously to the burned area the same day the burn is acquired will help keep the skin moist and relieve the pain and the unpleasant feeling of tightness so commonly noted the following day. Various burn ointments or aerosol sprays available without prescription can also be used. Some of these contain tannic acid or picric acid, long valued as burn remedies, while others contain surface anesthetics of the Novocaine family. These latter should be used only sparingly, for such local anesthetic agents can be quite toxic to the body if too much is absorbed, and one is often tempted to use them over broad expanses of skin area. Such preparations should be reserved for the most painful areas of the sunburn alone, and discontinued after one or two applications.

Any sunburn involving extensive blistering and severe pain should be seen by a doctor, if only to guard against troublesome or dangerous complications. Even mild sunburns can sometimes activate herpes simplex infections ("cold sores") around the mouth; blistering burns are vulnerable to secondary bacterial infections when the blisters break. But for those who suffer severe sunburns, prevention is by far the most sensible treatment. The best prevention for sunburn is a regular exposure to the sun for increasing periods of time on successive days, starting perhaps with ten to fifteen minutes' exposure the first day, twenty the second, twenty-five the third and so on. Even the individual with very fair skin who ordinarily "doesn't tan" can often accommodate to the sun in this fashion sufficiently well in a matter of a week at the beginning of the sunny season to be spared the plague of severe sunburn throughout the rest of the summer. The

second best approach to prevention is the use of one of the emollient "suntan oils" or lotions when exposed to the sun. Many of these lotions contain a chemical known as glyceryl para-amino benzoate, a substance which is highly effective in filtering out the burning rays of the sun sufficiently to prevent sunburn but not so thoroughly as to prevent the stimulus to tanning. Unfortunately, people who tend to have skin allergies frequently have allergic reactions to lotions containing this substance. But even in the absence of such reactions, these lotions do not afford complete protection and are often washed off when swimming or by perspiration. Thus it is wise not to rely too heavily on these preparations, and to reapply them often during the course of a day in the hot sun. Finally, any protective measures used should also include special protection for the eyes with tinted glasses or a hat.

To most people sunburn is more a nuisance than a hazard, but to some it can be a serious danger. Many fair-skinned people simply do not tan or accommodate to repeated sun exposures, and recurrently suffer from severe, painful burns. Individuals with vitiligo—a total absence of melanin pigment in patches of the skin—are especially vulnerable even to short exposures, and should always approach the sun with caution. Certain serious systemic diseases, including the connective tissue disease known as lupus erythematosus (see p. 403), may have acute symptoms triggered by exposure to the sun, and chronic overexposure to sun and wind is a well-recognized cause of certain kinds of skin cancer. Finally, tanning enthusiasts should recognize that they may eventually pay a price for the rich tans they acquire each summer; when overdone, exposure to the sun contributes to premature aging and wrinkling of the skin, with gradual loss of skin texture, elasticity and tone.

Frostbite. At the opposite extreme from sunburn, frostbite is a result of chilling surface areas of the body to the point that the skin and subcutaneous tissue become frozen. It occurs most commonly from moist rather than dry cold, and tends to affect areas that are exposed to direct wind or covered with tight damp clothing. Typically it "creeps up" on the victim without his realization because cold tends to anesthetize the skin. It is usually easily recognized, however, because of slight swelling of the affected area, a dead gray-white color to the skin, and increasing pain as rewarming begins.

In treating frostbite, it is important to remember that any mechanical manipulation of the frostbitten area can easily further damage skin and underlying tissue. In very mild cases—a frostbitten part of an ear or a spot on the cheek, for example—slow rewarming of the area by exposure to cool room air, or the application of cool to lukewarm moist packs, together with gentle massage of the skin *surrounding* the frostbitten area to stimulate circulation, will usually be sufficient to rewarm the tissue and restore circulation. There may well be peeling of the skin thereafter, but mild cases usually recover without incident. More profound frostbite, however, may require careful medical attention, since impaired circulation in the affected area can cause tissue death, gangrene or sloughing of tissue. Medical treatment depends upon slow rewarming of the area, with the surrounding environmental temperature kept low so that metabolism in the surface areas of the body will be slower and what available blood there is will be more adequate. Medications are given to counteract spasm of the blood vessels and induce them to dilate. In extreme cases, anticoagulants may be given to prevent clotting of blood in the vessels as normal circulation returns to the injured areas. Smoking, which induces contraction of blood vessels in the skin, should be avoided completely until recovery. If pain is severe during the recovery period, analgesic medicines may be necessary.

Two somewhat similar conditions—*immersion foot* ("trench foot") and *chilblain*—can occur in the absence of freezing temperatures. Immersion foot is brought on by prolonged contact of extremities, particularly the feet, with moderately cool or cold temperatures in constrictive clothing and in conditions of continuing moisture. It was recognized as a major disabling condition during World War I, when multitudes of soldiers spent cold, wet European winters in muddy trenches or bunkers without an opportunity to get their feet really warm and dry for days or weeks on end. The result was a cooling and constricting of the blood vessels in the skin and underlying tissue of the feet, particularly the toes, causing impaired circulation and then, soon thereafter, a sort of anesthetic gangrene that affected the toes or sometimes the entire foot, often making amputations necessary. In civilian life immersion foot is a threat only to construction workers out in the wet and cold all day, fishermen, or others exposed to the precipitating conditions. By far the best "treatment" is prevention; when cold, wet feet are unavoidable for prolonged periods, see that they are completely warmed and dried and that full circulation is restored at least every six to eight hours. Also wear thick wool socks with relatively loose-fitting boots, since wool can absorb a great deal of moisture and still keep the feet warm even when it is wet. Treatment of mild cases of immersion foot is the same as treatment for mild frostbite; in more profound cases, or cases of longer duration, expert medical care is necessary in order to help reduce or prevent gangrene.

A far less serious condition, chilblain, involves a reddening and itching or "burning" of the skin, usually of the legs, as a result of recurring mild exposure to damp cold. Certain individuals suffer from it seasonally with the beginning of cold, wet winter weather, while others are not bothered at all by the same conditions, which leads some authorities to suspect it is a sort of individual "sensitization" to chill, damp air. Characteristically, women are more frequently afflicted than men, presumably because of poor protection afforded by bare legs or nylon stockings. The discomfort can be relieved by application of emollient lotions and gentle massage and warming of the affected areas, but those subject to chilblain are wise to prevent it during winter weather by wearing light, well-fitting woolen clothing. Woolen slacks or pants suits provide ideal protection for women.

Miliaria (Heat Rash or Prickly Heat). An inflammatory skin reaction, miliaria occurs when the ducts from the sweat glands become obstructed. The sweat reaches the outer layer of skin cells but not the surface, thus causing minute blisters that itch intensely. It is often considered solely an affliction of babies, but it is also common in obese adults and in people who have chronic skin disorders that interfere with the function of their sweat glands. The condition disappears promptly if the stimulus to sweating is removed. Staying in a cool environment, taking a couple of cool baths a day during hot weather and use of light clothing are all helpful. The itching may be relieved by a cool bath containing a handful of oatmeal or corn-starch.

Intertrigo. A somewhat similar condition to miliaria, intertrigo or simply "chafing" occurs where moist, sweating skin surfaces rub together: in the armpits, groin, between the buttocks, beneath pendulous breasts or even in the interstices between the fingers and toes. These areas become red, abraded and macerated, and begin to burn and itch. Scratching simply aggravates the condition and leaves these areas extremely vulnerable to secondary infection with bacteria or skin fungi of the same family as those that cause athlete's foot and ringworm. Intertrigo in the groin, complicated by fungus infection, is sometimes called "jock itch." Treatment of simple chafing or intertrigo depends upon scrupulous cleanliness (one or more cool showers per day in hot weather, or a warm shower with thorough drying during cold weather), copious use of talc or dusting powder on the chafing areas, the wearing of cool, loose clothing which permits air circulation during hot weather and, when obesity is a factor, weight reduction. If a secondary fungus infection occurs, one of the antifungal agents such as Desenex powder or ointment, containing zinc undecylate, or half strength Whitfield's ointment with sodium salicylate will often be helpful. When chafing is a problem along with itching, a powder preparation is always more satisfactory than an ointment, which may tend to increase maceration rather than relieve it.

Skin Irritation from Chemicals, Water and Air. Many of the chemical substances with which we commonly come in contact can have either toxic or abrasive effects on the skin. Often these are simply irritating substances—acids such as vinegar, alkalis such as dishwashing compounds or bleaches, astringents such as anti-perspirant preparations, salty brines, etc.—which the skin can normally withstand under ordinary circumstances of minimal contact, but which can cause skin irritation when there is prolonged or frequent contact. The affected skin areas become roughened, reddened and itchy, and repeated contact with the offending agent becomes increasingly uncomfortable. A common example of this effect is "dishpan hands" due to frequent contact with harsh alkaline soaps in the dishwater. Similar symptoms may be caused by allergic reactions to various skin contactants, but in cases such as this, it is often a simple, uncomplicated chemical irritation. In addition, some substances such as antifungal ointments containing salicylic acid or preparations containing mercury which are sometimes used against skin parasites such as itch mites are actually poisonous and cause severe skin reactions.

The treatment of such conditions, obviously, is to discontinue contact with the irritating substance, whatever it may be, and then to avoid more than minimal future contact with it. Emollient hand lotions may be used to relieve the reddening, drying and itching of the skin. If large skin areas are involved, relief from itching may be obtained by applying calamine lotion or by bathing in water to which a cup of uncooked oatmeal has been added. These simple measures are usually all that is necessary; when the skin is severely abraded, weeping or painfully sore, secondary bacterial infection should be suspected, and a doctor's counsel sought.

All chemical irritants are not necessarily surface contactants; both plants and insects can introduce highly irritating chemicals underneath the surface layers of the skin. Even the lightest skin contact with *nettles,* for example, causes an intense burning sensation caused by a chemical irritant carried by minute stinging hairs covering the leaves of this plant. The sensation, although harmless, may persist for up to an hour or more. Many stinging insects—ants, bees, wasps, etc.—inject irritating substances such as formic acid into the skin with their stings. The pain of these stings can be relieved by ice packs followed by sodium bicarbonate paste, calamine lotion or other soothing applications. In some people, however, a stinging or biting insect may cause allergic reactions that are troublesome or dangerous all out of proportion to the injury itself (*see* p. 139).

Much akin to chemical irritation, and a very common condition winter or summer, is *chapping* of the skin—usually of the hands or the lips—due to intermittent exposure to moisture followed by cold air or hot dry wind. The cells in the outer layer of skin in the affected area absorb moisture and swell, then dry and desiccate; the result is reddening and cracking of the skin, sometimes even bleeding. Again, the best treatment is to avoid the conditions that cause chapping. Keep exposed areas of the skin dry, warm and protected from wetness and cold air. Use an emollient hand lotion every three to four hours when chapping occurs. Chapped lips, the bane of skiers, autumn hunters and sailing enthusiasts, can often be prevented by frequent applications of Chap Stick or some other emollient to the lips during as well as after exposure. Again, any evidence of secondary infection should be examined by a doctor.

Corns and Calluses. Certain skin disorders arise from continuing abnormal rubbing or pressure on localized superficial areas of the skin, resulting in a piling up of many layers of dead skin cells which form a lump or pad of tough, horny tissue. The most familiar of these lesions are *corns,* which form on the toes where tight shoes rub and may have a deep, pointed core of dead cells at their centers, and *calluses* which are broader, flatter pads of dead skin on the ball of the foot, the heel, or any other area subject to constant rubbing, such as the fingers and palms. Both calluses and corns are usually harmless, but they may be tender or sensitive to pressure, and occasionally can become extremely painful. Most such lesions can be treated with preparations containing salicylic acid, a substance that tends to dissolve the thickened dead skin, and corn plasters or callus pads are especially effective because the padding helps redistribute pressure and thus prevent enlargement of the lesions. Generally corns and calluses do not cause any serious trouble except in individuals who have impaired circulation to the feet due to diabetes mellitus or other circulatory system disorders. In fact, calluses offer a measure of protection to the often-used skin surfaces of the hands and feet, but when corns and calluses are annoying or painful, periodic attention by a chiropodist or podiatrist is worthwhile. Paring or trimming these lesions yourself can be hazardous, for just where dead tissue ends and living tissue begins is often difficult to distinguish, and too vigorous attempts at mechanical removal can lead to extremely painful mistakes as well as secondary infection. Of course, the best treatment of all to prevent corns or calluses on the feet is to wear properly fitted shoes.

Decubitus Ulcers (Pressure Sores or "Bedsores"). A much more serious skin affliction, these deep, ugly ulcerating sores can appear, often very rapidly, in the skin and underlying connective tissue, especially over a bony prominence, when adequate circulation to the tissue has been cut off for prolonged periods of time as a result of pressure. Sometimes huge in size, decubitus ulcers most commonly arise in bedridden patients who are generally unable or disinclined to move or turn in bed, so that the weight of the body is maintained on a specific area for hours at a time. The first sign of developing trouble is a reddening and shininess of the skin in the pressure area, usually anesthetic or without sensation, followed by a painless breaking down of the skin surface and ultimately by sloughing away of skin and underlying tissue to form a still-painless but repulsive-looking ulcerative pit. A similar kind of pressure ulcer may form even in a matter of hours due to inadvertent pressure over a bony prominence on some part of a patient's body in the course of a single prolonged surgical procedure, or due to excessively tight restraints used to keep an agitated patient from hurling himself out of bed.

Whatever the immediate cause and wherever bedsores appear, they can virtually always be prevented by alertness and competent nursing care, and their appearance usually indicates carelessness, negligence or incompetence by either the hospital nursing staff or the victim's family. Nurses are specially trained to recognize the situations that can lead to bedsores and to take regular and militant measures to prevent them, turning the patient from one side to the other frequently, using massage to help stimulate circulation and, when an area of the skin appears likely to break down, using sponge rubber doughnuts or other devices to take pressure off the threatened area. Families caring for elderly patients in bed at home should be carefully instructed by the doctor to recognize the circumstances that can lead to this condition, and to avoid it by taking these same preventive measures themselves. Such precautions are absolutely essential, since bedsores, once formed, tend to heal extremely slowly and very commonly become the site of secondary bacterial infection or even gangrene. Care of bedsores may require months of additional hospitalization, costly medication and costly nursing care—a sinful waste, considering that they can almost invariably be prevented by a minimum of concerned anticipation before they have formed.

Allergies and Allergic Skin Disorders

The skin conditions that can arise from external factors are many and varied, but even more numerous are those caused by disturbances in the body's "internal environment." Among them perhaps the most frequent, and often the most bizarre, are the skin conditions that accompany allergic reactions in the body. These allergic skin disorders can range from the most minor of nuisances to certain truly grave conditions that require speedy and expert medical treatment.

Virtually everyone has experienced some type of allergy, and at least one person out of ten has allergic reactions severe enough to be disabling, sometimes at brief but regular intervals, sometimes for more prolonged periods or even continuously. And although an allergic reaction does not necessarily involve the skin, fully half or more of all allergy victims have, as part of their disorders, some form of allergic skin manifestation. The symptoms are often very visible and very uncomfortable; even so, many people regard allergies as somehow "imaginary." This is, of course, nonsense, although some allergies unquestionably do involve emotional factors. Allergies are, in fact, highly distressing *physical reactions* that occur, often in very exaggerated form, when some "foreign" substance finds its way into the body. Many of these foreign substances, which are known as *antigens* or *allergens,* are protein materials in the foods we eat, in the pollens we breathe in from the air, or in animal danders from livestock and house pets. Other allergens are found in house dust, garden dirt, molds, or oils from certain plants, while still others are chemicals present in ointments, cosmetics, drugs and medicines. In fact, virtually *any* substance not normally present in the body can act as an allergen under certain conditions. People have been known to become violently allergic to such unlikely things as the plastic in their glasses frames or even their own cut hair after a visit to the barber.

These allergens are not usually toxic or poisonous substances in themselves. But just as it takes two to make a fight, a special kind of tissue response to one of these substances must take place within the body before it can later trigger the kind of dramatic internal battle which we experience as an allergic reaction. The symptoms of allergy occur as a result of a complex chemical chain reaction that is set in motion when a foreign substance that has already gained entry into the body—or has come in contact with it—has created a condition of *hypersensitivity* to its presence. At the time of first contact, the body, reacting to the invader, begins generating substances known as *antibodies* to protect itself. Then when the invader enters or contacts the body again, this antibody army is called out in force to "fight it off." Under ordinary circumstances this is a perfectly normal and healthy reaction, but in certain people this rallying of body defenses is so greatly exaggerated and occurs on such a massive scale that the reaction itself causes mildly annoying or even disabling allergic symptoms. The severity of these symptoms depends on the degree of overreaction that occurs in each individual case.

No one pretends to know everything that is involved in this hypersensitivity reaction. We do know, however, that somehow the antibodies formed against a foreign substance seek to change or neutralize the molecules of that substance to "take it out of circulation" and render it no longer threatening. This, of course, is the basis of the so-called *immune reaction* that we deliberately try to create when we immunize our bodies against invading viruses or bacteria. By purposefully introducing weakened polio virus particles into our bodies in a vaccine, for example, we stimulate the formation of antipolio antibodies, which then remain circulating in the blood for years, waiting to fight off live, virulent polio viruses that may come along later. Obviously, such a reaction is highly beneficial; in fact, it is one of the body's most vital survival mechanisms. But sometimes its effects are not so beneficial.

Another part of this complex body defense system involves the pouring out of a chemical substance called *histamine* from cells the allergens have invaded. Once released, histamine is a highly irritating chemical which causes the swelling of surrounding tissues with edema fluid, together with spasm or contraction of blood vessels in the affected area. It also causes intense itching in the region. This release of histamine does help isolate the foreign invader from the rest of the body until sufficient antibodies can be formed or rallied to take over the defense; but in the meantime the swelling, itching, inflammation and outpouring of fluid in the area cause many of the discomforts we know as "allergic symptoms." If this defense reaction were confined to truly threatening substances, allergies might be considered completely benign and useful, if annoying, body reactions. But for reasons unknown the body can react blindly and witlessly to many foreign substances that are not threatening at all. What is more, some people overreact to certain allergens so repeatedly and massively that the resulting allergic symptoms can become chronically crippling. In such cases, the body's defenses may literally become more dangerous than the invader.

There is no clear-cut pattern governing who will overreact and who will not. Heredity plays a part; in fact, there are families in which "everybody is allergic" and the tendency to allergy is passed on from parents to children. The function of the endocrine glands, especially the outer portion or *cortex* of the adrenal gland, is also an important factor; we know that hormones from the adrenal cortex have the remarkable capacity to counteract or nullify allergic reactions almost completely, if only temporarily. And there are often emotional or psychosomatic factors involved in allergic reactions. But no one really knows if these emotional factors are primary or secondary; that is, whether certain people have a poor ability to adjust to changes in climate, food or surroundings *because* of emotional upsets, or whether they are emotionally upset because they are physically such poor adjusters.

For all the complexities of allergic disorders, certain things are always true. First, the allergy sufferer develops symptoms only in response to those specific allergens which happen to cause him to overreact. In order for these allergic symptoms to occur, his body must first be sensitized to the allergen by a previous exposure, a process which may have happened without any warning and without any resulting symptoms. Once sensitized, however, the victim may then suffer a sudden and dramatic reaction to the allergen the next time it comes along. Finally, different individuals have different "target organs" which seem to bear the brunt of their allergic symptoms. In some the target organ is the bronchial tree, so that allergies produce symptoms of asthma—an obstructive, choking respiratory reaction. (*See* p. 491.) In others the nasal mucous membranes and the linings of the eyelids are affected, leading to symptoms of hay fever. (*See* p. 490.) Occasionally, in the case of allergies to drugs or medicines, the bone marrow can be the target organ; or gastrointestinal symptoms may result from an allergy to food substances. More rarely, a dramatic whole-body shock reaction may occur in which all target organs seem to be hit at once—the dangerous *anaphylactic shock reaction* that occasionally occurs in response to penicillin allergy and may be swiftly fatal unless vigorously treated within a few minutes of onset. (*See* p. 139.) But by far the most frequent of all the target organs seems to be the cutaneous system.

Urticaria (Hives). Hives are raised, red, intensely itching patches that appear on the surface of the skin in response to many kinds of allergens. Usually they arise gradually over a period of hours, but on some occasions they may arise so quickly that the victim can literally watch them appear. There may be a single hive, or multitudes of them all over the body. Commonly a number of hives may run together or "coalesce" to form so-called giant hives as much as several inches across. Aside from the itching, the victim often experiences a sensation of chilliness, sometimes accompanied by a low-grade fever and headache, and may even have nausea or vomiting. Local treatment of giant hives includes the use of calamine lotion (a soothing, chalky preparation sometimes containing a tiny amount of phenol to help reduce itching) or the application of a paste of bicarbonate of soda to the affected area, a heaping teaspoonful mixed in a few teaspoons of water. For extensive hives a tepid bath containing a cup of uncooked oatmeal will provide soothing relief. Other measures in treating hives include use of antiallergic medicines (*see* p. 391), followed by identification of the causative allergen and then subsequent avoidance of it, whenever possible. Hives may arise from virtually any allergen, but are most frequently due to allergic reactions to foods—seafoods, eggs and wheat are commonly implicated—or to any of a thousand medicines or drugs to which certain people develop allergies.

Another important allergy manifested by the sudden appearance of urticaria is the intense reaction certain people develop to *insect bites and stings*. Bedbugs and mosquitoes can be the offenders, but the worst reactions usually arise from the stings of yellowjacket wasps, hornets, and even honeybees. Any sting is painful and causes a raised, burning welt at the site, but some individuals become sensitized to the sting venom, and when stung later may rapidly develop a massive crop of giant hives all over the body. Occasionally such a victim may begin to swell up before the very eyes of onlookers, and in severe cases the skin reaction can be complicated by acute bronchial spasm, choking and shortness of breath, even shock and collapse—symptoms typical of an anaphylactic shock reaction.

Thus beesting allergies may be far more serious than a mere urticarial skin reaction; extremely severe or even life-threatening reactions can develop without warning and with frightening rapidity. Details of emergency care in such situations are described elsewhere (*see* p. 139), but it should be reemphasized here that a doctor should be called immediately, or the victim transported to a hospital emergency room to guard against possible devastating circulatory collapse and shock. The urticaria will subside at the same time that the deeper threat is being treated. Many doctors also recommend that victims of this kind of allergy keep an emergency treatment kit readily at hand wherever they go, particularly on camping trips or vacations where exposure is likely. These kits contain capsules of a potent antihistamine such as Benadryl to be taken immediately following any beesting, plus syrettes of dilute adrenalin solution for injection if a reaction begins, and a longer-acting antihistamine to help hold the fort until medical help can be obtained. Such an emergency kit should never be regarded as adequate treatment in itself, and a doctor's instructions for its use should be followed to the letter; but it might well provide a lifesaving stopgap until help can be obtained in the face of an exceedingly dangerous and often underrated kind of allergic reaction.

Eczema (Eczematous Dermatitis). Although people often use the word "eczema" as a sort of wastebasket term in speaking of any and all kinds of skin inflammations, to doctors the term refers specifically to an allergic skin reaction common to babies and small children in which certain areas of the skin become roughened and scaly, with intense itching, often break down into open, weeping sores and then become encrusted with dried serum. Typically, the affected areas are on the inside surface of the forearms, the backs of the knees or around the buttocks, but eczema may involve other areas as well. Scratching can introduce bacteria into these raw eczematous skin areas, which then become secondarily infected, sometimes severely enough to threaten the child's life. Eczema is most frequently an allergic reaction to foods in the baby's diet, but it sometimes occurs as a result of some unknown allergen. Even when vigorously treated the condition may persist for months or years, constantly restimulated by repeated contact with the offending substance, whatever it may be. Fortunately, the condition may often be controlled by local applications of ointments or lotions containing cortisone hormones, combined with antibiotic therapy if infection is present, under the direction of a doctor. The real problem in routing the condition, however, is to discover the allergens at fault and withdraw them from the diet.

Contact Dermatitis. Very similar to eczema in appearance and discomfort, allergic contact dermatitis is suffered by people of all ages, and may affect any area of the skin as a result of surface contact with an allergenic substance. Often various chemicals in cosmetics are the villains, and girls or women who tend to have allergic reactions are well advised to avoid cosmetics of any kind. The perfumes in lotions or colognes, or agents in deodorant or antiperspirant preparations, may also be at fault. Some people react to the dyes in clothing, or even to clothing fibers themselves, notably wool. Oddly enough, others seem to have allergic reactions simply to surface heat, cold or light, although physical antigens may also be involved. Treatment is the same as for eczematous dermatitis, and identification and avoidance of the offending substances is particularly important. Often the location of the rash provides the best clue to what allergenic substance might be causing it.

One of the most distressing of all forms of contact dermatitis is that resulting from surface contact with *poison ivy, poison oak* or *poison sumac,* plants that everyone should learn to identify and avoid. The leaves and stems of these plants exude oils that are extremely allergenic and produce a severe itching contact dermatitis with the formation of vesicles in the skin. When the vesicles burst, they ooze serum mixed with traces of the allergenic oils, which are then transferred to other skin areas by scratching. Mild cases can be treated with calamine lotion and sufficient will power to avoid scratching until the reaction clears up in a day or two. When the vesicles break, antiallergic ointments or lotions containing cortisone will help quiet the itching and promote healing. Antibiotics are prescribed when secondary infection appears as a threat. Very severe cases are often treated by injections or oral dosages of antiallergic medicines. Poison ivy, a widespread weed in many parts of the country, is especially pernicious; the oil may be carried in smoke from brush fires and

affect people for miles around. It is best to ignore any and all folk tales about treating poison ivy. Obviously the best prevention is to avoid contact, but if contact occurs, a doctor should be consulted before treatment measures are undertaken. Some of the most severe cases of poison ivy ever reported have occurred in people who ate portions of the plant in the misguided belief that this would prevent the condition, and were rewarded by contact dermatitis involving the entire *interior* of the mouth and gastrointestinal tract.

Drug Eruptions. The widespread use of new, potent drugs and medicines during the past half century has led to an ever increasing incidence of still another skin allergy manifestation: the drug eruptions that are now such a common part of the medical treatment scene. Some drug allergies involve no more than the development of simple urticaria on the skin, which tends to persist until the drug at fault is discontinued. In other cases, however, the disorder may take the form of a generalized rough, red papular rash affecting widespread areas of the body, sometimes characterized by itching, sometimes by a feeling of "tightness" in the skin, sometimes by scaling with or without itching, sometimes by all three combined. Although drug eruptions may seem largely indistinguishable from other allergic skin reactions to the victim, an experienced doctor can usually detect subtle differences in the appearance and behavior of these rashes, and when he is familiar with the patient's medical history, identification of the offending drug is usually not too difficult. The *sine qua non* in treating a drug eruption is, of course, discontinuance of the offending medication, but since deeper-seated allergic problems may also arise and must be guarded against, a doctor (preferably the doctor who prescribed the medicine) should always be consulted when a skin rash appears during a course of medical treatment. Indeed, most doctors will warn patients of the possibility of drug reactions and query them about any suggestive symptoms as therapy progresses, with intermittent laboratory studies to help detect hidden allergic manifestations. But the victim of any form of allergic disorder, especially drug allergies, also has a commonsense responsibility to acquaint himself thoroughly with the names and natures of drugs, medicines or other substances to which he knows he is allergic and to tell any new doctor he consults about them so that these allergens, or similar medications, may be avoided whenever possible.

The Diagnosis of Allergies. Most skin allergies can be accurately diagnosed by your family doctor or a dermatologist on the basis of case history and physical examination alone, and treatment can be instituted. Determining which particular allergen is at fault, however, may be a much more difficult problem and can sometimes require the most canny and intensive detective work. Doctors know a wide variety of substances that are frequently allergy-producing, and sometimes a very carefully detailed medical history, combined with experienced guesswork, will narrow the range of possible offenders to comparatively few. In other cases there may be no apparent direct connection between the allergen and the reaction it causes, or else the allergy may be caused by a mixture of different allergens all at once. In these circumstances pinning down the offender can be a real chore.

One important means of identifying offending substances is by means of *skin tests*—a technique in which the patient's relative sensitivity to a multitude of possible allergens is investigated by systematically introducing tiny amounts of the diluted allergens into the outer layers of his skin, usually on the soft skin of the forearm or on the back. Testing may involve scratching the allergen into the skin, or actually injecting a tiny bit of it just beneath the outer layer of skin cells. When a patient is not sensitive to a particular substance, there will usually be no skin reaction; but when he is, a marked patch of swelling, with redness and itching, will develop at the test site in a matter of a few minutes. Skin testing can be a bother, since it may involve as many as 70 separate scratch tests or more, done 8 or 10 at a time until the range of common allergens has been exhausted. But in difficult cases, there may be no other way to identify the offending substance.

If the patient is allergic to some food substance, the offending allergens can often be identified by reducing the diet to entirely non-allergenic foods, and then, one by one, adding suspect foods until allergic reactions are noted. The same program may be used to identify stubborn or occult contact allergens. By one means or another it is usually possible to identify the major allergens causing allergic symptoms in any individual, although the process may take a long time.

Treatment of Allergies. Once an offending allergen has been pinpointed, the best treatment is, of course, to avoid it. But what about such inescapable items as house dust, molds, beestings, pollens or common staple foods? And what if a serious allergic reaction has already occurred? In addition to local treatment of skin allergies with soothing lotions or pastes, two groups of medicines are especially helpful: the so-called *antihistamines,* which specifically counteract or neutralize the histamine poured out during an allergic reaction, and the *cortisone-like hormones,* which help suppress the whole allergic reaction. In many cases antihistamines alone are sufficient to reverse an allergic reaction, but virtually all of these drugs tend to make the patient sleepy or groggy and must be used with care if his everyday activities, including driving, require alertness and concentration. The cortisone hormones are far more potent drugs, often effective taken by mouth or injected when antihistamines fail, and are frequently added to ointments and lotions as well in order to treat skin allergies. But prolonged use in any form may cause serious metabolic side effects, including retention of salt and fluid in the tissues and temporary elevation of blood pressure. Thus all these drugs should be used only under careful and continuous medical supervision. Finally, in very acute allergic reactions, administration of the hormone epinephrine (adrenalin) or its derivatives often helps turn the tide of a massive overresponse to a drug or other allergen.

For certain kinds of allergies, most notably asthma and hay fever, it is sometimes possible to *desensitize* the victim; that is, help his body accommodate to the offending substance by injecting extremely tiny doses of the allergen into the skin layers in a regular series of so-called allergy shots, gradually increasing the amount of allergen as the allergic reaction tends to quiet down. Then by continuing this procedure with booster shots at longer intervals throughout a pollen season or a winter when contact with house dust and molds is unavoidable, the victim may be kept free of severe allergic reactions. This kind of treatment is not permanent, however—it must be repeated every allergy season—and is much less helpful in combating allergic skin reactions than in dealing with nasal or respiratory allergies. For the skin allergies, the "great tetrad" still remains the therapy of choice: identification and avoidance of the offending allergens; use of antihistamines and/or cortisone medicines by mouth or by injection to counteract the allergic reaction; application of soothing lotions or topical cortisone preparations to the skin to quiet itching and combat inflammation and swelling; and the prescription of antibiotic drugs when the skin is broken and secondary bacterial infection is present or threatens.

Other "Internal" Causes of Skin Disorders

Metabolic and Glandular. A number of diseases of the metabolism, or disorders of various glands involved in the body's biochemistry, cause skin manifestations that may be highly characteristic of the underlying disorder. For example, diseases of the liver are frequently accompanied by a marked yellowing of the skin and the whites of the eyes known as *jaundice.* This condition arises from staining of the skin and subcutaneous tissue by the yellowish green pigments of the bile produced by the liver, and usually indicates some disorder in which the normal flow of bile into the gastrointestinal tract is obstructed. Jaundice in itself is not a disease, but it never occurs normally, and whenever it appears a thoroughgoing health investigation is indicated without delay.

Other changes in skin pigmentation may arise due to hormonal or other chemical disturbances. *Adrenal insufficiency* or Addison's disease produces an odd bronze to black pigmentation in the skin, especially in the skin folds. *Cushing's syndrome,* due to excess amounts of adrenal cortical hormone in the body, is often accompanied by purplish streaks or striations in the skin of the lower abdomen, while *pernicious anemia* is associated with a lemon-yellow pigmentation of the skin due to release of pigments from destroyed red blood cells. Long-term poisoning with silver salts, rare as it may be, has been known to result in a permanent slate-gray pigmentation of the skin over the entire body.

Certain metabolic disorders can also cause changes in the growth, texture or appearance of the skin, even though these changes are, strictly speaking, symptoms of the underlying conditions rather than skin diseases in themselves. In *hypothyroidism,* for example, the skin becomes thickened, coarse, dry and scaly, and eventually puffy with an almost plastic sort of edema that is characteristic of the disease. *Diabetes mellitus,* on the other hand, is often accompanied by increased levels of cholesterol in the blood stream, and a skin condition known as *xanthoma*—the appearance of yellowish plaques of fatty material in the outer layers of the skin, especially in the soft skin around the eyes and eyelids—is commonly seen as a sign of this disease. There is no particular treatment for these conditions other than treatment of the underlying cause.

Malnutrition. The skin, in order to be healthy, must be nurtured just as any other body tissue, and severe general malnutrition is often reflected in loss of skin tone, premature aging and wrinkling, a characteristic wizened appearance, and a predisposition to skin breakdown, ulceration and/or infection. Such conditions are particularly noticeable in persons suffering long-chronic protein starvation. In addition, deficiencies of certain specific vitamins may cause highly characteristic skin lesions: for example, the thickening and flaking of the skin on the inside of the elbows seen in vitamin A deficiency, the cracking of the skin at the angles of the mouth in certain vitamin B deficiencies, the petechial skin hemorrhages characteristic of *scurvy* due to lack of vitamin C (ascorbic acid), or the sore, red, swollen tongue and generalized blister-like dermatitis of *pellagra* resulting from niacin deficiency, to mention but a few. (The major vitamin deficiency diseases, including their skin manifestations, are discussed in detail on pp. 890 ff.)

Emotional Disturbances. The "internal environment" of the body is not, of course, exclusively physical or chemical; disturbances of emotion (as distinguished from organic nervous system disease) can also cause a disruption of the "internal environment" and lead to certain symptomatic skin phenomena. Much has been written in the popular press about a mysterious and ill-defined disorder called "neurodermatitis" —presumably a pathological skin eruption arising solely from nervous tension or emotional distress. Many leading dermatologists, however, deny that any such condition really exists, contending that emotional distresses can indeed trigger the manifestations of many organic skin disorders but that "pure" emotional dermatitis is largely a folk myth.

There are, however, certain *factitious*—that is, "made up" or self-produced—cutaneous system disorders which can be caused by emotional disturbances. Most familiar of these is simple *nail-biting* or some other form of nervous fiddling with the nails or the skin of the fingers. Similar nervous habits include pulling, twisting, chewing or even swallowing bits of hair, all lumped together under the fascinating medical name *trichotillomania,* as well as cheek-biting and lip-chewing. They are most often seen in children, and any number of psychiatric explanations for these habits have been put forth. They may possibly stem from some specific emotional pressure or disturbance, like a problem at home or in school, or more generally from feelings of inadequacy. In children attempts to force an end to the habit by coercion or faultfinding almost invariably fail. Providing emotional support, spending more time with the child and expressing a true interest in his activities and progress will often do more than anything else to help him "outgrow" the habit. In severe cases when the habit persists and there is the possibility that the child will permanently disfigure himself, the counsel of a doctor or even a psychiatrist may be advisable.

A similar but much more serious condition are the forms of so-called *psychoneurotic skin abuse*—digging, picking or scraping the skin, sometimes to the point of creating infected ulcerations, particularly on the face, or rubbing, scraping or abrading the skin on other parts of the body. This habit may stem from anxiety about some already existing skin condition— acne, for example—but in general it, too, may stem from feelings of inadequacy or from an attempt to gain attention or sympathy, escape some unpleasant task or otherwise enjoy the dubious benefits of being "sick." The habit may be conscious or unconscious, but in many cases the victim is unable to stop it, even though he is aware of the permanent scarring that may result. Treatment of true psychoneurotic skin abuse lies in the province of a dermatologist, who can deal with any existing physical skin condition that may be a causative factor, and a psychiatrist, who can deal with its emotional causes. Parental warnings and even punishment are usually fruitless, and any evidence of this condition should be brought to a doctor's attention without delay.

Bacterial and Viral Skin Infections

A wide variety of generalized infectious diseases may affect the cutaneous system as well as other parts of the body. Indeed, in many cases the signs and symptoms of infection apparent in the skin—rashes, eruptions or other lesions— may provide very important clues to diagnosis. Most of these disorders, which range all the way from the "childhood rash" diseases and "strep" and "staph" infections to tuberculosis, smallpox and syphilis, are caused by bacteria, viruses or parasitic infestations and are described in detail elsewhere. (*See* Part IV, "Patterns of Illness: The Infectious Diseases.") But in addition, there are a number of other infectious disorders, some common and some relatively rare, that arise in and primarily affect the skin itself.

Acne (Acne Vulgaris, Adolescent Pimples). Perhaps the most trying of all the common infectious—or at least infected—skin conditions is plain, garden-variety acne (multiple pimples), which occurs almost universally during adolescence and may persist into adulthood. This infection (or numerous foci of infection) begins in the oil-producing sebaceous glands in the skin, particularly on the face, back of the neck and shoulders where these glands are the most numerous and active. The onset of puberty brings an increase in the normal production of sex hormones in both males and females, and one of these hormones—androgen—is especially active in stimulating the amount of oil produced by these glands and in causing the ducts to enlarge. The ducts then become plugged with dirt and waxy oil to form *comedones* or "blackheads." Certain bacteria which have invaded the glands before they become plugged tend to break down the natural oils and produce highly irritating by-products which cause inflammation in the area of the sebaceous glands—a perfect setup for the development of tiny focal areas of infection beneath the skin. These pinpoint infections create sufficient pressure within the sebaceous glands to rupture the ducts and allow pus and oily material to escape into the surrounding tissue just beneath the skin. The small pustules that form frequently come to a head and burst, releasing pus onto the skin which may, unless removed by cleansing, simply help spread the infection to nearby sebaceous glands. In extremely severe untreated cases, *sebaceous cysts*—pocket-like collections of oily material from sebaceous ducts —may form under the skin, and sebaceous glands may become so severely infected that they form small boils which damage the subsurface tissue and burrow through to the surface, forming little infective tunnels or fistulas. These ultimately result in chronically infected areas that heal only with permanent pitting and scarring.

Certainly there is no skin condition that causes more unhappiness, shame or embarrassment among young people, chiefly because of its high degree of visibility at a very sensitive and self-conscious age, together with the possibility of permanent skin damage. And certainly there is no condition that is surrounded by more folk myths and false beliefs. Both embarrassment and possible long-term damage can be minimized by exploding these myths and examining the truth about the causes and proper care of this condition. Some of the most prevalent false notions about acne include the following:

Acne can be prevented. Unfortunately, there is no treatment that will actually prevent acne in any significant number of cases. More than 90 percent of all adolescent boys and girls develop some degree of acne, no matter what precautions they take or what program of prevention they follow. However, proper care can *significantly reduce the severity* of the condition and help avoid the entrenched boils deep in the subcutaneous tissue that lead to scarring and pitting.

Acne results from uncleanliness. Not so. It can develop in individuals who take the most fastidious care of their personal hygiene. There are people, however, who have acne and who do *not* bother to keep their faces clean, and these are the ones who often develop the more severe cases.

Acne is a "giveaway" that the victim (boy or girl) has been indulging in sexual activities or masturbation. It is certaintly true that acne develops in both males and females at the time of increasing sexual maturity, and that the hormonal changes at this time precipitate the condition. It is also true that masturbation in some form is commonly practiced at this age, and that young people also begin to show an active interest in the opposite sex at this time, often involving some degree of physical intimacy. Nevertheless, sexual activities of whatever kind do *not* cause acne or aggravate the condition, any more than masturbation causes hair to grow on the palms of the hands.

Foods such as chocolate, candy bars, nuts and cola drinks always aggravate acne and should be carefully avoided. For many years doctors themselves have proclaimed this dictum, and apparently in some individuals one or another specific food may indeed have an aggravating effect on acne. But this is by no means universal, and recent studies, particularly involving the use of chocolate, nuts and peanut butter, indicate that none of these foods is consistently implicated. When acne is severe, it certainly does not hurt to avoid these foods one at a time for a two- or three-week trial period. It may help pin down any such food that actually does aggravate the condition in a given individual, but other than this no particular dietary restrictions are helpful.

Removing blackheads and pinching pimples will help reduce the amount of acne. On the contrary, attempts to remove blackheads by pinching or squeezing the skin or using hairpins or other such instruments may very well make the acne worse and lead to more severe and deeper infection than would result from simply keeping the skin clean and leaving the blackheads alone. If the comedones are black, this indicates that the face is not being kept adequately clean. Very large comedones occasionally appear, and it is very tempting to try to dig them out, but the best advice is to leave them alone. The same goes for pustules or so-called whiteheads; efforts to break and drain them are more likely to stimulate infection deeper in the skin than allowing them to dry, crust and be removed by gentle washing. The individual who develops scars and pits from acne is most often the one who is "taking the offensive" and traumatizing his skin severely in the process.

The foundation of successful control of acne, although it will not prevent or cure the condition, is meticulous and faithful attention to cleanliness of all parts of the body affected. Careful washing of the acne areas, particularly on the face, at least twice a day, with a mild soap and warm water will remove much of the skin oil and cellular debris on the surface of the skin which, combined with the dirt, acts to plug up the pores. Specially prepared skin soaps such as Fostex or Neutragena may be somewhat more effective in reducing the oiliness of the skin, and in addition, an antiseptic soap such as Septisol or Phisohex used once a day tends to reduce the number of bacteria living on the surface of the skin. Application of some astringent such as rubbing alcohol to the affected areas after washing and before retiring for the night will help keep the skin dry. These measures will not prevent acne, but they will at least minimize it and help prevent a mild case from becoming severe. Girls afflicted with acne should recognize that makeup of any kind, even the widely advertised astringent and cosmetic creams that are alleged to help control or conceal the condition, are really nothing more than foreign materials to be smeared on the face; common sense dictates that *all* such substances should be avoided except, perhaps, on rare and special occasions. Finally, a doctor's advice should be sought in dealing even with relatively mild cases of acne; too many parents either nag their children remorselessly about their appearance or else regard acne

as an inevitable evil and offer no help at all, unaware of how very important an adolescent's self-image may be to his security and self-confidence during these difficult years. At the very least a victim of acne will feel that the doctor is on his side, and his anxiety will be relieved by the knowledge that everything that can be done is being done.

The simple measures outlined above will generally keep most cases of acne under reasonable control. In more severe cases, the advice of a dermatologist is essential. He will prescribe the proper hygienic routine, including any drying and peeling lotions he thinks advisable. Often ultraviolet light treatments are helpful, but these should be used only under a doctor's supervision; home use of ultraviolet "sun lamps" can result in truly disastrous sunburns. In addition, various prescription medications may be indicated. Most dermatologists today treat severely infected acne with broad-spectrum antibiotics, especially tetracycline, in moderately high dosages until the infection is under control, and may then continue the medicine in low daily dosages for prolonged periods to maintain the effect. The cortisone-like hormones are occasionally prescribed, but when used alone the results have not been consistently satisfactory. Recently, however, these hormones used in conjunction with small amounts of the female sex hormone estrogen to counteract androgen have been remarkably successful in controlling severe cases of acne. The main problem with this treatment is that estrogen may produce some degree of *gynecomastia* (breast enlargement) in boys which can persist for some months after treatment is stopped. Ordinarily, however, this effect is so temporary and harmless, and so minor in comparison to the beneficial effects of the medicine, that it does not contraindicate treatment in truly severe cases.

Some years ago X-ray therapy was used vigorously in order to reduce the activity of the sebaceous glands, but fewer and fewer dermatologists favor this approach today because of lack of convincing evidence that permanent control will result and because of the reluctance to expose adolescents to any more radiation than is absolutely necessary. In most mild and even moderately severe cases, given time and the proper treatment acne will eventually disappear without permanent aftereffects. There is also a marked seasonal waxing and waning of acne, with the condition becoming worse during the winter and improving during the summer when the victim is exposed to more sunshine and dry air.

In very severe cases, however, there will be noticeable scarring. Minor degrees of scarring tend to recede with time and no treatment is indicated. But with severe scarring, particularly in a woman, a procedure known as *dermabrasion* can often be used with excellent results. The outer layers of the skin are carefully abraded or ground down to the layer of cells that regenerate new skin cells, thus removing much of the superficial scar tissue and allowing a smoother skin layer to regenerate. This is a procedure, however, that should be done only by a specially trained dermatologist, and only on carefully selected individuals, since it may not always be effective and may, in some cases, be particularly vulnerable to infection. Fortunately, active acne begins to recede in most people by the time they reach seventeen or eighteen years of age, and it is only rarely a problem extending into older age groups.

Rosacea. Similar in many ways to adolescent acne, but common chiefly among people of middle age, this condition apparently begins as an exaggeration of the normal flush reaction of the nose, cheeks, chin and forehead which occurs in response to ingestion of various foods or beverages. Very hot, very cold or highly spiced foods are implicated in some cases. Alcohol is frequently a factor, although rosacea also occurs in total abstainers. Other suspect substances include coffee, tea, nuts, chocolate, hot peppers and various drugs and medications—all of which suggest that allergy in some way plays a part in the disease. In severe form small focal infections appear in the region of the sebaceous glands, capillaries become noticeably enlarged in the affected areas, and scar tissue may form beneath the skin surface, sometimes markedly enough to result in an enlarged, roughened *rhinophyma* or "rum nose" like that of the late comedian W. C. Fields. In most cases rosacea is more of a cosmetic problem than a problem of infection. Treatment is generally unsatisfactory, consisting of avoidance of suspected stimulants to the condition, use of antibiotics to control infection and, in extreme cases, dermatologic or plastic surgery to remove scarring or correct deformity. Medical advice is important even in mild cases to rule out conditions such as tuberculous or syphilitic lesions of the skin, or lupus erythematosus, any of which may resemble rosacea in appearance.

Bacterial Folliculitis. Deep-seated staphylococcus infections in the skin and subcutaneous tissues, ranging from solitary boils or furuncles to more massive carbuncles, are discussed in detail in Part IV, "Patterns of Illness: The Infectious Diseases." These infections often arise from the invasion of hair follicles by the infective bacteria; minor infection and inflammation leads to itching, which helps enlarge and spread these lesions. Certain individuals, however, have chronic trouble with small, multiple boils repeatedly forming in hair follicles, especially in such hairy regions of the body as the back of the neck, in the armpits, in the groin or between the buttocks. In mild cases this so-called *bacterial folliculitis* can usually be controlled by antibiotic treatment of the active infection, coupled with scrupulous attention to skin hygiene—keeping the skin in these regions immaculately clean, using antiseptic soaps to help control skin bacteria, avoiding irritating chemicals such as astringent deodorants, and applying unscented talcum powder liberally to prevent chafing in naturally sweaty areas. Occasionally, however, folliculitis resists such a treatment program and recurs again and again in an area, leading to scarring and pitting of the skin, and occasionally culminating in extensive areas of both deep and superficial suppurating infection of a kind that is highly resistant to any kind of antibiotic treatment. Such a condition can be troublesome both to the doctor, who finds it exceedingly difficult to treat successfully, and to the patient, who becomes discouraged with therapy and may move from doctor to doctor, sometimes over a period of years, in vain search for relief. Nevertheless, the best hope for control, if not cure, is consistent treatment by a qualified dermatologist, followed up regularly and faithfully as long as the condition is active. Occasionally, when an area has been deeply involved for a prolonged period, so that the normal structure of the skin has largely been destroyed, the best approach to treatment is massive surgical excision of the infected area, followed by skin grafting, a procedure best undertaken by a plastic surgeon.

Pityriasis Rosea. Once classed as a skin disorder of unknown origin, this mild and innocuous, but peculiar, condition is now thought possibly to be viral in origin, although no specific causative virus has yet been isolated. It is an inflammatory disease, occurring most frequently in young adults, which is characterized by a skin rash that often begins with a single patch of reddened and raised skin appearing on the neck, back or chest. This initial lesion is followed in a few days by a more generalized eruption of these rosy-colored patches, oval in shape and usually involving the skin of the back or trunk or arms, generally more or less symmetrically distributed. This rash cannot be mistaken for any of the childhood rash diseases, and it may be accompanied by a mild headache and a slight degree of malaise; the lesions tend to itch, and new ones appear as the older ones disappear. A visit to the doctor is in order to help in the diagnosis of any odd skin eruption, but if pityriasis rosea is diagnosed, there is nothing to do but wait for it to go away, which it will usually do within two or three weeks and almost always within two months. The "infectious" theory of this disease is somewhat strengthened by the fact that individuals who have once had an attack rarely have it again. On the other hand, there has been no convincing record of epidemics of the condition occurring as one might expect if it were a virus-caused illness such as measles. The condition is quite harmless, and its main significance is that victims tend to worry about the often quite spectacular rash.

Lichen Planus. Another itchy inflammatory eruption of the skin called lichen planus can easily be confused with pityriasis rosea. Its cause is unknown, but it usually occurs in adults who are extremely tense, nervous and high-strung, characteristically after some severe emotional shock. Certain kinds of chemicals such as arsenic or drugs such as quinacrine used to protect against malaria may cause a rash outbreak much the same as lichen planus. The lesions are irregular, somewhat violet in color, and show an odd sheen on cross-lighting as though tiny mica crystals were resting on their surface. Almost all areas of the skin and mucous membranes can be involved. There is no effective treatment for this condition, which tends to clear up spontaneously for no apparent reason, although it may recur again and again. A great deal of help is achieved by seeking out and reducing sources of emotional tension and worry; in addition, medicines which produce a tranquilizing effect and others which help reduce the itching will keep the condition under control in most cases. If it recurs or persists for a prolonged period of time, it may be a considerable annoyance, but there is no evidence that any grave or permanent harm arises from it.

Verrucae (Common Warts). These frequently occurring benign tumors of the skin, familiar to almost everyone, are believed to be viral in origin—but if so, they must surely be one of the most curious viral infections known to man, for they behave like nothing else in the entire medical lexicon. Warts are particularly troublesome when they form on areas of skin where they get in the way, crack and bleed, and may be subject to secondary infection. When these growths occur on the soles of the feet, where they are flattened by pressure and surrounded by deadened epithelium, they form the exquisitely tender so-called *plantar warts*. Some say that warts are contagious, although reports of proven direct spread from one person to another under normal circumstances are both hard to find and hard to believe. Warts have nothing to do with handling toads, much as one hates to explode such a charming folk myth. The fact, however, that they occur and recur in the same area and may spread seems to offer some proof that they are at least mildly infectious.

In most cases the best possible treatment for warts is to ignore them, since they often come and go quite spontaneously without causing any trouble whatever. There is no reason to attack a wart simply because it is there, and attempts to remove it may stimulate the appearance of new ones and invite secondary infection. When a wart is in an awkward position or tends to crack and bleed or become infected, it is best removed by a doctor by means of electrodesiccation under a local anesthetic. Alternatively, use of various "wart-dissolving" chemicals such as podophyllin will often soften the wart sufficiently so that it can be curetted away, a particularly helpful way of dealing with plantar warts, which are not as readily treated by electrodesiccation because the resulting scar may end up being even more painful than the wart was. Oddly enough, one of the best ways of getting rid of warts, particularly in children, is by "hexing" them. This is one folk myth that seems to have a basis in fact, although no one is quite sure why. Exactly what form the hexing takes appears to be immaterial—whether painting the lesions with colorful dyes, touching them with unusual objects or "irradiating" them with heat lamps—as long as the victim believes that the procedure, whatever it is, will make the wart go away. Some skeptics insist that the "success" of hexing warts is purely coincidental with spontaneous regression of the tumors, but many doctors are as convinced of its usefulness as are their patients. Very recent studies suggesting that individuals can, in some circumstances, be taught to exercise a degree of voluntary control over such "involuntary" body functions as gland secretions, heat control and so forth make this "hexing" procedure seem far less suspect than one might ordinarily think.

First cousin to the common dry skin warts are the moist so-called venereal warts which may form in the anogenital region. The medical name for these lesions—*condylomata acuminata*—is considerably more fearsome than the warts themselves, which have no relation to venereal disease. They are harmless, although some people find them alarming. They are easily removed with painless desiccating medication such as podophyllin or by electrodesiccation under a local anesthetic.

Fungus Infections and Other Skin Parasites

Because the skin is usually warm, soft, relatively moist or oily, and generally accessible, it is readily infested not only with many insect parasites but with a wide variety of skin fungi that can become lodged in the outer cell layers and begin growing. Most of these fungus organisms belong to the same family, the *Tinea,* and resemble each other closely both in their growth patterns and in the kinds of infections they cause. They are best known, however, by common names assigned according to the areas of the skin involved. The two most familiar and troublesome of these infections, ringworm and athlete's foot, are commonly assumed to be quite different diseases, although the organisms that cause them can be distinguished only by an expert mycologist.

Ringworm Infections. These are often classified and named according to location—ringworm of the scalp (*Tinea capitis*), ringworm of the body (*Tinea corporis*), ringworm of the groin (*Tinea cruris*) and so forth—but all are essentially the same disease. It is most commonly seen among children, and is so highly contagious that it often appears in grade schools in epidemic proportions. Ringworm gets its name from the typical appearance of the lesions, familiar to most mothers: circular, roughened, reddish eruptions on the skin or scalp which gradually enlarge, scaling around the outer edges and tending to heal in the center of the ring as the active infection spreads at the periphery. The sores of ringworm itch intensely, and the affected child will often spread the infection on his own skin by scratching; in severe cases it may involve the whole body before it is brought under control. Also, characteristically, the hair follicles are temporarily damaged by the fungus, so that the hair falls out in the infected areas until the condition is eradicated. Thus children with ringworm of the scalp have a very typical and unsightly moth-eaten appearance. The fungus is frequently spread by house pets and infected objects as well as by direct body contact.

Ringworm can usually be diagnosed on sight because of the typical appearance of the sores; in the doctor's office the fungus can be seen to fluoresce under an ultraviolet lamp or "black light" in a darkened room, and in questionable cases scrapings of the lesions will reveal the infective organism when examined under the microscope. Many surface medications have been successful in treating the condition in relatively mild cases. For example, half-strength Whitfield's ointment containing salicylic acid can be purchased without prescription, and is effective when applied two or three times a day to the lesions. Treatment can also be effected by painting the sores with a violently colored red dye known as Castellani's paint (unpopular because it stains everything it touches) or a 5 percent solution of silver nitrate (unpopular because the painted areas turn black). In the past decade an antibiotic known as griseofulvin, which is taken by mouth, has proved to be extremely effective in treating widespread or stubborn cases. This medication may be used either alone or in combination with a cortisone ointment applied to the skin. Griseofulvin will usually eradicate the infection in a matter of three or four weeks, and subsequent prophylaxis by way of a single dose of the antibiotic taken once every three weeks or so will help prevent reentrenchment of the fungus. It will even, eventually, root out deep-seated ringworm infections of the fingernails and nailbeds (*see* p. 407), although months of treatment may be necessary. The affected skin areas return to normal without scarring when the fungus has been eradicated, and in the case of scalp infections the lost hair will slowly grow back—convincing evidence that a cure has been effected.

Athlete's Foot. This too is technically a ringworm infection (*Tinea pedis*) which is distinguished because it attacks the relatively moist areas between the toes, and presents some special problems in control and treatment. Once thought to be spread primarily by contact in public swimming pools and shower rooms, it now appears that the fungus simply exists in the environment, and that the occurrence of the infection and its severity depend more on a given individual's sensitivity to the organism than upon mere contact with it, which probably cannot be completely avoided by anyone. In mild cases, athlete's foot is confined to a mild itching and cracking of the skin between the toes, but occasionally it develops into a severe, red,

macerated, spreading, scaly and enormously itchy infection which can involve the whole foot including the toenails and may form vesicles of fluid which break and then become secondarily infected by bacteria.

Both surface medications and scrupulous attention to foot hygiene play an important part in treatment. The infected feet should be bathed three times daily with mild soap in warm water, carefully dried and then powdered liberally, especially between the toes, with a dusting powder preparation such as Desenex containing zinc undecylenate. The shoes and socks should also be well powdered. These measures alone will often quiet the infection. Alternatively, soaking the feet in a dilute solution of potassium permanganate, which a doctor may prescribe, followed by careful drying and then application of one of the surface ointments containing cortisone is also effective, but has the disadvantage that the permanganate stains the feet purple and blackens the nails while it is being used. Griseofulvin taken by mouth is also highly effective in eradicating severe or stubborn cases, and when secondary bacterial infection is present, broad-spectrum antibiotics may be necessary. The person who is susceptible to athlete's foot is very likely to have recurrent infections and should take special pains to keep the feet immaculately clean and dry at all times. This, plus regular light dusting of the feet and shoes with zinc undecylenate powder, will usually prevent any recurrent infection from becoming entrenched.

Insect Pests. In addition to fungus infections, the skin is a favorite target for a wide variety of parasites such as lice, chiggers, itch mites, ticks and bedbugs (*see* p. 269) and for biting or stinging insects such as bees, mosquitoes, flies, spiders, ants and scorpions (*see* p. 139). These insects may be simply pests, but some actually invade body tissue or spread serious infectious diseases. There are also some, notably scorpions and black widow spiders, that can inflict poisonous stings or bites, while others, especially stinging bees, may give rise to allergic reactions (*see* p. 389). Treatment generally consists of recognizing and avoiding these pests and parasites, and destroying them in their natural environment. When they have invaded the body, a number of medications can be used effectively to eradicate them.

Disorders of Skin Pigmentation and Growth

Freckles. More a normal variation of skin pigmentation than a disorder, freckles are nothing but small patches or spots of brown pigment found in the skin of fair-haired or fair-skinned people, most commonly on the cheeks, the bridge of the nose and the backs of the hands, but sometimes all over the body. Redheads in particular tend to be charmingly peppered with them, but even light-skinned Negroes often have freckles. The only real medical significance of the condition is that heavily freckled people generally do not tan very readily in the summer sun; their freckles merely become larger and darker, and they may sunburn severely and repeatedly. These people should be especially cautious of sun exposure and may benefit greatly from the use of sun-screening lotions. Freckles should not be confused with *chloasma,* a condition in older people in which pigmented spots appear, especially on the backs of the hands, as a natural part of the aging process. Much money has been spent on cosmetic preparations to "bleach out" or conceal these spots, but none is really very effective. Since the condition is totally harmless, it is far more realistic—and less costly—simply to leave it alone.

Moles. These sharply demarcated pigmented spots, often present at birth or appearing shortly after, are composed of clusters of cells in or beneath the skin which contain varying quantities of the skin pigment melanin. Unlike freckles, a mole or *nevus,* to use the medical term, is usually solitary; it may be large or small, flat or raised, and often has hair growing from it. Moles range in color from almost white or reddish pink through all shades of brown to an intense blue-black. Usually they are perfectly benign and either remain unchanged or regress in size as time passes, but on rare occasions certain kinds of moles may undergo malignant changes in their cells to form cancers, including the extremely dangerous *malignant melanoma* (*see* p. 406). Frequently a person with a perfectly

benign mole will wish to have it removed for cosmetic reasons, and this can usually be done very easily by a doctor in his office with the aid of a local anesthetic. Any mole should be called to a doctor's attention at once, and should probably be removed, if it becomes itchy, appears to change in size, color or shape, becomes ulcerated, or shows any sign of bleeding or crusting over. None of these changes need necessarily indicate malignancy, but it is still considered wise, in such cases, to have the mole totally excised and submitted for pathological examination. Prophylactic excision of moles is also recommended when they are located in some area that is regularly irritated—under a bra strap, for example, or beneath the elastic band of undershorts. *Never* try to pick or scrape off a mole yourself, however. Let a doctor do it.

Sometimes small, soft, white "dangling moles" are found hanging from the skin by short, narrow pedicles. Technically these are not moles at all but small benign skin tumors known as *neurofibromata* which may appear singly or in veritable crops any time after adolescence. They are utterly harmless unless they are somehow in the way, but can easily be removed by electrodesiccation, for cosmetic reasons, if desired.

Birthmarks. This is rather a vague term commonly used by people to describe virtually any abnormal skin marking present at birth. Some refer to hairy moles as "birthmarks," but doctors use the word specifically in reference to a variety of benign capillary blood vessel tumors or *hemangiomas* that are often present in the skin of newborn babies or appear shortly after birth. These may be located anywhere and appear in all shapes and sizes, varying from bright red to deep purple in color. One variety, sometimes called a "strawberry birthmark," tends to be sharply limited in size, with a raised surface, and has a puffy feeling to the touch. These birthmarks are perfectly benign and often go away by themselves. If they do not or if they seem to be enlarging, the pediatrician may treat them by the application of dry ice to the tumor surface. Following treatment the lesions usually blister, scab and peel away, leaving only the most inconspicuous of scars. Failing this, either X-ray treatment or injection of the tumor with a chemical to destroy the capillary walls within the growth may be employed. Surgery is rarely necessary.

The other major form of vascular birthmark, the so-called port wine stain, involves much larger areas of skin, is dark purplish in color and is flat to the skin surface. Often the face or neck is involved. These tumors are also physically harmless, but they do not recede or fade of their own accord and cannot be successfully treated. Sometimes it is possible to conceal them to some degree with cosmetics, but in general the best approach is to provide the affected child with emotional support and help him become accustomed to the condition. Perhaps the most important thing for parents to realize about vascular birthmarks of any kind is that they are no one's fault—neither the parents' nor the obstetrician's. Nor are they likely to be passed on by heredity, and they virtually never develop into cancer.

Vitiligo. One of the strangest disorders of skin pigmentation, really more of a cosmetic defect than any manifestation of systemic disease, is a condition known as vitiligo, the loss of pigmentation in various irregular and sharply demarcated patches of skin. It may vary from a single vitiliginous patch somewhere on the body to involvement of great amounts of skin surface in pigment loss. The cause of the disorder is unknown, but usually there is a family history of vitiligo, suggesting some hereditary element. Medically, the condition is harmless except for one thing: the depigmented patches of skin are usually extremely sensitive to sunlight, never tan and can sunburn severely when the pigmented part of the skin suffers no sunburn at all. Thus individuals with this condition should always use a sun-screening preparation on the vitiliginous areas when exposed to the sun. Aside from this medical concern, many victims of vitiligo suffer embarrassment at the cosmetic defect, particularly noticeable in Negroes, Caucasians with dark complexions and those who tend to tan deeply in the summertime.

A physical examination to rule out extremely rare physical causes for vitiligo is necessary, but beyond that there is not much that can be done, although a person may wish to mask vitiliginous patches on the face, neck or arms with the use of carefully color-matched cosmetic pastes or lotions. Vitiligo rarely recedes or goes away once it develops; sometimes it is slowly progressive, but in most cases it tends to remain unchanged for years at a time. Most people who have it simply learn to live in peace with it, always keeping one eye out for the sun.

Albinism. A rare but striking condition in humans, albinism is the complete absence of any pigment at all in the skin, hair or even the eyes. Victims of albinism have pinkish-white skin that does not tan, white to pale yellow hair and pink eyes. The condition is a hereditary defect, often associated with astigmatism, with no known remedy. It is not always complete, and partial albinism much resembles vitiligo except that the same depigmented areas are found present in successive generations. Like people with vitiligo, albinos must guard carefully against sunburn, but suffer more from the cosmetic curiosity of their condition than from any physical disability.

Other Minor Growth Abnormalities. Most of the minor skin abnormalities have no particular medical significance. Among the few that do, *wens* are cystic lesions that form within the skin, usually in or around the scalp, filled with an odorless, waxy material. They tend to enlarge, and removal is often sought for cosmetic reasons; also, since wens have been known to undergo cancerous degeneration, doctors are happy to remove them. *Sebaceous cysts* are inflamed, often infected, cystic enlargements of the sebaceous or oil-producing glands, frequently filled with a rancid-smelling oil that may drain to the surface. Again, surgical removal is often advisable. *Keloids* are abnormally large, thickened scars that occasionally form with the healing of burns, surgical wounds or lacerations. In some a single keloid may form with the healing of a wound while other wounds heal without keloid formation; in others, any scar becomes a keloid. Negroes are particularly susceptible to this condition. No one knows why they form, and they are completely benign, but unfortunately they tend to recur if surgically removed. In persons known to be susceptible, X-ray treatment to a wound immediately after healing is often successful in preventing keloid formation. Finally, *seborrheic keratoses* are benign, brownish skin lesions formed of heaped-up epithelial cells that look somewhat like warts and somewhat like moles, but actually are primarily signs of aging skin. They are unsightly, and old people tend to pick at them until they become infected. Although they do not become cancerous, they also do not go away spontaneously, and often slowly enlarge. A single lesion may easily be removed in a doctor's office; but if a person has many of them, as is often the case, he may wish to think twice before embarking on a program of surgical excision.

Major Disorders of Skin and Connective Tissue

Psoriasis. In addition to the many benign or superficial skin conditions, there are several diseases involving the skin or connective tissue which have more serious implications, either in terms of prolonged, chronic, irritating illness or even as threats to life and health. Among the former is a tenacious, recurring, disfiguring skin disease known as *psoriasis*. This chronic condition chiefly affects adults between the ages of twenty and fifty, and is believed to afflict as much as 3 percent of the adult white population, although it is uncommon in Negroes. Despite centuries of study and research, its cause still remains wholly obscure, and although it seldom causes any grave long-term physical harm—it has even been called a "disease of healthy people"—it has caused untold misery due to its sheer unsightliness and discomfort, all the more pronounced because it so often persists for years or recurs repeatedly just when it seems at last to have been brought under control.

The characteristic lesion of psoriasis is one or more raised, thickened red plaques that form on the skin, usually covered with a distinct whitish scale, and usually accompanied by some itching, although this is not a prominent feature. It often involves the scalp, particularly behind the ears, and the outer or extensor surfaces of the elbows or the knees, but lesions may appear on virtually any other part of the skin as well. The plaques tend to grow progressively larger and coalesce, often forming very extensive areas of involvement.

There is no single satisfactory treatment for psoriasis, which at best is unsightly and irritating and at worst quite debilitating. It is common for the disease never to clear up completely, although severe attacks sometimes improve spontaneously for a brief time before recurring, while in other cases vigorous treatment appears to quiet the condition completely for prolonged periods. The on-again, off-again nature of the disorder is such that few doctors ever dare proclaim their patients cured, yet there are unquestionably cases—usually those treated early, vigorously and persistently—in which permanent cures take place. Among approaches to treatment which sometimes succeed, one of the oldest involves the use of keratolytic ointments designed to eradicate the whitish scale from the top of the lesions, combined with ointments containing coal tar derivatives or, alternatively, mercury compounds. Many of these ointments are available without prescription, and even those remedies that are so widely advertised are perfectly acceptable, but they produce no miracles; in some cases they seem to help significantly, in others not at all. More recently the use of cortisone skin ointments has established an equally spotty record of success. Cortisone-like hormones taken by mouth or injected directly into the lesions are far more effective in causing the disease to retreat, but in most cases the condition flares up again as soon as such treatment is stopped, and cortisone treatment cannot be continued indefinitely because of the undesirable side effects these medicines sooner or later bring about. X-ray therapy to the lesions also helps reduce activity, but can be used only as an occasional adjunct to other forms of therapy because of the danger of cumulative radiation effects. Of all forms of treatment, perhaps the most consistently helpful is whole-body exposure to the ultraviolet rays of the sun, in conjunction with application of coal-tar ointments to the skin lesions themselves. This may be accomplished by sunbathing or by judicious use of home sunlamp equipment as prescribed and supervised by an experienced dermatologist. Whatever the mode of treatment, the key to success is dogged persistence, even while recognizing that under the most favorable circumstances imaginable the end result may not be entirely satisfactory or permanent.

Pemphigus. Whereas psoriasis is common and only rarely severely debilitating, *pemphigus* is a much more uncommon disease of the skin which is potentially fatal. Although the cause is a mystery, the major skin lesion is quite striking: the appearance of *bullae* or giant water blisters, sometimes tense with the water they contain, sometimes fluctuant, which appear on otherwise apparently normal skin or mucous membrane. If these blisters first appear in the mouth, they rupture very quickly to reveal an eroded painful base, but other mucous membranes such as the lining of the vagina are frequently affected, as well as any of the other skin surfaces of the body. Exactly what causes the formation of these lesions is not entirely known, but there appears to be a breakdown or degeneration of the connective tissue bridges which normally anchor the external epidermal cells to the underlying skin layer, and frequently skin can be slipped away from the body in strips like tissue paper simply by lateral pressure. Although there are a few other conditions which cause the development of water blisters—skin damage as a result of unaccustomed pressure, for example—the bullous involvement of the skin in pemphigus is usually far more extensive without any predisposing activity, and can readily be distinguished by skin biopsy and pathological examination.

If untreated, pemphigus can progress rapidly to a fatal termination in a matter of a few months, or may drag on for as long as five years. Death usually results from secondary bacterial infection of the lesions, or septicemia arising from such infections, although malnutrition due to inability to eat with lesions in the mouth, serious protein losses due to loss of body fluids into the lesions, or upsets in the electrolyte balance in the blood are also contributing factors. Vigorous treatment with ACTH or with artificial cortisone-like hormones helps reverse the progress of this disease, especially when it is undertaken early; and maintenance with these medications, often in relatively low doses, helps continue the suppression of the symptoms. Occasionally the disease seems to clear up permanently under such treatment, but more commonly it continues, although under sufficient control that normal activities may be resumed.

Lupus Erythematosus and Scleroderma. Two other grave generalized illnesses which are usually manifested by lesions of the skin or connective tissue are members of the mysterious family of collagen diseases that include acute rheumatic fever, rheumatoid arthritis and acute nephritis. Both these conditions, lupus erythematosus and scleroderma, are most common in women, with lupus appearing during youth or young adulthood and scleroderma later in middle life. Both are characterized by a degeneration, hardening and scarring of the normally elastic connective tissue that underlies the skin and is scattered in greater or lesser amounts throughout all the organs and interior spaces of the body. The job of this collagen, or elastic connective tissue, is to maintain the pliable elasticity of the skin and underlying tissue and to form a flexible stroma or matrix—that is, a soft tissue-binding substance—that helps maintain the form or shape of different parts of the body. Both diseases affect this tissue and are the result of unknown causes, but otherwise have markedly different manifestations.

Lupus erythematosus, loosely translated as "disease of the red wolf," probably got its name because of the characteristic appearance of a patchy red skin rash, sometimes with ulcerations, that appears in a typical "butterfly" pattern across the prominences of both cheeks and the bridge of the nose. This type of erythematous or red-colored lesion may occur elsewhere on the skin as well, including the palm of the hand, the fingertips, or in irregular patches all over the face, upper trunk or extremities. These lesions tend to heal while others form and frequently leave a darkened pigmentation in the areas of the skin involved. The first onset of the disease may be accompanied by a wildly fluctuating fever which behaves much like the fever of an acute infection, but in other cases it appears silently and insidiously, present for months or even years before a definite diagnostic pattern appears. It is known that exposure to sunlight seems to precipitate the formation of the lesions, and further exposure makes them more severe.

In one form, called *chronic discoid lupus erythematosus,* the disease is restricted to lesions in the skin and connective tissue under the skin, with marked rash, scaling and atrophy of the skin, but without any systemic or generalized symptoms at all. This form tends to be prolonged and chronic and seems to respond best to treatment with antimalarial medications such as chloroquine in relatively large doses, sometimes combined with creams containing cortisone-like hormones for local applications on the skin. In this form it also tends to fluctuate, getting worse and then better for a time, but then gradually recurring less and less frequently, leading many authorities to believe that it is a separate disease entity from the dominant form of the disease.

That more serious form, called *disseminated* or *systemic lupus erythematosus,* tends to attack collagen tissue in widespread areas in the interior of the body as well as in the skin, and is a much more severe condition with a much poorer outlook. Often the joint surfaces are involved, leading to symptoms ranging from occasional intermittent joint pain to very severe and acute arthritis in a number of joints at once. Connective tissue in the lung and pleura may be involved, or even the connective tissue in the heart; the spleen may be enlarged, and the kidneys also affected. Indeed, in many cases lesions appear in the kidney very similar to those of acute glomerulonephritis, suggesting that lupus, like the other collagen diseases, may arise as an "auto-immune" disorder in which tissues of the body have become sensitized to antibodies formed by the body to protect against some other condition, so that the body is, in effect, attacking itself.

Systemic lupus erythematosus can prove to be extremely difficult to diagnose, arising insidiously and turning up with first one odd symptom and then another without any apparent pattern. In other cases, when it appears as a severe feverish wasting disease with a characteristic facial skin lesion, the diagnosis is easy. Diagnosis is assisted by laboratory studies, in particular an examination of the blood for abnormal

white blood cells, spoken of as L.E. cells, which are found in almost all victims of systemic lupus at some time or another during its course.

In the absence of treatment, lupus may follow a widely varying course, sometimes acting as a long-term chronic and recurring disease that often seems to clear up completely for years at a time, while in other cases the disease follows an acute febrile course which can end fatally within a few weeks. Thus treatment of the disease must be planned on a highly individualized basis. In the disseminated form of the disease antimalarial drugs seem to have little or no effect, but the use of aspirin in large doses helps combat the inflammation, and cortisone therapy is extremely helpful—sometimes lifesaving in acute, fulminating cases of the illness. The victim of lupus may have to take small doses of the adrenocortical hormones for years to keep the disease under control, and attention should be paid to the development of dangerous secondary bacterial infections. Disseminated lupus erythematosus is still considered an eventually fatal disease, but with modern treatment methods its course may be so prolonged that the individual dies of totally unrelated disorders.

Scleroderma is much less common than lupus and usually occurs in women during the middle years. The onset is gradual with a slowly progressive, diffuse thickening and rigidity of the skin and subcutaneous tissues, often with marked fibrosis and scarring, thus accounting for the name of the disease, which means "hard skin." It is even sometimes known as "hidebound skin." In addition to the thickening of the skin, the tendons and joints may become affected, with the laying down of calcium deposits in the subcutaneous tissue, and there is often involvement of the internal organs, most particularly the intestinal tract, the heart or the kidneys. When the kidneys are involved, hypertension becomes a complicating factor. The disease is slowly progressive, but it is not as uniformly fatal as systemic lupus, and spontaneous recovery sometimes occurs. As in lupus, the exact cause of the disease is not fully understood. Unlike lupus, there is no specific treatment that seems to be of value; cortisone therapy may help slow the progress of the disease in its early stages, but rapidly becomes ineffective in controlling it.

Erythema Nodosum (Nodular Erythema). Another inflammatory skin disorder that seems vaguely related to lupus erythematosus and the other collagen diseases (although by no means as serious a condition) is a so-called nodular erythema that occasionally occurs on the front of the lower legs, as well as elsewhere on the body, sometimes as a discrete entity and sometimes in relation to acute attacks of rheumatic fever, lupus, glomerulonephritis or even severe allergic reactions. In fact, the condition has been connected with so many other different conditions—acute infections, drug reactions and tuberculosis have also been implicated—that no one can say exactly what causes it, if it actually has any one single cause. It is characterized by the formation of red, raised, tender nodules in the skin and connective tissue, most often on the legs. The disorder usually occurs in young adults, and the appearance of the lesions is frequently accompanied by fever and a vague but persistent aching in the joints of the legs. Untreated, the condition tends to persist for months, and may recur off and on for years, whether treated or not. Treatment involves bed rest, antibiotic therapy if acute infection is suspected as a causative factor and, in some cases, administration of cortisone hormones. Unlike the more clear-cut collagen diseases, erythema nodosum is not a grave, life-threatening condition even when relatively severe, and in most cases is more of a chronic nuisance than a serious health hazard.

Cancers of the Skin. The cutaneous system, just as any organ system, can be the primary site of the various uncontrolled, invasive cell growths known as cancer. When these tumors develop in the skin they can, if undiscovered or untreated, eventually become just as dangerous as cancers arising anywhere else, but the victim of a skin cancer has certain factors in his favor that other cancer victims may not. For one thing, skin cancers develop on or near the surface of the body; they can usually be seen, or felt, or both, at a very early stage of growth, so that expeditious diagnosis and treatment is possible. Second, once discovered, they are usually easily accessible to treatment—by surgical excision,

radiation therapy, or both—so the victim has an excellent chance to be cured completely. In many cases the mere excision of a small suspicious lesion for purposes of diagnostic examination by the pathologist constitutes a cure. Finally, the two most common forms of skin cancer, both arising from epithelial cells in the skin, tend to grow quite slowly, and either do not metastasize (that is, seed to distant areas) at all or else do so only after a fairly prolonged period of growth in the primary location. This means that recurrences of skin cancers that have once been adequately treated are far less common than with other malignant tumors.

Because of these factors, a higher percentage of skin cancers can be completely cured than almost any other kind. But much depends upon the patient if early diagnosis and treatment is to be achieved. Occasionally skin cancers are first discovered by doctors in the course of routine physical examinations, but usually these tumors are first noticed by the patients themselves as lumps, nodules, thickenings or even small ulcerating sores in the skin. Any change, thickening, swelling or growth in the skin that does not seem to resolve and go away *completely* in a matter of a week or two should be called to a doctor's attention. In particular any break in the skin, with or without bleeding, that fails to heal quickly and completely must be suspect, especially any sore that appears on the face, on the lip or in the mouth. Occasionally a cancer that has formed a surface ulcer will seem to heal, at first, after application of an antibiotic salve of the sort that can be bought without prescription, but such "healing" of a skin cancer is never complete and the lesion never completely goes away. Obviously, one cannot be continually apprehensive about every minor abrasion and pimple that appears on the skin, but any *persisting* lesion should at least be investigated. Early diagnosis of a skin cancer can mean the difference between complete, speedy cure and a long, chronic, destructive illness which may ultimately even destroy life.

By far the most frequent skin cancers are those which arise from epithelial cells and are known as *epithelial carcinomas* or *epitheliomas.* There are two main forms. The *basal-cell carci-*

noma arises from cells in the deeper layers of the skin and is a slow-growing, sometimes deeply invasive cancer which, curiously enough, only rarely seeds by way of the blood stream or lymph vessels to distant areas. It merely enlarges, invading and destroying tissue around it—skin, cartilage, connective tissue, even nearby bone. It first appears as a firm, flattened nodule in the skin which becomes painful only when it has enlarged enough for the center to break down and form an ulcer; even then pain may be minimal. But a basal-cell carcinoma never grows smaller and never goes away by itself. When discovered early, a doctor will usually surgically remove the entire lesion together with a wide margin of healthy tissue on all sides of it. Pathological examination will confirm the diagnosis and will also reveal whether any active cancer remains at the site. If the tumor is large, a bit of it may be removed for examination before definitive surgery is performed. An alternative to surgical excision is X-ray radiation, which kills the tumor cells but also destroys healthy tissue in the vicinity, making determination of the correct dosage a problem. Most physicians prefer clean surgical excision when this is possible. These cancers, which are sometimes called "rodent ulcers" because they gnaw away incessantly at underlying tissue unless completely destroyed, often develop on the nose, cheeks, forehead or ears, and in earlier times were often treated conservatively in hopes of sparing the victim facial disfigurement, especially in the case of women. Doctors today realize that this is no favor to the patient, and with advanced plastic surgery techniques to help restore physical features when necessary, wide and thorough excision at the very beginning is the rule.

The other common epithelioma is the so-called *squamous-cell carcinoma* which forms in the outer layers of the epidermis as a flat, roughened or ulcerating sore on the external skin or as a raw, whitish plaque on the mucous membrane inside the mouth. These cancers usually appear on exposed skin surfaces, and chronic and excessive exposure to sun and wind is definitely a predisposing factor. They also appear on the lips, especially in the case of

tobacco smokers, since various distillates from the tobacco or its smoke are believed to act as a carcinogen—that is, a stimulant to this tumor's development. If caught very early, these cancers may be completely destroyed by the implantation of tiny beads containing radioactive radon gas or by the use of radium. Larger tumors must be surgically excised. Squamous-cell carcinomas are potentially more dangerous than basal-cell carcinomas because sooner or later they metastasize; but they usually spread only as far as the nearest lymph nodes, which can also be excised by the surgeon. Even so, one can never be certain that this cancer has been completely destroyed, once it has been treated, except by waiting to see if a recurrence appears.

Most dangerous of all skin cancers—indeed, second only to leukemia as the most deadly cancer of all—is the *malignant melanoma* which can arise from the pigment cells deep in the skin. Often a malignant melanoma is first discovered as a change in a pigmented mole, usually one that is not associated with hair growth. Unlike other skin cancers, the melanoma grows swiftly and metastasizes widely and very early; the chance of discovering it while it is still amenable to cure by surgical excision of the original cancer is discouragingly small. Radiation therapy is of no help, and once the cancer has seeded to other areas it is virtually incurable. But even then, the spread can sometimes be slowed and months added to the victim's life by extremely wide surgical excision of all surrounding tissue, including both near and distant lymph nodes. Often this cancer begins on a toe, under a nail or elsewhere on the foot, and any pigmented area on the lower extremities should be suspected. Fortunately, savage as they are, melanomas are comparatively rare. All hope of cure or even significant palliation depends upon early discovery and treatment.

A very few skin conditions, while not yet actually cancerous, tend to develop into cancer often enough, sooner or later, that they are considered *precancerous* lesions and are usually removed when discovered in order to avoid later trouble. Strictly speaking, of course, a pigmented mole that develops into a melanoma is also "precancerous," but malignant changes occur in moles so very rarely that they are customarily left alone unless some change in them is observed. The most common precancerous skin disorder is the *senile keratosis,* a flat, warty lesion with a dry scale on the surface which tends, over a period of time, to peel and peel repeatedly. This lesion is very similar to seborrheic keratosis (*see* p. 401). It may even be a variation of the same lesion, except that it is often very tiny, occurs primarily on the skin of elderly people, and is constantly scaling from the surface. Occasionally a senile keratosis will scale itself away completely and not reappear, but if it persists, it should be excised. Because of its potential for cancerous change, any such lesion should at least be checked by a physician, who can differentiate it from other utterly benign conditions and recommend removal when he feels it is indicated.

Finally, the skin may become the site of metastatic cancers that have seeded there from primary tumors elsewhere in the body. Often these cancers appear as multiple growths or ulcerating areas, rather than as single lesions. Biopsy will often reveal where the original cancer is located, if this is not already known, and treatment will depend upon the nature of the primary tumor.

Disorders of the Nails and Nailbeds

Fingernails and toenails are composed of a specialized form of epithelium, hard and protective in nature, which arises from special generative cells located in the nailbeds deep beneath the cuticles. The plates of the nails, while tightly adherent to the tender living tissue beneath, are made up of thick layers of dead cells which have no blood supply and no nerve endings, but the tips of the fingers and toes they shield are exceedingly rich in both. Hence, any injury to a nail in the adherent portion is likely to be either very painful or highly irritating or both. The formative cells in the nailbed are constantly multiplying and forcing the dead nailplates forward toward the ends of the fingers or toes, and the free ends of the nails can grow to surprising lengths unless periodically trimmed. It is a general principle that any injury, infection or other

condition that damages or destroys the formative cells in the nailbed will cause long-term or even permanent deformity of the nail, whereas any disorder—no matter how extensive—that leaves these critical formative cells undamaged will, if curable, ultimately heal without any permanent nail deformity. Most of a nailplate may be sliced off or evulsed in an accident, for example, yet the nail will grow back to normal in time, but even a minor infection affecting the nailbed may cause permanent wrinkling, thickening or distortion of the nail.

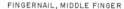

FINGERNAIL, MIDDLE FINGER

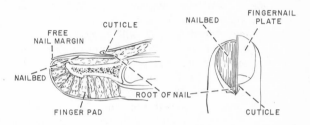

Figure 31–2.

Injuries to the Nails. Nails may be broken, cut, hammered, snagged or even accidentally torn off, and still presently be restored to normal just by natural growth. Most such injuries, however, are extremely painful, and most carry the threat of bacterial infection. The most common injury is probably a *hangnail*—a segment torn free at the edge of the nail, with the tear extending down into the cuticle, or a tear in the corner of the cuticle itself. Although hangnails may occur accidentally, most arise from picking, biting or other forms of nervous fiddling with the nails, and the best possible treatment is the hardest for the average person to manage: simply protect the hangnail from further injury with a small bandage, and then *leave it alone* until it has time to grow out or heal. Trim the free portion close with sharp cuticle scissors, but *never* attempt to pull a hangnail out by the roots, so to speak, and *never* dig into the cuticle with any instrument, because of the risk of introducing infection. Pain can be relieved, infection discouraged and healing promoted by soaking the finger or toe in hot water for 20 minutes three times a day, followed by clean rebandaging. If you cannot leave it alone, or if there is increasing pain or the appearance of pus at the corner of the nail, see a doctor, who can manage any minor surgery necessary with sterile instruments under sterile conditions.

Sometimes a hammer blow or other trauma will cause bleeding under a nail, seen as a discrete black or red-black splotch. Because of increased pressure beneath the nail, this kind of injury can be extraordinarily painful; if so, your doctor may elect to drill through the nailplate to allow the blood to escape. Otherwise, *leave it alone.* If the nailbed is not permanently damaged, the nail will presently grow out, carrying the clotted blood with it. Even a transitory resulting nail deformity will usually revert to normal with time. Other nail injuries should be treated as conservatively as possible. Trim a torn or snagged nail down to the quick but no further. If part of the adherent portion is peeled away, hot water soaks and clean dressings are indicated. Avoid salves or ointments, which trap bacteria beneath them and foster rather than prevent infection.

Ingrown Nails. Usually toenails are affected by this condition, which generally arises from a combination of improperly fitting shoes and improper trimming of the nails. A spur of nail at either edge may grow into, rather than over, the soft tissue of the toe folding around it. These growths, painful enough in themselves, usually become infected, leading to additional pain, swelling, inflammation and, often, the drainage of pus. Although many people with ingrown toenails limp along by themselves, picking away at them from time to time, treatment of this condition really requires medical attention, especially when infection is present. The ingrown portion of the nail can be surgically excised in the doctor's office and the wound packed with iodoform gauze or some other nonoily antiseptic. Extensive infection may require surgical drainage, followed by hot water soaks and antibiotic therapy. Once the nail begins growing out properly again, further ingrowing can usually be prevented by trimming the nails straight across (rather than in an arc following the curve of the toe) and by attention to better-fitting shoes.

Paronychia. The medical term for bacterial infection in the region around the nails, paronychia can be associated with the conditions mentioned above or arise without any connected injury or disorder. Strep or staph organisms are usually involved, and symptoms include localized swelling, redness, pain and, frequently, drainage of pus from between nail and cuticle. Treatment includes hot water soaks to encourage the infection either to subside or come to a head and drain, antibiotics taken by mouth, sterile dressings to absorb exudate and provide protection for the infected area, and, when indicated, surgical incision and drainage. In any but the most minor infection, self-treatment is unwise, as paronychial infections can be extremely stubborn, and any form of self-treatment involving tampering with the infected tissue will probably make things worse rather than better.

Onychomycosis (Ringworm of the Nail). This infection, caused by one of the fungi of the *Tinea* family, is notorious as the hardest of the ringworm infections to eradicate because it is so inaccessible to treatment. The fungus invades beneath the nail at the tip end, often involving multiple fingers and toes, and gradually erodes deeper and deeper into the nailbeds, until the entire nail may be affected. The infected part of the nail becomes an unpleasant brown color and tends to chip and crumble, with progressive wrinkling and thickening of the nails and, in many cases, considerable pain. Until the discovery of the antibiotic griseofulvin, onychomycosis would often persist for years, resisting every effort at treatment. Today, griseofulvin taken by mouth for an extended period of time —from two to six months or longer—will root out the infection, and the affected nails will grow back in normal fashion as long as generative cells in the nailbed have not been destroyed by the fungus. Recurrence can then be prevented by taking small single doses of griseofulvin once every three to four weeks. This antibiotic must be obtained with a doctor's prescription, but onychomycosis is still a stubborn enough condition that a doctor's supervision of treatment would be indicated in any event.

Thinness or Brittleness of the Nails. Any number of conditions can lead to excessive thinness, brittleness, pitting or unevenness of the nails—general malnutrition, chronic protein starvation, debilitating illnesses, thyroid gland disorders, various kinds of anemia or undue exposure to hot water and the defatting qualities of strong chemical detergents, to name but a few. Treatment, when indicated, requires identification and elimination of the underlying cause, but in many cases the condition is more a minor variation within the range of normal than a disorder or disease. When in doubt, consultation with a physician and a careful physical examination will help unearth any organic disorder that may be present. It was once fashionable for people to self-treat brittleness of the nails by eating quantities of gelatin, but exactly the same result can be achieved with an ordinary diet containing adequate quantities of meat or fish protein. Nails can be protected from the effects of detergents by use of rubber gloves for dishwashing, and from snagging or breaking by wearing gloves for gardening or other handiwork.

Hair and Scalp Disorders

Body hair, both on the scalp and elsewhere, is one of man's most prominent physical features, and we are quite naturally extremely sensitive to changes or apparent abnormalities in its growth, color or distribution, whether any true organic disorder is present or not. We tend to forget, however, that the hair undergoes a constant pattern of perfectly normal change throughout our lives from birth to old age, and that many of the things that happen to it are inevitable and simply cannot be altered. Hair, like fingernails, is another specialized form of hard epidermal tissue. It arises from tiny pockets of special cells, the hair *papillae,* buried deep beneath the surface of the skin. Once formed, rounded spindles of this tissue then grow out to the surface and beyond by way of a narrow sheath or *hair follicle.* Associated sebaceous glands beneath the skin surface constantly produce a natural oil which is released into the hair follicles and which, under conditions of normal health, helps keep the hair supple and flexible. The texture of the hair—fine or coarse, oily or dry, straight or curly—and its distribution—sparse or luxuriant—are both fac-

tors influenced by individual heredity, and further determined by the body's nutritional state, internal hormonal balances and various external factors that may be brought to bear. The natural animal functions of hair, including protection from cold and the dissemination of various body odors for purposes of olfactory identification or sexual attraction, are largely lost in human beings, so in one sense our hair is primarily window dressing. Nevertheless, like the skin, it plays an important part in our appearance; and as a tissue it may be subject to certain conditions which can be worrisome, even if they are normal, and certain abnormal conditions that may require medical care.

Normal Patterns of Hair Growth. A baby's hair is typically soft and downy, and even though a copious amount may be present at birth, it is often promptly lost, sometimes leaving the infant distressingly bald for months or even years—all within perfectly normal limits. Even a baby's hair may be damaged by external factors, such as being rubbed off the back of his head due to the friction of bedclothes. By early childhood the hair begins to take on its natural hereditary and racial characteristics. Innumerable variations in hair distribution may also become evident in childhood, ranging from a copious growth of dark body hair to an almost total absence of body hair at all except on the scalp. At puberty, the influence of increasing quantities of sex hormones is seen in the rather sudden development of hair under the arms, in the genital and anal region and, in males, on the face and neck. Often, too, hair color begins to change, with fair hair tending to become darker at the time of physical maturity. Baldness may begin to appear at any time from young adulthood on, and with the beginning of the middle years graying of the hair—loss of the normal hair pigment, a natural process—becomes more and more prominent. No one knows exactly why hair turns gray; heredity is certainly a factor, as attested by families in which almost everyone, male and female, tends to gray prematurely. Sometimes physical debilitation, chronic exhaustion or emotional shock plays a part, for reasons that remain totally obscure. The popular notion that hair can "turn gray overnight" is pure folklore, but there are indeed cases in which all pigment formation in the hair stops abruptly, so that the hair that grows subsequently is entirely white. Finally, with advancing age, the hair of both males and females begins to thin, becomes brittle and breaks off easily, so that the extremely aged may be left with only a few wisps.

Abnormalities of Distribution. Two opposite disorders involving the growth and distribution of hair are *hypertrichosis* (hirsutism or superfluous hair) and *alopecia* (baldness). The former in most cases is a hereditary or racial tendency or both; and just as there are men who have a heavy growth of body hair and may have to shave two or three times a day, there are others like the "lavender cowboy" of folk ballad fame who lamented that he could find "only two hairs on his chest" no matter what he did to grow more. Hirsutism, however, is usually a complaint of women, who may also display a wide variation in the growth of body hair. Very rarely, a tumor of the ovary, adrenal or pituitary gland (*see* p. 707) may be the cause of a sudden appearance, in a mature adult, of a quantity of body hair that was not there before, and any marked change from a previously normal pattern deserves careful medical examination. Surgical removal of such a tumor, when present, will also correct the abnormal hair growth. In addition, hirsutism may develop in an individual who has been taking adrenocortical hormones in relatively large doses for prolonged periods for the treatment of some other condition, since these hormones are very similar in structure to the sex hormones that normally help regulate hair growth and distribution. Occasionally such medication may have to be stopped when excessive hair growth indicates that normal hormonal balances are being too seriously upset. Most commonly, however, there is no disease or disorder involved in hirsutism, but rather a cosmetic concern which is as old as history. Ancient Egyptians regarded *any* form of body hair as repugnant, and women had themselves completely plucked from head to toe and then fitted with stylized wigs. Today we are not so extreme, but female facial hair and hair in the armpits and on the legs, all quite natural, are not in fashion, at least in this country.

Unwanted facial hair can be removed more or less permanently by destroying the individual hair papillae or follicles by means of electrolysis, a procedure that is tedious but perfectly safe if performed by a dermatologist. Hairiness on other parts of the body can be controlled by careful shaving, plucking or the use of depilatory agents. These latter preparations, however, can be highly allergenic and should be used with caution and discontinued at once if any evidence of itching or skin rash appears.

Alopecia, or baldness, is usually a normal, hereditary condition occurring among the males in families in which many men have been prematurely or markedly bald. Typical *male pattern baldness,* as it is technically known, usually begins in early middle age, occasionally at younger ages, with thinning of hair at the crown and a recession of the hairline in the front on either side of a "widow's peak." Gradually the thinned areas become bare, and the bare areas become confluent until nothing is left but a fringe of hair around the head above the ears. The process may move slowly or swiftly, and no one knows why it occurs; the hair papillae simply cease to grow hair, although the underlying scalp remains perfectly healthy in every other respect. Whatever the hereditary factor may be, it seems to be transmitted by the male sex chromosome, since women never suffer from pattern baldness, even though some may have a gradual thinning of hair or even extensive baldness in later years due to decreased circulation to the scalp and atrophy of the skin. Among men pattern baldness can occur in a variety of unpredictable forms; there are many bald men, for example, who are extremely hairy everywhere else. Some extraordinary myths have arisen with regard to this condition, but contrary to a surprisingly prevalent belief, bald men are not necessarily more virile or more intelligent than anyone else.

Even though baldness is a normal, and age-old, condition, for many men it is still a cause of considerable anxiety. Unfortunately, there is no form of medical treatment that can restore one single hair in cases of male pattern baldness.

Despite the advertising claims of so-called hair specialists, no medicine or treatment will have any lasting effect; and as dermatologist Richard L. Sutton, Jr., has pointed out, anyone who doubts this need only glance at an auditorium full of dermatologists at a medical convention. The repeated application of lotions or creams containing small amounts of male hormones such as testosterone may, in some instances, bring about a very modest temporary regrowth of hair in bald spots, probably through stimulation of such few hair papillae as still remain viable, but the effect will be short-lived at best. In addition, repeated applications of these medicines, even in small concentrations, may also lead to absorption of significant amounts of testosterone into the body, and this is one of the hormones which is known to contribute to the development of carcinoma of the prostate gland, particularly in men of late middle years who are already vulnerable to this kind of cancer. Thus any such treatments should be avoided unless prescribed by a doctor. What "hair specialists" *can* do is aid the individual in correcting or controlling seborrheic dermatitis of the scalp (dandruff), as well as conditions of excessive dryness or brittleness of the hair, in order to help eliminate any factor that contributes to a faster rate of hair loss than is necessary.

In addition, recent years have seen two developments that can offer the balding man avenues of relief if his condition is a cause of psychological discomfort. First, a variety of new techniques have been devised for transplanting hair-growing skin from areas where the growth is luxuriant to areas where it has ceased, or for implanting or "weaving" hair more or less permanently into the scalp in the denuded areas. These procedures should be undertaken only after consultation with a competent dermatologist, who can refer the patient to suitable specialists. Perhaps even better, the ancient art of making wigs and toupees today has entered a new era of skill and realism, and most men who are sensitive about their advancing baldness will find that they will, in the long run, spend far less money and obtain far more satisfactory results by investing in a truly well-made and individually fitted hairpiece than by paying for sundry medicines, treatments and the false hope offered by hair restorers.

Aside from male pattern baldness, alopecia will sometimes arise following a severe febrile illness such as typhoid fever or scarlet fever, as a result of nutritional deficiencies, or following nervous shock. In such cases the hair will usually grow back without treatment as long as the hair papillae in the dermis layer of the skin have not been damaged or scarred. On the other hand, if the hair loss is due to some organic decrease in circulation to the scalp, or to such conditions as senile atrophy of the skin, scarring and damage of the hair follicles by X-ray therapy, chemical or thermal burns, skin cancer, tuberculosis of the skin, scalp lacerations, ringworm of the scalp which has become secondarily infected with bacteria, or any other condition in which the hair papillae or follicles have been permanently and irreparably damaged, the baldness may be permanent.

Alopecia areata is the general medical term used for this kind of patchy hair loss, temporary or permanent, whatever the cause; but it is also used to describe a rare but peculiar disorder that occasionally arises in adolescents or young adults for totally obscure reasons. In this condition, patches of hair fall out here and there until, in many cases, the victim becomes totally bald. Drug reactions, feverish illnesses, emotional tensions and innumerable other things have been variously blamed, but there is no consistent connection; biopsy of the scalp usually indicates perfectly healthy, viable hair papillae which have simply stopped growing hair for the time being. There is no effective treatment, but in most cases, sooner or later, the hair grows back of its own accord. Occasionally the condition recurs, sometimes repeatedly—there is no pattern to it—but often a single attack is all there is to the condition, with eventual complete restoration of perfectly normal, healthy hair.

Scalp Disorders. Interestingly enough, the two most common skin diseases affecting the scalp— psoriasis and seborrheic dermatitis—however severe they may be, do *not* generally cause scarring of the hair follicles unless complicated by a secondary bacterial infection, and any hair lost with these conditions will generally grow back. Psoriasis is discussed in detail on p. 402. *Seborrheic dermatitis,* a chronic inflammation of the skin which is related in some way to both abnormal function of the sebaceous glands and the surface growth of certain bacteria, most commonly occurs in the scalp, beard and eyebrows and causes a flaking of the skin surface known as dandruff. The condition is generally harmless but unsightly, and is so persistent in some people that they eventually assume that nothing effective can really be done about it.

Most "dandruff-remover shampoos" in fact remove only a part of the surface scale and do nothing to correct the underlying condition. Dandruff can, however, be very effectively treated by means of weekly shampoos with preparations containing selenium compounds, available in full strength by prescription or in half-strength preparations over the counter in drugstores. In treating an active case of dandruff, the full-strength preparations are advisable. The hair should be thoroughly shampooed, including eyebrows and beard areas, and the shampoo should be left in contact with the scalp for a full five minutes before thorough rinsing, taking care not to get any of the preparation in the mouth. Because selenium is poisonous, it is best to rinse out a selenium shampoo (Selsun is the most familiar brand name) by means of reshampooing the scalp with regular soap, and later scrubbing the fingernails to remove all traces of the selenium. Except in rare cases of drug sensitivity to selenium, this procedure will, if repeated weekly for three to four weeks, resolve the most stubborn case of dandruff, and recurrence can then be prevented with once-a-month shampoos with the half-strength preparation. Any cases complicated by infection, sores, scalp rashes or tenderness should be under continuing medical supervision, but in most cases dandruff is persistent largely because the victim allows it to be. Equally persistent treatment will eradicate it.

Proper Care of Normal Skin, Hair and Nails

The cutaneous system plays a vital physiological role in the human body, but more than that, it is the one organ system that we can see, and that can be seen. Indeed, because the skin, hair and nails make up the façade we present to the world, we are continually tempted to "improve" upon them. These so-called improvements are as old as human history, and they have varied according to time, place and, above all, fashion. No sane person would ever think of grooming his liver; our concern with the body's other organ systems is to protect their normal function. But when it comes to the skin, hair and nails we sometimes actually interfere with healthy, normal function. Thus we shave hair from one area and urge it to grow in another, scrub off natural oils and smear on unnatural ones; we paint, pluck, curl, straighten, dye, bleach, clip, spray, pinch and pick. There is certainly nothing wrong with wanting to look our best, and many of these practices are harmless enough, even if enormously expensive and time-consuming. But where do you draw the line? Obviously when some practice is even slightly detrimental, no matter how flattering and fashionable it may seem to be. Commonsense precautions and care are no less important for the visible cutaneous system than for the body's invisible organs.

The Skin. The skin must be kept reasonably clean, of course, but most Americans are bath-crazy. Unless they bathe at least once a day they feel unclean, and the hands and face are diligently scrubbed even more frequently, always with soap. Detergents and soap get rid of surface dirt, but they also wash away the natural oils that lubricate and protect the skin—and they generally leave pathogenic skin bacteria happily untouched. Moderation would be healthier for the skin. Soaking baths or showers twice a week would remove most surface dirt splendidly; more frequent bathing should be brief and largely for purposes of comfort, using little soap. The parts that need washing—the groin, the genitals, the anorectal region and the feet—too often get a slap and a dash; children especially must be taught to wash these areas carefully. Lotions can be used to keep the skin from drying and cracking due to excessive washing; simple body lotions such as Alpha-Keri following the bath are not a bad idea providing the perfumes contained in them do not produce drug eruptions. Exceptionally oily skin may require more frequent bathing, but basically it is a natural human condition and in no way harmful. Special soaps and soap substitutes for bathing are in most cases medically beneficial only to the extent that they make you feel better; soaps containing bacteria-destroying chemicals are of some value as medication in treating such conditions as acne but, in everyday use, do nothing that ordinary soap will not do, and the chemicals they contain may be allergy-producing.

People spend extraordinary amounts of time worrying about sweating and body odor. During puberty both may indeed be excessive, due to hormonal changes going on in the body, and the adolescent is well advised to bathe frequently and, if necessary, use antiperspirants and deodorants. But strength of the various preparations available does not necessarily equate with effectiveness, and no scented spray or cream is a substitute for bathing the underarms and genitals. In adults regular bathing alone is often sufficient. All antiperspirant and deodorant preparations contain potentially irritating and/or allergenic chemicals, and use should be discontinued at once in the event of any kind of skin eruption. Many dermatologists, gynecologists and psychiatrists regard the recently marketed "feminine deodorants" as the ultimate in foppery. If simple attention to external cleanliness does not resolve a problem of genital odor, some underlying cause should be suspected and a gynecologist or other physician consulted. Foot odor, a surprisingly common complaint, can be controlled by maintaining physical cleanliness, changing socks once or even twice daily and absorbing perspiration with the liberal application of common unscented talc to the feet, shoes and socks.

Most women, as well as men in increasing numbers, use cosmetics of various sorts on the skin, and especially on the face. Dermatologists breathed a sigh of relief at young people's preference for "the natural look"—until enterprising companies began marketing "natural look" cosmetics. To give credit where it is due, cosmetics manufacturers have done a remarkably good job of eliminating the more irritating and allergenic chemicals from their products, but they are still

unnatural substances. They should be applied carefully and sparingly, and special care must be used to remove them. Remember that "cleansing creams" remove one foreign substance by substituting another. The recent burgeoning popularity of various "hormone cosmetics" and "wrinkle removers" should be viewed with even more suspicion; because of the potent hormones used in these preparations, they are potentially more dangerous than ordinary cosmetics and should be approved by your doctor before you use them.

The Nails. Keep nails clean and trimmed reasonably close—one-thirty-second of an inch beyond the end of the fingers in a smooth arc in the case of fingernails, one-sixteenth of an inch long and cut straight across in case of toenails. Most toenail problems stem from ill-fitting shoes. When tight, cramping shoes are necessary for show, remove them as quickly and often as possible; for everyday use wear shoes that provide plenty of room and comfort. Most fingernail problems result from snagging or breaking nails that are too long, or from biting or tearing instead of trimming them. Fingernail polish does little harm as long as you do not excoriate the nails getting it off. When long nails are desirable for cosmetic purposes, disposable plastic ones are inexpensive and a far better solution than growing the nails out to a point where they are vulnerable to snagging, breaking or cracking.

The Hair. Shampooing to maintain cleanliness is, of course, necessary, perhaps more so than general bathing. The natural oils of the hair collect dirt, debris, dust, mold, food odors and dandruff scales, and the longer the hair is worn, the more quickly it gets dirty. If you feel that special (and expensive) shampoos allegedly containing egg, beer, protein or some other substance make your hair cleaner, more supple and more attractive, use them; but otherwise soap is equally effective. If tonics, creams and sprays are necessary to hold the hair in place, they, too, should be used sparingly and washed off regularly. And any scalp irritation should be called to a doctor's attention.

Dyeing, color rinsing, bleaching, home setting or permanent waving all have deleterious effects on hair, and should be undertaken both with recognition of this fact and with caution. Again, most allergenic chemicals have been eliminated from hair dyes, but not all. Rinses color only the surface of the hair shafts so that the color washes away; the pigments in dyes are chemically or thermally baked into the hair shafts. Bleaches such as hydrogen peroxide, the most commonly used, make the hair more brittle and less able to withstand subsequent dressing or setting. Heat drying, permanent waving and the use of hot combs or curlers tend to dry out the hair and make it brittle. All should be used judiciously and as seldom as possible.

It should be said, finally, that the cutaneous system is marvelously equipped to take care of itself, if we would only let it. Minor blemishes and imperfections are perhaps to be expected, but preparations that promise medical benefits along with their cosmetic effects are no substitute for a doctor's advice. When it comes to altering the external appearance, common sense and moderation should be the rule. From a purely health standpoint, modifications should be minimal, irritating and allergenic substances should be avoided, and every individual should seek to complement rather than disguise the natural beauty of the skin, hair and nails.

32

Care and Disorders of the Teeth and Gums

Patients and doctors alike often make an illogical distinction between disorders of the teeth and gums and abnormal conditions affecting other parts of the body. Medicine and dentistry have evolved as such totally separate health care disciplines that the physician too often almost totally disregards dental diseases and tends to refer any patient with dental problems directly to a dentist, usually without any follow-up. Yet the teeth and gums, an important part of the cutaneous system, are intimately involved in the health and well-being of the entire body, and their proper care is a vital factor in the maintenance of overall optimum good health. Dental disorders can be unsightly, painful and chronically distressing, yet these conditions can be readily corrected—or prevented altogether—if a few simple fundamentals of dental care are observed.

The teeth have many functions in addition to the mastication of food. In lower animals they are found in an incredible variety of sizes, shapes and structures, ranging all the way from the fangs of a rattlesnake and the razor-sharp incisors of a beaver to the giant tusks of an elephant; and in each case they are uniquely adapted for use as weapons and even tools in addition to their function in capturing and chewing food. In man, they are used to grind food into small fragments in the mouth and mix it with saliva, the first step in the digestive process. But more than that, together with the tongue and lips, teeth are a necessary adjunct to normal speech; and of course clean, straight, healthy teeth are important to our overall appearance. Unfortunately, however, man's normal use of his teeth does not, in itself, keep them in healthy condition, as is the case with many lower animals. Bits of food lodge between them, they are easily accessible to invading bacteria, and without proper attention to dental hygiene we are vulnerable not only to tooth decay but to infection and other disorders of the surrounding gums and periodontal ("around the teeth") tissues.

Although the teeth originate from epithelial cells, and thus are properly part of the cutaneous system, they are composed of a tissue unlike any other in the body. They are *not* bone, but are formed of a highly compact crystalline substance known as calcium phosphate which is both harder and more brittle than bone. A typical tooth consists of two parts: the *crown,* the part of the tooth that extends above the gum line; and the *root,* which extends down through the soft tissue of the gums and is firmly anchored to the underlying bone by a substance known as *cementum.* The main body of the tooth is composed of *dentine* and contains a *pulp cavity* into which a tiny bundle of capillary blood vessels and nerves extends through a *root canal* from the underlying bone. In addition, the crown of the tooth bears a thick coating of dense crystalline calcium phosphate, much harder than dentine, known as *enamel*—a substance remarkably resistant to heat, cold or bacterial invasion. (*See* Fig. 32–1.)

Once a tooth erupts through the gum and

attains its full size it no longer continues to grow, although the jaw may widen to accommodate it. As compensation for this lack of growth capacity, human beings are born with

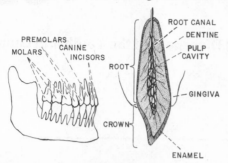

Figure 32–1.

two sets of teeth, the first an incomplete set of 20 *decidual teeth* (often called "baby teeth" or "milk teeth" because they begin appearing within the first year of life); the second a full complement of 32 *permanent teeth* which begin appearing as the decidual teeth fall out. The last of the permanent teeth do not appear until the jaw has reached full adult size. Not only do these teeth cease to grow once they attain their mature form; they have no capacity for self-repair such as other tissues do. A chipped or broken tooth stays chipped or broken as long as the tooth survives, and an area of bacterial decay in a tooth will never heal. Once erupted, a tooth remains in its position until it loosens and falls out—a normal process in the case of baby teeth—or as a result of decay and periodontal disease in the case of adult teeth. Over the years adult teeth do wear down, however, even to the point that some of the hard enamel coating eventually is ground away.

The teeth are named according to their position and function in the mouth. In front, in each jaw, are four *incisors,* flat-edged, wedge-shaped "cutting teeth." When the *occlusion* or "bite" of the teeth is correct, the upper incisors slide over the lower incisors and allow us to cut food with a scissors-like motion. Adjacent to the incisors, top and bottom, are somewhat larger and more prominent teeth, one on each side, known as *canines* because they are rounded, pointed and prominent like the long tearing teeth

in the front of a dog's mouth. These are sometimes known as "eye teeth" and were once believed to be somehow closely related to the eye sockets. Next to the canines are a pair of larger teeth on either side, top and bottom, that bear two points or *cusps* on each tooth and thus are known as *bicuspids.* These teeth are useful, together with the canines, in tearing and chopping fibrous foods, and since they appear earlier than the broad, flat, three- or four-pointed *molars* or "grinders," they are sometimes spoken of as "premolars." In the child the premolars are the last of the baby teeth; the three true molars on either side, top and bottom, have no predecessors and are all permanent teeth. The age of appearance of both the deciduous and the permanent teeth is listed in the accompanying table.

At the time of birth all 20 of the baby teeth are already forming within the gum, and the first of these to appear are usually the two middle lower incisors, which erupt between six months and a year of age. Very rarely a baby will be born with a fully erupted lower incisor, an unfortunate turn of events for the mother who wants to nurse. This is usually a superfluous tooth that will either fall out within a week or two or else should be extracted so that it can be replaced by the normal baby tooth that underlies it. The other incisors follow the first and are followed, in turn, first by the canines and then by the premolars, a process of "teething" that is usually complete by the time the child is two and a half to three years old. The appearance of each new tooth is likely to be somewhat irritating and uncomfortable to the child, heralded by a period of fretfulness. Contrary to popular belief, teething does not cause a child to run a fever, but when a fever due to an upper respiratory infection or a childhood rash disease occurs at the time a new tooth is nearly ready to emerge, the increase in metabolism due to the fever will often cause the tooth to "sprout" quite suddenly. At about the age of six the first of the true permanent molars or "six-year molars" appears; at about the same time, the baby incisors begin loosening and coming out, leaving characteristic gaps in the child's smile. The second or "twelve-year" molars make their first appearance at age

Normal Dentition

Tooth Name	Average Age of Eruption	Average Age Lost
Lower central incisors	6–12 months	5–6 years
Upper incisors	8–10 months	5–6 years
Lower lateral incisors	10–14 months	5–6 years
Canines	16–20 months	8–10 years
First molars	12–16 months	9–11 years
Second molars	20–36 months	9–12 years
Lower central incisors	6–7 years	Permanent
Upper central incisors	7–8 years	Permanent
Lower lateral incisors	7–8 years	Permanent
Upper lateral incisors	8–9 years	Permanent
Lower canines	10–11 years	Permanent
Upper canines	11–12 years	Permanent
First bicuspids, upper and lower	10–12 years	Permanent
Second bicuspids, upper	10–12 years	Permanent
Second bicuspids, lower	11–12 years	Permanent
First molars, upper and lower	6–7 years	Permanent
Second molars, upper and lower	12–14 years	Permanent
Third molars (wisdom teeth)	17–30 years	Permanent

ten to thirteen, about the same time that the last of the baby teeth have also been replaced. Often the new adult teeth appear abnormally large in the child's small jaw until the jaw itself has grown sufficiently to accommodate them.

Physical Abnormalities of Dentition

A number of disorders may arise as a result of physical factors in the eruption of teeth and their development within the growing jaw. In some cases these may be purely transitory anatomical abnormalities due to discrepancies between the time of tooth eruption and the growth of the jaw. In other cases hereditary factors may be at work to cause abnormalities, and physical injuries of one sort or another may also play a part. Sometimes these factors may be intermixed, and any abnormality of dentition occurring during childhood or adolescence should always be investigated by a dentist.

Extra or Missing Teeth. Although the child normally will develop 20 baby teeth (10 above and 10 below) and the adult a total of 32 (16 above and 16 below), the time of appearance of these teeth will not always necessarily follow the pattern noted above, nor will all of the permanent teeth necessarily appear. Sometimes baby teeth are lost unusually early or retained abnormally long. Quite frequently the loss of a baby tooth will not be followed immediately by the eruption of the underlying permanent tooth, and in some cases other permanent teeth erupting on either side of the delayed tooth will preempt the space, so that appearance of the tooth in the middle is further delayed and all the teeth are then crowded when it does erupt. When timing alone is at fault such crowding, which frequently results in adult teeth being turned slightly to the side or "crumpled," natural straightening will usually occur as the jaw widens. If, however, the jaw is abnormally narrow due to hereditary factors, the crowding may be permanent unless such mechanical aids as braces and retainers are used to prevent the late-appearing teeth from being crowded and twisted. Occasionally the problem will arise at the appearance of an extra baby tooth or adult tooth, so that extraction is indicated. Similarly, a baby tooth which persists abnormally long may, in some cases, best be extracted to make room for adult teeth beneath in seeking to erupt. Finally, a permanent tooth may be congenitally missing altogether, or congenitally deformed—abnormally small, for example. Such congenital abnormalities are not necessarily symmetrical, nor are they necessarily duplicated in both upper and lower jaws, so that a single extra or missing tooth in either upper or lower jaw can, if not treated adequately or in time, result in a moving of all the teeth in that jaw slightly out of alignment with their corresponding teeth in the other jaw.

For many years it was believed that physical manipulation of the teeth to correct the results of late or early eruption, crowding or congenital abnormalities—a dental specialty known as *orthodontia*—should be delayed until all the baby teeth had been replaced and the adult teeth erupted. Today orthodontists will often begin corrective measures at the age of nine or ten or even earlier if dental examination, X-ray studies and a review of the patient's family dental history all suggest that such manipulation is likely to be necessary. At the earlier age teeth are not as firmly welded into their sockets as they later will be, and thus correction of abnormalities is accomplished much more quickly and with better long-term results when the work is begun as early as possible.

In some cases missing teeth can be a boon. No one can tell for certain if the human jaw is continuing to narrow as a result of evolution, but a great many people today simply fail to develop one or more of the four wisdom teeth. In some cases the missing tooth may remain embedded in the gum as a "bud" or deformed tooth which just never erupts, and may be vulnerable to infection or abscess formation. In such cases surgical extraction is sometimes indicated. Since wisdom teeth are not really necessary for effective mastication, the person with one or more completely missing may be spared a great deal of trouble, since wisdom teeth often severely crowd the rest of the jaw, decay readily, and frequently have to be extracted anyway at some later date.

Impaction. A person with a full complement of wisdom teeth and a narrow jaw may suffer another physical abnormality: a tendency of the third molars to erupt too close to the second molars so that they jam together or impact. This can also happen to adult teeth in the front of the mouth. A dentist's attention to the teeth early in life is especially important in such cases, in order that the need for extractions or orthodontic treatment can be ascertained as soon as possible and the necessary correction initiated while the jaw is still somewhat plastic. Later the root system of wisdom teeth in particular may become so firmly anchored in the jaw that extraction can require major oral surgy. The decision to remove other teeth to permit an impacted tooth to erupt properly, or to use mechanical devices to hold the teeth on either side apart, must be made by the dentist based upon what he discovers in each individual case, and often an early consultation with an orthodontist is wise.

Malocclusion. This is a term used to describe an improper "bite" or meeting of the teeth of the upper and lower jaws, whatever the cause. Ordinarily the upper and lower teeth erupt and meet evenly, with each tooth in the upper jaw making proper contact with the corresponding tooth in the lower jaw. If for some reason the incisors in the upper jaw or lower jaw or both are crowded and thrust forward, so-called buckteeth result. Aside from their unfortunate appearance, buckteeth cannot properly perform the scissors action of cutting for which they were intended. Occasionally the entire upper jaw will contact and override the lower jaw slightly, a condition of "overbite," or the lower jaw will be thrust slightly forward so that occlusion is not correct, a condition of "underbite." Even more difficult, the early loss of a deciduous tooth, the impaction of a wisdom tooth or some other condition which leads to shifting of the teeth in one jaw slightly to one side or the other can result in a lateral or sideways malocclusion. Any malocclusion not only interferes with mastication but may cause excessive wear and tear to the teeth, gums or bone of the jaw and interfere with the overall appearance of the smile. Hereditary causes such as a narrow jaw may be at fault; so also may such physical factors as thumbsucking, mouth-breathing with the tongue habitually protruding between the teeth, or even habitual pressure of the tongue against the backs of the upper or lower teeth. There is no way for the untrained individual to guess whether a malocclusion will be temporary and self-correcting or permanent, but if one has crowded teeth or a small jaw, the likelihood is high that hereditary factors are at work and that orthodontic assistance will be necessary to correct the condition. The alert dentist who sees a child at six-month intervals for teeth cleaning or other preventive dental care will usually detect the development of malocclusion early and will recommend corrective measures to be taken when necessary.

Physical Injury and Wear and Tear. Everyone is vulnerable to physical injury to the teeth. When a baby tooth is knocked out or broken, little permanent harm is likely to result, since the tooth will be lost sooner or later anyway. Even so, a dentist should be consulted so that a broken tooth may be capped, if necessary, or so that the injured mouth may be properly cared for. Chipping, cracking or breaking an adult tooth, on the other hand, is a permanent injury and must be treated as such. The tooth that is broken off with the root still in place is particularly vulnerable to both pain and decay, and the teeth on either side of the injured one must also be prevented from shifting position. Occasionally a tooth may be chipped, a cusp may be fractured off, or some other injury may occur because the tooth has been weakened by previous decay. Reconstruction of such teeth—or replacement of them—is highly important, and any physical injury to teeth should be called to a dentist's attention as early as possible.

Diseases of Teeth and Gums

Caries. Certainly the most commonplace of all dental disorders is *caries* or cavities—small areas of erosion and decay beginning on the hard enamel surface of the teeth and gradually extending through to the somewhat softer dentine beneath. Caries arises from a combination of destructive factors, usually related to inadequate mouth hygiene and especially to the failure to brush the teeth regularly after meals. Bits of food lodged between the teeth spoil and support the growth of bacteria which, in addition to contributing to bad breath or halitosis, also produce acidic substances which cause roughening and erosion of the hard enamel surface.

These eroded areas then harbor bacteria which continue their growth and erosion, a process which may proceed for months or years in a given area before the enamel is finally pierced. The dentine of the tooth beneath the enamel is somewhat softer, and once decay enters this area it progresses much more rapidly. Unfortunately, the process usually remains entirely painless until the area of decay has extended deep into the dentine and is approaching the soft, pain-sensitive pulp within the central canal of the tooth. With still further neglect the decay may ultimately erode away the entire crown of the tooth and can extend down the root canal to cause a painful or destructive abscess of the root, or infection in the bone of the jaw. Thus caries may not only lead to complete destruction of the affected teeth but can, in extreme cases, cause multiple abscesses in the jaws with cellulitis of surrounding soft tissue and seeding of bacteria into the blood stream, or even osteomyelitis. To some degree the formation of caries depends upon congenital factors: some people have thinner or softer enamel than others and readily form cavities even early in life in their baby teeth, while others seem relatively impervious to this disorder, but sooner or later everyone becomes vulnerable unless regular hygienic measures are taken to keep the teeth clean.

The best protection against the ill effects of caries lies in periodic visits to a dentist so that cavities may be detected early. Dental examination, including X-rays, helps identify even the tiniest areas of decay. Treatment involves careful removal of all the decayed portion of the tooth and filling the resulting cavity with some inert substance such as gold or an amalgam of silver and mercury. Cavities should be filled even in the baby teeth of children, since decay of these teeth, left untended, can extend into the heart of the tooth, causing great pain and discomfort and may even form deep-seated abscesses that can affect the later normal development of the permanent teeth. Silver amalgam fillings are usually adequate for filling baby teeth, but when cavities appear in mature permanent teeth, the construction of close-fitting gold inlays to fill the eroded areas is often wise. The initial cost of gold inlays is considerably higher than for silver amalgam fillings, but the silver tends to chip and break away after a period of five to ten years, while well-fitted inlays will remain in place and prevent further decay for as long as twenty years or more.

Caries was once considered an almost inevitable dental disease about which little could be done by way of prevention. Today, however, we have available an excellent means of preventing the development of tooth decay. The application of certain fluoride compounds to the teeth by the dentist, beginning in childhood, and the use of fluoride-containing toothpaste, or the use of drinking water containing approximately one part per million of soluble fluoride salts, can provide the safest and most reliable protection. Fluoride acts to harden the enamel and render it far more resistant to decay than normal, and adequate fluoride treatment or the use of fluoridated water can reduce the incidence of caries by as much as 40 to 50 percent, even among people who neglect such commonsense hygienic measures as regular brushing and periodic cleaning by the dentist. Unfortunately the question of fluoridation of public water supplies has become a highly emotional issue in many communities. It is opposed by some who believe that because most compounds of fluorine are toxic in large doses, it follows that the addition of tiny amounts of fluoride to water supplies may cause harm. The fact is that innumerable communities have now been using fluoridated water for years without any evidence whatever of toxicity and with a marked reduction in the amount of tooth decay among their populations. Today virtually every physician and dentist in the country—the ones who ought to know best—stands foursquare in favor of fluoridation of public water supplies in any community in which the drinking water does not already contain an adequate amount of natural fluoride salts, and as more experience is gained in the use of this harmless and inexpensive means of protection against dental cavities, the scientific basis for opposition to it becomes weaker and weaker.

Even so, fluorides are not 100 percent effective in preventing caries, and research continues to find other even more effective means of prevention. Periodic cleaning of the teeth in the dentist's office remains one of the most important of all preventive measures. Under normal conditions a chalky plaque of material known as *tartar* forms on the surface of the teeth at the gum line, particularly between the teeth, over a period of time. This material cannot be effectively removed by brushing, and it forms an excellent harbor for decay-causing bacteria. Tartar should be removed mechanically by the dentist or his trained assistant at regular six-month intervals to prevent the conditions that lead to tooth decay. In addition, much experimental work has recently been done in the use of a hard plastic material impervious to bacteria to coat the teeth and thus prevent caries. No one is yet certain how effective such a substance will be in the long run, or how frequently application will be necessary, but such treatment in combination with other preventive measures holds out hope that carious teeth may become a progressively less common affliction in the future.

Pyorrhea. To many people this is a catchall term referring to any disease of the gums involving tenderness, swelling, retraction of the gums around the teeth and the production of a bad odor to the breath. To the physician or dentist the term refers more specifically to the advanced stages of a chronic inflammatory periodontal disease which begins as *gingivitis* or inflammation of the gums due to bacterial infection. Bacteria become lodged in the tartar plaque just below the gum line; the gums become inflamed, sore and swollen, with a tendency to bleed readily when the teeth are brushed. When left untreated the infection moves deeper into the gums and involves the bone in which the teeth are rooted, with destruction of the cementing substance that holds the teeth in place. As the soft tissue of the gums scars and retracts, the teeth become loosened in their sockets, or themselves begin to decay, or both. Pyorrhea can be prevented if the initial gingivitis is diagnosed and treated vigorously and persistently by the dentist by means of mechanical cleaning, treatment with antibiotics and surgical excision of scarred and chronically infected portions of the gum. But pyorrhea is largely a disease of neglect; the individuals who could benefit the most from early, vigorous preventive treatment are too often the ones who never visit a dentist or even bother with the most rudimentary measures of home dental hygiene. Thus the condition has often become long-chronic and deep-seated before the dentist ever sees it, so that teeth, gums and sockets are all damaged beyond the point of repair. In such cases total extraction of the teeth, healing of the gums and subsequent fitting of dentures or false dental plates may be the only possible remedy. Basically, the need for such radical treatment should be determined only by a qualified dentist who is committed to the restoration of normal dental health wherever possible. Most dentists seek to preserve the natural teeth whenever this is possible, but many people insist upon having diseased teeth pulled even when they could be saved by proper dental care. These are the ones who fall easy prey to the "denture salesmen" who are interested far less in optimum dental care for their patients than in selling dentures to anyone who will submit to full mouth extraction.

Even when dentures are truly necessary, it is wise to avoid any dentist or dental company that promises a fast, inexpensive job. No dental practitioner who is truly concerned with long-range optimum dental care of his patients advertises his work publicly, and ill-fitting, uncomfortable "assembly line" dentures are worse than useless. The preparation of properly fitting dentures requires a high degree of professional skill on the part of your dentist, together with his willingness to follow up his work as long as necessary to be certain that the final dentures are truly serviceable. Once teeth have been extracted and periodontal disease adequately cleared up, the gums must be given adequate time to heal and atrophy before satisfactory dental plates can be fitted; even then, periodic correction of the dentures may be necessary for a period of a year or two. In approaching such work, your best and most practical source of advice will be a legitimate family dentist who treats all kinds of dental diseases in patients of all ages in his community, with consultation with a physician or an oral surgeon when this is indicated.

Vincent's Infection. All forms of gingivitis are not necessarily the long-standing chronic infection described above. One notable form of acute gingivitis is Vincent's infection or Vincent's angina, also commonly known as "trench mouth" (*see* p. 218). (*see* p. 218) This is a sudden-appearing, painful ulcerative infection of the gums caused by two pathogenic bacteria—a nonvenereal spirochete living in close association with a short, cigar-shaped bacillus. The disease is quite contagious, but early diagnosis and dental treatment can effect a complete cure.

Methods of Dental Treatment

Half a century ago people regarded a visit to the dentist as an ordeal to be put off as long as possible and then undertaken only in the face of an emergency—a sudden toothache, a broken tooth, a lost filling or something of the sort. Today methods of dental treatment have advanced just as rapidly as medical or surgical methods, and the modern dentist's work, whatever its nature, is usually swift, thorough and quite painless, thanks to the use of various forms of local anesthetics and anesthetic aids. Much of dental treatment today is preventive or diagnostic. A thorough dental examination is not possible without first cleaning the scale or tartar from the teeth and polishing away food or tobacco stains which may obscure the presence of diseased conditions. This is often performed by a dental assistant in a separate preliminary visit and is rendered so painless with the use of a mild local anesthetic rubbed into the gums beforehand that even a child tolerates it well. Next a diagnostic examination by the dentist will reveal the presence of grossly decayed teeth or periodontal disease. Modern dental X-rays are not only an aid to the dentist in detecting malformed teeth, unerupted teeth, or disease of the roots or bony sockets of the teeth, but are also of vital importance in detecting caries in its earliest stage of development. On the basis of such an examination the dentist can then plan a program of treatment to restore teeth that have been damaged by decay, to extract any teeth that have been destroyed beyond salvage and to make possible the subsequent maintenance of optimum dental health with as little trouble and expense as possible. Local anesthesia skillfully administered can satisfactorily numb any area of the mouth that requires tooth repair, and high-speed, air-driven dental drills do away even with the irritating sense of grinding that was once so dreaded. Fillings, extractions, the fitting of partial plates or bridges to replace individual extracted teeth, or the preparation of full dentures when necessary can all usually be handled as office procedures. Minor degrees of malocclusion can sometimes be adjusted by removal of a hair's breadth of enamel at precisely the right point of contact. Misaligned teeth may be ground and capped for cosmetic purposes. Orthodontia—the correction of severe malocclusion or the straightening, spreading and proper aligning of teeth by means of braces, retaining bridges and other mechanical devices—is a highly technical dental specialty, and when such work is necessary your dentist may refer you to an orthodontist. Extensive surgery of the gums or bony sockets of the teeth, as well as difficult extractions, may best be done under general anesthesia, and oral surgery is another important dental specialty. Finally, the dentist, like the doctor, is licensed to prescribe antibiotics and other drugs for the treatment of periodontal disease and to provide advice regarding choice of toothbrushes, dentifrices, diet, fluoride treatments and other preventive measures designed to forestall dental disease before it makes its appearance.

But the dentist cannot do it all. Every individual can do his share to prevent diseases of the teeth and gums simply by instituting and maintaining simple measures of proper dental hygiene. A suitable diet is the obvious starting place. Calcium, plentifully supplied in milk, is necessary for healthy development and growth of teeth. Adequate supplies of dietary protein are important to the maintenance of healthy gums and bony tissue surrounding the teeth. Vitamin deficiencies, such as an inadequate supply of vitamin D, can affect the development of teeth as well as that of bone, particularly notable in such diseases as *rickets* (*see* p. 892). In children it is wise to curb too vigorous a sweet tooth, since candy lodged between the teeth provides an excellent medium for tooth-decay bacteria to grow, and the overwhelming majority of dentists vigorously oppose habitual use of any kind of carbonated beverages because of potential damage to teeth. These soft drinks contain not only sugar but a weak solution of carbonic acid as well, a chemical which actively erodes and dissolves tooth enamel. An occasional bottle of a cola drink or carbonated fruit soda will not do significant damage, but children who drink carbonated beverages habitually day after day run an exceedingly high risk of excessive cavity formation. Far safer and more sensible are the noncarbonated children's beverages such as Kool-Aid which may contain sugar but at least have no carbonic acid in them.

Beyond diet considerations, a regular program of proper brushing of the teeth and massage of the gums is important. Ideally the teeth should be brushed immediately after each meal in order to remove trapped food particles. If that is impossible, they should certainly be brushed morning and evening. The choice of dentifrice is relatively unimportant, except when a dentist recommends a fluoride-containing toothpaste; it is the brushing and not the dentifrice that makes the difference in the long run. A half-and-half mixture of bicarbonate of soda (to counteract acidity in the mouth) and salt, used as a tooth powder, will do fully as well as most commercial toothpastes for cleansing and polishing the teeth at one-twentieth of the cost. Toothbrushes with moderately stiff bristles are usually superior to very stiff brushes simply because sharp, hard bristles can abrade and damage the gums, and many dentists feel that the very soft bristles used in electric toothbrushes provide the best cleansing of all. A slap and a dash, however, will not suffice, no matter what toothbrush is used. Brushing should be continued for a minimum of two to three minutes, making sure that all surfaces of the teeth, front and rear, are thoroughly cleaned. Circulation to the gums can be stimulated by gentle rubbing with a fingertip at the end of the brushing operation. Unfortunately, no toothbrush yet invented is capable of reaching deep into the crevices between the teeth; to cleanse these areas dental floss is still far and away the best device. Most dentists discourage the use of hardwood toothpicks, whether flat or tapered, since it is possible to injure the delicate dentine of the teeth just below the gum line, but also because habitual use can actually tend to push the teeth apart and provide even more space in which food can lodge. Soft wooden toothpicks such as Stim-U-Dents are more satisfactory and will not generally do any harm. Recently marketed "water picks," which direct a fine high-pressure stream of water between the teeth, are also recommended as a means of cleansing hard-to-reach crevices.

Finally, remember that gum chewing is no adequate substitute for toothbrushing, much as it may refresh the mouth, and even the chlorophyll-containing chewing gums advertised to combat bad breath fail to remove the lodged and decaying food particles between the teeth or to cure the gingival infection which is so often the source of bad breath in the first place.

Any abnormality of the teeth and gums should of course be called to a dentist's attention immediately. Bleeding gums are an early indication that gingival infection may be starting; so also is swelling or tenderness of the gums. Sensitivity to hot or cold substances in a tooth may indicate that a cavity is penetrating the enamel and treatment is indicated. The occurrence of a toothache may be the result of cavitation of a tooth or of deep-seated infection around the root of the tooth or even an abscess in the bone. If a cavity is visible, or if a toothache occurs because a filling has fallen out, temporary pain relief may be obtained by applying oil of cloves, a natural local anesthetic, to the cavity—but any such occurrence is a signal that a dental emergency exists and the dentist should be consulted as soon as possible.

No amount of routine dental hygiene, however, can substitute for a periodic dental checkup. One often hears that such a checkup should be undertaken regularly every six months, but there is no particular magic about this time interval. The individual with a good diet, a faithful routine of proper dental hygiene, strong healthy teeth with firm enamel, and a history of few cavities may need a dental checkup (aside from cleaning at six-month intervals) only once a year or even at longer intervals, whereas a child with soft enamel, a poorly developed program of dental hygiene or a history of frequent cavities should be seen more often. The proper interval for each individual should be discussed with the dentist; ideally it will be planned to maintain optimum dental health at the lowest possible cost. But whatever the interval, the most important factor of all is regularity. By combining careful dental hygiene at home with regular periodic dental examinations, the teeth can be kept healthy and strong throughout life and the incidence of truly dangerous or destructive diseases of the teeth and gums can be reduced to a minimum.

The Special Sensory Organs: Eyes, Ears and Nose

In the long evolutionary chain which led to the development of man as the dominant creature on Earth, an early differentiation occurred between the "head end" and the "tail end" of moving creatures. The "head end" was the part that came first, responsible not only for gathering food through a "mouth" but also for exploring the terrain ahead, so to speak, to make certain that it was safe to move forward. Thus it is not surprising that even in the lowest of animals the major sensory organs—the eyes, the ears and the nose—became located in the forward part of the body or the head and remained there through higher stages of development, including man.

All three of these special sensory organs, although intimately connected to the brain by special cranial nerves (the optic nerve, the auditory or acoustic nerve, and the olfactory nerve, respectively), are located externally, and at least part of their structure arises from specialized external epithelial tissue. Thus, although we may not ordinarily think of the eyes, the ears and the nose as "cutaneous system organs" they are intimately related with that organ system. Each is in constant contact with the external environment. Each, to some degree or another, is subject to physical injury and especially vulnerable to infection, just as each may be involved in its own inherent major disorders. Finally, the continuing health and proper function of each can be enhanced by certain simple yet fundamental principles of normal day-to-day care, in terms of both preventing disease and avoiding unnecessary self-injury.

The Eyes

Among the highly specialized sensory organs, the eyes are by far the most complex in structure and function. What is more, the health of the eyes and the general health of the body are closely related. Their chief function, of course, is to bring clear, colored visual images of the outside environment to the part of the brain that responds to sensations caused by electromagnetic waves (light waves) that lie within the spectrum of visible light. Unfortunately, the eyes can be afflicted with a variety of disorders that interfere with that paramount function—disorders which lead either to significant impairment of vision or to partial or complete, temporary or permanent, blindness. But in addition, the eyes may also reflect a wide variety of other disorders in the body which have little or nothing to do with sight. Poets claim that the eyes are "the windows of the soul"; and while this may be only romantic hyperbole, it is not an exaggeration to say that the eyes are the windows of the body through which the physician may discover much of what is going on in some of the body's most inaccessible places. Simple examination of the retina of the eye by means of an ophthalmoscope provides the doctor with an excellent opportunity to assess the overall condition of the small arteries and veins throughout the body.

Evidence of the presence and degree of arteriosclerosis or hypertension can be detected merely by observing the retinal blood vessels, and certain other changes that can be observed here are characteristic of such diseases as uncontrolled diabetes mellitus or advanced kidney disease. Disturbances of focus or of the various eye reflexes may not only provide clues to disorders of the central nervous system or brain, but can aid the doctor in pinpointing exactly where in the nervous system these disorders originate. A continuous, slightly bloodshot muddiness of the eyes may suggest to the alert physician the possibility of chronic alcoholism; yellowing of the whites of the eyes is an early hint of jaundice due to liver disfunction or, occasionally, to the presence of primary pernicious anemia. Even something of the personality of the individual may be suggested by his eyes as a striking part of his facial expression: the direct, arrogant look, for example, that may bespeak defiance or mask falsehood or anxiety, or the downcast avoidance of gaze that can provide a subtle clue to depression.

To review all the disorders of the eyes would be impossible; few physicians other than ophthalmologists are equipped to diagnose many eye conditions, and most doctors promptly refer patients with serious eye disorders to a specialist. But there are a number of commonplace defects and disorders with which everyone should be familiar, so that he may recognize the conditions that require immediate medical care and, even more important, so that he may treat his own eyes and the precious gift of sight with the knowledge and respect that they deserve.

The Normal Structure and Function of the Eyes

The eyes are two slightly oval-shaped organs occupying the orbital cavities in the skull on either side of the bridge of the nose and held in place by surrounding connective tissue and fat. In the front they are covered by a very thin transparent epithelial membrane, the *conjunctiva,* which covers the exposed portion of the eye and then folds back to form the mucous membrane lining of the eyelids. In the rear the eyes are connected to the brain by thick trunks of nervous tissue containing fibers of the optic nerves; within the eye these nerve fibers diverge to make multiple connections with special light-sensitive cells in the internal lining of the back of the eye known as the *retina.* Since there are two eyes and two optic nerves, one might assume that each nerve connects with a single eye, but this is not in fact the case. Between the eyes and the brain, the nerve bundles carrying optic nerve fibers come to an X-shaped crossing known as the *optic chiasma* so that visual impulses from both eyes ultimately reach the visual cortex on each side of the brain. It is this sharing of images picked up by both eyes that accounts, in part, for our normally perfect binocular vision. The motion of the eyes within their sockets is controlled by *extraocular muscles—* bands of muscle connected to the sides, top and bottom of each eye and inserted into the eye socket. Three pairs of cranial nerves—the oculomotor, the trochlear and the abducens—control the contraction or relaxation of these muscles

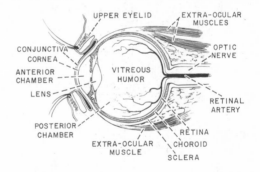

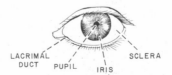

Figure 33–1.

and permit free synchronized movement of both eyes under normal conditions.

The eye itself is constructed remarkably like a fine camera. (*See* Fig. 33–1.) In the front, beneath the transparent conjunctival membrane, is a thicker translucent membrane known as the *cornea* which not only admits light to the interior of the eye but is also equipped with a rich network of pain-sensitive nerve endings to alert us when even the tiniest foreign body or chemical irritant touches the eye. This warning system is utterly essential, since the cornea must remain completely clear, uninjured and unscarred in order for vision to be possible. At its periphery the clear cornea is tightly interwoven with the white fibrous *sclera* which makes up the "white of the eye" and continues around the entire organ to form a supportive fibrous wall. Within the cornea the circular pigmented *iris*—the structure that gives the eyes their color—has an aperture or *pupil* in the center to permit light to flow through. The iris is equipped with tiny muscles which enlarge the pupil in dim light and diminish its size in bright light, thus controlling the total amount of light that enters the eye. Behind the iris is the *lens* of the eye, composed of a fibrous yet crystalline material unlike any other tissue in the body; ordinarily oval-shaped, the lens can be pulled out flat or allowed to become more spherical by the action of delicate muscles at its edges, so that the eye can focus the images of distant or nearby objects equally well on the light-sensitive retina in the rear. Finally, both the anterior chamber of the eye (the narrow portion between the cornea and the lens) and the posterior chamber (the larger portion between the lens and the retina) are filled with fluids—a thin, watery *aqueous humor* in the anterior chamber and a thicker, more gelatinous *vitreous humor* in the posterior chamber. Since the surface of the eye is exposed to air and drying, *lacrimal glands* or "tear glands" in the soft tissue surrounding the eye pour saline tears over the external surface constantly, and excessive quantities of this fluid are then drained through *lacrimal ducts* into the nasal passages for disposal.

The retina, of course, is the "business end" of the eye as far as reception of visual images is concerned. It is equipped with an intermixture of rod-shaped cells which are sensitive only to light and darkness, and cone-shaped cells, which are sensitive to different wavelengths of visual light

and thus permit color reception. Under ordinary daylight or artificial lighting conditions, both the rods and the cones function and we have clear color vision, but below a certain light threshold the cones cease to function so that in very dim light we perceive only shades of gray. Ordinarily we see the best when we are looking directly at an object, yet oddly enough certain kinds of images—those involving subtle motion, for example, which might be drowned out in the flood of images gathered by direct gaze—are actually picked up better "out of the corner of the eye" while the gaze is directed forward. Many a hunter has detected the nervous flick of a deer's ear in the brush by this so-called *peripheral vision,* and it is this capability which helps us avoid injury from flying objects approaching from the side.

Once visual images have reached the retina and are picked up by the rod and cone cells, they are converted into electrochemical nerve impulses of exactly the same nature as all other nerve impulses; but in some way that we still do not understand, the nerve cells in the visual cortex of the brain, located in the occipital lobes at the back of the skull just above the neck, have the capacity to arrange and interpret these impulses in such a way that we see—that is, become visually aware of—objects in the same size, shape and location that we feel them with our hands, for example. Obviously any disturbance in the conduction of electrochemical impulses from the retina to the brain can cause disturbance of vision even though the eye itself is functioning perfectly. Thus an injury to the visual cortex of the brain may disturb our ability to see. Similarly, damage to the fibers of the optic nerve or the optic chiasma due to the pressure of a tumor, for example, or to the destruction of the fatty myelin sheath coating the nerve fibers, a condition that occurs in multiple sclerosis, may blank out reception from a portion of the field of each eye and result in *hemianopia* or "half vision." If nerve fibers in one of the cranial nerves controlling the extraocular muscles are involved in injury or disease, coordination of eye movements may be affected and cause *diplopia* or "double vision"—a condition that can also arise from chemical poisoning or as a temporary disturbance due to acute alcohol intoxication. Under normal circumstances, however, we quite correctly relate perfect vision to the eyes themselves, and when disorders of vision appear, it is to the eyes that we look first for the source of trouble.

Structural Defects of the Eye and Surrounding Tissue

Because the eyes work much like roving stereoscopic television cameras, certain structural defects can result in blurring of the visual image, difficulty in accommodating when the vision is shifted from near objects to distant objects, and even disorders of color perception and the stereoscopic function. Most familiar of all these conditions are *errors of refraction or focus. Myopia* (near-sightedness) is a condition in which the distance from the lens of the eye to the retina is slightly too long, so that the focus of distant objects is blurred. Hereditary factors are a very common cause of near-sightedness, which may first appear even in childhood. In some cases the condition may be so extreme that the individual literally cannot see a clear image of anything farther than a foot or two away without the aid of thick corrective glasses. In *hyperopia* (far-sightedness), distance vision is excellent but near vision is impaired because the distance between the lens and the retina is slightly too short. Most infants are somewhat far-sighted during the first six months of life, a condition which usually corrects itself as the eye grows. The condition again appears quite commonly with advancing age and may require the person who has had perfect vision all his life to begin using glasses. *Astigmatism,* in which both near and far images may be blurred in much the same way that images seen through a window of poorly rolled glass are distorted, is caused by slight irregularities in the structure of the lens or, more rarely, the cornea. *Presbyopia* results from hardening of the lenses of the eyes due to advancing age, which makes accommodation from near to far vision difficult and focusing for very near vision almost impossible. These errors of refraction and focus can be readily detected by an ophthalmologist and can usually be corrected quite satisfactorily with properly prescribed glasses.

Other structural defects are not as easily correctable. *Color blindness,* usually an inherited defect, results from a malfunction of the color receptors in the retina, and may be so subtle that the victim does not even know the condition is present until some aspect of his behavior—an inability to distinguish stop-and-go lights, for example, or to select pleasing color combinations—calls attention to the fact that something is wrong. The most common form of color blindness is a partial or complete inability to distinguish between reds and greens; differences in shades are clearly distinguishable, and often the objects clearly have color, but the colors themselves cannot be readily distinguished. Less common and more subtle is color blindness for blues and yellows. Although neither condition is correctable, knowing that they exist makes it possible for the individual to accommodate himself quite successfully. So-called *night blindness* —the inability to distinguish subtle shades of gray under conditions of very dim light—may also, in some cases, be an inborn defect, but more often it is an early and correctable symptom of vitamin A deficiency which is improved markedly by dietary supplements of that vitamin.

Structural defects of the extraocular muscles may result in *strabismus* or "squint," in which the eyes do not converge properly on an image. In *medial strabismus* one or both eyes are drawn to the midline or "crossed"; in *lateral strabismus* (walleye) one or both of the eyes are drawn toward the outside, making stereo vision impossible; in *alternating strabismus* one or both eyes may either be crossed or pulled to the outside, depending upon the direction of the gaze. Very often the individual with strabismus has perfectly clear, sharp vision without any corrective measures having been taken simply because he has learned to accept visual data only from the "normal" or dominant eye, and simply to ignore the "out of focus" images from the other eye. However, depth perception is severely impaired in these individuals. Strabismus is not necessarily continuous; some people have no sign of it under ordinary conditions of eye use, but find that the squint appears when they are tired or have been using their eyes for prolonged periods —a condition sometimes known as the "lazy eye" syndrome. In such cases, and in many cases of consistent strabismus, correction can often be effected by the use of prescription lenses combined with muscle-strengthening exercises. These corrective measures are best carried out with children; with adults, or children in whom simpler corrective measures are not successful, correction or improvement of the strabismus may require surgical repair of the defective extraocular muscles.

Eye Injuries

Any severe injury to the eye—a scratch or laceration, or a thermal or chemical burn—or an injury to the surrounding area—a fracture of the orbit, for example—requires the immediate emergency attention of an ophthalmologist. If the eye has been injured by accidental contact with soap, detergents, acids, alkalis or other chemicals which cause severe pain, the simple first-aid measure of lavaging the eye repeatedly with clean warm water to wash out any remaining chemical, followed by covering the eye with a patch or a handkerchief (without pressure) until the ophthalmologist can be seen, may in itself save sight or prevent further damage. Under these conditions ointments and/or anesthetic eyedrops should never be used in the eye, since they may either mask the diagnosis or allow further mechanical damage to the already injured organ.

The most common of all eye injuries occurs either when a foreign body is trapped in the eye by accident or when the cornea is struck or scratched by some object moving so swiftly that the normal blink reflex is not fast enough to protect the eye. In either case there is immediate intense pain, together with copious watering of the eye and severe reddening or hyperemia of the conjunctiva. Occasionally, if a foreign body is visible and not embedded in the cornea, it can be removed by another person. The lower eyelid is carefully pulled down, the upper eyelid pulled up, and the foreign body removed, *not by a finger,* but by use of a sterile cotton swab such

as a Q-Tip moistened in warm water. *If the foreign body is found to be lodged or embedded on the surface of the eye, no unskilled attempt to remove it should be made,* since the preservation of the clear corneal membrane is essential to sight, and clumsy tampering in such a case can result in blindness.

Removal of a foreign body will usually result in speedy recovery from the pain, eye watering and injection of blood vessels. If pain continues, it may indicate that some part of the foreign body has been overlooked, or that it has scratched or pitted the cornea. When this occurs, infection in the abrasion is an extremely common complication, and it can be quite serious. If there is continuing pain or any question whatever that part of the foreign body still remains in the eye, an ophthalmologist should be seen on an emergency basis. Occasionally a neglected injury to the cornea can form a deep-seated *corneal ulcer* which always requires expert treatment at the hands of an ophthalmologist.

Since minor eye injuries can be an almost everyday occurrence, particularly among children, it is useful to follow a simple rule-of-thumb procedure in deciding when or even whether to take the child to an eye doctor. Any time a scratch or minor laceration of the eye is suspected, carefully inspect the eye, not only under the lids but also on the surface of the eyeball with the aid of side lighting with a flashlight, to see if any foreign body or abrasion is obviously present. If so, a doctor should be consulted. If nothing whatever can be seen, wash the eye gently with warm water, have the child close the eye and then cover it with an eye patch from a first-aid kit or even a folded handkerchief for a matter of an hour or two. If the pain increases during this time, or if it is not markedly relieved within two hours and completely gone within eight or ten, the eye should be examined by a doctor even though no obvious injury can be detected, since a corneal scratch or an early corneal infection or both are probably present.

Another common eye injury is the *flashburn* that results from the exposure of the eye to the ultraviolet rays from arc welding machines or sun lamps, or *snow blindness* caused by exposure to prolonged reflection of bright sun on white snow. These conditions are characterized by intense painful burning and itching of the eyes which may have to be controlled by anesthetic eyedrops or ointments prescribed by a doctor until the irritation of the lining of the eye causing the pain is quieted, usually within 12 to 24 hours. Prevention of flashburn or snow blindness by using adequate dark glasses or by avoiding direct gaze at electric arcs or the sun is by far the best "treatment" for this uncomfortable and sometimes serious condition.

Any blow or injury sustained in the region surrounding the eye is apt to cause hemorrhage in the soft tissue of the eyelid or beneath the orbit which may then evolve into a "black eye." As long as the eye itself is not injured, this condition is seldom very serious even though it may look perfectly horrid. The best way to prevent or minimize a black eye after a blow or injury is to apply an ice pack to the eye intermittently for the first 24 hours in order to shrink the blood vessels and reduce the amount of hemorrhage. Thereafter a warm (*not* hot) moist pack will help speed resolution of the "blackening" or ecchymosis. Quite often the blood in the soft tissue around the eye will drain down into the cheek, making the injury appear far more extensive than it actually is, and in some cases "blackness" will appear around the opposite eye as well. Unless there is such evidence of continuing internal bleeding as increasing and persisting swelling, pressure or pain, however, the condition will usually clear up in a matter of a few days.

Of course any serious physical injury to the eye itself—direct blows, lacerations, fractures in the bony orbit surrounding the eye, or tears or punctures of the eyeball—demand immediate emergency ophthalmic care. Often the most gross and destructive injuries to the eye can be successfully repaired by surgery and sight preserved or restored as long as the cornea itself is not irreparably damaged or the optic nerve completely severed or too grievously torn.

Eye Infections

Certain bacterial infections of the eye—especially conjunctivitis or "pinkeye"—are particularly common among children and should be given prompt medical attention. (*See* p. 205.) Special care must also be taken to prevent eye infections in the newborn infant. (*See* p. 880.) A chronic viral infection of the conjunctiva causes the very serious condition known as trachoma, fortunately rare in this country. (*See* p. 232.) *Blepharitis* is an inflammation of the margins of the eyelids with redness and thickening, together with crusting that looks much like dandruff. In fact, this condition almost always is associated either with an allergy or with seborrheic dermatitis (dandruff) of the scalp and eyebrows. It can usually be cleared up by eradicating the dandruff in the hair first and then treating the eye with an ophthalmic ointment containing surface antibiotics such as neomycin or gramicidin, together with a cortisone-like hormone ingredient.

Another eyelid infection is the so-called *sty,* a localized condition that is usually due to infection in an eyelash follicle. Ordinarily there is pain and redness in the local area, together with swelling; then a pocket of pus forms in the sty and ultimately the small abscess will "point" and drain. When a sty is just beginning, it can sometimes be aborted by using ointments or drugs of a combined antibiotic-cortisone nature. If the sty comes to a point—which may be hastened by the use of warm compresses over the eye for 10 or 15 minutes three or four times a day—but does not drain, it should be seen by a physician, who can incise and drain the lesion simply and painlessly, using antibiotic drops subsequently to prevent spread of the infection. Sties tend to occur regularly in certain children, and more rarely in certain adults, and often seem to be related to staphylococcus flora in the nasopharyngeal area.

Various bacteria or viruses may also cause infections not only of the conjunctiva lining the eyelid but of the cornea itself. These infections are all accompanied by a severe scratchy pain on the surface of the eye, together with reddening of the surrounding conjunctiva and sclera, sometimes swelling of the eyelids and excessive watering of the eye. Self-diagnosis and treatment of these conditions, commonly known as *keratitis,* are hazardous, since certain forms—notably that caused by the herpes zoster virus—can cause permanent scarring and opacity of the cornea with lasting visual impairment. Any persisting irritation of the eye should be seen by a doctor and treated by an ophthalmologist if necessary. Occasionally an inflammation of the conjunctiva may cause a chronic progressive enlargement of certain glands in the mucous membrane of the eyelid, leading to an unsightly growth known as a *chalazion* which most commonly appears near the inner corner of the lower lid. Often a chalazion will resolve spontaneously with the use of hot compresses and antibiotic-cortisone eyedrops prescribed by a doctor. If not, it can easily be removed by an ophthalmologist by means of incision and curettement under a local anesthesia.

Serious Eye Disorders

Blindness, partial or complete, may be the result of damage to the cornea or from changes in the lenses of the eyes involving clouding or opaqueness, a condition known as *cataract*. Other forms of blindness of varying degrees can result from increased pressure within the eyeball, damage to the retina, injury to the optic nerves, or a marked increase in intracranial pressure which results in swelling of the optic nerves at the point where they enter the eye. In the latter case sight may be restored by relieving intracranial pressure, but an injury or transsection of the optic nerve usually results in permanent blindness.

Corneal Blindness. Any of the conditions already mentioned—notably injury or a scarring infection—affecting the cornea in any way that renders it irregular or opaque may cause visual defects ranging all the way from indistinctness or dimming of vision to total blindness. Thus any disorder of the cornea must be regarded with the utmost seriousness and treated swiftly and skillfully. When corneal blindness does occur in the absence of any other eye defect, sight can sometimes be restored by means of a corneal transplant using a clear transparent cornea previously designated for donation by someone who has recently died. The victim of corneal disease must often wait a considerable time for a donated cornea to become available, but fortunately this particular tissue can be quite successfully transplanted with remarkably little of the "rejection reaction" typical of other tissue or organ transplants. Only a tiny patch of healthy cornea need be transplanted to make clear vision possible again, and today there are a growing number of people whose precious gift of sight has been restored thanks to the compassion of donors who have willed their eyes to eye banks. Procedures for willing one's eyes vary from state to state and locality to locality, but every ophthalmologist in practice can provide the information necessary to anyone interested in making this humanitarian bequest.

Cataracts. This condition, a progressive clouding or opaqueness of the normally crystal-clear lens of the eye, may occur congenitally during early life as a result of heredity or in later years due to degenerative changes related to age or to diabetes mellitus. The main symptom is a slow, progressive and quite painless loss of distinct vision, although awareness of light or darkness is usually preserved. In many cases cataracts are not complete; that is, they cloud only portions of the lens, and often frequent changes of prescription lenses aid the victim in maintaining useful sight for many months or years. Ultimately, if the cataract involves the entire lens, surgical removal of the lens may be necessary, a procedure which today can be performed quickly and safely on individuals of virtually any age. Following the surgical removal of cataracts, the focusing function of the lens must be replaced by properly fitted thick-lensed glasses, a small price to pay for the restoration of failing vision.

Glaucoma. Another prevalent form of blindness, which may range from slight impairment of the normal visual area all the way to complete and permanent blindness, may be caused by a chronic, progressive, destructive and usually relatively painless disease of the eye known as *glaucoma*. In most cases the cause of glaucoma cannot be determined, but the nature of the disease is clearly understood; there is an increase, sometimes rapid but more often gradual, in the fluid tension inside the eye due to the formation of more intraocular fluid than is able to escape through the tiny canals that normally drain it from the eye and help maintain a constant pressure balance within the eyeball. This intraocular tension may increase so greatly that sight is completely and permanently destroyed if the condition is not discovered early enough for effective treatment. The condition is all the more tragic because the vast majority of cases of glaucoma can be detected very early in the development of the disease by a simple, painless and remarkably accurate procedure in the doctor's office, using a pressure-measuring instrument known as a *tonometer,* long before any symptoms of visual loss have appeared. Proper treatment initiated at this point can almost always arrest the further development of glaucoma and save the sight of the victim. In these early stages the ophthalmologist may prescribe a medication which tends to dilate the canals that normally drain fluid from the interior of the eye. In many cases this is the only treatment necessary, although it usually must be carried out faithfully on a long-term basis. When the use of these medicines is not sufficient to reduce the tension within the eye, a specialized surgical procedure may be necessary to relieve the intraocular pressure and prevent it from building up further. Either or both of these forms of treatment, however, must be undertaken before irreparable damage to the optic nerve has permanently impaired vision. Although glaucoma frequently first appears in only one eye, it is common for it to appear in the other eye as well as the disease progresses. Thus the medication used for treatment is usually applied to both eyes from the beginning.

Eye Tumors. Fortunately these destructive growths, which usually begin in pigmented cells from the fibrous lining of the eye, are extremely rare. One such tumor is the highly dangerous malignant melanoma which may have its origin within the eye. (*See* p. 406.) Another major eye tumor is the *retinoblastoma* which develops as a cancer of the retina. In either case a rapidly progressive disturbance in vision, usually unilateral, and a sharp increase in intraocular pressure are the diagnostic clues. Treatment of these tumors is always surgical and usually involves removal of the afflicted eye and its surrounding

tissues as early as the diagnosis can be established.

Retinal Detachment. A much more frequent cause of partial blindness is *retinal detachment,* in which the visual lining of the inside of the eye becomes detached from the layer of tissue behind it. This detachment often occurs suddenly, and the victim begins to see strange flashing light patterns or "stars," followed by the sensation that a stage curtain is being pulled across the eye. If uncorrected or treated too late, retinal detachment can cause permanent vision loss in the affected eye. Early treatment by means of surgical reattachment of the retina can, in most cases, return vision very nearly to normal. In recent years special ophthalmoscopic lasers have been used with great success in cases in which the retina has just begun to detach; the area of early detachment can often be "tacked down" in place with the use of delicately controlled laser bursts, a sort of "spot welding" in which the laser beam is directed right through the pupil of the eye and precisely focused upon selected portions of the retina. If this procedure can be performed early enough, the need for surgical entrance into the eye may be obviated.

Proper Eye Care

Vision is beyond question the most precious of all our senses, and proper care of the eyes and avoidance of undue hazards should be matters of simple common sense. Obviously the eyes work best under proper lighting conditions, and undue eyestrain can be avoided by using light that adequately illuminates the field of vision but is directed or shaded to prevent glare. The eyes should also be protected from the glare of the sun by the use of dark glasses. The choice of darkened lenses is important; many dark glasses of the cheap plastic variety screen out all wavelengths of visible light sufficiently that the pupil expands but allow harmful actinic rays from the sun to pass into the eyes. Any dark glasses which seem to tire the eyes after a brief period of use should be discarded and replaced with glasses containing polarizing lenses. Color distortion can be avoided by using gray-colored lenses rather than green, brown, yellow or pink lenses which are often considered more fashionable. Eyestrain can also be avoided by the simple measure of resting the eyes briefly at hourly intervals when engaged in prolonged periods of work involving sharp visual acuity. This can be accomplished either by simply closing the eyes for a few moments or by breaking away from close-up work to move the eyes over distant objects for a few moments. Continuing overuse or strain of the eyes will often be accompanied by headaches, a feeling of tiredness about the eyes, or a sense of sleepiness—a natural warning that the time has come to close the eyes and rest them for a while.

Many nonprescription eyedrops are widely advertised to "relieve eyestrain," "rest the eyes," "cleanse the eyes" or "take the red out." Most of these preparations are simply saline solutions containing minute quantities of adrenalin-like substances that tend to shrink the capillary blood vessels in the lining and whites of the eyes; used occasionally they may indeed make the eyes feel better, but habitual use is not recommended. It is far better to relieve eyestrain by proper care and rest of the eyes than by the use of any external medication. Some years ago it was considered highly beneficial to wash the eyes out with a weak boric acid solution, and many homes still have the antiquated "eyecup" used for this purpose on the medicine shelf. Today most authorities consider the practice not only unsanitary but relatively useless, and worry about the additional threat of chemical irritation that is always present. If the eyes *must* be lavaged, it is now considered far better to do it with the use of copious quantities of clean warm water.

Even under perfectly normal conditions visual acuity may change with time, and it makes as much sense to have periodic eye examinations to assess the health of the eyes and help detect any disorders as early as possible as it does to have periodic medical and dental examinations. Too often, however, people are confused by the various names for "eye doctors" and specialists. The family doctor or general practitioner is, of course, acquainted with many eye disorders, but seldom has the equipment or the experience for

a thorough examination. The *ophthalmologist* is a fully trained doctor who has, after completing the basic medical and internship requirements, gone on to several years of specialized study of eye disorders. He is well equipped to perform complete eye examinations and to handle medical or surgical treatment of any disorders that may be found. Part of his eye examination involves testing visual acuity, measuring any defects found and prescribing corrective lenses when needed. The *optometrist* is also equipped and trained to measure visual acuity and to prescribe and adjust corrective lenses, but this is the limit of his function; unlike the ophthalmologist, he is not a trained physician and is not qualified to undertake the diagnosis or treatment of eye diseases. Finally, the *optician* is qualified to fill prescriptions for corrective lenses much as the pharmacist is qualified to fill prescriptions for medications ordered by a physician; he is also concerned with the fitting and fashioning of glasses frames, so that the prescribed lenses may be worn as comfortably as possible.

A bewildering variety of corrective lenses have been devised to help adjust defects in visual acuity, and these lenses must be changed as the qualities of acuity change. The notion that one's vision may be "improved" by corrective lenses to the point where they are no longer needed is largely valid only with young people. Even then it is more a matter of the eyes themselves acquiring their mature size and function than of any miraculous change brought about by the corrective lenses. With advancing age the eyes become less capable of accommodating to changes in near, middle and far vision; originally separate pairs of glasses were often kept on hand to be used for varying visual requirements, but today bifocal or even trifocal lenses build these variable qualities into the same pair of glasses and can be used by most people quite successfully after a period of adjustment.

Probably most controversial of all corrective lenses are *contact lenses,* tiny curved pieces of glass or plastic designed to be placed directly on the surface of the eye over the cornea with the use of lubricating eyedrops. Many thousands of people have found contact lenses to be entirely satisfactory and a happy, if expensive, substitute for ordinary glasses. But contact lenses are not without their problems: many find them continually irritating; they are infuriatingly easy to drop and lose; those made of plastic tend to become scratched; they must be removed at intervals throughout the day for replenishment of the lubricating fluid; and many people who attempt to wear them discover to their dismay that they simply cannot get used to them. The recent appearance on the market of contact lenses made of a softer, more flexible material may resolve some of these problems; meanwhile each person must make the decision for himself whether the attendant bother of contacts is balanced sufficiently by improvements in convenience or appearance to make them worthwhile. And, of course, they should be prescribed, and carefully fitted by a qualified specialist.

In spite of many recent advances in treating eye disorders, there are still those who are born blind or who become blind due to accident or illness at some time in their lives. Loss of vision is undeniably a grave abridgment of normal contact with the outside world, yet the many remarkable achievements of the blind bear heartening witness to the fact that blindness need not be totally disabling. Numerous organizations are devoted to training the blind in the special techniques needed to compensate for their loss, including the use of the Braille system, talking books and Seeing Eye dogs, to mention only a few. Loss of sight can be a severe emotional blow as well as a physical disability, but with time, determination and proper training, the blind are able to lead relatively normal, independent and productive lives.

The Ears

Hearing is second in importance only to vision among the human sensory powers. The ear is only slightly less complex than the eye as a special sensory organ, and subject to very similar injuries and disorders. The combination of binocular vision and binaural or stereophonic sound reception permits us to keep remarkably accurate tabs on our environment during all our waking hours. In addition, the ear serves as a warning system during sleep when visual contact with the world is temporarily suspended. Finally, aside from its function in hearing, it also serves as a center for maintaining the body's balance or equilibrium. Logically, then, disorders that affect the hearing often disturb equilibrium, and both are telling indications that something is wrong with the auditory function.

The Normal Structure and Function of the Ear

The human ear, an organ located bilaterally at the side of the head, is designed to collect sound waves from the environment and conduct them to a sensitive receiving apparatus embedded in the skull on either side, where they are converted into nerve impulses that are carried by the auditory nerves to the brain for interpretation. The major structures of this apparatus are divided into three general parts: the external ear, the middle ear and the internal ear. The *external ear* includes the *auricle,* a thin, convoluted cup of cartilage covered by skin, fibrous connective tissue and fat, which is tilted slightly away from the skull to act as a sort of "scoop" for sound waves, and the *auditory canal,* the narrow opening which leads to the deeper portions of the ear. Strictly speaking, the auricle is not essential to hearing at all, except to increase range and acuity, but because it is visible, its size and shape can be a cosmetic concern. The auditory canal is approximately an inch long and a quarter of an inch across and, like the auricle, is lined with

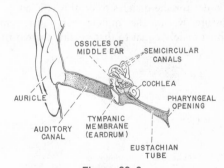

Figure 33–2.

skin and connective tissue; but it also contains a number of coarse hairs which serve to keep out dust, dirt or other foreign materials. In addition, the outer half of the canal is lined with tiny glands that secrete sticky ear wax or *cerumen* which further serves to trap foreign objects before they reach the sensitive oval-shaped *tympanic membrane* at the end of the canal.

This membrane, also called the *eardrum,* is a unique structure in the body, a tightly stretched oval of fibrous tissue less than one two-hundredths of an inch thick which separates the auditory canal from the small chamber known as the *middle ear* where the actual sound-receiving apparatus begins. Sound waves striking the tympanic membrane from the outside cause it to vibrate, with the vibration perfectly attuned to the rising or falling frequency of the sound. This conversion of the wavelike motion of molecules in the air into the mechanical vibration of a delicate fibrous membrane is the first step in the transformation of sound waves into the nerve impulses within the ear.

In the tiny middle ear chamber, barely a quarter of an inch across, the vibration of the eardrum is picked up by three minuscule bones or *ossicles,* by far the smallest bones anywhere in the body. These ossicles, called the *malleus,* the *incus* and the *stapes* (the hammer, the anvil and the stirrup) because of their distinctive shapes (*see* Fig. 33–3A), form a kind of three link chain from one side of the middle ear chamber to the other. They not only pick up and transmit the vibrations of the eardrum, but also help control their intensity, magnifying very faint vibrations and damping out excessive vibrations. In order for the ossicles to do this efficiently, air pressure within the middle ear must remain approximately equal to that outside the eardrum;

EXPLODED VIEW OF OSSICLES

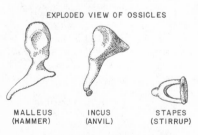

MALLEUS   INCUS   STAPES
(HAMMER)   (ANVIL)   (STIRRUP)

Figure 33–3A.

this is made possible by a narrow "pressure canal," the *Eustachian tube,* which extends from the middle ear down to the back of the throat.

When the pressure outside the eardrum exceeds that inside the middle ear, or vice versa, the act of swallowing or yawning will open the Eustachian tube and allow air to flow up or down the

SCHEMATIC OF OSSICLES & MIDDLE EAR

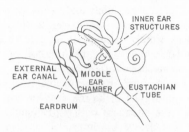

Figure 33–3B.

tube to relieve the imbalance. When this tube becomes plugged because of swelling or inflammation, or because of sudden atmospheric pressure changes, we suffer an uncomfortable sensation, as if the ears were plugged, and our hearing is markedly diminished until the pressure is equalized again as the Eustachian tube opens and we feel our ears "pop."

On the other side of the middle ear the ossicles are connected to a tiny *oval window* leading into another chamber, the *internal ear,* which is filled with a thin fluid. Here the mechanical vibrations of the ossicles are finally transformed into vibrations within this liquid. Two tiny organs are in contact with this fluid in the internal ear, but only one part, a spiraling series of tubes which closely resembles a snail shell and is called the *cochlea,* is concerned with hearing. Within the cochlea delicate sense receptors pick up the fluid vibration and transmit it as nerve impulses via the acoustic nerve and other nerve channels to the auditory cortex of the cerebrum located in the temporal lobes of the brain. The sound receptors within the cochlea are sensitive to vibrations ranging in frequency from as low as 16 cycles per second (deep bass tones) to as high as 25,000 or more cycles per second (high squeaky tones), but frequencies between 1,000 and 4,000 cycles are picked up the best. Sound waves with frequencies too low (*subsonic waves*) or too high (*ultrasonic waves*) for reception simply do not register as sound to humans, although they may be within the hearing range of many animals. It is possible, however, that subsonic and ultrasonic waves may have certain subtle psychological effects upon us. Some authorities contend, for example, that the low-pitched inaudible rumble of subsonic waves causes a curious sense of uneasiness or even alarm in the human mind, perhaps one source of the panic that seems to strike suddenly at the beginning of an earthquake, while ultrasonic waves created by machinery, whistles or traffic noises in the city may account, in part, for the irritability, jitteriness and nervous tension that so often afflicts urban dwellers. Any excess of sound in the audible range can also be psychologically as well as physically uncomfortable.

Thus sound waves are carried in an orderly fashion from external ear to middle ear to internal ear, delicately mediated by a series of small and sensitive structures. But this is not the only way that sounds can be transmitted. They can also be carried to the cochlea directly through the bone in which the internal ear is imbedded. Such *bone conduction* is not very efficient and ordinarily could be disregarded as an aid to hearing, but it does help the physician assess hearing loss in a patient. If the hearing deficiency is due only to a plug of wax in the ear canal, damage to the eardrum or a loss of vibratory capacity of the ossicles, sounds carried by bone conduction will be heard and interpreted perfectly well, whereas if the acoustic nerve or the auditory centers in the brain are impaired, sounds carried by bone conduction will not be heard any better than those received by the regular hearing apparatus.

A final structure in the internal ear, the *semicircular canals*—three curved tubes connected to the cochlea and lying at right angles to each other in three dimensional planes—have nothing to do with hearing, but are important to the body's balance and equilibrium. Special sensory receptors in these canals detect shifts in position of the head and send a constant flow of "position sense" impulses to the brain which help us maintain our physical equilibrium and prevent us from lurching and falling inadvertently. Any disorder involving the internal ear can disturb these sensors and cause a sense of dizziness or

vertigo, whereas constant bodily motion—on board a boat or in a moving automobile, for instance—may overload or "confuse" these position sensors, leading to the feeling of faintness, nausea and vomiting commonly associated with *motion sickness*. The semicircular canals do not react to gravitational pull on the body or to steady motion, but only to *changes* in motion or position. Thus the "dizziness" that may occur from acute alcohol intoxication, which continues even when sitting or lying perfectly still and becomes especially acute when the eyes are closed, is due to a toxic disturbance of the equilibrium centers in the brain itself and is not related to the semicircular canals at all.

Physical Abnormalities and Injuries to the Ear

Congenital defects may involve the absence, malformation or abnormal protrusion of the external ear, and a variety of defects of the middle or internal ear—absence or imperfect formation of the eardrum, congenital adhesions of the ossicles so they cannot vibrate, or malformations of the cochlea, to name but a few. The most frequent known cause of all these abnormalities is infection by the rubella or German measles virus during the early months of a pregnancy, but many congenital defects can never be clearly traced to any known cause. When the malformation involves the external ear or the external auditory canal, a remarkable degree of correction is often possible with plastic or reconstructive surgery, performed when the child is beyond the surgical risk period of infancy, and ideally after mature growth is attained, unless the abnormality interferes with hearing and thus must be corrected earlier. Treatment of congenital abnormalities of the middle and inner ear is not nearly as successful, which is particularly unfortunate because they are often the cause of partial or complete deafness. These portions of the ear are deeply embedded in the exceptionally hard, compact bone of the skull, and the possibility of correction depends upon both the exact nature of the defect and its accessibility to surgery. In such cases there may be no external evidence of any defect, and it may go undetected until the child is several months to a year old and the parents notice that he fails to respond to sound stimuli. Any suspicion that a child might have defective hearing during infancy should be immediately called to a doctor's attention so that diagnosis can be made and treatment, however limited, be instituted as early as possible.

The ears are far less vulnerable to injury than the eyes, since the working part of the ear is so well protected by bone. Lacerations of the external ear can usually be repaired surgically, often without leaving a trace of the injury. The "cauliflower ear" of the boxer is a result of repeated blows to the external ear which leads to progressive scarring and fibrosis over a prolonged period of time; this kind of recurrent injury is not ordinarily repairable. More threatening, in terms of hearing function, is damage or injury to the eardrum, which can be easily punctured by a sharp object thrust into the ear, torn by a sudden excessively loud noise, or ruptured as a result of sudden pressure changes, particularly when swimming or diving, or by a middle ear infection. Any rupture of the eardrum is painful because of the rich network of nerve endings located there, and infection of the injured eardrum is a serious complication which may lead to scarring or destruction of tissue. It must be guarded against with the aid of antibiotic therapy under a doctor's supervision. If infection can be prevented, or a middle ear infection properly cleared up, a torn, punctured or ruptured eardrum will usually heal spontaneously within a week or two following the injury with little or no permanent impairment of function. The rupture of an eardrum does not, as one might suppose, cause total deafness in the affected ear, but the hearing is definitely impaired until the ruptured area has healed and the membrane is tightly closed again.

By far the most common disorder is caused by a foreign body in the ear, and this should always be suspected when there is a sudden loss of hearing in one ear or the other. Children, who are fascinated by all the orifices of the body, often insert a stone, twig, bean, pea or some other foreign object into the external auditory canal and then are unable to retrieve it; vegetable seeds have actually been known to sprout in a child's ear before they were detected. Occasionally an insect will fly into the ear and become trapped, causing no end of irritation until it can be extracted. Among adults, certain individuals tend to have excessive quantities of ear wax which can, occasionally, form a solid plug that completely occludes the auditory canal. In any such case, the first and foremost rule is *do not try to extract the object yourself*. If the object is clearly visible it may be possible for someone else to remove it carefully. But if it is not or appears firmly embedded, see a doctor. If a foreign body is allowed to remain, intense irritation of the ear canal will cause progressive itching, pain and swelling; efforts at self-treatment almost invariably aggravate the condition, and may well convert a relatively minor problem into a major infection. The doctor can usually extract a foreign body with a small wire loop or curette, utilizing the excellent lighting and magnification of a simple office ear-examining instrument known as an *otoscope*. Any injury to the tissue of the ear canal can then be directly observed and appropriately treated. Often a foreign body, particularly a plug of ear wax, can simply be washed out by means of warm water squirted into the canal under gentle pressure from an ear syringe. Once a foreign body is removed, anti-inflammatory eardrops may be prescribed for a few days, but the irritation will usually improve within a few hours.

Infections of the Ear

The external ear canal can become infected from exactly the same kinds of organisms that cause other skin infections: staph or strep bacteria and fungi. Symptoms include itching, swelling of the ear canal tissue and intense irritation, as well as drainage of serum, blood or pus if the infection is severe. Diagnosis is made from microscopic examination or culture of infected material taken from the ear, and appropriate antibiotic therapy, in the form of either oral medication or medicated eardrops, or both, will usually clear up these infections promptly providing that treatment is instituted early. Certain fungus infections, however, can be quite stubborn once they become well entrenched, and may involve not only the auditory canal but the eardrum or even the middle ear. These will ultimately respond to treatment in most cases, but such infections must be followed up most persistently, sometimes over a period of months or even years, in order to completely eradicate them, and treatment is best supervised by the *otolaryngologist,* a specialist in ear, nose and throat disorders.

Middle ear infection or *otitis media* usually arises from invasion of the middle ear by bacteria or viruses carried up the Eustachian tube from the throat. Although these infections are more common among children, adults are by no means immune. The most characteristic symptoms are the onset of earache, fever, a feeling of pressure in the ear and often a distinct, annoying ringing in the ear known as *tinnitus.* Otitis media usually responds readily to treatment (*see* p. 196), but major complications may include a chronic middle ear infection and invasion of the inner ear by the infecting organism, both of which may permanently impair hearing. Extension of the infection into the mastoid area of spongy bone immediately behind the ear, a condition known as *mastoiditis,* was also a frequent complication before the era of antibiotics. Chronic ear infection remains an ever present threat, however, and any persisting pain or evidence of hearing disturbance should be investigated by a physician.

Disorders of the Equilibrium

Such phenomena as seasickness, carsickness or transitory dizziness due to wildly careening rides in an amusement park are familiar to everyone. All are a result of temporary disturbances of the equilibrium mechanism of the inner ear. More lasting and serious upsets of equilibrium may result from chemical poisoning or from the presence of a tumor such as the *acoustic neuroma,* a benign growth of cells in the acoustic nerve which, while not invasive or malignant, gradually destroys the nerve tissue by enlargement and pressure within the skull. Both equilibrium and hearing can be affected, but discovered early enough, an acoustic neuroma can sometimes be removed with marked recovery of both functions.

Most common of all disorders of equilibrium, however, and even today the most mysterious, is an odd condition known as *Ménière's syndrome* or recurrent vertigo. This condition tends to strike without warning during the early adult to middle years and seems to affect women somewhat more frequently than men. It is characterized by recurring attacks of ringing in the ears and vertigo or dizziness which progresses to nausea and, frequently, vomiting. There is a sense of fullness in the affected ear (often only one ear is involved) and some degree of hearing loss ranging from slight impairment to almost total deafness. Bone conduction of sound is usually impaired, suggesting that the acoustic nerve is involved in the disorder. In many cases the victim may also demonstrate *nystagmus,* an involuntary rhythmic jerking motion of the eyes when they are turned sharply to the right or left, again suggesting some disease process involving the cranial nerves or the brain stem. Attacks may last for only a few hours or may persist for days or weeks, only to clear up spontaneously and almost completely except for some residual hearing loss. Sometimes the disorder never recurs, but more often it appears again and again at highly unpredictable intervals.

No one is entirely sure what causes Ménière's syndrome; there may not be any common cause for all cases. Sometimes infection or inflammation of the semicircular canals, possibly viral in origin, seems related to the condition. Other causes that have been suggested include allergic reactions, head injuries that might have produced hemorrhage in the inner ear region, poisoning by bacterial toxin or various chemicals or drugs, or some form of nonspecific neuritis which affects the acoustic and other cranial nerves. Whatever the cause, victims suffering recurrent severe attacks often have a gradual progressive impairment of hearing over a period of time, but no other characteristic nervous system deterioration. Minor attacks of Ménière's syndrome are little more than transient irritating annoyances to the victim, with the vertigo and nausea easily controlled by small doses of such "motion sickness" medicines as Dramamine or Bonamine, or certain antiemetic tranquilizers that a physician may prescribe. In more severe attacks the victim may literally be unable to move without recurrent episodes of retching and vomiting so intractable that he cannot hold down either food or fluids for days at a time. In such cases hospital care may be necessary for administration of intravenous fluids and the use of gastric suction to keep the stomach free of secretions and help control the vomiting. Sometimes antibiotics are prescribed in hopes that a bacterial infection of the internal ear is at fault, but this therapy is by no means universally favored. When all other measures fail and only one ear is involved, it may be necessary to destroy the semicircular canals on the affected side by electrocautery to control the disorder. More recently, delicately focused ultrasonic waves have been used successfully for the same purpose in a way that the sound receptors in the cochlea are unaffected. Fortunately, such extreme cases of Ménière's syndrome are relatively uncommon, but even in mild cases progressive hearing loss remains an unsolved problem.

Hearing Loss and Deafness

In man the ears are auxiliary sensory organs, merely supplementing the more vital sense of vision, and hearing loss may arise so slowly and subtly that the individual remains unaware of it for a long time. To make the diagnosis of true hearing loss all the more difficult, many people with completely unimpaired hearing habitually "shut off" their response to auditory stimuli at times of concentrated thought, introspection or abstraction.

True hearing impairment can arise from a number of different causes. It is commonly differentiated as *conductive deafness,* in which the conduction of sound waves down the auditory canal to the eardrum, or through the middle ear, is partially or totally impaired, even though the nerve remains healthy; and *perceptive deafness,* in which the auditory nerve or the hearing centers of the brain are involved. Conductive deafness may arise from simple mechanical obstruction of the external ear canal by ear wax or a foreign body, from infection in the middle ear, from perforation and improper healing of the eardrum, or from *otosclerosis,* a disorder in

which the tiny ossicles in the middle ear become "frozen" rigidly together and thus cannot vibrate and conduct the sound waves to the inner ear properly. Such hearing losses may be markedly improved by correction of the underlying cause —removal of ear wax, for instance, or clearing up a middle ear infection. Otosclerosis can often be cured, or at least markedly improved, by the surgical separation of the adherent ossicles. This kind of surgery, of course, is highly specialized and is usually performed by an otolaryngologist. A common cause of partial conductive deafness in children is the overgrowth of lymphoid or adenoidal tissue in the back of the nasopharynx, with partial obstruction of the Eustachian tube. Improvement often follows surgical removal of the tonsils and adenoids. (*See* p. 194.)

Perceptive deafness due to destruction or impairment of the internal ear sound receptors, or of the auditory nerve, may result from such infectious diseases as meningitis, syphilis, mumps, measles or streptococcal infections. Other causes include destruction of nerve tissue due to brain tumors, meningeal tumors or acoustic nerve tumors; congenital defects; head injuries with hemorrhage into the inner ear; or even severe emotional trauma. Drugs or chemicals such as quinine, arsenic, mercury or the antibiotic streptomycin, which is used to treat tuberculosis, may all cause toxic destruction of the acoustic nerve. Finally, perceptive deafness may slowly develop as a more or less natural condition of advancing age, possibly because of impaired circulation to the inner ear or the acoustic nerve due to arteriosclerosis.

Hearing disorders of any sort can have a profound psychological effect upon the victim. Many people simply refuse to acknowledge hearing loss and needlessly cut themselves off from the world of sound around them because they will not recognize their impairment and wear a hearing aid. The individual who is born deaf may suffer even more dramatic secondary impairments; growing up from infancy in a world of silence, he can learn to speak only with intensive specialized training because of an inability to mimic normal speech sounds. Lip reading and sign language can be learned, however, as alternate means of communication. There are a number of special schools that train the deaf of all ages, and given the necessary educational and employment opportunities, many of the deaf lead full and productive lives.

Congenital deafness may be totally incorrectable, but hearing aids can be of great value to many who acquire some degree of conductive or perceptive deafness later in life. In general, hearing aids are of two kinds. One kind assists in the bone conduction of sound and is usually worn pressed against the skull in back of the impaired ear. The other kind, which aids air conduction of sound waves, is molded and fitted into the external ear canal. Today hearing aids of remarkably high quality have been miniaturized to be as inconspicuous as possible. Any impairment of hearing that becomes apparent either to the victim or to those closely associated with him should be evaluated by the family doctor or an otolaryngologist in order to determine the kind of hearing aid, if any, that will help resolve the problem. Commercial hearing centers in most major cities can then follow the doctor's directions in providing the optimum instrument for each individual's personal needs.

Proper Care of the Ears

Since most of the vital structures of the ear are deeply embedded in the bone of the skull, the normal ear requires comparatively little in the way of everyday hygienic care other than gentle cleansing of the entry to the external auditory canal with soap and water to remove excess wax and dirt, and careful cleansing behind the ear, an area all too often neglected. Digging into the external canal with a little finger, toothpicks, hairpins or other devices to dislodge wax and washing the ear canals with water pressure devices such as basting syringes or hypodermic syringes are both dangerous due to the risk of injury or infection. Ordinarily there is no need to clean out the deeper regions of the ear canal. Individuals who produce excessive amounts of cerumen, or people such as short-order cooks who work in an atmosphere laden with oil droplets that can gradually form an impaction in the ear canal, should schedule regular visits with their physician at whatever interval is necessary so that the ears can be cleaned under carefully controlled conditions.

The use of earrings or other ear adornments has been fashionable among women, and even men in some cultures, for many centuries. It is a perfectly harmless practice as long as the earrings do not disturb circulation or cause an allergic reaction. Very heavy earrings may permanently stretch the fibrous tissues of the ear lobes and should be avoided. Piercing the ears for earrings has been the subject of some controversy off and on for years. Even today many physicians regard ear piercing as a distasteful form of self-mutilation and refuse to perform the simple operation. But ultimately the decision for or against the procedure rests with the individual. Properly and professionally done, ear piercing involves little real risk. It can be performed under local anesthetic, or even with the aid of a simple device which pierces the ear lobe instantaneously without need of anesthetic. Once the piercing has been done, a strand of an inert metal such as gold must be left in position through the wound long enough for healing to take place and a narrow canal of epithelial tissue to form, a matter of approximately six weeks. This is *not*, however, a procedure that should be done by either a friend or a jewelry salesman. There is always some risk of infection and scarring. If you wish to have your ears pierced, it is best to seek out a doctor who is willing to do the job.

The Nose

In man the olfactory sense (the sense of smell) is by far the weakest, least developed and least useful of the normal senses. In contrast with certain lower animals, which depend heavily upon their sense of smell, sometimes to the exclusion of other senses, man's olfactory sense has become almost vestigial. Even so, diminishment of this sense can rob the individual of many olfactory pleasures and may also seriously impair his sense of taste, which is closely associated with the sense of smell. The olfactory sense may be impaired because of chronic nasal obstruction from one source or another, infection of the mucous membrane of the nose, or allergies affecting these delicate tissues. Often the correction of any of these conditions by proper medical or surgical treat-

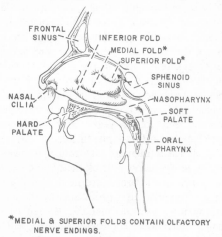

FRONTAL SINUS
INFERIOR FOLD
MEDIAL FOLD*
SUPERIOR FOLD*
SPHENOID SINUS
NASAL CILIA
NASOPHARYNX
SOFT PALATE
HARD PALATE
ORAL PHARYNX

*MEDIAL & SUPERIOR FOLDS CONTAIN OLFACTORY NERVE ENDINGS.

Figure 33–4.

ment will restore a flagging sense of smell remarkably. Heavy smokers often suffer olfactory impairment without even realizing it until they stop smoking and become suddenly aware of a marked improvement in their senses of both smell and taste. In addition, the olfactory sense can be impaired or distorted when a tumor presses on the part of the brain in which olfactory sensations are interpreted. Occasionally such a condition is first suspected when the individual begins to notice a constant or intermittent odd, disagreeable or noxious odor which seems to be present for no apparent reason and which others around him deny. As there is no normal condition in which this phenomenon is found, any evidence of it should be called to a physician's attention and an examination undertaken to find the cause of the problem.

Essentially the nose is a passage or opening in the front of the skull, divided in half vertically by a plate of cartilage into two nostrils or *nares* through which air can be drawn from the outside into the back of the throat. The nares are lined with thick folds of mucous membrane richly endowed with mucus-producing glands , so that the interior surface of the nose is always moist and serves to humidify air before it passes

into the bronchial tubes and the lungs. At the outer orifices the nares are guarded by a growth of coarse hairs which aid in preventing the accidental inhalation of insects or other minute foreign bodies, and the sticky mucous coating further serves to trap and hold such accidentally insufflated debris. The floor of the nostrils is closed off from the mouth by the bony plate of the *hard palate* in front and the soft mucous membrane of the *soft palate* behind. Sinuses or air pockets in the bones surrounding the nares open into the nasal passages to drain. The external part of the nose, a fleshy proboscis which represents the vestigial remains of the snout of lower animals (other primates have virtually lost this appendage), is lined with bone only for about half an inch at the upper portion and takes most of its form from a cartilaginous extension of that bone.

The entire back half of the interior of the nose, especially in the area above the soft palate, has a fine network of special olfactory receptors connected to the brain by means of the olfactory nerve. Essentially these are *chemoreceptors* sensitive to a wide variety of fine powders or dusts, gas molecules or oil droplets insufflated with the air that is breathed. Stimulated by the various chemicals in such substances, these olfactory receptors fire off nerve impulses which are carried to the olfactory cortex in the frontal lobes of the brain and are there interpreted as *odors*—sweet or fragrant, aromatic, pungent, musty, musky or acrid smells. Similar chemoreceptors on the tongue respond to sweet, sour, salty or bitter chemical qualities in foods, and together the two senses cooperate to create a surprisingly acute differentiation of combined smell-and-taste sensations.

But the nose has other functions in addition to providing the olfactory sense. It is, of course, an important aid to respiration, acting as a major air humidifier and allowing us to continue breathing while the mouth is occupied with chewing. Further, the nasal passages and the paranasal sinuses act in combination as echo chambers and resonators which markedly influence the tone, quality and timbre of the voice. In fact, the loss of the respiratory and vocalization functions of the nose is more disabling, in nasal injuries or disorders, than any loss of olfactory function.

Physical Defects and Injuries of the Nose

Cleft Palate. Most common of the congenital defects involving the nose is the cleft palate which may arise as a result of some disturbance to the fetus during the early stages of embryonic life. The nose and mouth initially form from three segments, one on either side which joins a third in the center and fuses to form the floor of the nose and the roof of the mouth, as well as the lips and the nares. Defective development may result in an imperfect fusion of both bone and mucous membrane in the palate on either or both sides, often associated with an external defect of the upper jaw and lip known as *harelip* —a misnomer, since the defect is always slightly away from the midline on either side or both. In extreme cases there may be a congenital absence of almost the entire palate, a condition which renders speech virtually impossible and leads to great difficulty both in breathing and in eating. More commonly the defect is less severe, but even a minor incomplete defect of the palate can result in some distortion of speech. Surgical correction of cleft palate and harelip is almost always possible today; it is usually initiated before the afflicted child is two years old and sometimes requires several progressive stages of repair before correction is completed. When a harelip is present, there will always be a small scar in the upper lip where the repair was accomplished, but there is no reason today for a child to grow up enduring the embarrassment and emotional distress once associated with these congenital defects.

Broken Nose. Obviously the external nose is vulnerable to physical injuries, blows, crushing or other forms of trauma, and a so-called broken nose is not an uncommon result of body contact sports in adolescence or of automobile accidents or injudicious disputes in adulthood. The bone in the upper part of the nose is actually broken in such injuries far less frequently than is assumed; very often a "broken nose" involves only tearing, breaking or dislocation of the nasal

cartilage, with no injury to the bone. Correct diagnosis can best be made as soon after the injury as possible, since nose injuries often result in an intense swelling which soon renders effective examination impossible. Treatment involves replacing fractured bone fragments or dislocated cartilage in normal anatomical position, followed by splinting to maintain that position and avoid further injury until healing can take place. Properly treated, a broken nose need not result in any permanent deformity, but too often these injuries are ignored or left untreated. In such cases improper healing and scar tissue formation may result in a far greater degree of twisting or visible distortion of the nose than the victim anticipates at the time of the injury. Later surgical restoration of a nose that has been distorted by previous injury is, of course, possible with modern plastic surgery techniques, but the process is apt to be far more painful and expensive than proper treatment at the time of the injury.

Foreign Bodies in the Nose. Nose picking is a problem that occurs almost exclusively among young children, either as a nervous habit or as an attempt to remove some obstruction. Most adults have sense enough not to stick things up their noses, including their fingers, and if there is some obstruction, either from internal secretions or from a foreign body, adult nares are large enough so that it can usually be snuffed back into the throat or effectively blown out. In children, however, the nasal passage is tiny, perhaps only a quarter of an inch across, and a tempting place to explore with a finger or insert such objects as beans, pencil erasers and bubble gum, all of which can easily become lodged and impossible for either the parent or the child to extricate. In any case in which a foreign body cannot easily and immediately be removed, take the child to an emergency room or a doctor's office. Usually removal with the use of proper forceps can be accomplished swiftly and painlessly under office conditions, but if necessary a brief general anesthesia can be administered to enable the doctor to do the job. A foreign body left in place for any length of time will cause irritation, pain and swelling of the nasal mucosa around the object, and can ultimately cause extensive and destructive infection. The sooner the foreign body is removed, the better.

Nosebleeds. A nosebleed can be an extremely irritating and perplexing problem, often inordinately frightening to the victim and sometimes very difficult to treat. Most nosebleeds arise as a result of rupture of a blood vessel in the nasal mucosa due to excessively forceful nose blowing, and once such a vessel is ruptured, the habitual nose blower will tend to rupture it again and again. A blow to the nose may also result in a nosebleed, but many times this phenomenon occurs quite spontaneously, particularly among people suffering from uncontrolled high blood pressure. Most difficult of all, although fortunately rare, are the nosebleeds that occur in individuals with some form of blood clotting defect, so that the natural clotting mechanism that would ordinarily stop a nosebleed is impaired or totally inoperative. Most run-of-the-mill nosebleeds can be effectively stopped by the victim himself. (*See* p. 134.) But if for some reason the bleeding cannot be stopped, or tends to recur repeatedly, or involves truly copious blood loss, medical aid should of course be sought.

Infections and Abnormal Growths

Since the nose is easily accessible to surface bacteria or insufflated viruses, infections in the nose are not uncommon. They are usually associated with infections involving other parts of the upper respiratory tract as well—head colds, influenza, or other infectious disorders discussed in detail in Part IV, "Patterns of Illness: The Infectious Diseases," and in Part VIII, "Patterns of Illness: The Respiratory Tract." The nasal mucosa is also a common target organ for allergic reactions, particularly to pollens, and many nasal infections are in fact a combination of infection complicating an allergic reaction. Common symptoms include itching, sneezing, irritation and the appearance of a clear, watery discharge from the nose which later may become purulent or thickened with excessive mucus production. (The diagnosis and treatment of such nasal allergies as hay fever are discussed on p. 490.)

Nasal Polyps. These soft tumorous overgrowths of the nasal mucosa may arise as a result of the irritation of chronic and recurrent infection or nasal allergies, or may simply appear for no known reason. They are perfectly benign tumors, in most cases, but can often grow large enough to obstruct partially one or both of the nares. Usually the victim himself cannot see them, but they can be detected by a careful examination by a physician or an otolaryngologist and can usually be removed quite easily under local or general anesthesia, depending upon the size and extent of the condition. Malignant tumors within the nose are quite rare, but can occur, sometimes as a cancerous change in an initially benign polyp, so that any nasal polyps removed are routinely presented for pathological examination no matter how benign they may appear.

Proper Care of the Nose

Many problems related to the nose are self-induced. Excessively traumatic blowing, nervous picking, tweezing away unwanted nasal hairs or excoriating the nose with unnecessary quantities of irritating nose drops or nasal sprays, all can cause chronic irritation of the nasal mucous membrane and lead to soreness, swelling, excessive mucus production or infection. Ideally, nose blowing should be confined to episodes of real need, and should be performed gently, one nostril at a time. Nose drops or nasal sprays certainly provide temporary relief from excessive nasal drainage during a head cold or the hay fever season, but should be confined to saline preparations, and even these should not be overused. Most saline nose drops contain adrenalin-like compounds designed to shrink the capillaries in the nasal mucosa, but prolonged or frequent use may so irritate this delicate membrane that these same capillaries tend to become excessively engorged as soon as the effect of the medication wears off, thus causing "rebound" nasal stuffiness and drainage that are worse than the original condition. Oil-based nose drops should be avoided altogether, since they may trickle down the trachea into the lungs and cause oil pneumonia. (*See* p. 488.) Any chronic or recurring nasal condition should, of course, be called to a doctor's attention, since the underlying cause may well be both identifiable and correctable. A slight misplacement of the nasal septum, the cartilage plate separating the nares, may, for example, cause excessive drying of one of the nostrils, which in turn leads to overproduction of nasal mucus. Such a condition may cause chronic nasal stuffiness, an annoying postnasal drip, or even the growth of nasal polyps. A deviated septum and the conditions it causes can be effectively treated either medically or surgically, but first it must be identified.

Much has been written—largely in vain—to induce people to breathe through their noses rather than their mouths. Realistically, however, most people usually breathe alternately through mouth and nose, or through both at once, unless an obstruction renders nasal breathing difficult or impossible. If anyone, child or adult, engages *exclusively* in mouth breathing, a search for an obstructive phenomenon in the nose should be made. But even the experts cannot fully agree whether mouth breathing is actually harmful or not, and no child should be subjected to the infinitely greater harm of persistent parental nagging simply because he prefers, consciously or unconsciously, to breathe through his mouth.

No discussion of the nose would be complete without some comment about plastic and reconstructive surgery of the nose undertaken for cosmetic purposes. Throughout history men and women alike have been dissatisfied with the size, shape or contour of their noses, without being able to do very much about it. Now that surgical techniques exist that make it possible to alter these features in almost any way desired, it is hardly surprising that people seek to take advantage of them. Assuming that no medical contraindications exist, the decision is really up to the individual, but it should be noted that the results of such surgery are by no means completely successful. Unsatisfactory results do indeed occur, even in skilled surgical hands, and may be irreparable. It is a surgical procedure, after all, with all the potential complications of anesthesia, infection or undesired scarring that may arise unexpectedly with any surgery. And it is usually very expensive. Finally, although social disapproval of cosmetic surgery of any kind is no longer a great concern, it is well to remember that it is virtually impossible to predict how pleasing a new nose or a "lifted" face may be physically or psychologically, both to the patient and to his family and friends. Certainly before any cosmetic surgical procedure is undertaken the individual should consult with family and friends, and then seek the advice of a skilled specialist.

34

Diseases of the Breast

Final in the consideration of special organs in the cutaneous system are the breasts or *mammaries*—skin-covered glandular structures that arise in both males and females from the epithelial tissue of the anterior wall of the chest. The breasts are remarkable organs in a number of ways. Although present in both sexes, they actually function only in the female, and then only during certain very limited intervals—during pregnancy and immediately following the birth of a baby. Their main purpose is to provide milk for the infant during his first few months of life, but more often than not in our society even this highly specialized function is deliberately suppressed by medicines and other foods are substituted. To many women, in fact, the breasts have become primarily a cosmetic concern; yet they can present a very real health problem as well, not so much because of disruption in their function but because certain prevalent breast disorders can be highly dangerous and even, in some cases, life-threatening. The difficulty for many women lies in distinguishing perfectly normal changes which occur in the breasts from time to time from abnormal conditions which must be called to a doctor's attention without delay.

Normal Changes in the Breasts

Perhaps more than any other organ, the breasts in both males and females undergo a number of obvious, but quite normal, changes at various times in life. Anatomically the breasts are composed of glandular tissue which arises during embryonic life from epithelial glands in the skin similar to the sweat glands. But this tissue has differentiated by the time of birth into a unique structure. As it develops on either side of the chest, this glandular tissue is embedded in an elastic meshwork of fibrous connective tissue and fat, loosely bound to the surface skin and underlying muscle. Rudimentary ducts from this glandular tissue converge in a special structure, the *nipple,* surrounded by a pigmented area of skin, the *areola,* and in this region the breast is more firmly attached to the skin. Oddly enough, about 5 percent of men and a slightly smaller percentage of women have one or more *supernumerary nipples*—small, flat or slightly raised pigmented spots, often mistaken for moles, located on the skin of the chest or abdomen along a line drawn from the armpit to the groin. These structures are virtually never functional and are perfectly normal and harmless when they occur, more of a minor anatomical curiosity than a concern.

In both male and female breast tissue is dormant throughout childhood, but at puberty an important change takes place. At that time, under the influence of hormones produced by the maturing sex glands, particularly the female sex hormone *estrogen,* the breasts begin to enlarge and mature. In the male, with less estrogen, this enlargement is very limited, but in the female it is quite marked, usually reaching a maximum at about age fourteen to fifteen, at which time both breasts and nipples achieve the mature size and shape that will be maintained, except during pregnancy, throughout the childbearing years. Often, however, adolescent girls notice a slight additional enlargement of breasts and nipples, accompanied by some tenderness, at the time of each menstrual period, a normal phenomenon which may continue for a period of several years. In about 40 percent of males there will also be a slight enlargement of breast tissue just beneath the nipple for a period of time during early adolescence, but this tumescence normally subsides within a year or two and requires medical attention only if it persists into late adolescence.

Many adolescent girls are concerned, even embarrassed, by breast development that occurs either earlier or later than they think normal; in some girls the breasts begin enlarging as early as age nine or ten, while in others enlargement does not occur until the age of fourteen or fifteen. Many girls are also concerned about the size of their breasts; those with small breasts may wish they were larger, and those with large breasts may wish they were smaller. However, most such individual variations in size, shape and time of development are within the limits of normal,

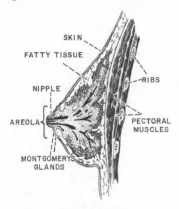

SKIN

FATTY TISSUE

NIPPLE

RIBS

AREOLA

PECTORAL MUSCLES

MONTGOMERY'S GLANDS

Figure 34–1.

determined by totally uncontrollable factors of heredity, race and overall body structure; and every girl should be reassured that these variations have nothing whatever to do with sexual

adequacy or her eventual ability to nurse her babies.

In the male all normal change in breast development comes to an end by late adolescence and no further changes are to be expected. In the female yet another period of normal change occurs with the beginning of a pregnancy. At this time the glandular tissue again begins to enlarge, often quite dramatically. The nipples and areolar areas also enlarge and become pigmented, and the special sebaceous glands encircling the nipple, known as *Montgomery's glands,* become prominent—an important early clue that a pregnancy has occurred. As the pregnancy advances, the breasts become engorged and tumescent, all changes in preparation for the milk-secreting function which normally begins within a few hours after delivery unless suppressed by hormone medication. In addition, most women have occasional drainage of thin, milky fluid or *colostrum* from the nipples throughout the last three months of a pregnancy, often stimulated by a hot shower or by sexual relations.

Breast changes after pregnancy and during the period of *lactation* or milk production are discussed in detail elsewhere. (*See* p. 847.) Once the baby is weaned, or the breasts "dried up" by medication, however, the breast tissue reverts to the approximate size and shape it had before pregnancy, although certain stigmata of the pregnancy may be permanent. The areola often remains larger and darker than before, *stria* or "stretch marks" may become visible in the skin, and the breasts will generally be somewhat more flaccid than before.

Except during recurrent pregnancies, most women see little or no further change in their breasts, other than some deposition of fat, until the time of menopause when menstruation ceases. At that time the glandular tissue of the breast slowly atrophies and the breasts become smaller, flatter and more pendulous. This final normal change becomes more marked with advancing age, but may be disguised somewhat in overweight women because the fat deposited in the breast area during earlier years tends to persist.

Abnormal Breast Conditions

All the changes discussed above are the result of natural, normal physiologic processes that occur in the body as life progresses. However, the breasts are also vulnerable to various changes that are not normal, caused by diseases and disorders which may first appear at any time from puberty on. To most women a breast disorder means only one thing: cancer—hardly surprising considering that cancer of the breast is such a familiar and serious threat. There are, of course, many breast disorders that are far less dangerous but still can be worrisome because they must be carefully distinguished from an early cancer. Most of these benign conditions are associated with *abnormal enlargement* of the breasts, with *pain and tenderness* of breast tissue, or with the development of a *lump or mass* in the breast, and any of these potential trouble signs should be called to a doctor's attention as soon as possible after they become apparent.

Abnormal Breast Enlargement (Hypertrophy). Ordinarily changes in breast size are limited to the normal range discussed above, but occasionally abnormal enlargement or hypertrophy can occur. When it does, it is usually due to some hormone imbalance arising elsewhere in the body. Growth of breast tissue is particularly stimulated by the female sex hormone estrogen produced by the ovaries, but overproduction of pituitary or adrenal gland hormones may also cause breast enlargement. Thus in any case of persisting enlargement, a physical examination is necessary to rule out such possible causes as estrogen-producing tumors of the ovary, hormone-producing tumors of the adrenal glands or the pituitary gland, or similar glandular disorders. (*See* p. 690.) Occasionally, an adolescent girl may develop breast hypertrophy as a result of abnormal sensitivity of the breast tissue to perfectly normal levels of estrogen. In such cases the enlargement is often irreversible and may, in some cases, lead to the later development of cysts or benign tumors of the breast.

Hypertrophy of the male breast, known as *gynecomastia,* may also arise as a result of hormone-producing tumors of the adrenals, pituitary gland or testicles. In addition, it may occur in elderly men owing to a normal decline in the production of the male hormone androgen at that period of life. In most cases the enlargement is confined to a small button-like mass of poorly developed breast tissue just beneath the nipple, and should not be confused with enlargement due to the deposition of fat which is commonly seen in obese middle-aged men. Cancer can occasionally occur in the male breast, too, so any mass or lump, particularly in the region of the nipple, should be called to a doctor's attention. When the gynecomastia is a result of some identifiable source of hormone imbalance, correction of the underlying disorder is followed by reversion of the breast to normal, but in cases in which the enlargement is merely a normal aspect of adolescent development, no treatment is indicated, and the gynecomastia can be expected to disappear spontaneously in a year or two.

Acute Mastitis (Septic Mastitis). Uncommon today, but serious when it occurs, bacterial infection of the breast occurs almost exclusively during the period of lactation following the birth of a baby, usually soon after nursing begins. Staph or strep organisms can invade the breast through abrasions or cracks in the nipple, or more directly by way of the milk ducts. The ensuing infection is accompanied by fever and chills, painful swelling, soreness and redness of the affected breast, and swelling of lymph nodes in the adjacent axilla or armpit. The victim becomes severely ill, even prostrated, and vigorous treatment is necessary to stop the spread of infection throughout the breast. Bed rest and extra fluids are mandatory, and breast feeding must be discontinued. High dosages of penicillin or other antibiotics are often required. At the same time, hormones are administered to suppress milk production and speed the involution of breast tissue, thus reducing breast distention, relieving pain and permitting speedier healing. Before antibiotics, acute mastitis often led to breast abscesses, blood poisoning, or a persistent, chronic infection, but these complications are uncommon today. Modern treatment leads to recovery within a week to ten days, but months may pass before the victim fully recovers her former strength and resistance, owing to the generalized toxicity that accompanies the infection.

Cystic Disease of the Breast (Mammary Dysplasia). This condition, usually of unknown origin, is characterized by the periodic formation of benign cystic masses, single or multiple, in the breast tissue during the years of sexual maturity. The breasts become diffusely lumpy, particularly in the upper outer quadrant, because of the intermittent growth and involution of irregular areas of breast tissue. Early symptoms involve little more than periodic swelling and lumpiness of the breasts, especially around the time of menstrual periods. This is followed by the development of small fluid-filled cysts in the breast, with thickening and fibrosis of the tissue surrounding the cysts. The condition is benign, and may remain stationary at this stage for prolonged periods, requiring no particular treatment, as some cysts shrink and scar and others form.

Occasionally, however, a larger cyst may form and persist as a distinct separate lump or "dominant mass" which, upon external examination, cannot be distinguished for certain from the tumor of an early cancer. When this occurs, a doctor must be consulted at once. Sometimes such a cyst will decrease in size at the end of a menstrual period or after a few days of conservative treatment with warm moist packs to the breast 30 minutes at a time four times a day. But if it does not, or if the doctor remains suspicious of the lesion, a *breast biopsy* must be performed to be certain that an early cancer is not present. This surgical procedure is quite simple, requiring only a few minutes, but both surgeon and patient must be prepared to proceed with more extensive surgery then and there if the lump proves cancerous. The biopsy specimen is immediately frozen, sectioned, stained and examined under the microscope by the pathologist while the patient is still anesthetized in the operating room. Three times out of four the growth proves to be benign. The surgeon then simply closes the biopsy wound and the procedure is over. If the growth is cancerous, however, everything is ready for the necessary

surgery without losing even a few hours unnecessarily.

Cystic disease of the breast varies greatly from one case to the next. Some women never develop cysts large or questionable enough to require biopsy diagnosis, while others may require repeated biopsies over the years, since the fact that one lump in a breast proves to be a cyst does not exclude the possibility of a cancer another time. Cystic disease is *not* believed to be a forerunner of cancer, or related to cancer in any way, yet women have been known to develop a benign cyst and a separate cancerous tumor at the same time. Years ago surgeons often treated patients with extreme cases of recurrent large cysts by *simple mastectomy*—surgical excision of glandular tissue of the breast—but such a procedure was highly unpopular for obvious cosmetic reasons. Today, however, with the development of silastic cosmetic implants to replace or augment breast tissue, treatment of cystic mastitis by means of simple mastectomy is on the increase. Many women, assured that use of a silastic implant will enable them to maintain a normal appearance and an attractive figure, prefer to undergo the necessary surgery rather than repeated biopsies when painful cysts and lumps recur. But in any case of cystic disease, careful follow-up examinations by the doctor at regular six-month intervals are necessary, and medical use of hormones for any condition is avoided if possible because they may stimulate cyst formation.

Other Benign Breast Tumors. Technically cysts are considered benign tumors because they arise from a benign overgrowth of breast tissue. Other noncancerous tumors of the breast may also develop from the glandular or ductal tissue in the breast, differing from cysts in that they are composed of solid tissue and are more likely to develop as single tumor masses than as multiple growths. Two quite common varieties in particular must be differentiated from malignant tumors. One is the *fibroadenoma,* a well-defined benign tumor which develops either from the fibrous tissue of the breast or from the milk ducts that enlarge during lactation. Usually this tumor forms a firm "dominant mass" or lump in the breast, but unlike a cancer, it is enclosed in a fibrous capsule, does not deform the breast, and is quite freely movable. It is not cancerous or precancerous, but must be removed for examination when it is discovered because there is no other way to be certain that it is not an early cancer. The other frequently encountered benign tumor of the breast, the *intraductal papilloma,* tends to grow from the milk ducts just beneath the nipple and may, in some cases, cause a clear or even bloody discharge from the nipple. Underlying tissue may be scarred, causing the nipple to become distorted. This tumor has long been an enigma to the surgeons, since it develops late in the childbearing years or after menopause and was once thought to be a precancerous lesion which might, if untreated, develop into a cancer. Surgeons doubt this now; in fact, statistics indicate that true breast cancers are only rarely associated with bleeding or nipple discharge. Today intraductal papillomas are merely removed for pathological examination, like other benign tumors, to be certain no cancer is present.

Another common benign breast tumor is the *lipoma,* a growth of fatty tissue somewhere in the breast. A lipoma has no medical significance except that it can sometimes mimic an early cancer, and thus it, too, occasionally must be removed for examination.

Cancer of the Breast

Malignant or cancerous breast tumors are totally different from benign cysts. Breast cancer is not a single disease entity so much as a group of different malignant growths that can develop from various parts of the breast, but the distinction between one kind and another is academic to the layman; all are dangerous, life-threatening diseases, the major cause of cancer death among women in the United States, and the leading cause of death from all causes in women between the ages of forty and forty-four. Most are *carcinomas*—uncontrolled growths of cells arising from epithelial tissue in the glandular structure of the breast itself, along the milk ducts or in the tissue of the nipple. All presumably start

from the abnormal growth of a single cell or a localized patch of cells, but sooner or later they begin to invade surrounding tissue and, ultimately, to seed cancer cells to distant areas, first to the lymph nodes in the axillae, and later to other parts of the body by way of blood vessels and lymphatics. And without exception, all are ultimately fatal diseases if undiagnosed or unchecked. Certain forms tend to grow, invade and metastasize more slowly than others and thus may give the victim and the surgeon a somewhat better opportunity for curative treatment, but these unfortunately are the rare ones. Far more common and dangerous is a swiftly growing *adenocarcinoma* which makes up more than 75 percent of all cases of breast cancer.

For this reason, it is the height of foolishness to temporize with *any* lesion of the breast which might be a cancer until it is proven otherwise by biopsy and pathological examination. And with a cancer, even a day or two saved between the time it is discovered and the time it is excised can make the difference between a cure and a lingering, chronic disease with an inexorably fatal termination. Thus it cannot be overemphasized that *a lump in the breast is never normal, it has no business being there, and there is roughly a 25 percent chance that it is a cancer.* In women past menopause, a single isolated lump in the breast will prove to be cancerous in an even higher percentage of cases.

Breast cancer is, in fact, one of the most frequently occurring of all malignant tumors; one out of every ten cancers develops in the breast. It usually appears in women during the years just before, during or after menopause, but may arise any time, and can occur in the male as well as the female. No one yet knows what causes it; possibly a virus may be at fault, but no scientific proof of this has yet been found. What *is* known is that the female sex hormone, estrogen, powerfully stimulates the growth of a breast cancer once it has begun, an important factor in treatment. Oddly enough, the disease appears far more commonly in women who have had few pregnancies and have never nursed than among multiparous ("many children") women. On the other hand, the widespread notion that breast cancer can arise as a result of injury or trauma to the breasts has no basis whatever in fact, nor has any clear-cut hereditary pattern ever been established regarding this disease.

Early diagnosis of cancer of the breast depends, obviously, upon discovery of a lump or mass in a breast, best accomplished by the woman herself in the process of breast self-examination, which is discussed below. In most cases definitive diagnosis must be made by means of breast biopsy in the operating room. Before a biopsy is performed, however, the physician will examine the patient carefully, since the location, size, shape, consistency and evidence of involvement of other tissue around the lump may provide a clue to the likelihood of a cancer. The axilla is examined for any evidence of enlarged lymph nodes. *X-ray mammography*—a special type of X-ray examination of the breast—has proven extremely helpful in recent years in making the diagnosis, and such exciting techniques as *acoustic holography,* still in the process of development, offer even greater promise for the future. Such examinations are not a substitute for breast biopsy, by any means; a solitary lump or nodule in the breast must be biopsied regardless of findings on physical or X-ray examination. But they do have value in helping prepare both the surgeon and the patient for what may be found in the operating room, and in helping the surgeon judge whether or not a cancer, if present, may already have spread to other areas.

In most cases when cancer is diagnosed at biopsy, the surgeon then and there will perform a *radical mastectomy*—the complete removal of the entire breast, the muscle layers covering the ribs beneath the breast and all of the lymph nodes in the axilla on the affected side. In addition, he may remove the chain of lymph nodes that lie along the underside of the ribs on the affected side in his search for any evidence of spread of the disease. Such widespread excision of tissue is necessary for two reasons. First, it has been found in thousands and thousands of cases that this radical surgery results in a higher percentage of cures than simple removal of the lump, or of the breast alone. Second, what is found during surgery provides information that is invaluable in planning further, sometimes life-saving, treatment. If careful pathological examination of the adjacent lymph nodes reveals no evidence whatever of any spread of the cancer to those regions, chances are very good that the patient will survive with no recurrence, or that any recurrence will be long delayed. If the nodes *are* involved chances are less good, but vigorous postoperative treatment of the disease can be planned right from the start.

The period following a radical mastectomy is admittedly difficult. Often a skin graft must be used to close the site of such an extensive excision of tissue, and removal of the axillary lymph nodes frequently results in swelling and edema of the affected arm for a prolonged period of time. But with expert nursing care, vigorous measures to avoid infection, and a program of physical therapy to aid in recovery of the use of the arm and reduce edema, the inevitable problems of this postoperative period can be minimized. Of course, such surgery is always emotionally traumatic, particularly to the woman who is still sexually active and deeply concerned about her physical attractiveness. However, untold thousands of such women, aided by their doctors and with the emotional support of their husbands and families, have found a way to adjust, knowing full well that the surgery, although radical, was the only possible avenue to a continued, comfortable and productive life. Breast prostheses and specially constructed garments help as far as appearance is concerned, but even more important is the knowledge that a deadly disease has been discovered and checked.

What are the chances for complete permanent recovery from a breast cancer following such surgery? Because recurrences may occur years later, even when no evidence of spread is found during surgery, physicians speak of "five-year cures" or "ten-year cures"—the time that elapses after the operation without evidence of recurrence—rather than of absolute cures. There are cases in which previous cancers have recurred fifteen or twenty years following surgery, but most patients with "five-year cures" have a very good chance of escaping any recurrence, and those with "ten-year cures" rarely have further trouble. On balance, the record for this kind of cancer is remarkably hopeful. One out of three victims who come to surgery today, including both those with very early cancer and those with an advanced cancer that has already spread, will remain free of recurrence five years later. Among those who show no evidence of lymph node involvement during surgery, almost 90 percent will reach the five-year point without recurrence, and most will achieve ten-year cures. Thus the woman who is diagnosed and treated early enough has an excellent chance of escaping any recurrence at all.

Even for those with more advanced or recurrent cancer of the breast the picture is by no means altogether gloomy. Over the years many ways to check the spread and further development of breast cancer have been devised, each approach effective in its own way. For example, because estrogen is known to stimulate the growth of breast cancers, various means of reducing estrogen levels in patients with recurrent cancer can be used. In some cases surgical removal first of the ovaries and then of the adrenal glands reduces estrogen levels enough to check progress of the cancer for months or even years. Because the male hormone androgen seems to balance or counteract the effect of estrogen, administration of this hormone often slows the cancer's growth. X-ray therapy is also effective, applied to target areas where recurrent disease has been discovered. Finally, a variety of potent anticancer drugs is available for use as needed. Each case is different, and the pattern of treatment will vary from patient to patient as the doctor seeks to block the cancer as long as possible at each stage while keeping the patient comfortable and active. With our present-day knowledge of this disease and the benefits of early diagnosis, skillful surgery and carefully planned and individualized follow-up treatment, recurrent breast cancer often behaves more like a prolonged, chronic illness than like the devastatingly fatal disease that most women imagine, and many victims can survive with it for years with only minimal discomfort. But for reasons unknown, others may pursue a swift, inexorable downward course and die from the disease within a few months.

Self-Examination of the Breasts

There is no question, however, that the best protection against the threat of breast cancer, bar none, lies in early detection of lumps or masses in the breast, and here no doctor can possibly help a woman as much as she can help herself. Surgeons know that fewer than 20 percent of all cases of breast cancer are first discovered by a doctor; eight times out of ten the first sign—a lump in the breast—is discovered by the woman herself in the course of *self-examination of the breasts.*

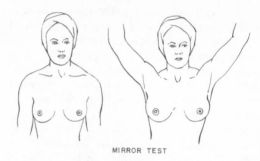

MIRROR TEST

Figure 34–2.

This procedure is so simple and effective that it should be performed regularly and faithfully at least once a month by every woman from the age of puberty on, and most particularly after menopause. The ideal time for this self-examination is approximately a week after the end of a menstrual period when any normal cyclic hormonal changes in the breasts have subsided. It is exactly the same sort of breast examination done by a doctor during a physical exam, except that it is performed by the woman herself, and when done regularly, the woman becomes so thoroughly familiar with the normal appearance and structure of her own breasts that she can easily detect any change from the normal that may occur between regular medical examinations. First, the breasts are inspected in the mirror, both with the arms held down and with them raised, to detect any sign of asymmetry, "dimpling" or denting of the skin, or change in the nipples. Next each breast is divided into imaginary quadrants and gently but methodically

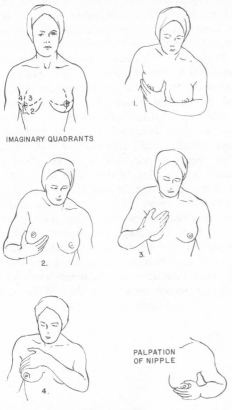

IMAGINARY QUADRANTS

PALPATION
OF NIPPLE

Figure 34–3.
Self-palpation of breasts.

palpated, quadrant by quadrant, for any sign of a lump or mass that was not present at the last self-examination. The woman soon becomes familiar with the slightly ropy or nodular texture of her own breasts, so that even a minor change will be apparent. Next the nipple is palpated for any abnormal lumps, and squeezed gently for any sign of exudate or blood. Finally, the armpit is palpated with the arm half raised to detect any swelling or soreness of the lymph glands in the axilla. The whole procedure takes less than 5 minutes, and simple as it may seem, it is more effective than anything else in bringing to light

any lump or enlargement that might be an early cancer.

Of course the mere discovery of some change in breast tissue during this self-examination is not enough. Any change should be called to a doctor's attention *immediately* so that definitive diagnosis can be made. Some breast cancers develop so quickly that the first signs can appear between one monthly self-examination and the next, and it is a supreme tragedy for a woman who has found a lump in her breast to delay seeing her doctor for weeks or months in the hope that the lump will go away. If it is cancer, it will not, and delay may allow the disease to advance until permanent cure becomes impossible. Finally, as important as self-examination is, periodic breast examinations by a physician are equally important, preferably at six-month intervals.

Cosmetic Breast Surgery

The breasts, like the other tissues and organs of the cutaneous system, are external and visible, and apart from their physical function, they inevitably play a role in a woman's overall appearance. That role has varied enormously throughout history and even in the last few decades. In the 1920s breasts were strapped down to achieve a "tomboy" look; later they were padded and supported in positions of unnatural prominence, and while that fashion still prevails, many young women today have chosen a more natural "braless" look. The breasts are also richly endowed with sensory nerve endings and as such play a role in sexual relations, in many cases no less important to the man than to the woman. It may very well be that this importance is exaggerated in our society, but whenever physical appearance or sexual attractiveness is at issue, the question of improving upon nature inevitably arises. Many women are dissatisfied in one way or another with their breasts, and both men and women quite erroneously relate breast size or shape to sexual capacity. Small-breasted women in particular may feel handicapped, and surgeons, particularly those specializing in plastic and reconstructive surgery, have found a solution. Today a truly remarkable variety of so-called augmentation or breast enhancement procedures can be performed, when desired, with reasonable success and safety. Most such procedures involve implantation of inserts—even balloons—made of silicone rubber, silastic or other comparatively inert foreign materials beneath the breasts. Some surgeons raise pads of fat from the lower chest wall or elsewhere for implantation beneath the breasts, and new techniques are constantly being explored. This in itself would suggest that no one procedure yet devised has proved to be ideal.

Is this kind of surgery really justified? No one but the patient herself can really say. The value of large breasts might be questioned, but the psychological discomfort that accompanies a physical handicap, real or imagined, cannot be discounted. Unfortunately, breast augmentation may not be the best solution; and any woman contemplating such surgery should first consult family and friends, and particularly a trusted medical adviser, to help her determine all the possible advantages and disadvantages. The long-term results of cosmetic breast surgery cannot be guaranteed, and the aftereffects may be as difficult to deal with psychologically as the condition it attempted to correct. The appearance of the breasts, when the normal aging process begins, must also be considered. Thus in most cases it is probably better, from the standpoint of long-term appearance and general health, to leave nature alone, unless compelling professional or personal circumstances make cosmetic surgery seem worthwhile.

The same surgical techniques that have made the various "breast augmentation" procedures possible have, however, proven extremely beneficial in medical rather than cosmetic areas. Women with breast hypertrophy, for example, can be truly burdened by disproportionately large breasts, and reconstructive surgery can often help reduce this handicap. Women's breasts are also highly vulnerable to trauma of all sorts, including lacerations in automobile accidents or blows which can lead to scarring and other deformities. Here again skillful reconstructive surgery may help restore a severely damaged breast to normal appearance. Finally, these same techniques can be employed following breast biopsies to help minimize any scarring or other minor deformities that might result from such very necessary procedures.

VIII

PATTERNS OF ILLNESS: THE RESPIRATORY TRACT

35. Respiration and Life   455

36. Chest Injuries, Mechanical Obstructions and Respiratory Tract Infections   464

37. Hay Fever, Asthma and Emphysema   490

38. Tumors of the Respiratory Tract   498

Of all the vital body functions upon which we depend there is none of which we are more consciously and immediately aware than respiration, the continuous and rhythmic process by which fresh air is drawn into the lungs and stale air expelled. This awareness of our breathing arises in part from the fact that we can voluntarily control the process to a certain degree; but even more, we are aware of respiration because of the immediate and compelling distress that we suffer any time some disorder interferes even briefly with the free flow of air in and out of the lungs.

Most diseases of the respiratory system do just that, in one way or another, and thus respiratory illnesses are among the most alarming and acutely symptomatic of all health disorders. Because of its unique physical structure—a hollow, expansible organ system supported and protected only by a thin cage of bone and muscle—the respiratory tract is particularly vulnerable to physical injury and mechanical damage to its function. Because the air tubes, large and small, are lined with a moist mucous membrane that constantly comes in contact with air from the outside, this organ system is especially vulnerable to infection. In addition, part of its normal defense mechanism—the production of protective mucus to keep the interior of the air tubes moist—can also lead to various forms of internal bronchial obstruction that prevents oxygen from reaching the delicate gas-exchange membrane that makes up the lung tissue itself. Other disorders may arise as a result of acute or chronic allergic reactions, or from the growth of benign or malignant tumors. But because so many respiratory system diseases produce early and easily recognizable symptoms, and because so many of these conditions respond readily to well-directed early treatment, it is doubly important not only to understand how disease processes can impair normal respiratory function, but also to recognize the significance of respiratory symptoms when they occur, so that medical aid can be sought before minor and correctable respiratory disorders can evolve into serious and crippling diseases.

Respiration and Life

Even in this era of ever accelerating biomedical research, no one yet has identified all of the links in the intricate chain of mechanical, physical and chemical events that constitute the process of life. Over the years, however, bits and pieces of the puzzle have fallen into place. Today we know of many factors essential to human life, and paramount to all others is the body's continuous, unflagging need for *oxygen.* The equation is simple: as long as fresh oxygen is available to every cell in the body at all times, life remains possible; without it, we die. Oxygen is the vital substance that provides us with internal body heat and the endless supply of raw energy our cells and organ systems must have to continue functioning. It is essential to innumerable of the biochemical reactions that occur within our cells which, taken together, we know as *metabolism,* and there is no known substitute for it.

Fortunately, we live on a planet that is fantastically rich in oxygen. As a free gas, this element makes up approximately 20 percent of the Earth's atmosphere at sea level, a quantity constantly replenished by green growing plants all over the world. Much of the Earth's crust is composed of oxygen compounds, and the water in our streams, lakes and oceans not only holds great quantities of oxygen in solution, but is itself a compound of oxygen and hydrogen. We face no oxygen shortage here; but to utilize the abundance of oxygen around us, our bodies must have some means of taking it in and transporting it to the cells and tissues. We must also have some means for expelling excess quantities of a major metabolic waste product—*carbon dioxide*—from the body into the atmosphere. This continuing exchange of atmospheric gases —the inhalation of oxygen and the expiration of carbon dioxide—is a process known as *respiration,* and it is carried on by the lungs and other tissues and organs that make up the *respiratory system.*

The Process of Respiration

The normal anatomical structure of the respiratory system was outlined briefly in an earlier section. (*See* p. 62.) Vital to the entire process of respiration is the function of a remarkable layer of tissue, the *respiratory membrane,* which forms a lining just one cell layer thick around the innumerable tiny air sacs or *alveoli* within the lungs. It is this filamentous layer of cells, far thinner than the thinnest man-made cellophane wrapper, with its many folds and pockets covering a surface area of more than 600 square feet, that permits oxygen that is pulled into the lungs from the atmosphere to "cross through" into the blood stream. It also permits carbon dioxide to pass out of the blood stream into the lungs, where it can be expelled. But far more is involved in the process of respiration than the function of this respiratory membrane alone. Other organs of the respiratory system must pull air into the lungs in the first place. Once oxygen is absorbed, it must be carried in the blood to distant parts of the body by the *circulatory system,* and carbon dioxide must be collected from the cells and brought back to the lungs by the same means. Finally, the operation of both the respiratory system and the circulatory system must be delicately monitored and controlled, day and night, by the action of exquisitely sensitive nerve control centers in the brain stem, a part of the *nervous system.* Ultimately it is the inter-working of all three of these major organ systems that makes the process of respiration possible and allows our cells and tissues the constant supply of oxygen necessary for life.

The Respiratory Tree. In order to reach the respiratory membrane, oxygen in the atmosphere must first be drawn into the lungs through the nose or mouth and passed down a series of branching conduits known as the respiratory tree. Air brought in through the nose or mouth is warmed and humidified by contact with the mucous membrane lining the nasal passages, the back of the throat above the soft palate, known as the *nasopharynx,* and the cavelike *pharynx* proper which forms the arch of the throat below the soft palate. Air is warmed, humidified and cleansed more effectively when it enters by the nasal route, but this means of entrance is narrower than the mouth, so that most people who breathe quietly through the nose under normal circumstances will unconsciously resort to mouth breathing when they need more air. As an additional protection against inhaling pathogenic bacteria into the lungs, the entire nasopharynx and pharynx are lined with soft, spongy lymphoid tissue, including the *tonsils* guarding the pharynx and the *adenoids* located on the upper surface of the soft palate in the floor of the nasopharynx. Aside from these protective mechanisms, the nose, mouth and pharyngeal cavity also serve as a resonating chamber, greatly affecting the magnitude and timbre of the voice.

In back of the soft palate, the nasopharynx and the pharynx join to form a downward funnel which directs inhaled air into the great air tube or *trachea,* the main trunk of the respiratory tree. This tube, approximately an inch in diameter and held open by rings of cartilage in its walls, lies in the midline of the neck in front just beneath the skin, subcutaneous tissue and

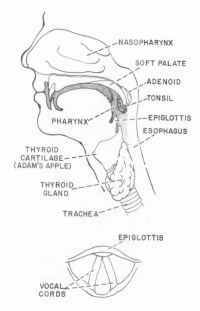

Figure 35–1.

neck muscles. Immediately behind it is the *esophagus,* which carries food from the mouth to the stomach, since the mouth serves for eating as well as for intake of air. The two tubes are separated by a small flap of tissue known as the *epiglottis,* which acts as an ingenious sort of flutter valve, blocking off the esophagus while air is being drawn into the trachea and closing the trachea during the process of swallowing food. This mechanism, which works automatically to keep food out of the trachea and air out of the esophagus, is not fail-safe, however. It is perfectly possible to swallow air; everybody does it inadvertently to some extent, and in extreme cases it becomes a nervous habit known as *aerophagia.* Similarly, food may be inadvertently inhaled or *aspirated* into the trachea, leading to a violent reflex action of coughing until the foreign material is expelled.

In the upper two inches of the trachea just below the epiglottis is a structure known as the *larynx* or voice box, an enlarged cartilaginous chamber which is palpable as the *Adam's apple* in the front of the throat. The larynx is equipped with two thin semicircular membranes, the *vocal cords,* which normally relax to allow air to pass, but can be stretched tight to vibrate as air moves past them when a person wishes to speak or make other vocal sounds. The vocal cords work most efficiently for sound production during the exhalation phase of respiratory movements, but less well modulated and controlled sounds can also be made during inhalation.

Below the larynx inhaled oxygen has a clear passage down the central column of the trachea to a point about five inches below the upper notch of the breastbone, where it branches into two *mainstem bronchi,* one of which leads into each side of the chest cavity. A few inches farther along, each of these bronchi begins to branch and branch again into progressively smaller bronchi; with each branching the supporting rings of cartilage become less and less significant until they disappear completely in the tiny tubules known as *bronchioles* which are composed entirely of elastic connective tissue and smooth muscle fibers. Finally, after many more branchings, each bronchiole opens into a cluster of tiny, elastic alveolar air sacs, and multitudes of these alveoli, lined with the moist, delicate respiratory membrane, make up the soft, spongy and expandable tissue of the lungs themselves. Thus the air brought in through the nose and mouth with each breath ultimately reaches the alveoli in the lungs, and from there oxygen molecules can pass through the respiratory membrane into the blood stream.

This entire respiratory tree, from the upper end of the trachea to the tiniest bronchioles, is lined with a membrane containing mucus-producing cells which help keep the whole system of tubules moist. In addition, the cells of this mucous membrane are equipped with tiny hairlike projections known as *cilia* which have the job of keeping the airways clean. These cilia are constantly in motion, waving or beating like a field of wheat toward the upper end of the respiratory tree and carrying inhaled particles and mucus up from the bronchioles into the bronchi and thence on up into the trachea, where they can be expelled by coughing, sneezing or clearing the throat. Many surgeons today believe that this action of the cilia in cleansing the respiratory tree is all-important to the maintenance of a healthy respiratory tract, and that it

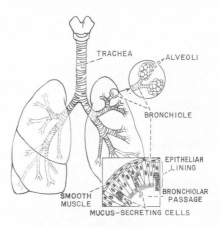

TRACHEA   ALVEOLI   BRONCHIOLE   EPITHELIAR LINING   BRONCHIOLAR PASSAGE   SMOOTH MUSCLE   MUCUS-SECRETING CELLS

Figure 35–2.

is only when the cilia in some areas are destroyed beyond recovery by chronic infection or recurrent contact with tobacco smoke that such destructive diseases as bronchiectasis (*see* p. 476) or lung cancer (*see* p. 500) can get their start.

The Mechanics of Breathing. Before oxygen can reach the respiratory membrane, however, it must be drawn into the lungs, and exhausted air must be expelled, in the rhythmic, bellows-like action of respiration or breathing. In addition, the lungs as well as the heart, which are among the most delicate organs of the body, must be well protected from accidental injury. Both the mechanics of breathing and the protection of the heart and lungs depend upon the physical construction of the *thorax* or chest cavity, a virtual miracle of structural engineering. The ribs encased in layers of muscle, the breastbone or *sternum,* and the upper vertebrae of the backbone form a strong but elastic "cage" for the lungs, the heart, the trachea and the esophagus. The sternum, which is attached to the upper six ribs in front by means of cartilaginous bridges, acts as a shield for the vital structures of the "life stem" or *mediastinum* running down the center of the chest. This "life stem" contains the heart, the trachea and mainstem bronchi, the pulmonary arteries and veins, the aorta and the vena cava—the great vein which runs up from the abdomen to enter the rear of the heart. All of these structures are arranged in a column or conduit beginning at about the level of the top of

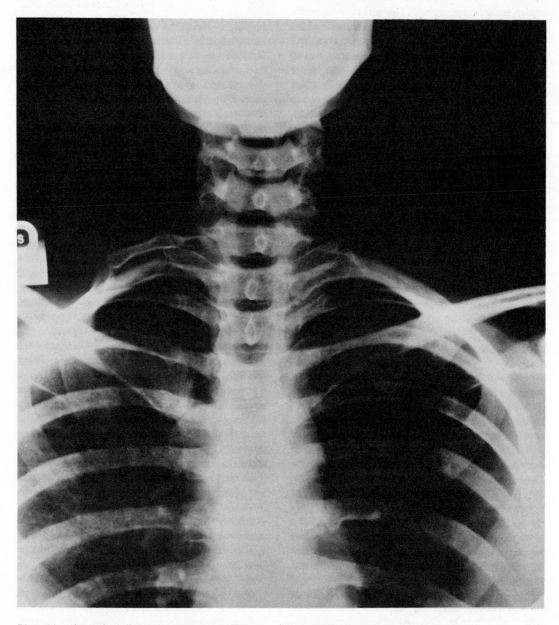

Plate 11　A cervical rib in a young woman. This short "extra rib" can be seen on the patient's right side, above the uppermost normal rib and articulating with the 7th cervical vertebra. This uncommon oddity can cause nervous and circulatory difficulty in the affected arm. A smaller rudimentary cervical rib is also present on the patient's left side.

the sternum and extending down to the *diaphragm,* the smoothly curving layer of muscle which forms the bottom of the chest cavity. This mediastinal column varies from three to six inches in diameter and is arranged just as an architect arranges the main electrical and plumbing conduits in a new house, in a centralized well-protected place. Thus these vital organs are shielded against shocks and blows so that their function is not impaired except in cases of severe penetrating or crushing injuries.

The thoracic cage, however, is not fixed in a solid piece, for it must enlarge and diminish as the lungs take in and expel air. Therefore, in addition to their elastic cartilage attachment to the sternum in front, the ribs are connected to the vertebrae in back by means of shallow ball-and-socket joints, so that each rib can move slightly up and down with the rhythmic breathing motions. Below the level of the sixth rib, the ribs themselves are shorter, with progressively longer cartilaginous bridges to the sternum; indeed, the twelfth and lowest rib has no cartilaginous attachment in front at all and for this reason is called the "floating rib." With no weight-bearing function to perform, the ribs are thin, curved and flattened bones, slightly flexible so that even severe blows to the chest can often be absorbed without fractures. Finally, they are bound loosely together with fibrous tissue and with strips of muscle spanning the space from one rib to the next, the *intercostal* ("between rib") *muscles.*

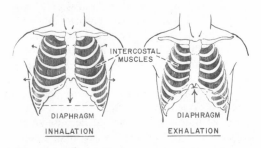

INTERCOSTAL MUSCLES

DIAPHRAGM
INHALATION

DIAPHRAGM
EXHALATION

Figure 35–3.

Breathing itself—the rhythmic filling and emptying of the lungs—is made possible in part by the action of these intercostal muscles pulling the ribs closer together during exhalation (thus diminishing the space within the chest cavity) and relaxing to allow the ribs to spread apart during inhalation (thus increasing the room within the chest). But even more important to respiration is the action of the diaphragm in coordination with the muscles of the abdominal wall. In its normally relaxed position, the diaphragm forms a curving dome that extends up into the chest cavity from the rear and then down to its attachment in the front just under the edge of the rib cage. When this broad, thin muscle contracts, its upward curve is flattened at the same time that the intercostal muscles relax, allowing the ribs to spread. This, in effect, sharply decreases air pressure within the chest cavity, so that air is pulled in as the lungs expand to fill up the extra space created. Once the lungs are fully inflated, the diaphragm relaxes, bulging up into the bottom of the thorax again and pressing air out of the lungs at the same time that the intercostal muscles contract and draw the ribs together. Toward the end of exhalation, still more air is expelled when the powerful striplike muscles that extend down the front of the abdomen tighten and press the abdominal organs up firmly against the diaphragm from below. Indeed, once normal exhalation is completed, still more air can be expelled from the lungs in a *forced exhalation* by further tightening of these abdominal muscles—exactly what happens, for example, when we cough or sneeze. Finally, the large *pectoral muscles* crossing the front of the chest from shoulder to midline further aid expansion and contraction of the chest cavity by their contraction and relaxation.

The Control of Breathing. Although breathing is largely a muscular function, the entire process is primarily controlled by a group of nerve cells located in the brain stem and known as the *respiratory center.* One might think that these cells would be specially attuned to the amount of oxygen in the blood stream, but this is not the case. Rather, it is the amount of carbon dioxide dissolved in the blood that determines, to a large extent, how fast or slowly we breathe. The nerve cells in the respiratory center are singularly sensitive to this substance, and when too much piles up in the blood these cells send off automatic signals that stimulate the respiratory muscles to do their work, so that breathing becomes deeper and more rapid. As a result, the excess carbon dioxide is "blown off" or exhaled by the lungs very quickly and its concentration in the blood stream falls sharply; but once it reaches a certain level, the respiratory center slows down its signals again, so that fewer and shallower breaths are taken until the carbon dioxide blood level builds up to normal again. Under most circumstances this automatic regulatory system works very smoothly and subtly, guaranteeing respiration at the proper rate of speed to maintain adequate oxygen flow into the lungs while simultaneously removing adequate amounts of carbon dioxide.

We are able, however, to override this delicate respiratory center control system and exercise voluntary control over our breathing, at least to a certain extent. It is possible, for example, to "hold our breath" for a brief period in spite of respiratory center signals to start breathing. This voluntary control makes underwater swimming possible, and permits us to stop breathing long enough to keep out noxious materials which we consciously detect contaminating the air. But it is also sharply limited, and in a crisis the respiratory center will automatically take over preemptory control. Thus it is impossible to commit suicide by holding one's breath; as soon as the higher brain centers are affected by oxygen hunger and increased concentrations of carbon dioxide, the individual loses consciousness, voluntary control of the breathing is also lost, and the respiratory center takes over to bring things back to normal.

The Respiratory Membrane. It is only when oxygen has been inhaled into the lungs and brought in contact with the respiratory membrane in the alveoli that the really vital function of the respiratory system can begin: the passage of oxygen through this membrane into the blood stream, and the simultaneous passage of excess quantities of carbon dioxide from the blood stream back into the lungs to be exhaled. However, oxygen does not diffuse into the blood as a free gas, but must be dissolved in moisture before passing through the membrane and into the capillaries. Similarly, carbon dioxide is dis-solved in the blood stream and diffuses through the respiratory membrane in a water solution before it is released into the alveoli as a gas. Thus the interior of the lung must always be kept moist, and the bronchioles and bronchi of the respiratory tree are lined with tiny glands which produce a thin, slightly sticky mucus to perform this function, as well as to help trap fragments of dust, smoke or other foreign materials inhaled with the air.

Special chemical reactions also help this simultaneous exchange of oxygen and carbon dioxide through the respiratory membrane. In the case of oxygen, a chemical substance known as *hemoglobin,* which is carried in the red blood cells, has the power to hold and bind oxygen. The lung capillaries are tiny blood vessels which, like the respiratory membrane itself, are only a single cell layer thick. They are so arranged that they lie in direct contact with the inside of the respiratory membrane throughout the lung. Each oxygen molecule passing through this double membrane into the lung capillaries is caught and bound by a hemoglobin molecule in a red blood cell and immediately swept away in the blood stream. Far more oxygen can thus be absorbed per unit of surface area of lung tissue than would occur if the absorption depended merely on the diffusion of a dissolved gas back and forth across the membrane barrier. The expulsion of carbon dioxide from the blood stream into the lung is similarly speeded by means of a biochemical reaction involving an enzyme called *carbonic anhydrase,* so that the dissolved carbon dioxide is almost literally "pushed out" of the blood stream through the respiratory membrane into the lung. Without this mechanism the period of time available for gas exchange with each respiration (about .6 of a second) would not be sufficient for the necessary amount of carbon dioxide to be expelled.

Respiration and Circulation. Because so much oxygen must be absorbed in so small a volume of space, the capillary bed supplying blood to the lungs is one of the richest in the body; virtually every fraction of an inch of the surface area of the respiratory membrane is in contact with a capillary blood vessel. These capillaries are fed by two pulmonary arteries extending from the heart, one to each lung, and are drained by four pulmonary veins, two returning to the heart from each lung. This special *pulmonary circulatory system* must carry just as much blood through the lungs in a minute as is distributed through all the rest of the general circulation in the same minute; and in a rapid and single circuit through the lung, oxygen-exhausted blood which is overloaded with carbon dioxide must simultaneously become oxygen-enriched and depleted of carbon dioxide waste, then returned to the heart ready for recirculation to the most distant cells.

Thus respiration and circulation work together with marvelous ingenuity. Indeed, the two processes are so closely interrelated that physicians often speak of the cardiovascular and the respiratory systems combined as a single great *cardiorespiratory system.* This terminology seems particularly appropriate in the case of modern heart surgery when both circulation of the blood and its oxygenation and the removal of carbon dioxide may be temporarily turned over to a *heart-lung machine.* In order to permit the surgeon sufficient time to make delicate repairs of the heart, the machine takes over the patient's vital circulatory and respiratory functions, prevents hemorrhaging, and keeps the surgeon's operative field clear of excess amounts of blood.

Obviously, then, the supply of oxygen to tissues in all parts of the body depends upon far more than just the respiratory system alone. It also depends upon the proper coordinated function of the circulatory system, the musculoskeletal system and the nervous system. Working together, these systems meet the body's widely varying needs of oxygen over a broad span of daily activities. Normally, an adult inhales and exhales in a smooth, unbroken rhythm approximately 12 to 14 times per minute, but during periods of strenuous activity this rate may increase quite automatically to 30 or more respirations per minute, a point at which we are virtually panting, while during deep sleep it may decline, equally automatically, to as few as 7 or 8 long, deep respirations per minute.

One of the most remarkable things about the process of respiration is the way it so effectively fulfills our need for oxygen with relatively little expenditure of energy. Ordinarily the amount of air drawn in and then expelled with each respiratory cycle is not very large—perhaps no more than 400 or 500 cubic centimeters, or somewhat less than a pint. During forced inspiration and expiration, the average-sized man can virtually double this so-called tidal flow of air, sucking in as much as a liter of air (1,000 cubic centimeters, or slightly more than a quart) and expelling the same amount with each breath. The maximum amount of air that can be sucked into the lungs in forced respiration will, of course, differ with each individual; a small man will be able to inhale less, a large man or a conditioned athlete considerably more than average. But for each person this volume of air is known as his *vital capacity,* and careful measurement of this quantity, usually surprisingly constant for each individual, can provide the physician with an extremely valuable gauge of the degree of damage or impairment to respiration that may be resulting from a wide variety of respiratory illnesses.

Oddly enough, however, most of the inhaled air never gets anywhere near the terminal air sacs making up the spongy mass of lung tissue, at least not directly. As it is carried turbulently into the bronchi and then fills the bronchioles, oxygen from the air reaches the terminal air sacs by a process of diffusion, and exhausted air containing carbon dioxide reaches the bronchioles and bronchi for expulsion by the same means. Thus, the air that is exhaled is not by any means "poisoned" or "dead"; it contains almost as much oxygen as the air that is inhaled, and only slightly more carbon dioxide. Recognition of this fact has led to the use of *mouth-to-mouth resuscitation* as a superior means of artificial respiration to provide oxygen to an individual who has stopped breathing due to drowning, asphyxiation or some other cause. Paradoxically, it was found that far more oxygen could be forced into such a victim's lungs by another person blowing his own expelled air directly into the victim's mouth than by the manual artificial respiration methods designed to "squeeze" air in and out of the lungs.

Even with the inhalation of fresh atmospheric

air, however, the actual amount of gases exchanged across the respiratory membrane during any one breath is surprisingly small. The oxygen content of atmospheric air is approximately 20 percent, and the air expelled from the lungs during exhalation still contains 17 to 18 percent of oxygen. Similarly, although inhaled air normally contains less than .5 percent carbon dioxide, the amount contained in exhaled air is only some 2 to 3 percent; and a sampling of the air from the alveoli themselves, where carbon dioxide concentration is highest, still measures only 5 to 6 percent.

Yet even these apparently small amounts of gases exchanged across the membrane breath after breath are quite sufficient to meet the needs of the body, and air passing through the respiratory system in one direction or another also enables us to speak, sing, whistle and even snore. Ordinarily respiration proceeds from the moment of birth to the moment of death without interruption, and with very little effort on our part, providing the respiratory tree is unobstructed and the tissues and organs that make up the system function without any impairment. Under certain circumstances, however, we can experience a variety of perfectly normal curiosities of respiration, many of them reflex responses designed to keep the airway open and clear for the free flow of oxygen. Any irritation of the nasal passages, nasopharynx or throat, for example, may trigger a sudden, violent expiratory burst or *sneeze* which helps expel irritating foreign bodies from the upper part of the respiratory tree. The accidental introduction of foreign material such as food into the trachea, or the accumulation of an excess of mucus in the bronchi, will stimulate *coughing,* a high-pressure, explosive exhalation caused when the respiratory muscles of the chest and the abdominal muscles tighten while the glottis is closed until enough pressure builds up in the thorax to force the glottis to pop open like a pressure valve and release a burst of air. When we are tired, bored or drowsy, yet refuse to succumb to sleep, our respiratory rate nevertheless slows and our respirations become shallow until we *yawn* as a normal reflex response to a piling up of carbon dioxide in the blood stream, an excellent hint

that it is time to suspend physical activity for a while. Occasionally, when something irritates the diaphragm or the phrenic nerve which controls it, that muscle may go into brief involuntary spasms which cause sudden, short, cut-off inhalations we recognize as *hiccups,* a matter of serious concern only if they occur while we are eating, with the attendant danger of aspirating some food, or when they continue for a prolonged period of time.

There are, however, other respiratory conditions that are not normal and that cannot be effectively handled by the body's reflex reactions or defense mechanisms. Obviously, respiration cannot proceed at all if something impairs the mechanical process of breathing. Physical injuries—fractures of the bony rib cage, penetrating wounds of the chest or crushing injuries, for example—can easily compromise the breathing mechanism and constitute a grave respiratory hazard. Even a relatively minor injury such as a single cracked rib may be so very painful that the rise and fall of the thorax during respiration is agonizing and makes the act of breathing difficult. Similarly, any kind of obstruction in the airway, whether it occurs in the nose and throat, in the trachea or anywhere else in the respiratory tree down to the tiniest bronchioles, can prevent the vital flow of oxygen to the respiratory membrane. Such obstructions are often caused by foreign bodies that become lodged in the respiratory tree, but the swelling of infected tissue in the throat or the plugging up of bronchi and bronchioles with excess mucus may also be seriously obstructive. Indeed, infection of the respiratory tract, whether it involves the air tubes themselves (upper respiratory infections) or the alveolar tissue of the lung, including the respiratory membrane (lower respiratory infections), constitutes the single largest and most dangerous group of respiratory disorders. But tumors and other tissue-destroying lesions in the lung can also be a hazard, impairing respiration either by infiltration of healthy lung tissue with cancerous growth or by outright destruction of that tissue by scarring and fibrosis. Certain respiratory tract disorders do not fit neatly into any of these categories—such conditions as inflammation of the pleural lining of the lungs known as *pleuritis,* the catastrophic collapse of a lung known as *spontaneous pneumothorax,* or certain less dramatic but equally dangerous conditions, including *atelectasis* (collapse of a segment of lung) and the scarring and fibrosis of lung tissue known as *pulmonary emphysema.*

Finally, a number of diseases and disorders which affect the body's ability to breathe do not have any direct effect upon the organs of the respiratory system, but rather result from damage or impairment of the other organ systems which are essential to the overall respiratory process. A brain tumor, for example, may cause pressure or damage to the respiratory center and lead to a disturbance of the pattern of breathing. Cerebrovascular accidents—hemorrhages or strokes—may also impair the respiratory center's function, causing temporary or permanent disturbance in the respiratory rhythm. In poliomyelitis, destruction of the nerve cells that control the activities of the voluntary muscles may cause paralysis of the diaphragm, and respiration must therefore be maintained artificially by means of a respirator or "iron lung" temporarily until the affected nerve cells recover, or even permanently if they do not recover. And such conditions as a pulmonary embolus, in which circulation of blood to the lungs is obstructed by a blood clot, or even the impaired circulation of congestive heart failure, can seriously compromise the respiratory process. Whereas none of these conditions is truly a disorder of the respiratory tract itself, any or all may hinder or even prevent the vital supply of oxygen flowing to the tissues and, if severe enough, may lead to serious illness, shock or even death.

Some respiratory tract conditions are commonplace and mild, others grave, but it is important to know what they are, how they come about, how they are recognized and treated, and above all, what can be done to prevent them, or to speed up healing and prevent recurrence once they are already present. And nowhere is this knowledge more important than in dealing with three groups of conditions to which the respiratory system is singularly vulnerable: physical injuries of the chest, mechanical respiratory obstructions and respiratory infections of all kinds.

Chest Injuries, Mechanical Obstructions and Respiratory Tract Infections

Physical injuries to the chest, mechanical obstructions of the airway or respiratory infections all may cause swift and severe respiratory embarrassment; infections alone are the most frequently encountered of all respiratory tract disorders. Knowledge of why these conditions are dangerous and what can be done about them often makes the difference between speedy recovery and prolonged illness.

Physical Injuries to the Chest

For all its built-in strength and elasticity, the chest is still vulnerable to injury and resulting hazard to respiratory function. Automobile accidents may result in the fracture of ribs, collarbone or sternum, internal injuries to the lungs or heart, or even open lacerations of the chest. Penetrating wounds due to bullets, knives or falls upon projecting objects can damage the lungs or heart and threaten life itself. Injuries may also affect nearby organs in the abdomen, neck, or shoulder girdle, and certain special complications often impair respiration further. Thus, any chest injury requires immediate medical attention and may constitute a major medical emergency.

Fractures. A fracture of ribs, sternum, collarbone or shoulder blade is as serious as any other fracture because of injury to the body's skeletal framework, and must be treated just like any other fracture to restore the structural integrity of the body. (*See* p. 300.) But chest fractures are especially hazardous because of the threat to

respiratory function. A chest injury may result in the fracture of one or more ribs on either or both sides; how badly respiration is impaired depends on the severity of the injury. One might crack a single rib without even recognizing it, suffering only from persisting soreness in the injured area for a few weeks. But if a rib is fractured through, it will cause severe pain because of tearing or stretching of the *pleura,* the delicate, pain-sensitive layer of epithelium that covers the lungs themselves and then folds back to form a slippery lining on the inside of the rib cage. In such a fracture the individual "splints" or involuntarily tightens the muscles on the injured side, since the pain is aggravated by respiratory movements. This kind of splinting, in effect, throws the burden of respiration on the other lung and may contribute to the development of bronchial infection or stasis pneumonia in the lung on the injured side. If a fractured rib is displaced, a sharp spicule of bone may actually penetrate the lung, allowing air to leak out into the chest cavity and forcing partial or complete collapse of the lung. Blood may also leak into the chest cavity, preventing full expansion of the lung. Such an injury may cause shock, pain and severe respiratory embarrassment.

Doctors rarely attempt to "set" broken ribs in the sense of replacing them mechanically in their normal position. If a partial or complete collapse of a lung results from a rib fracture, the air leaking out of the lung into the chest cavity may be removed by the surgeon with the use of a drain inserted between the ribs, permitting the lung to reexpand. Medicines are used to relieve the sharp pleuritic pain. As long as respiratory movements can be maintained, and the fractured rib held moderately stable by strapping the injured side of the chest, the rib will proceed to heal remarkably well even if the displaced ends of the fracture lie as much as an inch or two apart. The final healing may not be in perfect alignment, but that is not important; what is important is fixing the fractured rib into a single curved but flexible piece again.

Fractured ribs usually heal well, but many victims are alarmed at the time required for the pain to go away. Unfortunately, some pain will persist as long as the sensitive pleura in the area of the injury is irritated in the slightest. If the injury is under a doctor's care, with attention given to the possibility of such complications as lung collapse, pleuritis, effusion of fluid into the chest cavity, bronchitis or pneumonia, there is no need to be alarmed if episodes of pain recur for weeks or months. Complications are relatively easy to detect and can be treated effectively if they appear; and as the bone heals, the pain will gradually decrease even though months may pass before discomfort completely disappears.

More severe chest injuries can pose a greater threat to respiration. One of the most threatening is a crushing injury with ribs fractured on both sides, so that there is no solid structure anchoring the chest wall in the area of the injury. In this condition, known as a "flail chest," the injured segment of chest tends to be pulled inward during inspiration and pushed outward during expiration, exactly opposite from the normal movement of respiration. The lungs themselves are often damaged in such injuries as well as the ribs, and complications are common, so that there may be a prolonged period of touch-and-go and the victim must remain under close hospital observation. Respiratory support with a mechanical breathing device, and some means of immobilizing the flail segment of the chest wall may be necessary until healing of the ribs begins. Such an injury may also cause damage to the heart, with the added threat of irregularities of heartbeat or congestive heart failure. Modern surgery and respiratory support mechanisms have improved chances for recovery from severe crushing injuries of the chest immeasurably, if the victim can survive the shock and respiratory impairment during the first few hours or days following the injury.

Injuries to other structures surrounding the chest cavity may also affect respiration. A fractured collarbone, shoulder or shoulder blade may injure the pleura at the upper point of the lung or even involve the lung itself. Injury to the lower rib cage may not only fracture ribs but also cause internal injury to the spleen or liver, organs which lie in the abdomen up under the rib margin on either side. Injury to the ribs in back may also involve the kidneys. Obviously, injuries such as these also demand prompt medical attention.

Penetrating Wounds. Bullet wounds, knife wounds or impalement of the chest on sharp projecting objects may cause immediate internal injury to the heart or lung as well as damage to the ribs and always require immediate medical treatment. Most such injuries involve bleeding into the chest cavity or into the lung tissue itself, causing the victim to cough up bright red frothy blood. Blood in the chest cavity tends to pool below the lung and prevent it from expanding fully. If air leaks from the lung into the chest cavity, the lung will partially collapse, a condition know as *pneumothorax* or "air in the chest." Occasionally an opening into the chest wall will form a sort of one-way valve so that air is sucked into the chest cavity from the outside and then is blocked from escaping. Such a condition results in a rapidly developing *pressure pneumothorax*, which can collapse an entire lung in very short order unless the condition is discovered and this kind of "air suction" prevented by taping the wound tightly with several layers of adhesive tape, or even holding a piece of plastic wrap over it, gently but firmly, with the hand until medical aid can be summoned. Infection of the wound is another threat, and it may lead to scarring of lung tissue to the chest wall at the site of the injury, a condition known as *fibrothorax,* or the development of *empyema* (pus in the chest cavity) or a *lung abscess* within the lung tissue itself if infection cannot be blocked. These conditions may also occur in the

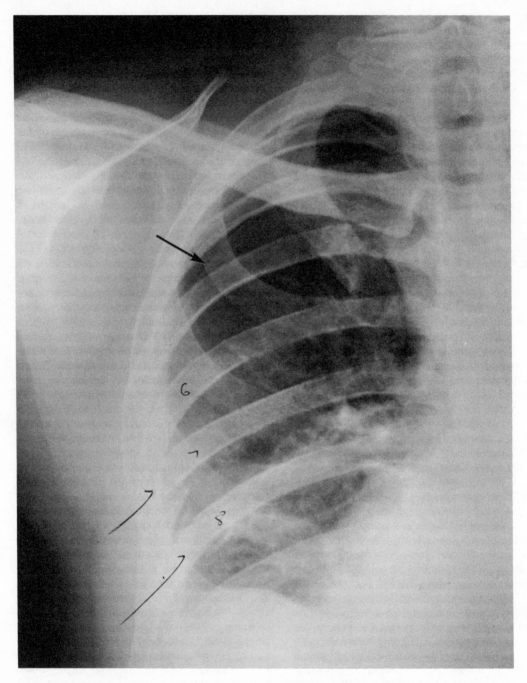

Plate 12a   Multiple rib fractures with partial collapse of the lung (pneumothorax) and a pulmonary effusion. Two fractures are marked, and the edge of the partially collapsed lung is indicated by the arrow.

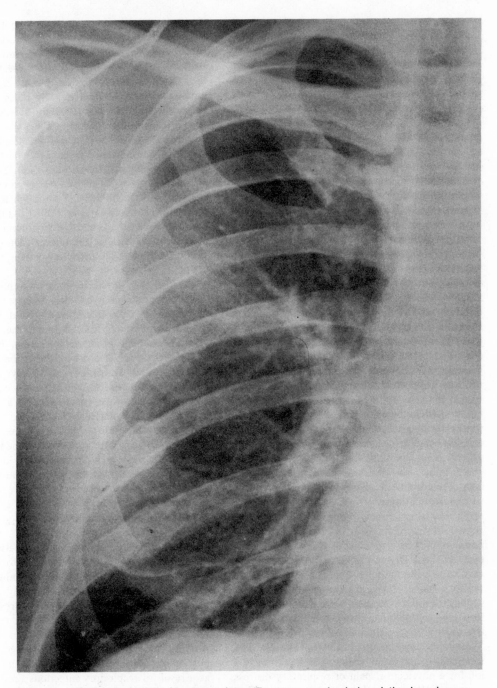

Plate 12b   The same patient four years later. Fractures are healed and the lung has re-expanded to fill the thoracic cavity.

absence of any chest injury as complications of primary lung infection. (*See* p. 480.) Finally, any chest injury, particularly a penetrating wound, is inevitably haunted by the specter of physical shock, a major threat to life which must be dealt with on an emergency first-aid basis even before medical help can be obtained.

Emergency First-Aid Measures. First-aid treatment of serious injuries is discussed elsewhere. (*See* p. 103.) Chest injuries, however, can pose a special problem. Medical aid should, of course, be summoned at once, but if the victim has to be moved before medical aid arrives, it must be done with extreme care to prevent further internal damage. Several people, if possible, should help move the victim onto a stretcher in such a way that his torso is not twisted or bent. In addition, an open wound of the chest must be temporarily closed, either with a tightly sealed adhesive tape dressing or with a piece of plastic wrap held over the wound by manual pressure. Meanwhile, the four emergency first-aid priorities must be instituted without delay. Hemorrhage must be controlled, if possible, by applying direct pressure over the wound. Mouth-to-mouth resuscitation should be started if the victim's breathing has ceased. External cardiac compression should be used to restore the heartbeat in the event of circulatory collapse, and first-aid measures for the prevention of shock should be initiated. In the case of a chest injury, however, any or all of these measures must be tempered with common sense to avoid inflicting more damage as a result of physical manipulations. For example, pressure control of hemorrhage, or external cardiac compression, may be impossible if the chest itself has been crushed. The best hope of saving the victim may be to abandon all else and transport him as swiftly as possible to a hospital emergency room, supporting his respiration with mouth-to-mouth breathing as effectively as possible until definitive medical treatment can begin.

Medical Treatment of Chest Injuries. The treatment of any kind of injury to the chest is a job for a physician if pain or respiratory distress is present. Whatever the injury, treatment first seeks to maintain normal respiration, then to support circulation and prevent or counteract shock, so that oxygen supply to the tissues is maintained while healing proceeds. Once those vital functions are stabilized, pain control is the next concern. Many of the most powerful analgesics tend to depress the respiratory center and thus must be avoided in treating these injuries, but surgeons have learned that excellent pain control can be obtained with the use of milder analgesics combined with various tranquilizing drugs, suggesting that the pain of chest injuries is much aggravated by apprehension. Pain control makes it possible for the victim to engage in periodic deep breathing and to cough up mucus that tends to pool in the bronchi during the shallow "guarded" respiration so commonly seen after chest injuries, an important factor in preventing such complications as post-injury stasis pneumonia.

Finally, the physician must watch out for various complications of chest injuries. Surgical debridement of a contaminated wound, followed by adequate drainage and antibiotic therapy, can prevent secondary bacterial infection. Blood or fluid collected in the chest can often be detected by X-ray and drawn off with a syringe and needle, a procedure known as *thoracentesis*. A rubber drainage tube equipped with a one-way flutter valve or water seal can be used to empty the chest cavity of air, allowing the lung to reinflate. Overall, with appropriate modern treatment, victims of even the most serious chest injuries have a far better chance for full recovery today than ever before in history.

Mechanical Respiratory Obstructions

Because the free exchange of air between the outside atmosphere and the respiratory membrane is so vital to maintain life, anything which obstructs this air flow, either partially or completely, not only causes immediate respiratory distress, but may also lead to serious complications or even death. The most common causes of respiratory obstruction are the blockage of some portion of the respiratory tree by mucus and pus as a result of respiratory infections (*see* p. 470) and the blockage of the smaller bronchioles throughout both lungs due to a condition known as bronchial asthma (*see* p. 491). Here we are concerned with the more sudden and dramatic mechanical obstruction of the airway that occurs when a foreign body is inhaled or aspirated, cutting off aeration of the portion of the lung that lies below the obstruction.

Tragic accidents have occurred from the aspiration of a large chunk of food that completely obstructs the trachea and leads to the sudden collapse and death of the victim from asphyxia. Such abrupt, total respiratory obstructions are major medical emergencies, and they are discussed in detail elsewhere. (*See* p. 114.) They are comparatively rare, fortunately, but the hazard of aspirating smaller foreign bodies into the respiratory tree is universal. Everyone, at one time or another, has suffered an explosive bout of choking and coughing because some food "goes down the wrong way." Children are particularly vulnerable to inadvertent inhalation of various foreign objects—small coins, peanuts, or bits of unchewed meat or gristle, for example. Often the foreign body enters a mainstem bronchus, and may ultimately wedge in a single side branch of one of these bronchi, so that air exchange with the rest of the lung remains possible. Sometimes an individual, following aspiration and a bout of choking and coughing, assumes that he has coughed up the foreign body, only to learn hours or days later that a portion of his respiratory tree is still blocked, with collapse of a segment of the lung beyond the obstruction.

Recognizing Foreign Body Obstruction. In most cases it is easy to recognize, or at least suspect, what has happened when an individual aspirates a foreign body. Even a tiny foreign object will stimulate violent choking and coughing which, in the vast majority of cases, helps dislodge the foreign material. Once the object has been coughed out, the cough reflex usually subsides, but if the mucous membrane of the respiratory tree has been irritated, further coughing may ensue. The violent coughing may, in itself, stimulate a gag reflex and vomiting, making it hard to determine whether a given bit of food or other foreign matter has come up from the stomach or has been coughed out of a bronchus. Coughing is inevitably followed by a deep inspiration which can, in some cases, help

wedge the foreign body more tightly into the bronchus. Thus, rather than assume that a foreign body has been expelled after an episode of choking, it is wise to have a doctor confirm that the obstructing object is gone by means of physical examination and chest X-rays. When a bronchus remains blocked, the gas in the alveoli below the obstruction is gradually absorbed, causing the segment of lung slowly to collapse, much like an exhausted bellows. This condition, known as *atelectasis,* can often be detected on a chest X-ray within a few hours of its occurrence. Sometimes the doctor can also identify an obstructed area of lung by changes in the breath sounds that he hears with a stethoscope.

Treatment of Foreign Body Aspiration. The sooner an aspirated foreign body is dislodged, the fewer complications are likely to ensue. Thus every effort should be made to help the victim get rid of whatever is causing his choking as quickly as possible. A sharp blow on the chest will sometimes help dislodge a foreign body. A child may be lifted bodily and tilted slightly downward so that gravity may help the expulsive force of coughing jar the object loose. An adult may accomplish the same thing by lying on the edge of a bed or couch with elbows on the floor, so that the entire upper torso is tilted downward. It is best not to hold a very small child (under two years of age) upside down to try to dislodge a foreign body; this maneuver may free the object from its original position in a bronchus only to wedge it into the narrow opening between the vocal cords in such a way that a partial obstruction becomes a complete obstruction. Since the child may be too weak for effective expulsive coughing, he should be transported immediately to the nearest hospital, even if the foreign body seems to have been dislodged. Finally, in any case of choking, keep the victim in such a position that if he vomits, any emesis will drain out of his mouth and will not be aspirated into his lungs to complicate the situation with the threat of an irritating chemical or aspiration pneumonia.

When a foreign body remains lodged somewhere in the respiratory tree despite efforts to jar it loose, the acute paroxysm of choking may subside, but episodic coughing will persist. Often the victim will feel that something is still lodged and will repeatedly try to cough it up. Pain may develop in the chest in an area coinciding with the part of the respiratory tree that the victim feels is still plugged. The appearance of a fever within a few hours, either alone or in combination with these other symptoms, strongly suggests that the obstruction remains, and the victim should see a physician without delay. A period of close observation may be necessary, and the doctor may have to search for the foreign body and extract it by means of an instrument known as a *bronchoscope*, a long, narrow, lighted tube which can be inserted into the trachea with the aid of a local anesthetic and used to examine the major bronchi.

Complications of Foreign Body Obstruction. Whether an obstructing foreign body is successfully expelled by coughing or must be mechanically removed, there is enough risk of secondary bacterial infection or bronchial irritation that a period of antibiotic therapy is usually advisable. When a foreign body remains lodged in a small bronchus, a lung abscess may even form below the area of obstruction. In any event, the victim of any severe choking episode should see a doctor to guard against the possible occurrence of a pneumonia or bronchitis even when the offending object is apparently coughed out.

Upper Respiratory Infections

Anyone who has ever had a bad head cold, a bout of tonsillitis, a severe case of bronchitis or pneumonia knows that respiratory tract infections are among the most uncomfortable and distressing diseases that commonly afflict man. They are also among the most readily recognized and diagnosed infections, partly because their symptoms are so obvious and partly because we are so extremely sensitive to *any* condition that interferes with breathing.

Until the mid-1930s, many respiratory tract infections were gravely dangerous, and pneumonia was the major cause of death in the United States. With the advent of sulfa drugs and antibiotics, pneumonia was toppled from its number one position, and today respiratory infections are more notable for their *morbidity*—

their capacity to cause distressing and/or disabling symptoms—than in terms of *mortality*—the power to cause death. These infections are legion, sometimes differing from one another to such a minor degree that only a specialist in respiratory tract disease can distinguish them. Many have already been described in detail elsewhere (*see* Part IV, "Patterns of Illness: The Infectious Diseases"). Here we can review them briefly, according to the part of the respiratory tract that is most commonly involved, and then discuss those other infections, both minor and major, that can also impair the vital respiratory function.

Bacterial or virus infections can involve all parts of the respiratory tree from the nose, throat and sinuses to the respiratory membrane of the lung itself. For convenience these infections can be divided into three major subclasses: *upper respiratory infections* which primarily attack the mucous membrane linings of the nose, throat and larynx; *bronchial infections* which involve the trachea and bronchi; and *lower respiratory infections* or "infections of the lung" which primarily affect the tissues of the lung itself, including the alveolar respiratory membrane and the connective tissue of the lung. This classification is not entirely arbitrary; although some upper respiratory infections may indeed become severe, or may ultimately extend to bronchitis or pneumonia, for the most part they are somewhat more superficial infections which do not directly interfere with the exchange of oxygen and carbon dioxide across the respiratory membrane, even though they may partially obstruct the air tubes with mucus or pus. Infections of the lung proper, however, can swiftly and directly prevent gas exchange across the respiratory membrane and thus tend to be much more dangerous.

Symptoms of Upper Respiratory Infection. Most upper respiratory infections begin with a typical feeling of dryness or scratchiness in the throat, irritation of the nasal passages, a sense of nasal stuffiness and a tickling irritation in the trachea or upper bronchi which stimulates a dry, irritative cough. When such prodromal or "beginning" symptoms commence, people speak of "coming down with a cold," but these symptoms soon differentiate according to the particular part of the upper respiratory tract involved. The nasal mucosa may become swollen and inflamed and begin to pour forth a thin watery discharge which soon becomes mucoid or even purulent. Sneezing often accompanies these symptoms, and there may be watering of the eyes and a feeling of pressure and pain in the sinus areas surrounding the nasopharynx or pharynx with increasing soreness and swelling of the back of the throat. If the larynx is involved, hoarseness soon becomes a prominent feature, and the dry bronchial cough becomes moist and productive as mucus is poured out by the membrane lining these air tubes. Often the senses of smell and taste are lost and the individual's voice changes markedly as a result of pharyngeal involvement or plugging of the nasal passages. A low-grade fever (up to 101° or more) often appears in this second stage of upper respiratory infection; the cough may become progressively more irritating, with a sense of "rawness" or tightness in the chest beneath the sternum. Untreated, these infections may clear up spontaneously within a day or two, but more commonly they last for a week or so, with the cough often persisting for several weeks before it finally clears up. In perhaps 10 to 15 percent of cases, severe untreated upper respiratory infections will progress to a more deep-seated bronchitis or even to pneumonia; consequently any upper respiratory infection that seems to persist for more than two or three days, or to become progressively worse, should be treated by a doctor.

Among the upper respiratory infections described elsewhere, the *common cold* (*see* p. 225) is by far the most prevalent. It is an irritative infection of the entire upper respiratory tract caused by any of a large family of closely related viruses and characterized by a runny nose, a scratchy throat and a superficial cough. The fever, if present, seldom exceeds 100°, and treatment is primarily symptomatic, since antibiotic therapy has no effect on the causative viruses. Most common colds clear up spontaneously within a few days, but many are complicated by secondary bacterial infection which may require antibiotic therapy to ensure speedy recovery. *Influenza* (*see* p. 228), which presents

upper respiratory symptoms similar to the common cold, is distinguished by additional symptoms of a more widespread systemic infection. These include a persistent nagging headache, a fever up to 102° or more, a persistent dry, hacky cough, and generalized muscle aches involving the back, the neck, the shoulders and the legs. Gastrointestinal symptoms such as nausea and vomiting may also be present. Influenza can vary markedly in its severity depending upon the strain of flu virus at work; some cases improve in two or three days while others persist for weeks, leaving the victim physically exhausted for a prolonged period following the attack. Again, treatment is symptomatic, but antibiotics may be prescribed to avert secondary bacterial infections. *Tonsillitis, adenoiditis* and *otitis media* (*see* p. 193) are common bacterial infections involving the tonsils lining the back of the throat, the adenoids surrounding the nasopharynx, and the middle ear, respectively. Vigorous antibiotic treatment of these infections, which can be identified by physical examination and bacteriological studies, will markedly shorten their course and bring speedy recovery. *Whooping cough* (*see* p. 187), a severely irritative bronchial infection caused by the bacteria *Hemophilus pertussis,* was once a dangerous killer of small children, but today it is usually prevented by vaccination in infancy, as is *diphtheria* (*see* p. 185), a virulent throat infection caused by *Corynebacterium diphtheriae. Scarlet fever* (*see* p. 183) is a severe throat infection due to a particular strain of streptococcus, once an extremely common childhood disease but now only rarely identified specifically because early antibiotic treatment tends to abort the infection before the typical scarlet fever symptoms and rash appear. Finally, many of the common childhood rash diseases (*see* p. 178), including rubella, rubeola, and chicken pox, as well as such viral infections as mumps (*see* p. 191), may cause mild to severe upper respiratory symptoms but can be differentiated from upper respiratory infections by the high fevers, skin rashes or other characteristic symptoms.

Sinusitis. Although many people ascribe to "sinus trouble" the nasal stuffiness and aching pain around the nose and beneath the eyes that so often accompany upper respiratory infections, and inaccurately speak of virtually any nasal infection as "sinusitis" whether the sinuses are involved or not, true sinus infections are, in fact, comparatively rare. They do occur, however, and those who are prone to them can suffer severely.

The sinuses in question are nothing more than hollow air pockets within certain bones in the front part of the skull which drain, by one means or another, through openings into the nasopharynx. The *supraorbital sinuses* are located in the bony ridge of the forehead just above the eye sockets, the *maxillary sinuses* in the cheekbones beneath the eye sockets on either side, and the *paranasal sinuses* deeper in the skull in the bones on either side and to the rear of the nose. These sinuses are lined with a thin layer of mucous membrane which keeps the air within them relatively moist at all times. The sinuses seem to act as resonators, together with the nasopharynx, to contribute depth and amplitude to the voice, and because they are connected to the nasopharynx by small passageways, it is possible for them to be invaded by bacteria. Inflammation and swelling of the sinus lining, together with the mucus and pus that form, can then obstruct ventilation and drainage of these air pockets, causing severe pain and pressure, particularly when a head cold is present. Other infections of the nose and throat may also lead to sinus infections, and the sinuses are particularly vulnerable to allergic reactions that may prepare the ground for secondary bacterial infection, a condition known as allergic sinusitis.

The treatment of sinusitis is much the same as for any upper respiratory infection: the use of nose drops to dry up the mucous membrane and open the drainage passages from the sinuses, aspirin for pain, rest, additional fluids and, when the infection is acute, antibiotics. But because allergies so frequently contribute to sinusitis, antihistamine medicines are also often helpful to establish drainage and relieve pressure and pain. A number of safe and useful nonprescription antihistamine preparations are available over the counter and include the same medications your doctor would prescribe, although in somewhat lower dosages.

Sinusitis is most often characterized by acute attacks, but some people develop *chronic sinusitis*—a continuing or recurring inflammation of the sinuses due to either infection or allergy, or both. Frequent "sinus headaches" and pain, often accompanied by a heavy nasal and postnasal discharge, are the common symptoms of this condition. In some cases, the swelling and engorgement of the mucous membrane lining the sinuses lead to the formation of nonmalignant growths of mucous membrane known as *polyps* within the sinuses; these may occur concurrently with nasal polyps (*see* p. 442) which fill the nasal passageways and block drainage of the sinuses. Chronic sinusitis, with or without polyps, can often be diagnosed with the aid of sinus X-rays; when polyps are present, they can be removed surgically and the affected sinuses drained as an aid to healing. In any case in which combined antibiotic and antihistamine therapy is not sufficient to quiet the sinusitis, the advice of an ear, nose and throat specialist should be sought to set up a program to relieve the disorder.

Pharyngitis. The part of the upper respiratory tract most vulnerable of all to infection is the nasopharynx—that part of the nasal and oral cavity above the soft palate and along the back of the throat. These areas, which are openly exposed to the outside air and to any contaminating bacteria or viruses that may come in, are surrounded by a ring of *lymphoid tissue* which lies in soft, spongy lumps all around the base of the pharynx. Lymphoid tissue, which includes the tonsils and adenoids, frequently becomes infected, and its vulnerability is increased by chronic drying due to mouth breathing, the irritation of tobacco smoke and the drainage of mucous material from the nose in cases of chronic postnasal drip.

Inflammation of this lymphoid tissue causes the dryness, scratchiness and soreness of the throat so commonly felt when any upper respiratory infection begins. But specific bacterial or viral infection may also center there, and in such cases the throat becomes bright red and sore. Flecks of pus may be seen exuding from crevices in the lymphoid tissue, and the throat grows raw as the underlying tissues of the pharynx become involved in the infection. When the tonsils and adenoids are repeatedly infected, enlarged and scarred, they may be removed surgically (*see* p. 194), but this is no guarantee that future bouts of acute pharyngitis will not occur. Bacteria or viruses can still find lodging in the nasopharyngeal region and cause severe infections.

Medical treatment of acute pharyngitis is both symptomatic and specific. Antibiotics such as penicillin, ampicillin or tetracycline usually work swiftly to destroy the bacteria causing the infection or prevent secondary bacterial invasion of the area during a viral pharyngitis. Aspirin can be used to control the fever characteristic of the infection, and the pain of the sore throat can be greatly relieved by gargling three or four times a day with a salt-water solution made from a teaspoon of salt in a half-cup of hot (not scalding) water. In severe cases a day or two of bed rest, additional fluids and a diet confined to soft, nonirritating foods will help speed recovery.

Occasionally acute pharyngitis will persist in spite of vigorous treatment and become chronic. In such cases throat smears and bacterial culture of the infectious exudate may help identify the offending organism and provide the doctor with a clue as to which specific antibiotic may be most helpful in eradicating the infection. In fact, antibiotic-resistant pharyngitis has become so common in recent years that many doctors prefer to make a throat culture routinely at the very beginning of any pharyngeal infection in order to identify the organism before starting antibiotic therapy, a practice that is becoming increasingly widespread.

Although pharyngitis is seldom a serious health threat today, the possibility of diphtheria (*see* p. 185) is always present, and must never be ignored in the case of any progressively severe sore throat accompanied by a fever. Frequently, a pharyngitis will extend down the respiratory tree to involve the larynx and trachea. A particularly unpleasant complication of acute pharyngitis is the so-called quinsy sore throat or *peritonsillar abscess*. In this condition the bacteria, usually streptococci or staphylococci, find their way deep into the soft tissue of the pharynx and there form a pocket of pus which may, if untreated, grow to the size of a walnut or larger and push a whole side of the throat forward in a bulge. The sore throat is agonizing; the fever is high and spiking and the victim becomes toxic and dehydrated. Sometimes a paratonsillar abscess can be aborted by vigorous treatment with massive doses of the appropriate antibiotic, but once formed, it must be lanced and drained of pus before healing can take place.

Laryngitis. Upper respiratory infections, whether viral or bacterial, frequently affect more than one area at once, and the larynx may be involved in any bacterial or viral infection of the upper respiratory tract. But the symptoms of laryngitis are unique. Whereas pain, a sense of dryness, and irritation or scratchiness are common in the nasopharynx when infection is present, since this area is richly endowed with sensory nerve endings, infection or irritation of the mucous membrane of the larynx is not as noticeably painful—but even slight laryngeal irritation can cause voice alteration from a minor degree of hoarseness to a total loss of voice as the infection progresses.

In typical laryngitis the hoarseness is first noticed in the morning and becomes worse during the day. If the victim continues to use his voice, vocal communication may be completely lost in 24 hours except for a sort of hoarse whispering. Persistent attempts to use the voice will lead to pain and rawness in the voice box sufficient to discourage the most compulsive talker.

Acute laryngitis is treated with additional rest, extra fluids, aspirin for fever or pain, expectorant cough syrup for coughing, and the use of antihistamines and antibiotics, much the same as any upper respiratory infection. In addition, *complete voice rest* is important. Even whispering causes subvocal vibrations of the inflamed vocal cords and retards healing. The cardinal rule is to stop talking until the laryngitis has cleared up completely, usually a matter of two or three days if other treatment measures are also pursued.

Laryngitis may also occur in the absence of infection as a result of marathon talking, shouting and other overuse of the vocal cords, or from continual irritation by dust, smoke or other

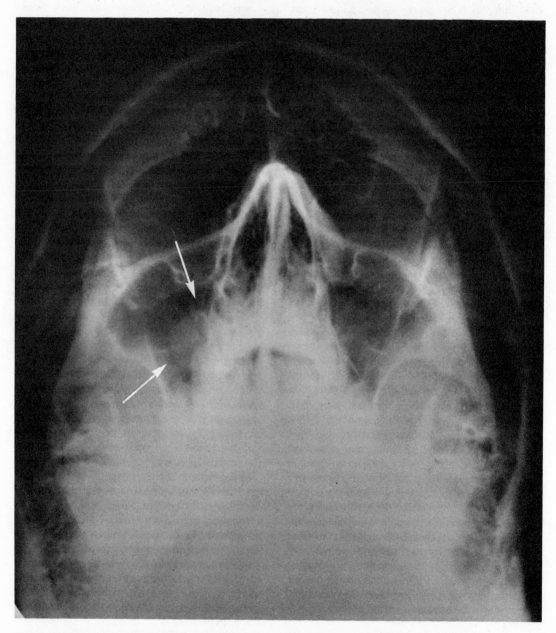

Plate 13   A large polyp is visible in the right maxillary sinus (see arrow). Patient's head was tilted back for this film to outline the maxillary sinuses on either side.

substances. Such mechanical or physical inflammation will usually respond well to voice rest for as little as 12 hours. Everyone has an occasional bout of hoarseness of this sort, but any such episode should be regarded with suspicion, particularly if the hoarseness appears excessive for the circumstances. *Any* hoarseness which persists for longer than a week should be called to a doctor's attention, as well as any progressive change in the resonance or timbre of the voice noted over a period of time. Sometimes *laryngeal polyps*—benign overgrowths of mucous membrane in the vicinity of the vocal cords—cause such changes and can easily be removed in a simple surgical procedure. But two other more serious conditions can also cause progressive and persistent hoarseness: *tuberculosis of the larynx* and *cancer* or *carcinoma of the larynx.* Both of these conditions can be treated and cured if the victim sees a doctor early enough. Tuberculosis is a serious bacterial infection that can affect many parts of the body (*see* p. 211) and if it first appears in the larynx, a thorough physical examination must be done to rule out tuberculosis of the lung or other organs. Laryngeal tuberculosis can completely destroy the vocal cords and voice box if untreated, but may be completely cleared up today with vigorous and persistent antibiotic treatment. Early cancer of the larynx can be diagnosed by means of a special procedure known as *laryngoscopy*—direct inspection of the inside of the larynx and the vocal cords by means of a lighted instrument—and with surgical treatment, it is one of the most commonly curable of all early cancers. (*See* p. 499.) If untreated, however, or if treatment is delayed because the victim of persistent hoarseness neglects to seek early medical advice, the condition may eventually prove fatal. Thus no one should postpone a doctor's examination if hoarseness recurs or persists without explanation.

Tracheitis, Bronchitis and Other Bronchial Infections

Infections of the upper respiratory tract, while sometimes severe and always uncomfortable, are rarely prolonged or threatening unless compli-cated by infection lower down in the respiratory tree. Unfortunately, many upper respiratory infections extend to involve the trachea, the main bronchi and the smaller branching bronchi and bronchioles which make up the tracheobronchial tree. Some authorities differentiate between *tracheitis,* involving the trachea alone; *tracheobronchitis,* in which the trachea and mainstem bronchi are involved, and *bronchitis,* involving any or all of the branching bronchi; but for all practical purposes the term *bronchitis* alone can be used quite correctly to describe any inflammation of the air tubes, acute or chronic, caused by infectious organisms or by physical or chemical agents. Such inflammation can result in severe illness, especially characterized by fever and coughing. In most cases the bronchitis occurs acutely (that is, suddenly) and is self-limited, eventually healing spontaneously with ultimate return of the infected tissue to normal. In some cases, however, *chronic bronchitis* may develop, considerably more serious because of the long-term damage to the bronchial apparatus that can result.

Acute Bronchitis. Often called a "chest cold," this condition usually occurs as part of a general acute upper respiratory infection, arising either from a common cold or other viral or bacterial infection of the nasopharynx or from a virus infection of the tracheobronchial tree itself with secondary bacterial invasion of the damaged tissue. The mucous membrane lining the trachea and the bronchi becomes inflamed and swollen, with an outpouring of a sticky mucoid or purulent exudate. These secretions tend to accumulate, interfering with breathing and stimulating the cough reflex. The coughing may be highly irritating and distressing, even painful, but it is essential if the bronchi are to be emptied of these sticky secretions. Thus it is seldom wise in this condition to use any cough-suppressing medicines or syrups, even for a while, unless they are specifically prescribed by a physician.

The early symptoms of acute bronchitis include a scratchy sore throat, a stuffy nose, low-grade fever, a sense of chilliness and a dry, non-productive hacking cough. In a day or two small amounts of sputum are coughed up, followed later by more abundant amounts of sticky, purulent mucus. In mild cases the acute symptoms may subside even without treatment after four or five days, but typically the cough persists for as long as two or three weeks. In more severe cases the victim may feel soreness or tightness in the chest in the early stages of the infection, and can often hear a squeaking or wheezing deep down in his chest during breathing. Even then, however, severe interference with breathing does not ordinarily occur. The most dangerous threat of severe acute bronchitis is the possible invasion of the lung tissue proper by the infecting organism, with resulting pneumonia, particularly in small children and elderly or debilitated persons. For this reason, most doctors treat all but the mildest acute bronchitis with antibiotics, more to protect against a secondary pneumonia than to eradicate the bronchial infection.

General treatment of acute bronchitis is much the same as that of any other upper respiratory infection. If the symptoms are severe, particularly with fever, chilling or chest pain, bed rest is advisable, and drinking extra liquids—as much as three to four quarts a day while fever persists—will help replace lost fluids and liquefy bronchial secretions. Aspirin will reduce fever and relieve discomfort, and an expectorant cough syrup which does not contain any cough suppressant will help loosen up the "dry cough" stage of the illness. Steam inhalation is helpful for the same reason. Commercial steamers or vaporizers, available at low cost at most drugstores, will keep the air in the room constantly humid; "cold steam" vaporizers are especially good because they eliminate the possible hazard of steam burns or scalding when used for children. But any means of humidifying the air, even a teakettle of water boiling on a hot plate in some inaccessible area, will work equally well. The same benefit in suppressing an irritating cough can be obtained in the bathroom by filling a tub full of hot water or running a hot shower with the door closed. The doctor may prescribe a cough-suppressant for occasional use to provide periods of relief from the coughing, if necessary, once sputum begins to come up. Finally, antibiotics may be indicated if the fever is high or the infection prolonged, and medicines to dilate the bronchial tubes help bring up sputum and permit more air to reach the lungs.

Chronic Bronchitis. In some individuals acute bronchitis does not clear up quickly, but persists or recurs over and over during the same season. Such a chronic bronchitis, often aggravated by heavy smoking or frequent exposure to irritating chemicals or gases, can become a prolonged and entrenched disease of the tracheobronchial tree. No single bacteriological agent is at fault, but the condition can result in slow but continuous damage to the bronchial mucous membrane. Over months or years the bronchi become scarred and narrowed, with increasing obstruction to air flow. The normal, natural cleansing action of the bronchi is chronically disturbed, secretions are retained, and bronchial drainage comes to depend upon a hacking cough. The victim becomes more vulnerable to pneumonia, particularly during winter months, or to a chronic obstructive condition known as *pulmonary emphysema.* (See p. 494.) In very severe cases death may result from progressive respiratory obstruction, or from terminal pneumonia or heart failure.

Obviously the best time to deal with chronic bronchitis is before it has become chronic. Any bronchial infection which persists should be treated until it has healed, and if some degree of chronic bronchitis is already present, each and every recurrence of acute inflammation should be given vigorous medical attention. A thorough physical examination is necessary to rule out such possible underlying causes as tuberculosis, lung tumor, bronchiectasis, silicosis or some other respiratory condition. In the presence of chronic bronchitis, smoking is a virtual guarantee that the condition will persist and get worse, and it should be discontinued to prevent permanent respiratory impairment.

Bronchiectasis. One long-term complication of chronic bronchial irritation is a condition known as bronchiectasis, in which the smaller bronchioles in one or more segments of the lung have been destroyed by infection, stretched and hardened into inelastic pockets where mucous exudate mixed with pus tends to collect. The condition is most commonly found in the bronchioles of the lower lobes of either lung, since gravity favors drainage into these areas. These collections of infected material keep the bronchial mucosa inflamed, sometimes even ulcerated, so that bleeding may originate here. In addition, adjacent areas of lung tissue also may become infected, abscessed or even gangrenous.

A victim of bronchiectasis usually has had chronic bronchitis and often a severe case of pneumonia, whooping cough or influenza at some time in the past. The disease is marked by an insidiously progressive cough, especially in the morning upon arising, late in the afternoon, and again at bedtime. Although many people with bronchiectasis have relatively little sputum, others bring up great quantities of foul-smelling material, particularly in the morning, which, when collected in sputum containers, will appear yellow-green in color and may even separate out into viscid layers of pus and mucus. Spitting up blood is not uncommon, and shortness of breath on exertion frequently occurs. If the disease interferes significantly with the absorption of oxygen, "clubbing" or swelling of the tips of the fingers and toes is sometimes seen, and the victim is extremely prone to recurrent acute respiratory infections, particularly pneumonia.

Treatment is primarily medical: the use of broad-spectrum antibiotics, bronchial dilators (often inhaled by way of an aerosol nebulizer) to help raise secretions, and such home-care procedures as daily *postural drainage* of the chest. This is accomplished by lying over the edge of the bed with the elbows on the floor so that the entire thorax is inverted, allowing gravity to help empty secretions which have pooled in the bronchiectatic pockets in the lower lobes of the lungs. It is best done early in the morning after use of a broncho-dilating aerosol, and should be continued for 10 to 15 minutes, then repeated in the late afternoon and again before going to bed at night.

Bronchiectasis is probably never completely cured, but progressive destruction of bronchioles can be halted. In exceptionally severe cases, isolated segments of the lung may be removed by surgery, a procedure now performed by general or thoracic surgeons throughout the world. Before surgery is considered, however, special X-rays are taken using radio-opaque dyes to show the bronchiectatic cavities so that the extent of the damage can be assessed. If large, multiple areas are diseased, surgical treatment may be impossible, since there is a limit to the amount of lung tissue that can be removed. Surgery works best when there is a single bad segment of bronchiectasis with only minor damage in other areas.

Acute Laryngotracheobronchitis and Croup. While bronchitis is rarely a fatal infection, one form of the disease is particularly dangerous because of its swift, fulminating course and indeed can be fatal when it strikes infants and small children. This is laryngotracheobronchitis, an acute bacterial infection which swiftly attacks the larynx, the trachea and the bronchi all at once. In some cases this infection may originate as a virus infection which prepares the way for a fast-moving bacterial invasion, irritating the tissues and lowering the victim's resistance to the attack. Whatever the causative organism, the disease is characterized by sudden onset of high fever, severe shortness of breath and an almost constant hoarse, "croupy" cough. At first the cough produces little or no sputum, but as the infection progresses, thick, sticky mucus begins coming up and the shortness of breath becomes so severe that the victim may show the gray-bluish pallor of cyanosis arising from oxygen hunger. The infection also causes such marked swelling of the mucous membranes of the larynx, trachea and bronchi that the swelling itself becomes obstructive. This, combined with mucus lodging in the larynx, can create such marked obstruction that the victim literally cannot get enough air, and death may ensue from suffocation before treatment has a chance to take effect.

This violent infection, which is particularly devastating to small children who simply do not have the strength for protracted bouts of fighting for air, is relatively rare. But diagnosis of the gravity of the condition is difficult for two reasons. First, the disease ordinarily strikes infants and babies who cannot tell the doctor how they feel; and second, the most characteristic symptom of the disease—the croupy cough—may occur so frequently during run-of-the-mill mild

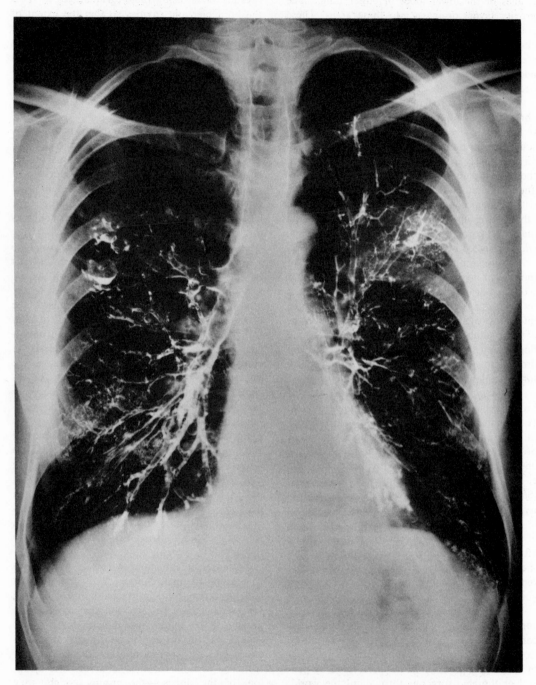

Plate 14a   Bronchiectasis as revealed by radio-opaque contrast medium in the bronchi. Note enlarged, saccular segments of diseased bronchi.

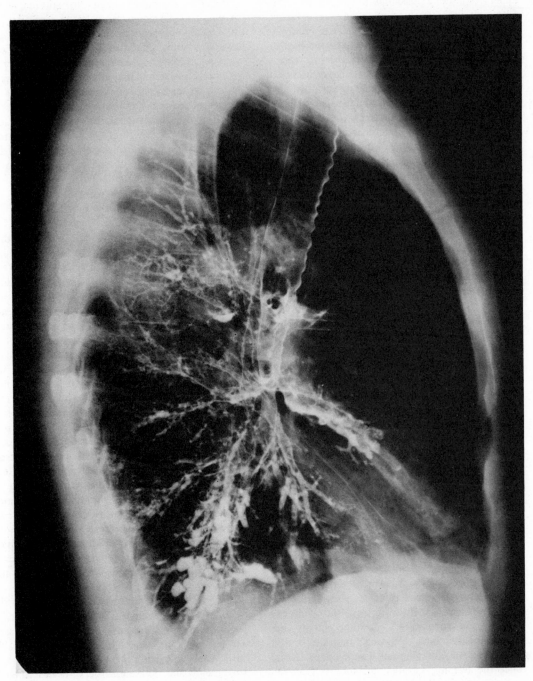

Plate 14b   Same patient, side view. Distended, sacculate segments of diseased bronchi are particularly notable in the lower lung field.

upper respiratory infections in infants and children that both parents and doctors can be deceived into treating the onset of the crouplike symptoms lightly. In addition, it may be hard to discern shortness of breath in a child who is crying at the top of his lungs whenever he is not coughing. Thus, differentiating an ordinary croupy cough from the rare, but gravely dangerous, onset of acute laryngotracheobronchitis can be extremely difficult, as reflected in the high mortality rate of this type of infection.

Doctors experienced in treating children's diseases are alert to this dangerous condition and regard *any* upper respiratory infection in which a croupy cough is a factor with respect and concern. The croup may stem from a variety of other less dangerous causes, but this is one situation in which it is advisable to assume the worst and summon a doctor. Even better, the child should be taken to the nearest hospital emergency room as soon as croup appears as a complication of a cold or other respiratory infection. There a "croup tent"—a vaporizer with a hood that fits over the child's crib—may be used to humidify the air and ease breathing in any form of croup. Oxygen can be administered if needed, together with bronchial dilators. Vigorous antibiotic therapy is indicated, and careful observation in the hospital will further protect the child from the consequences of sudden, acute respiratory distress. Occasionally, at the height of the infection, it may be necessary for the doctor to perform a *tracheostomy,* a surgical opening of the trachea below the level of the larynx, to permit insertion of a breathing tube. This is done when swelling of the vocal cords is so severe that complete obstruction of the airway is imminent. Prompt, vigorous treatment during the early stages of the illness may avert the necessity of this surgical procedure, but when it must be done it may prove lifesaving. After the tracheostomy has been performed and a breathing tube inserted, it must be kept free of mucus by frequent suctioning. The tube simply bypasses the inflamed, obstructed larynx so that the victim may breathe and cough more freely; once the swelling subsides, the tube is removed and the incision heals with a barely noticeable scar.

As the symptoms begin to subside, both parents and physician can relax to some degree, but close observation may be necessary for several days to guard against recurrence. Convalescence tends to be slow; fever and bronchial irritation with coughing may persist for weeks following the acute episode. This may be an inconvenience, particularly among teen-age or adult victims, but it is important that the patient understand the gravity of the illness, the unfortunate possibility of recurrence and the need for time to recover before attempting to return to normal daily activities.

Infections of the Lung

Upper respiratory infections, although they may cause partial obstruction of air flow, do not directly affect the respiratory membrane or hinder the exchange of gases across it. Infections of the lung tissue itself, however—the alveolar air sacs, the respiratory membrane and the surrounding connective tissue—are a different story. Here infections interfere directly and immediately with the normal exchange of oxygen and carbon dioxide, and thus strike at the very heart of the respiratory process, sometimes to such a degree that they are fatal.

One of the most serious of these infections of the lung, if undetected and untreated, is *pulmonary tuberculosis.* This devastating disease, caused by invasion of lung tissue by the tubercle bacillus, *Mycobacterium tuberculosis,* can lead to the irreparable destruction of large areas of lung tissue, and was once such a prevalent cause of death in the Western world that it was known as the Great White Plague. Modern diagnosis and treatment have sharply reduced the incidence of death due to tuberculosis, but even today the disease remains an ever present and world-wide health threat. (*See* p. 211.)

Perhaps even more threatening, because of the suddenness with which they strike, are a variety of bacterial or viral infections of lung tissue known as *pneumonia,* all of which are capable of severely impairing large areas of the respiratory membrane. These disorders are described in detail elsewhere (*see* p. 214), but a brief review here will place them in perspective with other

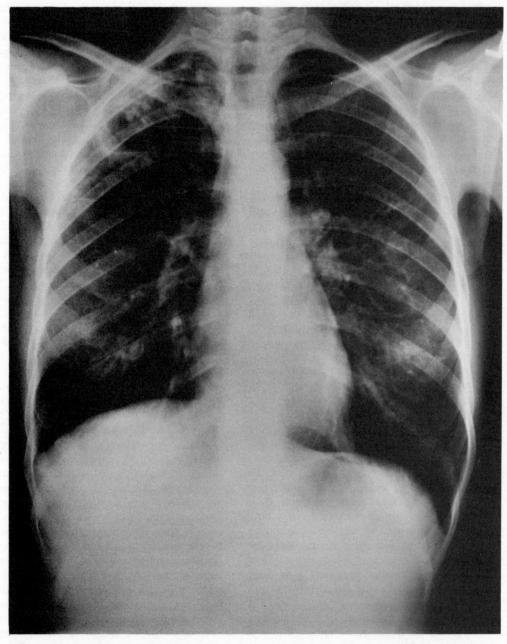

Plate 15   Pulmonary tuberculosis. Patches of infection are seen as cloudy areas in the upper portion or apex of the right lung.

diseases of the respiratory tract. Most infamous of the bacterial pneumonias is *lobar pneumonia,* caused by *Diplococcus pneumoniae* or, more rarely, by streptococcus or staphylococcus organisms. In this infection a whole lobe of the lung becomes involved in a fulminating infection which completely blocks the respiratory process in the entire area involved until the infection is brought under control. Occasionally lobes in both lungs are involved, a condition commonly known as "double pneumonia." Lobar pneumonia is an exceptionally severe, prostrating infection associated with a high spiking fever, the coughing up of bloody sputum, severe respiratory impairment and shortness of breath, and a prolonged convalescence. Once the top-ranking cause of death in the United States, it can now usually be swiftly controlled by antibiotic treatment but remains a serious life threat to infants and to elderly or debilitated patients.

Bronchial pneumonia, caused by a variety of different pathogenic bacteria, involves patchy areas of lung tissue surrounding the smaller bronchi and bronchioles, but both lungs are often affected simultaneously, so the disease can be almost as devastating as lobar pneumonia. *Viral pneumonia* is a diffuse infection of lung tissue throughout both lungs by certain viruses, usually a much less severe infection than the bacterial pneumonias but apt to run a longer course, with a very prolonged convalescence, because none of the antibiotics is effective in fighting off viruses. Less frequent but equally dangerous bacterial pneumonias include pneumonia due to organisms such as Friedländer's bacillus, *Hemophilus influenzae* bacilli, or the plague bacillus *Pasteurella pestis.* Finally, certain funguses may invade the lungs and cause severe pneumonias which can be extremely difficult to eradicate because no known antibiotic drug is effective in destroying the causative organisms. (*See* p. 276.)

Today most infectious pneumonias, if diagnosed early enough and treated vigorously with antibiotics, can be effectively controlled. But these infections attack one of the most delicate tissues in the body, and recovery is not always speedy. In addition, even with the most aggressive treatment and careful follow-up, certain serious complications may arise which are dangerous enough in themselves to deserve special mention.

Hydrothorax. In some pneumonias, when the lung tissue in contact with the pleura is involved, edema fluid may exude from the pleural surfaces and trickle down to fill the lower part of the chest cavity outside the affected lung, thus impairing the lung's capacity to expand to its fullest. This condition, known as hydrothorax, can usually be identified on X-ray after the pneumonia has run its course for several days—an important reason for taking repeat chest X-rays even when the infection is subsiding. When present, a hydrothorax can be drained by a simple bedside procedure known as *thoracentesis,* in which the doctor uses a local anesthetic and then inserts a special needle between the ribs in the lower rear portion of the chest to suck out the fluid. The amount of fluid that can collect is surprising; doctors know that as much as 100 cc.'s (approximately 3 ounces) must be present before it even shows up on the X-ray, and sometimes more than a quart is removed at a time. Drainage of this fluid, which is often contaminated with bacteria, not only allows the lung to reexpand but also helps reduce the chances of an even more difficult complication known as empyema.

Empyema. This is a purulent infection of the pleural lining of the lung and the chest cavity, often with a collection of pus in the area. Vigorous antibiotic therapy, either by mouth or by injection, and surgical drainage of the pus usually help quiet the infection, but not uncommonly the layers of pleura, which are normally smooth and able to slide over each other with the expansion and contraction of the lung, become covered with a fibrinous material that literally glues the lung to the inside of the chest cavity. This causes serious interference with respiratory movements—the lung tends to remain always expanded—and if the condition does not resolve itself, a surgical procedure known as *decortication* may become necessary. Once the active infection has healed, the surgeon makes an incision in the chest and literally peels the adhering lung away from the wall of the chest cavity. Fortunately, adequate treatment of the

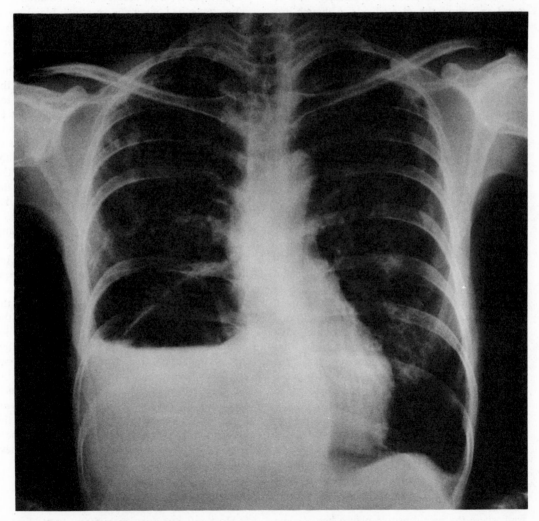

Plate 16   Hydropneumothorax (fluid and air in the chest outside the lung). Note the "fluid level" visible in the lower region of the right thorax.

empyema usually prevents this long-term complication and allows healing without surgical intervention in most cases.

Pleuritis or "Pleurisy." These are rather vague terms that describe any inflammation or irritation of the pleural lining of the lungs and the inside of the chest cavity, a particularly painful condition because the pleura is richly endowed with pain-sensitive nerve endings. The pain of pleurisy is a sharp, "cutting" or "scratchy" discomfort markedly aggravated by breathing movements, so the victims of pleurisy tend to guard or "splint" the affected side. Although it is a common complication of pneumonia, it may arise as a separate bacterial or viral infection in itself without any associated lung disease. The distinctive character of the pain is usually diagnostic, but the physician may also hear a characteristic squeaky-sounding *pleural friction rub* through the stethoscope when the patient breathes, rather like two pieces of leather being rubbed together. Pleuritis is treated with bed rest, mild analgesics for pain and antibiotic drugs; it will usually clear up within a few days under such a program.

Lung Abscess. This is an uncommon complication of certain kinds of bacterial pneumonias, especially those caused by Friedländer's bacillus or strep or staph organisms. Instead of healing with complete clearing of the alveoli in the affected regions, sometimes organisms become trapped in part of the lung and form a sealed-off pocket or abscess filled with pus. This is much the same as an abscess anywhere else in the body, often separated from the surrounding tissue by a tough coating of fibrous tissue that develops as the body attempts to isolate the infection. Lung abscesses may also occur as a complication of bronchiectasis when a distended and infected bronchiole becomes completely obstructed, making drainage impossible. Sometimes lung abscesses enlarge and form a direct channel between the end of the bronchiole and the pleural lining of the chest cavity, a so-called *bronchopleural fistula,* which often announces its presence at first by the sudden onset of severe aching pain at the localized spot in the chest wall where the pain-sensitive pleura has become involved in the infection. More commonly, however, a lung abscess may develop without symptoms except for intermittent fevers and chills and the evidence of an unhealing area of consolidation seen on a chest X-ray. The white blood count also tends to remain elevated and the erythrocyte sedimentation rate remains high, both indications of some continuing infective process in the body.

When a lung abscess is suspected, a return to intensive antibiotic treatment is indicated, sometimes at higher dosages than in treating the original pneumonia, because the circulation to a lung abscess is limited and very high blood levels of antibiotics are necessary to penetrate the area. Most frequently the abscess will drain spontaneously into a bronchus, and its contents will be coughed up by the patient. If the diagnosis has been uncertain, it may be confirmed then by the incredibly foul odor that literally permeates the room as soon as drainage begins. Unpleasant as it may be, drainage usually allows the abscess to heal, leaving only a small area of scar tissue in the lung. In the case of small or multiple abscesses, drainage may never take place; the lesions simply heal and scar more slowly as the body clears away the waste and debris of infection.

If a large lung abscess does not drain, and especially if the pleura is involved, surgical drainage of the abscess may be necessary. Indeed, if a large segment of lung tissue has been destroyed by abscess formation, the surgeon may open the chest and resect the diseased part of the lung in order to speed healing and avoid the complications that can arise from prolonged infection. One such complication is the possibility that a lung abscess will erode into a blood vessel and drain bacteria and purulent material into the blood stream, causing blood poisoning and spreading the infection to such distant parts of the body as the liver, the kidneys or even the brain. Speedy diagnosis and intensive treatment today are usually effective in avoiding these dangerous complications.

Other Inflammatory Diseases of the Lung

Most inflammatory respiratory tract diseases are caused by infectious bacteria or viruses, but other diseases, unrelated to infection, can also cause lung inflammation and, in some cases, long-term damage. These conditions arise from inhaling certain kinds of irritative dust, gases or other chemical matter which the body is unable to clear away under ordinary circumstances.

To some degree the inhalation of foreign matter is inevitable. An adult lung in a normally inflated condition fills a portion of the chest approximately a foot high, 6 inches wide and 8 inches deep; but if it were completely collapsed and all the air squeezed out, it would be reduced to a mass of tissue smaller than a fist. The entire lung is made up of thousands of tiny pockets of air, supported only by the thinnest cobweb of connective tissue, much as the air pockets in a sponge are supported only by thin strands of organic matter. Within the fibrils of this delicate connective tissue there are cells which engulf and retain particles of foreign material that come to the lung in the inhaled air—dirt and dust particles, tobacco smoke, soot and other insoluble debris. Thus, while the lungs of a newborn baby are a bright pink color, the lungs of an adult city dweller who has spent half his lifetime smoking have a mottled, black appearance. An adult nonsmoker who lives in a less polluted rural atmosphere will have lungs of a pinker color, but there will still be patches of sooty carbon and other debris scattered throughout. Up to a point this does no particular harm, nor does it take up any great volume of lung tissue. But that point is reached very quickly when the foreign matter is of a kind that in itself irritates and inflames lung tissue, or when a gradual accumulation predisposes the lungs to infection, degeneration or abnormal growth.

Silicosis. Among the irritative diseases of lung tissue are a group of conditions known as *pneumoconioses,* and the most common of them is silicosis, a widespread lung inflammation which arises, usually as an occupational hazard, among miners, wrecking crews and construction workers as a result of prolonged exposure to and inhalation of silicon-containing dust from rocks, powdered concrete, sand or gravel pits and similar sources.

In most cases silicon (not to be confused with silicone, a man-made chemical) is a comparatively inert element as far as the human body is concerned. It is usually bound up with other chemicals in the form of insoluble salts such as calcium silicate—simple sand. Ordinary contact with silicates has no ill effect; certain quantities are inevitably swallowed in food and pass on through the gastrointestinal tract with no harm. But when silicate particles are inhaled into the lungs in any quantity they lodge in lung tissues and cause a purely mechanical or irritative inflammation, leading eventually to an acute illness not unlike pneumonia. Silicosis is not an infection, and there is no effective means of combating the inflammation other than recognizing its presence and getting the victim out of contact with silicates that are causing it. With rest and relief from exposure, he will gradually recover from the acute inflammation, but the silicates remain lodged in the lungs, "boxed in" by little nodules of fibrous tissue which give the chest X-ray a permanent and characteristic mottled appearance. Even a small amount of involvement impairs the ability of the lungs to expand and fill with oxygen, and the greater the degree of the silicosis the greater the impairment of respiration. Over the long term severe silicosis can impair respiratory function by as much as 50 percent or more as a widespread net of abnormal fibrous tissue enmeshes the lung and severely limits its ability to expand and contract normally, a condition called *pulmonary fibrosis.* It can also lead to outright obstruction of various of the air tubules leading into the alveoli, contributing to *pulmonary emphysema.* Finally, victims of silicosis are also exceptionally susceptible to tuberculosis and other respiratory infections. Workers exposed to high concentrations of silicates on the job can and should wear protective breathing devices, and those in prolonged contact with even small quantities should take the precaution of frequent respiratory checkups.

A similar condition, *asbestosis,* occurs among workers in mines, factories or on construction jobs who inhale asbestos dust and fibers over a period of time. Still another known as *anthracosis* first became prevalent among anthracite coal miners in England, where the condition was commonly called "miner's lung." Better known

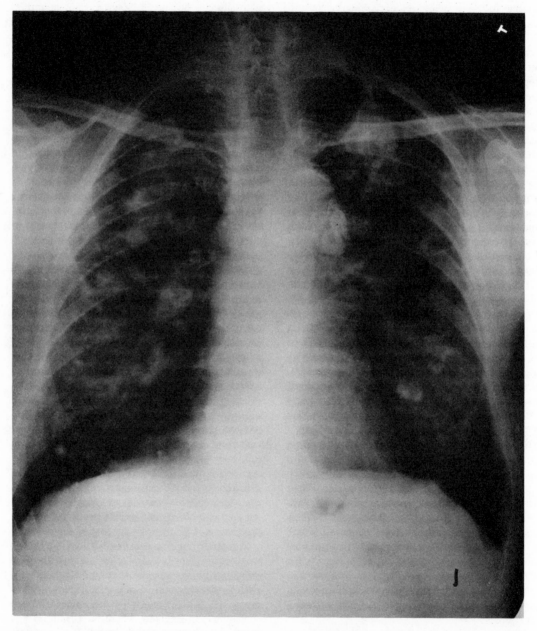

Plate 17   Advanced silicosis ("miner's lung"). Seriously involved areas appear as cloudy patches throughout both lung fields.

as "black lung disease" among coal miners of this country, it was once thought to be due to inhalation of coal dust, since victims of the disease, on autopsy, were found to have lungs peppered with black, grainy nodules of carbon. Most authorities today agree that the coal dust itself is not the troublemaker, much as it may discolor the lung tissue, but that the hard rock through which miners must drill to reach coal leads to silicosis. Other more obscure chemicals such as beryllium can cause similar kinds of inflammatory diseases.

Chemical Pneumonia. Inhalation of various irritative or poisonous chemicals and gases can cause inflammatory damage to the respiratory tract or even chemical pneumonia. Chlorine gas, for example, is highly irritating to any mucous membrane. When inhaled, it causes an acute inflammation accompanied by a severe outpouring of edema fluid into the bronchi, bronchioles and alveoli—in fact, anywhere the gas comes in contact with a mucous membrane. Thus the inhalation of any amount of chlorine gas may lead to a rapidly developing chemical pneumonia involving large portions of both lungs. Mustard gas, a chlorine compound used as well as chlorine gas as a weapon in World War I, was infamous not only as a respiratory poison but also for its blistering effects on the skin. Poison gases have now been banned as weapons of war, but many nations, including our own, continue to experiment with them as a part of their defense arsenals, and accidental exposure during manufacture, testing, transportation or disposal is a very real concern. Many poisonous chemicals and gases, however, do have legitimate commercial uses, and here, too, accidental exposure can pose a serious threat. Potential victims should take every industrial and personal precaution possible. In the case of chlorine gas, which is highly soluble in water, a water-soaked handkerchief held over the nose and mouth will provide at least partial protection, in the event of accidental exposure, until it is possible to get away from the gas. Even chlorine compounds used to purify the water in swimming pools can have irritative effects on the lungs and air tubes if any water is accidentally aspirated, similar to the irritation of the mucous membrane of the eyes so commonly noted after dips in chlorinated pools. Thus the chemical should be used with the utmost caution, following the directions that come with the product and erring on the side of too little rather than too much. Any excessive irritation noted from public swimming pools should be reported at once to the public park or public health authorities.

Another chemical irritant to the upper respiratory tract is ordinary tear gas used both in warfare and in riot control. This acrid and highly irritating substance, which is not as dangerous as chlorine, attacks primarily the mucous membranes of the eyes and nose and causes a copious outflow of tears. Deeper inhalation can lead to severe spasms of coughing, even to the point of vomiting, but the effect passes within a few minutes, and chemical pneumonia does not ordinarily result unless the victim already has an acute upper respiratory infection which the irritant gas merely aggravates. Again, considerable protection can be gained by soaking a handkerchief in water and holding it over the nose and mouth while passing out of range of the gas.

Severe chemical pneumonia can also result from inhalation of smoke from a fire. Damage to the lungs may be further exaggerated by the intense heat of smoke or air in a building that is on fire, and by the direct inhalation of flame, which literally sears the mucous membranes of the trachea and bronchi and can lead to an uncontrollable outpouring of mucus and edema fluid until suffocation results. In a fire it is wise to remember that both hot air and smoke tend to rise; the coolest and freshest air will almost invariably be at floor level, and you can protect yourself most effectively against smoke poisoning or heat damage to the lungs by dropping to the floor and, if possible, covering the nose and mouth with a water-soaked cloth. If a door must be opened in a situation where a burst of flame may occur, hold your breath and drop to the floor as quickly as possible. These simple precautions should be taught to your children and practiced during household fire drills. In case of an emergency they might very well prevent severe injury, prolonged illness or even death.

Another common form of chemical pneumonia is *aspiration pneumonia,* which can occur when an unconscious or debilitated individual, such as a baby exhausted from coughing or a very elderly person, regurgitates stomach contents and gastric juices and then inadvertently aspirates or inhales this acidic debris. The acid is very irritating to bronchical tissues, as well as to the alveoli themselves, and can cause an acute inflammatory reaction with an outpouring of mucus and edema fluid, often complicated by bacteria that were mixed in with the gastric contents. When such an accident occurs in a hospital and is detected in time, it is often possible to reduce the threat of pneumonia by using a rubber catheter, inserted through a nostril and down into the trachea, to suck up the debris before it can be inhaled more deeply. In a relatively strong, healthy individual coughing may suffice to raise much of the aspirated debris, but if the victim is a very sick child or an enfeebled elderly person, he may be unable either to cough effectively enough or to call for help, and aspiration pneumonia often becomes a terminal event in these age groups. In adults it is a common complication of acute alcoholism, when the victim has passed out and is totally unconscious at the time of regurgitation and aspiration. By far the largest majority of deaths of chronic alcoholics on the streets of our cities is due to aspiration pneumonia.

The threat of this condition is particularly great in a situation in which some medicine such as a general anesthetic, which may in itself stimulate vomiting, is to be used. Once a patient is anesthetized, or recovering from general anesthesia, aspiration of emesis can be a fatal blow in an otherwise perfectly safe surgical procedure. For this reason, surgeons adamantly insist that a patient take nothing by mouth, not even water, for a period of at least six to eight hours prior to the administration of anesthesia for surgery, even when the surgery is an emergency. It is only when immediate surgery is absolutely imperative to save a life that they will break this rigid rule. Thus everyone should be prepared, in the event of some sudden emergency illness, to outline for the physician or surgeon exactly how much and what kind of food was last eaten by the victim. Further, it is a very sound rule of thumb, when someone becomes suddenly and

unexpectedly ill, to withhold any food other than clear liquids—beef or chicken broth, etc.—for the first few hours of the illness, just in case it turns out to be a surgical emergency of some kind.

Oil pneumonia, a different kind of chemical inflammation of the respiratory tract, can occur suddenly and be extremely dangerous. Water or solid materials inadvertently aspirated into the bronchi cause choking, and the victim usually expels the material before it reaches the lung tissues. Oils, however, are far less irritating and can sometimes gain access to the trachea and bronchi without causing any significant cough reflex. Once the oil reaches the alveolar spaces of the lung there is no way for the body to clear it away, and a chemical pneumonia can result. Because of this risk, most doctors counsel their patients never to use oil-based nose drops or oily or greasy ointments or medications inserted into the nostrils for the relief of nasal congestion. (*See* p. 226.) It is the threat of oil pneumonia, also, which accounts for the common warning *not* to induce vomiting as a first-aid measure when someone has accidentally swallowed oily substances such as kerosene or gasoline. The likelihood of aspirating some of this material into the lungs is so great that emptying the stomach in such a case should be undertaken only by a doctor, if at all.

One final inflammatory disease of the lung that accounts for many deaths, especially among aged and debilitated people, is *hypostatic pneumonia* or "stasis pneumonia," an inflammation of the lung which can occur any time the victim is breathing very shallowly for prolonged periods, lying essentially still in one spot, and never really filling his lungs with air. The lungs, after all, are made to expand and contract, yet an aged person bedridden from some other illness may subsist on very shallow breathing, and great portions of his lungs fail to expand and contract at all with the movement of air. This is especially true if the patient is in pain, particularly chest pain, and actually resists filling his lungs with air. In such circumstances the inactive portions of the lung become highly vulnerable to infection by bacteria, and the bronchi may fill up with secretions which are not brought up by vigorous coughing. Segments of alveolar tissue then slowly empty of air and *atelectasis,* localized areas of collapse of the lung, takes place. Ultimately, bacterial invasion leads to a fast-moving "silent pneumonia" which can prove fatal before it is even detected.

Today doctors and nursing personnel are very alert to the dangers of stasis pneumonia, and if this condition develops, it is largely due to neglect of the cardinal rules of nursing care. This is one reason that physicians force patients out of bed for a period of time each day very soon after surgery and encourage movement of the patient even when he is largely immobilized, as with a broken bone. If an aged or bedridden patient is being nursed at home, his position should be changed as frequently as every hour or two so the different parts of his lungs are aerated properly even if he is not breathing deeply. This nursing procedure also has the additional benefit of helping to prevent bedsores. Furthermore, with the doctor's concurrence, the patient should be encouraged to breathe deeply for a brief period, even in the face of pain, so that at least three or four times a day he fills his lungs somewhere close to capacity. He should also be encouraged to cough up any mucus collecting lower down in his bronchial system, again even in the face of pain. With attention to these relatively simple nursing procedures the threat of hypostatic pneumonia can be greatly reduced.

Hay Fever, Asthma and Emphysema

Except in a few cases, infections of the respiratory tract are primarily irritative diseases, with obstruction of respiration only a secondary concern. There are, however, other disorders in which respiratory obstruction is the primary feature. These conditions, of course, include mechanical obstructions of the airway by aspirated foreign bodies (discussed in the previous chapter), but particularly notable are three other disorders; two of them are primarily allergic in origin, and the third most commonly afflicts the middle-aged or elderly as the result of some other chronic respiratory disease.

Hay Fever

Hay fever is a common and extremely uncomfortable obstructive disorder of the respiratory tract caused by an allergic reaction. Because so many manifestations of an allergy are related to the skin or the cutaneous system, the underlying causes and mechanisms of allergic reactions are discussed in detail in Part VII, "Patterns of Illness: The Cutaneous System." Briefly, however, allergic symptoms arise primarily from a natural defense mechanism intended to protect the body from possible damage due to the invasion of foreign protein materials known as allergens. These foreign materials may vary widely, ranging from the tiny particles of organic matter and mold spores found in ordinary house dust to myriads of different plant pollens carried in the air, animal hair and danders, a wide variety of different foods, various chemicals and metabolic

waste materials of invading bacteria, and the protein substance coating most virus particles. Oddly enough, the body's allergic reaction to these foreign materials is typically centered on certain "target organs." When the skin is the target organ, the allergic reaction may cause red itching welts known as *hives*. In the case of many allergens, however, particularly those that are likely to be inhaled—pollens, mold spores, house dust or animal danders—as well as a variety of allergenic foods, the respiratory tract becomes the target organ, and hay fever is by far the most commonplace allergic response.

This allergic reaction primarily involves the mucous membrane of the eyes, nose and upper portion of the tracheobronchial tree, and although extremely irritating and sometimes debilitating, it is not usually dangerous. In most cases hay fever is a pollen allergy, often so very specific that many victims develop symptoms year after year only upon contact with a single specific plant pollen. Others may be vulnerable to a dozen or more different pollens. No one knows precisely why one individual suffers from hay fever while another does not, but at least in some cases hereditary factors are involved; there are families in which virtually everyone suffers some degree of hay fever. Emotional tension may also play a part, since many hay fever victims are "sensitive" or emotionally overwrought. It is hard to distinguish cause and effect, however, since the discomfort of hay fever is often enough to make almost anyone emotionally overwrought.

Whatever the cause, the symptoms cannot be mistaken. Quite suddenly, with the beginning of the appropriate pollen season, the victim's eyes and nose begin itching and weeping and he starts

POLLENS ASSOCIATED
WITH HAY FEVER
(MUCH MAGNIFIED)

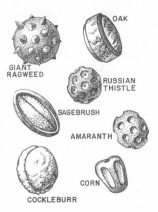

OAK

GIANT RAGWEED

RUSSIAN THISTLE

SAGEBRUSH

AMARANTH

CORN

COCKLEBURR

Figure 37–1.

to sneeze and cough, with a copious nasal discharge and a scratchy soreness of the throat. Infection is not usually a part of this syndrome, and there is seldom any measurable fever in spite of the name of the condition. Diagnosis is made by medical history and physical examination which reveals reddened, swollen nasal mucous membranes and, often, evidence of acute irritation of the entire upper respiratory tree. Diagnosis can often be confirmed by a therapeutic trial of one of the potent antihistamine medications, which may alleviate the acute symptoms almost miraculously in a matter of a few hours. Indeed, probably 80 percent of all hay fever victims require no other treatment than administration of antihistamines until the acute attack has subsided completely.

In other cases antihistamines are only partially effective, or else so many pollens are involved, spread out over such a long season, that more comprehensive treatment is necessary. The doctor may attempt to identify the specific pollens causing the reaction by means of skin tests, in which tiny amounts of various pollen extracts are injected beneath the skin of the back or the forearm and observed for the typical red-

ness and swelling of an allergic skin reaction, or by eye tests in which dilute solutions of pollen extracts are dropped in the eyes, which respond to the offending allergens by reddening and itching. Once the offending allergens have been identified, a serum containing extracts of these substances in very dilute form can be prepared and the victim "desensitized" with increasing doses of this serum injected under the skin on a regular weekly or biweekly schedule prior to the pollen season. This technique enables the body to accommodate gradually to the offending allergen without developing acute allergic symptoms, so that when the pollen season arrives the anticipated attack of hay fever is completely suppressed or markedly reduced. For reasons that no one understands, skin testing and desensitization do not always work with all hay fever victims; when they do work, however, they work extremely well and provide a means of regular annual prophylaxis against this aggravating condition.

Unfortunately, in a small percentage of victims, none of these treatment procedures is effective, and symptoms become so severe that treatment with such powerful anti-inflammatory substances as ACTH or the cortisone-like hormones is necessary to control the symptoms until the pollen season is over. Although research into the causes and treatment of hay fever continues, it seems likely that this affliction will never be completely eradicated; but treatment tailored to the individual needs of each victim can at least be effective in controlling symptoms in the vast majority of cases. There are no long-term or permanent ill effects of hay fever, and aside from the physical irritation and the trying effects on the victim's nerves, the condition rarely constitutes a serious or continuing threat to health.

Bronchial Asthma

Bronchial asthma is a disease in which the smaller bronchi and bronchioles are intermittently obstructed by large quantities of thick, sticky mucus secreted by cells in the bronchial walls. This is accompanied by contraction or spasm of the smooth muscle lining the walls of the bronchi and bronchioles, sharply reducing the size of these tiny air tubes, so that the victim has periodic attacks during which he has great difficulty breathing. And although this debilitating allergic disease, often chronic and sometimes even fatal, affects a great many people, bronchial asthma remains a mysterious condition, easy to diagnose but difficult to treat, and exceedingly distressing to live with.

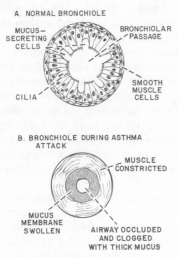

A. NORMAL BRONCHIOLE

MUCUS—
SECRETING
CELLS

BRONCHIOLAR
PASSAGE

SMOOTH
MUSCLE
CELLS

CILIA

B. BRONCHIOLE DURING ASTHMA
ATTACK

MUSCLE
CONSTRICTED

MUCUS
MEMBRANE
SWOLLEN

AIRWAY OCCLUDED
AND CLOGGED
WITH THICK MUCUS

Figure 37–2.

Unlike hay fever, bronchial asthma may result from allergic reaction to a wide variety of different allergens in addition to pollens. In many cases it can be traced to common house dust, mold spores, skin danders from house pets, various medicines or specific allergenic foods. The disease often appears first in early childhood as an apparent aftereffect of an acute attack of bronchitis or other upper respiratory infection. In fact, there is considerable evidence that childhood asthma is very frequently an allergic reaction to the by-products of upper respiratory tract bacteria, so that with each successive infection the child develops one or more attacks of asthma. Or it may occur first in older children or young adults, either suddenly or gradually, as a result of allergy either to extrinsic factors such as pollens, dusts and molds or to intrinsic factors such as bacterial by-products. Again, heredity may play a part, although familial incidence

of the condition is not nearly as marked as in the case of hay fever. Emotional factors and even endocrine disorders have been associated with asthma by various authorities, but no one has ever succeeded in defining a consistent, identifiable pattern to the part these factors may play. But in most cases the typical asthma attack is the same: the victim feels a sudden sense of tightening in his chest, followed by audible wheezing and coughing which progresses to serious respiratory impairment. As the muscles lining the walls of the bronchioles go into spasm and narrow the air passageways into the lungs, quantities of mucus are poured out by the mucus-forming glands of the bronchioles and it becomes harder and harder to move air back and forth. Characteristically, there is no problem *inhaling;* the problem is in *exhaling* the air trapped in the lungs, so that gradually, as the attack progresses, the lungs become distended, the alveolar sacs blow up like balloons, and great effort is necessary to force enough air out in order to inhale fresh air to replace it.

The duration and severity of asthma attacks varies widely. In some cases attacks never become severe, and clear up spontaneously in a matter of an hour or so; in other cases attacks may last six or eight hours or even a day or longer. In the presence of a long-standing chronic bronchitis, or in extremely severe asthma, the attack may persist for days on end, a condition doctors know as *status asthmaticus.* Whatever the length of an attack, and whether or not it is terminated by treatment, its end is characteristically heralded by coughing up great quantities of thick, sticky mucus, sometimes even in the form of small spiral plugs which perfectly outline the shape of the inside of the bronchi or bronchioles. As soon as the mucus starts to come up, breathing immediately becomes easier, and the victim, who often feels quite panicky at the height of an attack, experiences an overwhelming sense of relief at being able to get fresh air again.

There are many drugs and medicines which may help relieve an asthma attack, or even abort it before it becomes entrenched. One of the most dramatic antidotes is the injection of a small amount of diluted adrenalin solution; in some cases only a few drops of this medicine will begin to break up the attack within a matter of five or ten minutes. Individuals who have frequent asthma attacks, however, tend to become "adrenalin fast" after a while; that is, the adrenalin has less and less power to terminate the attack and other medicines become necessary. Another very useful drug, known as aminophylline, can be taken either by mouth or by injection. Unlike adrenalin, the effect of aminophylline does not diminish with frequent use, but other side effects may limit its use. But like adrenalin, the effect of aminophylline may diminish if the asthma victim uses it too frequently. Still other drugs contain adrenalinlike substances that are taken by means of aerosol spray. The asthma victim can use a spray nebulizer to create a cloud of the medicated substance in the back of his mouth and then, by inhaling deeply, introduce it into his lungs. Some of these aerosol medicines also contain so-called respiratory detergents which tend to soften and liquefy the mucous plugs, making them easier to cough up. Expectorant medicines such as potassium iodide, which can be taken by mouth, also have this effect. Finally, in severe cases, frequent acute attacks of asthma may be controlled by the administration of cortisone-like steroid hormones which have a tendency to suppress inflammatory reactions all over the body, particularly allergic reactions. With the use of various combinations of these medicines, together with the administration of oxygen, if needed, to help maintain oxygenation of the blood, victims of an acute attack almost always recover unless they are so weak and debilitated from other conditions such as pneumonia that the asthma attack is fatal. With medication they can also often remain free of severe attacks, with perhaps only relatively minor recurrences, for prolonged periods. There is no cure for the condition, however, and many victims suffer recurring asthma throughout their lives.

Obviously the best possible treatment for bronchial asthma is to discover the specific allergens causing the disease, and then take every possible precaution to avoid them. Sometimes the offending substances can be pinpointed simply from a detailed medical history. Since so many cases of asthma can be traced to house dusts, pollens or animal danders, it is wise for any asthmatic to get rid of any and all house pets, pay careful attention to dusting and maintenance of cleanliness in the home, discard all such notorious asthma-producers as thick, dust-catching carpets, feather pillows or overstuffed furniture (particularly if it is stuffed with horse hair), use an air filter device to cleanse the fresh air brought into the house, and eliminate any other possible sources of triggering allergens, including foods that seem to be related to subsequent asthma attacks. Sometimes skin testing can identify an unsuspected allergen, but this procedure is less likely to be helpful to an asthmatic than to a hay fever victim.

Any upper respiratory infection should be treated vigorously to prevent it from progressing, since these infections often trigger asthma attacks. Finally, attention should be paid to secondary factors that tend to intensify asthma: changes in climate, temperature or humidity, for example, periods of great fatigue or—a very common element in asthma attacks—periods of severe emotional distress. In fact, the emotional element is so strong in some cases of asthma that many people, including some doctors, erroneously write this disease off as purely psychosomatic. This, of course, is little comfort to the asthma victim, for his symptoms, no matter how strongly they may be influenced by emotional stress, can still be severe, frightening and dangerous, even if he is told that the attack is "all in his head."

What is the long-term effect of bronchial asthma on its victims? One often hears it said that an asthmatic child will "grow out of it" as he matures, and indeed it often happens that a child plagued with asthma at the age of six, seven or eight tends to suffer fewer and less severe attacks as he reaches puberty, and may in fact cease to have any trouble at all later in life. It is unlikely, however, that he has "grown out" of his allergy; what probably happens is that the allergy simply changes and manifests itself in other ways, attacking other target organs as time passes. And some children maintain their asthma throughout adolescence and into adulthood; it cannot always be counted on to go away.

Asthma that first appears in adults is even less likely to disappear, and although the victim gradually learns to sense when an attack is about to begin, and some may be very skillful in fighting it off or minimizing it, asthma can become a long-term, chronic bronchial obstructive disease that gradually works its damage in the form of permanent changes in the structure and function of the lungs. During the attacks the alveoli become repeatedly distended with air, and gradually lose their elasticity. The asthmatic begins to show a so-called barrel chest configuration as the walls of the bronchi and bronchioles thicken and the alveoli become more and more rigidly distended. When this occurs, even in the absence of an attack, the amount of air the chronic asthmatic can move in and out of his lungs is progressively impaired. With this decrease in air flow, he becomes more vulnerable to bronchial infections which further damage the smaller air tubes in the lungs and lead to chronic bronchiectasis. Or he may develop the permanent distention and obstruction of lung tissue known as pulmonary emphysema, in which movement of air in and out of the alveoli is reduced to the barest minimum necessary to maintain life.

These long-term effects can be minimized by early and vigorous treatment of asthma, and by the maintenance of a diligent program of medical management aimed at reducing the number and severity of attacks over the years. Perhaps the single most important factor in maintaining such a program is the patient's own realization that he suffers from a long-term, chronic disease that requires prolonged medical treatment and supervision which may never cure the disease but can at least reduce the amount of progressive damage to the lungs that would be inevitable without treatment.

Pulmonary Emphysema

This disorder of the lungs occurs most commonly, although by no means invariably, among people of middle age or older. It is characterized by enlargement and overdistention of the alveoli, as well as destructive changes in the walls of these air sacs, causing them to become fixed and rigid, incapable of the expansion and contraction necessary to the proper exchange of oxygen and carbon dioxide in respiration. Pulmonary emphysema usually develops slowly in the wake of some chronic obstructive disease of the respiratory tree, such as chronic bronchitis or bronchial asthma, and the damage to the alveoli may affect all parts of the lung equally or only one segment or lobe, depending on the chronic obstruction leading to the condition. In either case, just as an inflated rubber balloon never quite returns to its original deflated shape, and tends to become more and more permanently distended on repeated inflations, so the soft elastic tissues of the alveoli become thickened and permanently distended. Sometimes the walls between two or more alveoli break down, and healthy tissue in various areas of the lung is replaced by permanently distended, emphysematous blebs or air pockets that are virtually useless for respiration. In addition, mucus discharged by the bronchi tends to become trapped in the emphysematous areas and cannot be expelled by coughing, thus forming further obstructions to the effective exchange of oxygen. Eventually the victim of emphysema develops a chronic cough and wheezing, becomes progressively short of breath, and has greater and greater difficulty "clearing his chest" of normal mucus discharges.

As the condition progresses, the victim also displays a variety of physical changes. His lungs slowly increase in size because of hyperinflation and loss of the elastic quality of the lung tissue. The rib cage tends to assume the position of full inspiration, the diaphragm flattens, and the whole chest takes on a barrel shape. At the same time, the increased effort required for respiratory movements often leads to hypertrophy or enlargement of the pectoral muscles and the muscles between the ribs. Because of the need for increased blood pressure in the pulmonary arteries to pick up and circulate the diminishing supply of oxygen, the victim's heart is taxed and he is aware of shortness of breath varying from very mild distress upon exertion in the early stages of the disease to severe shortness of breath and even cyanosis at rest in more severe cases. When chronic bronchitis has contributed to the condition, coughing and wheezing may be almost constant, and in many victims the progress of the disease is markedly accelerated by concurrent bronchial asthma, repeated active bronchial infections, bronchiectasis or even chronic inhalation of noxious and irritating fumes. It is notable that heavy cigarette smoking is one of the most common factors associated with the early development of severe pulmonary emphysema, and the combination of heavy smoking with chronic bronchitis or bronchial asthma will almost invariably lead to severe trouble sooner or later.

Because the disease may progress very slowly over the years, and may well present few or no symptoms for a long period, early diagnosis of emphysema can be very difficult. Symptoms often begin to occur in the midst of repeated bronchial infections; the victim has increasing trouble with shortness of breath, more prolonged bouts of coughing, and greater difficulty in clearing up the infection. Once emphysema is entrenched, any other impairment of respiration, such as a cold or bronchitis, throws an almost intolerable load on the respiratory tract, and it is at times like these that the heart is taxed into heart failure, difficulty in breathing may become severe, and death can occur. In a great many victims, however, the condition may remain in this stage of severity for years, turning every respiratory infection into a nightmare, with prolonged periods required for recovery.

Early in the development of pulmonary emphysema various forms of treatment can relieve the condition or prevent its progress. Each episode of upper respiratory infection, particularly a bronchitis, should be treated vigorously with antibiotics to prevent prolonged obstruction of the bronchial tubes with mucus or thickening of the bronchial walls. Bronchial-dilating medicines such as aminophylline may be taken by mouth to help clear up secretions during acute attacks of bronchitis, and often the chest can be "kept open" by means of an aerosol bronchial dilator when active bronchial infection is not present. Careful attention to the so-called bronchial toilet at regular intervals during the day, particularly on awakening in the morning and before retiring, can help prevent bronchial secretions from accumulating. These procedures, similar to those discussed for bronchiectasis, include use of an aerosol to loosen sputum in the morning, postural drainage to allow gravity to help clear mucus from the bronchi, and a program of breathing exercises designed to expand as much of the lung as still is expansile, to strengthen the diaphragm and to improve aeration of the lungs as much as possible. In more severe cases heart failure and pulmonary edema may further complicate the exchange of gases in the lungs, and treatment of the heart failure with digitalis and other measures becomes necessary. In later stages, when shortness of breath is intractable and there is evidence that ventilation is inadequate to oxygenate the blood, various types of positive pressure breathing apparatus can be used to help improve the level of ventilation, remove carbon dioxide and increase the amounts of oxygen that can be absorbed by the lungs. Finally, the use of cortisone-like medicines may be helpful in reducing inflammatory reactions in the bronchi and in keeping the bronchial tubes and bronchioles dilated to permit as free an exchange of oxygen as possible.

Bullous Emphysema and Spontaneous Pneumothorax

Another form of emphysema is really quite a different disorder, characteristically affecting younger victims in localized portions of one or both lungs and occasionally leading to a kind of dramatic and frightening respiratory episode that is seldom seen in generalized emphysema. In this less frequent condition, the victim, who may be completely free of any symptoms of respiratory disease and have no history of previous respiratory tract troubles, develops localized areas of emphysema, usually in one or the other of the lower lobes and on the periphery of the lung. These may occur as a result of localized obstruction due to bronchitis or another previous lung infection, but it also may happen for no known reason. Whatever the cause, small areas of lung tissue break down, leaving thin-walled air pockets much like small balloons, ranging in size from a fraction of an inch to three, four, or more inches in diameter. Dead air is held under pressure in the pockets, and effective use of this part of the lung is destroyed. In medical terminology, these air sacs are spoken of as emphyse-

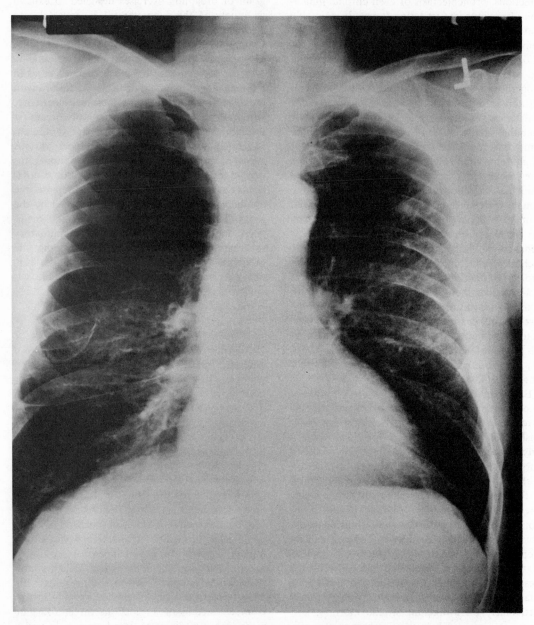

Plate 18   Bullous emphysema ("disappearing lung disease"). Tissue in the upper and lower regions of both lungs has been damaged or destroyed and appears abnormally translucent to X-rays. Functioning lung tissue can be seen in the middle portion of each lung field. Compare with normal chest X-ray, Plate 4.

matous bullae, and the condition is known as *bullous emphysema.*

A victim may have a single emphysematous bleb of this sort, or there may be multiple areas of the lung involved. In most cases there is no impairment of respiration at first, no particular hint of the presence of these areas, and no symptoms for prolonged periods of time, although sometimes the blebs are large enough to be seen on chest X-rays. (*See* Plate 18.) The main threat of this condition is that occasionally one of these sacs containing air under pressure will burst through the outer pleural lining of the lung, allowing air to escape into the chest cavity outside the lung and leading to a partial collapse of the affected lung itself.

This kind of accident, which may occur with no warning symptoms whatever, is known as *spontaneous pneumothorax,* and it can be an extremely frightening and threatening event. Typically there is sudden onset of sharp, pleuritic pain in the affected side of the chest; the victim is abruptly aware of severe shortness of breath and may take on the gray-blue coloring of the face characteristic of cyanosis or oxygen starvation. This sudden episode is often accompanied by shock and prostration due to the inexplicable pain and shortness of breath. The actual degree of lung collapse may be minor, but if the collapsed emphysematous bleb is in continuity with one of the bronchioles, a "ball valve" effect may take place. More and more air escapes through the ruptured bleb into the chest, but air is prevented from reentering the bronchial system; progressive pressure in the chest outside the lung begins to develop, causing greater and greater compression of the lung.

A spontaneous pneumothorax of this sort is, quite understandably, a serious condition, but with speedy medical treatment the chances for recovery are excellent. There is always a concern, however, that if a person has had one such episode, he may be vulnerable to another at some later time, and close attention should be paid to eliminating any contributing factors, such as cigarette smoking, chronic respiratory allergies, exposure to noxious fumes or other

conditions which can lead to episodes of bronchitis and secondary bronchial obstruction which may, in turn, aggravate the development of bullous emphysema.

Even more rare than bullous emphysema is a strange variant of the condition, thought by some authorities to be the same disease carried to an extreme. In this condition, known as "disappearing lung disease," the victim develops more and more emphysematous blebs, usually in both lower lobes of the lung, with many of these air sacs coalescing into larger and larger air pockets, sometimes measuring several inches across, separated by scar tissue. In extreme cases more and more of the total volume of lung tissue becomes involved in this kind of emphysematous degeneration, so that the useful amount of lung tissue gradually "disappears." In some cases this condition can reach a remarkably advanced state before the victim is aware of any kind of respiratory trouble at all; especially in young adults, accommodation to the "disappearance" of more and more lung tissue is so well handled that half or more of the total original lung tissue volume may be impaired before shortness of breath on exertion begins to make itself felt. What is more, the condition may spontaneously cease to progress at one stage or another, and the victim often has years of symptom-free life before trouble begins.

This is not the usual case, however; when the condition is discovered, it may progress either slowly or rapidly, with repeated episodes of pneumothorax or attacks of bronchitis accompanied by severe respiratory impairment, and sometimes both. Conservative treatment with medicines and bed rest is usually the first step, but the patient can frequently be helped a great deal by surgical removal of the damaged portion of the lungs so that the undamaged portion has more space in the chest cavity to expand. In any event, when "disappearing lung disease" is discovered, proper medical management requires frequent follow-ups with the doctor and the thoracic surgeon as well as the close cooperation of the patient in order to work out the best program of prevention of further trouble.

Tumors of the Respiratory Tract

Although infections, allergic conditions and obstructive disorders are by far the most frequent diseases of the respiratory tract, this organ system is also vulnerable in certain peculiar ways to the development of primary tumors, both benign and malignant. And because of the vast network of tiny capillaries spread throughout the lungs, they are also a very common site for the seeding of metastatic tumors arising from cancer cells shed by malignant tumors in other organs and ultimately trapped in the lungs to begin secondary growth. One respiratory tract tumor, *bronchogenic carcinoma,* is not only one of the most dangerous cancers known, but has recently been increasing in incidence so rapidly that it has become the fourth most common of all the life-threatening cancers—a phenomenon ascribed by many medical authorities to widespread cigarette smoking. Because of the great threat of this particular cancer, and because many other forms of respiratory tract tumors, both benign and malignant, can occur, it is imperative that everyone understand their nature and what can be done about them in terms of prevention and treatment.

Benign Tumors of the Respiratory Tract

Of the benign tumors or neoplasms that occur in the respiratory tract, most fall into the category of nuisance lesions. They do little real harm, nor do they impair respiratory function significantly. Nevertheless, because they often mimic certain malignant tumors or may be the

forerunners of others, they cannot safely be ignored.

Most common of these are the *polyps* or overgrowths of mucous membrane which develop in the upper nasal passages or sinuses as a result of chronic irritation or inflammation. Diagnosis and treatment of these tumors is discussed in detail elsewhere (*see* p. 442); it is necessary here only to reiterate that these polyps can, on occasion, undergo malignant degeneration, and consequently should be removed whenever they are discovered, a comparatively simple surgical procedure, and removed repeatedly if they tend to recur.

Another form of upper respiratory polyp is somewhat more serious because symptoms are so often similar to those of malignant tumors in the same area. These are the tiny polyps which can develop, again as a result of chronic irritation, in the larynx or even on the vocal cords themselves. The most notable symptom is the development of progressive hoarseness of the voice over a period of several months—exactly the same symptom most commonly seen with cancer of the larynx. Thus any change in the quality of timbre of the voice, or any hoarseness which does not clear up within a matter of a few days should be called to a doctor's attention. The presence of laryngeal polyps can be detected by a very simple examination of the larynx, and a biopsy will help determine whether they are benign or malignant. People often wonder why a biopsy is necessary when the growth is going to be removed surgically even if it proves to be benign. The reason is that the surgeon must do far more extensive surgery if a malignancy is found. (*See* p. 940.) Thus he must be as certain as possible of the diagnosis before definitive treatment is attempted.

Malignant Tumors of the Nose and Throat

A variety of cancerous tumors are known to occur in the nose and throat area of the upper respiratory tract. *Cancer of the lip* is particularly common among habitual pipe smokers and is believed to arise as a result of constant contact of a portion of the lip with the carcinogenic (cancer-causing) compounds from tobacco smoke that collect on the bit of the pipe. This disorder often first appears as an abrasion of the skin of the lip, usually painless, but with the subsequent development of a small raw area or sore which refuses to heal, or which breaks down repeatedly after healing. Diagnosis is made from the appearance of the lesion and from removal of a tiny fragment of tissue for biopsy. Cancer of the lip is relatively slow to develop, and once diagnosed, it can often be completely cured by radium treatments.

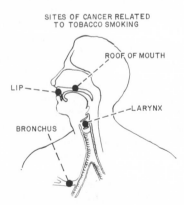

SITES OF CANCER RELATED
TO TOBACCO SMOKING

ROOF OF MOUTH

LIP

LARYNX

BRONCHUS

Figure 38–1.

Cancer of the mouth may develop anywhere in the mucous membrane lining the mouth. It is usually characterized by a small painful lesion which does not seem to heal, or by the appearance of the lesion itself—a rather flaky, white-surfaced sore, which is actually a very early

formative stage of cancer known as *leukoplakia* ("white plaques"). Smoking again is a suspected cause, and, again, diagnosis is made by tissue biopsy and treatment with radium is curative in the vast majority of cases. Indeed, with early detection these slow-growing malignancies provide an excellent illustration of how radiation treatment can be used to control or cure cancers: the abnormal cells in the cancer are far more readily damaged by radiation from radium or radon (a radioactive gas similar to radium in its radiation properties) than the healthy cells in the surrounding tissue, and the lesions are usually so shallow that radiation can penetrate all the cells in the tumor and destroy them, thus allowing healthy tissue to grow in the former tumor site very quickly. But if the cancer is undetected or ignored, and becomes larger or more deeply seated, radiation often can offer only palliation or temporary control. In such cases radical surgical excision may be necessary, with plastic surgery later required to reconstruct damaged areas of tissue.

Most dangerous and destructive of the malignant tumors of the upper respiratory tract is *cancer of the throat,* which usually also involves the larynx. As with most cancers, the precise cause of this malignant tumor is not known, but statistics indicate that it occurs by far the most commonly in individuals who have been heavy cigarette, pipe or cigar smokers over a period of years. The first symptoms are either the occurrence of a persistent sore throat or the onset of hoarseness which may begin with an upper respiratory infection and laryngitis but which does not clear up when the infection has healed. These symptoms may be related solely to a persisting upper respiratory infection or to the existence of benign polyps in the larynx; but if they do not clear up quickly under intensive treatment, they must be investigated without delay to rule out the possibility of cancer.

A simple physical examination may reveal suspicious-looking lesions in the back of the throat; but more frequently a somewhat more difficult examination by means of a *laryngoscope* is undertaken. With the patient under sedative medication, the use of this device allows the physician actually to look at the hidden areas of the inside of the larynx and back of the throat and at the same time to take a bit of tissue for biopsy if he finds a suspicious-looking growth or sore.

Untreated, cancer of the throat or larynx will continue to grow and spread, invading the soft tissues lining the throat and larynx and often causing increasing damage to the vocal cords. Ultimately it spreads into surrounding tissues in the neck or, by seeding through the lymphatic vessels, invades the lymph glands in the region. The disease becomes progressively more painful, rendering speech impossible and swallowing difficult, and after a course of a year or so is ultimately fatal.

Thanks to the fact that the cardinal symptoms of cancer of the throat or larynx are easily recognized and the source of the trouble easily examined, early treatment leads to a high percentage of cures. Treatment usually consists of a procedure known as *radical neck dissection,* the surgical excision of the primary site of the lesion plus a chain of lymph nodes in the neck, together with muscle and subcutaneous tissue that must be removed in order to get the nodes out. When the cancer involves the larynx directly, even in an early stage, the surgeon must also remove the voice box entirely. In this procedure the trachea is left open to the skin surface and the wound heals that way, permitting the patient to breathe directly through an opening in his throat. Clumsy as it may seem, a person soon becomes accustomed to this form of respiration. However, removal of the larynx also means that natural speech is no longer possible, and for many years it must have seemed to some patients that such surgery was as bad as or worse than the cancer. Then it was discovered that, with training and effort, these patients could learn a substitute form of speech. Air trapped in the nose and mouth is vibrated in the nasopharynx by the action of the tongue and the lips, which serve as substitute vocal cords. In addition, this form of speech is assisted by the regurgitation of swallowed air. The voice in this so-called *pharyngeal speech* is somewhat hoarse, but with practice words can be formed almost as quickly and coherently as in normal speech.

Even though surgical treatment must of necessity be extremely thorough, the fact that diagnosis can be made early renders this form of cancer one of the most hopeful in terms of cure. Even if there is recurrence at some time after surgery, the tumor tends to grow slowly, and its development can be sharply curtailed for a period of years by using radiation therapy and other medical means. Under these circumstances, it is foolhardy to postpone medical treatment for any reason. With early diagnosis and treatment, the larynx may be saved. Even if it cannot, the patient himself may be saved, and using substitute forms of respiration and speech, he can expect to continue a normal and healthy life.

Cancers of the Lung

Probably one of the most serious forms of cancer today, and one that is diagnosed more and more frequently each year, is cancer involving the inner lining of the bronchial tubes or lung tissue itself. The increased incidence of lung cancer is doubly tragic, first, because in many cases it is a *preventable disease,* and second, because it is exceedingly difficult to discover and diagnose early in its course of development. By the time symptoms and signs of the disease begin to manifest themselves, the tumor has all too often progressed beyond the point that a cure is possible.

"Lung cancer" is not a single disease entity; the lungs can be the site of a variety of different cancers, both primary (originating in the lung or bronchial tubes) and secondary or metastatic (seeded to the lungs from a primary cancer in some other organ of the body). Like the liver, the lung contains a vast network of exceedingly tiny capillary blood vessels; consequently when a cancerous tumor somewhere else in the body releases malignant cells into the blood stream, they will frequently become wedged in the lung capillaries and begin to grow. The lungs also have a rich network of lymph channels, another route by which cancer cells may travel. Thus it is not uncommon for a cancer originating in the breast, the stomach or the kidney, for example, to seed metastatic tumors, sometimes multitudes of them, in the lungs. Similarly, cancer originat-

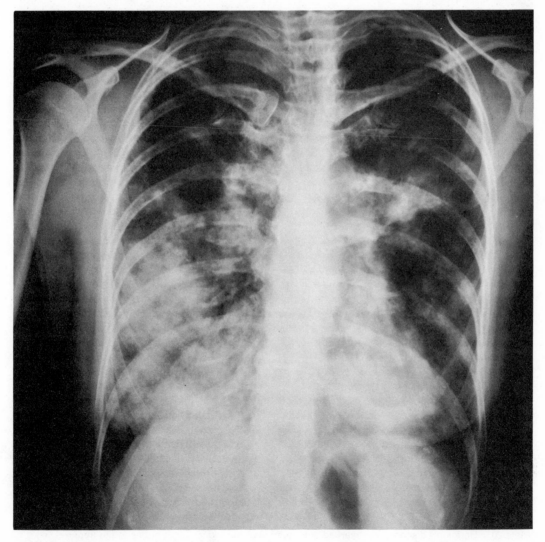

Plate 19   Metastatic carcinoma in the lungs. Multiple areas of disseminated tumor are seen
as cloudy patches in both lung fields.

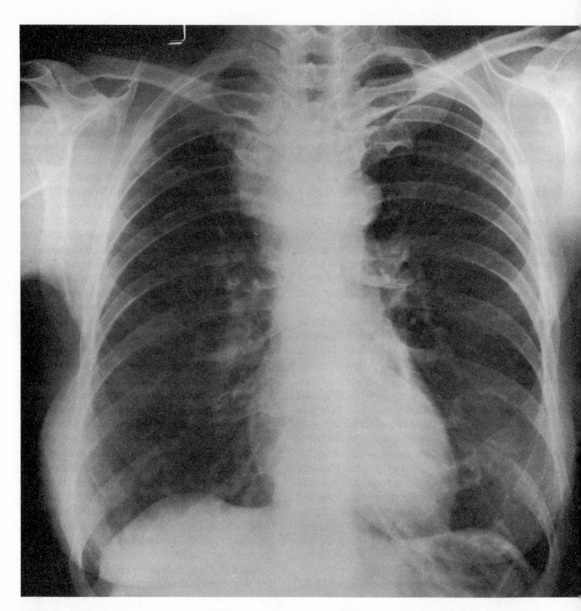

Plate 20   Hodgkin's disease, with marked enlargement of tumorous lymph nodes in the upper mediastinum.

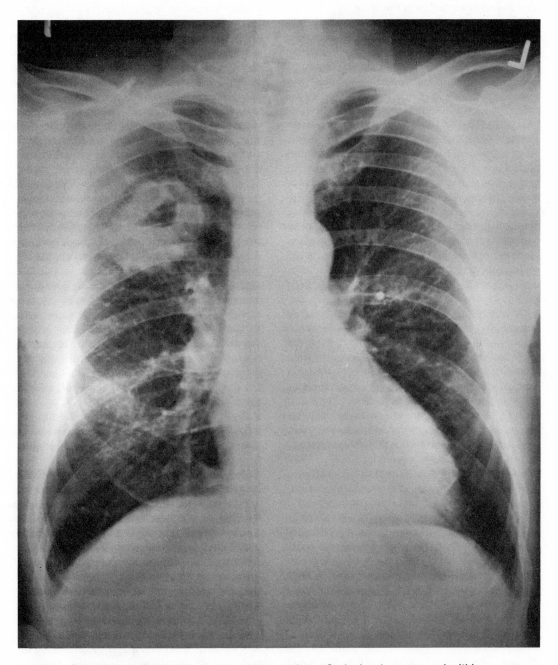

Plate 21   Bronchogenic carcinoma in the right upper lung. Cavitation has occurred within
the tumor because the cancer has outgrown its own blood supply and the center
has become necrotic.

ing in one lung readily spreads to the adjacent lung and to other organs in the body.

A metastatic cancer of the lungs frequently first appears on a chest X-ray as a scattering or so-called snowstorm of small gray shadows spread over both lung fields, and is usually a grave prognostic sign that a distant cancer has now reached a stage where it can no longer be controlled. In addition, various kinds of cancer of the bone marrow or lymph tissue, particularly Hodgkin's disease and some forms of leukemia, affect the lymph glands clustered in the central part of the chest. These glands may become so enlarged that the disease is easily recognizable on chest X-ray.

It is, however, a primary cancer in the lung tissue or bronchial tube lining which is today one of the most dangerous of all diseases afflicting man, and one which physicians and surgeons so far have had the least success in controlling. This is also the form of cancer that has been steadily increasing in frequency during the last 40 years and today is responsible for almost 10 percent of all cancer deaths. The statistical record of the disease is appalling: in 1930, fewer than 3,000 deaths due to lung cancer were reported in the United States; today the total has reached almost 65,000 deaths per year, most of them in men between the ages of forty and seventy, but with a steadily increasing incidence among women too. For years cancer authorities have speculated that this increase was directly related to heavy cigarette smoking, and by 1964 enough statistical evidence implicating cigarettes had been gathered to prompt the Surgeon General of the United States to state unequivocally that cigarette smoking is a major contributing factor in the development of lung cancer. Today we know that bronchogenic carcinoma occurs more than 20 times more frequently in men who are heavy cigarette smokers than it does in nonsmokers. Smoking, however, is not the only causative factor; the quantities of hydrocarbons polluting the air of our big cities from automobile exhausts and industrial wastes also contribute somewhat to the development of the disease, as evidenced by the fact that lifelong residents of congested city areas are five times more prone to cancer of the lung than lifelong residents of rural areas, quite aside from any relationship to cigarette smoking.

As with other forms of cancer, the major hope today for the victim of any kind of lung cancer is early detection and surgical removal of the cancer. Unfortunately these tumors very frequently develop in "silent areas" of the lungs where no physical signs or symptoms arise until the cancer has advanced beyond hope of cure. However, the occurrence of any of these cardinal symptoms—a persistent hacking cough, the appearance of even a small amount of blood in the sputum, unusual shortness of breath, a fever of unknown origin, chest pain, unexplained loss of weight or loss of appetite—means that a doctor's examination should be undertaken immediately, including careful chest X-rays for comparison with any earlier chest X-rays that may have been made. An early cancer of the lung can often be identified as a discrete coin-shaped shadow on a chest X-ray, the so-called coin lesion. Such shadows may be caused by some other condition—a localized tuberculous lesion, a small lung abscess, or a localized area of pneumonia, for example. Indeed, cancer of the lung is very frequently first detected when it is noticed that the lung of a patient recovering from a bout of pneumonia does not seem to clear as promptly as it should.

A variety of special diagnostic procedures can help establish the diagnosis or rule it out. In addition to ordinary chest X-rays, special kinds of chest X-rays known as *tomograms* may reveal a suspicious shadowy area in the lung in good focus at a number of different depths and help the doctor differentiate it from other normal shadows seen in chest X-rays. Fluoroscopic examination may also be useful. If fluid is present in the chest cavity, a sample can be withdrawn and analyzed for the presence of cancer cells. If a suspicious lesion is detected, a *bronchoscopy* may be performed, a procedure in which a lighted instrument is used to look directly into the trachea and the larger bronchi and to remove a bit of tissue for biopsy. Or a saline solution may be introduced into a suspicious-looking area and then recovered with a suction device for examination for cancer cells. Another common diagnostic procedure is the performance of a biopsy of the lymph nodes which lie at the base of the neck just above the collarbone or of nodes just under the breastbone; when a lung cancer first begins to spread, these particular lymph nodes are the most common site for the metastatic tumors to develop. If the tumor has already invaded these nodes, however, it may mean that the cancer has already spread too widely to hold much hope for surgical removal. In fact, between 65 and 80 percent of victims have the disease in such an advanced stage at time of diagnosis that they cannot be helped by surgery.

When diagnosis is made early, surgical exploration of the chest is necessary without delay. When the lesion is found, a biopsy can be taken of it then and there and the pathologist can report his tentative diagnosis within a matter of a few minutes. If the lesion is malignant, the surgeon can then proceed to remove it, usually by removing part or all of the afflicted lung, a procedure known as a *pneumonectomy*, necessary because even an early cancer may already have spread invisibly into neighboring regions.

Even with early diagnosis, the prognosis for lung cancer victims is very poor simply because the disease develops and spreads so rapidly. Untreated, the victim rarely lives more than a year, although survival times up to two years occasionally have been reported. With successful surgery an additional year or two of productive life may be gained; but few victims survive as long as five years postoperatively and fewer still as long as ten years. When the tumor recurs following surgery, or when it is already too advanced to permit surgical removal, various palliative measures may help reduce the size of the cancer temporarily and alleviate symptoms. These techniques include intensive radiation of the tumor, using high doses of X-ray focused on the area of the lesion itself, or treatment with radioactive cobalt. In addition, various anticancer medications such as nitrogen mustard or mechlorethamine can be administered intravenously. These anticancer drugs help suppress cancer growth primarily because they do more damage to the abnormal cells of the cancer than they do to healthy surrounding tissue. But they are extremely toxic and invariably make the patient seriously ill. All these measures can at best bring about only a temporary remission of the development of the cancer, and when the disease approaches its terminal phase, other medications may be used to alleviate pain and make the patient as comfortable as possible.

There are no new medical techniques on the horizon that offer much hope for improvement in this gloomy picture of treatment; the best hope of avoiding cancer of the lung, particularly among cigarette smokers and urban dwellers, lies in prevention or early detection. There is hardly a physician in the country who is not firmly convinced that cigarette smoking is a major cause of this form of cancer, and the profession has demonstrated this conviction not only by promoting antismoking campaigns, but also by the even more dramatic and convincing technique of giving up cigarettes themselves and urging their patients to follow suit. The story, they feel, is very simple: if you wait to stop smoking until a lesion appears on your chest X-ray, the chances are greater than 99 to 1 that you have already lost the struggle.

Even so, early discovery of lung cancer is vital, and cures *can* be achieved if the cancer is caught at the very outset. It has been demonstrated repeatedly that anyone, even the heaviest smoker, *can* stop smoking, given sufficient motivation to do so (*see* p. 590). In addition, *anyone who is or has been a cigarette smoker should have a chest X-ray taken at least every six months,* preferably in combination with a careful chest examination by his doctor. Cancer of the lung will probably continue increasing in incidence as long as people continue smoking cigarettes and polluting the air. But the more people who stop smoking now, and make sure they obtain chest X-rays at six-month intervals, the better the chance that the increasing incidence of this modern-day plague can be checked.

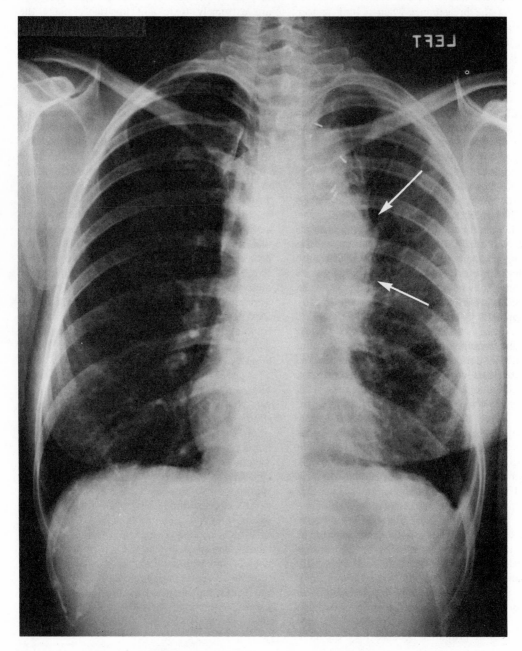

Plate 22a   A large inoperable carcinoma of the lung following diagnosis by exploratory surgery. Tumor could not be surgically removed and patient was referred for radiation therapy.

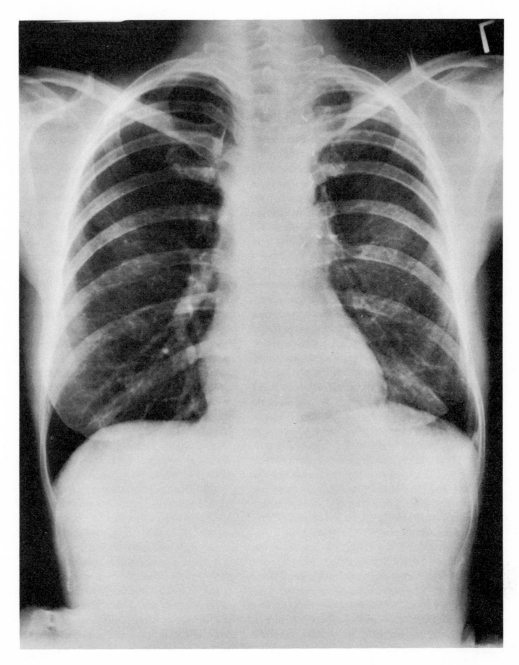

Plate 22b   The same patient 12 months later, following X-ray therapy of the cancer. Note the degree to which the tumor has diminished in size following radiation treatment.

PATTERNS OF ILLNESS: THE CARDIOVASCULAR SYSTEM

39. Disorders of the Blood and Blood-Forming Organs 511

40. Hemorrhage and Shock 533

41. Congenital Anomalies of the Heart and Blood Vessels 542

42. Inflammatory Diseases of the Heart and Blood Vessels 556

43. When the Heart Fails 573

44. Hypertension—The Silent Destroyer 582

45. Atherosclerosis and Coronary Artery Disease 592

Since time immemorial the heart has been inextricably associated with the very concept of life itself. Not only was it known to be essential to physical survival, but it was also regarded as the seat of the emotions. Courage, love and generosity all came from the heart, and even the soul was thought to be located there. Today we have a much more sophisticated knowledge of the heart and its less romantic, but no less important, function in the circulation of blood. Yet for all our knowledge, two of the most prevalent of all causes of death—atherosclerosis (sometimes called arteriosclerosis or hardening of the arteries) and hypertension (high blood pressure)—are diseases of the cardiovascular system for which medical science has not found a cure. What is more, many other defects and disorders of this vital organ system continue to take a heavy toll. Disease may affect the blood itself or the blood-forming organs; blood loss and attendant shock are ever present hazards when the cardiovascular system is injured. Congenital defects of the heart and blood vessels, as well as inflammatory diseases, can cause continuing illness and disability, and the threat of heart failure lurks behind a multitude of other disorders. Even so, this vital organ system has a surprising degree of resiliency and an amazing ability to adapt in the face of injury and diseases. Cardiovascular disorders may be deadly, but in most cases there are early warning signs which, if recognized and interpreted correctly, may enable the victim to forestall trouble. Thus an understanding of how this marvelously complex organ system functions, how it can be affected by disease, and how trouble signs can be recognized is of singular importance to everyone.

Disorders of the Blood and Blood-Forming Organs

Many of the organ systems that make continuing life possible do their work in sharply localized areas of the body and nowhere else. The lungs, for example, expand and contract within the confines of the thorax. Muscles operate in teamwork with specific bones and joints to move individual limbs, and the kidneys carry on their excretory function with remarkable economy in an extremely limited space. Even the cutaneous system, widespread as it may seem, is largely confined to surface areas of the body. Two major organ systems, however, extend to every part of the human body, and serve to bind all the other organs together in a continuous, integrated, functioning whole. One of these is the nervous system, and the other is the cardiovascular system, a vast and complex network of pumps, pipes, valves and tubules that endlessly circulates life-sustaining blood to every organ—indeed, to every living cell—throughout the body, a process that begins some months before birth and does not end until the moment of death.

The basic structures of the cardiovascular system, and of the blood which it circulates, are described in detail in an earlier chapter. (*See* p. 75.) Essential, of course, to the function of this organ system is the blood itself—a unique viscid fluid tissue which transports oxygen, nutrients, hormones and other substances to all the cells. The blood is carried to every part of the body by a system of tubes, first pumped from the heart up through the great arching aorta, then on through smaller peripheral arteries and branch-

ing arterioles into an intricate maze of capillary blood vessels that weave their way between the cells in the various organs and tissues. Ultimately these capillaries drain the blood into tiny thin-walled venules and thence into larger veins which empty into the great central vein or vena cava which returns the blood to the heart. In addition to moving through this *general circulatory system* to all parts of the body, pushed by the rhythmic beat of the heart, blood also travels through a separate, special capillary bed in the lungs, the so-called *pulmonary circulatory system,* where fresh oxygen is picked up for later distribution far and wide, and carbon dioxide is passed into the lungs to be exhaled from the body. Within this double system, worn-out blood cells are constantly being destroyed and removed from circulation in the capillary beds of the liver and the spleen, and fresh, new blood cells are constantly being supplied by the blood-forming tissues in the bone marrow and the lymph glands. But none of the circulating blood ever leaves this closed system of vessels unless injury or disease in some part of the body causes a leak. Even then certain proteins and cells in the blood immediately rally to form a gelatinous plug or clot to seal the leak, if possible.

Blood is, of course, circulated through this closed system by the pumping action of the heart, a powerful, muscular organ which receives blood in its hollow interior chambers and then rhythmically squeezes it out into the general and pulmonary circulation again in a ceaseless series of contractions or *heartbeats.* In an adult the heart contracts some seventy times a minute, on the average, under normal waking conditions. An infant's heart normally beats twice that fast. During sleep, however, the normal adult heartbeat may fall off to as few as forty contractions per minute, and at the peak of vigorous exercise may speed up to two hundred beats per minute, constantly adapting to meet the changing requirements of the body.

Indeed, the cardiovascular system is by far the most adaptable organ system in the body. It must function as a whole, continuously, in intimate contact with all the other organ systems, and particularly with the body's two major filtering systems: the lungs, which filter in oxygen; and the kidneys, which filter out soluble metabolic waste materials. Unlike such body functions as digestion, which occurs intermittently, the work of the cardiovascular system must go on smoothly and evenly, day in and day out, week after month after year, without significant variation. Clearly, efficient operation depends upon the adequate function of all of its parts at once, yet in any system composed of so many different parts in so many different places, breakdowns are bound to occur. And in fact, the cardiovascular system is vulnerable to more different diseases and disorders than any other part of the body. Some types of malfunction may be so minor that the system can go on functioning quite normally in spite of them, at least for a time, often without any symptoms whatever except during periods of extreme stress. Sometimes the system can adapt or *compensate* indefinitely for one or another type of malfunction, with other parts of the system working extra hard to make up for the loss. At the other extreme certain types of breakdown are so massive or so totally disruptive to the normal circulation of blood that death may result almost immediately unless something can be done to prevent it. Most serious cardiovascular disorders tend to give the victim some kind of advance warning so that preventive measures can be taken, and most heart and blood vessel diseases, if not always curable, are at least treatable to some extent. In this sense it can truthfully be said that disorders of the cardiovascular system, as frequent and various as they may be,

are often far more "fair" to the victim than the many diseases that strike swiftly and silently. But even minor disorders can have life-threatening consequences if they impede the system's one major, overriding function—the circulation of blood.

The Blood

Because of its peculiar nature as a fluid tissue, without any definitive shape or size, the blood has been regarded with awe and superstition since the earliest days of human civilization. Early medical history abounds with curious theories about the nature and function of the blood, virtually all of them wrong. It was not until the mid-1600s that the great English physiologist William Harvey finally proved that this peculiar red fluid was continuously circulated throughout the body in a closed system. A century later scientists using more and more powerful microscopes were startled to discover that blood was, in reality, a circulating suspension of free-floating cells, and it was only then that investigators really began to make sense of the structure and function of the mysterious cardiovascular system.

We still do not understand everything about the blood even today, but certain basic facts are clear. The normal adult has a total of eight to ten pints of blood circulating in his body at all times. And although blood is a tissue, it differs from any other tissue in the body in that its cells—about 45 percent of its volume—are not bound together but float about freely in a slightly viscid circulating fluid known as *plasma*. Plasma is more than 90 percent plain water, but it contains an amazing variety of dissolved chemical substances vital to the health and maintenance of the body. Many of these substances are *electrolytes*—dissolved salts and buffering acids—including ordinary salt or sodium chloride, and potassium, calcium, phosphorus and magnesium salts, and the ions of such acidic substances as carbonic acid, lactic acid and acetic acid. In addition, plasma contains quantities of blood proteins such as the albumin necessary to the body's health and nutrition, various forms of globulin involved in the body's immune defenses, and fibrinogen, the protein that is transformed into gelatinous fibrin when the blood clots. Plasma also carries hormones produced by the endocrine glands, nutritive substances such as the amino acids, sugars, and fatty acids derived from the digestion of food, metabolic enzymes and oxygen-laden red blood cells to the tissues all over the body, and it carries away such biochemical waste products as urea and creatinine for disposal.

The cellular elements of the blood include the red cells or *erythrocytes,* the white cells or *leucocytes,* and the platelets, sometimes called *thrombocytes* because they play a vital part in the formation of blood clots or *thrombi.* The red blood cells are perhaps the most familiar of these cellular components. Ordinarily an adult male has some 5,000,000 red cells in every cubic millimeter of blood and a woman approximately 4,500,000. Thus a single teaspoonful of blood (about 5,000 cubic millimeters) contains as many as 25 *billion* red cells. Obviously these red cells are too tiny to be discerned with the naked eye, but under a microscope they can be observed as small, identical disk-shaped bodies with depressed centers.

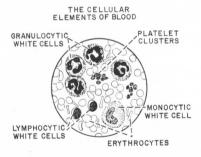

THE CELLULAR
ELEMENTS OF BLOOD

GRANULOCYTIC WHITE CELLS

PLATELET CLUSTERS

MONOCYTIC WHITE CELL

LYMPHOCYTIC WHITE CELLS

ERYTHROCYTES

Figure 39–1.

Under normal conditions, each red cell contains a quantity of *hemoglobin,* a complex protein substance containing iron as a vital constituent, which is capable of taking up or combining with oxygen in the lungs, where oxygen concentration is high, and then releasing it in the distant tissues where oxygen concentration is low. Among other things, hemoglobin is a *pigment* which appears bright red in a freshly drawn blood sample but has more of a yellowish

cast when seen under the microscope within individual red cells. When red cells are destroyed or broken up in the blood stream, a process known as *hemolysis,* the hemoglobin pigment is released into the blood plasma; and when a great many red cells are hemolyzed at the same time, as in certain blood diseases, the hemoglobin may stain the serum a dark yellowish brown color much the same as bile does. The iron in the hemoglobin, however, is carefully conserved by the body and reused in the manufacture of new red cells.

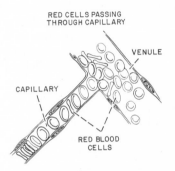

RED CELLS PASSING
THROUGH CAPILLARY

VENULE

CAPILLARY

RED BLOOD CELLS

Figure 39–2.

The red cells are not complete, self-sustaining units like other tissue cells. They do not have cell nuclei, and thus cannot reproduce themselves in the blood stream. They merely serve as floating containers for transporting oxygen-laden hemoglobin from the lungs to the distant tissues. As such they are constantly buffeted and banged around in the arteries and pushed through capillary tunnels hardly wider in diameter than they are; after a circulating life of approximately 120 days they finally disintegrate and are filtered out of the blood and destroyed in the capillary beds of the liver and the spleen. This means that quantities of new red cells must be manufactured at all times, a process that goes on in the spongy bone marrow in the pelvic bones, the breastbone and the rounded ends of the long bones. In these "blood factories" special "precursor cells" known as *erythroblasts,* equipped with nuclei, are constantly dividing and redividing to form young nucleated red cells. As these baby cells mature, they pick up hemoglobin molecules, lose their nuclei, and ultimately slip into the blood stream for circulation. Ordinarily, immature red cells never appear in the circulating blood, but when red cell production in the bone marrow is increased for some reason—to replenish the blood following a hemorrhage, for example—a few nucleated red cells may be found in a blood smear, and quantities of immature red cells may enter the circulation as a result of disorders such as "Rh disease" or *erythroblastosis.* (*See* p. 833.)

White cells in the blood are not nearly as numerous as red cells, numbering only 7,000 to 10,000 per cubic millimeter of blood under normal circumstances, and they have a totally different function. About three-fifths of the white cells, called *granulocytic leucocytes* or *granulocytes,* are formed in the bone marrow much as the red cells are, arising from special "precursor cells" known as *myeloblasts;* but they keep their nuclei when they are released into the blood stream and thus remain complete living cells. Other white cells known as *monocytes* also arise in the bone marrow, and with the granulocytes form a protective army of roving cells capable of attacking and destroying bacteria or other microscopic foreign invaders that find their way into the body. To accomplish this, white cells can even wiggle through minute pores in the capillary walls and move about through the tissues to fight invading bacteria. Many are often destroyed in battle, so to speak, and these dead cells are a major constituent of pus. No one knows exactly how the production of new white cells is regulated, but a bacterial invasion of the body is usually marked by a swift rise in the number of granulocytes in the blood, including many slightly immature cells, an important clue to the doctor that infection is present somewhere in the body.

Lymphocytic leucocytes or *lymphocytes* make up a third important group of white cells, some two-fifths of the total number. These are small white cells with very large nuclei, and they are formed not in the bone marrow like the other blood cells, but rather in the lymph glands scattered along the lymph channels all over the body. For many years the function of lymphocytes remained a mystery; they did not appear to engulf and destroy bacteria the way granulocytes

did, yet they often appeared in great numbers in areas of inflammation. Today researchers believe that they are intimately involved in the body's immunological defense mechanism, particularly important in fighting off various kinds of virus invaders. Indeed, in one kind of virus disease, infectious mononucleosis, the number of lymphocytes in the blood stream increases so markedly that their appearance there is an important diagnostic clue; and in certain forms of leukemia and lymphatic cancers, the liver, spleen and other organs may become literally packed with abnormal or immature lymphocytes.

A final cellular element in the blood is the *platelets,* which are not complete cells at all but merely tiny fragments of cell tissue from certain giant precursor cells known as *megakaryocytes* located in the bone marrow. As these giant cells mature there, they scatter their platelet fragments into the circulating blood. Platelets are much smaller than even red cells, and are found in the blood in numbers ranging from 100,000 to 300,000 per cubic millimeter. Under normal conditions they circulate just like other blood cells, but when the inner surface of a blood vessel becomes broken, diseased or roughened in some way, the platelets become sticky and cling to the damaged surface, disintegrating and releasing enzyme-like substances that trigger the blood's clotting mechanism to initiate the formation of a clot or *thrombus.* When the number of circulating platelets falls below normal for any reason, the clotting mechanism is severely impaired and capillary hemorrhages may occur all over the body, a condition known as *purpura.* Normally worn-out platelets are destroyed and removed from circulation in the spleen, but in certain abnormal conditions in which that organ does its job too effectively, it sometimes has to be removed surgically to keep the platelet level in the blood up to normal levels.

Taken as a whole, the blood performs a wide variety of vital functions. It carries oxygen, food and internal secretions to all the tissues of the body, and helps cart away and dispose of metabolic waste materials. As a great circulating reservoir for water, proteins and body salts, it helps maintain the body's temperature, regulates the fluid and chemical balance in the tissues and keeps the body's internal environment stable and unchanging, within very narrow normal limits, no matter what is going on in the environment outside the body. The blood plays a vital protective role in fighting infection and seals up leaks in the blood vessels by means of coagulation. Occasionally it can become an inadvertent carrier of such harmful substances as bacteria, viruses, parasites, cancer cells or various poisons; a bacterial invasion of the blood stream, for example—a condition known as *septicemia* or "blood poisoning"—can be an extremely dangerous, even fatal, complication of various infections. (*See* p. 206.) But in compensation, the blood can also carry medications to help combat such dangerous conditions.

Finally, because of its widely varied functions and its ready availability for examination, the blood serves the physician as a remarkably useful indicator of the body's condition of health. In a real sense the blood is the barometer of the body; innumerable diseases and disorders are reflected in readily detectable changes, gross or subtle, in its condition or composition, and blood examination today is probably the most important of all aids to diagnosis. And not the least common of the abnormal conditions that are often first identified by means of blood tests are certain disorders of the blood itself, or of the blood-forming organs.

The Anemias

Under normal conditions, the body has an ample number of red cells to supply all its tissues with the necessary oxygen, and as red cells wear out, sufficient new ones are formed in the bone marrow and released into the blood stream to keep the number relatively constant. But when something happens to reduce the number of circulating red cells much below the normal level at a given time, or to impair the manufacture of new ones, or to reduce the amount of hemoglobin carried by those cells, the result is the condition known as *anemia* (literally, "without blood"). And since an anemia from any source interferes directly with the normal and necessary supply of oxygen to the tissues, it is essen-

tial that such a disorder be detected as early as possible and vigorously treated.

Posthemorrhagic Anemia. Perhaps the most obvious cause of an anemia is sudden massive hemorrhage from a torn or injured major artery that can reduce the volume of blood in the body from the normal level of eight to ten pints to as few as six or seven pints in a matter of a few minutes. If the hemorrhage is controlled, and the victim survives the shock of the sudden blood loss, an anemia will result because the body can replenish the fluid portion of the blood much more quickly than its cellular components. Such an anemia will persist until sufficient new red cells have been manufactured to replace the loss, or until the condition is treated with transfused blood. Far more commonly, bleeding may occur slowly over a long period of time from some internal and unrecognized source such as a peptic ulcer, or from prolonged and extraordinarily copious menstrual flow. Again such a slow but steady drain on the blood supply may exceed the body's capacity to replace red cells fast enough, and anemia may result. In cases such as these there is nothing organically wrong with the blood-manufacturing process, and once the cause of the blood loss is identified and treated, the body can speedily replace the lost blood. Even so, this process may be aided by transfusions, if necessary, and accelerated by rest and a diet rich in iron and protein.

Iron-Deficiency Anemia. A related but more serious condition occurs when the body has insufficient iron to permit the manufacture of normal, healthy red cells. This may occur even without any loss of blood as a result of chronic nutritional deficiencies. The daily dietary intake of iron may be so low owing to a lack of meat or other iron-containing foods that it cannot keep up with the loss of iron that results from normal chemical processes throughout the body, or it may be insufficient to cope with a sudden new demand for iron such as occurs following a bleeding episode or when a woman becomes pregnant and her total blood volume must suddenly increase by some 15 percent in order to take care of the growing baby. Even the regular blood loss associated with perfectly normal menses can contribute to iron deficiency if a woman's dietary intake of iron is less than what is lost in the menstrual flow.

In any of these cases the net result is a so-called *iron-deficiency anemia,* a condition far more common among women than men because of the part menstruation so often plays in its development. Not enough new red cells are formed, and those that are formed are markedly smaller in size and contain less hemoglobin than normal. As a consequence, the entire body becomes slowly and chronically starved for oxygen, since there are not enough red cells or hemoglobin to supply normal oxygen requirements. The victim becomes weak and tired, fatigues easily and suffers from constant drowsiness or irritability. Often there is vertigo (dizziness) upon standing up from a sitting or lying position, and headaches are common. As an iron-deficiency anemia becomes increasingly severe, the heart must work harder to circulate such blood as there is as fast as possible, and the oxygen-hungry victim must breathe more rapidly and deeply in an effort to get more oxygen into the lungs. Often the burden becomes greater than the heart (which itself requires a great quantity of oxygen) can cope with and it begins to fail, further compounding the shortness of breath. The victim's normal resistance to any kind of stress declines and he becomes particularly vulnerable to infection. Ultimately, if the anemia remains untreated, he may die in heart failure, or his blood pressure may fall to shock levels followed by complete circulatory collapse.

Today an iron-deficiency anemia is rarely allowed to reach this critical stage, but treatment depends greatly on its severity at the time it is discovered. A mild anemia can often be treated by the prescription of a high-protein, iron-rich diet, together with supplementary iron. Often the cause of the anemia is plain—a new pregnancy or chronic dietary insufficiencies, for example—but even so a search must be made for contributing factors such as chronic bleeding from some hidden source. If the anemia has become severe, more heroic measures may be necessary, including treatment of impending heart failure, additional oxygen to aid respiration, and transfusions of whole blood or packed red cells. In times past

doctors often treated *any* kind of anemia with a shotgun blast of medicines, dietary prescriptions, supplemental iron, vitamins and so on, but it is now recognized that such treatment can actually mask or hide the presence of certain more dangerous kinds of anemia. Thus, today most doctors insist upon diagnosing the *kind* of anemia present, if possible, before starting any kind of treatment, and self-treatment of suspected anemia with vitamins or "iron tonics" without benefit of a medical examination is never advisable.

Pernicious Anemia. One kind of anemia that is totally unrelated to iron deficiency or blood loss was far more common 30 years ago than it is today, and was at that time extremely dangerous because its cause was unknown and there was no known cure. This anemia usually affected middle-aged or older people, and characteristically appeared so silently and became so progressively severe and so relentlessly unresponsive to treatment that it came to be called pernicious anemia.

This disorder comes on insidiously, and the earliest symptoms—a soreness of the tongue and an odd tingling in the hands and feet—hardly seem related to a blood disorder at all. Soon, however, gastrointestinal symptoms begin, including loss of appetite, weight loss, nausea and sometimes vomiting, diarrhea or attacks of pain in the abdomen. At the same time, the skin frequently becomes tinged with an odd lemon-yellow color, sometimes so striking that a doctor's suspicions may be raised by a single look at the patient. In advanced cases, typical symptoms of any severe anemia appear—weakness, fatigue, shortness of breath and even heart failure. In almost half such cases, marked degenerative changes occur in the nervous system; the victim has difficulty walking, especially in the dark, and develops a number of abnormal reflexes. In very severe cases when the anemia is profound, oxygen starvation of parts of the brain can cause sudden personality changes: the victim may become euphoric, or muddled and unable to remember, and may even begin to suffer from the sort of delusions often seen in severe mental illness. Prior to the discovery of the cause and cure of this anemia, the prognosis for its victims was invariably fatal no matter what was done, although the course of the illness often extended over several years.

Thomas Addison, an English physician, was the first to describe pernicious anemia as a clinical entity in 1849, and the disease is still sometimes called Addison's anemia. He discovered that patients suffering from this condition seemed to have no hydrochloric acid in their gastric juice, a point that is still important to diagnosis today. Other observers noted that there was often a family history of pernicious anemia, but no specific mechanism of hereditary transmission was found; examination of the patient's blood revealed that the total number of blood cells was markedly reduced even though the cell-forming bone marrow was actually overworking. The red cells themselves, however, were usually normal in size, or even larger than normal, with plenty of hemoglobin per cell.

Clearly the disease was quite different from an iron-deficiency anemia, but its cause remained a mystery until the late 1920s. The consistent gastrointestinal symptoms of the disease made researchers wonder if some defect in digestion might be at fault. Intensive studies conducted between 1926 and 1929 by various American scientists confirmed that sufferers from pernicious anemia seemed to lack some substance normally present in the cells lining the stomach that was necessary for the digestion and absorption of certain foodstuffs. This missing enzyme became known as the "intrinsic factor," but an additional 20 years of research were necessary to discover just what vital nutrient could not be absorbed when the "intrinsic factor" was missing. Finally the mystery was unraveled: victims of pernicious anemia were literally starving for one of the family of B vitamins, a substance known as cyanocobalamin or vitamin B_{12}, which could be taken into the body during digestion only with the aid of the "intrinsic factor" enzyme. There is still no way yet known to restore the missing "intrinsic factor" once it has been lost, but it was found that administration of adequate doses of vitamin B_{12} by injection, bypassing the digestive tract entirely, could not only cure pernicious anemia and prevent its recurrence as long as treatment was continued,

but also very effectively prevent the nervous system complications of the disease.

Today we know that vitamin B_{12} is vital to the proper manufacture of red cells, and that anyone deprived of it for any reason will develop pernicious anemia. But many foods, particularly meats, leafy vegetables and liver, are rich in the vitamin, and normally anyone eating a well-balanced diet will absorb as much as he needs. The "intrinsic factor" enzyme is the real culprit in the disease. When it is missing from the cells of the stomach lining for congenital reasons, the victim develops a primary pernicious anemia; if the cells containing the enzyme have been destroyed by tumors, peptic ulcers or other conditions affecting the upper gastrointestinal tract, the pernicious anemia is secondary. In either case it is seldom seen in advanced states today because it is usually caught and treated soon after the first symptoms occur, or even before symptoms, during routine health checks.

Pernicious anemia is not, however, the only condition caused by the lack of some vital nutritive substance, or the body's inability to utilize that substance. A deficiency of folic acid, a substance plentiful in green leafy vegetables, liver, mushrooms and yeast, can lead to an anemia similar to pernicious anemia. This so-called *folic acid deficiency anemia,* which frequently afflicts those who live on marginal diets, is treatable by prescribing additional folic acid in the diet along with vitamin C, which is necessary for its metabolism. Alcohol also interferes with the metabolism of folic acid, and chronic alcoholics are prone to develop this condition. A closely related condition is an uncommon disorder of the digestion known as *sprue,* in which a defect in the absorption of digested food by the victim's intestine brings about a lack of folic acid and a complicating anemia. Here again even small doses of folic acid will correct both the anemia and the diarrhea that is a particularly characteristic symptom of sprue.

Obviously, these deficiency anemias should be treated by *specific* therapy to replace the missing substance, rather than by the "shotgun" approach. Hence the importance of proper diagnosis. But often simply replacing the missing substance is not quite enough. If a person has an iron-deficiency anemia due to a constant, small but steady loss of blood from an undiagnosed and untreated bleeding ulcer, his condition may be temporarily improved by the administration of iron supplements, but unless the underlying cause of the disorder is also discovered and treated, the anemia will recur. Similarly, an iron-deficiency anemia is so much to be expected in the course of a pregnancy that most obstetricians prescribe additional iron supplements, together with other vitamins and minerals, to their pregnant patients almost as a matter of course; this sort of anemia will subside, all other things being equal, as soon as the baby is delivered and the mother's blood volume and eating habits return to normal.

Sometimes the underlying cause of anemia may be very difficult to track down. An alcoholic, for example, who conceals his drinking and refuses to acknowledge his illness even to himself may well become anemic owing to deficiency of iron, vitamin B_{12} or folic acid in his diet over a prolonged period of time as a result of his extremely limited food intake. In such a case the anemia can be treated, but it cannot be cured until the patient is willing to deal with the underlying cause. In cases in which congenital conditions or degenerative changes result in an anemia, however, it may not be possible to eradicate the underlying cause. Here continuous treatment is essential and achieves excellent results. Deficiency anemias that so frequently occur among the poor and undernourished peoples of the world perhaps present the greatest difficulties, for medical treatment, even when available, can be little more than a stopgap measure until the underlying social causes are corrected.

Hemolytic Anemias. There is yet another underlying cause of certain kinds of anemias, unrelated to dietary deficiencies. A variety of different anemias may occur as a result of abnormal destruction or *hemolysis* of red cells in the circulating blood. The resulting disorders are therefore known as hemolytic anemias. There are a number of conditions that can bring about this kind of blood-destruction anemia. Malaria, for example, can lead to excessive destruction of red cells because the malarial parasites multiply

within these blood cells and break them apart. This is one of the major world-wide causes of hemolytic anemia. (*See* p. 262.) More commonly in this country, hemolytic anemias can arise from blood transfusion reactions when mismatched blood is given to a patient or, in the case of infants, from Rh disease. (*See* p. 833.) Rattlesnake venom contains substances that destroy red cells, and certain poisonous foods may have the same effect. Chemical agents such as benzine can also cause hemolytic anemia.

These, of course, are acquired conditions, and once diagnosed, they can be treated simply by eliminating the blood-destroying element. Treatment is not that easy in the case of certain hereditary defects which can also cause chronic hemolytic anemias. In these cases, the cause of the anemia is literally built into the victim's body and cure of the condition is not possible. The anemia remains chronic throughout the victim's lifetime, often flaring up in "crises" of blood destruction which occur from time to time, rendering the victim intermittently extremely ill.

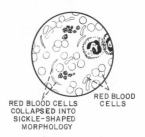

BLOOD SMEAR FROM
SICKLE-CELL ANEMIA

RED BLOOD CELLS COLLAPSED INTO SICKLE-SHAPED MORPHOLOGY
RED BLOOD CELLS

Figure 39–3.

Perhaps the most dramatic example of this form of the condition is *sickling disease* or *sickle-cell anemia*. While pernicious anemia occurs most commonly among members of the Caucasian race, sickle-cell anemia is almost exclusively a disease affecting Negroes. It results from a hereditary abnormality in the structure of the hemoglobin. Normal hemoglobin molecules consist of two pairs of protein molecule fragments bound together in a "double A" configuration by an atom of iron. But this structure is controlled by heredity, and occasionally an inheritable abnormality known as "S" hemoglobin is found. When this abnormal hemoglobin releases oxygen into the tissues, a very strange thing occurs: the red cells containing it tend to collapse into a crescent or "sickle-shaped" form instead of retaining their normal disklike shape.

Those who have inherited this "sickle-cell trait" from only one parent appear to have no trouble on account of it; they merely become "carriers" of the trait, capable of passing it on to their children. It is believed that some 8 to 13 percent of all Negroes in the United States carry this single-factor sickle-cell trait. But a person who receives the factor from both parents—approximately 1 percent of Negroes in the United States—develops a severe and strange form of anemia for which, today, there is no known cure.

The symptoms of sickle-cell anemia are as odd as the condition that causes them. For one thing, sickle-shaped red cells are mechanically unable to move through the narrow capillaries as readily as normal red cells. They form tiny plugs or blood clots known as thrombi in capillaries all over the body, obstructing the normal capillary blood flow and thus depriving various tissues of necessary oxygen and nutrient materials. In addition, sickle cells are extremely delicate and are destroyed in great numbers in the spleen far sooner than normal and far faster than they can be replaced. The result is a chronic anemia, often severe, marked by frequent wavelike episodes of widespread hemolysis of red cells. Such a "hemolytic crisis" is usually accompanied by acute joint pains and fever, and such severe abdominal pain, complete with vomiting, that the symptoms often mimic an acute surgical condition in the abdomen. The tiny thrombi of sickle cells may occur anywhere in the body, but they are particularly damaging in the central nervous system, where portions of brain tissue may be deprived of oxygen. Jaundice may appear during these "hemolytic crises" as the blood serum becomes stained by hemoglobin pigments from the hemolyzed red cells. In children both the spleen and the liver become enlarged, but in adults the spleen, damaged by multiple thrombi obstructing its blood supply, becomes scarred and atrophied into a useless lump of fibrous

tissue only a third its normal size. Gradually the heart becomes enlarged, and very few victims with a double-factor sickle-cell anemia live much beyond young adulthood. They usually die from thrombi completely obstructing circulation in vital organs such as the lungs or the brain.

Although sickle-cell anemia is incurable, the pain that occurs during a hemolytic crisis can be alleviated and heart failure can be treated when necessary. Blood transfusions are used only in severe crises because of the danger that transfusion reactions may cause additional hemolysis of red cells. The disease varies in its severity from one person to another; some sufferers have little more than a prolonged chronic anemia marked by comparatively rare hemolytic crises, and may live relatively normal lives for many years, but they must avoid travel in high altitudes or in unpressurized airplanes since the lower concentration of oxygen reaching their blood under these conditions tends to precipitate hemolytic crises. Others die in childhood or adolescence. Ultimately the best control of the disease today lies in its detection—the sickle-cell trait can be detected even in single-factor individuals by means of a simple laboratory examination—and in recognizing the possible consequences if individuals carrying the defect marry and have children.

Other hereditary defects besides abnormal hemoglobin may also produce hemolytic anemias. *Mediterranean anemia,* for example, is a hereditary condition which occurs most commonly among people living in the countries bordering the Mediterranean Sea. This anemia arises because the red cells are so abnormally thin that excessive numbers of them are destroyed in passing through the capillaries of the spleen, liver or lungs. The disease is most frequently found in children and is one type of anemia which can be effectively treated, at least for a while, by regular periodic blood transfusions. No other treatment is known.

In a more uncommon hereditary anemia known as *congenital hemolytic jaundice,* an inborn defect permits the red cells to absorb abnormal amounts of sodium along with excessive water. This makes the red cells swell from their normal flat disk shape until they become spherical, and are thus trapped and destroyed in large numbers in the spleen. The only treatment of value is removal of the spleen by surgery.

Fortunately, all of these "blood-destruction" anemias, with the exception of sickle-cell anemia among Negroes, are relatively rare. When discovered, they are usually best treated by a hematologist—a specialist in blood diseases with wide experience in the diagnosis and management of these illnesses.

Aplastic Anemia. Another rare but extremely dangerous form of anemia is the so-called aplastic anemia which occurs when some chemical poison or toxic physical agent acts to depress or even completely destroy the bone marrow's ability to make red cells. Most commonly any such substance also depresses white cell and platelet formation. The condition may occur suddenly, even explosively, and is frequently fatal. Such dangerous bone marrow depression can occur as a result of poisoning with chemical agents such as benzene, gold or arsenic compounds, drugs such as quinacrine used against malaria, chloramphenicol used as an antibiotic, or nitrogen mustard used as an anticancer drug. Insecticides such as DDT may also cause aplastic anemia, and this same condition is a common and dreaded feature of radiation sickness from overexposure to atomic reactions, hard X-ray treatments or even radioactive drugs such as radium or radioactive phosphorus used in treating other conditions. (*See* p. 143.)

Sometimes aplastic anemia occurs without any identifiable cause at all, but as we have learned more and more about unusual or "atypical" allergic reactions to foreign substances, it has become clear that almost *any* kind of medicine may, in certain sensitive individuals, cause a depression of the bone marrow's ability to form blood cells. Unfortunately, there is no way to tell in advance who may be abnormally sensitive to a given medicine. For this reason, doctors will rarely prescribe any medicine over a prolonged period of time without intermittently checking the patient's blood count, and will discontinue a medicine immediately, no matter how important it may be, if there is any sign of an unexplained anemia.

The only treatment for aplastic anemia is the replacement of blood cells by transfusions until the bone marrow has a chance to recover its normal blood-producing capacity. During that time medicines that may help stimulate marrow function—vitamin B_{12}, for example—may be used, and because of the blood's lowered capacity to stave off infections, antibiotics must also be administered. In some cases the marrow will eventually recover its function, but often it does not and death ultimately occurs as a result of infection. In cases of aplastic anemia in which all hope of natural recovery has been lost, surgeons have on occasion attempted to remedy the situation by transplanting healthy bone marrow taken from a donor's body into the bone of the anemia victim. So far these attempts have not been successful for long because the recipient's body tends to "reject" and destroy the foreign bone marrow, and many of the drugs used to counteract this rejection reaction tend further to depress bone marrow activity. Even so, as more is learned about the body's immune reaction to foreign tissues, there is reason to hope that bone marrow transplants may someday prove useful in combating persistent aplastic anemia.

Finally, a number of disease conditions not directly related to blood formation at all may nevertheless bring about anemias which can be extremely difficult to diagnose and very refractory to treatment. Such prolonged and chronic infections or inflammatory diseases as chronic bone infection, tuberculosis, recurrent rheumatic fever or rheumatoid arthritis all may lead to a severe *secondary anemia* which does not respond well to treatment until the underlying cause is discovered and corrected. Just why patients with these chronic conditions develop anemia is not completely understood. Their red cells appear normal in size and hemoglobin content, and the cell-producing bone marrow appears normal too, yet somehow not enough new red cells are manufactured to replace those normally destroyed in the ordinary course of events. It is as if the body has just so much energy to expend in the repair of damage, and if most of it is spent holding a chronic infection or inflammatory disease at bay, there is little left over for normal red cell production.

Similarly, over a period of time victims of

chronic kidney disease often develop an anemia so severe that it can become more immediately life-threatening than the kidney impairment. Anemia is also a frequent complication of cancer, especially when the malignancy has spread to the bone marrow itself, thus crowding out normal blood cell formation. Indeed, the appearance of an unexplained anemia in a patient with weight loss or an impaired appetite is often the doctor's first clue that a malignancy may be present.

All of these secondary anemias are difficult to treat effectively until the underlying cause has been dealt with. In such cases the anemia is, in effect, more a symptom of an underlying illness than a disorder in itself, yet it may become an increasingly troublesome secondary effect unless the underlying condition is identified. Mild cases of the more common forms of anemia occur quite frequently, and many people tend to be very casual about them or even ignore them. But there is no time of year or particular situation when anemia is "normal." It is always a disorder of a vital body function and should *never* be taken lightly, however mild it may be. Nor should it ever be self-diagnosed or treated, despite the thousands of patent vitamin preparations, "tonics," and iron supplements widely advertised and easily available without prescription. At best a self-treated anemia is likely to be a half-treated anemia; at worst, self-treatment may succeed in masking the real cause of the disorder, bringing about temporary relief of symptoms and a false sense of well-being while the underlying condition progresses dangerously. Even a mild case of anemia deserves a doctor's experienced attention and careful laboratory studies to determine its cause and the proper course of treatment.

Polycythemia: The Opposite of Anemia

Anemia is usually the result of decreased numbers of red cells in the circulating blood or a decrease in hemoglobin content, or both. The condition known as *polycythemia* (literally, "many blood cells") is just the opposite: too many red cells in the blood stream. The condition may result from some disorder of other tissues and organs in the body which causes the bone marrow to overproduce red cells, or from a disorder specific to the bone marrow itself. In the first instance, correction of the underlying disorder may automatically reduce the polycythemia; but where production of too many red cells is the primary disease, treatment depends upon reducing the number of cells already present in the blood stream, and then using medicines to slow down the rate at which they are produced in the bone marrow.

The simplest and least dangerous form of polycythemia occurs when the fluid portion of the blood is suddenly reduced without any comparable loss of red cells, so that the blood becomes much "thicker" than normal. This can occur as a result of dehydration of the whole body due to excessive vomiting or diarrhea, abnormal sweating, or reduced intake of fluids. As the fluid necessary to keep blood circulating is lost, the red cells become more concentrated and may form clots or thrombi and plug up tiny capillaries all over the body unless fluids are promptly restored. An adult afflicted with untreated cholera, for example, may lose several gallons of water in a single day due to violent diarrhea and can die from a "relative polycythemia" unless quantities of fluid are restored to the blood stream by means of intravenous infusions. Similarly, an infant with diarrhea and vomiting can dehydrate very swiftly unless fluids are replaced. Relative polycythemia is also a threat to victims of extensive burns, when a great amount of serum is lost due to seepage from the burned skin surfaces. Anyone lost or marooned can survive for weeks without food as long as plenty of water is available, but will die within 24 to 48 hours if his water supply gives out. Dehydration is, however, a well-known danger, and the condition is treated by restoration of appropriate amounts of water, dissolved salt and other electrolytes to the blood, usually long before the concentration of red cells in the blood stream becomes excessive enough to do damage.

Another kind of polycythemia may result when external factors cause a chronic decrease in the amount of oxygen in the arterial blood, thus stimulating red cell production. The human body can adapt to certain variations in oxygen supply. Natives of the Andes Mountains, for example, have polycythemia in direct proportion to the reduced amount of oxygen available in the air at such altitudes; the condition is "normal" for these people, who suffer distress only when they travel to lower altitudes. Similarly, people accustomed to low altitudes become short of breath, lethargic and easily exhausted by physical exercise when they travel to altitudes of 10,000 feet above sea level or more. Their bodies will gradually compensate for this change by producing more red cells, a form of polycythemia, and in most cases the symptoms of oxygen starvation will disappear without medical intervention. But those who cannot make this adjustment develop *chronic mountain sickness* and continue to exhibit all the symptoms of oxygen starvation. This condition is rare, however, and is usually related to some other organic condition which limits the body's ability to adapt.

Numerous internal factors may also deprive the body of the oxygen it needs and cause excessive production of red cells. Diseases of the lungs may reduce the amount of oxygen available for absorption into the blood to such a degree that polycythemia results; so also may a number of congenital defects of the heart or the great blood vessels that permit oxygen-exhausted venous blood to be shunted back into arterial circulation without going through the lungs for oxygenation. In such conditions the decreased oxygen content in the blood is somehow "detected" by cells in the kidneys which immediately release a hormone that stimulates increased red cell production in the bone marrow. As new red cells crowd into the blood stream, the victim's complexion turns a dusky reddish purple hue (sometimes frankly blue if a heart defect is present); he exhibits increasing shortness of breath, headache, fatigue and mental sluggishness—all symptoms consistent with impaired circulation—and may show red cell levels as high as 8 million to 10 million per cubic millimeter of blood, twice the normal number. After a period of time he also begins to demonstrate a strange physical change: the tips of his fingers become slightly enlarged and club-shaped, an important clue to the presence of polycythemia.

Polycythemia that arises as a result of some other organic disease or disorder is called "secondary," and treatment of the underlying cause relieves the excessive concentration of red cells immediately. Thus a child with chronic polycythemia due to a cardiac defect may show an abrupt increase in the oxygen concentration in his blood within minutes after a surgeon has corrected the defect, and the polycythemia may vanish of its own accord within a week or so after the operation. If a chronic lung disease such as emphysema or silicosis has caused a long-standing decrease of oxygen absorption followed by a secondary polycythemia, oxygen administration may be necessary any time some intervening condition such as bronchitis or pneumonia occurs to further decrease oxygen absorption.

Far more serious than the secondary form of this condition, however, is a chronic disease known as primary polycythemia or *polycythemia vera* ("true polycythemia"). No one knows what causes this disorder. Many hematologists regard it as a form of cancer, since it involves chronic overactivity of the blood-forming tissues in the bone marrow which, when untreated, floods the blood stream with far more red cells than normal and, to a lesser extent, more white cells and platelets as well. The disease usually appears at middle age or later, more frequently among Jews than gentiles and less frequently among Negroes than whites. It also develops in men more commonly than in women, and is accompanied by the later onset of true leukemia frequently enough to suggest some relationship between the two conditions.

Even when discovered and treated early, polycythemia vera is a prolonged and disabling chronic disease which is ultimately fatal if the victim does not die of some other cause first. There is no known cure, and most of the symptoms are related to three factors: a steady increase in the total volume of blood in the circulatory system; increased viscosity or thickness of the blood due to the presence of as much as 35 to 50 percent more red cells than normal per unit volume; and a decrease in the speed of blood flow through the capillaries because of excessive red cells and platelets, with resulting *thrombi* in many areas of the body. The victim complains of a characteristic "feeling of fullness," together with a constant dull headache. There may be itching of the skin (particularly after a hot bath), dizziness, excessive fatigue, shortness of breath and disturbance of vision. A dull bluish-red ruddiness of the complexion is commonplace, and many victims feel a sense of heaviness in the upper left corner of the abdomen due to enlargement of the spleen. As the disease progresses, severe and massive hemorrhage may occur from distended blood vessels in the lining of the gastrointestinal system, and blood clots forming in the veins and capillaries may cause strokes, kidney damage or scarring of the spleen and other organs.

Physical examination and laboratory studies reveal a red cell count as high as 10 million or more per cubic millimeter of blood when the disease is first detected, together with increased numbers of platelets and white cells. A variety of more subtle blood examinations—determination of the oxygen saturation of arterial blood, for example—helps differentiate this "true polycythemia" from a polycythemia resulting from some other cause. Once diagnosed, treatment is directed toward two goals: reduction of the excessive volume of blood by means of periodic bloodletting (one of the rare situations in which this venerable medical procedure is actually scientifically justified); and suppression of the excessive formation of red cells in the bone marrow by use of medications. The drugs first used for this purpose had the unfortunate effect of poisoning and impairing many other normal body functions as well, but today a man-made element, radioactive phosphorus 32 (P^{32}), provides a remarkably specific and safe means of therapy. Phosphorus is essential to normal bone maintenance, and most phosphorus taken into the body is first deposited in bone tissue. P^{32} given in tiny doses intravenously or by mouth was found to concentrate quickly in the bone marrow and to reduce the overproduction of red and white cells and platelets very sharply without interfering with other metabolic processes in the body. Unfortunately, the halflife of this radioactive element is comparatively long (some three months), and too large a dose can easily

oversuppress bone marrow production, with a resulting dangerous anemia and a drop in white cell count. Experience in the use of this potent medicine, however, has enabled hematologists to gauge the ideal dosage for a given patient with splendid precision. P^{32} is now used periodically, as sparingly as possible and in combination with small doses of other cancer-suppressing drugs such as nitrogen mustard, X-ray irradiation of the spleen, bone-marrow-depressing drugs, and the judicious use of bloodletting, in order to keep the number of red cells in the blood as close to normal limits as possible.

With such treatment, the patient with polycythemia vera can often look forward to years or even decades of a relatively comfortable life. Ultimately, however, the disease is fatal even with the best of treatment. Patients may die due to the formation of blood clots in vital areas of their bodies, the development of scarring and destruction of the bone marrow by fibrous tissue with a resultant fatal anemia, or the development of even greater overactivity of the bone marrow which leads to a fatal leukemia. But at least the disease is controllable for a time, and the vast amount of research that is now being directed toward the discovery of the cause of leukemia may also, in the long run, provide the knowledge and weapons necessary to control polycythemia more effectively and possibly even to cure it.

Leukemia

There is probably no form of cancer more familiar, or more dreaded, than leukemia, a disease particularly notorious for striking young children, and in many cases running its fatal course with almost unbelievable swiftness. There is also probably no other illness surrounded by more myths and misinformation. It is *not true* that leukemia afflicts only children; it has *not* been clearly established that the disease is inherited. It is also *not true* that nothing can be done when leukemia strikes and that the disease always kills swiftly. Nor is it true that "the white cells eat the red cells in the blood," a colorful description of the disease, but far from accurate. But it *is* true that leukemia can strike without warning at any age, and because help for the victim depends heavily upon his family's clear understanding of what is happening, it is most important for everyone to have accurate information about the true nature of this disease.

Leukemia is a "family name" for any of a group of slightly different cancers of the blood-forming organs, certain kinds swiftly fatal, other kinds chronic. Although children are frequently the victims of the disease, it occurs more frequently in young adulthood or in middle to old age. The kinds of leukemia that produce long-term, chronic illness which may respond well to treatment for prolonged periods are more common than the violently fulminating varieties that swiftly terminate life. It is true that leukemia does frequently strike with breathtaking suddenness, and the name of the disease, which means literally "white blood," is sometimes very apt—victims may become as white as a sheet, and a blood sample may look more like pink water than blood—but this picture of the disease is not by any means the most common.

Essentially leukemia is a cancer involving cells in the bone marrow, in the lymph nodes, or less frequently in the spleen or liver, and it behaves like any other form of cancer. The malignant cells in the bone marrow or the lymph nodes begin multiplying wildly and rapidly, far exceeding the normal steady growth necessary to replace white cells used by the body to help fight off infection. As new white cells are formed in ever increasing quantities, many are "spilled over" into the blood stream in far greater numbers than normal; the white cell count climbs from the normal ranges between 5,000 and 10,000 per cubic millimeter of blood to 25,000, 75,000, 150,000, or even 500,000 per cubic millimeter. When a smear of this blood is stained and examined under a microscope, almost all the white cells are found to be young or immature— "baby" cells, so to speak, which are practically never normally found in the circulating blood. And as the malignant cells grow and multiply, they also begin to crowd out the red-cell-producing cells in the bone marrow, so that the victim becomes anemic, sometimes massively so. In fact, shortness of breath, pallor, exhaustion, low-grade fever and other symptoms of a rapidly

advancing anemia are often the first indication that leukemia is present.

Because the cancerous cells also cause a decrease in the formation of blood platelets, capillary hemorrhages, spontaneous bleeding into the

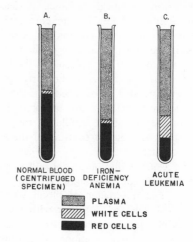

Figure 39–4.

tissues, and even spontaneous hemorrhage from larger vessels can occur. This is why one should always be concerned when a person, especially a child, seems to bruise too easily, and why victims of leukemia often look as if they had been beaten. In a child one should be particularly suspicious of frequent unexplained fevers, a persisting sore throat, bleeding gums, a rapidly increasing pallor, an unusual amount of bruising (numerous bruises appearing at the same time, for instance, without any apparent cause), excessive fatigue or a sudden decrease in physical activity. No one of these symptoms alone necessarily indicates leukemia, but they should be called to a doctor's attention immediately, since the earlier the disease is diagnosed, when present, the more effective the treatment will be.

Without treatment the leukemic white cells spread through the blood stream to lodge in the spleen and liver, which gradually become greatly enlarged and hardened by the abnormal cells with which they are packed; and as the disease progresses, white cells may also infiltrate many other body tissues as well. Ultimately the disease is fatal, with death resulting from the effects of prolonged severe anemia, from internal hemorrhage due to rupture of the spleen, from fever and exhaustion, or most commonly of all, from secondary infections that the body cannot fight off. Ironically, even though the victim's body may be virtually stuffed with white cells, nearly all of them are too young and immature to perform their normal function of destroying invading bacteria.

The various kinds of leukemia are classified according to the type of white cell which predominates, and according to whether the disease is in an acute or a chronic state. In children and elderly people lymphocytes are the predominating form of white cells produced. In children *acute lymphocytic leukemia* is the most common, with a life expectancy of less than a year from onset before modern treatment methods were developed. *Chronic lymphocytic leukemia,* a more sluggish cancer that may go on for some years, is more common among older people. Young adults more often develop either acute or chronic *granulocytic leukemia* centering in the bone marrow. Even without the benefits of modern treatment, the life expectancy in this form of leukemia can vary from as little as a few months in acute forms to more than twenty years in chronic forms.

Diagnosis of leukemia is rarely a problem. Apart from the telltale physical symptoms, many of which characterize one particular form of the disease, the most useful diagnostic aid is microscopic examination of the patient's blood. When leukemia is suspected following a blood test, a bone marrow examination confirms the diagnosis and determines the type and progress of the disease. This can be done quite easily in the doctor's office or hospital, using a small amount of a local anesthetic and removing a few drops of marrow from the breastbone or from the crest of the pelvic bone by means of a hollow needle for staining and microscopic examination. A pathologist can then determine precisely what kind of cancerous cells exist in the bone marrow and how many of the normal blood-forming elements still remain—an invaluable guide to treatment.

Other laboratory studies help determine the number of platelets present in the circulating blood and the effect of the growing numbers of leukemic cells on other organ systems and their functions. In some types of leukemia, for example, the level of uric acid in the blood stream is elevated because of the large numbers of white cells that are being formed and destroyed. Clotting times are usually normal early in the disease, but become abnormal later on as the platelet count decreases, and this, too, can be detected. Unfortunately, laboratory studies and research have yet to reveal the cause of the disease.

Recent studies have revealed that in about 90 percent of the patients with chronic granulocytic leukemia there is a consistent abnormality in the chromosomes of the leukemic cells with the presence of the so-called Philadelphia (Ph_1) chromosome. This suggests strongly that in that form of the disease, at least, part of the trouble lies in a disruption of the normal genetic coding structure in the cells, some abnormality of the DNA or RNA molecules in the cell nuclei. And more recently, studies have indicated strongly that human leukemia may be caused directly by one or more viruses capable of changing the structure of DNA or RNA in the nuclei of the cells they invade. If so, it may one day be possible to prevent leukemia with immunizations, much as polio can be prevented today.

So far no such breakthrough has occurred, nor is it considered imminent. But even though leukemia cannot yet be cured, and is virtually always ultimately fatal, recent research has yielded dramatic and effective new ways of treating the disease. And any leukemia will usually respond to one form of treatment or another well enough to allow the victim to enjoy a relatively normal life at least for a time. The nature and efficacy of the treatment used depends on the kind of leukemia present, and most particularly on whether it is acute or chronic. In slowly progressive chronic leukemia, proper treatment can increase survival time on the average to three or four years from the first appearance of symptoms, with the patient feeling relatively well throughout most of this time. One out of five such patients may live more than five years, and a few more than ten. Even in acute leukemia treatment may offer precious months or even years of comfortable, relatively normal life.

Without treatment the children who are the most frequent victims of this form of the disease could rarely survive more than four to six months from the onset of symptoms, and some might die in a matter of days. With modern treatment, more than 50 percent of these children survive for a year or more, and some may live as long as two years or more.

Any effective treatment of leukemia must suppress the wildly malignant production of immature white cells in the body without interfering too seriously with the normal production of red cells necessary for survival. In a chronic leukemia, X-ray therapy is often effective. The bone marrow, the spleen or the lymph nodes are bombarded with high doses of X-rays, usually focused on the areas of the body where the malignant cells are concentrated. This treatment can effect a dramatic decrease in the number of circulating white cells, and hopefully will produce what is known as a "clinical remission"— an abrupt disappearance of signs and symptoms of the disease—which may continue for as long as six months or more before the treatment must be repeated. In recent experiments lower dosages of X-rays have been used to irradiate the whole body of the chronic leukemia patient. Whether such treatment will prove more beneficial than "pinpoint" irradiation remains to be seen, but early results seem promising.

Similarly, some chronic leukemias can be treated with doses of radioactive phosphorus (P^{32}), which concentrates in the bone and suppresses cell production. This treatment may also bring about prolonged clinical remissions. In addition, a wide variety of chemical poisons have been developed which, when used in carefully controlled dosages, tend to poison the "sick" leukemic cells for varying periods of time without doing serious damage to normal cells. Because these are very potent drugs and the line between a safe, effective dose and a poisonous dose is extremely narrow, they must be used under the experienced supervision of a hematologist.

In acute leukemias the cortisone hormones produce prompt clinical remissions in a high percentage of patients, so these drugs are often chosen to begin treatment. Later, or even simultaneously, the whole range of antileukemic chemical poisons may be used, either shifting from one to another as the disease becomes more resistant or using two or more simultaneously to maintain control as long as possible. None of these methods is curative, but in most cases the disease can be checked for a while, sometimes for prolonged periods.

There are still many unanswered questions about leukemia, but two things are certain. First, the disease is by no means hopeless. Months or even years can be won, and in some cases victims undergo prolonged *spontaneous remission* of their symptoms at some point in the course of treatment. Second, medical researchers today are studying leukemia perhaps more intensively than any human affliction has ever been studied. There is little doubt that leukemia will be conquered sooner or later, and if it is indeed a virus disease, that day may come soon. Further, many researchers are convinced that the conquest of leukemia may well mark the beginning of the end of mankind's age-old struggle against all forms of cancer.

The Lymphomas

At least one type of leukemia, lymphatic leukemia, is primarily a disease affecting the lymph glands and the formation of one particular type of white cells, the lymphocytes. But a number of other diseases may also affect lymphoid tissue— sometimes called *reticulo-endothelial* tissue—of which the lymph glands themselves are composed and which is also found in the spleen, the liver and other organs in the body. Many of these disorders, known as lymphomas, resemble leukemia in certain respects, and have a number of cancer-like characteristics, yet differ enough from leukemia that they are considered separate disease entities. Some of these diseases are exceptionally rare, but at least two—lymphosarcoma and Hodgkin's disease—are encountered quite frequently.

Many people have trouble understanding the role of the lymphatic system and the lymph nodes scattered throughout the body, simply because this system, unlike other organ systems, has very few specific anatomical structures that can be easily visualized. Essentially it consists of a network of vaguely defined drainage channels throughout the body, running more or less parallel to the vessels of the circulatory system, but entirely separate from it. The purpose of these so-called *lymph channels* or *lymphatics* is to drain quantities of extracellular body fluid—mostly water containing body salts and nutriments—which has seeped out of the cells of various tissues, or through the capillary walls, and carry this fluid, known as *lymph,* back into the blood stream. There is no pump to propel lymph through these lymphatic channels; it merely trickles through, forced along by the pressure of contracting muscles in the extremities. At various places along the way, lymph passes through *lymph nodes,* nodules of lymphoid connective tissue which filter the lymph and also discharge into it the lymphocytes being formed. These lymph nodes are located at "junction points" scattered all along the lymph channels, and are also found in clusters in the groin, the armpit, the neck, the thorax around the mediastinum, and other places. Ultimately lymph finds its way into a thin-walled tube in the chest known as the *thoracic duct* which, in turn, drains into the vena cava. By diffusing into and out of the tissue cells and into and out of the capillaries, lymph acts as a sort of "overflow mechanism" for body fluid, important to the body in maintaining the right quantity of water within the cells and in the blood stream. In addition, lymph carries certain nutriments from the digestive tract, particularly digested fats and other fatty materials, both to the tissue cells and to the liver. Finally, the lymph channels serve as avenues through which lymphocytes can travel between the cells on their way to engulf and destroy invading bacteria.

The specialized reticulo-endothelial connective tissue making up the lymph nodes and scattered throughout the spleen and other organs has several functions. First, by filtering lymph draining from peripheral areas of the body, it helps contain and localize infection; lymph nodes characteristically become swollen and tender in regions where invading bacteria are at work. This lymphoid tissue is responsible for the formation of lymphocytes and also plays an important role, not yet fully understood, in the body's immune

mechanism, particularly in the manufacture of antibodies. And just as other kinds of tissue in the body have their special disorders, the lymphoid tissue in the lymph nodes and the spleen is subject to certain diseases.

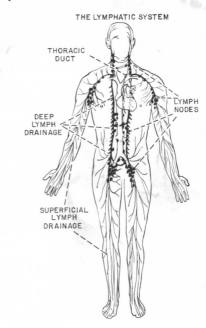

THE LYMPHATIC SYSTEM

THORACIC DUCT

LYMPH NODES

DEEP LYMPH DRAINAGE

SUPERFICIAL LYMPH DRAINAGE

Figure 39–5.

Lymphosarcoma. A malignant tumor which arises in the lymph nodes, particularly those draining the gastrointestinal tract, but sometimes in other lymphoid tissue as well, a lymphosarcoma spreads either by infiltration of malignant cells into surrounding tissues or by passage of those cells along the lymph channels to other lymph nodes. Early in the disease victims suffer rather vague, nonspecific symptoms including unexplained fever, sweating, loss of appetite and loss of weight. As the tumor grows, the affected lymph nodes become markedly enlarged and hard, and may cause symptoms due to pressure on the intestinal tract or on other internal organs. Sometimes the first sign of trouble arises when the intestine is obstructed because of the pressure of a massively enlarged lymph node against the intestinal wall. The spleen, the liver and the bone marrow are often invaded by tumor cells, and pathological fractures of long bones or compression fractures of the vertebrae are not uncommon. Anemia is a characteristic feature of the disease as a result of destruction of blood-forming cells in the bone marrow. The cause of this cancer is still unknown, but today doctors are increasingly suspicious that lympho-sarcoma and other cancer-like diseases of the lymph tissue may result from the action of certain as yet unidentified viruses. Lymphosarcoma is comparatively rare, but swift-moving when it occurs. Untreated, it will usually cause death within one to two years. It is incurable, but treatment with X-rays and such anticancer drugs as nitrogen mustard often causes shrinkage of the primary tumor mass, marked temporary relief of symptoms and prolongation of life for as long as five years or more.

Hodgkin's Disease. Similar to lymphosar-coma, but occurring far more frequently, Hodg-kin's disease is a chronic, slow-moving, cancer-like disorder which affects lymph nodes and other lymphoid tissue all over the body. Named after the British physician Thomas Hodgkin, who first described it in 1832, the disease is still an affliction of unknown origin. Usually it appears during young adulthood, affecting males about twice as often as females, but children are also frequently afflicted. In recent years researchers have come to suspect some unknown virus as a source of the disease. Virus-like particles have been discovered in the diseased cells, and a few cases have been reported in clusters among people living in close contact, suggesting an infectious agent of some sort, but there is, as yet, not enough evidence to confirm this suspicion.

Whatever the cause, the disease in most cases begins with a persistent painless enlargement of lymph nodes somewhere in the body—in the axilla, for example, or the neck or in the chest near the mediastinum. Gradually lymph nodes begin to enlarge all over the body; the spleen in particular enlarges and the liver and bone marrow are also commonly involved. Microscopic examination of affected lymph nodes reveals a characteristic giant cell in the lymphoid tissue, the presence of which is diagnostic. As the disease progresses, the victim develops intermittent fevers, weight loss, anemia and, oddly enough, a

severe and persistent itching of the skin. Later symptoms result from pressure of enlarged lymph nodes on the spinal cord, major blood vessels or the intestinal tract. If untreated, the disease slowly advances over a period of five to twenty years, often accompanied by a bewildering variety of changing symptoms, and ultimately leading to death due to destruction of various organs by the tumor-like masses. In this sense, and in that the growth of Hodgkin's tissue does not spontaneously regress or stop, the disease behaves like a cancer.

Fortunately, however, Hodgkins' disease can be effectively treated in most cases. The tumors are extremely sensitive to radiation; X-ray therapy makes the enlarged nodes shrink, relieves symptoms and slows down or stops the growth of tumor cells, sometimes for prolonged periods. When enlarged nodes are obstructing the intestine or other organs, surgical excision followed by X-ray therapy is often effective in controlling the disease for prolonged periods. Later in its course, anticancer drugs such as nitrogen mustard are effective. If the spleen seems to be destroying red cells too rapidly, surgical removal may be indicated, and the anemia that accompanies the disease is treated with transfusions. Cortisone hormones also help relieve pain, improve appetite and diminish fever. Such complex treatment is usually planned and carried out by a specialist with wide experience in dealing with the disorder. In skillful hands more than 65 percent of all victims of Hodgkin's disease survive in comparative comfort for longer than five years and many live as long as twenty or twenty-five years. Furthermore, if a causative virus can be discovered, there may be hope that an anti-serum will one day control or even cure the disease.

Certain other rare disorders of the lymphoid tissue are characterized by marked enlargement of the spleen and infiltration of lymph nodes with deposits of various abnormal fatty or lipid materials. In *Gaucher's disease,* a hereditary disorder, large quantities of a lipid known as *kerasin* infiltrate the lymph nodes and spleen. Although incurable, Gaucher's disease and its complications, including anemia and purpura, can often be controlled for prolonged periods of time by splenectomy (surgical removal of the spleen). Since victims of this condition are particularly susceptible to infection, continuing treatment with antibiotics may also be necessary. *Niemann-Pick disease* involves deposits of another lipid, *sphingomyelin,* in the lymphoid tissues, while *Hand-Schüller-Christian disease* is characterized not only by infiltration of these cells with lipids, but by actual destruction of bone in the skull and other tissues due to the encroachment of enlarging lipid-filled lymphoid tissue. Both of these two conditions appear during childhood and ultimately result in death, although treatment by means of X-ray therapy or splenectomy or both can sometimes be helpful. Both are extremely rare and are important primarily in that they must be differentiated from Hodgkin's disease, other lymphomas or leukemia.

Bleeding and Clotting Disorders

The cardiovascular system is essentially a closed circuit of organs and tissues through which the blood circulates to virtually every part of the body. But what happens when one of the vessels in this closed circuit springs a leak? Obviously the blood, which is circulating under considerable pressure, is going to escape with bleeding or hemorrhage as a result, whether the leak is outside or inside the body. When this happens, it is the blood itself which takes the initial steps necessary to repair the leak, for apart from its many other astonishing characteristics, it has the capacity to clot and plug up even a relatively large breach in a ruptured blood vessel. Further, this clot provides a fibrous bridge across which nearby tissues can grow to repair the leak permanently. Of course, in cases of massive external or internal hemorrhage, blood flow may be so copious that a clot cannot form or is continually washed away, and medical intervention may be necessary to check the blood flow or to repair the ruptured vessel surgically. But even then it is the blood's clotting mechanism which seals the leak and begins the healing process.

This clotting mechanism is a complicated chemical chain reaction that begins at the mo-ment of injury and involves in particular the platelets, a component of the blood, along with certain special blood proteins and a number of other enzymes and chemicals normally present in the injured tissue and the blood plasma. (*See* p. 79.) If the reaction proceeds as it should, a clot is formed in a matter of minutes and the healing process begins. But there are certain disorders which are characterized by excessive bleeding or hemorrhage, either because the blood vessels are fragile and break too easily or because clot formation does not take place as it normally should.

The Purpuras. A number of different disorders can cause an abnormal increase in the fragility of the walls of the tiny capillaries all over the body, with the result that these capillaries tend to break spontaneously, often for no apparent reason, allowing small amounts of blood to leak into surrounding tissues. In some cases the blood clotting mechanism may be unimpaired, while in others there may be an associated abnormality in the number or function of platelets in the blood. In any event, these disorders are marked by pain in the abdomen or in the joints, traces of blood in the stool, and the appearance of tiny pinpoint hemorrhages visible under the skin, so-called *petechiae* which later change into small "black-and-blue marks." Scattering of these spots all over the body is called *purpura.*

One form of purpura, once very common but now seen only rarely, results from *scurvy,* a disease caused by a deficiency of vitamin C or ascorbic acid in the diet, which often afflicted sailors on long ocean voyages who subsisted mainly on a diet of salt pork, potatoes and rum. Not infrequently an entire ship's crew died of scurvy, their bodies blotched with skin hemorrhages, their gums swollen and their teeth falling out. Then it was discovered that scurvy could be completely prevented simply by eating enough citrus or other fresh fruit containing vitamin C. A number of infectious diseases, notably meningococcal meningitis, streptococcal blood poisoning and others, are also characterized by the appearance of purpura.

Another strange condition, *thrombocytopenic purpura,* is due to a deficiency of platelets in the blood, which may occur for unknown reasons and leads to extraordinary spontaneous bruising and pinpoint hemorrhages beneath the skin and throughout the tissues. This disease, which occurs primarily in children or young women, may develop very slowly with sudden "showers" of petechiae in the skin and mucous membranes, followed by the formation of black-and-blue spots. Capillaries become so fragile that they burst spontaneously, and clotting is so impaired that extended bleeding may occur when blood vessels are damaged. This disorder tends to come and go, often never becoming severe enough to require active treatment. When it is severe, however, surgical removal of the spleen is often followed by a dramatic increase in the number of platelets in the blood, and about 70 percent of victims treated with splenectomy recover completely and permanently from the affliction. Cortisone treatment is also helpful in many cases. Today it is only rarely that a victim of idiopathic thrombocytopenic purpura is not benefited by either surgical or medical treatment. In a few cases, possible causes have been found, including exposure to various chemical poisons or ionizing radiation, but usually no source can be identified. So far, although the disease can be palliated and effectively treated, it cannot really be cured, at least not until its cause has been discovered.

Hemophilia. Of all the bleeding and clotting disorders, by far the most dramatic, dangerous and famous is hemophilia. Fortunately, the affliction is rare, and the overwhelming majority of men and women who have been told that they were "bleeders" or have "a long bleeding and clotting time" do not have true hemophilia at all; at worst, they may be suffering from one of several far less serious clotting disorders associated with deficiencies of various blood proteins required for good clot formation. These relatively minor clotting disorders seldom cause any more than mild annoyance and need treatment only when some form of surgery is contemplated.

True hemophilia is a different matter. This disease is due to a hereditary deficiency of one of the substances necessary in the formation of a normal blood clot, factor VIII or antihemophilic

globulin. The deficiency is "sex-linked"; that is, the gene that causes it is located on the sex-determining chromosome. Therefore males who

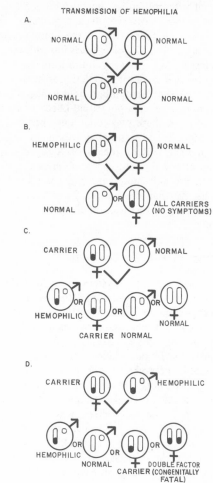

Figure 39–6.

have a defective sex chromosome suffer from the disorder, while females can be "carriers" of the defective gene and can transmit it to their offspring but never suffer from the symptoms themselves. Finally, the trait is recessive and thus appears only sporadically among the males in every other generation of afflicted families. Instances of hemophilia afflicting a male in a family with no previous history of the disease are extremely rare.

Symptoms usually appear in the infancy or early childhood of the afflicted males and continue throughout their lifetimes, which are often much shortened by the disease. The slightest trauma or cut results in bleeding which continues for prolonged periods without being stopped by natural coagulation of the blood. Even worse, bleeding also occurs internally in areas that normally can take quite a bit of wear and tear, such as the joints. Eating any irritating food may start bleeding from the gums that lasts for days, and both external and internal hemorrhages may occur spontaneously for no apparent reason. One of the most dreaded crises a hemophiliac faces is a nosebleed from vessels high in the nasopharynx where pressure cannot effectively be applied to stem the bleeding; such nosebleeds can continue for days, even to the point of exsanguination.

All victims of hemophilia are not afflicted to the same degree. Some may live virtually normal lives, displaying the tendency to hemorrhage only after tooth extractions, tonsillectomies or injuries in which blood vessels are torn or cut. Others are so severely afflicted that they may die from exsanguinating hemorrhage in infancy, sometimes as a result of such an innocuous procedure as circumcision. Among those who do survive, many develop progressive deformities as a result of bleeding into joints, fingers, tendons and other tissues. And unfortunate as the physical symptoms of this condition can be, both the hemophiliac and his parents may also suffer severe emotional stress. Even under the best of circumstances, they must be continually watchful; yet they know that no matter how careful they are, a minor accident may cause days and weeks of torment, possibly even death. And they know that the disease can never be cured. Learning to accept and live with hemophilia is certainly one of the most difficult aspects of the disease.

Until the mechanism of blood coagulation was understood, there was little or nothing that could be done to treat hemophilia. Today, although treatment is possible, it is only a "finger in the dike" until a given episode of hemorrhage subsides. It consists of administration of fresh blood by transfusion, or of fresh plasma, fresh frozen plasma or reconstituted flash-dried plasma, or concentrated quantities of human fibrinogen containing the antihemophilic globulin factor. All of these shore up the victim's clotting capacity temporarily, but all must be administered by inserting a needle in a vein, thus producing a new potential bleeding site. Minor episodes of bleeding can often be controlled by special clotting medications administered by the hemophiliac himself or his parents. The patient may also be fortunate enough to experience a temporary remission of the disease. Thus, with care and barring any uncontrollable hemorrhage, the hemophiliac may live for many years. Even major surgery can be performed in some cases, if an adequate blood supply can be maintained.

The only real "cure" for hemophilia, however, rests in preventing the affliction from being passed on from generation to generation. It goes without saying that a hemophiliac should not have children, for there is the possibility that his daughters may become carriers; nor should female carriers have children, for their sons may inherit the disease and their daughters become carriers. Carriers can be identified by laboratory studies, and when a family history of hemophilia is known to exist, every precaution should be taken to make sure its members are free of the defective gene before they have children.

Other Blood Clotting Defects. In addition to hemophilia there are a number of other rare blood-clotting defects also caused by hereditary factors. One of these is a deficiency of prothrombin, a substance normally present in the blood which is essential to clotting. Others are *afibrinogenemia* (total absence of fibrinogen in the blood) and the less dangerous *hypofibrinogenemia* (deficient levels of fibrinogen in the blood). Fibrinogen is a special kind of protein molecule normally present in blood serum and also essential to clotting. Along with hemophilia, these are *primary clotting defects* and can be distinguished from true hemophilia usually only by special laboratory studies. Like hemophilia they are treatable but incurable, and fortunately quite rare.

Secondary clotting defects are more common and arise as a result of some other disease or disorder. Vitamin K, for example, is needed by the liver in order to produce prothrombin; a vitamin K deficiency in the diet, which usually occurs only under starvation conditions, can lead to a secondary drop in prothrombin and reduced capacity of the blood to coagulate. A serious and destructive liver disease such as hepatitis or cancer of the liver may have the same effect.

Ironically, there are also a number of disorders in which the blood's clotting mechanism may work all too well, or work when it ought not to work, causing the formation of clots or thrombi in various parts of the body. Such a condition, a sort of "excessive tendency to thrombosis," is usually secondary to some other disorder, often of the blood vessels themselves. (*See* p. 514.) Or it may be caused by something as simple as enforced rest for a normally active individual, such as a woman recovering from delivery or a patient recuperating after surgery. In either case, clots may form in the veins of the legs, together with localized areas of inflammation and swelling, a condition known as *thrombophlebitis*. Patients are often forced out of bed and encouraged to move about as much as possible, even after a major surgical procedure, to stimulate circulation and thus help prevent the formation of thrombi.

The real danger lies not in the thrombi themselves, but in the possibility that they may break loose from their original location and be carried in the blood stream to some other site where they may pose a critical threat. A "moving thrombus," which is properly called an *embolus,* may lodge in a vessel supplying vital blood to the brain, causing a stroke, or it may travel to the lung to cause a pulmonary embolus which can be swiftly fatal. An embolus obstructing circulation to the heart may cause coronary thrombosis, the well-known "heart attack." If an excessive tendency to thrombosis is feared in a patient, however, there are medications that can be prescribed to retard the blood's clotting mechanism, just as there are others that are useful in speeding it up.

Other Disorders of the Blood or Blood-Forming Organs

A hereditary defect affecting the blood proteins but not the clotting mechanism is a congenital lack of gamma globulin, a condition known as *agammaglobulinemia* which is usually first detected in childhood. This defect robs the child of his ability to develop normal immune resistance to such invaders as viruses and bacteria. Consequently, he is extremely vulnerable to any and all forms of infection, responds poorly to treatment, and becomes reinfected again and again. The condition is rare, but it is also extremely difficult to diagnose. A child may suffer from several years of repeated infections before the diagnosis is made more or less by exclusion.

Agranulocytosis, a rare but devastating disease, is more often man-made than not. It is a condition in which the bone marrow ceases to form the normal number of white cells, or to form them at all. In most cases it is a result of hypersensitivity to some form of drug. Virtually any drug *can* cause the condition in a sensitive person, but it has been particularly identified with some of the potent bone marrow depressants used against leukemia, with certain of the tranquilizers, with certain antibiotics such as chloramphenicol and sulfonamides, and with drugs such as aminopyrine sometimes used to break high fevers. The condition often may begin weeks or months after the drug has been stopped, but more commonly it appears while the medication is still being used. This is one of the reasons why a doctor will not normally authorize repeated refills of a prescription drug without seeing his patient periodically and checking his blood count. Sometimes agranulocytosis may be temporary, clearing up as soon as medication is stopped, but often it remains doggedly permanent, in which case the outcome is fatal. The only treatment is caution, use of safe antibiotics to combat infection until the condition subsides (if it does subside) and patience. Agranulocytosis is also a primary aspect of radiation sickness when an individual has inadvertently been exposed to a massive overdose of X-rays or other radiation.

40

Hemorrhage and Shock

Probably the most common of all disorders of the cardiovascular system occurs as a result of a physical injury in which the skin is broken, a blood vessel is torn, and blood loss occurs. Often such bleeding is so minor that it can be ignored and the wound dressed with a Band-Aid until healing is under way. But occasionally more serious bleeding can occur. If the blood loss is severe, it can easily be complicated by some degree of shock and generalized circulatory impairment. The victim may grow chilly and suddenly pale; his body becomes covered with perspiration, his heart races, and he becomes short of breath, dizzy and mentally confused. He may lose consciousness and even die if the shock is accompanied by circulatory collapse, even though the blood loss may long since have ceased or been controlled.

Doctors speak of a blow, wound or injury to the body from some extrinsic force as a *trauma,* although the term, in its broadest sense, is also used to refer to a damaging emotional experience. *Hemorrhage* refers to any amount of bleeding, from the tiniest pinprick to the massive outpouring of blood that can occur when a major artery is severed. A hemorrhage may be external, when the injury tears the skin surface, or internal, as in the case of a crushing or bruising injury, or when some abnormal condition causes the rupture of a blood vessel somewhere deep in the body. The term *shock* is used to describe the strange chain of events often associated with trauma and hemorrhage, and although the word is also sometimes used in reference to

severe emotional distress, in the strict medical sense shock refers to the sequence of physiological changes, often overwhelming, which the body undergoes in response to blood loss, the impairment of proper circulation or severe pain.

The Control of Hemorrhage

The body has certain excellent built-in mechanisms to help control a hemorrhage when it occurs. When a blood vessel is torn, the muscle fibers in the walls of the vessel contract, thus pinching off the torn end of the vessel and automatically reducing bleeding. In addition, the clotting mechanism of the blood is set into motion in a swift chain reaction which forms a sticky gelatinous clot, further obstructing the outflow of blood. (*See* p. 79.) If the hemorrhage is internal, a further natural mechanism may act to control it: internal tissues are held in place by a network of connective tissue which is quite rigid, and when blood forces its way into the tissues, this rigid network tends to obstruct its movement and keep it in a localized area. Soon the tissue pressure increases sufficiently to press the broken end of the blood vessel and thus slow or stop the hemorrhage. Blood that escapes into internal tissues also clots and forms a gelatinous mass known as a *hematoma.* After a period varying from 24 to 72 hours, such a hematoma begins to dissolve slowly, and a watery fluid stained with hemoglobin pigments seeps to the skin surface or follows cleavage planes through the tissue until it is ultimately reabsorbed by the blood stream. A bruise or a "black-and-blue mark" visible through the skin is the characteristic sign of this process, and sometimes bruises appear in places far distant from the actual hemorrhage. For example, the victim of an injury to the lower leg just below the knee may find a black-and-blue mark forming at the back of his heel due to the seepage of pigmented fluid from a dissolving hematoma. Similarly, a person with a "black eye" often discovers a black-and-blue area forming below the *other* eye three or four days after the injury.

If the hematoma is very large, however, it may not dissolve completely, but may simply sit there for prolonged periods. In some cases the clotted blood ultimately forms a sterile abscess or pocket of brownish-black fluid which may eventually require surgical incision and drainage. In other cases fibrous tissue grows into the clot and it becomes "organized," literally assimilated into the tissue, and ultimately forms the basis for a permanent area of scarring. Often the healing of a wound involving a hematoma is much accelerated by surgical removal of the clotted blood.

Immediately after an injury in which there is significant loss of blood, the mechanism of shock may come into play, with a mass contraction of all the smaller blood vessels in the area of the injury, thus helping to stem the blood flow. This, however, is an extremely inefficient aid in controlling hemorrhage. In a sense, the body overreacts and shock itself may become a major problem and sometimes a threat to life.

How much blood loss can a normal human being tolerate without getting into serious trouble? The answer hinges more upon the speed of the blood loss than the actual amount lost. The normal volume of blood in an average-sized adult is approximately ten pints. If an individual suddenly loses as much as a pint of blood as a result of an injury, he may find himself weak, confused and exhausted; the loss of two pints in a brief period of time will be enough to put him into profound shock; and any greater loss may be fatal unless medical aid and blood replacement is immediately available. On the other hand an individual who is hemorrhaging a little bit day after day—from a bleeding ulcer, for

example—may actually lose as much as two-thirds of his normal blood volume over a long period of time without any more untoward signs or symptoms than evidence of a profound anemia. In this case, of course, some of the blood is being replaced by the formation of new blood cells in the bone marrow, and the fluid volume of the blood is partially replaced as well. But with a sudden hemorrhage, neither of these long-term body defenses against blood loss has time to come into play. As for the rate at which blood can be lost, if a major artery such as the femoral artery is severed, the victim may exsanguinate from uncontrolled hemorrhage in as little as two or three minutes; but in most cases an external hemorrhage of this sort can be detected and controlled by proper first-aid methods followed by medical or surgical attention.

Obviously it is of extreme importance to stop any copious external bleeding. The only thing which takes precedence is to make sure that the victim has an open airway, since he will quickly suffocate if his breathing passages are obstructed in some way. Fortunately, most hemorrhages are relatively easy to bring under control. First-aid measures including direct pressure over the wound, compression of an artery at a pressure point above the wound, and even, in some cases, the use of a tourniquet are discussed and illustrated in detail in another chapter (*see* p. 104). But in addition there are certain everyday hemorrhages which can be extremely awkward or difficult for a layman, and sometimes even a doctor, to control because of their location or some other complicating factor.

Nosebleeds (Epistaxis). Nosebleeds occur quite commonly, even chronically in some individuals, and can sometimes pose a problem in control. A nosebleed caused by a physical trauma, a punch in the nose, for example, will usually be self-limited and stop of its own accord without outside intervention. On the other hand, people who have stuffed-up or runny noses from an active upper respiratory infection may start a nosebleed by excessive nose blowing. Furthermore, if the respiratory infection is chronic, continual blowing may prevent broken blood vessels in the nasal passages from healing properly and nosebleeds may become recurrent.

Sometimes, however, nosebleeds are spontaneous, particularly among those with uncontrolled high blood pressure or, in rare cases, a clotting defect.

Many of the popular "home remedies" for controlling a nosebleed are actually not very effective. An ice pack on the back of the neck exerts no control over bleeding from vessels in the nose, although it is often a recommended procedure. Nor should the nostrils be packed with cotton or gauze by anyone other than a doctor; packing the nostrils tends to stretch the bleeding vessels open rather than close them. And the victim should *never* be put in a reclining position except temporarily while nose drops are being administered. The nosebleed may appear to stop but may actually continue for some time without being recognized simply because the blood is trickling down the throat and being swallowed instead of flowing out the nose.

Some simple measures *are* useful, however. The vast majority of nosebleeds occur from vessels in the front part of the nose. Thus one of the most effective ways to treat a nosebleed is to grasp the nose firmly between the thumb and forefinger and squeeze the nostrils together with some pressure. Hold this pressure position for five minutes *measured by the clock;* if you try to judge it without a timepiece, you will invariably release it too soon. Then gently release the pressure and avoid blowing or snuffing. Nine times out of ten this treatment alone will stop the nosebleed, but if bleeding resumes when the pressure is released, reapply it for another five minutes by the clock. During this time the victim should remain sitting up with his head tilted slightly forward. If the bleeding originates farther up in the nose, some blood may drain down into the throat, but in an upright position this occurrence will not go unnoticed.

Another aid in controlling a minor degree of nosebleed is the use of ¼ percent Neo-Synephrine or 1 percent ephedrine nose drops in a water-based solution. Lie on your back with your head over the edge of the bed and your nostrils pointed to the ceiling. Instill the nose drops in each nostril and then hold your head back for a long count of 15 to permit them to pool higher up in the nose. Then roll over and allow the nose drops to drain rather than swallowing them. These medicines have an immediate effect of shrinking capillary blood vessels in the nose and upper nasal passages—the reason they work so effectively in "opening up" a stuffy nose—and will help reduce the size of the bleeding vessel. This in itself, or used in combination with thumb and forefinger pressure, will usually stop a nosebleed.

More vigorous treatment is rarely necessary, but if it is, it should be left to a doctor. If a nosebleed cannot be stopped, or if the blood flow is extremely copious, prompt medical attention is, of course, indicated. Hospital emergency rooms are well equipped to deal with any hemorrhagic disorder. If nosebleeds are a recurring or chronic problem, however, or if they seem to occur for no reason, a thorough medical examination is necessary to investigate the possibility of high blood pressure or a clotting disorder.

Bleeding After Tonsillectomy and Adenoidectomy. One form of difficult hemorrhage is the excessive bleeding that occasionally occurs following performance of a tonsillectomy and adenoidectomy or "T and A." (*See* p. 194.) Occasionally such a hemorrhage may begin soon after a child has been taken home from the hospital following a T and A, or, more rarely, several days later when the soft "scab" that has formed over the tonsil bed following surgery peels away. In either case, the most frequent sign of bleeding is the sudden vomiting of a quantity of black "coffee-grounds" material—actually blood turned black by stomach acids—together with secondary symptoms of hemorrhage or shock such as pallor, sweating, shortness of breath, dizziness or fainting. Any such hemorrhage must be treated by a physician immediately, and parents should take the child to the hospital emergency room without delay, even while the doctor is being summoned. Fortunately, post-T and A bleeding is relatively uncommon today, but when it does occur it can be serious. In the hospital any degree of shock that is present can be controlled, and the bleeding vessels can, if necessary, be identified and ligated.

Scleral Hemorrhage. This kind of bleeding, in

which one of the capillaries under the sclera (the white of the eye) breaks and causes an unsightly red blotch under the eye, is more annoying than difficult or dangerous. It can arise for a variety of reasons, including injury or inadvertent abrasion of the sclera from a foreign body, as a side effect of high blood pressure, or sometimes from no discernible cause at all. It is very rarely, if ever, symptomatic of anything grave, nor is there anything very effective that can be done about it. An ice pack applied to the eye immediately following a known blow or injury may be helpful in preventing a scleral hemorrhage, but once one occurs, there is not much to do but to wait for it to go away, a process that may take anywhere from one or two days to a couple of weeks, depending upon the amount of blood lodged there. Such a hemorrhage does not interfere with vision in any way and need not be called to a doctor's attention unless it recurs repeatedly for no apparent reason or in conjunction with small capillary hemorrhages under the skin, a situation that suggests an underlying illness which should be investigated.

Hemorrhage from a Scalp Wound. Even a very tiny scalp wound can lead to copious bleeding which may be difficult to control simply because the blood supply to the scalp is so rich. Pressure points cannot be used because the blood supply reaches the head and scalp in symmetrical fashion from both sides, and any attempt to apply pressure on, say, both carotid arteries, will stop *all* blood supply to the head and lead to very rapid unconsciousness. The best way to control excessive bleeding from a scalp wound is *direct pressure on the wound itself* using a sterile bandage or clean cloth of any sort. If a scalp laceration is long or multiple, a pressure bandage applied with additional manual pressure over the wound will at least keep bleeding to a minimum and help prevent shock until the victim can be seen by a physician.

Bleeding Under a Fingernail. This limited sort of hemorrhage, which can be quite painful, is discussed in detail elsewhere (*see* p. 407).

Hemorrhage from a Varicose Vein. Here is a situation similar to a scalp injury, in which a relatively minor scratch or laceration can produce an alarming amount of bleeding. Varicose veins are simply veins, usually in the lower extremities, which have broken down structurally and dilated in size due to back pressure of blood being returned to the heart. (*See* p. 568.) If such a vessel just under the skin is torn, even by a minor scratch or scrape, there may be copious bleeding as the blood pooled in the vein above and below the injury wells out. The first rule, when this occurs, is *do not panic*. Veins deeper in the leg are quite adequate to carry the venous blood back to the heart, and such a superficial but copious hemorrhage can be easily controlled by compressing the injured vein immediately below the wound; that is, on the side of the wound *away* from the heart. If bleeding continues, place a sterile gauze dressing directly over the wound and then wrap the leg firmly but not tightly from the toes to the thighs with a four-inch elastic roller bandage or even pieces of old sheet torn four inches wide. If the toes turn blue or if tingling in the foot gives way to pain, the pressure is excessive and the bandage should be unrolled and rewrapped with somewhat less pressure. If a doctor cannot be reached, the wrapping should be removed after two to three hours and reapplied only if the bleeding begins to recur. This kind of hemorrhage is rarely dangerous and will usually stop spontaneously if the victim gets off his feet and raises his legs slightly above the level of his chest. But the person who suffers this kind of injury has more than just bleeding to worry about, since varicose veins tend to retard the healing of any lower leg abrasion. Such an injury combined with hemorrhage should be taken as a warning to see a doctor, have the severity of the varicose veins evaluated, and embark on a long-range plan to treat the underlying condition.

Rectal Hemorrhage. This type of bleeding often results from hemorrhoids (varicosed veins in the rectal area) or fissures in the rectum, but any bleeding from this area should invariably be investigated by a physician. For one thing, something other than hemorrhoids may be the source of the hemorrhage—a tumor of the rectum, for example. In addition, it is very difficult for the layman to locate and control a rectal hemorrhage. In the doctor's office this can be easily accomplished with no distress to the patient.

Excessive Menstrual Bleeding. This is a condition that worries a great many women unnecessarily, but it can be difficult for a number of reasons. It is often all but impossible for a doctor to determine objectively whether he is dealing with actual hemorrhage, in the accepted sense of the word, or merely with *menorrhagia,* the medical term for unusually copious menstrual bleeding, which may vary enormously even under normal circumstances. There can also be a problem determining whether the vaginal bleeding is actually menstrual flow at all, or whether it is *intermenstrual bleeding;* that is, abnormal bleeding which occurs between the end of one menstrual period and the beginning of another. If a woman, for example, has a long past history of regular and predictable periods, the differentiation is easily made, but if the woman presents a history of a grossly irregular and unpredictable pattern of menses, as is frequently the case, the question can be confusing indeed. It can be even more confusing in instances in which there may or may not be an early pregnancy involved. Finally, the issue can be further complicated by a number of factors, both physiological and extrinsic, which can cause variation in menses in the same woman from one period to the next.

Abnormal menstrual flow can be alarming, but many women are notoriously poor judges of how much more flow they are having than normal, are alarmed by any flow that seems more than normal, and vastly exaggerate both the amount of flow and its possible implications. Women who notice such an abnormality, and are sure they are not pregnant, often think they must have cancer, a frightening thought that can lead to increased blood pressure and heart rate, sleeplessness and general physical and physiological agitation—all of which, of course, tend to increase the abnormal flow. And while it is true that certain kinds of cancer *do* announce themselves through abnormal vaginal bleeding, such bleeding can also be caused by a number of other factors, many of which are far more likely than cancer.

What commonsense steps should you take, then, if you notice an abnormality in menstrual flow? First, be *concerned,* but not frightened. Most important of all: *observe very accurately what is happening.* Write it down if necessary, including how much abnormal flow you notice, why you consider it abnormal, when your last period ended and anything odd you noticed or can remember about it, what your regular or normal pattern of menses is, and whether or not you feel there is any chance you could be pregnant, and if so how advanced in pregnancy. Finally, try to think of any extrinsic or outside circumstances that might conceivably have had some effect on your menses: unusual emotional stress or physical activity, any medicines you may be taking or may have stopped taking, including oral contraceptives. Most women using "the pill" have experienced curiosities of menstrual flow at one time or another, not as a harmful side effect but simply because these medicines bring about a relative rebalancing of the hormones involved in normal ovulation and menstruation, and adjustments in dosage or even the particular variety of pill used may be necessary.

All the above suggestions, of course, are directed toward one goal: observing any abnormality and related information accurately enough to be able to help the doctor make a clinical diagnosis more rapidly and readily. Abnormalities in menstrual bleeding, as well as any nonmenstrual vaginal bleeding, do indeed require medical attention and, in certain cases, careful diagnostic studies or treatment. But the first step is always a commonsense reaction to any abnormal occurrence and careful, accurate reporting of what happened.

The Problem of Internal Hemorrhages

External hemorrhaging, because it is visible and accessible, only rarely presents problems in either diagnosis or treatment. Internal bleeding, whether due to an injury or to some disease condition, can be far more dangerous simply because it may not be readily detectable and, once it is detected, may necessitate surgical intervention to stop it. When the bleeding is due to internal injuries following an accident or other physical trauma, two clues suggest its presence: the onset of shock, together with an increase in pulse rate, a drop in blood pressure and such shocklike symptoms as pallor, sweating or shortness of breath; and the development of pain. When blood comes in contact with pain-sensitive membranes such as the pleural lining of the lungs, the peritoneal lining of the abdominal cavity, or the meningeal lining of the brain and spinal cord, it acts as a chemical irritant which causes these membranes to transmit very sharp pain sensations. Faced with either developing shock or localized internal pain, or both, in a patient who has been injured in an accident, the doctor will immediately suspect internal hemorrhage, locate the bleeding site and control the hemorrhage, even by surgical exploration if need be.

A wide variety of diseases can also lead to internal hemorrhage. Usually, however, the place and manner in which the bleeding is discovered, together with other clues, will help make diagnosis possible. Bleeding from a peptic ulcer, for example, occurs in the stomach or in the part of the small intestine just below the stomach, and the blood is immediately altered by the acid digestive juices so that it takes on a dark brown or black granular appearance. If the bleeding occurs in the stomach the patient may vomit, and the characteristic appearance of the vomitus, which looks like coffee grounds, is sufficient to identify the bleeding point as in or just below the stomach. If there is no vomiting, the blood is carried through the intestine into the colon and appears within a 24-hour period as a black, sticky material which looks like tar passed with the bowel movement. The passage of unchanged blood (that is, blood that is red in color) through the rectum, on the other hand, suggests a hemorrhage somewhere in the lower intestine or rectum.

Bleeding in the lungs is first noticed when blood is coughed up in the sputum, often very bright red and frothy. Such bleeding, known as *hemoptysis,* is never normal and should always be called to a doctor's attention even if only a small amount of blood is noted. It can arise from as innocuous a source as irritation from coughing during a severe case of bronchitis, or from more serious sources such as tuberculosis eroding a blood vessel in the lungs or bleeding from a bronchial tumor. Whatever the cause, such bleeding should never be ignored or allowed to pass without tracking down the source.

The same may be said about bleeding in the urinary tract, appearing either as gross blood in the urine or as microscopic quantities of blood detected by a urine examination. Again, a wide variety of conditions can lead to such bleeding—the presence of a kidney infection or inflammatory disease, the passing of a kidney stone, a tumor in the kidney or bladder, or even nothing more than cystitis or inflammation of the bladder. In any event, it too is *never* normal and should never be passed off without medical investigation to determine its cause.

Finally, surgical procedures are sometimes complicated by internal bleeding, and it is to guard against this that patients are so carefully observed in the immediate postoperative period, with regular checks of pulse rate and blood pressure. Any sign of rising pulse, falling blood pressure or other symptoms of shock will suggest postoperative hemorrhage to the surgeon and may necessitate reopening the wound to find and control the bleeding source.

The Problem of Shock

Shock is a potentially dangerous physiological condition that is often intimately related to injury and/or hemorrhage. It should not be confused with electrical shock or emotional shock, although both of these conditions can lead to physical shock when they cause injury, pain or severe emotional upset. True medical shock, in simple terms, is a state of circulatory failure or collapse in which there is insufficient return of blood to the heart, a sharp decrease in the pressure of blood in the arteries, and a continuing deficiency in the amount of blood actually flowing through the tissues of distant parts of the body. It is a condition which may result either from the loss of a considerable amount of blood during hemorrhage or from a massive overreaction of the body to an injury involving pain or fright and severe tissue or organ damage.

Typically the surface capillaries contract, slowing surface circulation, while larger and deeper blood vessels all over the body tend to dilate and "pool" blood, thus effectively reducing the amount of blood being returned to the heart. It is perfectly possible, in fact, for these vessels to pool so much blood for a short time that virtually *no* blood returns to the heart and the blood pressure in the arteries drops to zero. Shock may also occur when an individual is suffering from an overwhelming infection, from a toxic reaction to poisonous substances in the body, from dehydration (for example, during a prolonged and severe bout of gastroenteritis with both vomiting and diarrhea depleting the body fluids), from a severe allergic reaction or from a coronary heart attack.

Everyone has experienced some degree of shock at one time or another—the feeling of faintness and chilliness, the nausea sometimes followed by vomiting, the sudden excessive perspiration, the rapid but fluttery heartbeat and the wave of dizziness and instability that follow, for example, a mild but painful injury. What many people do *not* realize is that shock can involve far more than this sort of passing wave of physical reaction. In fact, shock and the degree of circulatory collapse associated with it can be so profound as to cause death, even when the injury or other condition precipitating the shock would not, in itself, be fatal.

In any case of injury, particularly when accompanied by blood loss, shock is a major threat and must be dealt with immediately. The emergency first-aid treatment of shock is discussed in an earlier chapter (*see* p. 111). But the most effective first-aid measures cannot get to the root of the problem. The definitive treatment of shock is a job for a physician in a hospital or in a medically staffed emergency unit or ambulance. Up to a certain point after the onset of shock, and before it becomes profoundly disabling, there are a number of measures a doctor can take to combat it long enough for the victim's body to "rebound" with its own natural defenses and adaptation to stress. First, pain and agitation must be controlled as quickly as possible, using narcotic drugs such as morphine or Demerol, or other potent analgesics. Second,

blood lost by hemorrhage must be replaced with transfusions; if transfusion is not immediately possible, at least the fluid volume of the blood can be restored temporarily by the use of intravenous infusions of dilute glucose or saline solutions, or for more prolonged periods by transfusion of blood plasma or the intravenous administration of one of the so-called plasma expanders such as Dextran, a colloidal solution similar in many ways to human blood plasma. At the same time, sagging blood pressure can be supported by the use of "pressor" drugs, medicines closely related to the natural hormone adrenalin or epinephrine. Finally, the physician must also be sure that any continuing bleeding is controlled, check carefully to be sure that there is no hidden internal hemorrhage to perpetuate shock, and proceed with other aspects of emergency treatment. In most cases these measures, taken together, will relieve shock and permit recovery, but in cases in which shock has gone beyond a certain degree of profundity, or has been present too long before definitive hospital care can be undertaken, it may become "irreversible": the victim goes on to die in shock regardless of what heroic measures are taken. In short, shock is a hazardous condition in which time is of the essence in beginning treatment.

Blood Transfusion and Donation

Hemorrhage with accompanying shock is one condition in which a blood transfusion—the intravenous infusion of blood taken from a donor—can be a lifesaving emergency procedure. In addition, whole-blood transfusions are extremely valuable in dealing with blood loss that may occur during childbirth or surgery, or in the treatment of severe anemias or any other condition in which the loss of red cells far exceeds the body's immediate reserve capacity to replace them. As a swift, convenient and reasonably safe means of replacing lost blood, blood transfusion has become a part of the standard operating procedure in every hospital. The history of blood transfusions is discussed briefly elsewhere (*see* p. 79), but much has been learned about blood typing and blood compatibility since Carl Landsteiner made his discovery of the A-B-O blood types in 1901. Today patients who require transfusions have their blood routinely typed and cross-matched with the prospective donor's blood prior to the transfusion to be sure that the transfused blood will be compatible with the recipient's own blood supply. An individual's blood type is controlled by heredity, and the major blood types—type O, type A, type B and type AB—are familiar to most people. Ideally, when blood is transfused, the donor's blood should be of the same type as the recipient's because when a different blood type is transfused a reaction may occur in which either the red cells from the donor's blood or the patient's own red cells become sticky and *agglutinate* into clumps, blocking up capillary blood vessels, with frequently fatal results.

Since blood types can be determined and matched accurately, such *transfusion reactions* occur only rarely today, but the supply of a given type of blood can be a problem because the different blood types are not evenly distributed in the population. Some 45 percent of the people in the United States, for example, have type O blood, and another 40 percent have blood of type A. Only about 10 percent have type B blood, and less than 5 percent have type AB. Fortunately, however, individuals with type A, B or AB blood in their veins can, in an emergency, receive small amounts of type O blood in a transfusion without too much risk of transfusion complications because the relatively small amount of type O blood given is rapidly diluted by the much larger quantity of blood in the recipient's own body. Thus the type O donor is sometimes called a universal donor, and the type AB recipient is called a universal recipient. Such "mixed type" transfusions, however, carry enough risk of troublesome complications with red cell agglutination that they are avoided in favor of transfusions of identical blood type whenever possible. Another possible transfusion difficulty can arise from incompatibility due to a quite separate blood factor known as the *Rh factor*. Problems involving Rh incompatibilities, most commonly related to newborn babies, are discussed in detail elsewhere. (*See* p. 833.)

A final problem that must be considered in the use of transfused blood is the threat of transmission of the virus of serum hepatitis, which may remain alive in the plasma of the victim for years after he has recovered from this disease. Attempts to purify or sterilize donated blood containing this virus by means of irradiation have not proved reliable, and today a prospective blood donor is asked to report any history of hepatitis or other liver diseases before his blood is taken. Even with these precautions, however, virus-contaminated blood occasionally slips through and causes hepatitis in the recipient, and today this has become a major reason why blood transfusions are used with caution and then only in cases of real need. If red cells are not vitally necessary, cases of hemorrhage or shock may better be treated by the administration of blood plasma, which can be effectively sterilized to destroy any virus that may be contaminating it without altering its effectiveness. On the other hand, in conditions such as profound, long-standing anemia, in which the victim needs red cells desperately but may not be able to accommodate to the infusion of a large volume of fluid without going into heart failure, it is possible to transfuse *packed red cells*—whole blood from which the cells have been allowed to settle and are subsequently used as a "concentrated red cell transfusion" with only a little of the plasma.

The immediate availability of either whole blood or packed red cells depends upon a well-organized system of "blood banks" whereby prospective donors can give blood at any time, and patients in need of transfusions can be supplied, without having to search to find a specific donor for a specific patient. Most of our cities have such blood banks operating on a 24-hour nonprofit basis. Banking of blood is possible because whole blood, withdrawn from a donor and mixed with an anticlotting agent such as sodium citrate, can be refrigerated and stored up to three weeks before the red cells begin to deteriorate significantly. Often friends and relatives of a patient who has received a blood transfusion are asked to donate blood to the blood bank to replace what was used; and in addition, service clubs and special community committees often hold drives to replenish blood bank blood when the supply is getting low.

In general any adult man or woman in normal

good health can donate a unit (500 cc.'s or slightly more than a pint) of blood with no untoward effects. Most blood banks will reject prospective donors who have a below-normal hemoglobin level, high blood pressure or a history of malaria, syphilis or hepatitis. In the case of donors who qualify, blood is painlessly withdrawn from a vein in the arm and drained directly into a sterile bottle or plastic container into which sodium citrate has already been placed. The procedure, which is supervised by a doctor or a registered nurse, takes a matter of about 10 minutes, and the donor is then asked to remain at rest for an additional half hour to recover from any degree of emotional shock that may have occurred as a result of the donation. Occasionally a donor will feel slightly faint or dizzy when standing up, even after this waiting period, but this feeling will pass in a matter of moments. Donating blood is an extremely important and praiseworthy community service, but no one should donate blood more frequently than once every three months, so that his body has ample time to replenish the slightly depleted blood supply.

Congenital Anomalies of the Heart and Blood Vessels

In order to perform its many vital functions, blood must circulate through virtually every tissue in the body, and although blood is a liquid, its circulation is far from random and uncontrolled. It moves through thousands of miles of circulatory tubing—the arteries, arterioles, capillaries, venules and veins—powered by the action of a very specialized muscle, the heart. Obviously any disease or disorder affecting the structure or function of the heart and blood vessels can impede circulation and may cause severe disability and sometimes even death.

The Remarkable Adjustment of Blood Flow

Perhaps the most unique characteristic of the cardiovascular system is its ability to adapt to the changing needs of the body. To compare it to the fixed, rigid pipes and the mechanical pump of a circulating hot-water heating system in an apartment building, however, is to do it a great injustice. For one thing, the heart, unlike a mechanical pump, does not always run at a constant speed, but will vary from one moment to the next, depending on the body's needs. The rate may fall as low as 45 or 50 beats per minute during deep sleep and increase to as many as 180 to 200 beats per minute or even more during a period of vigorous exercise. Further, blood vessels are not fixed and rigid like pipes; many of them can dilate and rebound rhythmically as blood surges out of the heart with each heartbeat. It is this rhythmic expansion and rebound of the arteries that we feel as the *pulse* when we

place a finger over an artery that runs close to the surface—the radial artery at the wrist, for example.

The heart may not be able to generate the pressure of a mechanical pump, but its pressure is certainly great enough to push large and continuing quantities of blood "uphill" when we are standing erect—from the heart to the brain, for example, by a fairly direct route, or from the body's lower extremities back to the heart by a much more circuitous route. Further, the pressure generated by the heart fluctuates in different parts of the body. If we had some magical means of inserting a pressure gauge in the aorta, the great artery that receives blood when it is first pumped from the heart, or the carotid artery that carries blood to the head, we would find that the pressure of the blood inside the walls of these arteries fluctuates with the heartbeat, increasing sharply to a peak as the heart contracts and squeezes blood into the artery, then falling off to a lower level during the period of relaxation before the next contraction. On the other hand, if the same pressure gauge could be inserted into the vena cava, the great vein extending from the lower abdomen to the heart, we would find a steady, unchanging pressure with no sign of a pulsation with the heartbeat.

Even more remarkable is the fluctuation and regulation of the *quantity* of blood circulating in the system in different parts of the body at different times. There is, for example, a wide variation in the quantity of blood delivered to the brain and to the stomach at different times during the day. Three or four hours after breakfast, when we may be engaged in some mental activity, the quantity of blood delivered to the brain is high, whereas that delivered to the stomach amounts to a comparative trickle. After a heavy lunch, however, the procedure is just the reverse. The supply of blood to the stomach is markedly increased, while arterial blood flow to the brain decreases—one reason that we tend to feel sleepy after a large meal.

Much of the remarkable adaptability of the cardiovascular system lies in the structure of the blood vessels themselves. The capillaries spread throughout the body are nothing more than microscopically tiny tubes just one cell layer thick without the capacity to expand or contract; they are so tiny, in fact, that blood cells must slip through sideways. The arterioles that carry blood into the capillaries, and the venules that carry blood away from them, are somewhat larger and have narrow layers of muscle fiber and elastic tissue in their walls. In the larger veins and the vena cava into which all other veins ultimately empty, these layers of elastic tissue and muscle are considerably thicker, and the veins are supported in position by a webbing of connective tissue. Furthermore, many veins, especially those in the lower extremities, are equipped with delicate internal valves which open to allow the blood to move toward the heart but close, preventing backflow, when the forward pressure of blood in the veins falls off.

In the larger arteries and the great aorta that

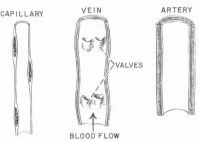

CAPILLARY   VEIN   ARTERY

VALVES

BLOOD FLOW

Figure 41–1.

arches up from the heart before branching into the major arteries to the head, abdomen and extremities, the amount of elastic tissue and muscle fiber in the walls is at least ten times

greater than in the walls of the veins. Thus these arterial vessels are normally quite rubbery, capable of expanding or stretching to receive a surge of blood pumped by the heart, then relaxing between heartbeats.

What this means, in brief, is that blood leaving the heart is conducted first through arteries which have the strength and elasticity to handle the surging pressure generated by each heartbeat. It then goes into smaller arterioles which can also expand or contract, allowing blood to flow more or less freely into the capillary system. In the capillaries the pulsating pressure of arterial blood is equalized into a steady flow which is then maintained as the blood passes on into the venules and veins, and ultimately returns to the heart. Finally, the heart chambers which receive and expel blood are themselves connected by means of a series of one-way valves so that, in normal conditions, the blood is constantly moved in a single uniform direction and cannot backflow from one chamber of the heart to another.

Essential to the continuing circulation of the blood, of course, is the heart itself, a surprisingly small and amazingly tough muscular organ, not much bigger than a man's clenched fist, which lies in the chest cavity slightly to the left of the midline. The heart walls are constructed of a singularly powerful, interwoven mesh of striated muscle fibers, woven in a spiral from top to bottom around a "skeleton" of fibrous tissue, and enclosing four hollow chambers for receiving and expelling blood. When the heart muscle is relaxed, these chambers can fill with approximately 200 cc.'s (about 7 ounces) of blood; once filled, the muscle contracts in a wringing motion, literally squeezing the blood out into the aorta and the pulmonary artery.

It is easy to imagine the heart as a pump—but it is a two-sided pump with an upper chamber and a lower chamber on each side. The upper chambers are comparatively thin-walled cavities, the *atria* or *auricles,* which serve as collecting places for blood returning to the heart; the lower chambers, known as the ventricles, have thick, powerful muscular walls and serve as pumping chambers. The right auricle and ventricle are concerned with receiving deoxygenated venous blood from the general circulation and pumping it into the pulmonary circulatory system for replenishment of oxygen and dumping of carbon dioxide; the left auricle and ventricle then receive freshly oxygenated blood from the pulmonary circulation and pump it out into the general circulation again. Even doctors tend to think of "the right side" of the heart and "the left side" of the heart operating independently of each other, and normally there is no direct connection between the chambers of the right side and those on the left, but of course both sides actually work simultaneously, rhythmically pumping and relaxing, to maintain circulation.

Powerful as it is, however, the heart could not consistently pump blood in the proper direction without the contribution of four one-way *cardiac valves.* When blood is returned to the heart by way of the vena cava, it enters the right auricle and is then admitted into the right ventricle through the *tricuspid valve* when the auricle contracts. When the ventricle starts to contract, the tricuspid valve snaps shut and blood is forced through the *pulmonic valve* separating the right ventricle from the pulmonary

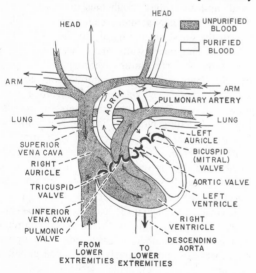

Figure 41–2.
Circulation of blood through the heart.

arteries. Once through the pulmonary capillaries, the blood is carried by the pulmonary veins back to the left auricle, and on through the *mitral valve*

(so called because it resembles a bishop's crown, or miter) into the left ventricle as the auricle contracts. When the ventricle contracts, the mitral valve snaps shut to prevent backflow, and the blood is forced through the *aortic valve* into the aorta and on through the general circulatory system again.

Thus the construction of the cardiovascular system itself not only maintains the direction of blood flow but also helps regulate its pressure. But the overall regulation of blood circulation, and of the heart's action as well, is a function of the nervous system. The *smooth muscle* fibers in the walls of the arteries, arterioles, venules and veins cannot be controlled voluntarily, but contract or relax according to involuntary nerve impulses carried by the *autonomic nervous system.* (*See* p. 48.) Although the "main headquarters" of this auxiliary nervous system is in the brain, there are certain special "secondary control centers" located elsewhere which are capable of taking delicate pressure and chemical measurements on a moment-by-moment basis, and thus exercising control over dilatation or contraction of the muscle in the blood vessels. One such center, the *carotid plexus,* is a gathering of nerve cells in the carotid artery in the neck at about the level of the lower jaw. These nerves are sensitive to carbon dioxide in the blood, and send involuntary signals to the respiratory muscles and the heart to increase their rates when the carbon dioxide level in the blood becomes a little too high, or to slow them down when it becomes a little too low. Other involuntary nerve centers monitor oxygen levels in the blood in various organs and tissues and control the expansion or contraction of the small blood vessels in areas which need more, or less, oxygen at a given time during periods of work or rest. Temperature sensors in the autonomic nervous system control expansion or contraction of arterioles and venules near the surface of the body to allow body heat to be lost or conserved as necessary; simultaneously, the sweat glands in the skin increase or decrease the production of perspiration, another means of body temperature control.

Perhaps the most singular of all the autonomic circulatory regulators, however, is the one that directly regulates or "paces" the heartbeat. The heart is equipped with a special *neuro-muscular conducting system,* a network of unique muscle fibers which are capable of conducting nerve impulses in much the same way as nerve fibers are. This network has its center in a small nodule of autonomic nerve cells located in the wall of the right auricle and known as the *sino-atrial node* or "S-A node." This node is also spoken of as the "cardiac pacemaker," for it regulates the rate of the heartbeat, acting on signals transmitted to it from the brain stem. When this pacemaker triggers a "heartbeat signal," the auricles immediately contract; instantly the signal is transmitted to the ventricles by way of the neuromuscular conducting system, and the ventricles contract. Then, following a brief *refractory period* while the cardiac muscle relaxes, another heartbeat is triggered.

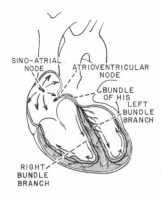

Figure 41–3.
Neuromuscular conducting system of the heart.

Normally the cardiac pacemaker triggers a heartbeat at a rate between 50 and 120 beats per minute, depending on the body's moment-by-moment need for oxygenated blood. Occasionally, however, the S-A node, or some other part of the conducting network, becomes damaged due to heart injury, inflammation or scarring following a coronary attack, so that signals cannot get through from the S-A node to the ventricles, a condition known as *heart block.* This does not mean that the heart stops beating under these circumstances; the ventricles continue to contract, but at a much slower rate than

normal, and without the capability to adapt to changing needs. In recent years medical engineers and surgeons have developed a device known as an *electronic cardiac pacemaker* which can be permanently implanted in the chest wall to substitute for the action of the natural pacemaker. People with electronic pacemakers can live perfectly normal lives, but must take care not to approach such devices as microwave ovens, diathermy machines or electronic blasting control mechanisms because electromagnetic waves from these devices can interfere with the electronic pacemaker's function.

Thus the circulation of the blood is carefully regulated and controlled by a whole series of mechanical and nervous system mechanisms. The truly amazing thing is the way in which all these mechanisms work together in splendid cooperation, completely outside our voluntary control. But if that cooperation breaks down, or if injury, infection, congenital abnormalities or degenerative changes affect the delicate structure and balance of the cardiovascular system, a wide variety of disorders may result.

Congenital Abnormalities of the Great Vessels

Very early in its development, the human embryo is little more than a three-layered sheet of precursor cells, all of which look much the same. Presently one layer of these cells begins to differentiate from the others to form the beginnings of the spinal cord and nervous system; another layer starts to form bone and muscle tissue, while the third layer forms the "hollow tube" of the gastrointestinal tract, as well as the heart and the blood vessels. By the time the human embryo is two to three months old, the basic shape and structure of the heart and blood vessels have been determined. From that "formative period" on, the cardiovascular system develops in more detail and to a higher degree of completion, but its ultimate structure is already set. In most cases, this development proceeds normally, but there are certain factors that can impede it. The virus of German measles, for example, can cross the placenta from the mother's blood stream, attack the fetus, and hinder, damage or destroy the normal development of the cardiovascular system. Various potent drugs or medicines can have similar damaging effects on the developing fetus. And finally, inherited genetic factors may lead to abnormalities in the structure or development of the heart and blood vessels.

Patent Ductus Arteriosus. One of the more common congenital anomalies of the cardiovascular system is not really an anomaly at all until some weeks after the baby is born, and then becomes symptomatic only if it does not take care of itself. In the human embryo the heart begins to beat and circulate its own blood at about the beginning of the fifth month of gestation, but at this time, obviously, the baby cannot breathe. The necessary oxygen is supplied from the mother's blood stream across the placenta, and is picked up by the baby's umbilical artery. Since there is no oxygen exchange in the baby's lungs, even though blood may pass through the rudimentary pulmonary circulatory system in the fetus, nature provides a perfectly normal by-pass or *shunt* between the venous blood entering the heart and the arterial blood leaving the heart. (*See* Fig. 41–4.) This arteriovenous shunt is nothing more complicated than a very short blood vessel, comparatively large in diameter, which connects the aorta just above its exit from the heart with the pulmonary artery just above its exit from the heart, thus effectively by-passing the pulmonary circulation. It is known as the *ductus arteriosus,* and it is utilized until the baby is born, expands his lungs, and begins breathing air. At that time, uninterrupted circulation becomes necessary for oxygenation of the blood. The ductus arteriosus ordinarily begins to diminish in size as the time of birth approaches and usually closes off and is absorbed within a few weeks after birth. In some people a fibrous strand may remain, but ordinarily even this disappears with time. In a relatively few individuals, however, the ductus arteriosus remains *patent* (that is, open) for several months after birth, and in some very uncommon instances it may remain open as a functioning arteriovenous shunt into adolescence or adulthood.

When this happens, trouble very gradually begins to occur, since a certain amount of ex-

hausted blood returning to the heart is shunted through the patent ductus and passes out with arterial blood without circulating through the lungs to pick up more oxygen. In a small child this causes very little difficulty, but by adolescence the defect begins to take its toll. The child does not get a normal supply of oxygenated blood, and his heart must work harder than normal to make up the lack. He tends to become short of breath, first only upon exertion, but later, progressively, even without exertion. The heart enlarges and by adolescence or early adulthood may go into heart failure from overwork. Often the child with this condition develops a grayish pallor, and observers at home or at school will sometimes see him break away from active play and squat down panting for breath

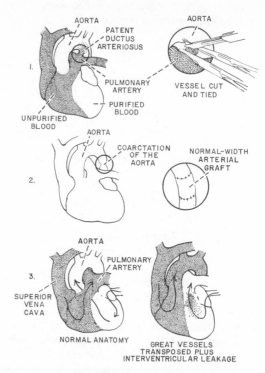

Figure 41–4.
Congenital abnormalities of the great vessels.

while his contemporaries continue with their games.

This condition is relatively easy to diagnose and is usually discovered by the family doctor during a childhood physical examination. The main diagnostic clue is the sound of a "machinery-like murmur," easily heard through the stethoscope: a continuing background rumble which is never present under normal conditions. X-rays and other studies, including cardiac catheterization (*see* p. 555), are usually done to confirm the diagnosis beyond doubt, since the condition requires surgical correction. The patent ductus is closed by means of ligatures, and then the connecting blood vessel is severed so that it can no longer conduct blood. Since the heart is not ordinarily entered at all, this is one of the least dangerous of all procedures in cardiac surgery. It is almost always successful, and the change in the sick child is most dramatic, with marked improvement in the oxygenation of the blood and relief of strain upon the heart becoming apparent within hours—sometimes even minutes—after the surgery. And once this congenital anomaly has been corrected, the child has as good a life expectancy as anyone else.

Coarctation of the Aorta. This is an even more common congenital anomaly, but it may not be discovered until the victim has reached maturity or even middle age. Some arrest during the fetal development of the heart and great blood vessels causes a narrowing or stricture of the aorta, usually just below the arch where the aorta curves down through the chest into the abdomen. It is as if someone had tied a string around the aorta at that point and pinched it slightly closed.

The effect of this stricture, known as a *coarctation,* is rarely noticed in early life, and there are no characteristic heart sounds or murmurs to reveal its presence. If the coarctation is narrow enough, however, it will ultimately result in the development of higher blood pressure in the arteries above the coarctation (that is, those supplying the upper trunk, the arms and the brain) than below the coarctation in the vessels supplying the abdomen, kidneys, digestive organs and legs. As adulthood approaches, this odd distribution of hypertension or increased blood pressure becomes quite marked: the blood pressure measured in an arm may be as high as 200/140, while at the same time it may be 110/70 in the leg.

Coarctation of the aorta is not a very common cause of increased blood pressure, but it occurs often enough that it must be suspected when hypertension appears, especially in a young patient. If blood pressure tests indicate the possibility of its presence, the coarctation can subsequently be identified by special blood vessel X-rays. It is one of the rare forms of high blood pressure which can be permanently cured—in this case by surgical correction of the coarctation. Blood is temporarily diverted from the defective portion of the aorta, and the stricture is removed, often with an aortic graft inserted to maintain the length of the artery where the defective segment was cut out. This procedure is usually well tolerated, with a dramatic drop in the increased blood pressure of the upper extremities and a permanent cure for the high blood pressure that was caused by the defect.

Transposition of the Great Vessels. Another congenital abnormality of the cardiovascular system, arising as a result of damage to the developing heart and blood vessels during the first trimester of gestation, is complete transposition of the great vessels. In this condition the aorta and the pulmonary artery develop in transposed or reversed position, with the pulmonary artery arising from the *left* ventricle and the aorta arising from the *right* ventricle. This anatomical defect separates both general circulation and pulmonary circulation into two completely closed systems. Blood from the left ventricle is pumped through the lungs and returns to the left atrium; then it moves back into the left ventricle and through the lungs again in a closed circuit with no opportunity to go on from there into general circulation. At the same time blood returning from the tissues enters the right atrium and passes into the right ventricle, from which it is immediately pumped directly into the aorta and back into general circulation again. Before birth when the baby receives oxygen through the placenta from the mother's blood supply, no problem arises, but as soon as the baby is born and the ductus arteriosus closes, there is no way to get oxygen, and the baby would very quickly suffocate if there were no open connections between the closed arterial circuit and the closed pulmonary circuit.

In most cases of transposition, the situation is not immediately fatal, since usually one or more shunts remain open between the two closed circuits. There may be defects or openings between the ventricles or the atria which permit *some* oxygenated blood to escape from the right ventricle into the left, and often the ductus arteriosus remains open as well. Even so, the baby will never obtain sufficient oxygen in his circulating blood with this condition. He will show increasing evidence of *cyanosis*, the purplish-blue skin color that results from poor oxygenation of the red blood cells, from birth onward, and within a few months will have marked evidence of shortness of breath, an enlarged heart, and often heart failure. Transposition is one of the most common of the conditions that cause the so-called blue baby, since the child never has the chance to develop the healthy, pink, well-oxygenated color of most babies.

Prior to the late 1930s and early 1940s, this congenital defect, together with many other defects of the heart, was regarded as hopeless; the only treatment lay in surgery involving the heart itself, a part of the body that had always been off limits to surgeons. Today with the great advances that have been made in cardiac surgery both in adults and in children, some victims of transposition of the great vessels can be saved. Nevertheless, it is still considered one of the gravest of all congenital abnormalities. Many victims die so soon after birth that there is not enough time to distinguish this defect from others and thus make the necessary preoperative diagnosis. In other cases, even when the child does survive for a while, he is in such poor physical shape that he cannot survive the surgery. Fortunately many children who are at first suspected of having transposition of the great vessels are found, upon preoperative studies, to have a less grave congenital heart or blood vessel defect; in that case, there is sufficient time to prepare the child for surgery, greatly increasing the odds of his survival.

Pulmonic Stenosis. This congenital condition is most commonly found in conjunction with other abnormalities, but occasionally occurs by itself. It is a defect in which the pulmonic valve, which provides for one-way flow of blood from the right ventricle into the pulmonary artery and thence to the lungs, is deformed, with a narrowed or *stenotic* opening, thus restricting the amount of blood that can be pushed through it. Occasionally the narrowing is not in the valve itself, but in the first portion of the pulmonary artery just outside the valve. This condition, when present alone, causes an increased pressure of blood in the right ventricle, with resulting enlargement of that heart chamber as it develops thicker and stronger muscle in its effort to push blood past the obstruction. Pressure of the blood in the pulmonary artery remains very low, and as the victim grows older there may not be enough blood flowing through the lungs for adequate oxygenation.

Diagnosis of this condition, which may remain without symptoms for many years, is generally made on physical examination when the doctor hears a characteristic "murmur" as he listens to the patient's heart sounds; X-ray and EKG studies help confirm the diagnosis. If the stenosis is severe, patients reaching adulthood often become short of breath, have episodes of fainting or pass out for no apparent reason, and presently develop heart failure. In milder cases there may never be any symptoms, or any impairment. If impairment is great enough that treatment is required, however, the condition can be greatly improved by surgery. The pulmonic valve may be cut or stretched or, if necessary, completely replaced by an artificial valve. In recent years such procedures have been highly successful in providing long-term relief for this condition.

Aortic Stenosis. This condition is very similar to pulmonic stenosis except that the aortic valve is narrowed to the point of obstructing blood flow, often by a constricting fibrous ring in the muscle of the heart just below the valve. The defect reduces the amount of blood that the left ventricle can pump out into general circulation with each heartbeat, so that it must beat faster and is always working under higher pressure than normal. Eventually this increased work load results in a marked enlargement of the heart. In most cases the victim remains free of symptoms for many months or years, even when the deformity is severe. Then, as the overloaded heart begins to fail, the victim notices increasing fatigue, shortness of breath even on very mild exertion, and episodes of fainting. Sometimes sudden, massive heart failure is the first sign of trouble: the heart works to its limit and then stops. Diagnosis again can be made during a physical examination when the doctor hears a characteristic heart "murmur," and confirmed by X-ray and electrocardiogram. As in pulmonic stenosis, correction of the condition involves heart surgery in which the valve is either stretched or cut open, or replaced by an artificial valve. Usually the decision for surgery is made, however, only if and when the patient begins to suffer symptoms or show evidence of approaching heart failure. Many people can live perfectly normal, active lives without requiring any correction of the condition, and any kind of heart surgery involves a significant risk in itself.

Congenital Malformations of the Heart

Congenital malformations of the heart that occur during the first three months of gestation are perhaps even more common, and potentially more serious, than malformations of the blood vessels, and in many cases they may occur simultaneously. For years no one had any explanation for the prevalence of these defects; then in 1942 an unusual observation was made by two physicians in Australia. The previous winter there had been an epidemic of German measles in Australia, an apparently innocuous virus infection which usually affects children but can also strike susceptible adults. Following this epidemic, Australian physicians noted a remarkable increase in the number of babies born with congenital heart defects. Subsequent studies proved beyond doubt that this "innocuous" virus infection, which causes no particular lasting harm to children or adults, nevertheless has the power to cross from the placenta of a mother into the blood stream of the baby she is carrying. When the fetus is in its most critical formative stages, between the first two and four months of gestation, the German measles virus

attacks embryonic cells and causes a wide variety of abnormalities in the way the heart and great vessels are formed. Indeed, the correlation between German measles in the mother during the first few months of her pregnancy and the development of heart defects in the baby is so high—more than 75 percent of all such infants are affected, according to some studies—that many physicians regard its occurrence as sufficient grounds to recommend interruption of the pregnancy.

What is the threat of these defects, what symptoms do they cause and what, if anything, can be done about them? Obviously, most congenital heart defects interfere in some way with normal circulation. Some are responsible for the so-called blue baby symptoms or cyanosis caused when the dark purple unoxygenated blood returning from the tissues and other organs is abnormally shunted back into general circulation without passing through the lungs for reoxygenation. With some heart defects cyanosis is present from birth; with others it may not appear until months or even years after birth, and then perhaps only intermittently when the child has been unusually active. But whether the defect causes cyanosis or not, virtually any abnormality of the heart's structure places an excessive burden on that organ, forcing it to do far more work than normal; consequently, symptoms of heart failure gradually begin to appear, even in small children. Finally, certain defects cause a persistent elevation of blood pressure in the pulmonary artery and the pulmonary circulatory system, a condition which can cause progressive and irreparable damage to the blood vessels of the pulmonary system and thus further increase the difficulty of adequately oxygenating the blood.

Tetralogy of Fallot. One of the so-called blue baby heart defects that can occur as a result of a German measles attack on the developing fetus, tetralogy of Fallot derives its name from the fact that not one but four different abnormalities are usually present at the same time. First, there is a narrowing or *stenosis* of the heart muscle just inside the outlet of the pulmonic valve through which blood is pumped from the right ventricle into the pulmonary artery for oxygenation in the lungs. Second, because the right ventricle must work extra hard to pump blood through this stenotic opening, it undergoes enlargement or *hypertrophy*. Third, there is a large defect or

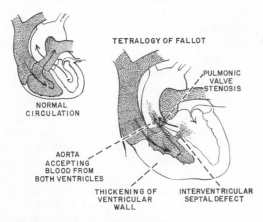

TETRALOGY OF FALLOT

PULMONIC VALVE STENOSIS

NORMAL CIRCULATION

AORTA ACCEPTING BLOOD FROM BOTH VENTRICLES

THICKENING OF VENTRICULAR WALL

INTERVENTRICULAR SEPTAL DEFECT

Figure 41–5.

opening in the muscular *septum* dividing the right ventricle from the left, so that the right ventricle, already working under extremely high pressure, squeezes some of the returned venous blood through the hole and directly into the left ventricle rather than into the pulmonary circulation. Fourth, the aorta is often improperly located, so that it overrides the right ventricle and allows unoxygenated blood to enter the outgoing arterial circulation along with the oxygenated blood returning to the left ventricle from the lungs.

Other Congenital Defects. Other structural defects of the heart and great vessels often parallel the four abnormalities found in tetralogy of Fallot. These defects are many and varied, but for all their variety, they usually involve one or more of the following patterns of abnormality.

Deformity, narrowing or other obstruction of one or more of the heart valves. The deformity may involve the valves themselves or occur in a part of the heart in their immediate vicinity. In either case, the valve or valves involved cannot properly open to permit normal blood flow, or else remain open so that blood can reflux or regurgitate back through the valve when it is not supposed to. When such a deformity is primarily

a narrowing of the valve opening, it is called *atresia;* when the valve itself is deformed, or fixed in a partially open or closed position so that it cannot function properly, the condition is known as *stenosis*. Both the *pulmonic valve* and the *aortic valve* are commonly subject to this kind of congenital malformation. Much more rarely, the tricuspid valve between the right atrium and the right ventricle can also be congenitally malformed. Stenosis of the *mitral valve* between the left atrium and the left ventricle, however, is almost always the result of a long-term inflammatory disease of the heart, particularly rheumatic fever, and rarely occurs due to embryonic damage.

Malposition of the great vessels is another common form of congenital heart defect, in which one or more of the great blood vessels entering or leaving the heart are improperly located during the time of fetal development. Such a defect may vary all the way from a slight *overriding* of the aorta across the dividing septum between the ventricles, causing some unoxygenated blood from the right ventricle to be pumped into the aorta along with the oxygenated blood from the left ventricle—a condition which may be relatively innocuous if the overriding is very slight—all the way to *complete transposition of the great vessels*.

Ventricular septal defects—literally holes in the muscle wall separating the right and left "pumping chambers" of the heart—are by far the most frequent of all congenital heart malformations. When such defects are present, blood is squeezed or shunted directly from one ventricle to the other, by-passing either the general or the pulmonary circulation. These defects arise during the early formation of the rudimentary heart when the developing baby has only one large ventricular chamber which is later divided in two by the development of the ventricular septum, a partition of muscle and fibrous tissue. A septal defect occurs when that "closing-up" process is impaired or incomplete.

Ventricular septal defects may be very tiny, perhaps smaller than the tip of a little finger, or they may be very large, permitting great quantities of blood to be shunted from one side to the other. Minor defects rarely cause trouble, at least during childhood, but larger ones soon have a marked effect. Because the musculature of the left ventricle is usually thicker and more powerful than that of the right ventricle, blood is first forced or shunted from the left chamber into the right with each heartbeat, thus short-changing the general circulation of the oxygenated blood it would normally receive, and forcing much more blood through the pulmonary circulatory system than it is built to handle. Often symptom-free at first, the marked increase in blood pressure in the pulmonary arteries presently leads to thickening and constriction of these vessels, which further increases the pressure in the pulmonary system until pressure in the right ventricle finally becomes higher than that in the left. At that point, the direction of the shunting of blood is reversed; unoxygenated blood from the right ventricle is forced into the left ventricle, and in severe cases cyanosis begins to occur, at first during vigorous exercise and then later even during minor exercise. Because of the extra load on both the right and the left ventricles, the heart muscle must hypertrophy and the heart chambers themselves dilate. The end result, in cases where the septal defect is more than about one-half inch in diameter, is severe—irreversible pulmonary hypertension, progressive cyanosis, heart failure and ultimately death if the defect cannot be corrected.

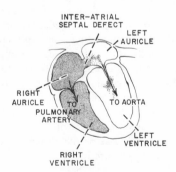

INTER-ATRIAL
SEPTAL DEFECT
LEFT
AURICLE
RIGHT
AURICLE
TO
PULMONARY
ARTERY
TO AORTA
LEFT
VENTRICLE
RIGHT
VENTRICLE

Figure 41–6.

Atrial septal defects are similar to ventricular septal defects, except that the hole or opening occurs in the thin muscular septum separating the right atrium or auricle from the left. These defects may also be very tiny, with little or no impairment of heart function, or very large, with the shunting of great quantities of blood from the left side to the right side of the heart beginning very early in life. Fortunately, the auricles act more as thin-walled collecting chambers than as pumping chambers; the pressure of blood in the auricles is not very high compared to that which develops in the ventricles during the contraction of a heartbeat. Thus any overload that occurs as a result of shunting of blood through an atrial septal defect develops more slowly than if blood were shunted through a defect in the ventricular septum. Many children born with this defect may have no symptoms at all for several years or only minor symptoms which progress slowly, providing ample time for study and evaluation as to the possible value of surgical correction. In about 15 percent of these cases, however, the atrial septal defect occurs low down in the septum, and is often associated with heart valve abnormalities as well. When this is the case, symptoms occur much earlier and much more severely, and attempts at surgical repair must often be considered within the early months or years of the child's life.

Any one or all of these various congenital malformations may be present in a given individual to one degree or another. Whether or not the defect or defects result in a "blue baby" depends partially upon the magnitude of the defect and upon the degree to which oxygen-exhausted venous blood returning to the heart is shunted into the left ventricle and recirculated without passing through the lungs. In many cases this does not occur until the child has lived long enough with the defect for it to begin to cause such permanent changes as sharply elevated blood pressure in the pulmonary artery. In addition, certain specific combinations of these defects occur frequently enough that they have been given special names. One such combination is the above-mentioned tetralogy of Fallot; another, known as *Eisenmenger's complex,* usually involves a large ventricular septal defect with severe pulmonary hypertension and the appearance, after a time, of cyanosis only during vigorous exercise.

The Decision for Surgery

Until 35 or 40 years ago virtually any congenital malformation of the heart or great vessels was an incurable affliction which in many cases sooner or later ended fatally. If the child survived infancy, the defect would retard his growth and limit his activities, make him excessively vulnerable to upper respiratory infections, and eventually lead to heart failure. That complication, of course, could be treated with the use of digitalis and other medicines, but at best these were only palliative measures and ultimately the victim would die during childhood or young adulthood. In the early 1900s pioneering surgeons did succeed in aiding or curing patients with patent ductus arteriosus by ligating and excising this vestigial connection between the aorta and the pulmonary artery, but the heart itself was still considered forbidden ground to the surgeon until the late 1930s.

Since then the whole field of cardiac surgery has been revolutionized; thanks to the pioneering work of a few men, surgeons all over the world have learned that the heart *can* be operated upon safely, many congenital defects *can* be repaired, and lives which would otherwise be forfeited *can* be saved. These surgical procedures are possible not only in adults, but even in tiny babies if the nature of the defect is such that surgery cannot safely be postponed. What is more, new surgical skills extend well beyond the repair of deformed tissue. Today they include the use of artificial materials or tissue grafts; artificial valves can be emplanted to replace damaged or deformed valves, various artificial fabrics can be used to close defects that are too large to be closed with the existing tissues, and various graft materials such as segments of aorta preserved in a tissue bank can be used to replace an abnormally narrow section of aorta.

Originally this kind of daring heart surgery was performed only when it was felt that the patient would surely die without it. Since the heart and lungs had to continue functioning throughout the operation, the surgeon often had no more than minutes or even seconds in which to work on the heart itself to effect his repairs; the mortality rate during surgery was exceedingly high, and some more extensive repairs remained impossible. Then during the late 1950s and early 1960s a revolutionary aid to such surgery was devised: the so-called *heart-lung by-pass machine,* a device through which the patient's circulating blood could be temporarily shunted during surgery, aerating and pumping it mechanically so that it did not have to pass through the patient's heart and lungs at all during the critical phase of the operation. This meant that the surgeon could literally disconnect the malformed heart from the patient's circulatory stream for a brief period, temporarily quiet the heartbeat with an electric current and then operate on a "dry" and unmoving heart. When the repair was completed, the heart and lungs could be "reconnected" to the circulating blood stream, the heartbeat restimulated and the blood flow returned to its normal channels. This remarkable device, now in wide use in hospitals all over the country, made it possible for the first time for surgeons to tackle really extensive repairs of the heart, particularly such lengthy and technically difficult procedures as closing septal defects or replacing malformed valves with artificial ones.

Even with the help of such mechanical aids, however, corrective heart surgery still poses a considerable risk to the patient, and its success depends upon both the doctor's diagnostic knowledge and his operating skills. Thus the decision to operate in any given case can be a very difficult one, made only after careful consultations among surgeons, pediatricians, internists, cardiologists and often other specialists with particular skills—radiologists, for example, who have a broad experience in interpreting diagnostic X-rays. New and startling diagnostic techniques have been developed to help the surgeon and his consultants pinpoint the diagnosis as closely as possible. Some of these procedures involve very little risk to the patient, but require great skill in interpreting the results. For example, techniques have been devised for introducing radio-opaque dyes into the patient's jugular vein and then taking a rapid sequence of X-ray films—ten or fifteen shots per second—to follow the passage of the dye through the chambers of the heart. Such a series of films, known

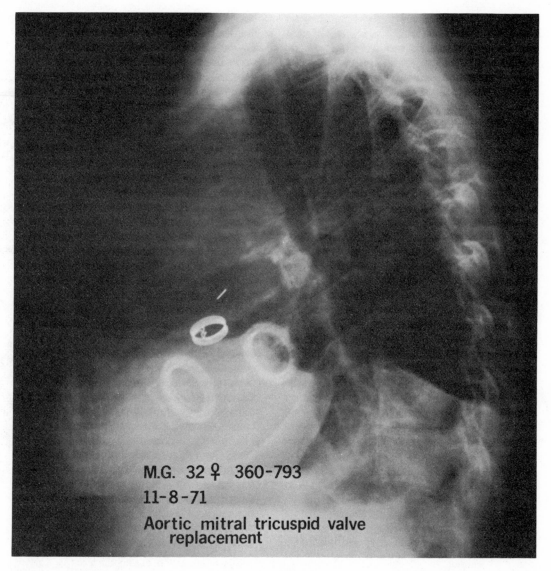

M.G. 32 ♀ 360-793
11-8-71
Aortic mitral tricuspid valve
replacement

Plate 23   Replacement of three heart valves in a single patient.

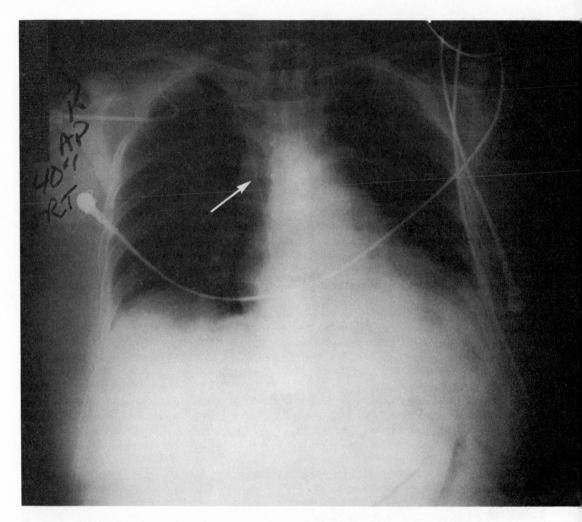

Plate 24　X-ray of a patient taken during cardiac catheterization. The very thin sterile catheter, indicated by the arrow, was inserted in the patient's right axillary vein and advanced until the tip entered the right atrium of the heart. The multiple leads of the electrocardiograph machine used to monitor the patient's heart action during the procedure are seen as thicker "wires" in this film.

as *angiograms,* requires skillful interpretation, but they often demonstrate beyond any question the nature and location of the congenital defect.

Cardiac catheterization—passing a small polyethylene tube or catheter into a blood vessel near the surface of the body until the tip of the catheter enters the chambers of the heart or even the pulmonary artery—is another procedure that provides indispensable diagnostic information. The actual concentration of oxygen present in various chambers of the heart can be measured by withdrawing blood samples through the catheter, and the comparative blood pressures in the various heart chambers or in the pulmonary artery can also be determined. This procedure, valuable as it is, also carries a certain risk, higher in the case of a very small patient than in the case of an adult. Thus, even the decision to perform a cardiac catheterization is undertaken with great care and consideration.

Today in most modern medical centers where cardiac surgery is performed, particularly in the case of children, the decisions for or against surgery are made with equal care by a conference of doctors, each well acquainted with the individual patient's case and each widely experienced in the treatment and outcome of patients with congenital heart lesions. Medical opinion is, in general, conservative when it comes to the risks of heart surgery. But the time may come when heart surgery is simply a matter of routine, and when the proper and optimum course of treatment for any given defect will be as clear-cut and well established as the optimum medical treatment for any number of other disorders. Until then, medicine will bend all of its resources and use its best minds, however divergent their opinions, in seeking to find the most successful approach to each individual case.

As to the prevention of congenital heart defects, the main thing to bear in mind is the danger of German measles in an expectant mother during the first three or four months of her pregnancy. Girls who have not contracted German measles well before they reach childbearing age should have a full course of German measles vaccine in their early teens to establish immunity to the infection. In addition, certain drugs or medications have been known to bring about congenital deformities of various types, and it is entirely possible that some may affect the embryonic development of the heart and great vessels too. Thus doctors generally urge their pregnant patients to avoid any and all medications that are not positively known to be free from any possible damaging effects, or may withdraw medicines they have been using to treat a patient as soon as they learn the patient has become pregnant, merely as an extra safety measure. With this kind of precautionary care there is reason to hope that the occurrence of congenital heart defects in the future will become increasingly rare and that the surgical techniques for dealing with such defects when they occur will render this kind of affliction less and less a hazard to health and longevity.

Inflammatory Diseases of the Heart and Blood Vessels

Like other organ systems, the cardiovascular system is vulnerable to a great number of different diseases and disorders. They stem from a variety of causes and affect the heart and blood vessels in a variety of different ways, but among them there is a group of diseases that share a certain characteristic in common, the special physiological condition known as *inflammation*. The cardiovascular system is probably less affected by inflammatory diseases than any other organ system, but the few such diseases that do strike the heart or blood vessels can be devastating, and the phenomenon of inflammation is at the root of the trouble.

The Phenomenon of Inflammation

Inflammation is so often the result of bacterial infection that we seldom think of it as a physiological phenomenon in itself, aside from the agent that causes it. The red, swollen sore throat of an upper respiratory infection is one manifestation of inflammation; so is the swelling, pain and sense of hotness in the vicinity of a boil, or the pain and swelling around an infected hangnail. But the redness and discomfort of an acute sunburn is also a result of inflammation, although no bacterial infection is involved, and the soreness and stiffness of an acute muscle strain is partly a result of inflammation.

What is this phenomenon, and what causes it? Perhaps the most obvious cause is *mechanical irritation*. Even if the skin, for example, is merely scratched without being broken, the irritation may cause slight pain and itching in the vicinity. The scratched area may also begin to swell as it fills slightly with tissue fluid, and the capillary blood vessels in the area dilate and engorge, further adding to the swelling and causing the skin to redden. Precisely the same sort of reaction, including swelling, redness, pain and itching, can be produced by *chemical irritation,* as when a drop of some caustic substance touches the skin. In both these cases, no bacterial agent is present, but, of course, the same phenomena occur when bacteria and/or their irritating toxins gain entry to the body. Inflammation can also be caused by an *allergic reaction* to some invading foreign material to which body tissues have previously become sensitive. And finally, in some cases, inflammation can occur spontaneously without any clear-cut indication of the cause.

Whatever the cause, and wherever it occurs in the body, inflammation displays similar characteristics and has certain very typical effects. First, blood vessels and capillaries to the affected area tend to dilate and become engorged with blood, one of the body's ways of increasing circulation to the area so that any irritating material present can be carried away by the blood stream. This engorgement of the blood vessels causes redness and is accompanied by a seeping of fluid from the capillaries into the tissue to form localized swelling or edema fluid in the area. At the same time, white cells are drawn to the area, an army of protective cells capable of ingesting or engulfing invading bacteria, if they are present, and destroying them before they cause further damage. If bacteria are present, the multitudes of white cells killed in the process of destroying the bacteria gather into a sticky semifluid mass known as *pus*. If the affected area is near the surface of the skin and if the seepage of fluid into the tissues in this area is extreme, pockets of fluid may form between the layers of the skin, causing the familiar *water blister* that occurs with a severe sunburn, for example, or with chemical or mechanical irritation of the skin.

At the same time, the increased pressure of fluid in the tissues tends to press the pain nerve endings in the area, causing first itching and then pain that may vary all the way from minor irritation to severe distress. If the inflammation is severe and prolonged, circulation to groups of cells in the area may be so impaired that they die as a result of oxygen starvation. This is a condition commonly known as *necrosis* of tissue, and it brings about a swift response: the body first attempts to dissolve and absorb the dead cells, and then attempts to repair the damaged tissue. Unfortunately, except in some specialized organs such as the liver, tissues cannot regenerate cells of their own kind, and a special type of cell known as a *fibroblast* grows into the damaged area. These fibroblasts form a thick fibrous network of cells in the region of injury and then gradually begin shrinking into a tough but disorganized protective web of fibrous tissue known as a *scar*.

Scarring is crude repair work, and often the scar tends to twist and distort the surrounding healthy tissue out of its normal shape. In areas of the skin this can cause some disfigurement, but normally there is enough elasticity in surface tissue that scarring does not seriously impair its function. In other parts of the body, particularly the internal organs, exact normal construction of tissue is essential for that tissue to fulfill its job and scarring can lead to disfunction. In the fibrous valves of the heart, for example, inflammation and subsequent scarring can twist and distort the shape of the valves so severely, over a period of months or years, that they can no longer open or close properly; the heart then can no longer circulate the blood efficiently, a condi-

tion that can ultimately lead to heart failure and death if the damage cannot somehow be repaired. Indeed, it is this scarring and distortion of the structure of parts of the heart or the blood vessels which make the relatively few inflammatory diseases of the cardiovascular system as gravely serious as they are.

Any inflammation which involves a significant amount of tissue in the body will also be accompanied by a generalized rise in body temperature which we know as *fever*. The exact reason that fever accompanies inflammation is not clearly understood. We do know that fever is associated with an increased heartbeat and an increase of all the body's metabolic processes including respiration and the amount of oxygen used in the tissues. Whether fever is simply an outward manifestation of this speed-up, or whether the speed-up actually generates higher body temperature, the presence of an inflammatory process somewhere in the body can always be suspected when an unexplained fever appears, and fever is a regular symptom of most of the inflammatory diseases that involve the heart and great blood vessels.

These inflammatory diseases may be *specific* —that is, related to actual bacterial infection of particular parts of the cardiovascular system—or *nonspecific,* inflammatory processes that can affect various parts of this organ system without any apparent cause. In either case such inflammatory disorders are described by the use of the suffix "itis" (meaning "inflammation of") tacked onto the end of the name of the afflicted part. Thus any inflammation involving the heart is spoken of as "carditis," while an inflammation of the great arteries is called "arteritis" and inflammation of the veins "phlebitis." As far as the heart is concerned, the inflammation can be present in three general areas: it may affect the *pericardium,* the fibrous sac surrounding the heart (*pericarditis*); the *myocardium,* the thick muscular wall of the heart itself (*myocarditis*); or the *endocardium,* the smooth satiny inner lining of the heart chambers or the arteries (*endocarditis* and *endarteritis,* respectively). When the fibrous heart valves themselves are involved in inflammation, the condition is often spoken of as *valvulitis.* Each of these cardiovascular structures can be affected by specific bacterial disease or by nonspecific inflammatory conditions, especially the serious condition known as rheumatic fever.

Bacterial Inflammations of the Heart

Bacterial Endocarditis. Bacterial infection of the various parts of the cardiovascular system is relatively uncommon, partly because the blood flows so swiftly through the system that bacteria have little opportunity to lodge and grow. Considering this, it is surprising that one of the most tenacious of all bacterial infections, and one of the most dangerous, is an infection of the inner lining of the heart, the endocardium. Usually caused by one of the bacteria of the streptococcus family, it can progress for weeks or months without being diagnosed and, until the era of antibiotics, was one of the few bacterial infections which was almost invariably fatal. In its uncommon acute form this infection is known as *acute bacterial endocarditis,* or ABE, a condition which even today may be fatal within a few days if untreated. In its much more common "slow" or subacute form it is called *subacute bacterial endocarditis,* usually abbreviated as SBE.

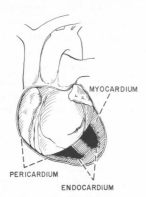

MYOCARDIUM

PERICARDIUM

ENDOCARDIUM

Figure 42–1.
The three tissue layers of the heart.

This infection is one of the hardest of all infectious diseases to diagnose simply because the infected organ is inaccessible and generally asymptomatic, and because the subacute infection usually runs a sluggish and indolent course without any dramatic initial symptoms. Often the only symptom, at first, is the appearance of a remittent or recurrent fever which appears and disappears for days or weeks, sometimes vanishing almost completely and sometimes spiking up to 103° or more. Although elderly people sometimes contract the infection, it usually attacks young adults and is one of the more serious illnesses that a doctor must consider when he is confronted with a fever of unknown origin. Very often the infection is acquired as a result of some minor surgical procedure that has inadvertently released a wave of bacteria into the blood stream; a tooth extraction, for example, in the recent past is a common factor in the victim's history, or a cystoscopic examination of the bladder. Increasingly in recent years, the disease has been caused by inadvertent release of bacteria into the blood stream following some kind of heart surgery; surgery that has broken the integrity of the inner lining of one of the heart chambers can provide a roughened healing area for the bacteria to lodge and grow. Most people who contract SBE or ABE have also previously had some structural defect or disease of the heart valves, so again there is roughened scarred tissue there.

The most common cause of ABE or SBE is the hemolytic or blood-destroying bacterial organism known as *Streptococcus viridans.* Once it becomes lodged on the inner lining of the heart, it begins to multiply and form rough, ulcerated spots for more bacteria to lodge in, and then to create "vegetations"—small nodules composed of fibrin and destroyed red cells, white cells and bacteria loosely attached to the heart's inner surface. The resulting inflammation is great enough to cause a fever, and as time goes on, the individual also begins to suffer the symptoms of anemia as red cells are destroyed; in addition, as a response to the feverish illness, his appetite falls off, and he finds himself becoming more and more tired and unable to cope with his everyday activities.

Presently bacterial emboli—tiny chunks of bacterial and fibrin material from the "vegetations"—break off and float into the blood stream. Too tiny to obstruct a larger blood vessel, those bacterial or "seed" emboli move with the blood until they reach a capillary bed through which they cannot pass—in the spleen, in the liver, in the kidneys, under the fingernails, in the retina of the eye or elsewhere in the body—where they lodge and the bacteria proceed to grow. By blocking blood flow through the capillaries, these emboli cause tiny *infarcts,* localized areas starved for blood and oxygen, and the tissue fed by the capillary dies and becomes necrotic. There are also localized hemorrhages in these infarcted areas, appearing like splinters (so-called splinter hemorrhages) under the fingernails, or like tiny hemorrhagic spots in the mucous membrane inside the cheeks. The doctor can often detect similar petechial hemorrhages in the inner lining of the eye upon examination with an ophthalmoscope. In other patients, bacterial emboli lodging in the spleen and causing infarcts may result in severe episodes of pain in the left upper quadrant of the abdomen; in still other cases, kidney function may, over a period of time, be increasingly damaged by multiple infarcts from these emboli, and frank blood commonly appears in the urine. As the vegetations continue to grow on the heart valves, there may be severe damage to the valves' structure, including twisting and scarring, perforation or even separation of one end of a valve, detectable by the appearance of heart murmurs that seem to change in the way they sound from time to time. More rarely, valve damage may result in the sudden onset of acute congestive heart failure.

Early in the disease diagnosis can be very difficult, and it is usually unwise to begin antibiotic treatment simply because it is suspected that some form of infection is present. The pattern of the fever, a history, perhaps, of previous valvular disease, the appearance of the hemorrhagic spots in the peripheral tissues and the pattern of progressive anemia and loss of appetite are all diagnostic clues, but these symptoms can also be caused by a variety of other conditions. The one most important diagnostic test, in the face of such symptoms, is a *blood culture*—withdrawing a sample of blood from the patient under sterile conditions, preferably during an episode of high fever, and then mixing the sampled blood in culture media of various

types in an attempt to grow and identify the bacteria. This is a more difficult procedure than taking a swab of the throat to culture; it may sometimes have to be repeated three or four times in succession, or even several times at longer intervals, before a positive blood culture can be found. Such a bacteriological study, however, not only helps clinch the diagnosis, but has the additional advantage that any organism grown from the blood can then easily be tested for sensitivity to a variety of antibiotics so that the one best suited for treatment can be chosen. In most cases the drug of choice even today is usually penicillin, since most streptococci are penicillin-sensitive, but resistant strains have developed and alternative antibiotics may have to be used.

Before the age of antibiotics, a diagnosis of subacute bacterial endocarditis was virtually a death sentence: 99 percent of its victims died, some succumbing to anemia and starvation, others to such severe kidney damage from septic emboli and infarcts that they died of kidney failure and uremia, still others dying in congestive heart failure because of severe damage to the heart valves. Today treatment with antibiotics in adequate dosages and for a long enough period can save some 85 percent of the victims of SBE. Truly massive doses of penicillin are used on a daily basis and continued for three to four weeks or even more. Alternative antibiotics include streptomycin, but dosages of this drug high enough to be effective against the bacteria can also cause permanent damage to the hearing of the patient. Thus, this is one disease in which the use of penicillin may well be continued even in the face of relatively severe allergic reactions to the drug, with the allergic symptoms suppressed by antihistamines or even the steroid hormones during the time the medicine is being used. Unfortunately, even though the infection is finally eradicated, the damage it has done to the heart valves or kidneys may be permanent. Thus, even with modern treatment, bacterial endocarditis is still an extraordinarily dangerous disease, and anyone with any kind of previous or current heart condition should be extremely wary of it. Such people are particularly vulnerable to contracting the disease as a result of surgery or dental operations, and the surgeon or dentist, if he knows of a history of heart disease, will often seek to protect his patient by administering antibiotics prophylactically both before and after such procedures.

Diphtheria Myocarditis. Bacterial endocarditis, acute and subacute, is by far the most common and dangerous of the bacterial inflammations that can affect the heart, but a number of other kinds of infection can also have cardiac complications. The powerful protoplasmic poison produced by the diphtheria organism *Corynebacterium diphtheriae,* for example, is spread in the blood stream to many parts of the body. One of the most sensitive parts of the heart is its muscular wall, the myocardium, and it can be seriously damaged by the diphtheria toxin. Weakened by this bacterial poison, the muscle cells in the heart wall become inflamed and swollen and can no longer contract properly, so that congestive heart failure often appears. Furthermore, the diphtheria toxin may damage the specialized muscular fibers that conduct the nerve impulses from the upper part of the heart (the atrium) to the lower part (the ventricle), thus causing a disturbance of the normal heart rhythm. If enough toxin is spread throughout the body, the victim may go into severe shock and complete circulatory collapse. In addition to normal treatment for congestive heart failure, this problem requires antibiotic treatment to destroy the diphtheria organism where it is growing in the throat and administration of antitoxin to prevent the toxin formed by the bacteria from further damaging heart muscle.

Meningococcal Carditis. In some cases the infectious organism that causes meningitis can also attack the heart, with resulting cardiac enlargement, some changes in the electrocardiogram, and occasionally heart failure. Treatment of this complication is the same as treatment for the infection elsewhere, with sulfonamide drugs or penicillin.

Viral Myocarditis. Finally, a number of viruses, including influenza viruses, poliomyelitis viruses, and others, can also affect the myocardium to one degree or another. Usually this kind of viral inflammation of the heart is mild and without any particular symptoms of significance, but occasionally there can be enough inflammation to weaken the heart and cause heart failure.

Rheumatic Fever and Rheumatic Heart Disease

Rheumatic fever is one of the oldest and strangest of all human illnesses, so variable in its symptoms and behavior that most laymen find themselves completely baffled when it comes to understanding it. Basically, rheumatic fever is an inflammatory disease attacking connective tissue in various parts of the body—the fibrous tissue that attaches the skin to underlying structures, binds the muscles and joints in their normal anatomical configurations, and holds all of the internal organs gently but firmly in their normal positions. In particular, it affects a fibrous protein material called *collagen,* a tough but elastic and somewhat gelatinous material that is a major component of connective tissue. It is, in fact, the collagen fibrils in connective tissue that enable the body to be a resilient, elastic and movable organism rather than a solid, immovable mass.

In rheumatic fever this collagen tissue tends to swell, become inflamed and lose much of its pliability. Since collagen material is scattered throughout all organ systems, rheumatic fever can affect virtually any or all parts of the body, including the connective tissue of the skin, the joints and all of the internal organs. Medically speaking, it is classified as a major member of the family of so-called *collagen diseases* which also includes rheumatoid arthritis, scleroderma, acute glomerulonephritis (a dangerous inflammatory disease of the kidneys) and lupus erythematosus. However, of all the areas of inflammation that may be involved in acute rheumatic fever, the only area where the damage caused by the disease is not reversible when the victim recovers is the heart, particularly the pericardium and certain of the valves separating one chamber from another. Because this damage is permanent, sometimes progressive, and very often the cause of death, rheumatic fever, in spite of its many other effects, can be considered one of the more serious causes of heart disease. And it is by no means a rare one. Typically it afflicts children and young adults, and according to one estimate as many as 1½ to 2 percent of all schoolchildren in the United States have rheumatic heart disease as a result of previous or still-active rheumatic fever.

What exactly is rheumatic fever? It is not actually an infectious disease, but most authorities now agree that this inflammatory disorder is a direct result of the body's reaction to earlier infection with one specific bacterial organism, known as the Lancefield group A, beta-hemolytic *Streptococcus viridans* organism. An attack of acute rheumatic fever can almost always be traced to a recent infection by this organism— an upper respiratory infection or scarlet fever, for example—which occurred and healed anywhere from two to four weeks prior to the onset of rheumatic fever symptoms. No one is entirely certain why the body should react differently to this strep infection than to any other; the best guess is that some product or products of the strep organism infecting the body have the power to act as an allergen and sensitize various tissues, particularly connective tissues, to its presence, so that when a subsequent strep infection occurs, the body suffers an exaggerated allergic reaction that takes the form of inflammation and swelling of collagen tissue. This theory is borne out by the fact that any individual who has once had an attack of rheumatic fever is thereafter extremely vulnerable to recurrent severe attacks of the disease a few days or weeks following each subsequent episode of infection by the offending strep germ. The theory is further substantiated by the discovery that these recurrent attacks of rheumatic fever can be prevented simply by administering small prophylactic doses of penicillin or sulfa drugs daily over a period of years following the victim's first attack of rheumatic fever, so that further strep infections are effectively prevented.

In most cases rheumatic fever begins with the sudden onset of a high steady fever and the development of acute arthritis, particularly in the joints of the knees, elbows or wrists. The affected joints become hot, red, swollen and intensely painful, but this form of arthritis is also typically *migratory;* that is, after initially affecting one or more joints, it tends to quiet down but then appear in another joint, and then in yet another. It was this characteristic pattern of fever and arthritis that gave the disease its name in the days when "rheumatism" was a vague term used to describe any chronic aching or swelling in the joints or tendons. Rheumatic fever, however, should not be confused with *rheumatoid arthritis,* a quite different destructive joint disease which is also one of the family of collagen diseases. (*See* p. 312.)

Along with fever and migratory arthritis so typical of rheumatic fever, small painless nodules frequently appear in the tendons in the vicinity of the joints, and a variety of transitory skin rashes also occur. But the most serious effect of the disease is inflammation of the connective tissue in the muscular wall of the heart, which drastically weakens its ability to contract and frequently triggers acute congestive heart failure at the peak of the attack. The pericardium is also affected by this inflammation, and the fibrous tissue of the heart valves swells up and produces fibrinous "vegetations" or "warts" on the leaflets of the valves or on the muscular strands known as the *chordae tendineae* that help control the movement of the valves. These inflammatory lesions heal and scar as adjacent areas become inflamed, and there is an increasing tendency for the affected valves to work incompetently. A doctor can hear the very fast "tick-tak" rhythm of the enfeebled heart trying to keep up, or even the galloping rhythm of frank heart failure, but "murmurs" also appear, abnormal additional sounds in the heart cycle caused by improper function of the valves. After a prolonged period of very severe rheumatic carditis, even if heart failure is successfully treated, the affected valves become severely scarred, twisted and even stenosed—that is, hardened—sometimes with a deposition of calcium in the scars; and presently the valves may completely cease to work properly. For reasons that no one understands, the inflammation most commonly affects the mitral valve separating the left auricle from the left ventricle, and the aortic valve separating the left ventricle from the aorta, so that permanent *mitral stenosis* or *aortic ste-*

nosis may throw a continuing extra burden on an already sick and feeble heart long after the acute phase of the disease has subsided, thus rendering the rheumatic fever victim a cardiac cripple for the rest of his life unless the damaged valves can be repaired or replaced.

A number of medical techniques are used to confirm diagnosis, including an electrocardiogram which reveals the irregularities of the heart action and laboratory tests that show an extremely rapid erythrocyte sedimentation rate and reveal the presence of antibodies to certain known streptococcus antigens. These diagnostic abnormalities revert to normal very soon after treatment is started and cannot, therefore, be used as a means of judging whether or not the active disease is subsiding. The only way to tell if the disease process has run its course is to discontinue medication; an immediate recurrence of symptoms signals the need to resume medication.

Treatment of rheumatic fever depends largely upon the severity of the disease. Because of the acute damage to the heart—or the threat of such damage—absolute bed rest for the patient during the acute phase of the illness is a must. When the patient is a small child, this may impose a considerable burden on both the child and his parents, but it is during the late convalescent period that the child is most vulnerable to the effects of heart damage, and even a brief period of activity may be enough to cause a debilitating or perhaps fatal episode of congestive heart failute. The arthritis is treated symptomatically with rest, hot wet packs and salicylates such as aspirin, which also help control the fever. Cortisone-like hormones are now also used to combat the inflammation, suppress symptoms of rheumatic activity, and help prevent the extension of valvular and heart lesions, thus decreasing the length of time the acute phase of the disease ordinarily takes to quiet down. A century ago an attack of acute rheumatic fever could keep a child in bed for six months; today even in a severe case convalescence may take only six to eight weeks.

The heart failure that may occur in conjunction with rheumatic fever can be accompanied by enlargement of the heart and must, of course, receive special treatment. Digitalis or a similar drug is used for this purpose, and again, absolute bed rest is essential with only a very gradual resumption of normal activities.

What are the prospects for the victim of an attack of acute rheumatic fever? The behavior of the disease is so extremely variable that it is all but impossible to make a general prognosis. In some cases acute congestive heart failure so severe that it does not respond to treatment may result in death in a matter of a few days or weeks. In other cases heart involvement may appear minimal, yet the later development of symptoms related to mitral or aortic stenosis gives unquestionable evidence that the heart *was* severely affected even though there were not any symptoms. In addition, the illness can recur as a result of a new strep infection, and each recurrence compounds the possibility of permanent damage to the heart, so that the long-term outcome depends heavily upon prophylactic antibiotic treatment to prevent further strep infections.

In any case, it is rheumatic heart disease that causes death from rheumatic fever, whether it occurs in the acute phase or later. Experts estimate that of all victims of rheumatic fever who sustain permanent heart damage, particularly valvular damage, the great majority will be dead within ten years no matter what is done. Thus it is that rheumatic heart disease is still one of the three most common causes of death from cardiac failure, the others being coronary artery disease and hypertension. However, recent statistics indicate that this heart affliction takes only one-half as many lives today as it did ten years ago. The main reason for this sharp decline obviously lies in the success of prophylactic or preventive treatment. Today any child who has been treated for an attack of acute rheumatic fever will be placed on a long-term continuing prophylactic dose of a streptococcus-destroying antibiotic such as penicillin or, in the case of individuals with violent penicillin allergies, sulfonamide drugs. So important is this prophylaxis, and so dangerous to children is the recurrence of rheumatic fever, that the United States Public Health Service, working in cooperation with the American Heart Association, makes the penicillin tablets for prophylaxis available at **no** cost to patients who require the medication but are unable to pay for it.

How long must prophylaxis be continued? There is no fixed rule, but many doctors today feel that the chance of recurrence of acute rheumatic fever after the age of twenty or so is small enough that prophylactic medication is often terminated in the patient's late teens. We do know that even the initial attack of acute rheumatic fever can be prevented if a strep infection is vigorously treated at the time it occurs, another reason why doctors urge patients, whenever they have upper respiratory infections, to have nose and throat cultures taken in order to determine if a strep organism is at work. In setting up a program of prophylactic or preventive care to avoid recurrence of rheumatic fever, however, the doctor must depend heavily on the patient's common sense, understanding and cooperation. The danger of recurrence is very real, but with doctor and patient working together in a practical and realistic program, that danger can be virtually eliminated.

Recent surgical advances have further contributed to the decrease in the death rate from rheumatic heart disease. In the late 1930s and early 1940s surgeons such as Charles Bailey of Temple University Medical School and others began to operate directly on the heart in attempts to reopen "frozen" or stenotic mitral and aortic valves in victims of severe rheumatic heart disease and restore them to function. In truly epoch-making surgical experiments, these men devised a technique whereby a tiny slit in the auricle of the heart could be incised, with a purse-string suture around it, so that the surgeon could insert a finger into the auricle without too much loss of blood and could then use the finger to pry open the stenosed flaps of the mitral or the aortic valve. Later a special kind of scalpel was devised to lie against the surgeon's finger as it was inserted so that a clean surgical incision of the valve leaflets could be made. Today the procedure, known as *mitral* or *aortic commisurotomy,* is performed by thousands of skilled surgeons all over the world on patients who might otherwise die of fatal heart failure because of stenosed valves resulting from rheumatic fever. More recently, it has been possible in

some cases to completely replace damaged heart valves with artificial valves with even better restoration of function, and this too may soon become a commonplace procedure.

Thus both prevention and treatment of rheumatic fever have progressed dramatically in the last few years. It is possible that some time in the future enough will be learned about the allergic nature of the disease that it can be prevented entirely, and when this time comes it will mark the end of yet another serious and crippling disorder.

Other Inflammatory Disorders of the Heart

Pericarditis. Inflammation of the tough, fibrous outer covering of the heart may occur either as an acute disorder or a chronic disease process. It may be caused by a variety of factors, among them rheumatic fever and bacterial infection from a tuberculous lesion in the lungs. A wide range of upper respiratory bacteria such as pneumococci, meningococci, streptococci or staphylococci may also be to blame as well as a number of different viruses. The former, when they directly affect the pericardium, can cause crusts to form on the inner surface of this sac and presently to fill the space between the pericardium and the heart itself. Finally, a great many cases of pericarditis seem to have no detectable cause at all; doctors speak of these cases as "idiopathic," meaning "occurring of its own accord."

When it occurs, pericarditis from any cause often mimics other heart disorders. If the outer surface of the pericardium lying in contact with the pleural lining of the lungs is inflamed, the condition can cause excruciating stabbing pain in the region of the heart, which is much like the pain of pleurisy, but which gets better or worse with breathing motion or changes in position. In other cases, the inflamed tissue may produce a thick fibrinous exudate in the space between the pericardium and the heart, which can become dry and scratchy enough that a "friction rub" can be heard through the stethoscope with each heartbeat—a strange, scratchy sound very similar to the sound of two hands rubbing together.

The most dangerous aspect of pericarditis,

however, is the accumulation of fluid, sometimes in great quantity, between the pericardial sac and the heart when the inflammation is acute. Because the pericardium is tough and inelastic, fluid forming inside this sac can literally squeeze the heart so tightly that it cannot adequately fill with blood and, in extreme cases, may cease to beat altogether. This squeezing of the heart due to pericardial fluid or effusion is called *cardiac tamponade.* It can develop very quickly, sometimes in a matter of a few hours, and must be diagnosed and treated without delay if life is to be preserved. Fortunately, it is possible to insert a hollow hypodermic needle through the pericardium so the effused fluid can be withdrawn without having the needle damage or even touch the heart itself. Further, the fluid so withdrawn can be cultured and subjected to other laboratory tests to help determine the cause of the inflammation.

If the cause is bacterial, vigorous treatment with antibiotics is required. When rheumatic fever is the cause, treatment of that condition will also help the pericarditis subside. Pericarditis with a fluid effusion that occurs as a result of severe underactivity of the thyroid gland responds almost miraculously to the administration of thyroid hormone.

In one form of chronic or long-standing pericarditis the pericardial membrane becomes thickened due to recurrent cycles of inflammation, healing, scarring, and outpouring of fibrous material, and may even become calcified as a result of the body's attempt to heal the disorder. The end result is a condition known as *chronic constrictive pericarditis,* in which the heart is slowly and progressively squeezed by the thickening membrane until it becomes less and less efficient in receiving blood and pumping it out. Once considered ultimately fatal, constrictive pericarditis today can often be cured by the simple expedient of surgically removing the pericardium completely. Since the original protective function of this fibrous sac has long since been lost in this condition, its surgical removal does no harm, the pressure on the heart is relieved, and the patient seems to manage perfectly well without a pericardium from then on.

Finally, pericarditis sometimes occurs in a localized area of the pericardium as a result of damage to the underlying heart muscle from a coronary thrombosis. In such a case, although it has very little significance in itself, the appearance of the pericarditis and the characteristic rubbing sound may help the physician judge the severity of the damage to the heart muscle.

Myocarditis. The most common cause of inflammation of the heart muscle itself is oxygen starvation which occurs when a coronary artery becomes plugged and a segment of heart muscle supplied by the artery is severely damaged and destroyed. Other causes of heart muscle inflammation are also known, including the myocardial inflammation that comes with rheumatic fever or as a result of various viral, bacterial or rickettsial diseases. Certain poisonous chemicals can also cause mild to severe myocarditis—carbon monoxide, for example, or drugs such as emetine.

When the myocardium becomes inflamed, several things may happen as a result: the weakened heart muscle tries to compensate by beating more rapidly; the heart tends to dilate or enlarge; and there is often a disturbance in the triggering mechanism that carries the impulse signal from the upper part of the heart to the ventricular muscle walls, causing abnormal rhythms to develop. Congestive heart failure is the great threat of myocarditis, and in severe cases even the most heroic measures to treat it may not succeed. Treatment of myocarditis includes both treatment of the congestive heart failure by means of digitalis, oxygen therapy, bed rest, and so on and also treatment of the underlying cause of the inflammation, if it is known. Only rarely does myocarditis appear as a disease entity in itself without some underlying cause, but occasionally a severe inflammatory disorder of the myocardium known as *Fiedler's myocarditis,* a disease of unknown origin, can cause severe and sudden intractable heart failure.

Inflammatory Diseases of Arteries and Veins

The blood vessels themselves can also be the target of various inflammatory diseases, both bacterial and nonspecific. Inflammation of the arteries, which is known as *angiitis* or *arteritis,* is comparatively uncommon except for a few rather special disorders noted below, but *phlebitis*—inflammation of the veins—is very common and may occur virtually anywhere in the body.

Syphilitic Aortitis. One of the most dangerous and destructive forms of angiitis is the inflammation of the aorta that can occur as a late complication of syphilis. In its tertiary stage this bacterial infection can attack virtually any organ system in the body including the heart and blood vessels. The syphilis organism can, for example, lodge in the wall of the heart and form a large, soft mass of inflamed and damaged cells which may so severely affect the heart's normal function that heart failure results; the organism can even form a perforation of the wall of the heart. Much more commonly, the organism takes up residence in the wall of the ascending aorta just above the heart, extending into but not beyond the aortic arch. As the thick, rubbery walls of this vessel are attacked by the bacteria, the elastic and fibrous tissue is gradually destroyed and the vessel wall, under the incessant pounding of the blood pumped out of the heart, begins to bulge out to form a tense, thin-walled *aneurysm.* If the aneurysm is undetected or untreated, sooner or later it will burst and the patient will die of a massive internal hemorrhage. Further, an aortic aneurysm may stretch the aortic valve so that it no longer functions properly, imposing an excessive burden on the ventricle, which is trying to push blood through a valve which is incompetent to hold it. The result of this can be enlargement of the heart and eventually heart failure.

The presence of an aortic aneurysm can sometimes be detected in a chest X-ray, and it is clearly defined by *angiography,* a process by which a radio-opaque dye is introduced into the arterial blood supply so that the damaged vessel is visible when X-ray pictures are taken. Antibiotic treatment of the infection will, of course, stop its progress, but the body has no way to heal the already destroyed tissue of the aorta wall. Formerly a person with an aneurysm simply lived with it as long as possible before the vessel finally burst, although he might sometimes die of some intercurrent condition before this occurred. Today it is commonplace for surgeons to support such an aneurysm with a patch made of some woven synthetic cloth such as Dacron, or even to cut out the diseased segment of the aorta altogether and replace it with an engrafted woven synthetic tube, often with extremely satisfactory results. An aortic aneurysm may also be caused by some other infectious agent or by a congenital malformation, but with antibiotics and surgical correction, where possible, the condition need not necessarily be fatal.

Thromboangiitis Obliterans (Buerger's Disease). This surprisingly widespread condition is characterized by inflammatory changes in the tiny arteries and veins in the extremities, most notably in the toes, with recurrent vascular spasm and blockage of these vessels with thrombi to such a degree that, in severe cases, the tissues fed by these peripheral vessels begin to die and become gangrenous. The condition appears most frequently in young males before the age of thirty-five, and is most commonly the result of heavy cigarette smoking, although trauma or exposure of affected extremities to wet or cold can precipitate acute attacks. Early symptoms include coldness, numbness, tingling or burning in the hands or feet, followed by progressively severe *intermittent claudication,* an aching pain in the muscles of the legs and feet during exertion which disappears as soon as the muscles are rested. Also, typically, arterial pulsation in the affected extremities is diminished or absent. There is no specific treatment for this disease, but progressive damage to the arteries in the extremities can be halted by giving up the use of tobacco in any form. The extremities must be protected from trauma and exposure; and physical therapy measures, including exercises to help reestablish arterial circulation to affected areas, are also helpful, particularly if the diagnosis is made before gangrenous changes have begun.

Other uncommon forms of arteritis include *Raynaud's disease,* a poorly understood condition in which arteries to the extremities, especially the hands, go into periods of spasm, thus episodically reducing blood flow and causing attacks of pain and cyanosis in the affected areas, and *periarteritis nodosa,* a rare form of

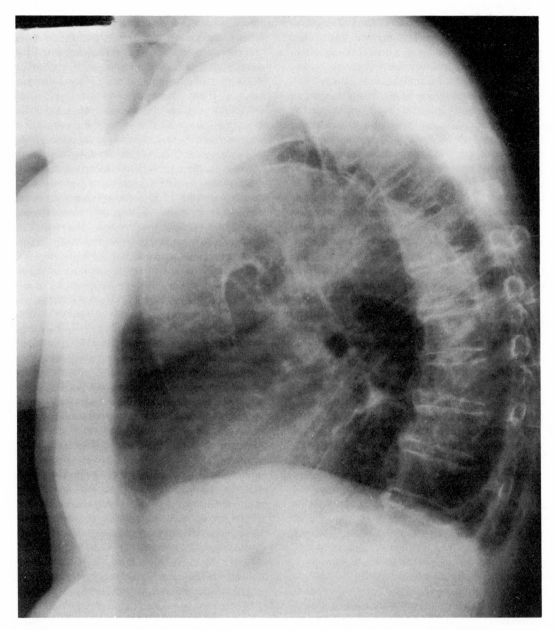

Plate 25   A large calcified aneurysm of the aorta due to syphilis. Film is taken from the side view, with vertebral column to viewer's right.

collagen disease in which the elastic connective tissue in the walls of smaller arteries all over the body tends to degenerate, sometimes causing widespread circulatory impairment. Administration of cortisone hormones is helpful, at least temporarily, but there is no known cure, and the disease often terminates fatally.

Phlebitis (Inflammation of the Veins). This commonplace and potentially dangerous inflammatory disorder most commonly affects the deep veins in the extremities, although it can occur anywhere in the body. It is often closely associated with the formation of a blood clot or thrombus in the area of the inflammation, in which case it is called *thrombophlebitis*. It can turn up without any apparent reason in virtually anyone, and the question of which comes first, the formation of a thrombus in a vein or the inflammatory process in the area, is moot. The condition is most common in people with severe varicose veins (*see* p. 568) and often develops as a result of trauma or injury to a varicose vein. It is quite common in pregnant women, whose venous return from the legs is impaired because of the pressure exerted by the baby against the great vein in the pelvis, but it can also occur quite easily in anyone who is very inactive, as in the case of a patient confined to bed rest for recovery from a severe illness. For some reason individuals suffering from cancer of the pancreas seem to be vulnerable to thrombophlebitis; thus the appearance of this disorder in any middle-aged or elderly person without any apparent cause will alert the doctor to investigate pancreatic cancer as one possible causative agent.

Whatever its cause, when thrombophlebitis appears it is usually characterized by a sudden onset of pain and swelling of the extremities in the region where the damage has occurred. The pain may be acute, and usually is exaggerated by hanging the leg down; and the inflammation of the vein may involve enough of the tissue around the area that the whole leg becomes hot, swollen, red and tender.

In most cases thrombophlebitis is best treated by bed rest, elevation of the afflicted leg, the use of hot wet packs on the inflamed area, and mild to strong analgesics to control the pain and discomfort. Starting such a regimen the moment any sign of vein inflammation appears will often help resolve the condition in a matter of a few days. Because the inflammation may be a result of bacterial infection, many doctors use penicillin in moderate doses in treating the condition; and when a doctor is concerned about the possibility of thrombus formation, he may use various medicines to sharply decrease the clotting power of the blood temporarily. In most cases the disorder will settle down promptly with proper treatment and bed rest, but there may be a prolonged convalescent period in which it is necessary to use an elastic bandage or a firm supportive stocking on the leg whenever the patient finds it necessary to be on his feet. Any sign of recurrence of the trouble indicates a return to bed rest and treatment again.

An important and very dangerous complication of this disorder occurs when a fragment of the thrombus from the inflamed area breaks off and is carried in the blood stream as an embolus. It may then pass through the heart and into the lungs, where it becomes a *pulmonary embolus*. A large pulmonary embolus that plugs a major vessel in the lung is very often fatal. Smaller pulmonary emboli may not be fatal, but can cause the sudden onset of chest pain and a degree of shock that seems far out of proportion to the size of the vessel that is blocked. Recovery from a small pulmonary embolus is possible, but in most cases a wedge of lung tissue is destroyed, leaving a thickened, tough rope of scar tissue that remains visible on chest X-rays.

Although the large veins in the leg or pelvis are the most frequent places where thrombi form, these dangerous blood clots can, in fact, occur in any number of different locations where circulation is slowed for one reason or another, or where the interior of the blood vessel has been roughened or damaged in some fashion, particularly by the changes of arteriosclerosis. Further, clots often tend to form where blood vessels divide or bifurcate. In older people with arteriosclerosis, for example, a large blood clot may occasionally form at the point where the abdominal aorta divides into two branches, the so-called iliac arteries, each supplying a leg with blood. Sometimes a clot in this "saddle" area will gradually grow larger until circulation to the legs becomes seriously impaired. Even organs such as the kidneys, supplied by arteries branching from the aorta higher up, may be affected. Only a few years ago such a saddle thrombus was beyond the scope of treatment, and at best the victim might suffer progressive gangrene in both legs due to oxygen starvation of the tissues. Today when a thrombus obliterates a major vessel, particularly an important artery, surgeons are sometimes able to relieve this dangerous situation by means of an extremely difficult operation known as a *thromboendarterectomy*. Essentially this procedure involves first temporarily blocking the circulation above and below the clot, and then carefully opening the artery and peeling out the obstructing thrombus together with the inner lining of the blood vessel to which the thrombus has adhered. The vessel is sewed up, the ligatures preventing blood from flowing through the vessel are then released, and the patient is treated with anticoagulant medicines to prevent formation of a new thrombus in the area. When the condition of the vessel prohibits removal of the clot, the obstructed area may sometimes be completely bypassed by an arterial graft made from woven synthetic fabric. Such operations can often prove to be lifesaving—just one more example of the way in which new, bold and radical surgical techniques have in the past two or three decades completely altered the outcome of many serious cardiovascular disorders.

The Problem of Varices (Varicosed Veins)

Among the most common of all cardiovascular system problems, varicosed veins are not always associated with inflammation, but are so commonly complicated by the occurrence of phlebitis or thrombophlebitis that one condition cannot easily be discussed without reference to the other. Most people quite naturally think of varicosed veins of the legs when the subject is mentioned, but *varices,* to use the medical term, can occur in many other parts of the body and in certain cases cause extremely painful and even dangerous trouble. In brief, varices are veins which, because of back pressure of blood, have been stretched, dilated and then twisted in a tortuous path as the muscle fibers in the walls of

the vessel break down, so that blood returning through these veins to the heart is slowed down and pooled in unnaturally distended portions of vein. Only the veins are vulnerable to this kind of stretching and distending, not the arteries. The reason lies in the anatomical structure of these vessels. The arteries, all the way from the aorta to the smallest arteriole, have thick, rubbery walls composed of comparatively heavy layers of muscle and elastic tissue. These walls can thus expand with the force of each heartbeat, then spring back to normal size again. But blood flow from the capillaries into the venules and veins is quiet and steady, and the veins, although also equipped with some muscle and elastic tissue in their walls, need far less resilience and therefore are much thinner.

In general the larger and deeper veins in the extremities are well supported by powerful bundles of muscle and held in place by tough connective tissue. These veins are also equipped with delicate flaplike valves at intervals along their interior length to prevent blood from "regurgitating" or backflowing as it is "pushed uphill" to reach the heart. But some veins do not have such good support to help them withstand the back pressure of blood. The veins just under the skin in the lower leg and thigh, for example, have very little support, and will often begin to fill and stretch with backed-up blood as an individual reaches his late thirties and early forties. Once this process begins, it creates a vicious circle: as the veins are stretched, the valves to prevent backflow no longer close properly to do their job effectively; more back pressure then occurs, which further stretches the veins and breaks down their interior valves. Thus, progressively over a period of months or years, varicose veins in the legs become more and more prominent and presently begin to cause symptoms.

Certain conditions greatly accelerate this process. For example, varicose veins in the legs will often develop rapidly in the course of a pregnancy, simply because the enlarged uterus containing the baby presses down on the great iliac veins carrying blood from the legs back to the vena cava, thus creating extraordinary back pressure in the leg veins. This situation can cause varices to appear in some women as early as age twenty, especially in small, thin, light-weight women who have comparatively less connective tissue and muscle in their legs to support these veins. After a first pregnancy is over, the varicosities seem to disappear in most cases, but the damage has begun, and ensuing pregnancies will cause further damage unless artificial support for the legs is provided to keep these veins from overfilling. Indeed, sometimes varices are so severe in pregnancy that veins in the legs, thighs and even the genital region may become massively enlarged. Men also may develop lower-leg varices, but seldom earlier than mid-adulthood, and even then less frequently than women, since they are not subject to the contributing factor of pregnancy.

Certain other veins are also vulnerable to varices. The veins draining the tissues around the lower end of the colon and rectum are subject to marked back pressure when individuals strain excessively to move their bowels. Thus they become varicosed, and the stretched or varicosed segments are frequently pinched, twisted and inflamed so that blood clots form within them. Varicosed rectal veins are known as *hemorrhoids,* and when blood clots form, with pain, swelling and inflammation in the area, the condition is known as *thrombosed hemorrhoids.*

Another disorder, less common but far more dangerous, is the formation of varices in the abdominal veins draining the upper part of the stomach and the lower part of the esophagus. This condition occurs when a great part of the liver, into which these veins usually drain, has been damaged and scarred by severe hepatitis, or cirrhosis of the liver due to chronic alcoholism or some other disease so that blood cannot flow through properly. When this happens the back pressure of venous blood causes the portal vein leading to the liver to grow extremely large and further backs blood up into the esophageal veins, where varicosities may occur. These so-called *esophageal varices* are particularly dangerous, for they lie just under the thin mucous membrane of the upper part of the stomach and connecting esophagus, where excessive stomach acid can easily help ulcerate the varicosed veins and ultimately erode through. When this occurs, it may cause a massive hemorrhage which tends to continue because the back pressure of blood in the portal vein keeps the broken varicosed vessels open. The location of the hemorrhage makes it difficult to control by pressure or other means; thus, bleeding esophageal varices is one of the most serious of late complications of infectious hepatitis, for example, or cirrhosis of the liver.

The symptoms and treatment of these various forms of varices depend upon the situation in each individual case, but early diagnosis and close cooperation between doctor and patient in a program of treatment are essential no matter what the individual circumstances.

Varicosed Veins in the Legs. Many individuals develop fairly severe and advanced varicose veins before they begin suffering noticeable symptoms—aching of the lower legs after prolonged periods of standing, together with some puffiness and swelling of the ankles due to fluid which has seeped out of the blood stream into the tissues because of the sluggish flow of blood through these vessels. Occasionally the first symptoms of trouble will come in the form of thrombosis or clot formation in one of the varicosed veins, often accompanied by acute phlebitis (*see* p. 567) in the vein at the site of the thrombus, with heat, swelling and soreness following soon after. This is a dangerous complication, since clots in these large distended veins may all too easily break free. Thus any localized sore, swollen, warm area in the vicinity of a varicosed vein should be called to a doctor's attention without delay for proper treatment.

Other symptoms and complications of varicosed veins in the legs may also require medical treatment. When varices are present, the simplest scratch, scrape or abrasion of the skin of the lower leg, particularly overlying the shinbone, may cause an open sore which requires weeks or even months to heal. Thus anyone who finds a scratch or abrasion of the lower leg to be healing far more slowly than normally expected should interpret this as a clue that varices may be present even if they are not yet visible. A varicosed vein close to the surface is also extremely vulnerable to hemorrhage when it is accidentally injured. And finally, in individuals with severe and advanced varices, an area of skin tissue on the leg may break down from inadequate supplies of oxygen and nutriments to form an open, weeping *varicose ulcer* which, rather than tending to heal, may become larger and larger unless treatment is undertaken. Every physician has seen neglected cases, particularly among elderly people, in which both legs from the knees down are studded with such ulcers, constantly vulnerable to infection or to further injury, and not uncommonly the forerunner of gangrene in a leg unless proper treatment is instituted.

Prevention is by far the best approach in dealing with varices in the legs, since the progress of this condition can be markedly slowed down with proper attention. The best prevention in relatively young adults is to provide external pressure on the lower leg and, if necessary, the thigh, by means of supportive hose or wrappings. At the first hint of development of varicose veins, pregnant young women should purchase one of the several kinds of supportive hose available and wear them whenever they are on their feet. The protection provided by supportive hose may vary, chiefly because "ready-made" sizes seldom correspond exactly to individual measurements. Also, they seldom reach high enough to provide support to the upper thigh; only recently have supportive panty hose become available, and these are strongly recommended. Regardless of these drawbacks, however, supportive hose do provide at least some protection, and if worn throughout a pregnancy and for two or three months after delivery, changing sizes if need be, a great deal of the damage from varicosities of pregnancy can be prevented.

Men with varicose veins are even more refractory than women to the idea of wearing supportive hose, although their use, or the use of an elastic bandage to wrap the legs from the instep of the foot up to or above the knee, will compress varicose veins and prevent them from getting progressively worse. For many people with severe varicose veins, individually made supportive stockings have also proven helpful. These custom-tailored elastic stockings, manufactured from a pattern the physician or his office nurse fits to the individual patient's leg, can be made to maintain a scientifically balanced pressure for support all up and down the leg.

For many people with mild to moderate varicose veins, these conservative measures may be entirely adequate to control the problem for years, and control can often be maintained by using supportive hose only in times of stress; that is, during a pregnancy or during working hours when a person must stand on his feet for long periods. For elderly people with severe varicose veins and varicose ulcers, healing sometimes can be encouraged by applying a rubbery gel-like material over a stockinette to the foot and lower leg like a boot, thus providing firm but gentle support that can be worn for as long as a week or ten days at a time without changing.

In many cases, however, the best possible therapy for deteriorating varicose veins in the legs is surgery to correct the basic problem. In years past, surgical treatment involved methods which were not altogether successful, but today most surgeons favor a quite extensive procedure in which virtually all of the superficial varicosed veins are not merely tied off but actually stripped away from their flimsy moorings in the soft tissue under the skin and removed completely. Quite adequate drainage of the tissues of the leg is still provided by the deep veins. Although vein stripping requires a month or two of careful postoperative supervision until the healing of the numerous small incisions and the areas from which the veins were stripped has taken place, the results of this procedure are surprisingly satisfactory; not only is the desired cosmetic effect achieved, but this unsightly and potentially dangerous condition cannot recur.

Rectal Varices or Hemorrhoids. Varicosed veins in the leg are often visible long before any symptoms occur. But with varicosed veins in the rectal area—*hemorrhoids* or "piles"—the first sign that a disorder may be present is more often the sudden onset of severe rectal pain, rectal bleeding, or both. Either or both of two groups of veins may become varicosed: the external hemorrhoidal veins in the area just outside the circular anal sphincter muscles, and the internal hemorrhoidal veins in the mucous membrane just inside the anus. Blood clots may also form in either area, obstructing the already sluggish flow of blood, together with the onset of acute pain in the rectal area and swelling and distention of the tissue around the blocked vessels. External hemorrhoids are usually visible, but even careful self-examination may not reveal the source of the distress if only the internal veins are involved. Similarly, bleeding from ulceration or abrasion of these blocked veins may arise from a site that can be observed only by a physician with the aid of examining instruments specially made for the purpose. With such an examination he can also assess the severity of the varices, and then plan the course and form of treatment best suited to the individual patient.

Early medical attention to any rectal distress is important for a variety of reasons. For one thing, disorders other than hemorrhoids can cause both rectal pain and rectal bleeding. A crack or *fissure* in the mucous membrane of the rectum, for example, can cause the sudden onset of excruciating rectal pain, especially severe at the time of a bowel movement. A rectal fissure may also bleed, or bleeding can come from some disorder farther up in the colon completely unrelated to hemorrhoids—from a polyp, a tumor or cancer, ulceration of the colon or a number of other things. Self-treatment for hemorrhoids without benefit of a careful diagnosis may therefore not only be useless, but dangerous as well.

Even when hemorrhoids are present self-treatment with the use of various widely advertised patent medicines will rarely bring about any basic correction of the underlying condition. Most of these nonprescription preparations contain mild surface anesthetics and astringent ingredients in a cream or oil base which can indeed reduce pain due to mild hemorrhoids and may well help the victim over an uncomfortable episode of pain or bleeding; but they will not, as the advertisements imply, bring about any miraculous cure. The real danger is that use of these medications without a doctor's advice may induce the victim to limp along with his condition until he gets into serious trouble—a large thrombosed hemorrhoid, for example, which produces pain that patent medicines cannot relieve.

Advertisements for these preparations invariably seem to imply that surgical treatment of hemorrhoids is some kind of dreadful procedure that should be avoided at any cost. This, of course, is nonsense. Surgery is not by any means *always* the best treatment for hemorrhoids, particularly in early cases in which conservative medical measures have not yet been attempted. In such cases, no conscientious doctor will recommend surgery until conservative methods have proved ineffective, or until the condition has progressed to a point that further attempts at conservative treatment will be a waste of time and money. Proper medical treatment is relatively simple and effective, when the symptoms are not too severe or the hemorrhoids have not become too large. It consists chiefly of temporary dietary restrictions to remove irritating roughage that can aggravate the condition, the use of simple physical measures such as hot sitz baths to soak the entire perineal and rectal region, and finally, the *proper* use of local medications containing surface anesthetics and astringent medications, either by means of rectal suppositories or, much more effectively, by proper local application of a salve or ointment form of medication. In self-treatment, the victim may apply such medications to the external hemorrhoidal area, but completely fail to bring the medicine in contact with the internal ring of hemorrhoids where the pain and bleeding originate. Effective application of these medications requires that the patient use a rubber finger cot and deliberately work the ointment into the entire anal canal, a procedure that is very easy to master with the proper instructions.

Very frequently a person who has been getting along well with conservative treatment for months or years may have a severe thrombosis of a hemorrhoidal vein, with sudden onset of pain and acute swelling. When this occurs, the doctor may elect to lance the hemorrhoid in his office, using local anesthesia, to bring about prompt relief simply by opening the thrombosed vein and removing the clot. But when this occurs, the time to consider surgical treatment is at hand.

When the condition has reached this point (as it may, eventually, even under the best of medical treatment), surgery may offer several advantages. It is not a prolonged or dangerous procedure, and above all, it can very often cure rather than merely palliate this annoying disability. It involves the simple surgical removal of the varicosed veins in the external and internal ring of the rectum, taking out the scarred and thrombosed tissue and then ligating the vessels so that new varices cannot form. Of those who are in need of surgical treatment, more than 75 percent heal quickly, with complete relief of their symptoms, and manage without a recurrence for many years. Even the remaining 25 percent have relief of symptoms for a period of time and can then often manage with conservative treatment of any recurrence. Today the surgery requires one to two days of hospitalization, and perhaps three or four days of any significant postoperative pain and discomfort. In any case, a doctor should be consulted as soon as the disorder arises and his advice carefully followed. Hemorrhoids are palliable only up to a certain point and, contrary to popular belief, are not a condition that one has to suffer with, considering the modern treatment facilities available.

Esophageal Varices. When acute or chronic disease destroys quantities of liver tissue and causes severe scarring, blood vessels through the liver are also destroyed and blood destined for the liver backs up under considerable pressure into the portal vein and from there into the veins around the base of the esophagus. These veins, never intended to stand up to much back pressure, are very thin-walled and lie just inside the mucous membrane near the surface; with any degree of back pressure over a period of time, they become varicosed and extremely vulnerable to ulceration or attack by chemicals in the gastric juice. The rupture of one or more of these veins can cause a dangerous, and possibly fatal, hemorrhage. Unfortunately, there may be no warning symptoms of this condition other than episodes of heartburn or mild indigestion—conditions that are often ignored or self-treated with antacids. Any episode of bleeding in which either bright red blood or black material resembling coffee grounds is vomited requires immediate medical attention. A history of liver disease will alert the doctor to the possibility of esophageal varices, and gastrointestinal X-rays often help clinch the diagnosis.

Hemorrhage from esophageal varices can sometimes be adequately controlled by inserting a special kind of rubber pressure bag down the esophagus into the stomach, inflating the bag with air, and then pulling it up against the upper end of the stomach to compress the bleeding vessels. This may control a hemorrhage which might otherwise be fatal, but it does nothing to relieve the underlying condition. And indeed, the sort of damage to the liver which precedes the development of esophageal varices is usually irreversible; it will get worse and worse until surgical intervention is attempted.

Surgical treatment of esophageal varices has not, so far, been strikingly successful; a number of different procedures have been developed to deal with the problem, each of which has provided a measure of relief in some cases, and occasionally for prolonged periods of time, but also has serious disadvantages. Fortunately, this disorder is relatively rare, but at least modern surgical procedures can help ameliorate the dangerous threat of the illness, whereas three decades ago it almost invariably ended in fatality.

43

When the Heart Fails

The human heart is a thick-walled, muscular organ with the specific task of pumping blood to and from virtually every organ and tissue in the body. The force necessary to perform this job is generated by a rhythmic, alternating contraction and relaxation of the heart muscle, familiar to everyone as the "heartbeat." The rate of this contraction varies from about 40 to 120 or more beats per minute according to the body's needs at different times of the day or night, but the amount of blood that the heart pumps with each contraction—known to doctors as the "cardiac output"—ordinarily will vary only slightly from one hour to the next, and this output of pumped blood must be continued without letup in order to maintain normal circulation.

Thus the heart has no opportunity to rest except for the momentary relaxation between heartbeats, and it has been estimated that it beats an average of three billion times during a normal life span. Naturally, it is subject to gradual degenerative changes due to wear and tear and aging, but everything else being equal, the heart performs its vital function admirably well. There are, however, a number of abnormal conditions that can impede this function and cause the heart to fail. The term "heart failure" is a broad one, but in general it is used to describe any condition in which the heart, because of overwork, injury or disease, fails to pump enough blood with each heartbeat to maintain the necessary cardiac output. The heart's failure may be gradual or sudden, but the end result is the same: progressive impairment of the circula-tion of blood, a succession of distressing symp-toms, and ultimately death if the failure cannot be promptly and effectively corrected.

To the layman "heart failure" suggests some-thing sudden and catastrophic, and the old say-ing that "everybody dies of heart failure eventu-ally," although not exactly medically accurate, further suggests that heart failure and death are somehow irrevocably intertwined. But this is not always true. Far more often heart failure ap-pears gradually, in varying degrees, and then slowly becomes progressively worse unless some-thing is done either to correct the underlying cause or to shore up the deteriorating function of the heart. In many cases, it is possible to completely reverse the development of heart fail-ure and add many years to the patient's life, providing that he recognizes the first symptoms as a warning to begin an orderly, continuing program of health care.

The Causes of Heart Failure

Generally speaking, heart failure can be caused by any circumstance or condition that places an excessive strain on the heart muscle. Under normal circumstances, the heart is often able to adapt itself or "compensate" for any temporary extra burden simply by beating faster, as it does during periods of strenuous exercise. But if that burden is continual, or excessive, the heart eventually becomes overtaxed beyond its capacity to compensate and begins to fail. A number of congenital abnormalities can place

573

the heart under an excessive strain from the moment it starts beating in the embryo. Similarly, although later in life, the heart may begin to fail or "decompensate" as a result of long-standing high blood pressure or hypertension; in this case, small arteries and arterioles are abnormally constricted and the heart must constantly push the blood against a greater pressure barrier than normal, eventually wearing itself out. The thrombosis or plugging of one of the coronary arteries feeding the heart muscle can severely damage a section of the heart wall with resultant heart failure. By the same token, a disorder that causes damage or structural change in any of the heart valves can also place an excessive burden on the heart and contribute to heart failure. Rheumatic fever, for example, not only can cause severe inflammation and weakening of the heart muscle itself, but can also cause thickening and scarring of the valves, followed by heart failure. Bacterial infection of the interior of the heart and the valves can do the same thing.

Indeed, heart failure can result from disorders far removed from the heart itself. A severe anemia, for example, may force the heart to work overtime pumping inadequately oxygenated blood around the body faster, ultimately exhausting itself. The disease known as *beriberi,* caused by chronic deficiency of the B vitamins, can cause such a weakening and flabbiness of the heart muscle that a dangerous degree of heart failure may occur. If the heart is already weakened from some other cause, a **chronic infection** with recurrent fever can cause it to fail by forcing the overall rate of the body's metabolism—including the heart rate—up 10 or 15 percent above normal. Excessive thyroid gland activity leading to an overall marked increase in the metabolic rate of the body can have the same effect.

Symptoms of a Failing Heart

When the heart first begins to fail, from whatever cause, it does not just stop beating. It simply begins beating ineffectively, so that there is generalized impairment of the circulation of the blood all over the body. It is not the heart alone which is affected when failure begins, but

virtually every other organ system as well, and it is because of this that the early symptoms of heart failure may appear to have nothing whatever to do with the heart.

Even a slight reduction in blood flow to various body tissues, for example, means that blood flow through the kidneys will also be slowed down. When this happens, the kidneys work less effectively to filter fluid, dissolved wastes and other materials from the blood, and especially tend to retain salt (or more precisely, sodium ions) in the blood, which in turn causes retention of more fluid in the body than normal. Similarly, reduction in the amount of blood circulating to the brain can cause a disturbance in brain function and can interfere with such vital processes as the automatic regulation of respiration simply because of oxygen starvation of the brain's respiratory centers. Even as the heart works harder and harder to maintain its excessive load, beating faster and faster but pumping less and less blood per beat, blood tends to pool and back up in various capillary beds throughout the body, and the excess retained water seeps out of the capillaries and into the tissues. The liver can become swollen and overfilled with blood, with further swelling because of water retention; and congestion of blood in the lungs, with seepage of retained water, can interfere with breathing. Instead of a light, air-filled buoyant organ, the lung literally turns into a wet, soggy sponge. It is because of this phenomenon of congestion of the lungs, the liver and other tissues with sluggishly circulating blood and retained fluid that slow, progressive failure of the heart is called *congestive heart failure.*

The symptoms connected with this condition vary widely from person to person and depend upon how profound the heart failure is at a given time, but in general they all fall into a recognizable pattern, depending upon the degree of severity.

Shortness of breath or dyspnea. Probably the earliest noticeable symptom of congestive heart failure is shortness of breath or breathlessness upon exertion, or, to use the medical term, *dyspnea* (literally, "difficult breathing"). Typically, this symptom appears insidiously, but then grows progressively more difficult to ignore; the

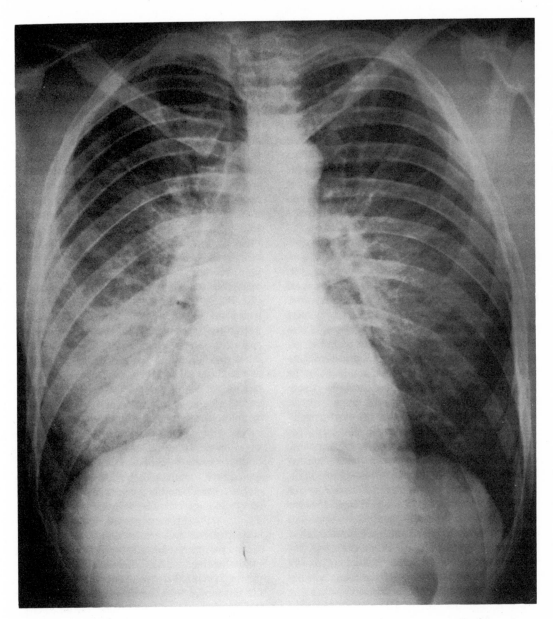

Plate 26   Congestion of the lungs and borderline enlargement of the heart as a result of congestive heart failure. Compare lung fields and heart shadow with normal chest X-ray, Plate 4a.

victim gradually becomes aware that exertion which seemed to be effortless a month or two before suddenly becomes a strain. He may find, for example, that he can no longer climb a flight of stairs without becoming unexpectedly winded by the time he gets to the top.

Increased heart rate. Another sign of trouble which frequently accompanies shortness of breath is the onset of very rapid heartbeat upon mild exertion, with the heart rate climbing sometimes as high as 140 to 160 beats per minute and then slowing back down to normal over a much longer period of time than usual. This rapid heartbeat, known as *tachycardia,* may be intermittent in early congestive heart failure, but can become the rule rather than the exception as the struggling heart tries to compensate for the poor job it is doing by pumping blood with more frequent contractions. This soon becomes a vicious circle; the heart may beat more frequently, trying to "keep up" with the body's circulatory needs, but the actual output of blood per contraction diminishes sharply the faster the heart beats, with the result that the total amount of blood passing through the heart in a given interval of time is actually less than before heart failure began.

Edema of the extremities. A third important sign of early congestive heart failure is the appearance of unusual amounts of fluid in the tissues, fluid which has seeped through the capillary blood vessel walls into the tissues, partly because blood is flowing through those capillaries more slowly than normal, and partly because the kidneys are no longer functioning properly to expel excess salt and water from the blood. This so-called edema or fluid in the tissues may first come to the victim's attention as a sudden and inexplicable gain in weight. By the time four or five pounds of excess water has seeped into the tissues, there will be noticeable puffiness of the ankles, especially late in the day or evening, but it generally disappears during sleep at night. Before long the amount of fluid that has gathered in the dependent or "hanging down" extremities can be detected by pressing the shinbone near the ankle with a finger, which leaves a temporary "pit" or depression. This "pitting edema" is evident when as little as five

or six pounds of excess water are retained, and it becomes worse as more water is held within the body. It is not at all unusual for as much as twenty pounds of water or more to be retained, with noticeable swelling from edema all over the body; and although various diuretic medicines can be used to help the kidneys expel retained salt and water, as soon as the medicine is stopped the edema will promptly return if the underlying problem is heart failure. Hormone imbalances, primary kidney disease, high blood pressure and a variety of other conditions can also cause a similar edema. Thus the appearance of edema does not necessarily indicate congestive heart failure, but it is one of a number of possible diagnostic clues.

Nocturnal breathing distress. As heart failure becomes more severe, other telltale symptoms may signal its presence. A person who normally sleeps flat on the bed with only a single pillow may awake coughing and choking, and have difficulty clearing "phlegm" from his throat. He may then discover that he can find relief either by getting up and walking around or by propping himself up on two or more pillows to sleep. This shortness of breath that seems related to the physical position of the body is called *orthopnea* and occurs because of increasing congestion of blood in the pulmonary vessels and impairment of breathing space in the lung by fluid that seeps out of the blood vessels into or around the air sacs. Even more dramatic and frightening is a symptom bearing the formidable name of *paroxysmal nocturnal dyspnea,* the sudden onset of acute shortness of breath that occurs some hours after the victim has gone to bed at night and wakes him from sleep with a racing pulse and a sense of imminent suffocation. These sudden acute episodes of nighttime dyspnea may last for only a few mintues or for as long as an hour or more, and are usually relieved when the victim sits up in bed, gets up and walks around, or sits upright near a window to relieve his apparent craving for "fresh air." He is, in fact, literally craving air of any kind, for these episodes occur when fluid exudes from the pulmonary blood vessels into the air sacs and actually fills the breathing apparatus of the lung.

Swelling and soreness of the liver. Finally, an

early acute episode of congestive heart failure will often cause a marked backing up of blood in the venous system. The heart is unable to move this blood efficiently, and there is a resultant congestion of the capillaries of the liver with blood and with fluid exuding from those capillaries into liver tissue itself. When this happens the liver swells to some degree within the fibrous capsule that surrounds it, so that the edge of the liver can be felt in the upper abdomen just below the ribs on the right as a firm tense mass. The swelling causes an aching pain in the right upper abdomen which can be quite severe and is sharply increased by any external pressure.

Ordinarily, in early heart failure, this congestion and swelling of the liver is a temporary and reversible process which goes away as soon as the heart failure is effectively treated. But in the individual who has repeated episodes of acute heart failure without effective treatment, or who suffers from long-standing chronic progressive heart failure, the congestion and swelling can actually cause permanent damage to the liver cells, literally destroying them one by one so that eventually the liver begins to shrink and atrophy, with scarring and permanent disfunction. It is this kind of progressive damage which accounts for the large number of people with chronic and severe heart failure who ultimately die from liver failure.

Treatment of Early Heart Failure

Many doctors regard heart failure, from whatever cause, as one of the relatively few very serious and threatening conditions which is "fair" to the victim, for he almost invariably has many warning signs of impending trouble, if he knows what to look for, before things have progressed to the point of severe disability that must be treated on an emergency basis. Furthermore, in most cases early congestive heart failure, or even more chronic heart failure of a mild or moderate degree, can be effectively treated, whether or not the underlying cause has been diagnosed and whether or not that cause, if diagnosed, can be corrected. That is why it is vitally important to recognize the symptoms of early heart failure and seek immediate medical

help. Treatment can often be instituted in the doctor's office without requiring hospitalization and can be carried on with the patient going about his daily schedule or, at worst, taking bed rest at home. Dealing with early heart failure most commonly involves the following steps:

Physical examination and laboratory data. Early congestive heart failure does not ordinarily appear out of the blue; usually there is some underlying cause, and when emergency measures are not required as a matter of life or death, it is imperative that a thorough physical examination and certain laboratory studies be undertaken before active treatment is begun. There is a two-fold purpose behind this approach. First, treatment and even reversal of the heart failure will be of only temporary advantage if some grave or chronic underlying cause of the condition is overlooked and left untreated. To treat heart failure that results from long-standing or severe high blood pressure without detecting and effectively treating that condition is like trying to shore up a leaky dike with a few sandbags. Some temporary relief may be obtained, but the continuing effect of hypertension will soon overwhelm any protective measures. Similarly, heart failure that has resulted from damage to one or another of the heart valves will not respond well to treatment unless the underlying cause is also treated. If a portion of the heart muscle has been weakened by coronary thrombosis, absolute bed rest and a very careful treatment program for the coronary may be necessary at the same time that heart failure is being treated. In short, every possible underlying cause of heart failure must be checked off the list, and the earlier the better.

Another reason for such a diagnostic workup at this point, even if the underlying cause cannot be found, is simply to establish a *baseline evaluation* of the patient's overall physical condition, particularly the condition of his heart and lungs. If treatment is given before diagnostic studies are made, and it is effective in reversing the many profound physiological changes that accompany heart failure, it may mask how severe the heart failure really was, and may even obscure clues to the underlying causes. For example, if the heart failure resulted basically from some inflammatory process that affected the mechanism that triggers the heartbeat, causing the heartbeat to become irregular or *arrhythmic,* effective treatment may easily quiet the arrhythmia and "convert" the heartbeat to a normal rate. But it might then be extremely difficult to assess what kind of arrhythmia was present to begin with and thus prepare in advance for any possible recurrence.

Where heart failure is concerned, the physical examination should be careful and thorough to seek out possible causes, assess symptoms and determine the nature and extent of the disorder. Aside from such routine laboratory studies as blood counts and urine analyses, the examination should include blood chemistry examinations to assess the function of the kidneys, the liver and the heart muscle itself. Chest X-rays help evaluate the degree of congestion in the lungs and reveal any significant degree of heart enlargement that may be present. An electrocardiogram may tell the doctor if an unrecognized coronary attack is contributing to the heart failure, and will also identify heart enlargement and reveal disturbances in the rhythm of the heartbeat. If an underlying cause of the heart failure is discovered, treatment can then be instituted at the same time the heart failure is treated, with a far better chance of being truly effective. And even if no underlying cause is found, at least the physician and the patient can feel confident that nothing has been overlooked and that treatment of the heart failure will not in itself obscure some contributing condition.

Digitalization. For well over 200 years digitalis, a potent medicament found in the leaves of the common foxglove plant, has been known as one of the most beneficial of all of the natural plant herbs and drugs because of its value in treating heart failure. Records of the use of foxglove leaf date back to medieval times, and foxglove was recommended in various printed pharmacopoeias in Germany and England as early as the 1500s and 1600s. The first scientific study of this medicine, however, and the first detailed account of its almost magical effect in treating "dropsy" (swelling of the ankles and even more massive edema of various organs as a result of heart failure) was made by the English

physician William Withering in 1785 in a clinical work entitled *Account of the Foxglove.* Withering realized that some substance in the foxglove leaf, which he was unable to isolate or identify, had the effect of slowing down rapid heart rate and of causing *diuresis,* a marked increase in urination accompanied by reduction in the amount of edema fluid present in the ankles or in the lungs. Later this natural herb was found to contain a powerful sugar-like substance or glycoside named *digitoxin,* so called because it could have severely toxic or poisonous effects unless the dosage was carefully regulated.

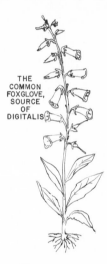

THE COMMON FOXGLOVE, SOURCE OF DIGITALIS

Figure 43–1.

For many years digitalis was prepared for use either by extracting the active principal from foxglove leaves with alcohol to form a tincture of digitalis, or simply by drying and grinding up the leaves and administering them in tablet form. Even today many doctors continue to prescribe standardized preparations of digitalis leaf in gray-green tablet form on the theory that overdosage can be more readily detected by various side effects than if the purified glycoside itself is used. Purified preparations of digitoxin are more often used, however, and experience with this medicine is so widespread that overdosage is seldom a threat. Furthermore, electrocardiograms, introduced around the turn of the century, can show the effect of digitoxin on the heart so that it is possible to monitor dosage by this means.

Today we know that the digitalis glycoside is a potent protoplasmic poison which acts particularly upon the heart muscle cells. How then can it be beneficial to a failing heart? Curiously enough, the "toxic" effect of small amounts of digitalis on the heart is to slow down or prolong each contraction slightly while at the same time improving the strength and quality of the contraction. Thus instead of contracting at 120 or 130 beats per minute and pumping only perhaps one-third as much blood per contraction as normal, the heart under the effect of digitalis slows down to 70 or 80 contractions per minute, with each contraction longer and stronger than before, so that with each heartbeat the proper amount of blood or possibly a little more is pumped. Furthermore, the "rest period" between contractions is also slightly prolonged by digitalis, so that instead of beating itself frantically into deeper and deeper trouble, the heart's overall function is improved and its efficiency markedly increased.

The effect of digitalis is particularly striking when the failing heart is beating very fast and feebly with an irregular type of rhythm known by doctors as *auricular fibrillation*. Patients with this condition may be extremely short of breath even at complete rest, with pulse rates as high as 240 beats per minute before digitalis is administered. After a few hours without any apparent effect, the digitalis may then suddenly "convert" this fast hammering arrhythmic pulse quite suddenly to a normal rhythm of 80 or so beats per minute, with almost immediate relief of the dyspnea and a marked improvement in the patient's sense of well-being and physical comfort.

Other Drugs Affecting Heart Action. Digitalis is an invaluable drug, the mainstay of treatment of any form of heart failure, often restoring a failing heart to normal function by its own action alone. Once the pumping action of the heart has been stabilized and made more efficient, circulation to the other organs is immediately improved, congestion of the liver begins to clear up, the pileup of blood in the lungs leading to pulmonary congestion and edema fluid is relieved, and even the kidneys begin to function more normally again to evacuate retained salt and water. But in special cases other drugs also have a highly beneficial effect in treating heart failure, used mostly in conjunction with digitalis. When the heart failure involves an arrhythmia which is not corrected by digitalis, another more potent cardiac drug known as *quinidine* may be used to help restore and maintain normal cardiac rhythm. This drug, however, is more toxic than digitalis, and more variable in its behavior. Thus it is usually prescribed today only with great caution under the direction of a doctor with long experience in its use.

When pain is associated with heart failure, a variety of medicines can be used to relieve the distress. There is a very special kind of pain that often accompanies impairment of blood circulation to the heart muscle, a severe chest pain known as *angina pectoris* which usually occurs only when the victim is exercising and his heart is unable to supply blood fast enough even to meet the oxygen demands of the heart muscle itself. This type of pain is also often associated with arteriosclerotic heart disease (*see* p. 592), but when a person develops angina in the midst of heart failure because of overwork of the heart, a variety of drugs may help dilate the coronary blood vessels, thus permitting more adequate blood flow to the heart and reducing the anginal pain. Of these, *nitroglycerine* is perhaps the quickest-acting and most widely used. It is exactly the same chemical that can be a powerful explosive, but when used as a medicine it is administered in extremely tiny amounts—$\frac{1}{150}$ of a grain, for example—in a small white sugary tablet which is usually held under the tongue to dissolve and be absorbed directly into the blood stream. In this amount and this form, of course, there is no threat of explosion.

Other discomforts associated with congestive heart failure include abdominal ache due to a tense swollen liver, and a sense of congested fullness in the chest which, together with shortness of breath and a fast, irregular heartbeat, is often extremely alarming to the victim, who sometimes describes it as a "sense of doom" or a feeling of "imminent death." The apprehension this sensation causes actually makes the heart failure worse, since any frightening experience makes the heart beat faster. To counteract this discomfort and sense of alarm, a powerful narcotic such as morphine is commonly given by injection. In some cases doctors prefer to use one of the milder narcotics such as Demerol for this purpose, but many cardiologists with a great deal of experience in handling the problem feel that morphine is almost specific to this job and will accept no substitute.

Sometimes a patient may have an unusual accumulation of tissue fluid even after treatment with digitalis, and in this case certain so-called *diuretic* drugs are prescribed to force the kidneys to expel excess salt and water. These drugs may either be taken by mouth or be administered by injection according to individual need. Certain older diuretics contained mercury compounds which temporarily interfered with the ability of cells in the kidney tubules to reabsorb and retain water, but these comparatively toxic preparations have been largely replaced today by extremely potent drugs capable of draining away as much as five or six pounds of water in the course of 24 hours with far less risk of damage to the kidneys.

Other Treatment Measures. In very mild early cases, heart failure may be treated with the appropriate medications while the patient is up and about carrying on his normal activities. In other cases, however, supportive measures may also be required to help speed recovery and prevent recurrence. Adequate *rest* is one such measure, not necessarily total bed rest, but at least periods of daytime relaxation and full uninterrupted nights of sleep. The patient should also avoid any excess physical demands on his heart. Since a great many people suffering from heart failure are also moderately to markedly obese, and since obesity can be a very strong contributing factor, a weight-reduction diet rich in protein and low in carbohydrates is usually prescribed. Few people recognize the enormous physical burden they impose upon themselves by carrying around 15 or 20 extra pounds of fat; not only must the heart do extra work to supply the muscles that carry this load, but the fat itself, although essentially useless tissue, contains many miles of capillaries which still must be supplied with blood. Losing extra poundage may well be the single most effective measure that can be taken to relieve a failing heart of a deadly excess load.

Finally, in more severe cases of failure, or in cases in which swelling of the ankles or pulmonary edema is a prominent symptom, restriction of dietary salt may be beneficial, since it will reduce the amount of salt in the blood stream and thus the amount of water the kidneys can retain. Few heart failure patients are required to eliminate salt from their diets completely, but a great many Americans habitually oversalt their food and can simply reduce their salt intake with very little effort.

Many victims of early heart failure are amazed at the sudden increase in energy, tolerance of exercise and general feeling of well-being that an appropriate program of treatment can achieve. But it should be reemphasized that such remarkable results are possible only when the disorder is diagnosed in its early stages, and when doctor and patient cooperate closely in the treatment program.

The Congestive Heart Failure Crisis

All too many patients with heart failure do not seek medical help soon enough; they may be unaware of the telltale symptoms, or may have learned to "live with" their condition until, suddenly, something precipitates a heart failure crisis, an acute episode of heart failure in which the victim becomes abruptly and markedly sick and emergency measures must be taken to save his life, regardless of the underlying cause.

In a congestive heart failure crisis, the symptoms of early heart failure are greatly magnified and intensified; the victim suddenly begins to gasp for breath, his heart races, his blood pressure falls dangerously low, and his lungs become so full of edema fluid that it is virtually impossible to breathe. Panic aggravates the crisis, and unless the victim receives prompt emergency treatment, he may well die of suffocation or circulatory collapse before his heart function can be brought under control. In general, treatment consists of a crash program of the same measures that can be used to ease the symptoms of a less serious attack. Morphine or some other narcotic drug may be used to quiet the victim's apprehension and slow down his frantic breathing efforts. He may be placed in an oxygen tent, and the edema fluid aspirated from his trachea by means of a long rubber tube attached to a suction machine. Digitalis-like drugs can be administered intravenously for rapid action to quiet the frantic heartbeat and stimulate diuresis, while medicines such as aminophylline are used to dilate the victim's bronchioles and allow more oxygen to reach his lungs. In some cases tourniquets may be placed on three of the four extremities and rotated every ten minutes to trap quantities of blood in the limbs, thus temporarily removing it from circulation and reducing the load on the heart. If the congestion of blood is severe and persistent due to the heart's inability to circulate it properly, a procedure known as a *phlebotomy* may be performed, in which a vein is opened and a pint or more of blood removed from the circulation, again to relieve the overloaded heart—one of the rare instances in which the ancient practice of "bloodletting" is really useful.

These and other measures, taken almost simultaneously, very soon have a beneficial effect in most cases. The crisis passes and the patient begins a gradual but progressive recovery with the return of normal heart function and circulation, along with a marked improvement in respiration and kidney and liver function. Recovery may take as little as a day or so, or as long as several weeks, but meanwhile studies and tests can be undertaken to determine the underlying cause of the heart failure, and a longer-term program of treatment can be initiated to prevent or minimize any recurrence.

In most cases congestive heart failure is a *reversible syndrome*—a condition that can be ameliorated and reversed, even when it occurs in severe and sudden episodes, if the underlying cause can be diagnosed and treated soon enough. The fact remains, however, that multitudes of Americans die every year of diseases of the heart or the circulatory system that may ultimately result in heart failure, particularly inflammatory heart diseases, arteriosclerosis and hypertension. In recent years massive research efforts have been directed toward discovering the causes of these cardiovascular diseases and their possible cures. One day the symptoms of heart failure may occur far less frequently than they do today, but until then they will remain urgent indications of some underlying disorder that demands immediate medical investigation and treatment.

Hypertension—The Silent Destroyer

Almost everyone has heard of the dangers of "high blood pressure," but very few really know much about this shadowy affliction, and what little they do "know" is probably only half true. Yet every day hundreds of people die from abnormal blood pressure conditions, and one major end result of disorders of high blood pressure—hypertensive heart disease—claims more than 100,000 lives every year in the United States alone.

The maintenance of normal blood pressure within the arteries and veins is one of the human body's most vital physiological functions. In cases of circulatory collapse or massive hemorrhage, one of the earliest danger signs is a sudden fall in blood pressure, indicating that insufficient blood is being forced through the capillary beds throughout the body to provide adequate oxygen to the tissues. Yet physicians have known for centuries that blood pressure that is *too high* over a prolonged period is one of the major silent destroyers of human life, a dangerous disorder which day by day and year by year pounds away at the very structure of the heart and the circulatory system.

In most people blood pressure is maintained at a normal range, and will remain so all their lives; but in some, as a result of a variety of factors, blood pressure begins to creep above normal in young adulthood, a condition that is heralded by few or no symptoms. This was once regarded by physicians as a comparatively harmless change in the body without particularly grave significance, hence the term "benign essential hypertension" that was used to describe it.

Today we know that that "benign" blood pressure elevation is by no means harmless, but is actually the first stage in a prolonged disease process which, if not controlled early, can cause permanent changes in the anatomical structure of the heart and blood vessels, and can grow progressively worse until it emerges as "malignant" hypertension which continues totally out of control until the victim dies.

Medical research has taught us a great deal about hypertension in recent decades. We have learned, for example, that benign essential hypertension and malignant hypertension, once considered two separate disorders, are really two different stages in the same dangerous disease. We have come to understand many factors that contribute to hypertension, and have found many weapons, both medical and surgical, to combat and control it. Today those with normal blood pressure can take certain positive steps to see that it remains normal; and if it is already abnormally high, there are steps that can be taken to help minimize the damage it can do. Perhaps more than in any other long-term disease, close cooperation between physician and patient is necessary to combat early hypertension, but the reward for such cooperation can be lifelong control of a dangerous disease and the addition of decades to the life expectancy.

Normal and Abnormal Blood Pressure

Measuring blood pressure is a simple and familiar procedure in any doctor's office, and next to measurements of temperature, pulse and respiration rate is the most common item of information recorded in a patient's medical records. Blood pressure measurements are taken by wrapping a thin rubber bladder enclosed in a cloth cuff around the patient's upper arm, and then squeezing air into the cuff by means of a rubber bulb until it begins to feel uncomfortably tight. This instrument, known as a *sphygmomanometer,* is designed to compress the main artery of the arm gently and firmly until blood flow through it is momentarily blocked. Then, by listening with a stethoscope as air is released from the cuff a little at a time, the doctor can detect the exact point at which the pressure exerted by the heart is just sufficient to force blood past the gentle obstruction the cuff has created. This pressure, which is measured by the number of millimeters of mercury it can support in a long glass tube, or on a pressure dial, represents the *systolic blood pressure*—the maximum force the blood inside the artery exerts against the blood vessel wall with each heartbeat. By listening further as the cuff pressure is released, the doctor can also measure the point at which the blood exerts the *least* amount of pressure against the vessel wall, which occurs when the heart is relaxing before another contraction. This measurement is the *diastolic blood pressure.* The two pressure readings are then recorded together with the higher systolic pressure written over the lower diastolic as 110/80 or 155/105. Many people erroneously assume that the systolic pressure is the more significant measurement, but actually the diastolic pressure is a far more sensitive indicator of the presence of high blood pressure. During periods of stress, excitement, fright, or physical exercise, the systolic pressure may rise high above its normal level without having any significance; but if the diastolic pressure is even slightly above the normal range, particularly at rest, it is a serious and worrisome sign that hypertension is present.

Why should there be any pressure of blood within the circulatory system in the first place? The answer was discovered by the English physiologist Sir William Harvey in the mid-1600s when he proved that the human heart and blood vessels form an endless, closed system of pipes through which blood is circulated again and

again, driven by the rhythmic pumping action of the heart. The pressure arises from the force of the pumping and from the push of the blood against the vessel walls with each heartbeat. As one might expect, the closer to the heart the pressure in the arteries is measured, the higher it will be: blood surges out of the heart into the aorta in the chest under very high pressure with each contraction, while the same blood upon reaching the tiny capillary blood vessels in the toes will move under very low pressure.

Healthy blood vessels are tough, but they are not rigid; they are made of flexible, elastic tissue that can yield a bit with each heartbeat. What is more, layers of muscle lining the blood vessel walls can contract and narrow the channels, or relax and dilate the channels through which the blood travels. The heart may also beat faster or more slowly according to special demands of the moment. Thus, from day to day, or even from moment to moment, the normal pressure of blood inside the vessels may change. If someone is suddenly startled, for instance, his heartbeat will speed up, his blood vessels will contract, and his blood pressure will increase sharply for the moment. On the other hand, when he is asleep his heartbeat will drop to its lowest ebb for the day, and his blood pressure measured at that time will be lower than even the "normal" range measured at rest while he is awake.

This capacity of the heart to beat faster or more slowly according to demand, and of the arteries and arterioles to dilate or contract to meet changing needs of the body, is part of a delicate regulating mechanism. It permits additional circulation of blood in areas when extra oxygen is required, yet reduces the flow to a minimum during periods of rest. A number of factors, however, can cause the smaller arterioles all over the body to contract and remain contracted far too much of the time—factors as widely different as malfunction of the kidneys or excessive nervous tension. Such conditions, acting by themselves or in combination with each other, can lead to a chronic resistance to the normal flow of blood in the arterioles, and thus may result in the abnormal condition known as high blood pressure or *hypertension.* If, on the other hand, the arterioles remain abnormally dilated and flaccid, an opposite condition known as low blood pressure or *hypotension* may occur.

What is the normal range of blood pressure? It differs with age, but not by any rigid formula. In healthy children blood pressure may easily be as low as 85/55 with average normals of about 90/60. For adults normal blood pressure may range all the way from 100/80 to 135/90. Most doctors agree that when a person's systolic pressure exceeds a level of 135, or the diastolic pressure reaches a level of 95, the blood pressure must be regarded as suspiciously high, and a pressure of 140/100 would be abnormally high for anyone.

Of course the blood pressure varies in the course of an average day's activities. Emotions such as fear or anger may temporarily elevate it. Various hormones that are normally produced by the body can affect it, and many medicines are capable of artificially increasing or decreasing blood pressure. Indeed, blood pressure is a dynamic reflection of everyday patterns of living, rising or falling to meet the body's needs, and a single abnormal measurement does not necessarily mean anything. It is only when blood pressure remains *consistently* too high or too low on repeated measurements that a doctor will consider it "abnormal."

False Ideas About Blood Pressure

Because blood pressure is related to general health in ways which are sometimes difficult to understand, a number of very strange ideas and old wives' tales have grown up about it. It is often said that blood pressure should normally measure "100 plus your age," and that "low blood pressure" is a dangerous condition. Neither of these notions is true. People *do* tend to develop high blood pressure as they approach middle age, especially harried businessmen and nerve-racked housewives, but there is no rule-of-thumb increase in normal blood pressure according to age. A blood pressure of 140/100 is just as abnormal for a man of sixty-five as it is for a girl of eighteen.

Nor is *low* blood pressure particularly dangerous, in itself. In a few unusual circumstances—in a case of shock following an injury, for ex-

ample, or during a severe hemorrhage, or in the presence of a few rare diseases—low blood pressure may be truly abnormal and constitute a threat to health. Low blood pressure may occasionally even cause symptoms. Some people notice a momentary spell of dizziness when they stand up quickly from a sitting position as a result of a sudden, but perfectly normal, sag in blood pressure which quickly stabilizes as soon as the shift in body position is completed. This phenomenon is known as *orthostatic hypotension,* and it may be greatly exaggerated as a side effect of various kinds of medicines. Blood pressure can also sag when one is tired, hungry, overheated and/or forced to stand in one position for a prolonged interval without moving. It may cause a spell of dizziness or even fainting, but it can be easily corrected simply by sitting down and placing the head between the knees for a few moments. None of these instances of "low blood pressure" is evidence of disease or disorder. The fact is that most people who have "low blood pressure," far from being sick, are extremely fortunate. The *real* danger arises not when blood pressure is too low but when it is too high—*even a little too high.*

The Onset of Hypertension

Although everyone's blood pressure fluctuates, if on repeated readings it is found to remain steadily and consistently too high, then it can become a real threat to health. It is estimated that from 5 to 15 percent of the entire adult population of the United States is afflicted with some degree of high blood pressure, with approximately twice as many women affected as men. It is also estimated that hypertension is present in an accelerated or so-called malignant form in some 1 to 5 percent of these individuals. The term "malignant" as used here has nothing to do with cancer, but merely refers to an advanced and irreversible stage of hypertensive disease in which blood pressure is dangerously high and cannot adequately be brought under control.

In most victims of hypertension, there is rarely any sudden or dramatic change at first; in fact, there may be no early symptoms at all. But from the very beginning the presence of high blood pressure imposes a dangerous strain on all parts of the circulatory system. A vicious circle is set up. Gradually, and often for unknown reasons, the small arteries and arterioles all over the body begin to contract, offering more resistance than normal to the flow of blood. As a result of this, the heart, which is forced to pump blood at higher than normal pressures, gradually begins to enlarge as its muscular walls thicken to handle the overload. The tough, elastic walls of the great arteries and the smaller arterioles then gradually lose their elasticity because of the heart's high-pressure pounding, and soon can no longer "bounce back" normally from the force of the heartbeat. In some parts of the body, particularly in the liver, the kidneys, or the arterioles feeding the retina of the eye, this damage gradually becomes "fixed" or permanent; the vessel walls harden and thicken, narrowing the channel for blood, offering progressively greater resistance to blood flow and forcing the heart to work even harder.

As months or years pass and the high blood pressure continues, or more commonly increases, certain symptoms and clues to damage begin to appear. The hardened arterioles occasionally burst under the constant hammering of excessive blood pressure, so that tiny hemorrhages appear in the tissue. These can frequently be observed, for example, in the vicinity of the small arterioles in the retina of the eye; or they may occur in the brain, causing impaired vision or repeated small episodes of brain damage usually so small that no specific neurological changes can be noted, but large enough that tiny bits of brain tissue are destroyed by repeated pinpoint hemorrhages. In other parts of the body, damage to arterioles in the kidneys begins, and the overworked heart begins to tire and fail. But even as the disease becomes moderately severe, symptoms may be relatively inconspicuous. Some victims may suffer from "morning headaches," a dull aching pain in the back of the head that is present upon arising but disappears once the person is up and about. Other symptoms may include dizziness, excessive nervous irritability or even vomiting. But these symptoms are not always present to herald the disease.

More often than not, hypertension is discovered by a doctor, quite unexpectedly, in the course of a routine office examination. For this reason, blood pressure measurement is a standard procedure and offers the best means of early detection, the time when the disease can often be controlled and prevented from developing further.

The Causes of High Blood Pressure

Even today doctors are not entirely sure what causes the onset of this insidious affliction, at least in most instances. In certain cases a specific cause can be found and corrected, thus alleviating the trouble, but this is rare. Occasionally, for example, an artery supplying one of the kidneys is found to have been abnormally narrowed or obstructed from birth, a condition that has been found to cause severe generalized high blood pressure. Today this disorder, known as "Goldblatt kidney" or "Goldblatt hypertension" after the man who first demonstrated that obstruction of the kidney artery could produce artificial hypertension in laboratory animals, can be corrected by delicate surgery in which the obstructed portion of the artery is removed and the vessel closed again in normal configuration. But only a fraction of 1 percent of all victims of hypertension suffer from this correctable abnormality.

Again, a certain kind of hormone-producing tumor of the adrenal gland can cause severe fluctuating hypertension. This tumor, known as a *pheochromocytoma,* is not cancerous, and can be surgically removed if its presence is detected, with resulting cure of the hypertension. Similarly, hormone-producing tumors of the thyroid gland can also cause hypertension which can be cured if the tumor is removed. But in 90 percent or more of cases of hypertension, no specific identifiable cause can be found to account for the development of the disease. Rather, a number of very general and nonspecific "contributing conditions" seem to be related to high blood pressure for reasons that are not clearly understood. Among these factors are a *family history of hypertension, obesity, excessive cigarette smoking, excessive intake of salt with meals,*

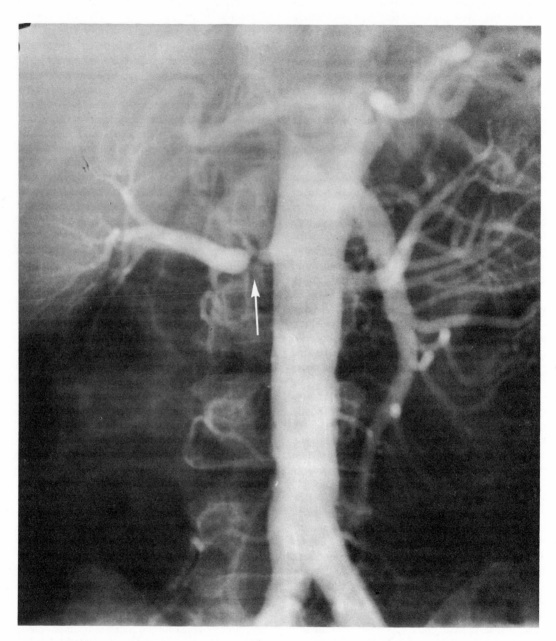

Plate 27 Constriction of a renal artery, as revealed by angiogram. Radio-opaque dye was used to make visible the abdominal aorta and renal arteries supplying the kidneys. Such an obstruction to the blood supply of a kidney can cause a severe but curable hypertension.

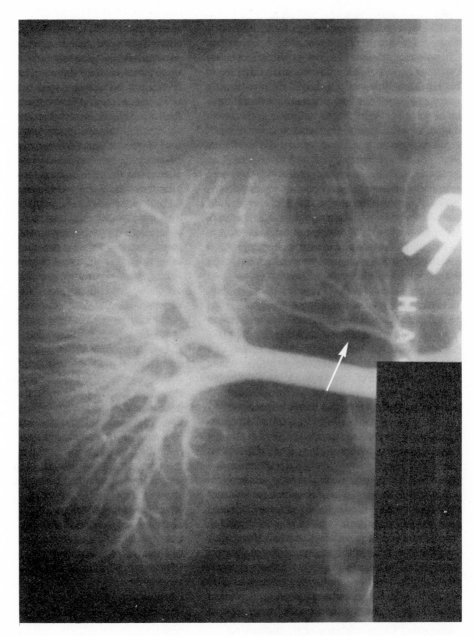

Plate 28 A pheochromocytoma—a functioning tumor of the adrenal gland—is revealed indirectly by means of an angiogram. Although the tumor, located above the upper pole of the kidney, is invisible to X-ray, its presence is betrayed by abnormal blood vessels (see arrow) supplying the tumor.

and—perhaps more important than any of the others—*chronic physical and emotional tension.*

Probably no single one of these factors, in itself, strongly influences the development of high blood pressure. Hypertension is not, for example, a markedly hereditary disease; the fact that a parent or grandparent had the disease does not necessarily mean that it will occur in other members of the family as well. Hypertension is indeed *more likely* to occur in an individual from a family where there is a history of the disease, but this may not involve heredity at all. It may simply be a reflection of the way a given family lives and the amount of physical and emotional tension present there. Similarly, high blood pressure cannot be stopped by weight loss, discontinuance of smoking, or abstaining from salt—but it may be markedly improved.

Most confusing of all is the very strong role of emotional tension in the development of high blood pressure. Some have spoken of hypertension as "a disease of civilization," and certainly it appears far more frequently today in our tense, competitive and complicated society than it does among members of quieter and simpler societies. Although the direct relationship is not understood, it may very well be that the physical and emotional pressures of modern life "wind up" an individual like a watch spring, increasing the adrenalin levels in his blood stream to an abnormal high at all times as if he constantly had to be prepared either to fight or to flee. Part of this reaction to tension is a generalized contraction of the muscular walls of all the small arteries in the body; and as this unconscious and uncontrollable state of overwound-spring tension continues, the high blood pressure necessary to circulate the blood whittles away at the strength and structure of the blood vessels. Early discovery and treatment can reduce and minimize this kind of damage, but for all too many people the damage has already reached dangerous levels before it is discovered.

Dangerous Complications of Hypertension

What happens if blood pressure is allowed to climb abnormally high, and to become progressively higher, without treatment or control?

Already mentioned is the effect it can have upon the heart, causing first enlargement as the muscle walls thicken in an effort to handle the extra load, and finally culminating in *congestive heart failure* which may be extremely difficult to treat because the basic underlying cause is not under control. Further, small arterioles and capillaries all over the body can break and hemorrhage under the continuing pressure. When the vessels in the retina of the eye are so affected, vision may be permanently impaired, and if the underlying high blood pressure is not controlled, blindness may ensue if the victim does not die of some other cause first.

Another serious complication of severe hypertension is *cerebral hemorrhage,* the bursting of a blood vessel in the brain, either large or small, which can cause the sudden collapse, loss of consciousness and neurologic damage of a cerebrovascular accident (CVA) or "stroke" (*see* p. 360). Sometimes such a hypertensive stroke causes only minor damage and the victim may recover most of his normal function, given time and patience, but sooner or later, if the hypertension is uncontrolled, a stroke will occur large enough to cause death. Further, hypertension is a potent contributing factor to the development of *atherosclerosis* which, in turn, can lead to serious circulatory difficulties in the kidneys, the brain, the arteries in the extremities, and even to *coronary artery disease* and *coronary thrombosis* (*see* p. 592).

Perhaps the most serious of all complications of hypertension, and the one which accounts for the greatest number of deaths from this disease, is the gradual loss of kidney function resulting from damage to the tiny arterioles in the kidneys over a period of years, and the development of a condition known as *uremia* when the kidneys finally cease to function at all. This does not happen suddenly; the damage begins with the earliest appearance of hypertension and becomes slowly worse. First the kidneys lose their capacity to concentrate urine; then, gradually, they lose their power to filter out nitrogen-containing waste products, so that these poisonous chemicals begin piling up in the blood stream. Blood may also seep from the kidneys into the urine, causing a severe anemia. By the time uremia develops, hypertension is so entrenched that few medicines can help bring it under control, and even if it does respond to medication, the drop in pressure may even further impair the capacity

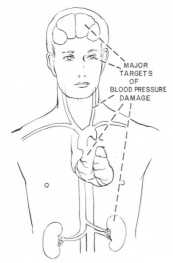

MAJOR
TARGETS
OF
BLOOD PRESSURE
DAMAGE

Figure 44–1.

of the kidneys to do their job. The uremia becomes worse and ultimately the victim dies after a prolonged and painful illness.

In the advanced stages of hypertensive disease, when control has not been established or maintained, more than just the smaller blood vessels are affected. Changes in the artery walls themselves become permanent, and a so-called fixed arterial hypertension ensues. This marks the turning point from "benign" hypertension to its accelerated "malignant" stage. From this time on, blood pressure in certain victims begins a steep and relentless climb to higher and higher levels, and the damage to the blood vessels all over the body, particularly in the kidneys and the brain, is fiercely accelerated. As this stage progresses, the hypertension becomes refractory to any sort of treatment; it can perhaps be slowed by one maneuver or another, but only temporarily.

As little as fifteen years ago this "malignant" phase of hypertension was seen quite frequently; today, fortunately, it has all but disappeared from our population, rarely occurring in areas where adequate medical facilities are available.

The reason for this change is simple: early detection and rational preventive treatment of early hypertension have succeeded in most cases in controlling the progress of the disease. A widening knowledge of the nature of hypertension and a variety of new medications that make it possible to keep hypertensive disease within bounds have also contributed to this change—one of the greatest and yet least known medical achievements in the last 25 years.

Preventive Treatment of Hypertension

Obviously, treatment of hypertension depends first upon its detection, usually in the course of a routine physical examination. But there are four important preventive measures that can be taken to minimize the chances of developing the disease in the first place, or to help reduce high blood pressure to normal if it is already present and prevent its progressive damage. In fact, these measures have proved to be so beneficial to long-term good health that they should be practiced by everyone, hypertensive or not.

Weight Control. Far too many people are overweight, particularly those with hypertension. There may be no cause-and-effect relationship, but obviously extra pounds mean an extra burden on the heart. Without question weight control actively favors reduction of high blood pressure to normal levels or helps prevent the development of the disease. Your doctor can tell you what your weight ought to be and can suggest a sensible program of *gradual* weight reduction. Fad diets or crash programs almost never work in the long run; the weight lost this week is gained back the next. For lasting benefit any reducing program should help a person break the habits that have contributed to continuing overweight and establish in their place new eating habits that will reduce weight to the proper level and maintain it there without much fluctuation. Most good reducing diets, of course, restrict the *total amount* of food eaten, yet provide the *kinds* of food that relieve hunger the longest and supply the necessary balance of nutriments and vitamins, particularly proteins. Thus, such a diet will reduce or discontinue excessive sugars and starchy foods, in favor of meat and other high-protein foods, fresh fruits and salads. But weight reduction to help maintain normal blood pressure may be a lifetime affair. A person should select a diet and eating habits with which he can live comfortably, without much change, forever—and then stick to them.

Salt Control. Reduction in the total intake of salt (or more precisely, sodium-containing chemicals including table salt) is a significant factor in reducing high blood pressure or preventing its occurrence. A great many people, including most hypertensives, use far more salt than necessary. The simplest way to reduce salt intake is to see that food is adequately salted as it is prepared, and then leave the salt shaker off the table. To the confirmed salt addict, everything will taste flat and insipid for the first few days, but if he persists, he will soon discover a variety and subtlety of flavors in his food that had previously been completely drowned out by salt.

Smoking Control. A heavy smoker, particularly a cigarette smoker, subjects his heart and circulatory system to an excessive burden every time he inhales a cigarette. This is particularly true of the early hypertensive, for one of the effects of the nicotine absorbed from tobacco smoke is to constrict small blood vessels and thus cause an elevation in blood pressure. That elevation may not be very much, but when blood pressure levels are already above normal, even a little is too much, and smoking constitutes a very real and progressively dangerous threat.

Smoking can be a psychological addiction, and as such difficult to give up, but it is not a physiological addiction, and contrary to popular myth, anyone with sufficient will power and motivation can stop the habit. It may very well cause some discomfort and irritation at first, and the compulsion to smoke may give way to a tendency to overeat, which must be carefully avoided. But it is far better to suffer these small discomforts *before* the physical conditions that smoking aggravates have progressed to the stage where it becomes mandatory to give it up or where it is already too late. A desire for continuing good health, rather than the fear of death, should be more than ample motivation to stop smoking. In seeking to prevent or control high

blood pressure, it is best to stop smoking completely, but for those who cannot or will not stop altogether, even reducing the amount of smoking is a help.

Control of Physical and Emotional Tension. There is no question that physical and emotional stress is one of the chief contributors to hypertension in the early stages of the disease, before fixed changes in the blood vessels conspire to keep blood pressure elevated whether tension is present or not. Indeed, high blood pressure and physical and emotional tension so frequently go hand in hand that doctors speak of "the hypertensive personality": the active, hard-working, hard-driving man or the tense and nervous woman who never seems to be able to relax either at work or at play. Of course, our fast-paced society, with its emphasis on competition and achievement, makes some tension almost impossible to avoid, but there are many people who never slow down whatever the circumstances. Their drive may very well make them leaders in their businesses, professions or communities, but ironically, it also lays them open to the dangers of hypertension. More often tension and worry combined make real achievement all but impossible, but the end result is the same.

There is very little hope that people like these can change their personalities overnight, or even at all; nervous tension has deep psychological roots. But they can, and must, relax and slow down from time to time. Many do not, unless it is on a doctor's specific orders when their condition makes it imperative. But it is infinitely better to recognize the dangers of hypertension, not to mention the several other disorders that can be traced, at least in part, to physical and emotional stress, and slow down before it is too late. It is not difficult to do: recognize those situations that can cause nervous tension and avoid them, or if that is not possible, learn to take them in stride, whether at home or on the job. Get plenty of sleep, relax after a hard day's work and on the weekends, and take real vacations, not the kind that are as exhausting and nerve-racking as everyday life. There is no reason to become even more anxious and nervous if a slight degree of hypertension is discovered, but there is reason to cut down on strenuous physical activities and avoid emotional strain of every sort. Modifications like these are easy and practical to make; they do not require any drastic changes. As a matter of fact, they will not only help prevent hypertension and prolong life, they may also immeasurably increase the joys and satisfactions of that life.

The Treatment of Hypertension

Preventive measures are sometimes not enough to check the progress of even early hypertension. In this case, the doctor may elect to prescribe any one of a number of modern drugs to reduce elevated blood pressure and keep it within the normal range. Among these medications are simple sedatives, not taken as sleeping aids but rather in very small doses during the day to take the edge off emotional tension. Similar in effect, but less likely to induce drowsiness, a wide variety of mild tranquilizing medications can also be used, either by themselves or in combination with such sedatives as phenobarbital taken in small doses.

Other medications that are highly effective in dealing with early hypertension are the diuretics, drugs which help the kidneys do a more effective job of ridding the body of excess fluid that has been retained in the tissues. A number of the so-called saline diuretics, which increase the urinary excretion of salt and with it quantities of water, also have a direct effect in lowering blood pressure. These preparations are among the most effective and popular of all antihypertensive medicines, particularly because they so rarely have untoward side effects.

When hypertension has progressed from its early mild stages to a moderate and fixed level, more potent drugs must be used as a combative weapon. The most commonly utilized class of these drugs, of which methyl-dopa is an example, slows down the nerve impulses to the muscular walls of the arteries and arterioles, thus reducing the amount of constriction and lowering the pressure necessary for the circulation of blood. For even more severe hypertension, in which rapid lowering of blood pressure and more potent control is necessary, still other drugs like Apresoline may be used.

Of course all of these medicines should be taken only under a doctor's guidance, and in the dosages he prescribes. Often when medicine is used to control hypertension it is undertaken on a lifelong basis, and the patient is sometimes tempted to experiment. But one medicine may be far too potent, another far too mild, and there is always the risk of uncomfortable or even dangerous side effects. It is up to the doctor to prescribe the proper drug and check its effectiveness. It is also his province to determine the length of time treatment should be continued, how often blood pressure should be checked, and the frequency of physical examinations to assess any ill effects of the disease.

Finally, there are certain kinds of hypertension, particularly blood pressure that is dangerously high and refractory to treatment with medications, which can be treated by surgical interruption of the autonomic nerve pathways that moderate the involuntary constriction of muscle in the arteriole walls. One such procedure known as a *splanchnicectomy* involves opening the abdomen and removing the autonomic nerve ganglia that lie along either side of the spine on the back wall of the abdomen. This kind of surgery was much more frequently used a decade or so ago than today, before many of the modern medicines were available, and even then it was not effective consistently enough to be used as a routine procedure. Today candidates for operations of this sort are carefully picked and relatively few, but on a selective basis surgery can still provide one more weapon in the arsenal against this disease.

Most important of all, however, is intelligent cooperation between the hypertensive patient and his doctor, to help keep blood pressure normal and to minimize the amount or kind of medicine necessary for control. Even with the use of medications, it is imperative that the patient maintain weight control with a proper diet, reduce salt intake, give up smoking, and avoid physical and emotional stress. With cooperation and reasonable care, the hypertensive can expect to lead a long and comparatively normal life with a minimum of time and energy devoted to keeping his blood pressure under safe control.

45

Atherosclerosis and Coronary Artery Disease

The process of aging is a complex, and puzzling, phenomenon. The human organism is in a continual state of change, but sooner or later the changes that are generally a welcome part of "growing up" are superseded by those less welcome changes that accompany "growing old." No one knows just why these changes come about. We do know that from the beginning of life body-building and body-destroying reactions occur simultaneously in the human organism. With the passage of years the body-destroying processes begin slightly to outweigh the body-building processes and we start to show the effects of "aging." Hair begins to gray, eyesight begins to fail, skin begins to wrinkle, and just as there are external evidences of deterioration and aging, so there are deep internal physical changes that begin to occur in the mid-twenties and thereafter at an accelerating pace until the body can no longer sustain life at all. And one of the most universal and implacable changes associated with aging is a physical process of deterioration, shared by virtually everyone, which is commonly known as *arteriosclerosis*.

The name of this condition and its more commonly used nickname, "hardening of the arteries," is slightly deceptive, for it implies a single specific change or disorder. But arteriosclerosis actually results from any of a number of processes associated with age which cause the blood vessels, and particularly the arteries, to lose their elasticity; it can be caused by the gradual diminution of elastic tissue fibers in the artery walls, the deposition of calcium in those walls, the

aging and scarring of tissues surrounding the arteries, the deposition of fatty materials in the artery walls, or several other factors. It is, however, the deposition of fatty substances in the walls of the arteries, followed by the laying down of calcium in these same areas, which in many people goes *beyond* the limits of "normal" aging and becomes, in fact, a disease process. A typical plaquelike deposit of fatty materials and calcium in the wall of a large artery is called an *atheroma,* and the formation of such plaques, by far the most common of all disease processes associated with arteriosclerotic changes, goes by the more specific medical name of *atherosclerosis*. It is also this particular one among many sclerotic changes which ultimately leads to damage to the kidneys, the brain, the arteries in the extremities, and even the dangerous and frequently fatal blocking of the coronary arteries which is known as *coronary thrombosis,* one manifestation of coronary artery disease.

The Formation of Atheromas

The earliest changes of atherosclerosis first appear in susceptible men in their late twenties or early thirties, and somewhat later in women. At this time streaks of fatty material are deposited in the walls of the arteries, just inside the inner lining of those vessels. These streaks are composed of a combination of body fats, often in tiny droplets, several forms of a waxy fat material known as *cholesterol,* and certain protein molecules combined with glycerine-like chemicals in the form of so-called *triglycerides.* None of these substances is the same as dietary fats, which are broken down by digestion into simpler components in order to enter the blood stream. Some of those components aid in the nourishment of the body, but others are changed, particularly in the liver, into the different fatty or "lipid" substances that can be deposited in the vessel walls and lead to the formation of atheromas. As these fatty deposits enlarge, they break down the fibrous and elastic tissue of the artery walls and often form swellings in localized areas within the arteries that tend to obstruct circulation. Atheromatous plaques in the smaller arteries can, in fact, actually reduce the size of the opening through which blood is carried by as much as 60 to 70 percent.

These fatty plaques have an even further ill effect on the arteries where they appear. The normal cells of the artery walls, like other cells in the body, require a capillary blood supply to keep them alive and healthy. As the atheromas enlarge they cut off the capillary blood supply to areas of the artery wall, causing oxygen starvation of these tissues and sometimes inflammatory reactions. Presently small ulcers form on the inner linings of the vessels, allowing the waxy material of the fat deposit to pour into the orifice of the vessel. In younger people these atheromatous plaques consist of a sticky, waxy stuff with the consistency of moistened, compressed Parmesan cheese, but as these plaques persist and enlarge, calcium is also deposited in the area, probably as a result of the body's attempt to heal the chronic inflammation there. Gradually the vessel walls become hardened and stiffened, often like pipe stems, with only a tiny passageway through which blood can still move. Ultimately fibrin is laid down on the roughened, ulcerated inner surface of the blood vessels, and small blood clots or thrombi form, further blocking the passage of blood. None of this happens suddenly, but over a long period of time the vessel may become almost completely occluded, with the blood forming abnormal channels through the occluding thrombus in order to maintain some circulation.

This process can occur in any of the arteries, but those most commonly affected are the coronary arteries supplying the heart, the cerebral arteries supplying the brain, and the peripheral arteries supplying the lower extremities. As these vessels become progressively obstructed, the heart muscle, the brain tissue or the tissues of the lower legs and feet become more and more starved for oxygen; and when any unusual demand is placed upon these organs, symptoms begin to occur. When cerebral arteries are blocked, symptoms may vary all the way from a minor degree of "absent-mindedness" or forgetfulness to a massive stroke due to total occlusion of an artery. This can lead to results much the same as in strokes due to cerebral hemorrhage: there can be permanent damage or impairment of various parts of the brain tissue, which leads to impairment of brain function and, quite often, to death. Narrowing of the coronary arteries leads to episodes of severe chest pain which occur when the victim attempts to be more active than normal, a condition known as *angina pectoris,* and obstruction of one of these coronary vessels by a thrombus can cause a "coronary heart attack" or, more accurately, acute coronary thrombosis, with resultant severe damage to a segment of heart muscle and possibly even sudden death. Obstruction of the arteries to the extremities can lead to a peculiar kind of severe pain in the muscles of these oxygen-starved areas which occurs when they are over-exercised but disappears when they are at rest, a condition doctors speak of as *intermittent claudication.* In extreme cases, gangrene can develop in the toes or other portions of the lower extremities when obstruction of blood flow becomes too great.

In most cases the development of atherosclerosis is a slow, progressive, chronic process which is remarkably silent and symptom-free. Just as we normally do not notice the appearance of wrinkles from day to day, the "interior aging" of atherosclerosis goes unnoticed until the sudden occurrence of one of the resulting symptoms: the heart pain of angina pectoris, a stroke, an episode of coronary thrombosis or some other complication. Nor is there any particular laboratory study that helps the doctor diagnose this condition in its early stages, although reduced pulsations in the peripheral arteries suggest the presence of the condition in middle-aged adults. When chest X-rays are taken of elderly people, the deposits of calcium in long-standing atherosclerotic areas of the aorta can sometimes be seen, but since calcium deposition is a late phenomenon, this does not help with early diagnosis.

Factors Contributing to Atherosclerosis

Even though the diagnosis of atherosclerosis can usually be made only when symptoms of its complications appear, many factors are known to contribute to the development of this condition. Hereditary factors, for example, influence the progress of the illness, although the exact hereditary mechanism is not known. Individuals who tend to become overweight and then doggedly remain so seem more vulnerable than those who are fortunate enough not to have a weight problem. Further, there is some evidence that hereditary control of the way dietary and "metabolic" fats are handled by the body may result in a definite predisposition to the condition. In short, there are doubtless those who by their hereditary makeup are more vulnerable to, and more likely to develop, atherosclerosis earlier than others.

It has also been established that certain other diseases or disorders can accelerate the deposition of fatty materials in the arteries. For example, victims of diabetes mellitus show a marked tendency to develop an exaggerated degree of atherosclerosis much more prematurely than normal; indeed, one of the most dangerous aspects of diabetes is the development of arteriosclerotic cardiovascular disease at a very young age. Even though diabetes can be controlled by medication once the diagnosis is made, the degree of atherosclerosis that has already occurred before treatment begins is not reversible.

No one yet is entirely certain what role dietary fats play in the development of atherosclerosis, but most specialists in heart disease are convinced that certain kinds, particularly animal fats which are made up of so-called saturated hydrocarbons which harden at room temperature, are a very real contributing factor. Further evidence that diet can affect the development of atherosclerosis lies in the fact that during periods of privation and starvation, as in Germany during World War I and the Scandinavian countries and Holland during World War II, the clinical frequency of this disease declined. Also, death rates due to atherosclerosis and its complications in men aged forty to fifty-nine are approximately 8 per 1,000 in the United States and western Europe compared to 1 per 1,000 in Japan, China, Ceylon, Chile and the Indonesian islands, where diets are modest and low in fats. These low rates in the Orient cannot be attributed to race, since Japanese living in the United States show rates of coronary disease approaching those of Caucasians in this country.

Many physicians believe that a sedentary life with very little regular exercise is also a contributing factor in the development of this disorder, perhaps simply because exercise promotes better circulation in general and helps develop "standby" or collateral circulation to areas which might otherwise be starved for oxygen because of formation of thrombi or occlusion of vessels by atherosclerosis. Many heart specialists believe that heavy tobacco smoking over a long period of time speeds the process of atherosclerosis; certainly statistics indicate that the heavy cigarette smoker is more vulnerable to coronary artery disease and other arteriosclerotic manifestations than the nonsmoker, but once again a cause-and-effect relationship, whatever it may be, has not been definitely established. Finally, individuals with high blood pressure are known to develop atherosclerosis earlier and more rapidly than individuals whose blood pressure remains normal—or at least to suffer from complicating disorders earlier and more severely. But whether this is a result of the abnormal beating that the hypertensive's arteries take or whether the hypertension actually promotes the development of atherosclerosis has not been definitely determined.

Coronary Artery Disease

Although atherosclerosis may remain silent for years as it develops, several of its complications are not only distressingly symptomatic but exceedingly dangerous. Most of these complications result from gradual obliteration of arterial channels or from ulceration of the interior walls of the arteries, so that thrombi form, obstructing blood flow to certain critical organs. Of all the arteries affected by atherosclerosis, none are more vulnerable than the *coronary arteries* supplying the heart muscle itself, and no complication of atherosclerosis is more grave or, in the long run, more frequently fatal than the atherosclerotic changes which cause coronary artery disease.

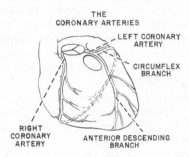

THE
CORONARY ARTERIES

LEFT CORONARY ARTERY

CIRCUMFLEX BRANCH

RIGHT CORONARY ARTERY

ANTERIOR DESCENDING BRANCH

Figure 45–1.

Coronary Insufficiency. In most individuals with atherosclerosis, the coronary arteries are among the earliest to develop atheromatous plaques, and often are the first to display the symptoms of impaired circulation. There are three coronary arteries supplying the heart, but because these vessels are very small (no more than one-fourth inch in diameter at the largest), symptoms of insufficient blood flow may first appear in the early or middle thirties. In many individuals the first evidence of trouble occurs not as a result of any sudden blockage of these vital arteries, but rather as a result of gradual narrowing and progressive diminution of circulation to the heart. This narrowing process may go on slowly for years, and may never become symptomatic; indeed, it is not unusual to discover in a post-mortem examination of a middle-aged man who dies of some other cause that his coronary arteries are so narrowed by waxy-like fat and calcium deposits that only a trickle of blood has been passing through, yet the man never had symptoms. In most, however, symptoms do begin appearing anywhere from the mid-thirties with increasing frequency to the age of sixty or seventy, at which time 70 to 80 percent

of all individuals are affected. The groundwork for coronary symptoms and even attacks in the late thirties and early forties is laid between the ages of twenty and thirty in many people, as revealed by studies of American soldiers killed in Korea, in which it was discovered that 40 percent of well-nourished men twenty to thirty years of age already showed some involvement of the coronary arteries.

Angina Pectoris. The most common symptom in these gradually progressive cases is a characteristic severe crushing pain felt in the chest under or slightly to the left of the breastbone when the victim is in the midst of active physical exercise or has become violently angry or emotionally overwrought. This sort of pain, due to *myocardial ischemia*—that is, the sudden starvation of the heart for oxygen because of a temporary deficiency of blood—goes by the name of angina pectoris (literally, "chest pain"). Characteristically coming on during exertion, excitement or anger, the pain vanishes just as quickly when the situation related to it subsides, but while present it may be severe enough to be almost totally disabling. At its peak the pain often is felt not only in the chest but also up both sides of the neck and frequently down the inside of the left arm all the way to the wrist. This pattern of so-called referred pain is so typical that doctors regard it as an important diagnostic sign. It should not be a cause for unnecessary alarm, however, because it can arise from other sources as well. Many individuals, for example, suffer very similar episodes of pain due to acid indigestion after a particularly rich meal. But in most cases the pain of acid indigestion can be distinguished from angina pectoris by the simple expedient of taking a mild antacid such as Tums, milk of magnesia or even bicarbonate of soda. If the pain disappears almost immediately, it is probably not angina pectoris at all. Furthermore, acid indigestion pain is seldom triggered by physical activity, as is angina pectoris, and conversely, rarely goes away when activity is stopped.

In many individuals angina pectoris first appears in a very mild degree, and then becomes progressively worse over a period of years, perhaps controlled by medications as the severity increases, until the impairment of coronary circulation is so great that ordinary controls are no longer effective. In other victims the angina may appear quite suddenly and severely at a late stage in the disease condition, sometimes almost as a herald of impending coronary thrombosis. In the former case probably more than just narrowing of the coronary arteries by atherosclerosis is involved. Along with atherosclerosis there is often inflammation and irritation of the walls of the arteries, and many people experience angina pectoris as a result of spasm of the irritated arteries—a muscular phenomenon rather than a true blocking or obliteration. For these people in particular there is a specific medication which swiftly relieves anginal pain by relaxing spasm of the coronary artery walls and dilating the vessels. This medicine, oddly enough, is nitroglycerine, taken in minute doses by allowing the tablet to dissolve under the tongue, since the active ingredient is damaged or destroyed by gastric acids if swallowed. Within a matter of minutes the nitroglycerine dilates all of the arteries feeding the heart, thus providing a flood of fresh oxygenated blood to the heart muscle and relieving the pain almost miraculously. The drug may also cause a temporary pounding headache because it dilates the arteries in the brain as well, but this side effect can be minimized by carefully regulating the dosage and using only the amount necessary to relieve the angina. Nitroglycerine is neither narcotic nor habituating, and does not produce tolerance; in other words, it can be used repeatedly, as often as necessary over a period of years without losing its effectiveness. But the frequency with which it is used is often an indication to the doctor of the progressive seriousness of the disease; when a patient who initially required only one or two nitroglycerine tablets a day gradually is forced to increase the dose to ten or fifteen a day, the doctor can be quite certain that the coronary atherosclerosis producing the angina is becoming progressively and seriously worse.

It is important for the victims of angina pectoris to understand that it is not a temporary or passing condition which time or medicine will heal, but rather the symptom of atherosclerosis, a long-standing disease process which is intricately related to heredity, individual physical makeup, dietary habits and many other aspects of the victim's way of life. As a symptom, it may be markedly improved by treatment; but unless steps are also taken to combat the underlying atherosclerosis, the angina will, in most cases, become progressively worse until one of the coronary vessels becomes completely blocked by a thrombus, causing an acute coronary thrombosis and *infarction* or tissue destruction of the part of the heart muscle supplied by the vessel, or until circulation is so impaired that the whole heart muscle is weakened beyond its capacity to recover and goes into heart failure and/or severe disturbances of the rhythm of the heartbeat. In either case, death can result.

The onset of anginal symptoms is no reason to despair, however, particularly if the symptoms are just beginning. For one thing, there is great individual variation, and the amount of anginal pain and distress that one suffers is not necessarily directly related to the severity of damage to the coronary arteries. In many early cases of angina, much of the pain may be caused by spasm of the coronary blood vessels and actual damage to the vessels may not yet be severe. Even if the damage is moderately severe, there are a number of things which the early angina victim can do, working in close cooperation with his physician, to slow the progress of the underlying disease and to postpone the grave terminal complications, sometimes for decades.

Medical consultation and proper treatment are a must simply because the onset of angina *is* a grave warning of serious potential danger ahead, and it may be possible to postpone permanent ill effects. The first step is a thorough physical examination with special attention to the condition of the heart and blood vessels. Electrocardiogram tracings will help the doctor determine the degree of severity of the damage to coronary arteries, particularly if a previous electrocardiogram is available for comparison, since these tracings show characteristic changes when the heart muscle is *ischemic;* that is, starving for oxygen as a result of inadequate blood supply. If the doctor feels it is advisable, he may record a patient's electrocardiogram first at rest, and then again after a period of mild to moderate exercise, in order to determine a baseline for medical management of the problem. In a more vigorous kind of exercise tolerance test, familiarly known as a "step test," a patient steps rapidly up and down from a stool until his heart is working significantly faster than at rest. Here a doctor's judgment is necessary, however, since too vigorous exercise can conceivably do damage. Any such physical evaluation should also include X-ray examination of the chest, careful recording of the blood pressure, an evaluation of kidney function (since kidneys, too, can be involved by atherosclerosis) and a number of blood studies including an examination of cholesterol level in the serum.

With a careful baseline drawn, a rational and practical regimen of treatment can be worked out. If the patient also has high blood pressure, every effort should be made to reduce it to normal levels and keep it there by medication or other means, since high blood pressure can accelerate the progress of atherosclerosis. If the angina victim is a cigarette smoker, he should give up smoking, since one of the physiological effects of nicotine is to induce spasm or constriction of the smaller arteries and arterioles all over the body, including those in the heart. If obesity is a factor, a sensible program of weight loss will be of lasting benefit; but whether or not weight loss is necessary, most physicians urge a specific dietary regimen, substituting polyunsaturated vegetable fats for animal fats and reducing the total intake of carbohydrates in favor of protein. Such a diet program will help in weight reduction, but it should be undertaken not as a "crash program" but rather as a permanent change in eating habits. None of these measures will reverse or repair the damage already done to the coronary arteries, but they can, in combination, help slow down the progress of atherosclerosis, and if weight reduction and control of high blood pressure are maintained, they may reduce the frequency of anginal attacks quite significantly.

Medication also has its place, particularly nitroglycerine or other nitrite preparations prescribed in carefully regulated dosages for use as needed to control pain. Finally, and perhaps most controversial of all treatment measures, is the matter of physical exercise. Until quite recently many physicians felt that deliberately undertaking physical exercise when the patient was unused to it could provoke anginal attacks and even pose a more serious threat. And there are, doubtless, a great many victims of severe angina who should not take the risk. Certainly anyone with angina pectoris should carefully avoid any sudden exercise load at irregular or extended intervals; the threat of precipitating a coronary thrombosis is just too great. On the other hand, a relatively young person with early angina can benefit greatly from a steady program of modestly increasing daily exercise designed to build up tolerance to exercise gradually and safely. Many cardiologists believe that such a program also helps develop the collateral circulation; that is, it helps enlarge the small auxiliary arteries that feed parts of the heart muscle and thus gradually improves the circulation even though no change in the obstructed coronary arteries takes place. In short, as long as an exercise program is not strenuous enough to tax an undernourished heart, it can be highly beneficial not only in preventing the progress of atherosclerosis in one who does not yet have symptoms, but also in improving the cardiovascular condition when coronary insufficiency or angina pectoris is already present. The question of what kind and how much exercise is one that can properly be answered only by a physician thoroughly familiar with an individual patient's medical history and physical condition. Fad exercise programs or any degree of physical activity above the normal should *not* be undertaken without a doctor's advice.

A variety of other conservative measures may help relieve angina pectoris and prevent its progress. Adequate rest on a daily basis is extremely important. Removal to a mild climate may be worth considering, in some cases, since angina can be precipitated by sudden forays out of a warm house into a bitter cold winter atmosphere. Sometimes an overall reduction in the pace of the patient's life is indicated as well as a reevaluation of priorities to enable him to preserve energy that has previously been squandered.

Such a conservative program of proper diet,

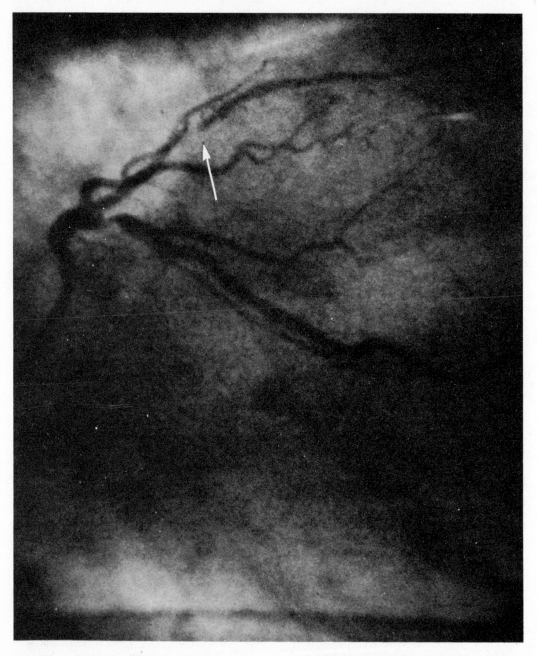

Plate 29a   Partial obstruction of a coronary artery due to atherosclerosis. Flow of blood through the artery to the heart beyond the obstruction is greatly diminished. Vessels are visualized by coronary angiogram.

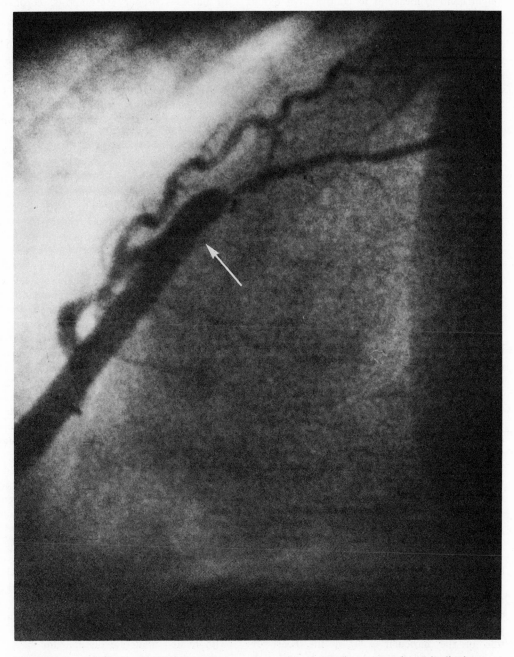

Plate 29b   A similarly obstructed coronary artery with circulation restored surgically by grafting a segment of the patient's own saphenous vein to bypass the obstruction.

weight control, measures to control high blood pressure, no smoking, and sensible exercise, carried out with continuing medical supervision and cooperation between doctor and patient, may not only relieve the pain and disability of angina pectoris and delay the further progress of atherosclerosis after it has become symptomatic, but in many cases may even prevent symptoms from occurring in the first place. It is only common sense, then, that these measures should be a part of everyone's normal health routine. Far too many people wait for the symptoms of progressive atherosclerosis to appear before they do anything about it. What is more, there are cases in which angina pectoris becomes progressively more severe and disabling in spite of any conservative program to control or minimize it. In such patients surgeons have recently had considerable success in relieving pain and restoring circulation to the heart by means of coronary artery surgery. In this kind of operation, in which the heart-lung by-pass machine must be used to take over the circulation and aeration of blood while the surgeon works, the obstructed segments of coronary artery may be removed completely and replaced by grafts made from the patient's own saphenous vein, a superficial vessel in the leg which the patient can do without. These surgical techniques are still being developed today, and only those patients with intractable angina are considered candidates for the operation, but results thus far have been so encouraging that it seems likely that surgical treatment of angina will become increasingly important.

Acute Coronary Thrombosis

Coronary insufficiency and angina pectoris, both complications of gradual atherosclerosis, are slow to develop, but quite a different situation arises when a major branch of one of the coronary arteries becomes suddenly and completely blocked, abruptly depriving a whole section of the muscular wall of the heart of oxygenated blood. Such a blockage or *occlusion* is frequently caused by a blood clot or thrombus that becomes lodged in an arterial vessel already narrowed by atherosclerosis. Known by a variety of names—coronary thrombosis, coronary occlusion, myocardial infarction or just a "heart attack"—this condition can occur without warning, and if a major coronary artery is involved, it can be a prostrating and even fatal event.

A coronary thrombosis is often associated with the middle-aged or elderly, but the fact is that it can strike a victim who is still relatively young and may have had no previous symptoms of any kind of heart disease. Indeed, there is a sort of deadly inverse ratio between the age of the victim and the outcome of an attack: it is the relatively young man in his mid-thirties or early forties, with no previous history of heart disease, who is most likely to be struck dead by a major coronary thrombosis the first time it occurs, while the older victim is more likely to have a milder attack from which recovery is possible. Statistically, however, coronary thrombosis is relatively uncommon before the age of thirty-five, and throughout the population in the United States and western Europe, the areas recording the highest incidence of arteriosclerotic heart disease, only about 3 percent of all "first coronaries" are fatal. The peak incidence of this particular kind of heart attack is in the age group between forty-five and fifty-five, and it seems likely that most individuals who have lived to the age of fifty-five or sixty without any evidence of a coronary thrombosis either have relatively minor atherosclerosis which may not lead to coronary attacks until a more advanced age, or else have over the years developed sufficient secondary or "collateral" circulation to their heart muscles that coronaries, when they occur, have less severe results. The incidence of coronary attacks is about ten times as great among men as among women, partly because women seem to be protected against the early onset of atherosclerosis due to hormonal influences during their childbearing years, and partly because the predisposing factors—high blood pressure, severe physical and emotional pressures, insufficient rest and exercise, a rich diet with related moderate obesity, and heavy cigarette smoking—are found more commonly in men than in women.

Typically a coronary thrombosis occurs in an overweight man either at rest (such as in bed at night after a heavy meal) or in the midst of extreme and unaccustomed exercise such as shoveling snow. The first symptom is usually the sudden onset of severe chest pain felt directly under the breastbone, most commonly described as "crushing" or "squeezing," accompanied by sudden shortness of breath, pallor, profuse sweating and a highly distressing subjective sensation frequently described as a "sense of impending death." Unlike the pain of angina, the pain of a coronary thrombosis does *not* ease up with rest, but persists either unchanged or growing progressively worse for a period of some hours if treatment is not started very quickly. The doctor usually finds the victim prostrated and sometimes unconscious from severe continuing chest pain, clutching his chest, gray of face, with cold clammy skin, blood pressure that has fallen to shock levels and a faint, weak rapid pulse. In some people the symptoms begin fairly mildly, and may be mistaken for a gastrointestinal upset—"heartburn" or acid indigestion— but the pain of a coronary will not be relieved by antacid medicines, and "heartburn" which does not respond quickly to such simple measures should be regarded with suspicion, and a doctor summoned.

When a branch of a coronary artery is plugged with a thrombus, the area of heart muscle that it feeds is deprived of oxygenated blood and the muscle cells begin to die. Thus that section of muscle is unable to contract normally or carry its normal work load. If the damaged area is large enough, the entire heart may stop completely or go into an irregular twitching rhythm known as *fibrillation* with immediate profound shock and sudden death as a result. If the area involved is smaller, however, shock will still be present, together with severe pain, but the rest of the heart is able to carry a minimum load and maintain the general circulation. When the victim survives the initial shock of the attack, he may still suffer later from acute shortness of breath as a result of heart failure which arises because the uninjured heart muscle cannot maintain adequate circulation; indeed heart failure may become a major complication a few hours after the coronary occurs. Further, a blood clot may form inside the heart, attached

to the area of damaged muscle. If this happens, a portion of the clot may later break loose and jam one of the pulmonary arteries, causing sudden death from pulmonary embolus. This is such a common late complication of coronary thrombosis that in modern treatment of this kind of heart attack every effort is made to reduce the coagulating ability of the blood drastically from the very beginning of the attack to prevent the formation of such a thrombus.

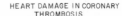

HEART DAMAGE IN CORONARY THROMBOSIS

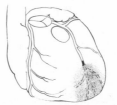

Figure 45–2.

The death of muscle cells due to coronary thrombosis does not happen all at once, and if there is good circulation to the muscle immediately surrounding the damaged area from coronary vessels that have not been blocked, the heart can continue to pump. But during the next several days the affected segment of dying muscle gradually becomes soft and pulpy, reaching its weakest point about ten days after the heart attack. At this critical time even a slight extra demand on the heart may cause the injured heart wall to rupture, if enough heart muscle has been damaged or destroyed. More often, however, a slow process of healing begins. The heart muscle cells do not regenerate, but fibrous tissue grows into the damaged area and gradually forms a scar. Over a period of months and years following recovery, this scar will become firmer and smaller but it will never completely go away.

An electrocardiogram series provides a startlingly clear picture of the changes that take place in the heart muscle after a coronary attack. An electrocardiogram (EKG) is a measurement or "picture" of the electrical impulses generated by the contractions of the heart muscle. Normal contractions are characteristically smooth and rhythmic, but after a coronary attack, the electrocardiogram shows a disruption of this smooth flow and usually reveals a so-called current of injury which can give the doctor an invaluable clue to the location and extent of heart muscle damage, and even which of the coronary arteries is involved in the attack. As healing slowly takes place, EKG tracings gradually revert almost to normal, but will always show the disruption of current caused by the scarred area of heart muscle. Even a coronary thrombosis so mild that it went unrecognized still inevitably "leaves its footprints" on the electrocardiogram.

ELECTROCARDIOGRAMS

A. NORMAL

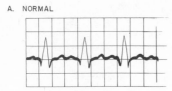

B. CURRENT OF INJURY- CORONARY ATTACK

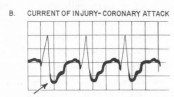

C. SCARRING - OLD CORONARY

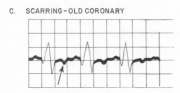

Figure 45–3.

Even though most victims of an initial coronary attack survive, it can be a frightening experience. There is almost nothing that can be done in the way of routine first-aid measures to help the victim. Medical aid should be summoned at once if a coronary attack is suspected or if the victim's condition even remotely mimics the symptoms of an attack. If the victim is conscious, he should not be left alone or permitted to move, and steps should be taken to reassure him and keep him warm to alleviate shock. It is

preferable, even in cases of a mild attack, to wait for an ambulance to transport the victim to a hospital under medical supervision, but if this is not possible, he must be moved with the utmost caution, since even slight exertion can deepen the severity of the attack. The most important thing, however, is to summon or reach medical aid as quickly as possible. It may mean the difference between life or death, or the degree of recovery possible after the attack.

A coronary thrombosis requires the highest quality of professional care. One of the doctor's first concerns is the use of medicine to relieve the victim's pain and apprehension, since both these factors contribute heavily to the very dangerous degree of shock the victim may be suffering. In addition, administration of oxygen will be started as quickly as possible in order to relieve the shortness of breath so often accompanying these attacks and to enrich the oxygen level in the blood that reaches heart muscle. Both of these measures may be instituted even before the victim arrives at the hospital.

Once in the hospital a number of additional measures will be taken promptly. A series of EKGs will be run, along with other laboratory studies, to help the doctor determine the location and extent of heart muscle damage, essential information in planning the most effective course of treatment. Anticoagulant medications such as Dicumarol are also commonly administered to prevent the formation of dangerous blood clots within either the heart or the large veins of the legs. For the first ten days or more, depending on the severity of the attack, the patient is kept on a strict nursing regimen known as a "coronary routine" in which he is permitted to do virtually nothing for himself. Thereafter, the doctor will want a coronary patient to be up and moving about, to some degree, as soon as possible, but how soon depends on when he regains his strength and when his heart has healed sufficiently to tolerate any more than the most minimal activity. The decision rests with the doctor. Many patients are allowed limited activity within as little as two weeks after an attack, while others may have to stay in bed for as long as two months. The average hospitalization period is approximately a month to six weeks, and there is a further convalescent period at home of a month or more in order to permit the heart full recovery. From that point on, both the doctor and particularly the patient must concentrate on preventing a recurrence, which can happen all too frequently and pose an even more dangerous threat than the first attack.

The Acute Coronary Care Unit. Even under the best of circumstances, many coronary victims—particularly those with histories of previous coronaries or younger individuals with their first coronaries—simply die in the middle of an acute attack, often in the first hour or so from the onset of symptoms. Many such deaths have been a result of cardiac rhythm disturbances brought about by the acute injury of the attack, even when the amount and degree of heart muscle injury are such that the heart could well recover, given sufficient time. Recognition of this fact has led to the establishment of acute coronary care units in most major hospitals in the country—specially equipped hospital receiving areas, manned by physicians and a highly trained nursing staff, in which the victim of an acute coronary attack can be continually observed and the behavior of his heart monitored second by second to detect and counteract any potentially fatal rhythm disturbance the moment it occurs. In such units lifesaving cardiac pacemaking, for example, can be instituted in a matter of minutes. Respirators can be used as needed in an instant, as well as medications or cardiac resuscitation. Thanks to these specialized care units, countless lives are now being preserved that would have been lost only a decade ago, and many communities have extended these acute coronary care concepts to emergency vehicles staffed by specially trained personnel. These vehicles are equipped to broadcast a patient's condition by means of telemetry to a doctor at the hospital emergency room, even while he is en route to the hospital. The doctor can radio back medication orders or instructions for pacemaking or defibrillation to the emergency car staff as needed, and thus keep the coronary victim under guided medical care from the moment the emergency unit reaches his home. There is little question today that increasing use of this kind of emergency program, both in the hospital and in the traveling emergency vehicles, will soon become routine procedure in virtually every community in the country, saving multitudes of coronary victims who would otherwise die in the critical acute phase of a coronary attack.

Ultimately, however, prevention is the best possible solution to the threat of coronary artery disease, and much can be done to prevent coronary episodes once a diagnosis of severe atherosclerosis has been made. Both coronary artery disease and coronary thrombosis are the end result of chronic and progressive atherosclerosis, a disease process that affects arteries and arterioles all over the body. Nothing can be done to reverse the damage already done by this disease, but preventive measures can be taken to slow down its inexorable progress and possibly delay a recurrence of these life-threatening complications for many years. These measures are, of course, the same as those described earlier for victims of coronary insufficiency or angina pectoris: the patient must give up smoking completely and permanently; if he is overweight, he must take off the extra pounds and keep them off; he must maintain a low-calorie diet rich in protein but low in fats (especially animal fats) and carbohydrates; if hypertension is a complicating factor, it must be controlled by avoiding any unnecessary emotional and physical stress or, if necessary, by medications; ample rest is an absolute necessity; and, finally, after recovery of the damaged heart muscle, a carefully controlled program of physical exercise should be undertaken regularly. Perhaps most important of all, the patient must take a new look at his entire way of life, reevaluate the things that are important and the things that are not, and take the steps necessary to reduce physical and emotional strain in every way possible. Doctor and patient must work together in this preventive program, but obviously the major responsibility lies with the patient. A brush with a coronary attack is not pleasant, nor is the possibility of a recurrence cheering to contemplate, but the two in combination are usually enough to convince a patient, perhaps even more than his doctor's advice, that these essentially simple changes in his pattern of living may very well save his life.

Immediately after recovery from an attack, a

coronary patient must, of course, be very careful, but once the injured heart muscle has healed and he has regained his strength, there is no need for him to become a "cardiac cripple" who regards the possibility of recurrence with such fatalism that he does nothing to try to prevent it or, at the other extreme, becomes so incapacitated by fear and caution that all of the savor goes out of his life. The rule of moderation applies here perhaps better than anywhere else; the patient must make peace with his condition but at the same time do everything he can to prevent a recurrence. Then even if there is a recurrence, the deck will be stacked in his favor. Medical records show, in fact, that many victims of coronary thrombosis, among them President Dwight D. Eisenhower, successfully survived recurrent attacks and, by modifying their living patterns, went on to lead extraordinarily rich, long and productive lives.

The Fight Against Atherosclerosis

No one can be certain what promise future medical research may hold for the victims of atherosclerosis and coronary artery disease. Much of what has been learned in recent years is in the realm of probability rather than fact, and as is so often the case when science tackles a complex problem, new information has led to even more unanswered questions.

For example, there has been a great deal of research and study to try to determine the exact role of cholesterol in the body's metabolism and, more specifically, in the development of atherosclerosis. Hopes were high that some basic answers might emerge from this research, but the problem, unfortunately, is not that easy. While cholesterol is still believed to be an important factor in the development of the disease, and its reduction in the diet an important factor in preventing its progress, researchers have unearthed half a dozen quite different fatty or "lipid" substances in the body, including the triglycerides, that seem to be far more active than cholesterol in the formation of atheromatous deposits in artery walls, and the family of fatty substances known as *phospholipids*, some of which play a critical role in the structure and function of

nerve tissue. What is more, it was found that there is not necessarily any *direct* relationship between the intake of cholesterol or other fatty materials in the diet and the development of atheromatous lesions in artery walls. In fact, if cholesterol and various triglycerides are withheld from the diet in an attempt to lower the serum level of fatty materials, the body simply manufactures these materials by means of chemical reactions, in the liver and elsewhere, using carbohydrate and fatty building blocks already present in the body. Indeed, in a diet that is kept *too* low in fat, the triglyceride level in the blood serum is actually increased to a higher level than if moderate amounts of fat are consumed.

The search for medicines or drugs which might hinder or block the formation of these fatty substances has to date been quite disappointing. One type of drug was discovered that did seem to lower blood cholesterol levels, but it had to be withdrawn from general use because of untoward side effects. Other substances have proved either less effective or too costly. In another line of approach, researchers have recently found that the thyroid gland has a great influence on the way fats are handled and disposed of in the body, and early studies have suggested that the use of additional thyroid hormone by coronary-prone individuals over a long period of time may slow down or prevent the development of atherosclerosis. It has long been known that a metabolic condition known as *myxedema*, resulting from an extremely low production of thyroid hormone, is associated with rapidly progressing atherosclerosis, and that both conditions can be relieved by the administration of thyroid extracts as a medicine. There is even some reason to suspect that a person who has had myxedema and then is treated with an adequate level of thyroid hormone not only stops developing atherosclerosis, but may even reabsorb some of the fatty material already deposited in his arteries. But again, definite answers are not yet available, and this must still be regarded as an interesting and hopeful theory which has not, as yet, been proven.

A truly scientific study of a long-term disease process like atherosclerosis is also complicated by the fact that the laboratory animals frequently used in medical research simply do not develop this disease under normal conditions. Only the small primates—monkeys, for example —have a disease process anything like it. Thus man himself is the "laboratory animal" that must be studied closely for the final answers. At best, then, clinical research into the causes and prevention of atherosclerosis and its complications in humans is a long, slow and often frustrating process, a matter of putting together a huge, complex jigsaw puzzle only one small piece at a time.

Meanwhile, other investigators have been dealing with coronary artery disease much more directly, particularly in patients who have suffered such severe damage to all of their coronary arteries that they are literally living on the razor's edge and are certain to die very soon unless something dramatic can be done to relieve the condition. In such cases cardiovascular surgeons have sought new ways to supply blood to the endangered heart muscle. One technique involves the artificial abrasion of the pericardium surrounding the heart, or the outer surface of the heart itself, in order to stimulate the development of new blood vessels to help replace the damaged old ones. In another procedure, the surgeon removes damaged or occluded segments of the coronary artery and replaces them with grafts made from segments of the patient's own saphenous vein, a vein in the leg which is not vital to life. This latter operation has proved remarkably successful in providing the oxygen-hungry heart muscle with an adequate supply of blood.

More recently, individuals with intractable coronary artery disease, whose hearts have been irreparably damaged by myocardial infarctions due to coronary thrombosis, have had their damaged hearts removed entirely and replaced with young, undiseased hearts transplanted from donors who have died from unrelated causes— traffic accidents or brain injuries, for example. The long-term benefits or widespread applicability of this still highly experimental technique cannot yet be fully evaluated. The surgeons who have pioneered these operations are very enthusiastic about their eventual success, once surgical techniques have been perfected and once we have learned to control or prevent the body's rejection of these "spare parts." A few recipients of transplanted hearts have survived as long as three years or more, but many have eventually died because their bodies rejected the "foreign" heart. Some studies have indicated that transplanted hearts also may become atherosclerotic very rapidly, another problem that must be controlled. Thus, only with far more experience and year-by-year evaluation, coupled with the improved techniques necessary to overcome complicating problems, can we be certain about the long-term value of these operations.

Efforts to develop purely artificial, mechanical hearts—self-contained pumping machines which can be grafted into the chest to take over the whole function of a mortally damaged heart— are the object of another line of intense surgical research. Thus far, initial attempts to provide an artificial ventricle for pumping blood, for example, are still too recent for proper evaluation, and a completely mechanical heart implant has not yet been devised that meets all the necessary criteria to make this a hopeful or useful procedure. Many surgeons working in this area feel that a completely artificial heart is more likely to be perfected and prove permanently suitable than transplanted human hearts with their inherent problems. Both techniques are still in their infancy, however, and as revolutionary as they may seem to be, it is well to remember that many of today's safe, successful and even routine surgical procedures were not long ago considered totally impossible to perform.

The final answers to atherosclerosis and coronary artery disease are not yet in hand. These conditions are still widespread, and with hypertension, cancer and the final enemy, old age, they will in all probability remain among the four major causes of death in the Western world for many years to come. But there is reason to hope that the massive amounts of medical research devoted to their study will someday soon begin to bear fruit, perhaps even in our lifetimes.

PART

X

PATTERNS OF ILLNESS: THE DIGESTIVE TRACT

46. Digestive Function and Disease   609

47. Inflammatory Diseases of the Digestive System   630

48. Peptic Ulcer Disease and Intestinal Cancers   648

49. Diseases of the Pancreas, Liver and Gall Bladder   660

The ingestion and digestion of foodstuffs, their assimilation within the body and the elimination of unusable wastes are all functions of the human digestive system. Although the system is essentially a one-way tube passing through the body, these functions are extremely complicated and are performed by a number of complex and delicate organs and tissues. They involve both mechanical and chemical reactions which, in turn, depend upon the secretion of gastric juices and enzymes, and the presence of certain hormones and vitamins. The whole process is further regulated by voluntary and involuntary activities of the nervous system, and without the circulatory system to carry its end products to every living cell, the process would be useless. The complexity and interdependence of the system is perhaps best reflected by the variety of diseases and disorders that can impair its functions, and the variety of symptoms, some vague and mysterious, but many all too common and familiar, that these malfunctions can cause. Certainly we are more aware of digestive functions, both normal and abnormal, than of any other process in the body. But more important is an understanding of just how the digestive system works, and the kinds of illness that affect it as well as the symptoms they cause, if digestive disorders are to be prevented or effectively treated once they occur.

Digestive Function and Disease

No one could survive for long without taking in fluids and foods, converting them into the nutriments basic to the function of every living cell and, finally, ridding the body of wastes. These are the essential operations of the human digestive system; yet this is only the beginning of the story, for as simple as these operations may seem, they are carried on by a number of organs and tissues far more diverse in their structure and function than those of any other system. It is hardly surprising, then, that the digestive tract is the site of a greater variety of disorders and diseases than any other organ system of the body, extending from halitosis to hemorrhoids, with consequences ranging from the mildest temporary "stomach ache" to the sudden death that can follow the rupture of a gangrenous appendix with subsequent peritonitis. And associated with these disorders is an equal diversity of disagreeable symptoms—nausea, vomiting, cramps, gaseous distention, diarrhea, abdominal pain and many more.

As complex and important as the digestive system is, however, we can do without the function of many of its parts perfectly well for brief periods of time, and can even dispense with some parts altogether without suffering any particular discomfort or lasting damage. Our needs for food and fluids can be supplied temporarily by means of intravenous feedings, for example, by-passing the digestive tract entirely for days at a time. The gall bladder can be removed completely without seriously impairing digestive function, as can two-thirds of the stomach. Life can be maintained with as little as one-quarter of the liver in functioning condition, and from 40 to 50 percent of the small intestine and virtually all of the large intestine can be removed surgically, if necessary. Yet diseases of these selfsame, apparently "expendable" organs can make us thoroughly and chronically miserable, and when they do, paradoxically, the digestive system may function much better without them. Thus successful medical treatment does not always necessarily depend upon restoring normal or near-normal function, as it does with the body's other organ systems, and the reason for this is surely related to the amazing adaptability of the digestive system.

The Digestive Assembly Line

The digestive system is essentially a hollow, twisting tube or tunnel, extending from the mouth to the anus, through which fluids and food are passed in orderly assembly-line fashion from one processing station to the next. (*See* p. 84.) This tube is variously called the digestive or gastrointestinal (GI) tract or the alimentary canal. Some 900 years ago the Anglo-Saxons referred to it as the "gut" and, curiously enough, associated it with bravery and courage, possibly because they observed that nausea, vomiting or involuntary evacuation of the colon sometimes occurred in the presence of acute fear or panic; the terms "gutlessness" and "intestinal fortitude" or "gall" still have similar connotative meanings today. A modern surgeon also refers to it as the "gut," but without any reference to courage. The major component parts of the digestive tract are the mouth and pharynx, the esophagus, the sac-like stomach, a length of some 20 feet of small

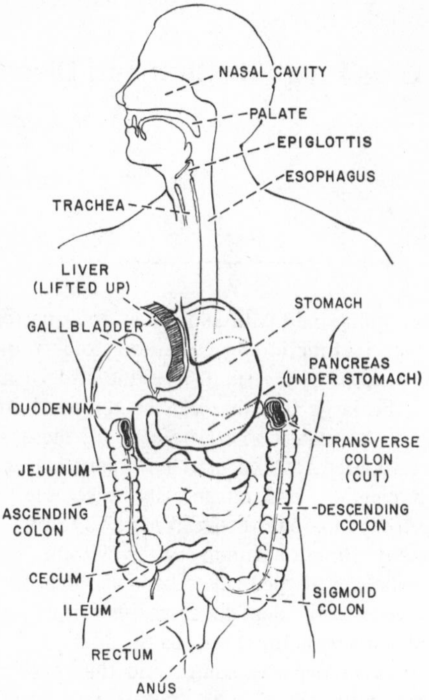

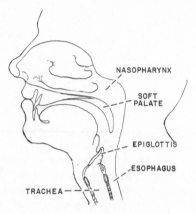

Figure 46–1.
The digestive system.

intestine, and another 5 feet or so of large intestine or colon. There are, in addition, several other organs and glands, including the pancreas, the liver and the gall bladder, that are not properly a part of the digestive tube but manufacture digestive juices that pour into the tube, and thus play important roles in the digestive function.

The "assembly-line" nature of the body's food-processing procedure or *digestion*, the main function of the digestive system, is not particularly complicated. The *mouth* and *pharynx* serve mainly as a receptacle for food materials, an area where they are softened and moistened and where larger fragments are torn apart by chewing. The *salivary glands*, located in each cheek just in front of the ear (the parotid glands) and in the lower jaw underneath the tongue (the submaxillary and sublingual glands), are stimu-

lated to produce saliva by either the odor or the taste of food, and the saliva itself then enhances the taste of food by dissolving various chemical constituents to which the taste buds located on

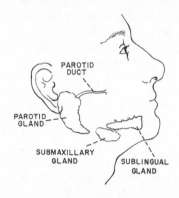

Figure 46–2A.
Structure of the mouth and throat.

the top and sides of the tongue react. An enzyme in the saliva known as *ptyalin* even begins the digestive process by starting to break down starches in the food into simpler components. Not many years ago it was thought that this function of the saliva, aided by thorough and complete chewing, was extremely important to the digestive process, and everyone was exhorted

Figure 46–2B.
The salivary glands.

to chew all ingested food to a pulp before swallowing it. Today we know that neither of these functions has any great importance, other than to moisten food slightly and break it down into smaller pieces so that it can be swallowed and passed down the relatively narrow esophagus. The person who wolfs down his food in great unchewed chunks ultimately manages to digest it just as efficiently as someone who chews each bite 27 times.

The *tongue* contributes greatly to our enjoyment of food by registering intermixtures of salt, sweet, sour and bitter flavors by means of the taste buds, several thousand of them, each equipped with special sensory nerve endings. These "flavor signals" from the tongue, combined with the "odor signals" from the nose, account for our sense of taste. The tongue also contributes to the act of swallowing, a semi-involuntary act which occurs when food contacts the *uvula*, the tag of tissue hanging down from the back of the soft palate. This contact triggers a contraction of muscles in the pharynx and the base of the tongue that forces food back and into the upper end of the esophagus, while another flap of tissue, the *epiglottis*, moves to cover the adjacent opening to the trachea and prevent food from inadvertently going down the windpipe.

The *esophagus* is a long, narrow and rather finicky tube that connects the mouth and pharynx with the stomach, passing down the neck and chest, through a natural opening in the musculature of the diaphragm, and terminating at the top of the stomach in a sort of circular "purse-string" muscle, the *cardiac sphincter,* which opens and closes to allow food to pass. Once in the *stomach,* a J-shaped organ about ten inches long that lies horizontally in the upper abdomen, food is mixed thoroughly with quantities of acidic gastric juice produced by special cells in the wall of the stomach, as well as with certain enzymes including *pepsin* which helps begin the breakdown of meat fibers into protein molecules and their component amino acids. The muscular walls of the stomach churn to aid in this process, but the real work of digestion occurs not in the stomach, which acts more as a receptacle, but in the *duodenum,* the upper ten inches of the small intestine. The two are separated by a powerful muscle, the *pyloric sphincter,* which, again, opens and closes to allow food to pass. The acidic food-and-fluid mixture in the

stomach is released into the duodenum a little at a time, stimulating the secretion of digestive juices from the pancreas, the liver and the lining of the small intestine itself. Secretions from the *pancreas,* which empty into the duodenum through the *pancreatic duct,* are highly alkaline and contain powerful enzymes which contribute to the final breakdown of protein and carbohydrates and, to a lesser extent, fats. *Bile,* manufactured by the *liver,* reaches the duodenum by a more circuitous route, traveling from the liver by two *hepatic ducts* which unite to form the *common bile duct.* The *gall bladder* is also connected to this duct and serves to store and concentrate the bile, which is released during digestion and acts in the breakdown of fatty materials in the intestines. The presence of fatty materials in the duodenum causes the gall bladder to contract and squeeze its concentrated contents of bile into the common bile duct and thence into the duodenum.

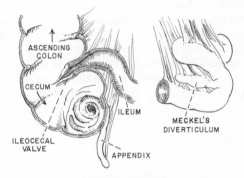

Figure 46–3.

At this point the long passage of digesting food down the small intestine begins. Once food materials have been broken down into simpler substances the body can use, they are absorbed by the *villi,* tiny finger-like projections that line the small intestine in a sort of velvety nap. The villi are rich in blood and lymph vessels, and digested food materials are absorbed and transported through these vessels to every living cell in the body. This process takes place almost exclusively in the small intestine, although some food materials, chiefly alcohol, are absorbed into the blood stream directly from the stomach.

Starches and complex sugars, which have been broken down into simple sugars such as glucose, are absorbed into the tiny capillaries in the villi. Protein materials, now in the form of some 20 different kinds of amino acids, are also absorbed in this way. But fats, most resistant of all foods to digestion, are ultimately split into component fatty acids and absorbed chiefly by the lymph vessels in the villi.

By the time the food reaches the large intestine or *colon,* little remains other than water and indigestible fragments of fiber, gristle, seeds, etc., but even here a lively population of intestinal bacteria attack the remains of the food, a sort of final filtering in search of useful material. These normal colon bacteria also contribute to the production of vitamin K—a vital link in the clotting mechanism of the blood—which is absorbed through the walls of the colon into the blood stream. The first part of the colon, which is normally located in the right lower quadrant of the abdomen (*see* Fig. 46–1), is a pouchlike receptacle known as the *cecum,* separated from the lower end of the small intestine by a flap of tissue, the *ileocecal valve.* It is from the cecum that the *vermiform appendix,* the site of acute appendicitis, protrudes like a tail. As the debris from digestion passes through the cecum and on along the colon, any excess of fluid is reabsorbed

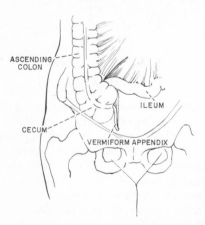

Figure 46–4A.

and the remaining detritus is packed into a semisolid mass in the *rectum*—technically the lower eight or ten inches of the colon—ready for

evacuation. At the end of the rectum is the *anal canal,* approximately two inches long and terminating in the *anus,* which is equipped with both

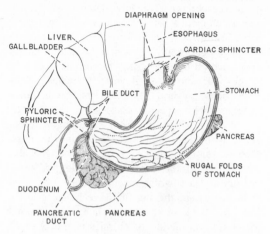

Figure 46–4B.

internal and external sphincter muscles that can be voluntarily controlled to help prevent untimely evacuation of fecal matter.

Disorders of Digestion

Obviously quite a number of different functions take place on the digestive assembly line, and quite a number of different organs are involved in the process. There is, however, a considerable "margin for error" built into the process, so that a disease or disorder that affects only a small part of the system may go virtually unnoticed at first. On the other hand, those disorders, even very minor ones, that interfere with the overall digestive process, rather than with just a particular part, can be acutely symptomatic.

For example, a highly important part of the digestive function is the mechanism by which ingested foods are moved along the digestive assembly line. This motion is made possible by the peculiar muscular structure of the walls of the digestive tract; two separate layers of muscle encase the gut from top to bottom, one layer longitudinal and the other circular. This muscle is beyond the control of the will and normally will contract when stimulated by the presence of food, or even at a time when food *ought* to be present. The wavelike muscular contractions, known as *peristalsis,* squeeze ingested food down the entire length of the digestive tract, and any disorder that interferes with these contractions, or obstructs the passage of food material in some way, can profoundly affect the whole digestive process. Similarly, any disorder which in any way impairs the absorption of digested food materials through the intestinal lining can defeat the chief purpose of digestion. These so-called malabsorption diseases are relatively few and rare, but they are seriously debilitating when they occur.

Digestive tract organs, like all other parts of the body, are also liable to bacterial or viral infection and parasitic infestation, but there are a number of other inflammatory conditions of the upper or lower intestine which are not necessarily related to invading organisms at all. Certain highly prevalent inflammations of the digestive tract, for example, are caused at least in part by the oversecretion of digestive juices. Such disorders can range all the way from the simplest and most innocuous attack of acid indigestion to the dangerous and sometimes fatal peptic ulcer disease. In addition, the digestive tract is vulnerable to the development of cancers, particularly in the stomach, the pancreas, or the colon. Fortunately, these cancers very frequently cause early symptoms, or can be detected in the course of a routine physical examination or on X-rays, and it is in the treatment of such cancers that modern medicine has made some of its greatest strides in the struggle to conquer this kind of disease.

Proper digestion also depends upon the secretions of various glandular organs such as the pancreas and liver, as well as on the function of the gall bladder and the bile and pancreatic ducts which store or carry these secretions. Some of the most serious disorders of the digestive system are those which afflict these secreting organs or prevent digestive secretions from reaching the intestine. And, finally, certain anorectal disorders may be relatively unimportant to the digestive function, but are of decided importance to the victim and can be among the most aggravating and painful of all digestive tract illnesses.

Most diseases and disorders of the digestive system are unquestionably physical, but there are also others which, while they may cause unmistakable physical symptoms, nevertheless have very strong emotional or psychosomatic overtones. No one knows why the digestive tract is so vulnerable to the effects of such nonphysical disorders as fright, anxiety, neurosis, or physical and emotional tension. But the distinct connection between digestive function and various emotional states has been recognized for centuries, both in man and in animals, sometimes to the degree of extreme physical disability. For example, the secretion of gastric acid in a dog's stomach and the motility of his digestive tract come to a standstill if he is suddenly frightened, angry, physically attacked, or otherwise disturbed. We may chuckle at the claim by some dairy companies that their products are superior because they come from contented cows, but the fact is that a *discontented* cow does not graze and digest its food properly, and thus produces milk of poorer quality and in smaller than normal amounts. Thankfully, there are relatively few things that make a cow discontented.

Human beings suffer a very similar interrelationship between emotional tension and digestive function. When we become angry or frightened, we "lose our appetite"; when we are physically exhausted or emotionally tense, we tend to hypersecrete gastric acid and suffer such annoying symptoms as indigestion, heartburn, sometimes even nausea and gaseous distention. One of the most prevalent and disabling of all human illnesses, peptic ulcer disease, almost invariably has a strong factor of emotional tension involved in its development; and a number of other digestive illnesses are either related to emotional tension at their onset or are aggravated and complicated by the effects of emotional tension. This does not by any means imply that such diseases are all "mental" and therefore not real. There is nothing unreal about the seriously debilitating symptoms that they sometimes cause. Nevertheless, emotional tension does play such a critical role in their development that they cannot be effectively treated without dealing with both the physical symptoms and the emotional factors that contribute to the illness.

Thus, the digestive system is not only vulnerable to a great many different kinds of physical illness, but is also a sort of psychosomatic stamping ground in the human body—a "target organ system" where the effects of physical and emotional tension very commonly make themselves felt. Even today the true nature of many digestive diseases is not fully understood, yet it is an area in which modern medicine has made perhaps the greatest strides of all in diagnosis and effective treatment.

Disorders of Digestive Motility

At one time in the not too distant past, the movement of the bowels on a regular schedule was considered an infallible bellwether of the health or disorder of the digestive system. Mothers watched their children like hawks to see that they remained "regular," and laxatives at one end and enemas at the other were forced upon perfectly healthy youngsters who happened to have slightly sluggish bowels. Even grown men and women regarded their own bowel movements with apprehension; at the first hint of constipation, laxatives and "roughage foods" were consumed, and if evacuations were too frequent or loose, there was bismuth-with-paregoric to fall back on.

Much of that concern was based on ignorance; it was then a prevalent theory that all sorts of vile toxins and poisons would be absorbed back into the body if fecal matter were allowed to remain impacted in the colon for too long, and the uncomfortable, distended and heavy feeling that so often accompanies constipation was cited as confirmation of this theory. Today we know better and regard constipation as more of an annoyance than a danger. But we also now know that many disorders of the digestive system are indeed accompanied by disturbances in the normal movement of food, not only in the colon but in the esophagus, the stomach and the small intestine as well. Some disorders, for example, can cause the motility of the stomach or the intestine to cease temporarily, and very real

distress results unless normal motility is restored. In fact, any condition which in any way obstructs the flow of food materials through the digestive system will very quickly be followed by acute symptoms and sometimes very serious consequences. Motility is absolutely essential for continued healthy digestive function, and although the degree of motility varies throughout the day, and from day to day, any disturbance in the normal pattern is soon called to our attention by a variety of symptoms—nausea, vomiting, distention, abdominal pain, cramps, constipation or diarrhea—and relief comes only when motility is restored.

Normal Motility Disorders. Certain phenomena associated with peristaltic movement of the digestive tract, although noticeable, cannot be considered disorders or abnormalities. The familiar "lump in the throat," for example, is an odd sensation associated with emotional responses such as fear, anxiety, nostalgia, sadness or sense of loss. This sensation is partly due to involuntary peristaltic action in the upper end of the esophagus, while part is also engendered by a sudden increase in heartbeat. Similarly, there is a normal touch-sensitive reaction known as the "gag reflex" which induces us either to swallow or to gag when some foreign material touches the uvula and the back of the throat; in some individuals this reflex is triggered by attempting to swallow *any* unfamiliar substance or by a real or imagined aversion to some food. Hence the child who literally cannot eat his spinach, or the person who cannot swallow even the smallest pill unless it is crushed up in a teaspoon and mixed with a bit of water.

Certain other reflexes related to digestive function are also familiar and perfectly normal. When we smell delicious food being cooked, we tend to salivate, but the same stimulus triggers active peristaltic churning of the empty stomach which creates a sensation commonly recognized as hunger. "Hunger pangs" may become quite acute, but if unsatisfied for a prolonged period of time, the peristaltic activity causing the sensation usually subsides. The sensation of thirst is related to the activity of the salivary glands which, when the body's water content is at an acceptable level, keep the pharynx moist. But when water content decreases, salivation also decreases and the pharynx dries, stimulating thirst. In addition, individuals occasionally feel a sense of food "sticking" in their throats, usually an indication that a morsel of swallowed food is too large or insufficiently moistened. In some cases there may be quite severe pain in the midchest if the food swallowed actually is too large to pass through the esophagus comfortably, and as in any other part of the digestive tract, the stretching of the esophageal tube is detected by special sensory nerve endings and transmitted as a pain signal.

Our awareness of normal peristaltic activity, however, is not confined to the throat, esophagus or stomach. Everyone tends to swallow a certain amount of air with his food, some a great deal more than others, and this air mixed with food is carried along the digestive tract by peristaltic activity, accounting for the familiar gurglings and rumblings which occur in the stomach or intestine. Belching is one way of expelling this swallowed air; but if great quantities are swallowed, or foods are eaten which tend to generate intestinal gas, some of it is quite normally expelled as gas or *flatus* from the anus.

Finally, some kinds of intestinal motility, while not strictly speaking "normal," serve a useful purpose, often as a defense mechanism. Reverse peristalsis, or vomiting, occurs when the wavelike muscular activity in the walls of the digestive tract suddenly changes direction, ejecting the contents of the stomach into the mouth. Although any number of other factors can cause this reaction, it most often occurs when one has ingested some food or other substance that is highly irritating to the lining of the stomach.

Disorders of Motility in the Upper Digestive Tract. There are a number of disorders that may result from an interruption or an obstruction of the motility of the esophagus, stomach or upper intestine. Some of these disorders are minor, others much more serious, but even though all are accompanied by relatively familiar symptoms, they are not normal and, in many cases, demand medical attention.

Esophageal spasm, for example, occurs occasionally if a swallowed bit of food is so large that it is arrested at some point in the esophagus.

Such a spasm can be quite painful until it is relieved by taking water to help ease the chunk of food down or, conversely, until it is regurgitated. Esophageal spasm is usually no more than a transitory annoyance that can stem from either physical or emotional factors; however, occasionally a child is born with a congential narrowing of part of the esophagus, a condition known as *esophageal atresia,* and suffers this spastic pain whenever food is swallowed. In such cases careful and gradual mechanical dilatation of the esophagus may relieve the defect, providing all of the neuromuscular mechanisms needed for peristalsis are intact. If the nerves that stimulate peristalsis are also absent, a surgical procedure may be necessary to remove the abnormal segment of esophagus, replacing it with a portion of the small intestine.

Esophageal spasm may also result when some caustic poison is ingested and causes a chemical burn of the esophageal lining. When the injury heals, it tends to scar, making the damaged part of the esophagus somewhat rigid and less able to expand to accommodate swallowed food. In such cases, mechanical dilatation of the damaged or *stenosed* area of the esophagus may be required. Many modern medicines can also be highly irritating to delicate mucous membranes, and if they are taken with insufficient water, they can actually burn or ulcerate the esophageal lining. Even common aspirin can cause an extremely painful burn of the esophagus if the tablets are taken dry and become lodged partway down. Such a burn may result in a continuing aching pain felt in the chest somewhere below the throat, with marked increase of pain when anything, even water, is swallowed. An esophageal burn may take several days to heal, and it is necessary to confine the diet to soft or liquid foods in small quantities until healing takes place. Thus it is far better to avoid this kind of problem by being certain that medicines are taken with ample water.

Similar to esophageal spasm is a condition known as *cardiospasm,* in which the cardiac sphincter, the circular muscle separating the esophagus from the stomach, goes into spasm, usually as a result of irritation from excess gastric secretions. The pain of cardiospasm can be sharp and severe, but will ordinarily respond to a dose of antacid medicine. Drugs of the atropine family are also often prescribed, but they seldom prove any more effective than a simple antacid.

A *hiatus hernia* is a surprisingly common and often serious disorder of motility in the upper digestive tract. In this condition, which is also known as esophageal hernia or diaphragmatic hernia, the lower end of the esophagus and the upper portion of the stomach tend to push or *herniate* upward through the diaphragm so that the upper part of the stomach is actually above the diaphragm in the thoracic cavity. The disorder may result from congenital weakness of the muscle fibers of the diaphragm in the region where the esophagus normally passes through into the abdomen. It may also stem from an injury, or it may come on gradually through the stretching or relaxation of the muscle fibers in this area. Hiatus hernia may afflict women who have had several babies, because of the abdominal stretching and the increased abdominal pressures that are present during labor and childbirth. Obesity, advancing age and chronic coughing are also contributing factors. Two different types of hiatus hernias can occur. Most common is the so-called *sliding* type in which the esophagus just seems too short and remains permanently above the diaphragm, holding the top part of the stomach with it. Less common is the so-called *rolling* or *paraesophageal* type of hernia, in which the esophagus remains attached to the stomach below the diaphragm, but a part of the stomach pouch rolls up through the diaphragm alongside the esophagus.

In recent years gastroenterologists have become convinced that hiatus hernias are far more prevalent than was once believed, but often are not detected simply because the great majority of them are completely asymptomatic. When symptoms do occur, they are mainly a result of irritation of the delicate mucous membranes of the esophagus by regurgitated stomach acid that the esophageal lining is not normally in contact with. Thus the most common early symptoms, when any at all appear, are those of gastric hyperacidity, including *heartburn*—an uncom-

fortable searing sort of pain that seems to start in the upper abdomen and work its way up to the back of the throat—a certain amount of dull

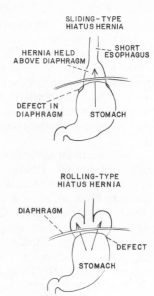

Figure 46–5.

pain in the upper abdomen, and a feeling of fullness which begins soon after eating and then spontaneously goes away after a few minutes to an hour. Sometimes there is belching or hiccuping as well. These symptoms, which are caused by the sloshing or regurgitation of acid gastric juices into the esophagus due to the position of the herniated part of the stomach as well as to increased intra-abdominal pressure, are often worse when the victim is lying down, and are relieved when he stands up. Once they appear, symptoms tend to become progressively more severe, and presently may be triggered by food or drink of all kinds; the heartburn and cardiospasm may be relieved temporarily by taking antacids, but tend to recur again with each meal. If the irritation of the lower esophagus is sufficiently great, there may be frank bleeding from the raw eroded tissue, sometimes accompanied by vomiting of blood. With repeated episodes of ulceration and erosion occurring over a prolonged interval, the lower end of the esophagus may become severely scarred, and stenosis (hardening) and stricturing (narrowing) may occur. In advanced cases, surgical treatment may be the only solution.

Diagnosis of a symptomatic hiatus hernia depends upon a series of X-rays of the upper gastrointestinal tract for which the patient ingests a suspension of radio-opaque material such as barium sulfate. He is then examined under the fluoroscope by the radiologist, who by changing the patient's position and applying pressure to the abdomen can often demonstrate the portion of the stomach herniating through the diaphragm into the chest. The fact that a hiatus hernia is found on X-ray, however, does not necessarily mean that it is the sole cause of the symptoms or the bleeding. A thorough examination of the entire esophagus, stomach and small bowel must be performed by X-ray to rule out some other source of the symptoms, particularly if there is evidence of bleeding. Other diagnostic procedures include testing to detect acid gastric juice in the lower end of the esophagus when pressure is applied to the abdomen and direct inspection of the esophagus with a long, narrow lighted instrument known as an *esophagoscope*.

In the vast majority of cases, hiatus hernia can be treated conservatively in order to relieve the distressing symptoms. Since these are due to irritation or inflammation of the lower end of the esophagus, a condition that is aggravated by overfilling the stomach at mealtime, bland, non-irritative foods are prescribed in frequent small feedings—perhaps as many as six a day rather than three larger meals a day—with a good antacid used at regular intervals between meals. If obesity is a contributing factor, weight reduction is important, and if a chronic cough is also present, it should also be investigated and treated. Finally, the patient should try to avoid exercise that involves bending forward, as this movement tends to increase intra-abdominal pressure and push the stomach up through the diaphragm more readily. Carried out faithfully, such a treatment program will relieve symptoms in most cases, and if they do not later recur, nothing more need be done. In short, a hiatus hernia is a physical defect, but it is not one which has to be surgically repaired just because

it is there, and it is not a precursor of some more serious condition as long as it remains without symptoms.

If conservative treatment fails, if symptoms recur, or if there is a recurrent complication such as bleeding from the irritated segment of the esophagus, then surgical repair of the hernia is indicated. In theory the surgical task is relatively simple: the surgeon brings the herniated part of the stomach down below the diaphragm and then closes the defect in the diaphragm by suturing the diaphragmatic muscle snugly around the esophagus. In fact, however, the surgery is major in scope because this area is relatively inaccessible and the surgeon must make a wide incision either in the abdomen or through the thorax in order to reach the region of the disorder.

In some cases surgical repair is complicated by the discovery of a relatively short esophagus or an esophagus scarred and hardened by repeated inflammation and healing. Recently surgeons have sought to resolve this problem by removing the damaged part of the esophagus and using a segment of the middle portion of the small intestine, known as the *jejunum,* to replace it. This is a very extensive surgical procedure, but so far it has achieved remarkably good results. Even in uncomplicated cases surgical treatment is not always entirely successful, but perhaps 80 percent of the patients so treated are relieved of symptoms and recurrences permanently, or at least show marked improvement in terms of fewer symptoms and less frequent recurrences.

Acute gastric dilatation is another disorder of motility of the upper digestive tract which is probably far more common than was once suspected. The neuromuscular mechanisms that make intestinal motility possible are very delicate, sensitive to many stimuli, and often respond to abnormal stimuli by "freezing in their tracks," as if they operated under a standing order of "when in doubt, stop." Thus, during the first 72 hours or so following major abdominal or pelvic surgery, motility of the stomach and upper intestine comes almost to a complete halt. This cessation of motility is a useful indicator to the surgeon, for the resumption of so-called

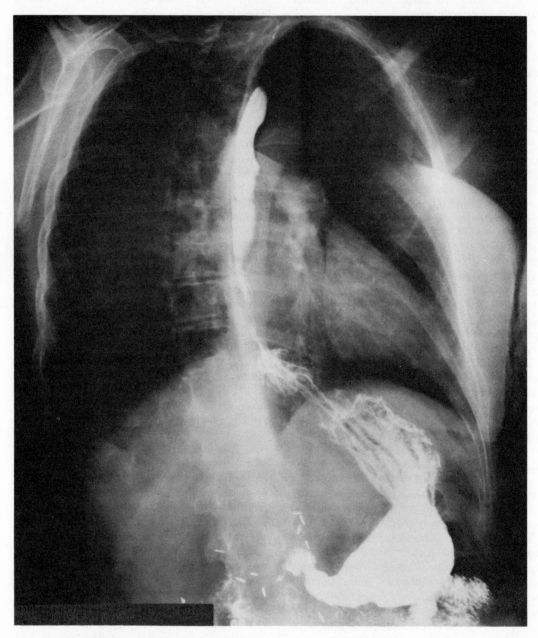

Plate 30   Severe scarring and narrowing of the lower segment of the esophagus. In this case
the condition arose from prolonged irritation of the esophagus by regurgitated
gastric acids associated with a hiatus hernia. (See Chapter 46, p. 618). (X-ray courtesy of David B. Hurlbut, M.D.)

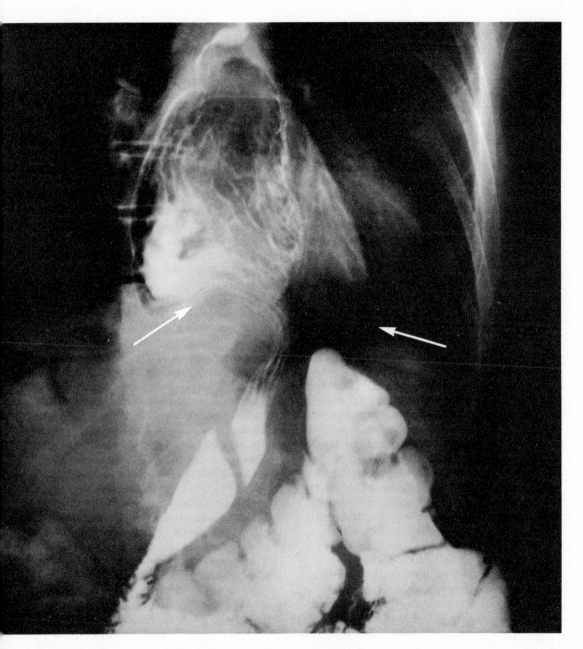

Plate 31   A huge hiatus hernia. Much of the stomach, lined with radio-opaque barium sulphate suspension, is pushed above the diaphragm. Approximate level of the diaphragm is indicated by the arrows.

bowel sounds following surgery is usually a sign that there are no internal complications and that the patient is on the road to recovery. Unfortunately, most patients tend to swallow air whether or not they are taking any food or fluid by mouth, and since the stomach begins pouring out gastric juice as a result of increasing distention caused by the swallowed air, the whole upper gastrointestinal tract may become acutely and painfully distended with gas and fluid. To avoid this situation, which can result in a serious loss of body fluid and electrolytes if unchecked, and may even lead to shock or death, surgeons today almost invariably pass a narrow rubber or plastic suction tube known as a *Levin tube* down the esophagus and into the stomach as part of the patient's preoperative preparation, and then leave it there to remove gas and secretions until bowel tones return.

But gastric dilatation is not a condition limited to postoperative patients. It can also happen to anyone who subjects his stomach to noxious substances that cause irritation of the gastric lining, or who ingests far more food at a time than the stomach can comfortably hold. The victim of acute gastric dilatation typically becomes ill following a large holiday dinner or a party at which quantities of unusual and spicy foods were consumed. Alcoholic beverages, notorious as gastric irritants, are often part of the picture, causing inflammation of the stomach lining so that too much food eaten too fast along with a number of drinks may be the overpowering blow that signals the cessation of gastric motility. The condition comes on quickly and the victim becomes aware of a sense of overfullness, a feeling of distention in the upper abdomen, and then progressively severe pain, accompanied by an urge to vomit but an inability to do so.

In many cases acute dilatation of the stomach is not this extreme and may be markedly relieved simply by taking a teaspoonful of bicarbonate of soda mixed in half a glass of warm water—one of the rare instances in which bicarbonate of soda is to be recommended as an antacid. It brings relief not only by neutralizing excess stomach acid but also by reacting with it to form carbon dioxide gas which can be expelled by belching, carrying quantities of swallowed air along with it. In fact, a mild case may subside before it becomes particularly painful. The victim should not delay too long, however, in seeking a doctor's aid if the pain and distention become acute or if a single attempt at relief with bicarbonate of soda does not produce prompt results. The trouble is that a vicious circle may be established: the stretching of the stomach walls causes increased irritation which further diminishes gastric motility, and the stomach dilates still more from swallowed air and an outpouring of gastric secretions. In such severe cases a doctor's attention is needed quickly, since the victim may well go into shock, and the stomach must be evacuated by means of a Levin tube or a stomach pump. Once the pressure is relieved, adherence to a light diet of nonalcoholic fluids and soft bland foods in small quantities will allow the timid and overtaxed stomach and intestine to recover and hesitantly begin motility again. Obviously, common sense dictates that the best treatment is prevention; sensible eating habits are invariably preferable to a rendezvous with a stomach pump.

Motility Disorders in the Small and Large Intestine. Scientists find it convenient to divide the small intestine into three segments: the *duodenum* or first segment, which joins the stomach and is slightly less than a foot long; the *jejunum* or middle segment, which is about eight feet long and is the "digestive" portion of the intestine; and the *ileum* or "absorptive" portion, which is about twelve feet long and narrows finally to join the large intestine. A number of motility disorders of the small intestine fall more in the category of normal reactions to stress than in the category of disease. Surgical manipulation of the bowel, for example, causes a cessation of intestinal motility. So also do a variety of emotional states including sudden surprise, fright, anxiety or any situation of stress or threat. When intestinal motility slows down or stops, there may be symptoms of abdominal distention as loops of the bowel become filled with gas; the intestine appears to be temporarily paralyzed, and indeed this condition is often spoken of as *paralytic ileus*. While such a condition is normally transitory, periods of prolonged stress such as military conflict, preparation for college examinations or chronic emotional tension may lead to intermittent episodes of intestinal irritation on the one hand and paralytic ileus or distention on the other.

The large intestine or colon is also influenced by such real but ephemeral emotional tensions. Even such a simple and innocuous thing as changing from familiar to unfamiliar surroundings may precipitate an intestinal motility reaction. The most common symptoms of these reactions are diarrhea and constipation. Both conditions can vary widely in severity, but they are symptoms that stem from any number of causes, and while some relief can be obtained by treating the symptoms, it is also necessary to discover and treat the root cause.

Diarrhea is a familiar symptom of a variety of digestive disorders. It may be stimulated by viral or bacterial infection of the intestine, or infestation with intestinal parasites, but a number of other disease conditions in the body completely unrelated to the digestive system may also cause diarrhea as one of the symptoms—diseases such as kidney failure, Addison's disease, acute thryoiditis, congestive heart failure or lead poisoning, to mention only a few. Finally, diarrhea may be largely a reaction to emotional stress or an irritative reaction to various foods. So-called tourist's diarrhea is often the result of a combination of emotional, irritative and infectious factors. (*See* p. 255.)

Diarrhea is never a normal occurrence in the body, and when it is persistent, efforts should be made to investigate the cause. In most cases it arises because something irritates the intestine and causes abnormally increased motility, so that stools are passed before excess fluid can be reabsorbed in the colon. Many common laxatives are intestinal irritants and act on this principle. More rarely, as in cases of cholera (*see* p. 258), some infectious agent attacks the lining of the small intestine in such a way that its normal capacity to absorb substances into the blood stream is reversed, and instead body fluids are drawn out of the blood stream and into the intestine in great quantity. Vast amounts of fluid can be lost very quickly in this way, posing the serious threat of *dehydration*. Whichever factor

is at work, if diarrhea is too frequent or too prolonged, it can lead to a sharp loss of body fluids and dissolved electrolytes such as salt, potassium chloride or magnesium. Most adults can tolerate considerable dehydration and salt depletion due to diarrhea without any dangerous or lasting effect. In a severe case of intestinal flu, for example, an adult may lose as much as ten or fifteen pounds in the course of a few days, almost all of it water from the body's tissues. But that fluid can be very rapidly regained in a matter of two or three days. In an infant or small child, however, the loss of body fluid and electrolytes due to diarrhea can very swiftly reach dangerous proportions; indeed, one of the most common causes of death in infants and children is acute dehydration that occurs from diarrhea which may itself stem from a perfectly innocuous cause. These children's lives could be saved simply by recognizing that diarrhea can cause a child to become dangerously dehydrated in a matter of a few hours, and by seeking medical care *before* the telltale symptoms begin to appear. (*See* p. 865.)

People have the impression that diarrhea has some beneficial effect in terms of ridding the body of harmful agents. Perhaps so; certainly irritating foods or spices in the intestine are expelled, and diarrhea can also rid the body of offending organisms. But the danger of dehydration effectively outweighs any benefit the diarrhea may produce, and when diarrhea is copious or persistent, whatever its cause, a doctor should be consulted.

The classical symptomatic treatment for mild diarrhea is the administration of a bland bulking agent such as a suspension of kaolin, a chalky or powdery substance, and pectin, a vegetable gel. This suspension is the basis of most of the antidiarrhea medicines available over the counter. For more persistent diarrhea another old standby is tincture of paregoric—or more accurately, camphorated tincture of opium—which will slow down diarrhea because of the long-recognized ability of opium or opium derivatives such as morphine to suppress intestinal motility very sharply. More recently a number of newly developed drugs which contain no opiates have been developed to suppress diarrhea by interfering temporarily with the transmission of involuntary nerve impulses to the intestinal muscle. One such neuromuscular blocking agent, diphenoxylate hydrochloride, combined with atropine (also capable of reducing intestinal motility) and prepared under the brand name of Lomotil, has proven highly effective. In some people it brings about a temporary cessation of intestinal motility as suddenly and effectively as if someone had thrown a switch. Lomotil is particularly useful, under a doctor's guidance, in stopping infant diarrhea that threatens to produce dehydration, and it was the medicine taken along by the Apollo astronauts on their Moon voyages, a situation in which diarrhea might have been both uncomfortable and inconvenient.

Constipation lies at the opposite end of the spectrum of intestinal motility, or lack of it. Everyone has suffered from this annoying condition, in which the stools are excessively dry and the evacuation of the bowel occurs at longer than normal intervals and then only with difficulty, leaving the individual with a sense of incomplete emptying. In most cases constipation, if it is really present at all, is far less important than most people think it is; there is no natural law that says a person must have a bowel movement every day, and considering the wide variety of foods we eat and our often erratic eating habits, it is hardly surprising that some bowel irregularities result. Various factors may contribute to the condition: dehydration of the body during a feverish illness, for example, or emotional disturbances that affect normal intestinal motility. When one does suffer constipation to the point of being uncomfortable, it is easy to compound the problem by worrying about it, and the frequent use of laxatives to stimulate evacuation can all too often lead to a situation in which the bowels will not move at all without chemical stimulation. On the other hand, excessive straining at stool in cases of constipation can be dangerous; it increases both the blood pressure and pressure within the abdomen quite markedly and has been known to precipitate strokes or coronary attacks.

Often constipation can be relieved by eating naturally laxative foods such as bran flakes, baked beans or fruit, and drinking copious quan-

tities of water. If the condition occurs frequently, or if, as in a pregnant woman, there is some mechanical reason for constipation to become a bother, the use of a bulking agent such as Metamucil is a better solution than frequent resort to a laxative. Such agents, usually taken in the form of a powdered gel mixed with a small amount of water, tend to absorb water and expand in size, mixing with the fecal matter as it forms, and helping stimulate a normal defecation reflex when the soft but bulky mass reaches the lower end of the colon. If a laxative must be used, a simple and mild one such as milk of magnesia taken at night before retiring is preferable to the more potent household standbys such as castor oil, cascara or Epsom salts.

For all of this, persisting or recurring constipation should not be ignored without first checking out possible causes. Constipation in children is more often a figment of the mother's imagination than a disorder of the child's colon, and may indeed be made significantly worse by the mother's worry about it. Nevertheless, there are occasional children who have some physical basis for constipation. For example, a child might have a congenital condition in which a segment of the bowel does not have the neuromuscular connections necessary for intestinal motility, and this "nonenervated" segment of the colon stands as an unmoving ring or stricture behind which fecal matter tends to pile up. This condition, known as Hirschsprung's disease or *congenital megacolon,* may go undiagnosed for years, and the colon above the inert segment gradually becomes massively dilated. The child will have bowel movements infrequently, suffer from continuous discomfort due to distention between bowel movements, and evacuate an enormous quantity on the rare occasions when bowel movements do occur. The presence of a megacolon can usually be determined quite readily by examination of colon X-rays, and the condition can be cured surgically by removing the inert segment of bowel and suturing the active segments above and below it together again.

Occasionally in adults constipation is a result of some mechanical obstruction in the colon, such as a tumor, or of some disorder of the anorectal area such as thrombosed hemorrhoids, a fissure or a fistula which makes bowel movements so painful that the victim habitually avoids them for as long as possible. In cases of chronic or recurrent constipation, careful examination of the anorectal area and of the lower segment of the colon with a proctoscope is indicated. Colon X-rays should also be taken to help identify disorders higher up in the colon. In the absence of any illness that might be causative, most cases of constipation can be resolved quite readily by embarking upon a program of good eating habits combined with regular bowel habits.

Patent laxatives and enemas should be avoided except in the case of bedridden patients whose bowel habits are greatly disrupted. One complication of constipation which occasionally occurs to a patient who is suddenly put to bed to recover from an illness is the formation of a *fecal impaction,* a hard, dehydrated lump of feces which cannot be evacuated and which prevents evacuation of new fecal matter entering the colon. Fecal impactions may be softened by use of an *oil retention enema,* installation of several ounces of mineral oil into the rectum, to be held for an hour or more to soften the stool before evacuation.

Irritable colon or *irritable bowel syndrome* is a vaguely defined but very commonplace disorder that occurs somewhere in the no man's land between diarrhea and constipation. The condition is also sometimes called spastic colon, hypertonic constipation, intestinal neurosis or even nervous indigestion. It has been estimated that this annoying condition accounts for fully 50 percent of all disorders of the digestive system, and some authorities maintain that, aside from the common cold, irritable bowel syndrome is responsible for more of mankind's minor disabilities than any other single entity. Oddly enough, most people have never heard of it, and although virtually everyone has suffered from it at one time or another, certain individuals develop attacks of it so severe and so recurrently irritating that medical attention is necessary. Unfortunately, symptoms are so various that the disorder can mimic virtually any other digestive tract disturbance known, and

victims of the disorder often have a discouragingly long and tedious history of repeated diagnostic workups done by a long succession of different doctors, none of whom succeeds in pinpointing the actual cause of the distress. This is not entirely the fault of the physician, for irritable bowel syndrome is perhaps the most completely functional or psychosomatic of all digestive tract disorders. Its victims are often tense, nervous, anxious and irritable, which makes them vulnerable to the condition in the first place, and often unwilling to persevere with the diagnostic studies and therapeutic programs that might ultimately resolve it.

The symptoms of irritable colon may be diverse, but most common are episodes of abdominal pain of varying degrees. It is usually a diffuse pain which is felt first here and then there in the abdomen and characteristically is relieved, at least temporarily, by passage of gas or a bowel movement. In some cases the pain may be severe and may on occasion mimic pain arising from more serious causes. Thus, when the pain arises from distention and gas in the part of the colon that lies in the upper left-hand corner of the abdomen, it may be felt in the left chest, left shoulder or even down the left arm, very similar to the heart pain of angina pectoris. It may also occasionally mimic the pain of a kidney stone that occurs in the small of the back and down into the groin, and there is no question that irritable colon syndrome accounts for a number of "negative" appendectomies that are performed because the pain so closely mimics appendicitis.

In addition to pain, the syndrome may also include constipation or diarrhea or both, interspersed, often with a pattern of frequent small, semisolid bowel movements mixed with quantities of mucus. At the same time the victim may have unexplained episodes of nausea, excessive belching, even occasional vomiting and loss of appetite. But the single most characteristic feature of this condition is that its onset or recurrence tends to coincide with peaks of stress or emotional tension in the victim's life, and symptoms frequently subside spontaneously when the emotional stress abates.

Diagnosis has to be made by excluding other possible causes of the symptoms, since there are no signs and symptoms that are pathognomonic (that is, diagnostically specific) of irritable colon. Experienced physicians often suspect it just on the basis of the patient's history and the relationship between attacks and emotional tension. Once the diagnosis is made, treatment must be geared to the patient's degree of discomfort. In many cases little more than the doctor's reassurance that nothing grave is afoot is needed to relieve a great deal of the anxiety that contributes to the illness, and this, combined with the patient's own insight that discomfort is a relatively harmless physical reaction to emotional stress, may obviate any other form of treatment.

When symptoms are severely uncomfortable, symptomatic treatment can be of great value. A diet regimen to avoid irritating foods, the use of a bulking agent if constipation is a feature, or the judicious use of occasional antidiarrhetic medicines if diarrhea is a feature, all can do a great deal to relieve the severity of the symptoms. Sedatives or tranquilizers or both are sometimes an aid in taking the edge off emotional tension and anxiety, but should be used most carefully under the close supervision of a physician, since victims of irritable bowel syndrome tend to be of a personality type that may form a dependence on such medications. In really severe and refractory cases, psychiatric consultation and psychotherapy are sometimes the best approach. At the same time, victims of this condition should make positive efforts to modify their living habits, seeking to eliminate sources of emotional stress if possible. The condition tends to be chronic, but except in severe cases symptoms occur at longer and longer intervals and are reduced sharply in severity by the simple measure of reassurance and occasional symptomatic treatment.

Intestinal Obstruction

In many ways the digestive tract is the most tolerant and long-suffering of all organ systems in the human body. It patiently accepts such various assaults as highly spiced or chemically irritating foods and distention from overeating; it accepts harsh laxatives and all sorts of irrita-

tive enemas, and generally, except for an occasional mild reaction, it goes on quietly doing its job.

There is one thing, however, that the digestive tract does *not* tolerate well, and that is the presence of an obstruction somewhere along the line. Such conditions as acute gastric dilatation, paralytic ileus or megacolon, described above, can indirectly cause acute and profound illness on account of either obstruction or cessation of intestinal movement; but certain of the most dangerous of all disorders of the digestive system are directly related to mechanical obstruction at some point in the intestinal channel.

An *inguinal hernia* is perhaps the most common form of obstruction to the flow of materials through the intestine. A *hernia,* or as it is more commonly known, a "rupture," occurs when any organ or tissue protrudes through an opening in the walls of a cavity in which it is normally contained. The soft material in the center of an intervertebral disk, for example, may "herniate" or protrude through the cartilaginous capsule that normally contains it and cause abnormal pressure on spinal nerves, a condition known as a herniated or "slipped" intervertebral disk (*see* p. 325). Similarly, infants may suffer an *umbilical hernia* when the muscle and connective tissue of the abdominal wall fail to close in the umbilical region after birth, allowing a loop of intestine to protrude through a small hole or defect—usually a congenital condition. Abdominal hernias may also occur postoperatively when the fibrous and muscular layers of a surgical wound separate before they are fully healed and allow abdominal contents to push through. In most hernias the protruding organ is contained by a layer of tissue—the peritoneum, in the case of abdominal hernias—which forms a *hernia sac* and controls the protrusion to some degree. The outer skin and superficial connective tissue also help contain the hernia, but all of these tissues stretch under pressure, allowing the hernia gradually to become larger and larger.

An inguinal hernia occurs when the tissues of the lower abdominal cavity just above the groin on one side or the other become sufficiently weakened, stretched or torn that a tissue defect or hole appears internally and allows a loop of intestine to protrude through the aperture into the soft tissue of the groin, just above and outside the pubic bone. In some cases the defect is somewhat more to the side so that the protrusion of bowel occurs in the direction of the top of the leg and is called a *femoral hernia;* but often the surgeon cannot be entirely sure whether the hernia is femoral or inguinal until he is in the process of repairing it.

Why is this particular spot so vulnerable to tissue breakdown and the development of a hernia? For one thing, a weak spot remains there due to the embryological development of the child, particularly the male. When the fetal testicles are formed they are located in the lower abdomen, and at some point in the later development of the fetus they descend into the scrotum along a sort of a tunnel known as the *inguinal canal.* Once the testicles have descended, this inguinal canal usually closes and obliterates itself, but in many cases an area of tissue weakness remains. And indeed many children, particularly male children, are born with *congenital inguinal hernias,* frequently present on both sides and not uncommonly associated with one or both testicles undescended. (*See* p. 875.)

Since this weakness exists low down in the abdomen on either side, it may be further aggravated by the pull of gravity on the contents of the abdominal cavity. Heavy lifting, chronic coughing, straining to urinate or straining at stool may also increase the pressure on muscles and tissues of the abdominal wall, weakening them even further. In fact, hernias most commonly occur in those involved in heavy lifting, in relatively obese people who pay too little attention to the muscle tone of their abdomens, and in individuals who have the bad habit of straining mightily to evacuate their bowels. Although inguinal hernias are probably 20 times more prevalent in men than in women, they occasionally occur in women who have stretched and weakened the muscles and tendons in the inguinal region with multiple pregnancies.

Sometimes an inguinal hernia protrudes through a very large defect, and in this case it may pose relatively little threat, since a loop of bowel can readily slip back and forth through the defect. Most often, however, the defect is relatively small, sometimes no more than a half-inch in diameter. It is in such cases that a loop of bowel can be forced through the defect by a sudden strain or other increase of abdominal pressure, and then become trapped so that food materials passing through that portion of intestine are effectively obstructed. A corner of the bladder or even a bit of abdominal fat might also be forced through the hernia opening and be trapped. Anything caught in such a hernia that cannot be pushed back is said to be *incarcerated,* a condition that soon leads to pain in the inguinal area, often with a palpable lump in the groin. If circulation to the incarcerated segment of bowel, bladder or other tissue is cut off, the hernia is *strangulated* and gangrene may develop in the trapped tissue within a few hours. If a loop of bowel is involved, the typical symptoms of intestinal obstruction soon appear. There is gaseous distention above the obstruction, nausea, often vomiting, and steadily increasing pain which may begin as intermittent cramping but soon becomes constant. In the course of a few hours, the *peritoneum,* the fibrous tissue that lines the abdomen and is just as sensitive to mechanical and chemical irritation as the pleura lining the chest cavity and the lungs, shows definite signs of *peritoneal irritation:* the victim becomes extremely sensitive to any touch or pressure, involuntarily guards the area of the incarcerated hernia by tensing muscles, and begins to feel pain more and more sharply localized to the injured area.

If the victim of an incarcerated inguinal hernia seeks medical help very soon after the incarceration occurs, the doctor can often reduce the hernia manually. With the patient lying on his back with his legs and hips elevated ten inches or so above the level of the shoulders, and sedated to help him relax tensed abdominal muscles, the doctor applies gentle massaging pressure to the herniated mass until it is coaxed back through the defect into the abdomen again. If he is successful, the patient may experience dramatic relief of the pain and distention within a few minutes. Even so, the physician will observe him for a period of some hours to be sure that no damage was done to the incarcerated loop of intestine. Then he will recommend surgical repair of the hernia defect as soon as possible to avoid a recurrence of this dangerous condition.

Only a small percentage of inguinal hernias, however, are first discovered as a result of an obstructive episode such as this, and manual reduction, if possible, is at best only a temporary measure. By far the majority are discovered on routine physical examination, often to the surprise of the patient, and surgical repair is the most effective form of treatment. Years ago when major surgery of the abdomen was considerably more risky than it is today, and when many people, particularly in rural areas, rarely saw a doctor at all unless someone was being born or dying, corset makers and medical appliance manufacturers did a land office business in trusses—devices made of spring steel, covered with leather and shaped like a belt with a large leather knob or pad at one end that could be seated over the hernia to apply pressure and keep the bowel from passing through the defect and incarcerating. Ugly and uncomfortable as the trusses were, some hernia sufferers wore them day and night for years rather than submit to surgery. Even with a truss, it was not uncommon for the hernia to grow larger and larger until it extended far down into the scrotum or into the soft tissue at the top of the thigh. The stretched surface of the skin was, of course, extremely vulnerable to injury and infection, and the danger of internal injury and gangrene was always present. In those days death from incarcerated hernias was a frequent occurrence.

Today there is no reason to risk such a tragedy. Most physicians agree that a hernia should be repaired surgically as soon as possible after it is discovered, whether it is symptomatic or not. Trusses are considerably more sophisticated than formerly, but even so, they are recommended only when surgery is considered too hazardous. There are many people who resist the idea of major surgery to repair a condition they did not know they had and which seems to be causing them no trouble. But most eventually realize that surgery is preferable to the pain, physical incapacity with or without a truss, and the possibly fatal complications of an incarcerated hernia.

Repair of an inguinal hernia, known as a *herniorrhaphy,* is considered a major operation because it is necessary to suture and close the peritoneum, even though the surgeon approaches the hernia from outside and below the abdomen. Once he has found the defect and the small sac of peritoneum that contains the intestinal protrusion, he can reduce the hernia, remove the sac and repair the peritoneum, and then proceed to repair the defects in the tendons, ligaments and muscles overlying the herniated area, layer by layer. The procedure sometimes takes as little as 25 or 30 minutes, and the patient is encouraged to get up and move around, particularly to walk, on the first postoperative day. Aside from fairly severe soreness in the groin area for a few days postoperatively, and some residual aching or twinges that may continue for three or four weeks, the recovery period is in the neighborhood of six weeks before the patient can return to his normal activities without fear of recurrence.

There are two other conditions, both of them in the nature of accidental occurrences rather than structural defects, which can lead to obstruction of the small intestine with the same symptoms and complications of an inguinal hernia. The first of these, known as *intussusception,* is a condition in which a portion of the small or large intestine telescopes on itself and can, if not released, cause strangulation of that segment of the bowel and complete obstruction. This disorder is relatively common in babies, and in adults often occurs at the location of a polyp or tumor, especially in the colon. All the symptoms of intestinal obstruction—abdominal pain, nausea, vomiting, distention and gas—are present, and as complete obstruction occurs, the patient's increasing pulse, increasing white blood count and rising temperature may indicate a deteriorating condition which requires surgical exploration of the abdomen. Occasionally the site of an intussusception can be found by means of a lower bowel X-ray, for which a barium enema is introduced per rectum; if this diagnostic procedure is done early, it will occasionally reduce the intussusception all by itself. More often, however, the condition becomes a surgical emergency, in which case an exploratory operation or so-called *laparotomy* is performed and the damaged segment of bowel removed.

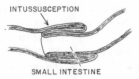

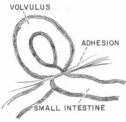

Figure 46–6.

A similar sort of accident is the occurrence of *volvulus,* a condition in which a segment of the bowel, usually the small intestine, becomes looped and twisted, obstructing the intestine much the same way as twisting a garden hose obstructs the flow of water. Volvulus frequently occurs as a result of the presence of fibrous bands or adhesions in the abdomen, a commonplace residual from previous abdominal surgery. Again, volvulus may resolve itself, but if the looping is severe enough to cut off circulation, it can soon become gangrenous, cause a great deal of swelling of the tissue of the intestinal wall and evolve into a surgical emergency. In this case, the only approach to treatment is opening the patient's abdomen and resecting the damaged loop.

Other conditions can also cause partial or complete intestinal obstruction or impairment of the ability of a segment of intestine to carry a normal peristaltic wave. Such an obstruction can be produced by tumors either within the intestine or pressing on the intestine from outside, or from scarring and stricture as a result of infection or other inflammatory disease of the intestine. Occasionally a blood clot or thrombus may lodge in a major artery or vein supplying a portion of the intestine, destroying its circulation

and causing that segment of the bowel to become infarcted. Even impacted foreign bodies or large gallstones which have found their way into the intestine can cause partial obstruction.

Thus, both disorders of motility and obstructions in the digestive tract stem from a variety of causes and range in severity from the mildest of intestinal upsets to truly dangerous conditions, all of which are heralded, at least at first, by similar symptoms. A question often asked is just how can the layman tell which is which. Since the symptoms are so similar, it is often their pattern and persistence that spells the difference between a mild and a serious disorder. Occasional gas pains, cramps and other discomforts in the abdomen occur from time to time to anybody and should not occasion serious worry; often complete relief is obtained by taking a mild antacid such as Tums, Rolaids or various "seltzer" preparations, or by having a bowel movement. Persisting or worsening abdominal pain and distention, however, are not likely to occur in the normal course of events. Neither is nausea or vomiting normal, particularly if persistent and repeated. Any of these symptoms which persist and recur for several hours, or which occur in combination, can be warnings of trouble and should be called to the attention of a doctor.

Disorders of Absorption

The whole purpose of digestive system function is to take the various food materials that we eat—meats and other proteins, sugars and starches, fats, vitamins, minerals—into the body, subject them to mechanical and chemical processing to break them into more simple substances, and finally to absorb these breakdown products, together with vitamins and minerals in the diet, into the blood stream for use in the metabolic processes necessary to sustain life, rejecting only a small indigestible residue which is carried out of the body by way of the colon. Just as any condition which obstructs the passage of these food materials through the digestive tract is sooner or later reflected in symptom-producing disorders, so any condition which interferes with the absorption of digested food materials into the blood stream from the small intestine will also lead to trouble. For example, certain of the vitamins—chemicals which are found in our foods and play a vital role in the body's nutrition—are *fat-soluble* and are normally absorbed through the intestine into the lymph vessels, dissolved and intermixed with acids from the fatty foods we eat. Both vitamin A and vitamin D fall into this fat-soluble category. But external factors can influence the absorption of these necessary vitamins into the body. In an individual who is habituated to using quantities of mineral oil as a laxative, enough fat-soluble vitamins may be soaked up by the mineral oil and carried out in the stool before they can be absorbed that serious vitamin deficiencies can develop. This, of course, is not a "disease" of the body; once such a deficiency is diagnosed and the cause identified, the deficiency can be corrected simply by changing to a non-oily laxative or learning to dispense with laxatives altogether.

Sprue is one disorder of absorption that does arise from an intrinsic malfunction in the body. It is an insidious disease of unknown origin which sometimes occurs during adulthood or middle age, developing so slowly that the victim may be in trouble before any definitive diagnosis is made. The first symptoms, which often appear very stealthily, are an increase in gas production in the colon, expelled through the rectum as flatus, and a gradual loss of appetite. Presently the victim notices increasing weakness and loss of weight, together with the onset of semiformed and extremely bulky and frothy light-colored stools which may be found to contain large quantities of fat. At the same time the victim may notice an increasing soreness and redness of the tongue, an early sign of vitamin deficiency. While the abdomen becomes unusually distended or prominent, the rest of the body may slowly become emaciated in severe cases, and the victim grows apathetic and listless or depressed. Anemia often develops, and small capillary hemorrhages under the skin appear due to a deficiency of vitamin K, one of the key factors in the blood-clotting mechanism. At one time it was thought that sprue was strictly a tropical disease, and one form of the disorder does appear characteristically among people in tropical climates, but we now know that a nontropical variety of the disease also afflicts people in temperate climates. There is also a childhood disorder of absorption, very similar to sprue, which is known as *celiac disease* (*see* p. 893).

No one knows exactly what causes sprue, but some authorities suspect that it is an inborn defect, particularly in childhood cases, which impairs the ability of the small intestine to absorb digested carbohydrates and fats. Others cite some type of infection, as yet unidentified, as the source of the condition, while still others blame dietary deficiencies. Whatever the cause, the symptoms arise from the inability of the intestine to absorb essential nutriments, including such necessary vitamins as A and sometimes B_{12}, from digested food. Another important chemical known as *folic acid,* which enters into the metabolism of food products within the body, is also poorly absorbed, and the anemia that appears with sprue is very similar to *pernicious anemia* (*see* p. 516) except that there is no concurrent decrease in the amount of acid formed in the stomach.

For a long time treatment of sprue was most unsatisfactory, primarily because no one understood exactly what substances were being lost due to malabsorption and thus had no idea what substances needed replacement. Even today treatment is not always satisfactory; it depends primarily upon careful adjustment of the diet, administration of additional vitamin A, B vitamins and folic acid, and elimination of certain foods which, for reasons unknown, seem to make sprue symptoms worse. Among these foods, in particular, are those including a substance known as gluten which occurs in rich supply in such common cereal grains as wheat, oats and rye. Additional dietary supplies of such substances as calcium and potassium are also given in treatment. Recovery from the illness under this complicated diet-plus-medication plan is often very slow, but today it can frequently be speeded up by the administration of cortisone hormones which often produce very dramatic and prolonged remissions of symptoms. A few people who have developed sprue and are treated early in the disease recover completely with no recurrence of symptoms, but in most cases recurrence is the rule, and dietary and medical regimens must often be maintained for prolonged periods. In most cases control rather than cure is the best that can be achieved, and until research has revealed far more about the cause and nature of this odd disorder, probably no form of treatment will be completely effective.

Other malabsorption symptoms can appear not because of any built-in defect or disease of the body, but as a result of surgery which has necessitated removal of part of the stomach and/or large segments of the small intestine. In most cases of such "surgically created" malabsorption disorders, the surgeon is well aware of the deficiencies that may occur and will guide patients in dietary measures designed to replace various nutriments that may be partially lost. On the other hand, there are cases in which such surgery is performed for the deliberate purpose of reducing absorption of nutriments, a rather extreme approach to the treatment of dangerous and otherwise intractable degrees of obesity. Few surgeons will consider such a procedure, however, until all other approaches to weight reduction have been exhausted.

Once a physical disorder of the digestive tract has been diagnosed, it is not, in most cases, difficult to treat. If, however, psychological factors combine with physical factors to cause a digestive disorder, or if psychological factors are alone responsible, treatment can be more difficult. The digestive tract is very often a "target organ" for the expression of emotional tension, fear or anxiety; in fact, many people take some degree of pride in having "sensitive stomachs" or "delicate digestion" and often complain that they suffer from "nervous indigestion." These same people also tend to be the ones who suffer an "abdominal reaction" to almost any other illness. Their symptoms are real enough, however, and if they, too, recur or persist, they demand patient and thorough medical investigation.

Perhaps the most important thing to remember is that the digestive system *is* "delicate." Its healthy function depends in general upon the overall good health of mind and body, and in particular upon sensible, regular eating and bowel habits. Under these circumstances, the system does a remarkably good job of taking care of itself; it demands only commonsense care and respect, not excessive worry or misguided attempts at home medication with harsh laxatives, enemas and other assaults. If disorders do occur, only the simplest, mildest and safest of home treatment measures should be tried. If they fail, and the symptoms recur or persist, it is just as foolish to ignore them as it is to try even more potent home medications. That is the time to consult a doctor who will investigate the causes, both physical and psychological, and prescribe the proper treatment.

Inflammatory Diseases of the Digestive System

A variety of inflammatory diseases can afflict the digestive system, often in strange and unfamiliar ways. Inflammatory conditions caused primarily by the invasion of pathogenic bacteria or viruses, as well as by parasitic organisms, are discussed in detail in Part IV, "Patterns of Illness: The Infectious Diseases." These diseases range all the way from the mildest episodes of one-day "stomach flu" to such life-threatening infections as bacillary dysentery or typhoid fever. But in addition to these, there are a number of inflammatory conditions which are not primarily bacterial in origin but arise from other factors, both organic and emotional. Some of them, such as regional enteritis, are unfamiliar; others such as appendicitis are perhaps too familiar. All, however, represent breakdowns or alterations in the physical structure of the digestive tract which, if not treated early and vigorously, can cause severe digestive disturbance and, in some cases, thoroughly dangerous illness.

Acute Gastritis

Probably most familiar of all the inflammatory conditions of the digestive tract, well known to almost everyone by its symptoms if not by its proper name, is acute gastritis, which means simply acute inflammation of the stomach. It can arise from a variety of sources, but most cases are caused by immoderate ingestion of alcoholic beverages (alcohol is highly irritating to the mucous membrane lining the stomach, particularly when taken undiluted), excesses of hot, spicy foods, other gastric irritants such as coffee or strong tea, and foods that are mechanically irritating—popcorn, for example. Everybody has eaten food that is so physically hot—like a pizza directly out of the oven—that it blisters the inside of the mouth, and such food can also literally burn the inside of the esophagus or stomach. In addition, there are a variety of medicines—common aspirin, sulfonamides, antibiotics, quinine and various other drugs—capable of causing serious chemical irritation or even burns of the stomach.

The symptoms of acute gastritis may vary from relatively minor discomfort due to distention, "acid indigestion" with heartburn or acid belching, and a sense of shortness of breath (often due to overstuffing) to outright pain in the upper abdomen, nausea, vomiting and upper abdominal cramps, depending upon the amount of the irritating substance taken in and the degree of irritation it causes. Typically, acute gastritis turns up suddenly and sometimes quite violently a short time after ingesting the irritating substance, and may be of brief duration, often symptomatically relieved by vomiting. This sudden onset, combined with a history of injudicious eating of irritating substances, is usually the tip-off that gastritis is at fault and not something more serious. Mild cases can be treated with small doses of a nonconstipating antacid, preferably in liquid form, such as milk of magnesia, or aluminum hydroxide gel (Aludrox, Gelusil or Maalox). One-half ounce to an ounce of half-and-half milk and cream is an effective substitute, with the capacity to soothe the irritated gastric lining with a bland demulcent and absorptive coat. When symptoms are markedly relieved by these steps, the diet should be restricted to small amounts of bland food, preferably liquid or semisolid, such as unseasoned eggs, milk, clear soup, or light buttered toast for a period of 12 to 24 hours following the episode.

Occasionally acute gastritis can be extremely severe, with little relief of symptoms from home remedies; in such a case medical attention should be sought and it may be necessary to empty the stomach by artificial means to get rid of the irritating substance. In any event, such acute episodes usually settle down without any further complications unless irritation is so great that the stomach perforates, creating a gastric emergency of quite different magnitude and requiring immediate surgical attention.

Less common but far more dangerous is acute *corrosive gastritis,* usually caused by accidental swallowing, often by children, of strong acids or caustic alkalis, iodine, or oily substances such as kerosene, turpentine, paint thinner or gasoline. Among the most dangerous of such substances in the average home are various powerful cleaning detergents and automatic dishwasher compounds, drain openers and ammonia, almost always left on open shelves within easy reach for a child. All these substances cause immediate and aggravated distress when taken into the stomach and demand swift and knowledgeable first-aid action. (*See* p. 116.) Such action can literally save the victim's life and can minimize damage to the mouth, esophagus and stomach that might otherwise take months or even years of difficult and painful medical treatment.

Chronic Gastritis

Acute gastritis usually occurs fairly swiftly and, except in the case of poison ingestion, also subsides swiftly without recurrence as long as commonsense precautionary diet measures are taken. But gastritis can also occur in a chronic form. In this condition either long repeated exposure to gastric irritants or other unknown factors result in a continuous or recurrent pattern of indigestion, distention after meals, flatulence, belching, heartburn and other forms of "indigestion," not necessarily acute or alarming in nature, but persisting. Certainly any such prolonged pattern of symptoms should be investigated, since it can signal the presence of a number of potentially more serious disturbances. But often the only organic change found with this chronic symptom complex is either a thickening of the mucous membrane lining the stomach, sometimes so marked that great folds of stomach mucosa can be identified in X-rays, or, in other cases, a shrinking or atrophy of the gastric mucosa.

Usually chronic gastritis represents no serious threat, and can be controlled by the use of antacids, bland foods in the diet, and careful avoidance of irritating substances such as alcohol and coffee. The condition worries doctors, however, first because these recurring symptoms, often ignored as unimportant by the patient, may well mask the development of other illnesses such as peptic ulcer and gall bladder disease; and second, because they may occasionally be the first clue to the development of a cancer in the stomach or another disease frequently related to stomach disorders, pernicious anemia. Oddly enough, the symptoms associated with chronic gastritis, particularly in older people, are more often a result of inadequate rather than excessive acid formation in the stomach, and symptoms can frequently be relieved by the prescription of small quantities of dilute hydrochloric acid as a medicine at mealtimes. But typically, both cancer of the stomach and pernicious anemia are also closely associated with diminution or absence of acid formation in the stomach; therefore the doctor caring for a patient with chronic gastritis will very wisely require periodic checkups so that any change can be detected early.

Most people who suffer from acute or chronic "indigestion," however, do so quite needlessly as a result of atrocious eating habits. They could put an end to their discomfort by following a few simple rules: eat an adequate breakfast and a moderate but nutritious lunch and dinner, balancing food intake throughout the day; make a point to eat at least *some* food at the cocktail hour along with cocktails, and have a moderate meal soon afterward; eat highly irritating or spicy foods only rarely and then in reasonable amounts; use a mild antacid to combat hyperacidity between meals, but be sure that its use is not excessive or habitual. Finally, if digestive symptoms do persist in spite of these common-sense measures, consult a doctor.

Regional Enteritis

A rather diffuse and variable inflammatory disease of the small intestine, regional enteritis is often considered an affliction of early middle age; but in as many as half of its victims, the trouble begins even earlier, between the ages of twenty and thirty. It is usually nonspecific—that is, not related to any specific bacterial infection—and may attack one or many areas of the small intestine, particularly the lower end or *ileum,* sometimes extending into the upper part of the large bowel or colon. The inflammation appears to begin in the lymph vessels under the mucous membrane of the intestine, but soon involves all the layers of the intestinal wall with swelling, dilatation of the blood vessels and infiltration by many white blood cells, followed by the development of fibrous scar tissue as the body tries to heal the lesion. These areas of inflamed intestine frequently become permanently thickened, hardened and inelastic, and the condition may later be complicated by the development of shallow ulcerations in the inner lining of the intestine, the formation of abscesses due to secondary bacterial infections, or the appearance of *fistulas,* scarred tunnel-like openings through the tissue which may extend from one part of the intestine to another or may even open into the abdomen. Often as much as one or two feet of the lower end of the intestine is involved, and it is not uncommon for multiple areas to be involved all at once. The affliction may appear quite suddenly in an acute form or may become a chronic disease with frequent recurrences and progressively severe symptoms.

There is no single known cause that accounts for the incidence of regional enteritis, but many authorities consider it to be an excellent example of a disease in which very real physical change and damage to body tissue are closely related to physical and emotional tension, continuous worry, pressure or conflict. How large a part emotional factors play in the development of the disease varies greatly from one individual to another and is often exceedingly difficult or even impossible to differentiate. Many gastroenterologists regard regional enteritis as primarily a physical affliction which is merely aggravated to some degree by emotional factors; but many psychiatrists take the extreme opposite view, maintaining that victims of the disease are people filled with anger, resentment and hostility, who are unable to express or "externalize" their conscious or subconscious feelings and thus must "internalize" them, with a very real, distressing and often recurrent chronic physical lesion appearing as a direct result.

Whatever the cause of the condition, the symptoms and natural history of regional enteritis can be thoroughly uncomfortable for the victim. In most cases symptoms include the development of cramping pain and colic in the mid-abdomen, accompanied by a change of bowel habits from the normal pattern of defecation once or twice a day to the passage of small, loose, bowel movements from three to six or seven times a day. When the disorder is acute there is often fever, sometimes quite high, with steadily increasing abdominal pain which may be felt primarily in the right lower quadrant of the abdomen and can often be confused with the pain of acute appendicitis. In a more chronic form the pain may not be so severe, or may wax and wane, with a loss of appetite, a persisting mild fever and, presently, weight loss of some degree. Occasionally during an acute attack or an acute recurrence of a chronic condition, symptoms of intestinal obstruction develop, with a sharp increase in abdominal pain and distention, followed by vomiting. In the chronic form of regional enteritis, partial obstruction may also occur periodically with milder episodes of cramping pain and vomiting which then proceed to subside, only to recur again. In many cases the onset is so gradual that the patient seeing a doctor is unable to pinpoint any specific acute episode. Usually the disease does not seem to bear any relationship to eating habits, and acid indigestion or peptic ulcer symptoms are absent

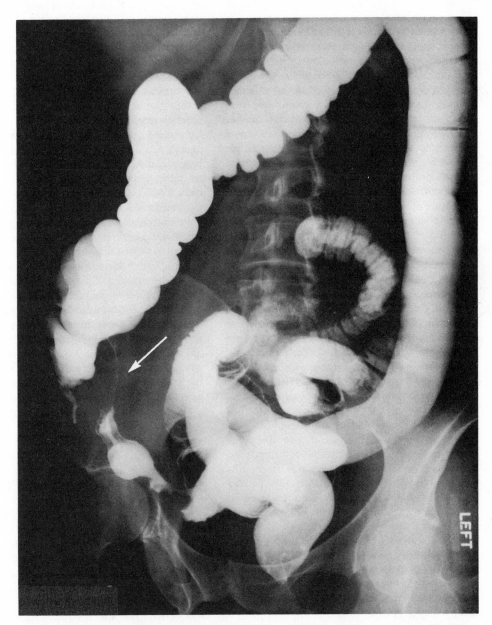

Plate 32   Regional enteritis (Crohn's disease) as revealed by barium enema. A diseased, scarred segment of the small intestine, itself invisible to X-ray, can be identified by the narrow ribbon or "string" of radio-opaque barium sulfate suspension passing through it (see arrow).

unless a peptic ulcer is also present independently.

The doctor may suspect the diagnosis from the patient's history, but in most cases diagnosis is established by X-ray examination in which the same barium sulfate suspension ingested for an upper GI series of X-rays is allowed to pass through the small intestine with hourly X-ray films checking its progress. On the other hand, diagnosis may also be made by *laparotomy* (exploratory surgery) when a patient with a sudden attack comes to surgery, because the doctor cannot rule out acute appendicitis and dares not wait long enough for GI X-rays, which take time and which might, if appendicitis is present, actually precipitate further trouble.

Treatment of the disease must be tailored to each individual patient's symptoms and history. A single acute attack may well subside on a program of bed rest, a special low-residue diet, supplemental vitamins, and medicines such as tincture of belladonna, which helps relax cramping muscle spasm in the smooth muscle of the intestine. Occasionally, when diarrhea is present, tincture of paregoric or other antidiarrheal medicines, except bulking agents, may be of help. Some doctors use antibiotics, even in the absence of evidence of bacterial infection, but others consider the risk of further irritation of the intestine by the drug to outweigh any possible benefit. In acute cases or acute exacerbations of chronic cases the cortisone-like hormones have also proven helpful. But any treatment program may well have to be continued for a long period, sometimes as much as six months or more. In some chronic patients a prolonged vacation or change of scene helps quiet down the affliction; and where potent emotional conflicts seem to be seriously involved, psychiatric consultation or some form of psychotherapy may help alleviate symptoms. In any case of a single acute attack, total recovery is possible with no recurrence whatever, but the general pattern of the illness is that of recurrence and progressively severe chronic disease.

Surgery for removal of the affected area of bowel is not always the best treatment for this condition, unless a life-threatening complication such as intestinal obstruction, perforating fistula or massive bleeding intervenes. Indeed, some experts feel that surgical intervention is contraindicated, except on an emergency basis, because it may actually *increase* the rate of recurrence, and statistics show that a new area of intestine becomes involved in recurrent enteritis following surgical treatment between 50 and 75 percent of the time.

Regional enteritis can be a thoroughly disabling disease; it has been known to strike children in emotionally disturbed homes and to force medical students out of training. Treatment of acute recurrences, combining medication and diet, may at least render the condition tolerable, but the best overall approach to treatment when the disease is chronically disabling is a multifront attack, with a carefully programmed diet and medication regimen, even when acute symptoms are not present, surgical consultation in the event of emergency complications, and a serious attempt to root out contributing emotional factors—attempts, ideally with psychiatric guidance, to eliminate emotional conflicts and trouble spots in the patient's life, or to find personally and socially acceptable ways to "externalize" these conflicts. Such an approach can consume time, energy and money without any guarantee of complete success, but because the disease so often causes chronic and progressive discomfort, disability and ultimately a threat to life, comprehensive treatment is well worth the effort.

Ulcerative Colitis

Chronic ulcerative colitis, even more than regional enteritis, seems consistently to be a physical manifestation of some personality disorder or emotional pathology. Many gastroenterologists are convinced, after long experience with this disabling and discouraging disease, that its victims are individuals who so thoroughly despise themselves, their lives and their bodies that they seek literally to destroy themselves. But other equally experienced authorities disagree sharply with this view, maintaining that the raw, bleeding ulcerating lesions of the disease appear in the colon as a result of some yet unknown physical process: infection by an unidentified virus, for example, or an obscure hypersensitivity to certain foods, or even as a result of some obscure immune process in which the body manufactures antibodies against its own mucous membrane lining the colon. Supporters of this view maintain that the disturbed emotional state of victims of the disease is not a reflection of their normal personalities, but rather is the result of long and chronic suffering from the effects of the disease. But whatever the cause, and whatever part emotional factors play in either cause or effect, it is certain that chronic ulcerative colitis is a grim affliction which can resist every effort to cure it.

The disease ordinarily involves a slow and progressive chronic inflammation of the mucous membrane of the colon, sometimes localized in the lower end, sometimes involving almost all the large intestine and even the lower end of the small intestine. The mucous membrane swells, becomes edematous and then hemorrhagic, and abscesses begin to form, gradually breaking down into raw weeping ulcers, large and small, secondarily infected with bacteria and oozing blood and pus. As the disease progresses, the breakdown of tissue extends into the muscular layer of the intestine; still later the body's attempt at healing fills the bowel wall with fibrous and scar tissue, gradually impairing the colon's major physiological function, the reabsorption of water from digested food material. The disease can begin at any age, but it starts most commonly during young adulthood, equally distributed among men and women. In some cases the onset is acute, with the sudden appearance of severe cramping pain, bloody diarrhea, fever, distention of the colon and, sometimes, perforation with resultant peritonitis. In such cases the disease can move so swiftly that the victim may die from peritonitis or profound toxemia even before the condition can be diagnosed. Far more commonly, however, ulcerative colitis begins stealthily with mild lower abdominal cramps, increased urgency to move the bowels, and slowly progressing diarrhea until the victim has continuous severe cramps and 20 or 30 stools a day, with a constant feeling of bowel urgency both day and night. The watery stools are frequently mixed with pus, blood and mucus; there

may be a spiking fever that appears and disappears; and often the victim suffers a sudden total lack of appetite, nausea and vomiting, leading frequently to rapid and progressive weight loss.

Typically colitis is a disease of spontaneous remissions and exacerbations—recurrent mild or severe attacks which come and go irregularly, often without any apparent relationship to treatment. Sometimes a single attack may seem to arrest itself and heal, with no recurrence of symptoms for months or years, but structural damage done by that attack will persist in the form of scar tissue and changes in the mucosa, easily abraded and tending to bleed readily. As the disease progresses, the attacks tend to become more severe, causing more and more permanent damage to the colon, so that frequent watery stools become the rule rather than the exception even during periods when active symptoms are quiet.

Complications of the disease range from the merely irritating and annoying, such as the development of hemorrhoids, painful cracking of the mucosa of the anus or the formation of abscesses around the rectal area, to such highly dangerous complications as acute hemorrhage when a major vessel in the colon is eroded away, perforation through the wall of the bowel with resultant peritonitis, obstruction of segments of the colon due to damage and scarring in local areas, or the development of polyps that tend to degenerate into malignant tumors. Indeed, cancer of the colon all too often occurs in individuals who have suffered from ulcerative colitis for prolonged periods—in some studies as many as 5 to 10 percent. Although one out of four people is said to recover completely after a single attack of ulcerative colitis, a high percentage of the rest suffer repeated incapacitating attacks which may ultimately lead to partial or complete invalidism.

Diagnosis of the disease is usually indicated by the history of its onset, and examination of the lower end of the bowel by proctoscopy will usually confirm diagnosis. Further confirmation is obtained from examination of X-rays of the colon. Other diseases and disorders can be ruled out by various laboratory tests and X-rays.

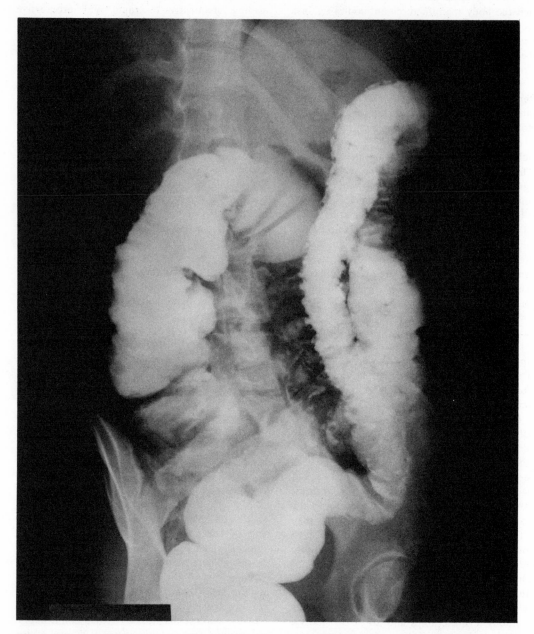

Plate 33   Ulcerative colitis, as revealed by barium enema. The affected segment of the colon
is narrowed, scarred and ragged in appearance; it has lost the normal smooth,
saccular appearance of the healthy portion of the colon.

Treatment will depend upon the severity of the attack and the presence or absence of complications. But just as the cause or causes of this disease are not known, neither is there any known cure or any combination of treatment programs that seems to help consistently. The basic principle of any treatment is to allow the diseased colon to rest as much as possible, to restore nutritional balance when it has been upset by the presence of the disease, and to provide supportive care to assist the patient to regain strength and help his natural body defenses go to work in combating the disease. In addition, treatment is concerned with the relief of symptoms—pain, diarrhea, the constant urge to defecate—as much as possible. Except in extremely severe cases when food should be restricted to clear fluids, modern treatment generally provides a selective diet of foods aimed at encouraging the appetite, avoiding only very cold liquids or food or drink known to be laxative or otherwise irritative to the colon.

In treating symptoms, often a period of bed rest and mild antispasmodic medicines to control intestinal motility may be sufficient to relieve the cramping pain and control diarrhea. Tincture of belladonna is one such medicine that is useful and nonaddicting. Tincture of paregoric can also be used, although in chronic diseases such as this most doctors avoid any regular use of narcotics, even in low dosages, because of the risk of addiction. Sedatives and tranquilizers also help allay apprehension and perhaps contribute to "cooling off" the emotional tension that is so often a factor in the disease. Although usually there is no specific bacterial organism present, antibiotic treatment is frequently used, particularly in severe and toxic cases in which secondary bacterial infection of the damaged bowel may be a factor, and sometimes dosages of penicillin or tetracycline bring very dramatic improvement. Unfortunately, response to antibiotic treatment is inconsistent, even in the same patient; it may seem to help a great deal in one attack and have no effect whatever in a subsequent attack.

The discovery of the anti-inflammatory properties of cortisone-like hormones or ACTH, a substance that stimulates the body's own formation of steroid hormones, has opened a new avenue for treatment; today these medicines are frequently helpful in acute and severe phases of the disease or in patients who have failed to show any significant improvement with more conservative medical treatment. Cortisone treatment is, however, a double-edged sword. While such hormones may help quiet the inflammation and resolve an acute attack, or prevent it from recurring if a low maintenance dose of the medicine is carried on, discontinuance of treatment is often followed by an acute recurrence of the disease; and since the use of these hormones for prolonged periods is so often accompanied by a variety of unfortunate side effects, they must be prescribed judiciously under the watchful eye of an experienced physician.

Finally, psychotherapy is often a valuable part of conservative medical treatment, and the development of a close doctor-patient relationship is a key factor in its effectiveness. Patients with this disease tend to be emotionally vulnerable and highly dependent, however, leaning heavily on the physician treating their condition and hypersensitive to any action on the part of the physician, friends or family which they may regard as rejection or withdrawal. Thus really effective psychotherapy should be undertaken by a psychiatrist who has had a great deal of experience in managing this kind of patient. As with any other form of treatment, the results are inconsistent; while psychotherapy may help one patient immensely, it may have no effect whatever on another.

Among those patients who do respond adequately to conservative medical treatment and those in whom the colitis tends to improve spontaneously, some 75 percent manage to get along for prolonged periods of time without surgery. The *degree* of remission or control by medical treatment may vary from patient to patient, and undoubtedly some who might benefit from surgery never are seen by a surgeon. On the other hand, surgical intervention in cases in which patients can manage moderately well without it has a rather unimpressive record, as frequently followed by recurrent severe disease as not. Thus surgical treatment today is considered only in two general groups of patients:

those with extremely acute and severe colitis in which massive hemorrhage or a threat of bowel perforation creates a surgical emergency; and those patients whose response to medical treatment has been very poor and whose condition is leading them into chronic invalidism.

Some years ago surgeons were reluctant to tackle the acute fulminating case of the disease on the grounds that the patient was often too sick to undergo an operation; more recently careful use of antibiotics, transfusions, attention to electrolyte balance through intravenous infusions, and other medical techniques have greatly improved the patient's capacity to survive surgery, and the operation can now be performed with a much lower risk of mortality. Furthermore, surgical techniques have improved to the point where a surgical approach is considered much earlier than it once was; most authorities no longer wait until the patient is so ill that surgical risk would be unconscionably high. Often these patients are treated and followed over a period of months or years in regular consultation with a surgeon, so that if surgery is finally elected he is fully informed about the patient's condition.

Even when medical treatment is successful, the surgeon may be called upon for the relief of certain local symptoms, such as the removal of thrombosed hemorrhoids or the treatment of a painful anal fissure. Surgical treatment of the disease itself sometimes involves merely the excision of a diseased segment of the colon, if only a part of the colon is affected, and particularly if it is acting as an obstructive lesion. More often, however, the entire colon is removed, followed by one of two procedures—either the connection of the lower end of the small intestine to the rectum so that normal evacuation is possible even though it will always be in semifluid form, or the complete removal of colon and rectum and the performance of a so-called *ileostomy,* in which the lower end of the small intestine is brought out through the abdominal wall where it is permanently fixed and attached to a removable bag to collect the fecal drainage. When this procedure was first introduced, it was often difficult to manage and keep clean, and was massively embarrassing to a patient already very

emotionally vulnerable. But over the years new surgical techniques, as well as more sophisticated procedures for attaching and removing the bag, have rendered this a far more acceptable operation, and the formation of so-called ileostomy groups or clubs of individuals who have undergone the operation has often provided additional emotional support and understanding.

How successful is surgical treatment when it is undertaken? If there were a clear-cut answer, the whole question of medical versus surgical management of colitis would be vastly simplified. All that can be said, really, is that results vary all the way from massive relief and long-term eradication of the disease to far less effective control. The trend today is toward earlier surgery in patients who have not been ill long or who are in better physical condition for the procedure. It is hoped that this trend will lead to fewer operative deaths and a higher percentage of long-term control. On the other hand, the hope of obtaining good or better control of the disease by medical rather than surgical means has not been abandoned. In either case, perhaps only time and careful evaluation of results can better help physicians assess which approach will be the most effective in individual cases.

Today the prognosis for any victim of this disease must still be very guarded. Relatively few enjoy a complete remission of symptoms with no further recurrence, but on the other hand, fewer remain as severely afflicted as was once the case, thanks to the benefits of combined medical and surgical treatment. Until we can discover the real causes of the disease—and until we know much more about how emotional factors affect various "target organs" such as the colon—the best that can be hoped for is reasonably good control and a reduction in the percentage of victims who become chronic invalids. A permanent cure for this disease is still not in sight.

Appendicitis

Among the most familiar and common of all inflammatory diseases of the digestive system is acute appendicitis. Oddly enough, medical historians have found that this disease seemed to appear only rarely prior to the late 1800s and then began to occur more and more widely until the mid-1930s, when it began slowly to fall off again. No one understands why this should be so, or why the disease seems to strike more frequently in developed nations than in undeveloped ones, and more frequently among urban dwellers than among those in rural areas. Certainly its occurrence seems mysteriously quixotic, following no family pattern and sparing no age group, although it is more common among children and young adults than it is among the middle-aged and elderly.

Acute appendicitis is an inflammation of the *vermiform appendix,* a small wormlike sac or closed tube attached to the cecum, the bulbous part of the large intestine in the area where the small intestine and the large intestine join. The appendix serves no purpose in the body as far as anyone knows; possibly it is a nonfunctioning remnant of a digestive tract organ possessed by some early evolutionary ancestor of man, although what that organ's function might once have been also remains a mystery. We do know that certain of the apes have a similar structure, as do domestic pigs, but that it is not found in lower animals.

Generally the appendix, though functionless, is inoffensive enough, but it does form a small dead-end pocket in the large intestine. Ordinarily it does not contain fecal matter, but occasionally fibrous detritus can become lodged in it, sometimes impacted so firmly that the circulation to the appendix is obstructed. A similar obstruction can also occur when some indigestible item such as a raspberry seed becomes lodged in the appendix. In fact, two of the earliest cases of appendicitis recorded in medical history both involved obstruction of the appendix by straight pins which had been ingested by the victim. When such foreign matter becomes lodged in the mouth of the appendix, bacteria within the appendix are able to grow in the tissues that are deprived of their food and oxygen supply, and a suppurative infection begins which can very quickly involve the entire interior length of the appendix and, frequently, the outside surface and the surfaces of adjacent structures as well. Once this process has begun, it soon reaches a point of no return after which, even if the obstructing material were dislodged, the infection would continue, proceeding to gangrene and ultimately to perforation of the appendix with spilling of infected material into the abdomen, leading to peritonitis.

Thus appendicitis is almost always a one-time disease, progressing either to general peritonitis and death or to the formation of a walled-off appendiceal abscess unless the course of the disease is interrupted by surgery. There is a popular idea that certain individuals have "chronic appendicitis" with repeated mild attacks, but most surgeons discredit this, maintaining that attacks of symptoms ascribed to "chronic appendicitis" are, in fact, a result of other disease processes.

The most demanding and consistent symptom of acute appendicitis is abdominal pain, which usually starts as vague, generalized discomfort felt all over the mid-abdomen, but gradually becomes localized in the right lower quadrant of the abdomen, the site of the appendix in most individuals. As the pain changes from vague and crampy to localized and constant, the victim often becomes mildly nauseated, and one or two half-hearted episodes of vomiting are typical in the course of the disease. A low-grade fever usually develops, seldom higher than 99.5° or 100°, and the white cell count in a blood sample characteristically shows a sharp rise in the course of a few hours. As the inflammation in the appendix begins to spread to adjacent structures covered by the peritoneum, the pain becomes progressively more severe, sometimes excruciating; it is aggravated by movement of any kind, and there is an involuntary tightening of the muscles of the overlying abdominal wall, a phenomenon known as "guarding." Because stretching and pressure within the gangrenous appendix are temporarily relieved when the organ perforates, sudden relief from the pattern of constantly increasing pain is usually an ominous sign that the appendix has burst. With modern surgery this does not necessarily mean that the victim will die; it simply means that the infection is free to spread beyond the localized area. Thus recovery and healing will be slower following surgery, and there is greater likelihood of shock, toxicity and other complications than if surgery is performed before the appendiceal rupture occurs.

Curiously, this "classical" sequence of symptoms occurs only occasionally, and when it does doctors speak of a "textbook case" of appendicitis. There may be many variations from this pattern in individual cases. Sometimes, because the appendix lies underneath the cecum in certain people, the pain may be felt more in the back than in front, or it may never clearly localize. Also, since the bowel is movable, in a certain number of people the appendix may be located part of the time in the upper right quadrant of the abdomen, or even in the lower left, and the pain may be felt in those areas. Thus appendicitis cannot be ruled out simply because pain is not localized at *McBurney's point,* an area in the middle of the right lower quadrant where it is most frequently felt. Furthermore, there are other conditions which may produce similar symptoms, or at least some of them, with sufficient frequency to throw even the astute surgeon off. Diverticulitis is one such condition, and a kidney infection may also cause symptoms mimicking appendicitis, so that a urinalysis is a critically important diagnostic test. If the urine is full of pus cells, suggesting the presence of a kidney infection, the surgeon may be hesitant to accept the diagnosis of appendicitis, even though appendicitis may also be present.

In women several pelvic disorders can also mimic appendicitis. Girls in puberty often have pain associated with such a minor disturbance as the rupture of a Graafian follicle of the ovary, the small, fluid-filled vesicle in which an ovum is forming. In older women the development of a tubal pregnancy may give rise to all the signs and symptoms of acute appendicitis at a time when a certain small amount of hemorrhage takes place; and an acute inflammation of one of the Fallopian tubes, a condition known as acute salpingitis, may also be impossible to differentiate.

In fact, the diagnosis of acute appendicitis can be extremely tricky, and the surgeon may find himself impaled on the horns of a dilemma. He cannot always be certain that appendicitis is causing the trouble, yet he knows that if appendicitis *is* the diagnosis and he temporizes too long, the patient may be in grave danger of rupture and peritonitis which will surely prolong his recovery and may even pose a threat to his life. It is for this reason that surgeons quite frequently elect to proceed with surgery even though they are uncertain of the diagnosis, and this is also why statistics show that between 5 and 10 percent of the appendices removed in appendectomies are completely free of any evidence of infection or disease. Much has been made of this, and uninformed laymen have taken it as evidence that surgeons are too eager to operate. Physicians, including pathologists, take a different view: a surgeon who has too few "negative" reports on the appendectomies he performs may be criticized by his colleagues for waiting too long and taking too great a risk of perforation and peritonitis in patients who *do* have acute appendicitis.

Diagnosis of acute appendicitis is especially difficult in children and adolescents who are generally unaccustomed to any degree of abdominal pain and consequently may overreact when it occurs, misleading both parents and doctors. Thus because acute appendicitis does indeed occur quite frequently among this age group, the surgeon must exercise an extremely fine degree of judgment. Parents, too, must recognize that in a small percentage of cases an appendectomy may prove to have been "unnecessary" postoperatively, but preoperatively all the available evidence indicated otherwise. In short, it is far wiser to risk a wrong diagnosis than the life of the patient, whatever his age. In any case, an appendectomy in skilled hands is a relatively uncomplicated surgical procedure involving very little morbidity and only the most occasional mortality. If, however, the surgeon waits too long, the appendix may rupture, finally confirming diagnosis, of course, but then surgery is much more difficult, recovery much slower and the possibility of mortality much higher.

Children frequently have "stomach aches" for one reason or another, but parents who are in the habit of reaching for the laxative bottle whenever a child complains of any kind of abdominal discomfort should remember one important fact: if the stomach ache is a result of acute appendicitis, administering a laxative may cause an acutely inflamed appendix to perforate. *Laxatives should never be given to anyone suffering from abdominal pain except upon specific directions from a physician.* Nor should voluminous enemas of warm or soapy water be given, since these too can be highly irritating to the bowel and increase the threat of perforation. However, if the child's medical history suggests that constipation really is a factor in abdominal pain, the use of a small-volume, prepared chemical enema, such as a pediatric-size Fleet's enema obtainable at most drugstores, is relatively safe, and may well lead to evacuation of a constipated stool and marked relief of the abdominal pain and distention. But even this home treatment measure should not be undertaken if the pain is severe and constant. In such a case a physician should see the child first and direct the use of enemas or any other medication.

The treatment of acute appendicitis is surgical, and the earlier in the course of the disease the better. The surgeon enters the abdomen on the lower right, making an incision through the skin, subcutaneous fat and the peritoneum, but separating and holding aside abdominal muscles. The appendix is located and removed, taking care that its infected contents do not spill out. The intestine is then repaired and the incision in the other tissues is closed and heals quickly, leaving only a small scar. A few decades ago this surgery was usually done under inhalation anesthesia, and the patient was then restricted to bed for several days in the hospital, followed by a three- to four-week convalescence. This approach, however, has been found to contribute to complications rather than prevent them. Many surgeons now prefer the use of a spinal anesthesia, long demonstrated to be splendidly safe and free of the many unpleasant complications which can follow inhalation anesthesia—bronchitis, pneumonia, collapse of a portion of a lung, vomiting and aspiration of vomitus. And today the otherwise normal and healthy patient recovering from appendicitis is got out of bed as soon as the anesthesia wears off and is encouraged to be physically active as soon as possible.

At present, convalescence in the hospital rarely exceeds a week, and the patient can usually go back to his normal activities within two weeks of surgery.

Since acute appendicitis can be such a serious threat unless surgical relief is available, and since surgery is so free of complications, many people wonder why appendectomies are not performed *before* an attack. Perhaps almost every surgeon has encountered at least one request for this kind of prophylactic surgery, particularly from those planning long trips to remote areas of the world. There are two reasons why no reputable surgeon today would recommend such a procedure: first, the odds that any given individual will develop acute appendicitis remain very small, even though the disease is common enough; and second, although an appendectomy is remarkably safe, there is, nevertheless, a certain risk involved, and no surgeon with good judgment is willing to take even that small risk on the offhand chance of preventing an illness which is not too likely to occur anyway. It must be said, however, that any time a surgeon has occasion to open a patient's abdomen, particularly in the lower portion, for some other reason, he will routinely perform an appendectomy along with whatever other procedure is under way, as long as the patient's condition during the operation warrants taking a few extra minutes. Thus any woman who has had a Caesarian section, a hysterectomy, surgery for removal of an ovarian cyst or any of a dozen other conditions will also have the added benefit of an appendectomy if her physical condition permits. Curiously enough, a number of women are either never told of this by their surgeons or else forget about it, for every doctor has seen patients apparently suffering from acute appendicitis who have the scars of earlier surgery on their abdomens and who literally do not know whether their appendix is there or not, necessitating a swift search through their medical records to find out.

In any other situation, however, prophylactic surgery to prevent appendicitis is not recommended. But the person going on a trip that will take him well beyond the reach of medical aid should by all means carry a supply of one of the broad-spectrum antibiotics such as tetracycline, and be prepared to start taking full therapeutic doses in the event that severe abdominal pain occurs. Such self-treatment should not, however, be undertaken without prior consultation with a doctor. Treatment of appendicitis with an antibiotic is not ordinarily a good practice; in fact, it may be hazardous, and every effort must be made to obtain medical help in the event of an attack. But an antibiotic may well be better than nothing at all in a true emergency.

Diverticulitis

When symptoms of "acute appendicitis" occur in individuals of middle or advanced age, and particularly when recurrent episodes of relatively mild pain and fever occur and then seem to resolve themselves, the source of trouble may not be appendicitis at all but a very similar condition known as diverticulitis. In a certain number of young adults, perhaps 5 to 10 percent, and in a higher percentage of older people, the muscular wall of the colon tends to relax and permit small, saclike pouches or *diverticula* to form, little dead-end pockets some one-fourth to one-half inch deep that protrude through the wall of the colon. Ordinarily diverticula appear in great numbers rather than singly, and can be readily seen on colon X-rays.

The mere development of diverticula in the wall of the colon is not a sign of any serious disease and in most cases is completely harmless; the diverticula themselves cause no symptoms, do not interfere in any way with the function of the bowel, and require no treatment or even concern. Occasionally, however, one of them may become plugged with fecal matter or with a fragment of undigested food and develop a suppurative inflammation almost identical in nature to appendicitis, although on a somewhat smaller scale. Even the symptoms are similar—generalized abdominal pain which finally localizes in the area of the infected diverticulum, accompanied by nausea, sometimes vomiting, a slight increase in temperature and an elevation of white cell count in the blood. Indeed, acute diverticulitis occasionally may follow exactly the same course as appendicitis, with the diverticulum becoming gangrenous and ultimately perforating the wall of the colon. More often, however, the pain does not become as severe as appendicitis, clear-cut signs of peritoneal irritation are not present, and the condition does not progress to a "point of no return." Simple bed rest, a liquid diet and the use of a broad-spectrum antibiotic will very often quiet a case of acute diverticulitis within a day or so.

If the patient has had X-rays of his colon taken previously, the discovery of diverticulosis preexisting the episode of distress will be a great help to the surgeon in differentiating that condition from an early appendicitis. In any case colon X-rays should be taken to determine, if possible, whether or not diverticula exist. When they do, and when the condition recurs, the surgeon may elect to operate and resect the segment of the bowel containing the diverticula. Similarly, if symptoms during an acute attack progress to a point where the surgeon worries about the possibility of perforation or hemorrhage, he may perform an exploratory operation, either removing the inflamed portion of the colon then and there or at least establishing drainage of the infection as a first step with later definitive surgery to remove the abnormal segment of colon.

One anatomical curiosity which deserves mention here, although its involvement in disease is comparatively uncommon, is the presence of a fairly large "blind tunnel" or tube which is attached to the small intestine and is known as *Meckel's diverticulum.* (*See* Fig. 46–4B.) This structure, a remnant of an embryonic duct normally present at a certain stage in the development of the fetus, ordinarily disappears completely within a few weeks after birth. Occasionally, however, it persists and remains as a fibrous cord, often hollow and lined for some distance with intestinal mucous membrane. A Meckel's diverticulum may cause an obstruction of the small intestine or become obstructed and/or infected itself, following a course and causing symptoms virtually identical to those of acute appendicitis. In fact, very often it is diagnosed only during surgery planned as an appendectomy. When this happens, surgical re-

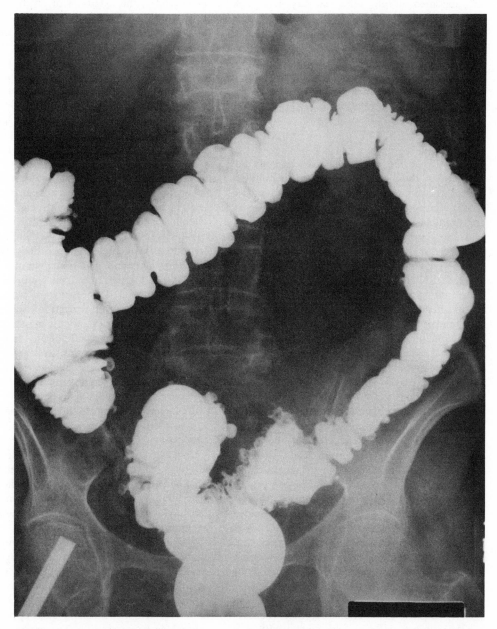

Plate 34   Diverticulosis of the colon. The diverticula can be seen as small outpouchings
scattered from one end of the colon to the other. One area of active inflammation
or diverticulitis can be identified near the lower end of the colon.

moval of the diverticulum is usually indicated. In addition, since the structure serves no purpose, the surgeon who has occasion to explore the abdomen during other surgery will look for a Meckel's diverticulum and remove it if it is present, even when it is causing no symptoms or disease. The mere discovery of such a structure on X-ray, however, is not ordinarily considered a reason for surgical intervention unless symptoms occur or the abdomen must be opened for some other reason.

Peritonitis

Virtually all the vital organs of the body are covered by thin, tough but glossy membranes which serve to separate them from surrounding structures and protect their integrity. The *pleura,* for example, covers the surface of both lungs and also lines the inner surface of the thorax. The *pericardium* is another such protective tissue layer covering the heart, and the *meninges* form a similar protective covering around the brain and spinal cord. The *peritoneum* lines the entire interior wall of the abdomen, front and back, and covers all the abdominal organs as well, both protecting them and helping suspend the abdominal viscera loosely in position. In addition, a thin double layer of peritoneum called the *mesentery* secures the intestines to the rear wall of the lower abdomen and carries blood vessels, lymph channels and nerve fibers to the intestines.

Although doctors often speak of the "peritoneal cavity" or the "peritoneal space," it is not really a space at all, since the peritoneum covering the abdominal organs comes in close contact with the peritoneum that lines the abdominal walls. However, the peritoneum secretes a clear, sterile lubricating fluid into this space which permits a considerable degree of friction-free movement of the abdominal organs, necessary both in digestive motility and in normal body movements. But like the pleura covering the lungs, the peritoneum is richly supplied with extremely sensitive nerve endings so that whenever a foreign substance comes in contact with it, a particularly sharp, constant and excruciating pain results. Virtually any foreign substance irritating

the peritoneum or penetrating the peritoneal space—because of perforation of one of the digestive tract organs with leakage of its contents, hemorrhage, the extension of an infection, or a penetrating wound from the outside—will cause an acute inflammation of this delicate membrane, which is known as peritonitis.

Other than peritonitis caused by a penetrating abdominal wound, this condition usually occurs as a complication of some other disorder of the abdominal organs and is classified either as chemical peritonitis or an infected peritonitis. *Chemical peritonitis* occurs as a complication of a number of digestive tract diseases—perforation of an ulcer of the stomach or duodenum, for example, which allows highly irritating digestive juices to escape into the peritoneal space. However, many other body fluids can also cause chemical peritonitis. Blood from hemorrhage of a tubal pregnancy or from any other source is an irritating chemical to the peritoneum. Rupture of the urinary bladder which permits urine to escape into the peritoneal space creates a chemical peritonitis, as does leakage of blood into the peritoneal space from a ruptured spleen, one of the "internal injuries" that can occur from a blow to the abdomen without any sign of external injury. In cases like this, leakage of irritating body fluids into the peritoneal space can cause a chemical irritation and inflammation of the peritoneum without necessarily being contaminated with bacteria. However, in most cases bacteria are also present, compounding the inflammatory process with infection. *Infected peritonitis* occurs when an infected appendix or diverticulum ruptures, or when there is contamination of the peritoneal space by perforation of the colon in ulcerative colitis, for example, or even when the peritoneum is soiled by bacteria in the course of abdominal surgery.

Whatever the source of the peritoneal inflammation, the major and immediate symptom is severe and excruciating pain, often so severe that it is accompanied by extreme degrees of shock. Thus when an ulcer perforates, the victim may be subjected to constant steady pain severe enough to be prostrating. The entire abdomen is tender and stomach muscles tighten to guard the area, often making the abdominal wall almost "boardlike." Any movement at all intensifies the pain, and the victim tends to lie very still, breathing only shallowly, and may bring up his knees or hunch his shoulders to relieve the irritated peritoneum of any stretching due to physical position. The onset of peritonitis is commonly accompanied by acute nausea followed by vomiting, but as the inflammation continues and spreads, the motility of the intestine decreases and a certain amount of abdominal distention from gas occurs. When the condition is severe and widespread, the victim's temperature begins to rise, his pulse increases, he begins chilling, and the white cell count in a blood sample may increase sharply. Frequently the pain is severe and constant enough that the victim knows something very serious has happened, and he may become extremely apprehensive, sometimes even irrational.

In the days before effective antibiotic and other treatment measures were available, it was not at all uncommon for victims of peritonitis, whatever the cause, to proceed into profound shock and die. But in many cases natural body defenses came to their aid. As a result of acute inflammation the peritoneum produces a quantity of thick sticky fibrinous material which would often succeed in "walling off" the area of leakage from a perforation or infection by gluing loops of intestine and other abdominal viscera together and thus localizing the disease process. If untreated, this localized area of peritonitis might well later proceed to form a *peritoneal abscess,* but at least it provided some degree of protection against generalized spread of the irritating process with increasing pain, shock and death.

The treatment of acute peritonitis today, in most cases, is primarily centered on treating its cause. Thanks to the use of antibiotics, increased knowledge of how to maintain fluid and electrolyte balance, and increased surgical skills, the once high death rate from this disease has been sharply reduced. But even so, when the condition results from some underlying disease, mortality is still approximately 10 percent—far too high to risk this dangerous complication. Furthermore, even among those who survive

acute peritonitis, the formation of abscesses can produce a source of further complications and recurrent disease which may be extremely difficult to prognosticate. Certainly when peritonitis is a result of perforation of one of the organs, the earliest possible surgical intervention is necessary to repair the damage, followed by massive antibiotic therapy and alert attention to any signs of later abscess formation. But the best treatment of peritonitis, by far, is early diagnosis and effective treatment of the conditions that can lead to it as a complication.

Anorectal Disorders

Although few people actually *like* to be sick, there are many who delight in talking about their various abdominal afflictions, and especially their operations, to anyone who will listen. But one category of inflammatory disease which afflicts vast numbers of people with pain, discomfort, annoyance and embarrassment is rarely a topic for cocktail or dinner conversation: the variety of disorders that can affect the anorectal area. For evidence of the widespread prevalence of anorectal disorders, we need only glance at a neighborhood drugstore's large and varied supply of nonprescription medicines intended for treatment of such conditions. And it is precisely *because* many anorectal disorders seem both relatively minor and embarrassing that so many people endeavor to treat these problems themselves, often unsuccessfully or incorrectly, thus prolonging an otherwise curable condition, or even masking the symptoms of a possibly more serious disorder.

One kind of common anorectal disorder, thrombosed internal or external *hemorrhoids,* is discussed in detail elsewhere. (*See* p. 570.) Many people suffer from hemorrhoids without ever requiring or seeking medical advice, but in others the symptoms can become severe enough to drive them to a physician. Similarly, the pain, discomfort, bleeding and change in bowel habits which so often herald the onset of such grave conditions as carcinoma of the rectum are likewise usually severe enough to encourage the victim to see a doctor. But other more minor conditions can also cause prolonged discomfort, often quite needlessly if the victim would only seek proper medical attention.

An *anal fissure,* for example, can be a source of agonizing pain, often recurrent with each bowel movement, under circumstances that frequently lead to chronic nonhealing. This condition begins as a minor crack or tear in the mucous membrane lining the rectum or the anal canal, often due to passage of an abnormally large constipated stool or a stool containing some indigestible abrasive material that scratches the mucosa in passing. Tissue in this area tends not to be prone to infection, but such an injury may nevertheless result in mechanical inflammation, with swelling of the surrounding tissue, some bleeding, and severe pain whenever the tissue is again stretched. Subsequent bowel movements then act as a chronic irritant so that the fissure does not adequately heal; ultimately the region may well become chronically swollen and indurated, building up scar tissue as the body tries repeatedly and unsuccessfully to heal the fissure. Often the pain at the time of defecation is severe enough that the victim prolongs the interval between bowel movements as long as possible, which results in larger, harder, more abrasive stools which further traumatize the area.

Any number of proprietary ointments, creams or suppositories are available for symptomatic treatment of an anal fissure. They often contain drugs which act as temporary surface anesthetics for relief of pain, and in all justice, such conservative treatment may lead to eventual healing. Too often, however, the fissure persists, sometimes enlarging, until it demands medical attention.

Obviously one commonsense measure to help promote healing of an anal fissure is adherence for a period of time to a diet that contains mostly fluids and low-residue foods to reduce the size and bulk of stools, and simultaneous use of a water-absorbing bulking material such as Metamucil which will tend to keep the stools soft. Laxatives may render the stools soft or watery enough to prevent stretching of the fissure, but they also induce more frequent bowel movements, and thus are of little benefit in treating this annoying condition. Any of the "liquid weight control" diet preparations which supply adequate protein and carbohydrate to maintain nutrition without providing bulk can be a help in overcoming the pain and distress of an anal fissure, and will also help promote healing in a matter of a few days. Virtually anyone can manage for two or three days on such a program, and then move on to a selected diet of low-residue foods for several days longer. Surface medications, particularly those with an oily base, tend merely to coat the lesion and make healing more difficult; these should be avoided entirely or used most sparingly only when necessary for pain. However, *any* condition that causes rectal bleeding, even in small amounts, should be called to a doctor's attention. It may only be a fissure, but other possible causes should be thoroughly investigated.

Sometimes when fissures have been present for a prolonged time, the rectal orifice may actually become *stenosed* or hardened due to a build-up of scar tissue, making it prone to further mechanical damage with every bowel movement. In such cases the problem can often be relieved in the doctor's office by means of a series of rectal dilations intended to stretch the tissues under controlled conditions to make room for the passage of normal-sized stools. In other cases the condition may be severe enough that surgical removal of the fissure and surrounding scar tissue is indicated, with care exercised to keep stools soft and infrequent until the surgical wound has healed.

An even more distressing disorder is *fistula-in-ano,* a condition in which an abrasion in the wall of the anal canal becomes infected, and the infection over a period of months or even years may form an abscess which ultimately bursts, creating a tunnel through to the skin surrounding the anal area. Such a fistula may develop with relatively little pain or discomfort and first be noticed because of a persistent drainage of fecal matter through the tunnel, soiling the region around the anus and any clothing in contact with it. Most authorities agree that a fistula, once started, will never heal by itself. Sometimes it is a source of continuing or recurrent pain, but even in the absence of pain the only way to correct the condition is surgical removal of the fistula and closure of the opening inside the anal canal. Such a procedure generally requires brief hospitalization and an anesthetic, but contrary to the fears of many people who believe that any or all rectal surgery must be agonizingly painful during the recovery and convalescent period, there is only mild temporary postoperative discomfort.

Anal pruritus, chronic or recurrent severe itching in the area of the anus, can arise from a variety of causes and often can be relieved only when the cause is identified. Virtually everyone suffers occasional mild itching in this area, and it can usually be relieved by thorough soap and water cleansing. There is absolutely nothing abnormal about this, but it *is* abnormal to suffer chronic or recurrent itching so severe that the skin is abraded or that painful scratching is necessary to relieve it. To compound the trouble, many victims use oily or greasy proprietary medications which tend to macerate the sensitive skin in the area rather than promote healing. In most cases pruritus can best be controlled by careful daily cleansing in a shower or tub followed by application of a drying agent such as a mild fungicide powder, talc, or some other powder preparation. Intestinal pinworms are a frequent cause of anal pruritus, and examination for this pest should be undertaken if the pruritus does not clear up quickly or if it recurs, since it will recur as long as pinworms are present. Pruritus is particularly common in patients who have been taking a full dosage of broad-spectrum antibiotics in treatment of some other condition, partly because of the looseness of the stools that follows such treatment and partly because of the appearance of irritating fungus overgrowths such as *Candida albicans* or "thrush" in the perianal region. Abrasive or highly spiced foods may also be sufficient to trigger pruritus in this area. Often merely avoiding these foods for long enough for the pruritus to disappear is all that need be done.

The major decision to be made when anal pruritus is present is whether or not it is severe enough to warrant consulting a doctor. Often the best rule to follow is to take particular pains with personal hygiene, use soothing powder in the area after it is well dried following a shower, and avoid irritating foods for several days to encourage healing. If the condition persists or recurs, it is then time to have a doctor examine the area in order to rule out any more serious condition that could be present.

When to see the doctor can, in fact, be a difficult problem in the case of a great many different kinds of digestive tract disorders. The symptoms of a chemical peritonitis may well be so dramatic and painful that no one can ignore them, but very often less disabling symptoms of digestive tract diseases *are* ignored for too long, to the victim's later grief. No one wants to call a doctor about every mild episode of gastritis or diarrhea, but it is well to remember that any recurrent or chronic symptoms related to digestive function are *never* normal. Anyone who is afflicted with such symptoms should seek medical help and make a concerted effort to find the cause and eliminate it. If no pathological cause can be found and the trouble continues, the patient should at least take the precaution of repeated medical consultation at reasonable and orderly intervals, since a condition which seems purely "psychosomatic" one month may within another six or eight months subtly progress to involve physical change. Treating both the physical changes and the emotional factors that influence digestive tract disease is a complex and difficult branch of medicine, but the medical profession includes a large number of physicians who have years of training and experience in dealing with precisely this kind of problem. There is still much to be learned in this area of disease, but with present-day understanding and experience there are few conditions that cannot be treated and markedly improved by judicious medical observation and care.

Peptic Ulcer Disease and Intestinal Cancers

For many years it has been fashionable to talk about peptic ulcers in a half-joking manner, even to consider an ulcer some sort of a bench mark on the long climb to success in our competitive world. But for the people who actually develop ulcers—some three million or more Americans each year, 15 people out of every 1,000—ulcer disease is no laughing matter. For those who ignore early symptoms, or in whom the developing ulcer is "silent" or relatively asymptomatic, the sudden occurrence of one of the serious complications of the disease—massive internal hemorrhage, for instance, or intestinal obstruction—may catapult the victim into an acute surgical emergency without warning, and well over 10,000 people in this country die each year from ulcer disease or one of its complications. "Fashionable" or not, a peptic ulcer is nothing to joke about. Yet commonplace as it is, most laymen are either confused or misinformed about peptic ulcer disease and even doctors still regard it as very much of a mystery in many respects.

The Nature of Peptic Ulcer

Just what is a peptic ulcer, and what causes it to form in the first place? Essentially a peptic ulcer is a crater-like open sore that forms somewhere in the mucous membrane lining the upper portion of the digestive tract, most commonly in the duodenum, but sometimes in the wall of the stomach itself or in the narrow canal between stomach and duodenum called the *pylorus*. The most obvious immediate cause is the presence of

excess amounts of hydrochloric acid and a digestive enzyme called pepsin, both of which are normally secreted by special glandlike cells in the lining of the stomach and are useful in the digestive process, but which in some individuals, under certain circumstances, are secreted in vastly excess quantities.

When there is little food to be digested in the stomach or duodenum, these excessive secretions begin acting on the digestive tract lining itself, corroding one or more areas in the lining of the stomach or the duodenum and forming one or more shallow, open sores. Prevented from healing by these same secretions, such a sore, known as a peptic ulcer, gradually grows deeper, eroding into the muscular wall of the stomach or duodenum, exposing sensitive pain nerve endings, sometimes eating through the walls of blood vessels or even completely perforating the stomach or duodenum, thus allowing gastric acid and bacteria to escape into the peritoneal space in the abdomen. Some peptic ulcers can become very large, as much as three-fourths of an inch in diameter and half an inch deep. As with any other open sore, the body attempts to heal a peptic ulcer as soon as it forms, and often evidence both of the processes of healing and of further erosion is found present in the same lesion. Unfortunately, a large, deep ulcer tends to heal by scarring, and if an ulcer has been present for a long period of time in a narrow or constricted area such as the lower end of the stomach or the upper end of the duodenum, recurrent scarring together with swelling of the tissue in the vicinity of the ulcer may bring about an obstruction of the digestive tract, a very dangerous complication of peptic ulcer disease.

The relationship between excessive secretion of gastric acids and the development of peptic ulcer has been known for many decades, but this relationship alone does not completely explain the disease. Why is it that one person may fall victim to such excessive gastric secretion while another person does not? No one knows, exactly. We know that normally the interior of the stomach is coated with a mucus-like secretion which seems, under most circumstances, to protect the stomach lining from self-digestion in spite of the fact that normal amounts of these gastric secretions are capable of initiating digestion of virtually any kind of protein material put in the stomach. One theory holds that in certain people some kinds of emotional pressure and tension tend to suppress the normal production of this mucinous protective coating, and that these are the people who ultimately develop peptic ulcer disease. Precisely *how* an emotional state can act to suppress a body defense mechanism in this fashion is by no means clearly understood, but there is unquestionably a strong emotional factor involved in peptic ulcer disease —strong enough, in fact, that successful control of the disease depends not only upon physical treatment but also upon success in eradicating or modifying the emotional tensions of the patient.

Certain facts about peptic ulcer are clearly recognized. First, it is predominantly (though not exclusively) a male affliction; on the average, three out of every four victims of the disease are men. Second, the incidence of peptic ulcer in the United States and other advanced nations of the world is rising steadily and alarmingly; in the past 20 years, it is estimated, the occurrence of peptic ulcer disease has quadrupled, afflicting more and more women as well as men. No doubt part of this increase is a reflection of improved diagnostic techniques, and the fact that more people suffering from persistent "acid indigestion" consult a doctor today than was the case 20 years ago; but most authorities agree that the major part of this increase is very real—not only are more cases of

peptic ulcer disease diagnosed, but many more people acquire the disease than formerly. Third, peptic ulcers may occur at any time from infancy to old age, but by far the majority of victims first encounter trouble during their thirties and early forties. And a great many of these people, although they embark on medical treatment programs for their disorder, tend to have recurrent trouble, sometimes to the point of suffering a lifelong chronic illness.

Perhaps the most confusing fact about peptic ulcer disease is its strange relationship to the victim's emotional state. This most emphatically does *not* mean that peptic ulcer is "all in the mind," or in any way imaginary, or even primarily a neurotic disease. Peptic ulcer is a very real physical affliction, and there is nothing the least bit imaginary about an open, ulcerating sore in the wall of the stomach or duodenum. But doctors with wide experience treating the disorder see an unmistakable correlation between certain personality types and the development of this condition. They speak of the "ulcer personality": the tense, hard-driving perfectionist, the man who takes all his obligations perhaps too seriously, the worrier who is intensely involved emotionally in everything he does and who seems never to be able to relax. These authorities point out that in people of this personality type peptic ulcers typically tend to develop, or to recur, at times of extreme emotional stress— when the heat is on, so to speak—and to recede or even heal themselves when emotional pressures are relieved.

There is other evidence, too, to support the "stress" theory of ulcer disease. Whereas it was once thought that peptic ulcers always took a prolonged period of time to develop, we now know that they can develop with amazing rapidity under intense conditions of stress. During World War II in London it was discovered that individuals could develop peptic ulcers from scratch, even dangerous perforating ulcers, in as little as 24 hours following a night spent in an air raid shelter. Such "stress ulcers" are commonly recognized today, although we know that they often heal almost as quickly as they form once the extreme stress situation is relieved.

Other authorities, however, maintain that the

"stress" theory of peptic ulcer disease has been vastly overrated, and point to the large numbers of apparently easygoing and happy-go-lucky individuals who develop ulcers. Thus far neither side can satisfactorily answer the key question: do people develop ulcers because they are tense and irritable, or do they become tense and irritable because they have developed ulcers? All that can be said for certain is that emotions unquestionably play a major role in this disabling disease complex.

Symptoms and Diagnosis of Peptic Ulcer

The symptoms of peptic ulcer often follow a predictable pattern, but they can also be extremely deceptive. Many people with typical and recurrent "ulcer symptoms" never do actually develop an ulcer, while many other disorders of the digestive tract, including gall bladder disease, liver diseases or simple gastritis (inflammation of the stomach), can so closely mimic the typical "ulcer syndrome" that diagnostic differentiation can be a major problem. Beyond doubt the most common symptom of peptic ulcer is pain, sometimes quite severe, other times intermittent and merely annoying, centered in the pit of the stomach just below the ribs. Usually the pain of peptic ulcer is relieved by food, but then tends to recur a few hours after a meal or during the night after the stomach has been empty for a while. Some people describe their ulcer pain as a "gnawing hungry feeling," while others may be gripped by extremely painful cramps in the upper abdomen.

In some 30 percent of cases the ulcer is "silent," located in an area where relatively few nerve endings are involved, and the victim must take warning from less dramatic recurring symptoms such as heartburn, excessive belching or a sour taste in the mouth, all of which may be temporarily relieved by taking antacids. In cases in which the ulcer tends to obstruct the digestive tract because of scarring or swelling, symptoms may include vomiting, sometimes with brown "coffee-ground" flecks of blood in the vomitus. And if an ulcer is bleeding significantly, the stools may become black and sticky like tar. Any such symptoms demand the immediate at-

tention of a doctor, since they may be the first warnings of an impending emergency situation. But even patterns of continuing or recurring upper abdominal pain, heartburn or the queasy feeling of recurrent indigestion deserve investigation. A peptic ulcer is far easier to treat, or to prevent altogether, when symptoms are brought to a doctor's attention early in the game.

If the symptoms of an ulcer are so variable, or so similar to symptoms of other conditions, how can a doctor tell whether an ulcer is present or not? The overall pattern of the patient's symptoms, combined with the details of his medical and personal history, is a great help; but by far the most effective aid to diagnosis is an X-ray examination which may reveal not only the presence of an ulcer but its location as well. The location is very significant in itself, for a lesion in the duodenum, at worst, will probably not be anything other than a peptic ulcer, but a lesion located in the stomach can sometimes be an early cancer in disguise.

Most peptic ulcers can be identified by means of a special fluoroscopic X-ray examination, commonly spoken of as an "upper GI series" because it involves a number of "spot X-rays" of the interior of the entire upper gastrointestinal tract. For this examination the patient enters a darkened fluoroscopy room and is given a quantity of a chalky liquid containing barium sulfate to swallow. The esophagus, stomach and duodenum do not normally appear in an X-ray examination, but this "contrast medium" is opaque to X-rays, and thus throws a shadow picture that reveals the interior of the upper digestive tract. The radiologist watches the fluoroscope screen for any sign of the telltale crater of an ulcer or the muscle spasm that often occurs in the vicinity of an ulcer, as the barium sulfate moves through the upper digestive tract, and at the same time he snaps a succession of spot X-ray pictures for permanent record. By pushing the upper abdomen in order to be sure that the barium coats the entire lining of the stomach and duodenum, and from his long experience with the normal pattern of peristaltic motions in these regions, the radiologist can usually spot an ulcer. He will also check to see if a hiatus hernia is present, one condition that can mimic peptic ulcer, and be on the lookout for any evidence of impairment in the way material in the stomach is emptied into the duodenum. This type of X-ray study takes about ten minutes to complete, and in most cases the radiologist can report his findings to the doctor immediately after the examination if he has seen evidence of an ulcer. The X-ray films, when developed, confirm the presence and location of the ulcer, and are kept on file for reference when later examinations are made to check the effectiveness of treatment.

If the ulcer is located in the stomach, other laboratory tests and special examinations may be necessary. A sample of gastric juice may be withdrawn through a narrow tube inserted into the stomach and its acidity tested; if a peptic ulcer is present, gastric acidity is usually significantly higher than normal, whereas if the lesion is an early cancer, there may be little or no acid in the gastric juice at all. If this proves to be the case, a procedure known as *gastroscopy* may be performed, in which a long, narrow lighted tube is passed down the esophagus into the stomach to permit the physician actually to examine the inner lining of the stomach and if necessary take a biopsy of the questionable lesion. At the same time, "gastric washing" may be performed by inserting a sterile saline solution into the stomach and then withdrawing it by suction for centrifuging and examination for cancer cells. If the lesion proves to be malignant, it is a serious matter, although much less serious than if the cancer remained undetected, since cancer of the stomach, caught early enough, can often be cured.

Medical Treatment of Ulcer Disease

Everyone has heard mock-humorous tales of the trials and inconvenience involved in medical treatment of an ulcer—stories of grown men eating baby food, drinking gallons of cream and popping pills into their mouths every hour on the hour. There was a time when those tales were no exaggeration, but medical treatment of ulcer disease today is not as rigorous and troublesome as it used to be. Unless an ulcer is first discovered because of some serious complication such as perforation or massive bleeding,

most ulcer specialists today favor a fairly simple and conservative medical regimen for treatment, reserving the more drastic surgical treatment for the small proportion of cases in which medical treatment fails, or in which the ulcer recurs with threatening complications.

The primary goals of medical treatment of peptic ulcer are simple: first, allowing the ulcer to heal; and second, preventing the development of a recurrent ulcer. To achieve these goals, therapy seeks to accomplish four things:

1. To neutralize excessive digestive acid with frequent regular doses of an antacid medicine.

2. To reduce the *total amount* of acid formed in the stomach with the use of medicines that slow down gastric secretion and, at the same time, help relieve ulcer pain by reducing motility and muscle spasm in the stomach and duodenum.

3. To provide several small, frequent meals throughout the day, rather than two or three large ones, so that the digestive juices have something other than the ulcer to work on, while avoiding such irritating substances as alcohol, coffee or highly spiced foods and such relatively indigestible substances as deep-fried foods, cabbage or onions.

4. Perhaps more important than anything else, to reduce the level of emotional tension, stress or pressure that has prepared the ground for the patient's ulcer in the first place.

Such a therapeutic program may take several slightly different forms. The use of antacids is always a key part of the program, since excessive quantities of digestive acid are always present and can be neutralized only by hourly doses of antacid between meals. Frequent small meals, perhaps four or five a day, further aid in this program. The insistence upon excessively bland and soft foods that was once a prevalent part of most ulcer diets has been relaxed considerably. Doctors have since realized that success of an ulcer treatment regimen really depends heavily upon the patient's faithful adherence to the program for weeks or sometimes months at a time, and that a diet that is imaginative and offers more variety is easier to maintain than a diet that the patient soon comes to hate. Today in the modern ulcer diet most foods can be eaten in

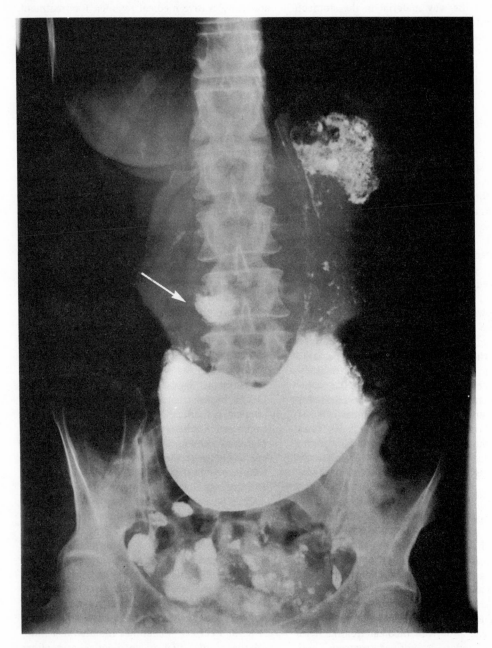

Plate 35a   A large duodenal ulcer is revealed by a patch of barium sulphate contrast medium trapped in the ulcer crater (see arrow). Note the distended, over-filled stomach shadow, indicating that the ulcer is obstructing the stomach outlet.

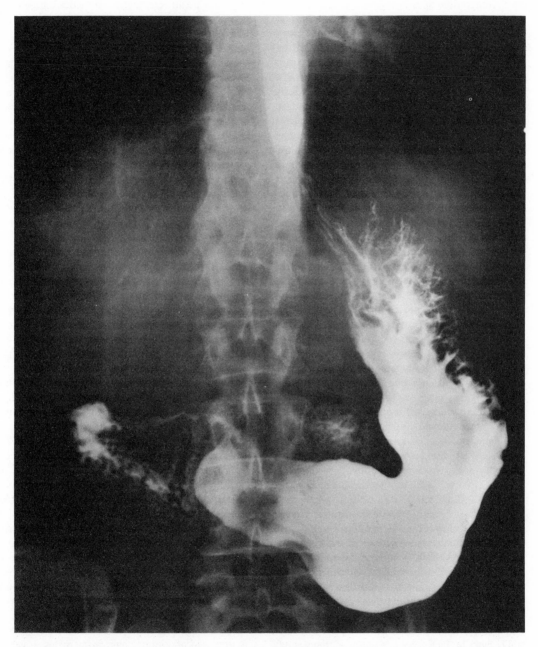

Plate 35b   The same patient with the ulcer healed. Shadow of the stomach is normal. The
             duodenum shows some loss of its normal contour due to scarring.

moderation, avoiding only the obviously irritating or indigestible ones.

Such a medical regimen, continued faithfully for six to eight weeks, will usually result in very rapid relief from the distressing symptoms of an ulcer within the first week or so and will ultimately lead to healing of the ulcer in most cases. Later recurrence can usually be prevented by continuing the program of active treatment in modified form, combined with the patient's own efforts to slow down, relax and avoid, or react more realistically to, situations that cause emotional tension and stress. Often more frequent rests and recreational breaks can contribute to this change, as can a reappraisal, with the doctor's guidance, and with the help of family, friends and business associates, of what things are important and what things are not.

It is not easy, of course, for the ulcer patient to remake his personality or alter his life style, even on a doctor's orders. But drastic change is not always necessary. Faithful adherence to medical treatment, diet and minor but realistic changes in attitudes and values are usually enough to help stave off recurrent ulcer trouble. Often it is the patient's own insight into the causes and the possibly life-threatening complications of the disease that motivates the necessary changes. Certainly the popular notion that ulcers *always* recur is false; many ulcer patients heal completely and are never bothered again. But ulcers *do* recur and even become a chronic condition, and in such cases, it is often the patient himself who is responsible.

The Unfortunate Few

In a small proportion of patients—roughly 10 percent—the conservative medical treatment discussed above fails to bring about healing of an ulcer, or else the ulcer recurs, or complications such as bleeding, obstruction or perforation enter the picture. In such cases, surgical treatment is necessary. Uncontrollable hemorrhage, or perforation of the wall of the upper digestive tract, can, in fact, create a surgical emergency even in the case of a first ulcer, although it is far more common in recurrent or chronic cases. Many people regard surgical treatment of ulcer

disease as a sort of "last ditch" procedure to be avoided at all costs, but statistics show that surgery has proved highly beneficial in treating the refractory, chronically recurring or dangerously complicated cases.

Just what kind of surgical treatment is performed depends a great deal on the surgeon; there are half a dozen different procedures in use today, each with certain advantages and disadvantages. Most surgeons prefer to perform a *vagotomy,* a disconnection of the vagus nerve which leads to the stomach and stimulates the secretion of gastric juice, combined either with removal of much of the acid-forming part of the stomach or with *pyloroplasty,* a procedure to reduce cramping and spasm of the pylorus. An older procedure still used by many surgeons is an operation called a *subtotal gastrectomy,* in which the lower two-thirds of the stomach, where most of the gastric acid is formed, is removed, even if the ulcer itself is located below the stomach in the duodenum. Oddly enough, normal digestion can proceed perfectly well without these gastric secretions. Following subtotal gastrectomy the part of the stomach remaining may be reattached to the duodenum directly, or to the small intestine below the duodenum, in effect by-passing the duodenum altogether; this latter procedure is called a *gastrojejunostomy.* In some cases the vagus nerve may also be disconnected in the course of these procedures.

The fact that such a variety of surgical procedures is in use today obviously suggests that no one procedure is universally ideal, or free of postoperative complications. A small number of patients on whom a subtotal gastrectomy has been performed will suffer a tendency to regurgitate whenever more than a small amount of food is taken. When a vagotomy has been performed, approximately one out of every six or seven patients suffers a curious syndrome surgeons speak of as "dumping." This "dumping syndrome" has nothing to do with regurgitation or throwing up; rather, it involves some degree of nausea and abdominal pain after meals, together with excessive sweating and sometimes diarrhea. It occurs most commonly in highly emotional patients, and in individuals who have lifelong histories of "headaches" prior to their ulcer surgery—people with "hair-trigger nervous systems," so to speak. Today, however, careful postoperative treatment spares most patients from these annoyances; and in fact, all the common surgical procedures for ulcer disease give at least relatively satisfactory results most of the time.

Even so, surgeons continue to explore new techniques that will give even better results. Some new approaches which appeared highly promising at first have later proved disappointing. For example, in the early 1960s a special technique was devised for freezing the inner lining of the stomach by means of a balloon filled with ice cold alcohol. In theory, this technique was intended to destroy the acid-forming cells in the stomach by freezing, and thus allow ulcers to heal without surgery. At first this radical new departure in ulcer treatment seemed extremely promising; long-chronic ulcers healed and patients were spared the necessity of surgery. But unfortunately, within a few years it was discovered that the "healed" ulcers seemed to recur, and the freezing procedure has now largely been discarded. On the other hand, it has been found that *cooling* the stomach to a certain degree by means of this technique is still very useful in helping slow down otherwise uncontrollable bleeding from an ulcer.

With such a complex illness, is there any possibility that peptic ulcer disease will be "conquered" in the future? Probably not; in fact, as emotional tensions in our society increase, we can well expect a continued increase in the incidence of ulcer disease. This annoying and dangerous affliction may always be with us; but with early diagnosis and sensible, conservative treatment aimed not only at temporary relief of symptoms and healing but at prevention of recurrence as well, there is at least reasonable hope that peptic ulcer will become less of a threat.

Carcinoma of the Stomach

Curiously enough, the uncomfortable digestive symptoms that may or may not be caused by peptic ulcer disease have had one beneficial side effect. They cannot easily be ignored, and investigation of these symptoms in recent years has often led to the early detection and treatment of another far more dangerous upper gastrointestinal disease—carcinoma of the stomach, one of the most frequently encountered of all cancers. Just as a higher incidence of diagnosed peptic ulcer disease has resulted from an increasing tendency to seek medical help for apparently minor digestive disturbances, so the incidence of diagnosed carcinoma of the stomach has also increased; but these cancers have been discovered earlier and their greater incidence has been accompanied by increased numbers of cures or long-term palliative control.

Carcinoma of the stomach, like any other cancer, occurs as a result of a change in the normal growth pattern of cells in the stomach lining; at some point, for reasons unknown, one cell or group of cells begins to multiply rapidly, escaping the normal growth-control influences of the body and spreading to invade the surrounding tissue. In the case of carcinoma of the stomach, the initial lesion soon reaches a point of uncontrolled local growth that is so rapid that blood supply to the area is impaired and the early cancer tends to break down to form an ulcer very similar in appearance to a benign peptic ulcer. Indeed, there is a suspicion, as yet unproven, that a benign peptic ulcer that has formed in the wall of the stomach may in some cases actually develop into cancer.

There are, however, some very distinct differences between the "ulcer" of a stomach cancer and a benign peptic ulcer. For one thing, carcinoma of the stomach is almost always associated with a marked *decrease* or even an absence of acid gastric secretions. For another thing, the "ulcer" of stomach cancer will not completely heal under the medical regimen used for peptic ulcer, even though pain, heartburn and other symptoms are temporarily relieved. It may *partially* heal, or improve, but will not go completely away. Finally, carcinoma of the stomach is frequently associated with three other danger signs that are uncommon with a benign peptic ulcer: an unusual loss of appetite, unexplained weight loss, and the development of anemia, at least in part as a result of a continuous small

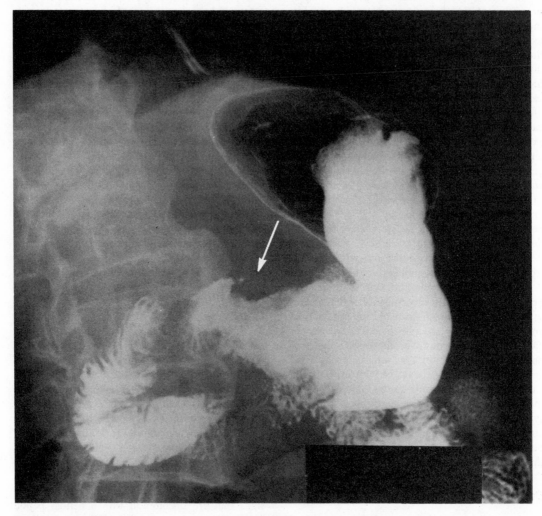

Plate 36   Carcinoma of the stomach. This tumor, itself invisible to X-ray, is revealed to the radiologist by the roughened, ragged and scarred stomach margin seen at the region of the arrow.

amount of bleeding from the cancerous lesion in the stomach. In fact, the relationship between a detectable anemia and a still-hidden early carcinoma of the stomach is so striking that upper GI X-rays should always be taken before a newly discovered anemia is treated, and the stool should be examined for telltale traces of blood, particularly if there has been any weight loss or falling off of appetite, or any upper digestive tract symptoms.

The only effective treatment for carcinoma of the stomach is surgical removal of the cancer together with surrounding tissues which may have been invaded by the tumor cells, and the sooner the better. Cure of this disease depends on early detection and surgical removal before the point has been reached that cancer cells have seeded into the blood stream and lodged in the liver or elsewhere in the body. If treated early enough, cures are possible, but most surgeons are cautious about speaking of such cures except in retrospect. Rather, they speak of "three-year cures" and "five-year cures"; that is, individuals who have survived for three or five years after surgery with no evidence of any recurrence.

Left untreated, the disease is invariably progressive and fatal, running a natural course of from nine months to two years, with death ensuing as a result of starvation due to obstruction of the stomach by growth of the tumor, or by anemia or hemorrhage, or a combination of both. But with early detection and effective surgical treatment, a great many people survive as long as five years and frequently much longer, and in most cases these salvaged years are comfortable and productive. Unfortunately, this record has not been found to improve much in the past 20 years, and it seems likely that the final answer to truly effective treatment and cure of this disease, like that of many cancers, must await a major breakthrough in our understanding of the nature of malignant diseases and perhaps totally new approaches to control or cure.

Other Digestive Tract Cancers

The stomach is not by any means the only place in the digestive tract that cancers can originate, although certain parts seem to be more resistant to this disease than others. For reasons that no one understands, cancer only rarely arises anywhere in the small intestine, and it practically never develops in the upper third, including the duodenum. It is true that the walls of the duodenum or upper small intestine can be invaded by cancers that originate in such adjacent organs as the stomach or the pancreas, but this one segment of the intestine seems remarkably resistant to the development of primary cancerous growth. This is the reason that doctors often seem relieved when they find that a patient's newly developed ulcer is in the duodenum; there, at least, the lesion is most unlikely to be a cancer masquerading as a peptic ulcer.

Other areas are far more vulnerable. Cancer may arise in the mouth, in the tongue or in the esophagus. Cancers of the mouth, the palate or the tongue are usually detected early, because any persistent swelling, ulceration or soreness is quite noticeable and is usually called to a doctor's attention promptly. Diagnosis is confirmed by biopsy of the lesion, and treatment by means of surgical excision or localized radiation with radium or radon usually is curative. Cancer of the esophagus is a more difficult problem. Symptoms tend to appear gradually; any persisting and progressive dull soreness felt deep in the throat or chest upon swallowing should arouse suspicion, particularly if there is increasing difficulty swallowing larger chunks of food. The condition can be diagnosed by careful X-ray examination, followed, if necessary, by *esophagoscopy*—direct examination of the esophagus by means of a gastroscope. Once diagnosis is confirmed, treatment is surgical, in most cases involving excision of the lesion and the adjacent areas of the esophagus, followed by implantation of a segment of the jejunum to substitute for the missing segment of esophagus. This is an extremely difficult operation to perform, however, and statistically the overall success in treating this form of cancer is poor compared to other digestive tract cancers.

Cancer of the Colon. Cancers that originate in such "auxiliary" digestive tract organs as the pancreas, the liver or the gall bladder, discussed in the following chapters, are relatively uncommon. Unfortunately, the same cannot be said for the large intestine, which is a frequent site of cancer all the way from the cecum, the bulbous upper end where it is joined to the small intestine, down to the rectum and anus. In general, however, the tissue of the colon appears increasingly vulnerable to the development of cancer the closer it is to the anal orifice, and the great majority of cancers of the colon have their origin in the lower twelve inches or so of the large intestine. This means that a great many cases of carcinoma of the colon can be detected early enough to permit successful treatment.

Detection usually occurs during a routine physical examination by means of two simple office procedures: a rectal examination performed by the doctor, using a surgical rubber glove in order to feel with his finger the area of the rectum just inside the anus; and the use of a lighted instrument called a *proctoscope* which can be inserted into the rectum, permitting the doctor actually to examine the lower ten inches of the colon by direct visualization. Early cancers farther up in the colon beyond the reach of the proctoscope can also often be detected by means of an X-ray examination. A radio-opaque barium sulfate suspension in the form of an enema is injected to fill the entire length of the colon, and then any evidence of abnormal contours or structures within the interior of the colon is revealed by X-ray. Cancer of the colon or rectum rarely occurs in younger age groups, but most physicians recommend proctoscopy as part of the routine physical examination of anyone over the age of thirty-five or forty. It is a simple procedure, requiring only that the patient take a mild laxative the preceding night and then use a warm tap-water enema a few hours before the examination to cleanse stool from the lower end of the colon. The examination is performed in the doctor's office and, while slightly uncomfortable, is over in a matter of a very few minutes. Patients who dislike this examination are generally more upset by the apparent indignity than by any discomfort, but most patients realize that a slight degree of both is worth the high degree of protection the examination provides against one of the more common cancers.

The cardinal signs of developing cancer in the large intestine are simple enough for anyone to recognize and take warning from: first, any change in bowel habits, particularly accompanied by the passage of frequent stools or stools of a markedly narrowed diameter; second, the appearance of blood with the bowel movement, particularly intermixed with the stool; and third, the development of pain or discomfort associated with evacuation. Any or all of these symptoms may also occur due to other perfectly benign reasons. Both blood in the stool and pain on defecation, for example, can be a result of a fissure or tear in the mucous membrane of the rectum or due to thrombosed and bleeding hemorrhoids; other conditions can produce bowel movements more frequent than normal, stools of narrower diameter, recurring diarrhea alternating with constipation, and other changes in bowel habits. Nevertheless, the appearance of any of these cardinal symptoms is a signal to see a physician for a thorough diagnostic examination.

Treatment of carcinoma of the colon involves the surgical removal of the segment of the bowel in which the tumor is located, together with resection of the adjacent mesentery and lymph glands to which the cancer may already have spread. When the tumor is found high up in the colon, the surgeon can often perform an "end-to-end anastomosis," that is, suture the segment of colon above the lesion to the segment below, thus preserving the rectal area so that the patient can continue normal anal evacuation. When the lower part of the colon or the rectum is involved in the cancer, however, a colostomy may be necessary, in which the upper end of the colon is carried out to an opening made in the abdominal wall, and the patient uses a colostomy bag for bowel evacuation. Because this cancer can so often be visualized directly through the proctoscope or detected so readily by X-ray studies, it is often diagnosed in the course of a perfectly routine physical examination long before any symptoms have appeared. Consequently it is a cancer which may in many cases be cured and in other cases treated effectively enough to enable the patient to enjoy years of relatively normal life.

Another reason that cancer of the colon or rectum can be caught early is that in many cases the cancer develops first as a perfectly benign *polyp* or overgrowth of mucous membrane somewhere in the lower end of the colon. Rectal or intestinal polyps may be single or multiple and can be detected by the same diagnostic procedure used to detect cancer. Small polyps are almost always completely without symptoms, but as they grow they may cause bleeding, partial obstruction of the free evacuation of stools, or even pain—precisely the same symptoms that so often occur in malignant cases. In addition, many studies have shown that a certain percentage of benign polyps will undergo malignant change at some point. For this reason, when one is found on proctoscopic examination, even a small one, X-ray studies are then undertaken in an effort to discover any others that may be located higher up in the intestine, and the doctor may recommend that they be biopsied or removed. Removal is usually a simple procedure that can be performed in the doctor's office and does not require hospitalization or convalescence. In patients who have multiple polyps of the colon or develop them recurrently, particularly those with a history of cancer of the colon or rectum among parents or grandparents, more elaborate surgical treatment may be advisable, perhaps even resection of the segment of colon containing the polyps. This, of course, is essentially a medical and surgical decision. But the major responsibility for early detection is up to the patient, even in the absence of symptoms. Periodic and regular physical examinations, including digital rectal and proctoscopic examinations, are certainly the most important aspect of preventive medical care, and the surest way of detecting physical disorders of the lower colon *before* they have become symptomatic or have progressed to a potentially more dangerous stage.

Diseases of the Pancreas, Liver and Gall Bladder

It is in the duodenum, the ten-inch section of small intestine immediately below and connected to the stomach, and further down in the small intestine, that the body's major biochemical digestive reactions take place. The digestive functions of the duodenum and small intestine are made possible because of certain digestive juices and enzymes produced by two organs in the abdomen adjacent to the digestive tract, the *pancreas* and the *liver.* The secretions of both these organs are carried from their place of manufacture to the duodenum by means of ducts, and any disease that materially affects the secretory function of either organ, or that somehow prevents their secretions from reaching the intestinal tract, can result in grave disruption of digestion, often with death as a result if the disorder cannot be corrected or healed. A third organ, the *gall bladder,* acts primarily as a receptacle and storage pouch for digestive secretions formed in the liver, but it, too, is vulnerable to diseases and disorders that can disrupt digestive function as well as present a threat to life. The gall bladder, like the stomach, can be surgically removed when it threatens life or normal function without severely affecting the digestive process; the liver may continue to function effectively even after much of it has been destroyed by disease; but the pancreas cannot be materially damaged or tampered with surgically without serious repercussions and the need to replace its vital secretions if normal digestion is to continue.

The Pancreas

Of these three organs, the pancreas is perhaps the most interesting. Essentially it is a glandular structure composed of masses of secretory cells called *acini* supported by a fibrous and fatty matrix. These cells pour secretions into tiny collecting tubules which connect with larger tubules and finally empty into the *pancreatic duct,* which, in turn, empties into the duodenum. These "external" secretions of the pancreas, so called because they are poured into a collecting system of tubes rather than being absorbed directly into the blood stream, contain great quantities of alkaline substances which serve primarily to neutralize the hydrochloric acid of gastric secretions mixed with the food that passes from the stomach into the duodenum.

In addition, pancreatic secretions contain a number of enzymes capable of extremely powerful action upon complex food substances. For example, the enzyme *trypsin* breaks down protein foods into their component protein molecules, and then further breaks the protein molecules into molecular components known as *proteoses* and, ultimately, *peptides.* These peptides are further broken down into amino acid fragments, and it is these fragments that are absorbed through the wall of the small intestine into the blood stream and from there enter the cells as protein building blocks. Another potent enzyme known as *amylase* is capable of breaking down starches and complex sugars into glucose and other simple sugars which are assimilable in the small intestine and are used by the cells in the production of heat and energy. Finally, *lipase,* another pancreatic enzyme, acts upon fats to break them down into fatty acids which can also be absorbed into the blood stream through the walls of the small intestine. The production of all these secretions is governed by a complex triggering system. When acidic gastric juices mixed with food enter the duodenum, they stimulate the release of a certain enzyme from the wall of the duodenum which, when it reaches the pancreas, stimulates the secretion of pancreatic enzymes. Thus, the production of one enzyme depends upon the influence of another, so that a breakdown anywhere along the line can seriously impair the entire digestive function.

In reality, the pancreas has a dual role. In addition to the acini which produce and carry off the external pancreatic secretions, the pancreas contains a quantity of totally different cells, known as *Beta cells,* which produce the enzyme *insulin,* needed throughout the body as a catalyst in the biochemical reactions whereby simple sugars are oxidized to produce heat and energy. Insulin is not collected in any series of tubules, but rather is absorbed directly into the blood stream, and thus is considered an "internal" or *endocrine* secretion. The production and use of insulin has nothing whatever to do with the process of digestion; the pancreas just happens to be the organ in which these cells are located. But diseases and disorders impairing the function of the pancreas often lead to destruction of Beta cells as well as the acini, and thus may cause *secondary diabetes mellitus,* commonly known as sugar diabetes. Far more often, however, the Beta cells in a perfectly healthy pancreas may cease to function properly quite spontaneously, leading to *primary diabetes mellitus,* an extremely complex and fascinating condition. Both forms of this disease are discussed elsewhere. (*See* p. 696.) Here only those pancreatic disorders which directly affect the digestive function are considered.

Diseases of the Pancreas

The pancreas is probably one of the least familiar organs of the body, and considering its importance, it may seem relatively unimpressive —a small glandular organ shaped rather like a fox tail, hidden back against the rear wall of the abdomen underneath the stomach and duodenum, perhaps seven inches long, three inches wide and one-half inch thick. Interestingly enough, in spite of its vital double function in the body, the pancreas is not a paired organ like the lungs, the kidneys or the adrenals, nor is there any great quantity of it to spare as is the case with the small intestine, nor does it have the capacity to regenerate itself when damaged or injured as the liver has. If some disease or disorder strikes the pancreas and knocks it out, it cannot be repaired or replaced, and its vital functions must be carried on by artificial means in order to preserve life.

As with most organs of the body, there are certain kinds of disorders to which the pancreas is vulnerable. Developmental abnormalities or genetic factors may, for example, result in a deformity or shortage of pancreatic tissue. Most authorities recognize that diabetes mellitus, caused by inadequate insulin production of the Beta cells in the pancreas, is a disorder very strongly influenced by genetic factors, if not directly inherited. Another grave disorder of the pancreas is *congenital fibrocystic disease,* which also occurs in a strong hereditary pattern and typically afflicts the victim in infancy and childhood. (*See* p. 893.) The pancreas is also vulnerable to inflammatory disease which may or may not be a result of infection by bacteria or viruses. And finally, malignant tumors may engulf the pancreas, the most common of which is singularly virulent and dangerous.

There is, in fact, no really mild or inconsequential disease that affects the pancreas, with the possible exception of mumps, which may occasionally be complicated by *mumps pancreatitis.* When this happens, cells in the pancreas are attacked by the mumps virus with resulting inflammation and swelling, but by and large, the condition is seldom grave, even though permanent destruction and later scarring of a certain amount of glandular tissue in the pancreas can result.

Acute Pancreatitis. The most common inflammatory disease of the pancreas, acute pancreatitis, can be a grave and sometimes devastating affliction. It is not associated with bacterial or viral infection; in fact, for years physicians remained totally in the dark about the cause of this disease which seemed to strike out of the blue, leading to death in some 50 percent of acute cases and to a pattern of chronic recurrence in a great many of those who survived.

Today acute pancreatitis is believed to result either from an accidental backup of bile into the pancreatic duct, with inflammation triggered when the bile reaches the cells of the pancreas, or else from obstruction of the pancreatic duct itself, causing the backup of pancreatic juices and ultimately the activation of those juices in the pancreas so that a process of self-digestion begins. Physicians still do not know exactly how obstruction or premature activation of pancreatic juices triggers the inflammation of the pancreas, but it is known that more than 50 percent of the victims of acute pancreatitis also have concurrent obstructive disease of the biliary system—gall bladder stones, for example, or stones lodged in the common bile duct. In addition, a large number of victims of acute pancreatitis are alcoholics whose attacks often follow prolonged bouts of heavy drinking—suggestive that alcohol in excess in a relatively empty upper digestive tract succeeds in activating pancreatic juices which then, in effect, turn on the very tissue that produced them.

It is also believed today that acute pancreatitis may occur in a wide range of severity, some cases so mild that the disease goes unrecognized, other cases more severe but never diagnosed. In its most acute form, however, the disease can cause massive destruction of pancreatic tissue, together with swelling of surrounding tissues, sometimes intractable hemorrhage, agonizing pain, shock, circulatory collapse and death.

The most characteristic symptom of acute pancreatitis is the sudden onset of severe abdominal pain usually felt high in the abdomen and referred into the back. Unlike the cramping intermittent pain of intestinal obstruction, this pain is usually constant, and it may be so severe that large doses of potent pain-relieving drugs fail to relieve it. The use of morphine or other opium derivatives is doubly contraindicated, however, because these drugs tend to cause muscle spasm at the outlet of the pancreatic duct and thus aggravate obstruction, and because the disease so often occurs in dependent persons like alcoholics that the danger of addiction is extremely great. Furthermore, the pain tends to be steady and persistent for days or weeks, depending on the severity of the inflammation and the amount of tissue destruction that occurs. In addition to the pain, the victim usually has a low-grade fever of 100° to 101° and a sharp elevation in white cell count in his blood. Unfortunately, all these symptoms are similar to those of other abdominal disorders such as certain types of gall bladder disease, perforating peptic ulcer or even appendicitis. They present an apparent picture of an acute surgical emergency, and surgeons are frequently trapped into exploratory abdominal surgery before the diagnosis is made.

One feature of the disease, however, helps confirm a diagnosis: in the first 24 hours or so of symptoms, backed-up digestive enzymes such as amylase and lipase may be absorbed in great quantity into the blood, so that careful laboratory examination reveals a sharp increase of amylase and lipase levels in the blood serum while the acute attack is in progress. Such a laboratory finding is extremely valuable in achieving fast and accurate diagnosis of acute pancreatitis, and has very frequently been the major factor in preventing unnecessary surgery which may aggravate the severity of the disease.

Medical treatment of acute pancreatitis is limited to relieving pain, providing intravenous feedings, and using a nasogastric tube to keep the stomach sucked dry of secretions which might further trigger the inflammatory reaction in the pancreas. In addition, antibiotics such as penicillin or tetracycline are given by injection to prevent secondary bacterial infection of the damaged part of the pancreas, and various drugs in the belladonna-atropine group may be given to reduce spasm in the smooth muscle of the intestine and pancreatic ducts. Medical management also includes the administration of calcium compounds, since pancreatic juices attacking fatty tissue in the abdominal cavity react with the fat to form soap, a process which uses up large amounts of calcium. In severe cases, further supportive care may include blood transfusion in the event of hemorrhage, the administration of insulin if enough of the pancreas has been destroyed to reduce normal insulin levels, and careful nursing. As an extreme measure, surgical drainage of secretions from the inflamed gland may be attempted, combined with lavage of the abdominal space to clear away irritating pancreatic secretions and sometimes surgical correction of biliary obstruction if it is found to be present. Any surgery in this condition, however, carries a very high mortality rate and is not performed unless physician and surgeon alike are convinced that the patient will die without it.

In severe acute attacks of this sort, the disease can be fulminating and terminate in death in a matter of a few hours, no matter what anyone does. Victims with milder attacks frequently recover, some even permanently. There are, however, an unfortunate few who suffer relapses or recurrences, as the pancreatitis turns from an acute and violent disease to a chronic, smoldering inflammation which repeatedly flares up and cools off, destroying a little pancreatic tissue at a time, perhaps over a period of years. In many such cases, replacement therapy is necessary to provide insulin as well as pancreatic enzymes to aid digestion.

A few precautions can be taken, in the case of one who has had an attack of acute pancreatitis and recovered, to help prevent recurrences. If a careful physical examination and X-ray studies indicate the presence of biliary tract obstruction or disease, surgical treatment to remove a gall bladder full of stones or to detect and remove a stone lodged in the common bile duct may forestall the circumstances that could lead to a recurrent attack of pancreatitis. Avoidance of alcohol in any form will also increase the odds against recurrence. Unfortunately, once a pattern of recurrent attacks of the disease becomes entrenched, the victim is involved in one of the most unpleasant of all chronic illnesses, and one of the most difficult for the doctor to treat successfully. No one program of treatment is effective for all cases, and dependence or addiction to narcotics is an ever present threat, since medication for pain must be used so frequently.

Tumors of the Pancreas. Both benign and malignant tumors of various sorts may arise in the pancreas, most commonly in the middle or older years. One of these is an overgrowth of Beta cells in the *islets of Langerhans,* the portion of the pancreatic tissue that produces insulin. This very rare "islet cell tumor," usually benign, may be completely free of any symptoms except that it liberates excessive quantities of insulin into the blood stream. The disorder is discovered when the apparently normal, nondiabetic victim begins having bouts of *hypoglycemia* (very low blood sugar)—literally, episodes of insulin shock without taking any excess insulin. Once diagnosed, this "functioning" tumor (a term used to describe tumorous overgrowths of secreting glandular tissue in which the cells in the tumor continue to produce the secretion in larger and larger quantity) can be cured by surgical exploration and removal. Only very rarely does it prove to be malignant, showing characteristics of metastatic spread to the liver by way of the regional lymph nodes.

Another rare benign tumor of the pancreas, which, for reasons unknown, seems to produce extraordinary ulcer-forming tendencies in its victims, was first described in 1955. Victims of this unusual tumor characteristically have a marked increase in gastric secretion and acidity, and tend to form ulcers that are highly resistant to all forms of treatment. These growths are spoken of as "ulcerogenic" tumors of the pancreas, although so far not enough is known about them to be certain of a cause and effect relationship between the tumor and the ulcers. When this condition is recognized, the ulcer disease can sometimes be treated effectively by removal of the tumor-bearing portion of the pancreas, or when this is technically impossible, by performance of a total gastrectomy (total removal of the stomach).

By far the most common tumor of the pancreas is a malignant neoplasm known as *carcinoma of the pancreas,* a cancer that makes up from 1 to 2 percent of all carcinomas. It rarely occurs before middle age, and its highest incidence is in people between sixty and seventy years old, with more than twice as many men affected as women. A large majority of these carcinomas form in the head of the pancreas, the portion nearest the intestine, and nearly all of them arise from wild growth of the cells lining the pancreatic ductules or from the secreting glandular cells themselves. Because of the location of these tumors, they often spread to involve the neighboring bile ducts, and the first symptom in about one case out of four is the mysterious appearance of a painless jaundice as a result of obstruction of the bile ducts. In other cases pain is the most frequent presenting symptom, constant and "boring" in type, usually felt in the upper part of the abdomen and extending into the back. All too often, however, the tumor develops asymptomatically for months or even years, so that by the time pain begins to occur, massive spread of the cancer into the liver, the peritoneum, the lungs or the diaphragm may already have taken place. Many victims suffer nothing more than a very mild and annoyingly persistent indigestion, apparently too minor to warrant visiting a doctor. In addition, for reasons no one clearly understands, carcinoma of the head of the pancreas seems to be associated with the occurrence of thrombophlebitis of the leg veins, and occasionally the sudden appearance of sore, painful thrombosed veins in the legs is the first sign of trouble. As the disease progresses, weight loss, loss of appetite and jaundice appear.

Because the course of the disease is so often asymptomatic, early diagnosis is seldom possible, and even laboratory studies of a screening variety offer very little help. Only in a small proportion of victims is the cancer diagnosed early enough to be operable, and even among those, very few survive as long as five years after surgery. Thus in most cases only palliative treatment is possible and the disease usually runs its fatal course in a matter of a few months following diagnosis.

The Liver

Of all the organs making up the digestive system the liver is by far the most diversified in function, and for that reason is truly vital to continuing good health. (*See* p. 87.) Actually, the liver's direct contribution to the digestive process, the formation of pigmented bile salts that aid in breaking down dietary fats into fatty acids for absorption, is of comparatively minor importance. Far more significant are some of its less well understood functions, including the formation and storage of a complex carbohydrate food material known as *glycogen* from biochemical processing of simple sugars absorbed from the intestine, the filtering of old red blood cells from the blood stream and the conservation of the pigmented substance in those red cells which is later used in the manufacture of bile pigments, and the biochemical manufacture of fatty compounds known as *cholesterol* and *triglycerides,* an important step in the body's metabolism of fatty food materials. The liver also manufactures prothrombin necessary to blood coagulation, as well as various blood proteins, acts as a storage depot for amino acids, iron and other vital substances, and serves to destroy or detoxify many potentially harmful chemicals, including various medicines that may be taken.

Like the pancreas, the liver is an organ which is not paired, but it does have a remarkable capacity to regenerate its cells when damage has been wrought by infection or other destructive influences. Furthermore, the normal liver contains such an excess of liver cells that it has been estimated that the body could survive if only one-quarter of the liver remained undiseased and functioning. However, this means that in destructive disorders of the liver a great deal of damage can be done before the presence of the trouble is recognized, even though certain biochemical laboratory tests might have revealed the disorder earlier if symptoms had directed the physician's attention to possible liver trouble.

The liver is able to perform its many vital functions because of a unique double circulation system. Like any other organ it has an arterial blood supply, in this case by way of the hepatic artery which branches from the lower aorta near the place where it enters the abdomen. This artery branches into arterioles and capillaries which, in turn, lead into hepatic venules and veins which return blood from the liver to the heart. Completely separate from this system, which provides a nutritive blood supply to the liver, is the so-called *portal circulation system.* In this system the great majority of the veins that drain other parts of the digestive tract—the stomach, the duodenum and the small intestine in particular—and contain the absorbed nutriments that have resulted from the digestive process do *not* feed directly into the vena cava for return to the heart, but rather drain into a large vessel known as the *portal vein* which then carries this venous blood through a completely separate network of capillary blood vessels in the liver. It is only after passing through the portal network that this blood is finally returned to the general circulation again, and it is from the blood in this portal network that the liver draws the metabolic raw materials for its many biochemical manufacturing processes.

Thus, in a way, the liver is doubly vulnerable to diseases or disorders related in any way to circulation—bacterial or viral infections carried by the blood stream, for example. Cancer cells released from distant sites and carried by the blood stream also frequently lodge and grow in the liver. In fact, cancers arising almost anywhere in the digestive tract most often spread first to the liver. Another disorder related to circulation is *passive congestion* of the liver caused by congestive heart failure when blood backs up in the liver and damages liver tissue if not properly relieved. These and other liver disorders may lead to pain and tenderness in the upper right quadrant of the abdomen as a cardinal symptom. Disease may also interfere with other manufacturing and storage functions of the liver, upsetting the body's delicate chemical balance. Thus diagnostic tests of the blood, urine or feces can frequently be used to detect liver disorders in the absence of more obvious symptoms. But there is one symptom that may arise with a number of liver disorders that is so striking and unmistakable that it can hardly be overlooked. This is the appearance of jaundice.

Jaundice is not a disease itself, but it is a symptom not to be taken lightly. In most cases it is first seen as a yellowish-green tinge that appears in the sclera or white of the eyes and in the mucous membrane of the mouth. This color change occurs when bile that is produced by the liver is prevented from draining normally into the duodenum for use as a digestive juice, usually as a result of some disease or disorder that obstructs the drainage tubules. When this happens, the yellow-green bile, which takes its color from the bile pigments it contains, tends to back up in the liver and gall bladder and presently is absorbed into the blood stream and carried to distant parts of the body, staining all organs and tissues it touches. At the same time, the kidneys work to filter excess quantities of bile pigments out of the blood stream, so the urine takes on a distinctive reddish brown or coffee color which, when diluted, appears more yellow-green or yellow-orange. Finally, when jaundice is due to obstruction of the biliary ducts, which prevents bile from being emptied into the duodenum as it normally is, it may be accompanied by very light yellow "clay-colored" stools, or even stools that are a pasty gray-white color, since bile pigments that account for the normal brown color are absent. As jaundice becomes more severe, the color of the entire skin may turn a distinctive yellow and, in profound jaundice, even a yellow-orange color.

When even a hint of jaundice appears it must be taken as a yellow danger flag signifying that something may have gone seriously wrong with the function of the liver, gall bladder or bile ducts. It does not *always* mean liver disease, however; a similar jaundice can also arise as a symptom in certain diseases such as hemolytic anemia, in which blood cells are destroyed or hemolyzed in great quantities, but that form of jaundice can be readily differentiated by special blood tests. Nor is jaundice necessarily an *early* symptom of liver or bile duct disease; a considerable degree of elevation of bile pigments in the blood stream must already have occurred before obvious staining of the tissues makes itself apparent. The important thing to remember is that jaundice *never occurs normally.* Diagnosis of its cause and assessment of its seriousness are a physician's responsibility.

Whatever its cause, the chances of nipping potentially serious or fatal illness in the bud rests heavily on early medical consultation.

Diseases of the Liver

Cirrhosis. Perhaps the most familiar of liver diseases is a condition caused by widespread damage to liver tissue, usually over a prolonged period of time, which leads to a permanent form of scarring known as cirrhosis of the liver. Although cirrhosis may occur as a result of a number of different disorders, by far the most common form in this country and in Europe stems from chronic, long-term protein starvation that arises as a secondary effect of alcoholism.

Actually, this class of liver disease with its devastating consequences is prevalent throughout the world, albeit for different reasons. It is estimated that in the United States and Europe cirrhosis in some form is found in from 2 to 3 percent of all post-mortem examinations, although it is by no means the cause of death in all these cases. In the Western world it occurs most commonly between the ages of forty-five and sixty-five, and in men two or three times more frequently than in women. It is also notably more frequent in persons of Irish and Italian stock than in other Caucasians. In other parts of the world—the Orient, the Near East and throughout Africa—the incidence of cirrhosis is significantly higher, found in up to 10 percent of all post-mortem examinations, but here the disease is by far the most common in children and is known as *kwashiorkor*. The nutritional deficiency factor in victims of this age group is emphasized by the name, which has been loosely translated to mean "the disease of the red devil of jealousy," so called because in Negroes with the disease the hair often becomes bleached to a reddish cast, and the disorder characteristically first makes its appearance when the child-victim is necessarily weaned from his mother's breast to make room for a new baby, and consequently must change from the protein-rich diet of mother's milk to the typical native diet of carbohydrate foods such as yams, sweet potatoes or cassava root, all notably poor in protein. The disease, however, can occur at any age when the victim's diet is depleted or completely free of protein.

Most laymen associate cirrhosis of the liver with excessive intake of alcohol, and one oftens hears it said that "drinking is bad for the liver." But this is an oversimplification, and not quite accurate at that. Aside from the intoxicating quality of alcohol, it is a relatively simple carbohydrate which can be taken up in the digestive system and used by the body; but unfortunately, alcohol cannot be converted into vital protein by any biochemical process. Thus in a great many excessive drinkers, the immediate energy demands of the body can be met by the alcohol intake, and if enough is consumed over a prolonged period, the individual ceases to feel hungry for other foods, and indeed may not eat at all for days at a time. This means that the body, either chronically and constantly or intermittently, is robbed of protein, and particularly the protein amino acid constituents known as *choline* and *methionine,* which are a normal and vital part of the diet. And in the face of this prolonged protein starvation, liver cells begin to die.

What, exactly, is cirrhosis of the liver? Essentially it is the end result of a long process involving destruction of liver cells, together with a deposition of fibrous connective tissue and extensive scarring as the damaged tissue seeks to heal and regenerate. Ultimately, the liver shrinks in overall size and there is progressive diminution of the amount of liver tissue that can actually function. As this scarring process proceeds, circulation of blood in the liver, both its normal nutritive circulation and the circulation by way of the portal vein, tends to be gradually limited and closed off, so that as the disease progresses the blood pressure in the portal vein steadily rises. This leads to such late symptoms of long-term cirrhosis as the development of *ascites*—a collection of fluid in the abdominal cavity outside the digestive tract as a result of high portal vein pressures and the subsequent osmotic loss of water into the abdomen—as well as the development of enlarged veins or varices in the region of the esophagus and severe engorgement of the veins draining the small intestine.

Symptoms of this usually prolonged and chronic process may be relatively few or absent for a long period of time. If the cause is chronic alcoholism combined with haphazard eating habits, the victim usually develops a gradual loss of appetite and a tendency to be nauseated or to vomit when food is taken in, which results in a considerable weight loss. He may also feel physically weak and often mentally dull or confused; there may be discomfort on account of pressure and abdominal distention, or some degree of pain, and low-grade fever may be present. As the disease progresses, jaundice may appear because of destruction of ductules in the liver that would ordinarily conduct bile into the duodenum. Even so, many victims postpone seeking medical help in an effort to conceal their alcoholism. When they do seek help, two things in addition to any jaundice present may tip the doctor off to the diagnosis: the discovery of tiny capillary lesions on the skin of the upper body, descriptively spoken of as "spider nevi" or "spiders," and the typical rough or "hobnail" feeling of the liver which can actually be palpated below the rib cage on the right. Also, a victim of the disease at this point may suffer from various bleeding phenomena, particularly nosebleeds, since the damage to the liver results in a diminished production of the special blood proteins and enzymes needed for the normal clotting of blood. In addition, if esophageal varices develop because of portal vein hypertension, there may be massive hemorrhage due to a rupture of these veins, with the vomiting of frank red blood or the passage of tarry stools composed mostly of digested blood.

Diagnosis is not difficult in most moderately advanced cases, but earlier diagnosis very often is. In some clinics doctors perform needle biopsies to obtain fragments of liver tissue for microscopic pathological examination by inserting a needle through the skin of the abdomen into a palpable liver edge. Success of this procedure, however, depends upon great skill and experience and thus is not yet universally approved. Early diagnosis is, however, of extreme importance; if cirrhosis of the liver is not recognized or treated until the appearance of such late symptoms as jaundice or the formation of ascitic

fluid in the abdomen, so much of the liver will have been permanently damaged that a "point of no return" is reached and little can be done to reverse its progress. In that case, victims of the disease tend to follow a downhill course of survival ranging from one to five years with death eventuating from liver failure, intercurrent infections which the body cannot adequately fight off, or the most dread of all complications and the most common cause of death—rupture and hemorrhage from varicose veins of the esophagus or stomach as a result of increased portal vein pressure. But before this "point of no return" is reached, the presence of some degree of cirrhosis of the liver does not necessarily mean a severe shortening of life, particularly if active treatment is begun to stop the progress of the disease.

Treatment normally emphasizes the use of a diet rich in protein materials, particularly choline or its biochemical equivalent, methionine. Such a diet includes eggs for breakfast, meat with lunch and supper, and milk at each of the three meals. In addition, extra quantities of the major vitamins are beneficial. Any form of alcohol in the diet is literally poison, and alcoholism as a concomitant and predisposing disease must be treated as vigorously and effectively as possible. Unfortunately, if the patient is an alcoholic, faithful adherence to a no-alcohol and protein-rich diet may be exceedingly difficult to achieve, as alcoholism is one of the most cruelly refractory of all human illnesses. Indeed, knowledge of the impending threat of cirrhosis can all too often precipitate the patient into greater depths of alcoholism. Thus treatment at a time when it can still be effective demands not only the skill and ingenuity of the physician and the whole-hearted cooperation of both the patient and his family, but sometimes the assistance of psychiatric consultation. The chronic alcoholic who has eggs, meat, milk products and other proteins in his daily diet on a consistent basis may well suffer many other ills due to his alcoholism, but cirrhosis of the liver can be avoided.

In the areas of the world where kwashiorkor in children is prevalent due to grossly insufficient protein, the disease can be stemmed and life prolonged by introducing adequate protein-bearing foods into the diet. As simple as that may sound, in underdeveloped areas it can be a social problem that involves powerful cultural components; even if foods containing adequate protein are made available, they may still be rejected by the victims of the illness as strange and unnatural substances, differing widely from their traditional food. This problem has already been encountered in India where wheat has been rejected in famine areas by the population whose traditional staple food is rice. Only major national and international attention to education, advanced agricultural techniques and improvement of native diets will be able to check the present incidence of kwashiorkor, and in those countries where a burgeoning and uncontrolled population growth is also a factor, the situation will perhaps become worse before it becomes better.

Certain other conditions can result in cirrhosis of the liver, and both the treatment and the prognosis of the disease depend upon accurate identification of the specific cause. Thus in patients who suffer a chronic obstruction of the biliary system due to stones and/or inflammation or infection, a so-called *obstructive cirrhosis* or *biliary cirrhosis* may occur as a result of back pressure of the bile in these ductules suppressing and ultimately destroying liver cells. Carcinoma obstructing the bile ducts or the presence of parasites infesting the ducts can also cause cirrhosis. In addition, *toxic cirrhosis* can occur when liver cells have been severely damaged by some external liver poison. Perhaps the most dangerous of these chemical poisons are the chlorinated hydrocarbons such as carbon tetrachloride, a common ingredient in home dry cleaning fluids, spot removers and fire extinguishers for use against electrical fires. An amazing amount of this substance can be inhaled even with a fairly brief exposure, and the danger cannot be overemphasized. Carbon tetrachloride has no place among household cleaning supplies, and it should not be used at all except by individuals fully knowledgeable of the necessary means of self-protection. Phosphorus and arsenic compounds also act as liver toxins, sometimes leading to a much more gradual degree of liver injury than the chlorinated hydrocarbons.

Finally, a variety of drugs and medicines which are ordinarily tolerated by the body can occasionally cause drug reactions in which severe liver damage occurs, probably as a matter of individual sensitivity. The sulfonamide drugs and many of the antibiotics fall into this category, and these medicines should never be used without a physician's prescription or continued for prolonged periods without careful observation and the use of laboratory studies to detect any sign of drug reaction.

Perhaps the most dangerous and disheartening of all forms of cirrhosis is "post-necrotic cirrhosis" which occurs as a residual effect of the massive destruction of liver cells that can occur in the course of *infectious hepatitis* or *serum hepatitis*. These disorders are discussed in detail with other infectious diseases. (*See* p. 200.) Here it is enough to note that in very severe cases of hepatitis massive quantities of liver cells may be destroyed, and in the body's effort both to combat the infection and to repair the damage, the typical scarring and poorly organized regeneration of liver cells can gradually cause the development of a grave degree of cirrhosis which cannot be reversed. The amount of liver destruction caused by toxic substances or infectious hepatitis often can be held to a minimum by early diagnosis and by the strictest adherence to rigid medical programs involving rest, adequate diet and careful protection from intercurrent illnesses. In some, the infection may be so severe that even these measures do not help, but in most cases liver damage and the threat of later post-necrotic cirrhosis can at least be held to a minimum.

Liver Failure and Hepatic Coma. To further complicate the already complex problem of diagnosing and treating various types of acute or chronic liver disease, physicians must also be alert for the development of a progressive comatose state which may appear at any time that damage to the cells and function of the liver is severe, or when an extra burden such as intercurrent infection is thrown on the body in the face of borderline liver function. *Hepatic coma* is a condition that usually develops while a patient is already under a doctor's care, but there are cases in which it may first appear in those with undiscovered liver disease, and may first come to a doctor's attention because relatives or friends of the victim are alarmed by an increasing degree of apparently inexplicable behavior. No one is entirely sure why the symptoms of hepatic failure occur as they do, or what causes them, but in most cases the victim has an increase in the amount of ammonia in the blood stream, and it is generally thought that hepatic failure is heralded by ammonia intoxication because the liver is unable to function well enough to convert the ammonia absorbed from the digestive tract into another organic compound known as urea which is ultimately filtered from the blood stream by the kidneys.

The onset of hepatic failure may be swift or relatively slow, with the victim often going through a period of confused behavior, apathy, inexplicable loss of memory and other symptoms suggesting some type of brain intoxication. Certain abnormal reflexes appear at this time also, indicating hyperirritability of the nervous system, and electroencephalograph changes are often found present on examination. During a prolonged period of onset there may also be loss of appetite, and a degree of confusion or stuporousness may appear and increase with the intake of high-protein foods. If untreated, or all too often in spite of treatment, the victim's state of stuporousness will gradually progress to a frank state of "unwakable sleep" or coma.

In some cases treatment can help alleviate various factors precipitating the coma, such as replacement of blood lost by hemorrhage from esophageal varices or the use of various medications to lower the blood ammonia level. In addition, of course, a search must be made to discover the underlying cause of the liver failure, if it is undiagnosed, and to correct it if possible. But in any event, the individual in hepatic coma needs supportive nursing care, and medical attention should be sought immediately upon any sign of the development of this disorder. Early treatment can often help reverse the condition, but in some cases the underlying liver-destroying disease has already progressed too far and hepatic coma is often a terminal state.

Cancer of the Liver. Both primary and secondary cancers can develop in the liver; indeed primary cancer of the liver accounts for a relatively large number of cancer deaths (from 5 to 20 percent) in such Asiatic countries as Japan, China, Malaysia and the Philippines. These cancers are far less common in Europe and the Americas, for reasons unknown. Overall there is a much higher incidence among individuals with cirrhosis than among those who have had no previous liver disease. Once a primary carcinoma has made an appearance, the clinical course of the disease lasts only a few months in most cases, although surgical removal of carcinoma is occasionally successful. Modern surgeons have experimented with liver transplants, as yet without notable success, but it is conceivable that as surgical knowledge and techniques improve, more radical surgery of primary liver cancers will become possible, replacing lost function by transplanting a healthy liver, and thus brightening the currently dim prospects for recovery from this disease.

Secondary cancer in the liver, spread either from nearby digestive tract organs such as the stomach, gall bladder or pancreas, or from other abdominal cancers, occurs with great frequency. When it is detected, it is generally clear evidence that the cancer has spread beyond the point that cure is possible, but in many cases surgical removal of the primary tumor may afford considerable relief of pain, prolongation of life, or both. While such surgical treatment and medical supportive care may not be able to cure the disease, it may well give the patient several more months and sometimes even years of relatively comfortable life.

The Gall Bladder

The gall bladder is a small, hollow, pouchlike organ, ranging from three to six inches long and approximately two inches in diameter, which lies adjacent to and underneath the liver in the central part of the abdomen. It is connected to the digestive tract by means of a rather short, stubby and thick-walled *cystic duct,* a collecting tubule perhaps one-half inch in its interior diameter. Ordinarily this duct does not communicate directly with the small intestine, but rather meets and joins the hepatic ducts which drain bile

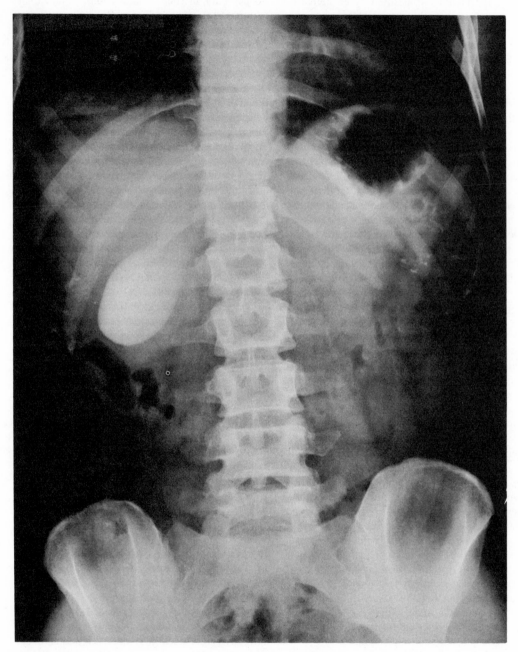

Plate 37a   A normal gall bladder, visualized as an oval shadow of radio-opaque dye in the patient's right upper abdomen.

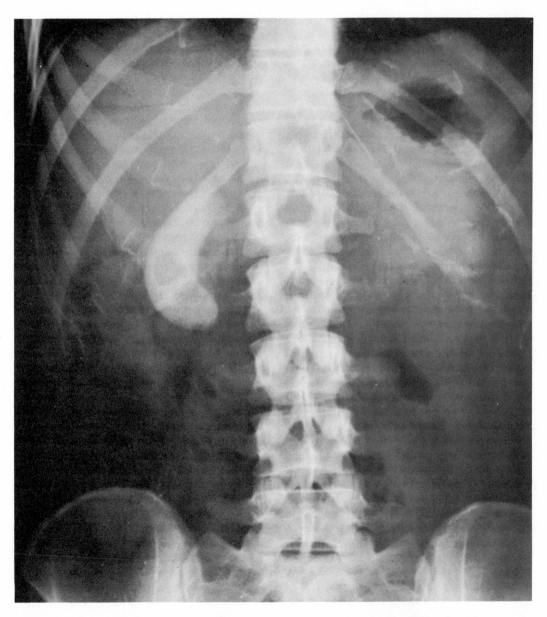

Plate 37b   A diseased gall bladder containing two large and many small radiotranslucent stones. The stones appear as dark areas within the gall bladder shadow.

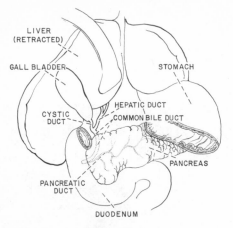

Figure 49–1.

from the network of ductules throughout the liver; together they form the *common bile duct,* a somewhat larger tubule which opens into the intestine very near the place where the pancreatic duct enters the intestine. (*See* Fig. 49–1.)

The gall bladder itself does not contribute any digestive secretion; rather, it acts as a receptacle for the collection of *bile,* the alkaline and extremely bitter-tasting digestive secretion manufactured by the liver. In addition to storing bile as it is formed, the gall bladder acts to concentrate the bile some five to ten times by reabsorbing part of its fluid content. Then when stimulated by the presence of fat in the digesting food poured into the duodenum, the gall bladder contracts, emptying the concentrated bile into the common bile duct which, in turn, empties into the duodenum.

Oddly enough, although the gall bladder has a function and purpose, it has long been known that the human body can do perfectly well without it; therefore, if it becomes diseased in any way, it can safely be removed by surgery. In some cases when this is done, the common bile duct itself becomes somewhat enlarged and acts as a storage receptacle and concentrating organ for bile, but in other cases it does not and digestion proceeds just as well with unconcentrated bile pouring into the intestine directly from the liver. On the other hand, disorders which impair the function of the gall bladder can cause thoroughly unpleasant symptoms and sometimes even pose a threat to life unless they are properly treated.

Diseases of the Gall Bladder and Bile Ducts

In general, disorders afflicting the gall bladder and the bile ducts fall into one of three categories: inflammation or infection of the gall bladder, known as *cholecystitis;* obstruction of the gall bladder or the common bile duct due to the formation of stones, called *cholelithiasis;* or cancer of the gall bladder.

Cholecystitis and Cholelithiasis. The occurrence of a gall bladder inflammation and the presence of gallstones are so closely interrelated about 90 percent of the time that it is convenient to consider them both at once, although it is perfectly possible to have one condition without the other. No one knows for certain why one person forms gallstones and another does not, but there is little doubt that the presence of chronic inflammation of the gall bladder is a contributing factor.

Gallstones in most cases are single or multiple hard nodules of cholesterol, one of the components of bile, which, in some people, apparently precipitates out in the gall bladder during the process of concentration of the bile. When gall bladder inflammation is present, small bits of inflammatory exudate—white blood cells, epithelial cells and fibrin, for example—serve as nuclei around which cholesterol and another chemical substance known as bilirubin settle. Other stones may contain calcium salts. The stones tend to form in middle life, most commonly in overweight women who have had one or more pregnancies. Incidence is much higher among women than among men, and much more common among Caucasians than among Orientals or Negroes, facts which have led to the diagnostic "4 F's" popular among young medical students—fair, female, fat and forty.

When the stones form, those containing calcium carbonate or calcium bilirubin (one of the bile salts) become radio-opaque and can be detected on X-ray films taken of the abdomen. Cholesterol stones do not show up on normal X-ray films, but become visible on X-ray plates as translucent shadows in the gall bladder when a special radio-opaque dye is taken by mouth, digested and later excreted. Stones as large as one and one-half inches in diameter have been detected in the gall bladder, or multitudes of tiny stones may be found, sometimes lying in distinct layers, one on top of the other, the heavier ones sinking to the bottom, the lighter ones floating on top.

The presence of gallstones in itself does not necessarily mean that there will be symptoms; doubtless many people live out their lives with gallstones without even realizing it, and every doctor knows at least one patient who has resisted the idea of surgery when gallstones were discovered and succeeded in avoiding serious illness for years. In most people, however, gallstones and the inflammation in the gall bladder which is so often present concurrently can cause a variety of different symptoms. Most common are excessive flatulence and belching, acid indigestion and rather vague complaints of feeling overstuffed and uncomfortable, especially after meals. Certain foods characteristically seem to trigger these symptoms: pork, cabbage and fried foods, for example.

Quite a different situation occurs when a gallstone becomes wedged or impacted in the cystic duct and causes a typical colicky "gall bladder attack" or *biliary colic.* The most frequent symptom is severe pain, usually felt high in the abdomen, beginning abruptly several hours after a heavy meal. The pain comes in waves which seem to increase sometimes to agonizing proportions and then ease off, only to recur again. The pain is caused by stretching or spasm of the smooth muscle in the gall bladder or the cystic duct, and it is often accompanied by profuse sweating and sometimes vomiting as well. If infection of the gall bladder is present, complicating the obstruction, gangrene may develop and the colicky pain progresses to a continuous acute abdominal pain, the onset of fever, chills, and ultimately the rigid guarding of abdominal muscles that alerts the surgeon to the presence of an acute surgical emergency. If a gall bladder attack is not complicated by infection, the attack may last for a few hours or even less, and then apparently clear up, only to recur anywhere from days to months later.

Often in the midst of an attack of biliary colic, jaundice will appear temporarily, owing to a backup of bile and the absorption of bilirubin and other bile salts into the blood stream, and the urine may darken and stain with the yellow-green bile. If the stone moves down the cystic duct and becomes lodged in the common bile duct, a much more profound jaundice occurs, often with the patient turning a bright yellow, his urine a dark yellowish-brown color and his stools changing from the normal brown color due to bile pigments to a light yellow or sometimes even gray color, indicating that the bile salts are not reaching the intestine at all.

Diagnosis of a gall bladder attack caused by gallstones may be very difficult in some cases because the symptoms mimic those of peptic ulcer or intestinal obstruction. Usually the diagnosis can be confirmed if the patient has had a history of periodic attacks of pain that have cleared up by themselves in the past, intermittent darkening of the urine or lightening of the stools, the appearance of jaundice during an attack and other telltale symptoms. The diagnosis can be confirmed by X-ray examination revealing the presence of gallstones, if the stones can be seen. Occasionally the cystic duct may be completely blocked by a stone, or the gall bladder so chronically diseased that it has lost its function of collecting and concentrating bile, in which case no shadow of the gall bladder can be seen on X-ray and the doctor can only ascertain that the patient's gall bladder is "nonfunctioning," whether stones are present or not. Another type of X-ray examination involves the injection of a radio-opaque dye intravenously, permitting visualization of the bile ducts that come from the liver and sometimes revealing the presence of stones there. Since attacks of biliary colic occasionally occur in the absence of any gallstones at all, it is sometimes necessary to engage in a period of prolonged watchful waiting and repeated examination before the diagnosis of gallstones can be made. This so-called *biliary dyskinesia* without gallstones can present a difficult diagnostic challenge before cholecystitis or cholelithiasis can be ruled out.

In the face of gall bladder attacks, with or without the complicating presence of stones, conservative medical treatment has very little to offer other than temporary control of symptoms. Various medications can be used to reduce the pain of biliary colic, ranging from mild analgesics to the potent narcotic painkillers, and pain is often relieved in part by the use of medicines that relax smooth muscle spasm, the source of much of the discomfort. During acute attacks, however, this kind of medication must be used with a great deal of judgment, since there is a real possibility of masking the pain of acute cholecystitis until the gall bladder has become gangrenous or has burst. If that happens, an acute but controllable surgical disease can become a life-threatening generalized peritonitis.

When there is infection involved, a variety of antibiotics can be used to control bacterial contamination, and if this is a major factor, they may be of great importance in cooling off an acute attack. There are even some medicines which are capable of stimulating the production of bile and thus "flushing out" the gall bladder, sometimes helpful in reducing obstruction due to a collection of very fine sand-grain-sized stones or even smaller debris that may be plugging the bile ducts. But there is no medicine that can effectively "dissolve" gallstones, reduce their size, or protect against recurrent attacks. Once a diagnosis of stones in the gall bladder, with or without inflammation or infection, has been made, the only definitive treatment is surgical removal of the organ as well as removal of any stones that have been impacted in the cystic duct or the common bile duct.

With definitive diagnosis of this condition often so difficult, and delay in surgical treatment so dangerous because of complicating changes, one might assume that surgeons would undertake exploration of the abdomen and removal of the gall bladder immediately, even on the basis of strong suspicion, as is frequently the case, for example, with suspected appendicitis. But surgeons do not proceed in this way in the case of acute gall bladder attacks, for a very significant reason: the surgery required is extremely difficult. It requires a high degree of skill, and it carries a very real risk. It has been said that the surgeon removing a gall bladder is "working at the bottom of an inkwell," for this organ is lo-

cated deep in the upper abdomen, hidden beneath the bulky liver and attached by the stumpy cystic duct and the common bile duct to the duodenum, which lies deeper yet against the back wall of the abdomen—just about the most inaccessible place one could find in the human body for the surgeon's fingers to reach. Furthermore, if stones are found in the gall bladder during surgery and any part of the patient's history indicates apparent obstruction of bile as well, it may be necessary not only to remove the gall bladder but also to open up and explore the common bile duct to be certain that no stones remain impacted there to give continuing trouble. Such a "common duct exploration" amounts to a separate major operation in itself, materially increasing the operative risk to the patient and even then offering no guarantee that every obstruction can be found and removed. To be as thorough as possible, however, in any case in which the common bile duct is opened the surgeon will usually perform an X-ray examination known as an "operative cholangiogram" then and there with the patient still on the operating table before closure is begun. In this procedure a special T-shaped tube is inserted into the common duct; through the tube a radio-opaque dye is injected into the duct, filling the entire bile-collecting system all the way down to its entrance into the intestine. X-ray pictures are then taken and developed on the spot in an attempt to detect any impacted gallstones that may have been missed. Thus the surgeon tries to make certain that every possible obstruction has been removed before he begins closing the patient's abdomen. The T-tube must be left in place and carried out through the wound in order to drain excess bile that is formed in the immediate postoperative period before the opening in the common duct has had an opportunity to begin to heal. Then at a certain point postoperatively the T-tube drain is removed.

In cases of proved gallstones, removal of the gall bladder usually effects a cure, and the operative mortality rate is well below 1 percent in the hands of experienced surgeons, with a slightly higher fatality figure related to operations on the common bile duct. As with many other surgical procedures, however, the age and general condi-

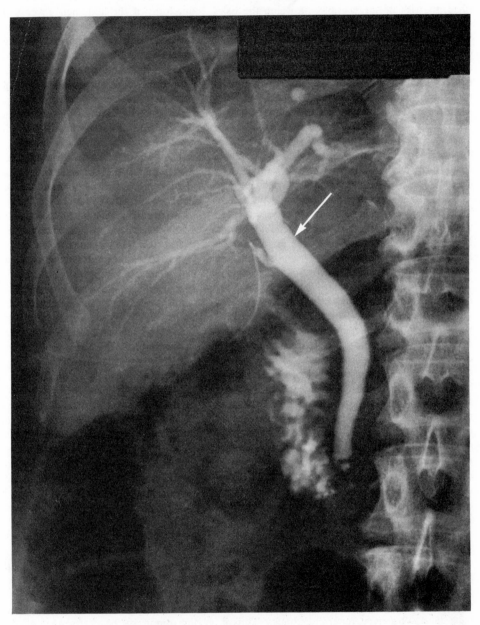

Plate 38   An operative cholangiogram, a special X-ray study conducted during gall bladder surgery to outline the common bile duct after the gall bladder has been removed. This film reveals a single small gallstone (see arrow) which remained lodged within the common bile duct—a source of future trouble had it not been detected and removed.

tion of the patient are extremely important factors. In an aged patient who is also malnourished, the risk of surgery may outweigh the risk of complications as a result of the gallstones. When a patient is being prepared for surgery, a diet high in protein and carbohydrates and relatively low in fats is necessary for a period of time to improve his general physical and nutritional state. Whether surgical treatment is being planned or not, control of the diet is of great importance for any patient with gall bladder disease. Foods such as fats and eggs should be eliminated from the diet, while greasy or fried foods, pork and pork products, rich salad dressings, cheese, spicy foods, cabbage, onions, sauerkraut and alcoholic beverages should either be reduced or eliminated because they appear most likely to cause recurrence of symptoms. Following surgical removal of the gall bladder, however, special diets are generally not necessary beyond the immediate postoperative period —an encouraging consideration for anyone who is faced with the need for gall bladder surgery.

Acute cholecystitis without gallstones is relatively uncommon but does occur, often as a result of bacterial infection and particularly as a complication of typhoid fever. Indeed, living typhoid bacilli have been recovered from the center of gallstones known to have been present for years; for some reason the gall bladder seems to be a favorite "hiding place" for typhoid bacilli, even if the victim has never developed symptomatic typhoid fever. Other infective organisms include the various colon bacteria, staphylococci, streptococci or pneumococci. The main dangers of cholecystitis, with or without stones, is the threat that increased pressure in the gall bladder, softening of the wall or frank gangrene may lead to perforation and peritonitis. In older people such a dangerous course is not uncommon. However, a first attack of acute cholecystitis may occur at any time from the age of twenty on, and although it may subside without surgical intervention, the victim will almost always have subsequent recurrent attacks. Thus it becomes a matter of surgical judgment whether or not to intervene and remove the gall bladder even when no stones are present.

Attacks of acute cholecystitis are accompanied by pain, especially in the right upper quadrant of the abdomen, fever which may rise as high as 104°, nausea, vomiting, sometimes abdominal distention and often muscle spasm and "guarding" of the abdominal muscles in the right upper quadrant of the abdomen. Prominent jaundice usually indicates that an obstruction is present in the bile ducts, but slight jaundice may occur due to associated liver damage which can result from spread of the infection from the gall bladder to the liver.

Cancer of the Gall Bladder and Bile Ducts. Although comparatively uncommon, malignant tumors can begin in the gall bladder proper, in the cystic duct leading from the gall bladder, or in the common bile duct. Statistically, carcinoma of the gall bladder usually arises in people with gallstones, and most authorities agree that chronic irritation of the gall bladder or cystic duct due to the presence of gallstones and related infection is a major factor in the development of malignant disease there. This also accounts for the fact that carcinoma of the gall bladder is more common among women than among men, since women are more vulnerable to the development of gallstones.

As with any cancer, carcinoma of the gall bladder or bile ducts can be effectively treated only if it is discovered early in its course. The major symptoms of this disease consist of the onset of dull, constant pain and tenderness in the right upper portion of the abdomen, very frequently accompanied by some degree of jaundice, since the tumor tends to obstruct the bile ducts as it grows. Often a cancer beginning in the gall bladder spreads by direct invasion into the duct system or into the liver itself. Like carcinoma of the pancreas, it may be relatively free of any symptoms until the disease is well advanced, but unlike carcinoma of the pancreas, this kind of cancer can often be effectively controlled for a significant period of time if discovered early enough that surgical removal of the tumor can be performed. As diagnostic and surgical skills have improved, there are increasing numbers of cases in which victims of the disease have survived for as long as five or ten years following surgical removal of the cancer, some with reasonable hope of a complete cure. In general, "radical" or widespread removal of all the structures in the vicinity of the cancer, often including the pancreas and the duodenum, offers the best hope of prolonged benefit if not a cure.

Rare as this kind of cancer may be, it again draws attention to the importance of investigating, *without delay,* any persisting or recurring digestive symptoms, however minor they may seem.

50. The Mighty Midgets 681

51. The Major Endocrine Gland Diseases 690

The body's different organ systems usually vary in size and weight according to the importance of their functions—with the notable exception of the endocrine system. These tiny bits of glandular tissue tucked away in obscure corners of the body, with a total weight of only a few ounces, exercise such profound chemical control over so many functions that they are considered the "master control system" of the entire human organism. The endocrine glands mystified ancient anatomists; they had no idea what possible function these seemingly insignificant tissues performed. Today we know that the endocrine glands, including the thyroid, the parathyroids, the "islet cells" of the pancreas, the adrenals, the male testes and the female ovaries, and the pituitary, produce powerful chemical agents known as hormones which are released directly into the blood stream, travel to distant sites and perform virtual miracles of biochemical control. The patterns of body growth, the overall rate of biochemical reactions, the body's ability to utilize food materials, its capacity to rally its defenses against emergencies and adapt to stressful situations, the development of its reproductive organs and the control of its sexual functions, all are directed primarily by hormones from the endocrine glands. Needless to say, disease or malfunction of any of these glands can have a profound influence on the normal development and general health of the body. Thus a knowledge of the often mysterious ways in which the endocrine glands work is important to an understanding of some of the most fascinating and complex diseases in the medical lexicon.

50

The Mighty Midgets

Throughout history a long succession of medical fads and fancies have been swept into popular use by doctors and patients alike in the (usually) forlorn hope that some new technique, drug or chemical might prove to be the long-awaited panacea for all the ills of mankind—a sort of Rosetta Stone that would suddenly unlock the mysteries of every disease. For example, at the very beginning of the era of modern medicine, in the late 1600s and early 1700s when William Harvey was investigating the circulation of blood and learning to measure blood pressure, there was the widespread conviction that an excess of blood in the body had many deleterious effects, and ailing patients were systematically bled as a means of treating every condition from carbuncles to coronary artery disease. During this time more blood was shed in doctors' infirmaries than on any battlefield, and although the procedure, by pure chance, actually *did* help occasional victims of congestive heart failure, far more often it merely speeded the patient along the road to an early grave. From the 18th to the 20th century, the fads of hypnotism and autosuggestion, introduced respectively by the Austrian doctor F. A. Mesmer and the French pharmacist Émile Coué, enjoyed enormous popularity as cures for every ailment. Still later the liver became the scapegoat for multitudes of health problems and "liver pills" were eaten by the thousands.

After the first decade of the 1900s, medical thinking became a little more scientific, but the discovery of vitamins—chemical substances which appeared necessary in certain quantities to the body's normal function—led to the widespread belief that the lack of these curious chemicals was at the root of most, if not all, illnesses. And finally, in the 1920s and 1930s, certain even more mysterious chemical substances, the *hormones,* were singled out for special attention. It was discovered that hormones played an important role in many body functions, and any number of these substances, particularly those that appeared to be related to sexual function, were used more or less willy-nilly. Women were given "hormone treatments" when their menstrual periods were too short or too long, or when they ceased altogether, while men endured everything from hormone injections to transplantation of the sex glands of monkeys as a means of restoring vigor and waning potency. Widespread abuse of these substances has since dwindled, but even today there remains an aura of mystery about hormones and a vague conviction that they have strange and miraculous powers in treating illness.

Oddly enough, this conviction has considerable basis in scientific fact. Hormones, which occur in a baffling variety of chemical forms, do indeed seem mysterious in their action, in part because they cause effects in the body that are far removed from the areas in which they are produced, and in part because such tiny amounts of them exert such dramatic effects. On a weight-for-weight basis they are by far the most potent substances manufactured anywhere in the body.

But just what are hormones? Where do they

come from, how do they reach the areas in which they take action, and what effects do they have? Most of the hormones are manufactured in certain special glandular organs located in various parts of the body, and each hormone has a particular effect or group of effects on very specialized aspects of the body's physiology. The glands that manufacture the hormones, however, are distinctively different from most glands in the body. The salivary glands, for example, manufacture saliva and empty it into the mouth through tubelike ducts, while the pancreas manufactures digestive enzymes and discharges them into the intestine through the pancreatic duct. But the glands that manufacture hormones have no ducts to carry their products from one place to another. Rather, they are supplied with singularly rich networks of arteries and veins, and the hormones are absorbed directly into the blood stream and carried to distant sites. These special "ductless" or "internally secreting" glands are called *endocrine glands* from the Greek word meaning "to separate," and their secretions are called *hormones* from the Greek word meaning "to set in motion" or "to spur on." And this is precisely what hormones do. Originally it was believed that they were formed only in the endocrine glands, but later the term was also applied to various chemicals which are not produced by special glands but which nevertheless are required to excite or regulate a number of physiological activities. All these substances are, in a sense, the "chemical messengers" of the body, dispatched to "inform" various tissues and organs of the activities necessary to normal, balanced function.

A number of the more prominent ductless glands have been known to exist since the beginning of the Christian era, and certain specific diseases resulting from overproduction or underproduction of various hormones have also been known since antiquity. But a direct connection between the impaired function of these glands and the various endocrine diseases was not made until the mid-1800s. In 1849 the German scientist Arnold Berthold came up with the first experimental proof that such a thing as an internal secretion or hormone existed. It had been commonly known that castration of a

rooster would cause a shrinking of its comb and wattles until it soon became indistinguishable in appearance from a hen; Berthold showed that if the removed testes were transplanted into some other part of the rooster's body, the expected change in the rooster's comb did not occur. At approximately the same time the English physician Thomas Addison (1793–1860) described a strange and fatal illness characterized by anemia, weakness, abnormally low blood pressure and an odd brown pigmentation of the skin. When victims of this disorder were examined at autopsy, it was found that their adrenal glands, located like small caps over the upper ends of each kidney, had been destroyed by disease. This particular condition came to be known as Addison's disease, but it was not until the early decades of the 1900s that physicians recognized that the disease was a direct result of underproduction of certain hormones by the diseased adrenals.

Today dozens of different hormones have been discovered and studied, and the study and treatment of hormone-related diseases, known as *endocrinology,* is one of the most fascinating and difficult of all medical specialties. It would be impossible here to undertake a detailed description of all of these hormones, but certain of the endocrine diseases are so common and so widespread that everyone should understand the functions of the main hormone-producing glands and learn something of the two main types of hormones: those which have a direct effect upon tissues and organs outside the endocrine system; and those, more recently discovered and understood, which act primarily upon other endocrine glands themselves to stimulate or inhibit the production of hormones.

The Endocrine Glands and Their Hormones

The Thyroid Gland. The existence of the thyroid has been known since the time of Christ. The name "thyroid" comes from the Greek word meaning "shield" because of the gland's shape and position in the front of the throat lying across the trachea. To locate the thyroid, place your thumb and forefinger on either side of the windpipe just below the Adam's apple and then swallow; you will feel the soft glandular structure move up and down under your fingers. Disorders of the thyroid, such as "goiter," cretinism, overactivity (hyperthyroidism) or underactivity (hypothyroidism), were also known to exist for

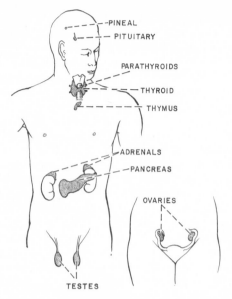

Figure 50–1.
The endocrine glands.

centuries before anyone connected them in any way with the gland's major function, which is the manufacture and storage of the thyroid hormone, *thyroxin,* a substance which regulates the speed at which biochemical reactions progress throughout the body—the so-called *basal metabolism rate* (BMR). So exceedingly important is the role of thyroid hormone in regulating the body's biochemistry that the production of thyroxin itself is carefully regulated on a day-to-day or even hour-to-hour basis by other hormones produced in the pituitary gland. (*See* p. 686.)

The Parathyroid Glands. These little nodules of glandular tissue, usually four in number, lie in the throat immediately behind the thyroid gland and are sometimes embedded in it. Their real importance was not fully understood until surgeons in the late 1800s and early 1900s began excising the thyroid gland in treatment of thyroid diseases and inadvertently removed the parathyroids at the same time. Indeed, ridiculous

as it may seem, these tiny glands were first discovered in 1850 by Sir Richard Owen, a British physician, in the process of dissecting an

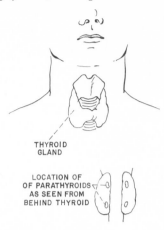

Figure 50–2.

Indian rhinoceros which had died in the London zoo; but they were not discovered in man until 1863. Today we know that the parathyroids secrete a hormone known as *parathormone,* which has the task of controlling the metabolism of calcium and phosphorus within the body, thus powerfully influencing the formation of bone tissue.

The Pancreas. In addition to secreting potent digestive enzymes which are carried by way of a duct to the intestine, the pancreas also contains small clusters of special cells which have a completely different function, the manufacture and secretion of the hormone *insulin,* which is not carried to the intestine through the pancreatic duct but is absorbed directly into the blood stream. These cell clusters are called the *islets of Langerhans,* and the so-called *Beta cells* within these islets produce insulin, which has a vital regulating role in the way the body cells utilize simple sugars as a source of energy. The common and once devastating disease known as diabetes mellitus comes about as a result of inadequate production of insulin in the Beta cells of the pancreas, whereas a much less common disorder in which an overproduction of insulin takes place results in a condition known as hypoglycemia—literally, "low blood sugar."

The Adrenal Glands. The two adrenals, which are lodged like caps over the upper poles of the kidneys and are thus sometimes called "supra-

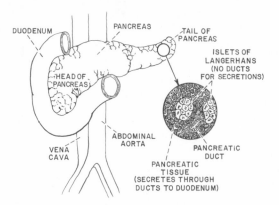

Figure 50–3.

renal glands," were first described in the mid-1500s by the Italian anatomist Bartolommeo Eustachio, who illustrated them in an anatomy textbook that was published a century or more after his death. Study of the function of these glands began in the mid-1800s, and it was soon found that they were formed of two quite different kinds of cells: a central area of gray-colored cells known as the *medulla,* and surrounding that a thick, firm layer of whitish tissue called the *cortex.* Further research revealed that each part of the gland produces different hormones. The adrenal medulla produces *epinephrine,* sometimes also called *adrenalin,* a hormone

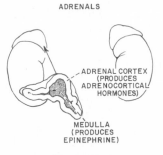

Figure 50–4.

which plays an important role in preparing the body to face serious physical threats and emergencies. One major action of epinephrine is to

speed the release of sugar stored in the form of glycogen both in the liver and in the voluntary muscles, thus providing an extra supply of "instant energy" in situations in which the individual is frightened, in pain or faced with the necessity to either fight or flee under some physical or emotional stress. Even more important, epinephrine stimulates production of an almost identical hormone known as *norepinephrine* or *noradrenalin* by involuntary nerve endings of the autonomic nervous system in the lungs, the capillary blood vessel walls or other viscera. Thus epinephrine and norepinephrine act in concert to speed up the heartbeat and the rate of respiration, to make the blood vessels in the skin and other surface areas of the body constrict, to increase the blood pressure, to supply additional blood to the brain, and to relax the bronchial tubes so that more air can reach the lungs quickly—all actions which prepare the body to defend itself in times of stress, and which even influence emotional feelings of strength and courage. This close interplay between the actions of the adrenal medulla and the autonomic nervous system is just one of many ways in which chemical or hormonal influences in the body work together with the nervous system to exercise a widespread moment-by-moment regulation of many physiological reactions—cooperative functions so important that they are sometimes spoken of as *neurohumeral* (i.e., "nerve-body") reactions.

The function of the adrenal cortex—the part of the gland wrapped around the medulla like bark around a tree—was largely a mystery until the early 1930s when it was discovered that extracts of adrenal cortex contained more than 30 different hormones, all with the same basic chemical structure, known as *steroids,* one of which became familiar to the world as *cortisone.* It was found that cortisone and other adrenocortical hormones exercised an effect on the retention or loss of sodium, potassium and phosphate salts in the body and helped keep the body fluids in proper balance. Later it was found that these hormones also regulate the body's ability to adapt to sudden environmental changes such as those causing shock or injury. In fact, another reciprocal hormonal reaction was identified: epinephrine released by the adrenal medulla in times of stress stimulated another ductless gland, the pituitary, which is located in close contact with a portion of the brain, to produce a hormone known as *adrenocortical stimulating hormone* (ACTH), which then acted to stimulate production of cortisone by the adrenal cortex and further prepare the body to cope with or adapt to abrupt changes in the environment. In addition, the adrenocortical hormones were found to help regulate the production of sex hormones, and to aid in suppressing the pain and swelling that accompany inflammation in the body. It was this latter effect which led, in 1949, to the first use of cortisone in the treatment of such inflammatory diseases as rheumatoid arthritis and rheumatic fever, often with seemingly miraculous results.

The Gonads. The term gonads is the generic name used to describe the so-called sex glands, the ovaries in the female and the testes in the male. Here again is an instance of endocrine glands which have more than one function: the formation of germ cells—ova in the female, sperm in the male—that make reproduction possible; and the manufacture of certain "sex hormones" which help regulate the reproductive process, particularly in the female, and account for the development of *secondary sex characteristics* in both male and female at the time of sexual maturation or puberty. In the male the testicular secretions are known as *androgens* or *androgenic hormones,* from the Greek words meaning "male-producing," and two in particular seem to be the most active, one known as *androsterone* and the other as *testosterone.* Both have the word "sterone" in their names because they so closely resemble the chemical structure, if not the action, of the steroid hormones of the adrenal cortex. Testosterone is some ten times as potent as androsterone, and both bring about distinctive changes in the young male at puberty: an enlargement and maturation of the genitals, deepening of the voice, the growth of the beard and of axillary and pubic hair in a characteristic male pattern, a spurt in the growth of muscle and bone, causing the male to become physically larger and more powerful than the female, and the development of both physical and emotional readiness for sexual activity,

which is sometimes spoken of as the *libido* or "sex urge." In the female the ovarian sex hormones are known as *estrogens* or *estrogenic* (literally, "estrus-producing") *hormones* because in lower animals these are the secretions which account for the female's periodic readiness to accept the male's sexual attentions during periods of estrus or "heat"—a pattern of reproductive function that humans do not display. The main estrogens in the human female are *estrone, estradiol* and *estriol,* all again similar in chemical structure to the adrenocortical steroid hormones, and all working together to bring about many of the physical and emotional changes that characterize the female at puberty: the development of breasts, the growth of pubic and axillary hair in a characteristic female distribution, the deposition of body fat that leads to the smoothly rounded shape of the mature female figure, and the maturation of the reproductive organs in readiness for the onset of ovulation and menstruation and for adult sexual activity.

It would be reasonable to assume that these sex-maturation hormones are the exclusive property of only one sex; that is, that the androgens are formed *only* in the male testes and the estrogens *only* in the female ovaries. Oddly enough, this is not the case at all. The fact is that both kinds of sex hormones are normally produced in both male and female, but they are produced in varying quantities depending upon the sex of the individual. What is more, additional supplies of both hormones, and especially of the androgens, are also produced in the adrenal cortex of both male and female. However, *far more* androgens than estrogens are produced in the male testes and adrenal cortex, while in the female it is estrogen production that predominates. It is the relative predominance of the sex hormones from both these sources that accounts for the varying degrees of physical (but not necessarily psychological) "masculinity" or "femininity" that differentiates the sexes or individuals of the same sex. This also accounts for certain "masculinizing" or "feminizing" changes that can occur when sex hormones are used in treatment of diseases such as cancer of the breast of the female (*see* p. 448) or of the prostate gland in the male (*see* p. 741), or when a tumor of the adrenal cortex, for example, results in the production of abnormally large amounts of androgenic hormones in the female.

Finally, the male and female sex hormones play an important role in maintaining the capacity to generate reproductive cells. Therefore, when the production of androgens or estrogens begins to fall off with advancing age, the ability to produce sperm or ova also declines. In the male this is usually a gradual process that extends over a period of years; beginning in the late forties or early fifties there is a slow but progressive diminishment of sperm production and a concurrent decrease in the man's interest in, and capacity for, sexual relations. In most men these changes may not be complete until seventy, eighty or more years of age, but in some the process seems more abrupt than in others, perhaps during the fifth or sixth decades, and is sometimes referred to as the male climacteric or male menopause. In women a decline in the natural production of estrogens from the mid-forties on brings about a more readily definable change at the point when ovulation ceases completely, and the woman experiences a comparatively abrupt end to menses. This phenomenon, known as *menopause* or "change of life," is occasionally accompanied by a variety of physical and emotional disturbances which may require medical treatment. Because the functions of the ovaries and testes, and the hormones they produce, are so inextricably connected with the reproductive process, these disturbances as well as the other diseases and disorders of the male and female sex glands are discussed in Part XII, "Patterns of Illness: The Urinary and Genital Systems."

The Pituitary Gland. For all their importance to sexual maturation and function, the male and female sex hormones are not by any means the only hormones that have roles to play in the human reproductive process. The formation of sperm cells in the male, for example, does not occur solely in response to the androgenic hormones, but also as a result of the action of hormones produced by quite a different endocrine organ, the pituitary gland. In the female, certain special hormones produced by the ovaries do bring about the cyclic changes of menstruation and other changes that occur with pregnancy, but all these changes are indirectly triggered by the maturation of an ovum or egg cell, which again is a result not solely of the female sex hormones but also of yet another pituitary gland hormone. The pituitary influences the function of other endocrine glands as well, and is, in turn, influenced by their functions in a complex reciprocal cycle that helps regulate and balance a multitude of vital body functions. Obviously, then, this gland is not only the most important endocrine, it is one of the most important organs in the human body.

The pituitary, about the size of a hazelnut and located at the approximate anatomical center of the head, is certainly a remarkable—and powerful—fragment of tissue. This tiny organ was known to the very earliest anatomists, but it was not until the late 1800s that anyone had even the remotest idea of its function. Clearly it is one of the best-protected of all the glandular structures in the body, resting in a small pocket in the sphenoid bone, the bony plate which passes through the skull from one side to the other, forming part of the floor of the eye sockets and the roof of the nasal passage and serving as a resting place for the forward portion of the brain. Even early anatomists recognized that the pituitary gland was made up of two distinct portions, an anterior lobe and a posterior lobe, and later investigators found quite different kinds of cells in these two lobes. Today we know that these two parts of the pituitary actually develop from two very different primitive tissues in the embryo and perform quite different functions, but it was not until the first two decades of the 20th century that researchers began to sort out and make sense of the truly staggering number and variety of functions that the pituitary has.

The action of the posterior lobe of the gland is by far the simpler to understand. Essentially it is engaged in storing and releasing certain hormones that have direct and specific effects on other parts of the body. The most important of these is a hormone known as *vasopressin* which stimulates the contraction or constriction of the muscle layers in the walls of capillaries and arterioles and thus helps maintain blood pressure. Vasopressin also has a specific effect on the cells in the kidney which are responsible for limiting the total amount of water that is lost in the urine independently of dissolved body

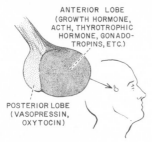

PITUITARY GLAND

ANTERIOR LOBE
(GROWTH HORMONE,
ACTH, THYROTROPHIC
HORMONE, GONADO-
TROPINS, ETC.)

POSTERIOR LOBE
(VASOPRESSIN,
OXYTOCIN)

Figure 50–5.

wastes. The other major posterior pituitary hormone, *oxytocin,* stimulates the contraction of the uterine muscles at the time of labor; in synthetic form it is frequently used by obstetricians to induce active labor or to help control the contraction of the uterus after delivery of the placenta and thus to control post-partum bleeding. These two hormones were once thought to be formed in the cells of the posterior pituitary gland proper, but more recent evidence suggests that they are probably formed in the nerve cells of the *hypothalamus,* an area of the brain directly connected to the posterior pituitary, and then merely stored by the gland.

Although the anterior half of the pituitary gland lies immediately adjacent to the posterior portion, it acts as an entirely independent organ, and its function is much more complex. It was characteristic of research into the functions of the endocrine glands that the first breakthrough in identifying a given gland with a chemical substance it produced often arose from a study of diseases or disorders caused by the overproduction or underproduction of that substance. Thus it was the study of certain growth disorders that led investigators to suspect that the anterior pituitary gland was a growth center for the whole body. Eventually it was learned that one of the hormones produced there is the *growth hormone,* sometimes called the *somatotrophic* ("body-nourishing") *hormone,* because it acts directly, without any influence on other glands,

to regulate and control the growth of the bones, muscles and all other body organs from infancy on. General bodily growth normally stops at maturity simply because the natural supply of growth hormone dwindles to a trickle at that point in life; but abnormal overproduction of this hormone at any time leads to certain characteristics of overgrowth of the bones and body, while underproduction leads not only to a sharp limitation in physical growth, but in some cases also causes arrested maturation of the sexual organs and functions. Abnormal childhood obesity can also be a related condition, and this may well be the reason that many chronically obese adults who cannot control their weight by dieting often excuse their failure by saying, "It must be glandular." True pituitary obesity occurs so rarely, however, that it can safely be disregarded as a serious factor in adult obesity.

This direct action of an anterior pituitary hormone on other organs and tissues, however, is really only part of the story of the function of this tiny but powerful gland, and perhaps the least important part. In addition to the growth hormone, the anterior pituitary also produces a whole family of hormones which are completely different from the ones that operate directly on various "target" organs. These hormones act as very powerful regulators of the functions of the other ductless glands; they are, in effect, the chemical messengers that tell the other endocrine glands when to speed up or slow down production of their specific hormones. The anterior pituitary is, in a very real sense, the body's "master" gland.

For example, the *thyrotrophic hormone* manufactured in the anterior lobe of the pituitary enters the blood stream and exerts a powerful stimulating influence on the thyroid gland, causing it to increase its production of thyroxin. Then when this hormone reaches a certain level in the blood stream, it in turn acts on the anterior pituitary to *inhibit* the production of any more thyrotrophic hormone for a while; not until the level of thyroxin in the blood stream again drops below a natural "balance level" is this inhibition overcome so that more thyrotrophic hormone is once again formed by the pituitary to stimulate production of more thyroxin. The

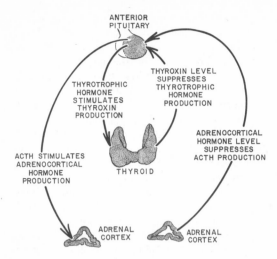

Figure 50-6.

same holds true for the *adrenocorticotrophic hormone,* often abbreviated as ACTH, which is formed in the anterior pituitary gland and then travels in the blood stream to the cortex cells of the adrenal gland, where it stimulates the production and secretion of all the adrenocortical hormones. Again there is a reciprocal relationship; when a certain level of adrenocortical hormones is reached in the blood stream, these hormones act to inhibit the production of any more ACTH in the pituitary until that level falls back below normal again.

It is this kind of reciprocal balance that makes it possible for the body to produce various powerful hormones in precisely the right amounts necessary to normal function, as well as to adapt very quickly to sudden extraordinary demands for one or another of these hormones. It also helps explain the extremely close and (at first glance) confusing relationship between the pituitary and the gonads in the production of germ cells for reproduction in both male and female, and the normal cyclical pattern of ovulation and menstruation in women. In addition to the so-called trophic or stimulating hormones mentioned above, the anterior pituitary produces a whole family of *gonadotrophic hormones* which have very specific roles in stimulating certain activities of the gonads, and which rise or fall in the blood stream in reciprocal relation-

ship to the level of androgenic or estrogenic sex hormones. One of these gonadotrophins from the anterior pituitary, called the *follicle-stimulating hormone* (FSH), has the job of stimulating nests of cells in the ovary, known as follicles, to prepare them for the production of egg cells. Then a second gonadotrophin, called the *luteinizing hormone,* stimulates the final maturation and release of the ovum by the ovary. This event in turn stimulates the cells in the ovary adjacent to the place where the ovum was formed to produce the hormone *progesterone,* which acts on the interior wall of the uterus to prepare the tissue there to receive and nurture the ovum if it is fertilized by a sperm.

The next step in this chain of events depends entirely upon whether or not conception occurs. In addition to preparing the uterus to receive a pregnancy, progesterone also inhibits the production of more FSH by the anterior pituitary, so that ovum production is temporarily halted in the ovary. If the egg cell just formed is not fertilized by a sperm, progesterone production in the ovary gradually ceases, until the prepared uterine lining degenerates and begins to slough off, resulting in the onset of normal menstrual flow some 12 days after ovulation has occurred. As progesterone levels dwindle, FSH production in the pituitary is resumed, and this hormone then stimulates the ovary to begin preparing another ovum. Thus the whole fertility cycle in the female occurs as a chain reaction of hormone functions triggered by the anterior pituitary gland.

In recent years it has been shown that small quantities of synthetic forms of progesterone can be used by a woman in daily doses to inhibit FSH production more or less indefinitely, so that ovulation cannot occur as long as the hormone is taken—the basis for "the Pill" as a highly reliable means of contraception. When progesterone is used cyclically in conjunction with synthetic estrogens, the woman's body is "fooled," so to speak, into preparing the uterus for a pregnancy even when no ovum has been formed, so that women taking the Pill have an apparently normal cyclic flow month after month without ovulating or becoming vulnerable to pregnancy. (The Pill and other contraceptive measures are discussed in greater detail on p. 917.) In the male FSH stimulates the cells in the testes that are responsible for the formation and maturation of the male germ cells or sperm, and the luteinizing hormone triggers the formation of testosterone in other testicular cells. These, however, are continuous rather than cyclical functions and, of course, explain why the mature male is normally capable of fertilizing ova at any time, while the female is capable of conceiving for a period of only 48 to 72 hours immediately following the release of each ovum, which occurs only once every 28 days or so.

But what happens if an ovum is fertilized? In that event the whole sequence of hormonal functions in the female is sharply altered, with the anterior pituitary gland again deeply involved in the change. The fertilized ovum becomes implanted in the uterine lining prepared for it. Progesterone production by the ovary continues, aided by the action of yet another pituitary gonadotrophin which is known as the *lactogenic hormone* because it also works in harmony with the estrogens to stimulate the breasts in preparation for later milk production. Meanwhile FSH production by the pituitary remains inhibited, and the anticipated menstrual flow does not occur—usually the first clue to the woman that a pregnancy is present. Soon a placenta develops to help nurture the growing baby, and this maternal organ also produces progesterone and, in addition, a gonadotrophin of its own, called *chorionic gonadotrophin,* which further stabilizes the pregnancy. It is the appearance of this particular "pregnancy hormone" in the woman's blood stream and urine that is the basis for most pregnancy tests, since it never appears except in relation to a pregnancy. In summary, the functions of the gonads and the pituitary gland in the regulation of the entire reproductive process are so intimately intertwined that it is impossible to say which is the more important, and obviously a malfunction of either at any stage along the way can have serious disruptive effects.

The Pineal and the Thymus. No roster of endocrine glands is complete without brief mention of two glandular structures in the human body which may possibly have some endocrine function: the *pineal gland,* located at the base of the brain about an inch and a half behind the pituitary; and the *thymus gland,* found in the front of the thorax just beneath the breastbone. No one is entirely certain what role either of these glands performs in humans. The pineal gland in birds is believed to exercise some regulating function on body temperature, but no such function in humans has yet been identified. Some authorities believe that the thymus gland has a part, during human infancy, in developing immune mechanisms in the new baby's body, but this function soon seems to be lost, and the thymus normally dwindles away or atrophies by adolescence or young adulthood. Thus, for the most part, these structures are considered unimportant except in rare instances when one or the other is the site of tumor formation. A benign or malignant tumor of the pineal, known as a *pinealoma,* may be dangerous if it takes up space and presses against surrounding brain structures, even if cancerous spread does not occur; unfortunately, because of its location, such a tumor is exceedingly difficult to remove. Tumors of the thymus, known as *thymomas,* are more common, and some authorities believe that they are related to the muscular disease known as myasthenia gravis. (*See* p. 289.) In some cases, victims of this disease have been markedly aided by surgical removal of the thymus gland.

It is not difficult to see, from the amazing number and variety of functions performed by the endocrine glands, that overproduction or underproduction of certain hormones, or diseases that damage or destroy the tissues in these glands, can produce a wide range of illnesses or abnormalities in the body. And the fact is that certain endocrine diseases are among the most serious, as well as the most common, afflictions to which human beings are vulnerable. But thanks to our gradually broadening understanding of how the endocrines and their hormone secretions work to control a vast number of body processes, even the most serious of these endocrine diseases today can be cured or at least controlled.

The Major Endocrine Gland Diseases

The endocrine glands, like every other body organ, are subject to a wide variety of diseases and disorders. They can become involved in inflammatory reactions owing to bacterial invasion or from some nonspecific cause. They may be damaged or destroyed by such infections as tuberculosis or syphilis. They can develop tumors which may cause either overproduction or underproduction of hormones. They may also become involved in infection, tumor growth or scarring that occurs in adjacent parts of the body. Whatever the disorder, the end result is the same: a disruption of the body's delicate physiological balance, which, in some cases, may occur for completely unknown reasons.

It might seem strange that diseases and disorders involving a total of only a few ounces of tissue can result in grave and widespread disability or even death. But if the human body has an Achilles' heel, it is surely the endocrine system, since the hormones it produces are so vital to normal function. Thus, even the most minor abnormality in hormone production may lead to a serious disorder.

Diseases of the Thyroid Gland

Goiter, the swelling or enlargement of the thyroid gland, was known to occur in certain areas of the world for many centuries. In fact, a slightly swollen neck was sometimes considered a mark of beauty in women when fashion favored the full and voluptuous feminine figure. However, goiterous thyroid swelling could, in extreme cases, become as large as a baseball or even larger, and the condition was found to be related to certain confusing and highly uncomfortable symptoms. In some areas, usually mountainous or inland countries like Switzerland or the middle western United States, goiter seemed to be accompanied by listlessness, mental slowness, below-normal body temperature, a tendency to fall asleep far more readily than usual at odd times of the day, a thickness of the tongue and slurring of speech, dryness and coarsening of the hair with considerable hair loss, a sort of puffy swelling or edema of the cheeks, hands and other parts of the body, a slow heartbeat and a strange sensitivity to coldness. But oddly enough, in other parts of the world, individuals with goiters were often troubled by quite the opposite symptoms: a flushing of the face, excessive sweating, marked nervousness and hyperirritability, a rapid heartbeat and often a prominent bulging of the eyes, a condition that gave rise to naming this disorder *exophthalmic goiter.* Finally, there were some people with goiters who had no symptoms of either kind.

This was a baffling situation indeed; yet it proved to be perfectly logical when more was learned about the thyroid gland and its function in the production of *thyroxin,* a sort of "master control" hormone which helps regulate the rate at which many biochemical reactions occur in the body. Thyroxin was discovered to be a unique substance; like many other hormones it is a protein, but it can act as a hormone only if the protein is linked up with ions of iodine, which exist only in trace amounts elsewhere in the body but are concentrated in the thyroid gland. In parts of the world where there was little or no natural iodine in the diet—mainly those mountainous areas with iodine-depleted soil and areas far from the sea, which contains most of the Earth's supply of iodine that can be ingested by eating fish—the thyroxin produced by the thyroid gland was ineffective for lack of iodine to activate it. In an effort to meet the deficiency of active thyroxin in the body, the thyroid gland would begin to enlarge and produce more and more of the thyroid hormone protein, thus leading to a goiterous enlargement of the thyroid gland; but since the thyroxin had no iodine to activate it, symptoms of underactivity of the thyroid, or *hypothyroidism,* appeared, including a slowing down of the rate of all biochemical and other metabolic reactions in the body, a slowing of the heartbeat, a dulling of the mental processes and the puffy edema which gave hypothyroidism its medical name, *myxedema.* This condition, however, appeared only in adults or teen-agers; babies born in the same area often suffered from much more dramatic symptoms: stunted growth and development, severe mental retardation and such abnormalities as a thickened protruding tongue, scanty growth of hair, and marked ugliness of the facial features—a condition known as *cretinism.* By the late 1800s study of cretinous children and adults with myxedema had revealed beyond doubt that these two conditions arose from the same cause: a marked poverty of active thyroid hormone due to a lack of sufficient iodine in the diet. If the condition became severe during infancy, the child developed cretinism; if it did not become severe until adulthood, myxedema was the result. Both conditions were treated with remarkable success by the addition of small amounts of iodine to the diet, either taken as a medicine or, later, provided by mixing trace amounts of iodine compounds in common table salt.

This, however, proved to be only half the battle, for goiter accompanied by nervousness, irritability, fast heartbeat and protuberant eyes is a condition quite the opposite of hypothyroidism. Such goiters developed in victims who had adequate iodine in the diet, but in whom, for one reason or another, the thyroid gland had begun enlarging and pouring out abnormally large quantities of iodine-activated thyroid, with a resultant marked increase in all the body's metabolic processes. These people began to suffer from restless overactivity and weight loss in the face of marked increase in appetite, to develop high blood pressure and even heart failure because of the increased load upon the heart, and to suffer from so-called thyroid storms or thyroid crises: episodes in which all these symptoms became suddenly more severe, sometimes even fatally so, as a result of minor infections, sudden emotional strains or physical shocks such as surgery. This symptom complex was particularly well described by the Irish physician Robert Graves in the year 1835, and is still often referred to as *Graves' disease;* other names for it, in addition to the already mentioned exophthalmic goiter, are *hyperthyroidism* and *thyrotoxicosis* ("thyroid poisoning"). Treatment of this form of goiter proved to be a much more difficult task, since medicines had to be found to block the formation of thyroxin, and surgery to remove part of the thyrotoxic gland involved the risk of fatal thyroid crises at or immediately following surgery. Only recently have really safe and effective drugs been found for treatment.

Either of these conditions—hypothyroidism due to marked iodine deficiency or hyperthyroidism with marked overproduction of the thyroid hormone—is often diagnosed today just on the basis of the sharply contrasting symptoms together with evidence of an enlarged thyroid gland. The picture is confused, however, by the fact that it is quite possible for either hypothyroidism or hyperthyroidism to arise *without* any discernible enlargement of the thyroid gland under certain circumstances. Underactivity of the thyroid gland, for example, can result not only from lack of sufficient iodine in the diet, but also from atrophy or shrinking of the thyroid gland as a result of acute *thyroiditis* (inflammation of the thyroid) when thyroid tissue has been damaged and scarring takes place, or following vigorous treatment of acute hyperthyroidism with drugs designed to decrease thyroid activity, or even just following the physical strain of a long and exhausting illness. Hypothyroidism without enlargement of the thyroid gland occurs predominantly in women, often about the time of menopause. On the other hand, overactivity of the thyroid may occur even without marked enlargement of the gland if the whole gland is involved in overproduction of thyroxin, under conditions of severe emotional stress, or in cases in which a small tumor of thyroid tissue has formed and produces thyroxin at a rate far in excess of normal. In some such cases a definite nodule can be felt in one portion of the thyroid gland and the condition is known as *nodular goiter,* but in other cases overproduction may occur before a nodule can be found on physical examination.

Obviously, with such a bewildering variety of conditions to deal with, it was extremely important to find some way to measure accurately the amount and rate of thyroxin production in order to help with the diagnosis of thyroid disease. One of the first methods devised was measurement of the *basal metabolism rate* (BMR)— actually a measurement of the amount of oxygen used by a patient during a brief period of time when he is at rest, warm, relaxed and comfortable. Under these so-called basal conditions the normal person uses, on the average, a certain amount of oxygen per pound of body weight— an amount that varies remarkably little from one normal individual to another. A victim of hypothyroidism, however, has a metabolism rate so markedly slowed down that he consumes far less oxygen than normal during the test period, while the hyperthyroid individual, with his metabolism keyed up far above normal rates, consumes far more oxygen than normal. For many years this means of measuring thyroid activity was the best laboratory test available, even though results could be thrown off by a variety of factors. The patient who feels ill, frightened, nervous or keyed up during the test, for example, can easily register a high BMR reading even though his actual thyroid function is perfectly normal.

Thus today other more accurate means of measuring thyroid function are commonly used. One such test is a measurement of the amount of iodine bound up with proteins in the blood serum, the so-called *protein-bound iodine test*

(PBI). This test is quite accurate, since the only organic compounds in the entire body which normally contain iodine are the large molecules of *thyroglobulin,* combinations of thyroid hormone and large proteins known as globulins that are stored in the thyroid gland, and the much smaller molecules of active thyroid hormone circulating in the blood stream. Thus by measuring the iodine content of the blood, the thyroid hormone content can also be measured. In addition, today it is possible to judge the activity of the thyroid gland by administering a very small dose of a radioactive form of iodine (I^{131}) and then measuring how much of this radioactively tagged dose is actually trapped in the thyroid gland for use in manufacturing thyroid hormones within the first 24 hours. This "I^{131} uptake test" not only provides a remarkably accurate measurement of underactivity or overactivity of the thyroid gland, but can also enable the doctor to identify a "hot spot"—an area of tissue within the thyroid gland which is manufacturing much more thyroid hormone than other parts of the gland, sometimes the first clue to the presence of a small tumor.

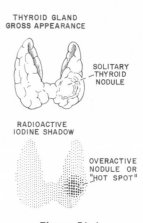

THYROID GLAND
GROSS APPEARANCE

SOLITARY
THYROID
NODULE

RADIOACTIVE
IODINE SHADOW

OVERACTIVE
NODULE OR
"HOT SPOT"

Figure 51–1.

The goal of treatment of either hypothyroidism or hyperthyroidism is the restoration of the patient's thyroid hormone production to the normal or *euthyroid* state. Prolonged hypothyroidism can lead not only to generalized physical and mental sluggishness, but also to the rapid development of arteriosclerosis and a markedly increased risk of coronary artery disease. Prolonged hyperthyroidism, on the other hand, can become a grave or even fatal illness as the victim literally exhausts himself and goes into congestive heart failure or dies in the midst of a crisis or "storm" of thyroid-induced overactivity of the body's chemical processes. If deficiency of thyroxin is a result of lack of iodine in the diet, the condition can often be sharply relieved by the administration of small quantities of iodized salt as a medicine. In fact the routine use of iodized salt in the diet can, for the most part, prevent this condition from occurring very commonly, even in the "goiter belt" regions mentioned earlier. In adults suffering hypothyroidism due to iodine deficiency, treatment with iodine brings about a slow but steady reversal of symptoms over a period of time as thyroxin production gradually increases. In children potential cretinism can be very dramatically reversed to normal if the condition is diagnosed early and iodine therapy started at once, but in long-standing cases recovery may be slowed or even limited by a degree of irreversible mental retardation.

In cases in which the thyroid gland itself is incapable of making enough thyroxin, iodine or no iodine, it can be replaced by the administration of extracts of beef thyroid or synthetic thyroid hormone. In the case of overactivity of the thyroid, the production of excess thyroxin must first be slowed down with one of the drugs which actively "poisons" the thyroid gland or inhibits the manufacture of thyroxin; several such medicines are known today and may be administered alone or in combination with additional iodine. Such treatment can often result in a sharp reversal of symptoms to normal within a matter of days. If hyperthyroidism is accompanied by a sizable goiter, or if thyroid overactivity recurs after successful medical treatment has been terminated, surgical removal of a large portion of the thyroid gland, a procedure known as *subtotal thyroidectomy,* may be indicated. However, overactivity must once again be slowed down to normal prior to surgery, and excellent medical and nursing care is required following surgery because recovery is often complicated by highly unstable activity of the part of the thyroid gland that remains, and a thyroid crisis or "storm" can occur unexpectedly even after much of the gland has been removed.

Alternatively, hyperthyroidism is sometimes treated by administering radioactive iodine sufficient to partially destroy the thyroid gland so that only a small part of the gland remains able to manufacture thyroxin. In cases in which one or more nodules of tissue can be felt in the thyroid gland, the usual treatment is surgical removal of the majority of the thyroid gland, including the part containing the nodules, because experience has indicated that nodular or cystic areas in the thyroid are at least potentially malignant and may develop into cancer. If a "cold" or non-hormone-producing nodule is identified in the thyroid by means of an I^{131} uptake test, the likelihood that the nodule may prove to be an early carcinoma is quite high, and immediate surgical excision may be indicated. A "hot" nodule that produces excessive thyroid hormone is most often benign, although there is no way to be certain without surgical removal. Indeed, the threat of cancer in this organ is great enough that many authorities favor surgical removal of any cystic or nodular area in the thyroid gland whether the patient has any other symptoms of thyroid disease or not. Other physicians favor a somewhat more conservative approach, conducting a trial of medical treatment to reduce the size of the goiter if possible before recommending surgery. If a nodule in the thyroid seems to be growing rapidly, however, if there is a family history of thyroid cancer, or if the nodule proves to be "cold," even the most conservative physicians agree that surgical treatment is imperative. Fortunately the most common form of malignant tumor of the thyroid tends to grow relatively slowly and to spread first to the nearby lymph nodes in the neck before metastasizing to distant parts of the body. Thus if any evidence of malignant change is found during surgery or detected in microscopic examination of removed portions of the thyroid, meticulous surgical removal of all the lymph glands and connective tissue in the neck in the area of the tumor must be undertaken and may often produce a cure in cases in which the cancerous growth is early and localized.

Thyroiditis is another kind of disorder of the

thyroid gland. In some cases it appears as an acute inflammatory or infectious disease with sudden symptoms of pain, swelling and redness of the front of the neck, together with spiking fever, increased white blood cell count and pain on swallowing. Frequently there has been a recent previous infection of the teeth, throat or upper respiratory tract, and in rare cases the inflammation in the thyroid may progress to the formation of abscesses. The disease is treated like any acute infection, with bed rest, application of an ice collar or warm compresses to the neck to help control pain, and the administration of penicillin or another of the broad-spectrum antibiotics.

In another form of thyroiditis, the onset of symptoms is similar to those of acute thyroiditis but they develop over a period of days instead of hours and the course of the disease is longer, lasting for several weeks in the absence of treatment. This slower, or subacute, form of thyroiditis is often accompanied by destruction of the hormone-manufacturing cells of the thyroid gland, and it may be followed by hypothyroidism once the thyroiditis clears up. The course of the disease and the severity of the symptoms may be dramatically diminished by X-ray therapy to the thyroid. In general, antibiotic treatment does not influence this type of thyroiditis.

Finally, chiefly in women between the ages of thirty and fifty, sometimes younger, a very gradually developing *chronic thyroiditis* may appear without any previous history of infection or other thyroid disorder. The cause of this condition, which goes by the name of *Hashimoto's struma,* is unknown, but the disease usually results in a slowly developing, firm, smooth goiter and evidence of slowly diminishing manufacture of thyroxin. The main symptoms of this chronic thyroiditis are due to pressure caused by the enlarging mass of thyroid gland in the throat, and these pressure symptoms may become troublesome enough to warrant surgical removal of the gland. Often, however, early cases may improve markedly with the administration of thyroid extract or synthetic thyroid hormone; similarly, if the disease ultimately leads to hypothyroidism, treatment with replacement thyroid hormone may be indicated. Although this may

be a long-term and sometimes troublesome disorder, there is no evidence that it leads to the development of cancer or any other condition more serious than hypothyroidism. In another form of chronic thyroiditis, an extremely rare condition known as *Riedel's struma,* the thyroid gland becomes enlarged and very hard, with marked irreversible destruction of the thyroxin-producing cells. Sometimes in this condition thyroid enlargement is sufficient to require surgical removal of the gland, with subsequent treatment with synthetic thyroid hormone to replace the loss of the natural hormone.

Diseases of the Parathyroid Glands

The two main disorders of parathyroid gland function are directly related to abnormalities in the production of parathyroid hormone in these tiny but important structures. Probably the most common of these disorders is underproduction of parathyroid hormone, a condition called *hypoparathyroidism* or *parathyroid tetany.* This condition almost always arises from intentional or accidental surgical removal of the parathyroid glands, which are hard to distinguish from thyroid tissue and are very often taken out or damaged in the course of such thyroid surgery as a thyroidectomy. Indeed, in the early days of thyroid surgery, before parathyroid function was understood, a common postoperative complication was the appearance of increased neuromuscular excitability which resulted in jerky spasms of the muscles of the hands, feet or face. Sometimes these symptoms were accompanied by breathing difficulty because of spasm of laryngeal muscles, and in severe cases the muscle spasms progressed into convulsions and sometimes ended in death.

We know now that all these symptoms can occur as a result of a sudden lowering of the amount of calcium present in the blood serum, and they can be successfully treated by the administration of calcium compounds given either intravenously or by mouth, as the case demands. In normal individuals the parathyroid hormone has two main effects: it causes the excretion of phosphorus from the body by way of the urine; and it helps maintain a normal level of calcium in the blood serum, probably by mobilizing calcium from bone tissue after dietary calcium taken in with such foods as milk has been laid down in the bone. If the parathyroid glands are removed or severely damaged, there is a sudden drop in the amount of parathyroid hormone available to handle these regulating jobs; calcium from bone tissue can no longer be brought into the blood serum, and calcium already in the serum is lost in the urine, while phosphorus piles up to abnormally high levels because its excretion by the kidneys is suddenly sharply diminished.

As soon as the danger of removing the parathyroid glands was known, surgeons began taking special care to find the parathyroids and save or preserve at least one or two of them when a thyroidectomy had to be performed. If symptoms of muscle spasm, low serum calcium and high serum phosphorus appeared anyway, to a mild degree, the condition could be treated by the administration of small daily doses of calcium and vitamin D, with restriction of phosphorus-containing foods in the diet. Administration of parathyroid extract from cattle may also be used during an acute occurrence of symptoms of hypoparathyroidism, but it is usually not suitable for chronic or continued use because the body soon ceases to respond to it. Synthetic forms of vitamin D together with certain medicines that block muscle spasm can be used as effective long-term substitutes.

The other situation in which hypoparathyroidism arises occurs when a surgeon has intentionally removed most of the parathyroid glands because of abnormal enlargement of those glands and overproduction of parathyroid hormone—a condition known as *hyperparathyroidism*—or because of the necessity to remove a parathyroid gland tumor. Overproduction of parathyroid hormone occurs most commonly as a result of excessive hormone production by a benign tumor of one of the glands known as a *parathyroid adenoma*. Sometimes, however, hyperparathyroidism results from a generalized enlargement of the parathyroid glands due to unknown causes. The result of an oversupply of this hormone is the development of an excessively high level of calcium in the blood serum,

combined with a normal or slightly low level of serum phosphorus. The excess of calcium can produce such symptoms as generalized muscle weakness, loss of appetite, nausea and constipation, and an increase in urine production as a result of the body's attempt to unload excess calcium from the blood serum. Indeed, the increased excretion of calcium sometimes leads to the formation of calcium kidney stones, and occasionally the first clue that something is wrong with parathyroid function is the sudden onset of kidney colic or the passing of a kidney stone. In addition, high serum levels of calcium can interfere with the transmission of the tiny bioelectrical waves that trigger the heartbeat, so that irregularities of heart rate and abnormalities on the electrocardiogram sometimes appear. Finally, if the hyperparathyroidism is severe and has been present for a prolonged period of time, more and more calcium is leached from bone tissue, causing the bones to become weak and often leading to bone pain and *pathologic fractures*—spontaneous fractures of such bones as the long bones of the leg without any apparent trauma or cause.

Oddly enough, one of the more common manifestations of hyperparathyroidism, particularly when it is due to a hormone-producing parathyroid adenoma, is the occurrence of chronic duodenal ulcer disease that proves extraordinarily refractory to normal conservative treatment. Although the exact relationship between the two conditions is not yet clearly understood, this combination of disorders occurs frequently enough that investigation for a possible parathyroid tumor is now made in any case of persistent ulcer disease, particularly if the patient also has a history of kidney stones.

In any case, hyperparathyroidism has to be differentiated from other conditions which might result in increased calcium levels in the blood stream—excessive intake of vitamin D or calcium-rich foods such as milk, for example, or increased calcium levels due to various kinds of cancer which invade bone tissue and release calcium. Usually, however, the differentiation can be made with the aid of careful blood chemistry and serum enzyme studies, combined with X-ray examinations of the skeleton.

Hyperparathyroidism is almost always treated surgically. If a single parathyroid adenoma is found, simple removal of this benign tumor may be all that is required to reverse the symptoms and cure the disorder. In cases of generalized enlargement of parathyroid tissue the surgeon may remove all but a very small part—perhaps one-half of one—of the parathyroid glands. For a while after such surgery, maintenance treatment with increased quantities of vitamin D plus supplemental calcium in the diet helps overcome the sharp drop in parathyroid activity, and this replacement therapy can usually be abandoned after a few months. Malignant tumors of the parathyroid glands are found only rarely and can be treated surgically if diagnosed early enough.

Diseases of the Pancreas

Diabetes Mellitus. One of the most prevalent of all the serious chronic diseases that occur in North America and Europe is the glandular disorder known as diabetes mellitus (from the Greek words meaning, literally, "the passing through of honey"), or more commonly "sugar diabetes" or just "diabetes." It is estimated that as many as two out of every hundred people in the population of the Western world develop diabetes mellitus at some time during their lives. There are some one and a half million people with recognized diabetes in the United States alone, and another half-million or so in whom the disease is in its early stages and has not yet been discovered. A considerably lower incidence of diabetes is found in India, China, Japan and other countries where chronic obesity is less common and where the average diet is not as rich in carbohydrates and fats as in this country. Heredity is also a powerful factor in the development of this disease; it is estimated that there is a family history of diabetes in as many as 50 percent of all cases, and the incidence of the disease increases sharply in middle-aged and chronically overweight people, more often in women than in men. People do *not* develop diabetes as a result of overindulgence in sweets, a common misconception. The disease can appear at any time in life and tends to be more severe the younger the victim is when symptoms begin.

Diabetes usually results from an insufficient amount of the hormone insulin, which is normally produced by special secreting cells called Beta cells located in the islets of Langerhans, small clusters of tissue scattered throughout the pancreas. These islets are not connected in any way to the pancreatic duct system and have nothing to do with the digestive enzymes produced by the pancreas; rather, they release insulin directly into the blood stream. Alpha cells, another kind of secreting cell, surround the clusters of Beta cells in each of the islets and produce the hormone glucagon, which is totally different from insulin and actually tends to counteract its action. In the normal person the production of insulin in the Beta cells and glucagon in the Alpha cells of the pancreatic islets helps regulate certain of the most important of all biochemical reactions in the body: those in which simple sugars and other digested carbohydrates, as well as digested fats, are consumed by tissue cells all over the body in the production of heat and energy.

Ordinarily the regulation of these biochemical processes involves a delicate balance of insulin and glucagon in the body. This balance may shift from hour to hour or even from minute to minute, constantly changing as new food materials are digested and made available, as the body develops an increased need for quick energy, and as the body's "reserve stores" of energy-producing carbohydrate in the form of glycogen—a complex carbohydrate substance manufactured and stored in the liver—is either built up in surplus or depleted as the body's energy needs wax and wane. Under normal circumstances we have no awareness whatever of this metabolic balancing act; we may notice only such gross reflections as "developing an appetite" when our energy stores dwindle from fasting or are expended during exercise, or we may feel slightly sluggish and sleepy after a full meal. But we have two ways of judging that the metabolism of carbohydrates is progressing as it should. The first is by measuring the concentration of glucose ("blood sugar") in the blood stream, which ordinarily remains remarkably constant at about 100 milligrams of sugar for every 100 cc.'s of blood, rising only slightly after a rich meal (perhaps to 130 or 140 milligrams) and sagging slightly (perhaps to 80 or 90 milligrams) when we are hungry. The second is by testing for any sign of glucose in the urine. Under normal conditions no sugar can be detected in the urine, but when the blood sugar is extremely high (about 200 milligrams per 100 cc.'s of blood), the excess glucose begins "spilling over" into the urine and can be easily detected by simple laboratory tests.

Normally the balanced production activity of insulin and glucagon keeps glucose levels in the blood stream stable even in the face of a sudden marked increase in the amount of carbohydrate in the diet. Digested sugar, largely in the form of glucose, is absorbed from the intestine and carried directly to the liver by way of the portal vein, and there it is pulled out of the circulation and stored as glycogen. Then when energy requirements increase, the hormone glucagon slowly breaks down the stored glycogen into glucose again and the liver releases it by driblets into the blood stream, while insulin aids in the absorption and utilization of this glucose by the cells of the body. But if something is wrong with the insulin-glucagon balance—an inadequate supply of insulin, for example—such energy-burning cells in the body as brain cells or muscle cells are unable to obtain and utilize enough glucose as rapidly as necessary. They then register a "hunger" signal which stimulates glucagon to convert the liver's glycogen into sugar immediately, which then floods the blood stream and spills out in the urine. In such cases the blood sugar level climbs much higher than normal, particularly after a meal, and then declines much more slowly, perhaps never returning to the normal level at all.

This chain of events is extremely useful to the physician in the diagnosis of early diabetes. After an overnight fast, the patient is fed a large dose of simple sugar by mouth, thus flooding his system with glucose. By testing blood sugar levels at hourly intervals thereafter, it is possible to assess the patient's *tolerance* to large quantities of glucose administered all at once. In the normal person, the body's response to such a "glucose tolerance test" shows a modest rise in blood sugar level immediately after the glucose is taken, and then an abrupt fall to normal levels an hour or so thereafter. But if the blood sugar spikes up to a markedly high level after the glucose is taken and then declines only slowly toward normal levels, there is very strong evidence that something is out of order with the patient's insulin production. This test can provide the first measurable clue to the development of an early stage of diabetes as much as weeks or months before any other symptoms appear. It is somewhat too time-consuming, clumsy and costly, however, for routine use during regular physical examinations, so many physicians use a modification as a screening test. The patient is asked to eat a normal hearty breakfast and then present himself for a blood sugar examination just two hours later. If the level of blood sugar is within the normal range at that time, it is unlikely that diabetes is present; however, if it is well above normal range, the full glucose tolerance test must be performed to rule out the possibility of diabetes.

What exactly does insulin do to help the cells of the body make use of the glucose that comes to them in the blood stream? Insulin itself was isolated in 1921, and twenty years later it was theorized that the hormone somehow counteracted an enzyme reaction that inhibited the cells from utilizing glucose. But even the complete blueprinting of the incredibly complicated insulin molecule, a task finally accomplished in 1955 by British biochemist Frederick Sanger and his associates after eight years of painstaking research, did not finally answer the question of how insulin actually works. Today the best guess is that it does not enter the cells or affect the breakdown of glucose directly at all, but rather attaches itself to the cell walls to permit glucose to pass through more readily. Thus, when glucose appears in the blood stream in great quantity following a meal, insulin is produced in the pancreas, circulates through the blood stream to the tissues all over the body, and throws open the cell membrane doors, so to speak. Glucose enters the cells and is metabolized, its concentration in the blood is sharply lowered, insulin production is once again inhibited, and the remaining insulin is destroyed until the next rise in blood sugar triggers more insulin formation. It would follow logically, therefore, that any condition that reduces the amount of insulin manufactured in the pancreas, or that acts in some way to destroy insulin's effectiveness in permitting glucose to enter the cells, will result in a pileup of sugar in the blood stream and the disruption of all the chemical reactions involving the utilization of glucose throughout the body. And this is precisely what seems to happen in the case of diabetes.

In its most common form diabetes has an insidious onset in moderately overweight individuals beginning in the mid-thirties or early forties, the incidence evenly divided between men and women. In this age group the disease may be well entrenched before any of the symptoms begin to appear; in fact, it is most commonly discovered during a routine physical checkup by detection of sugar in the urine. (Occasionally women will tend to "spill" a little sugar into the urine during pregnancy as a result of biochemical changes in their bodies at that time, but this phenomenon is not related to diabetes and usually disappears when the pregnancy is over.) When symptoms of diabetes do begin to appear, they may be mild enough to go unrecognized for some time. First, the victim may notice that he is urinating progressively more frequently and more copiously than usual; at the same time he finds himself drinking greater and greater quantities of water to quench an unusual thirst. Simultaneously with these changes, there is a marked increase in appetite between meals, at night, and even shortly after a full meal. The victim may begin to eat much more than usual, but oddly enough, this steady increase in food intake does not result in any weight gain; in fact, a gradual but steady weight *loss* often appears.

Other symptoms are slightly more subtle. There is a characteristic fruity odor on the breath, sometimes marked muscular weakness and easy exhaustibility, or itching of the skin. As the diabetes progresses, one or a combination of these symptoms usually brings the victim to a doctor, but occasionally a new diabetic will go unrecognized until the breakdown in carbohy-

drate metabolism leads to a pileup of abnormal concentrations of various acidic compounds in the blood stream. Then *diabetic acidosis* occurs and becomes progressively severe, with symptoms of nausea and vomiting, dizziness, deep stertorous breathing and finally outright coma. This is by far the most dangerous acute complication of diabetes, since the victim of diabetic acidosis may die very quickly if emergency treatment is not immediately undertaken. It is all too easy for those unfamiliar with the symptoms of diabetes to confuse the coma of diabetic acidosis with unconsciousness from acute alcoholism, and the sweetish odor on the breath of the diabetic further compounds the confusion. It is for this reason that diabetics are urged to keep some form of identification on their persons, describing their condition and the steps that should be taken in case of an acute attack. It is for this reason, too, that aid should be summoned for anyone found unconscious, even though it may appear that he has merely "passed out" from alcohol intoxication. There is no first-aid treatment of any value in dealing with diabetic acidosis; the victim must be transported to a hospital and a doctor's care without delay so that swift definitive treatment can be started as soon as possible.

A great many victims of diabetes, particularly those in their middle years, never develop symptoms of this severity and may well suffer a mild degree of unrecognized diabetes for years, even though a simple urinalysis test would reveal the condition. But there are long-term complications that arise in anyone who has *any* degree of diabetes for any length of time. The physical changes due to this illness are not restricted to those that arise from an excessively high blood sugar. Untreated, the disease characteristically causes a marked increase in the rate of the development of arteriosclerosis, for example, and impaired circulation may lead to high blood pressure, a vulnerability to strokes or other cardiovascular diseases, and the development of gangrene in the extremities. Arteries in the kidneys are particularly affected, whittling away at the ability of kidney tissue to do its job. The nervous system may also be affected, leading to the symptoms of nervous disorders as well as changes in the personality. Another common complication of diabetes is the development of *cataracts*—an opaque haziness that develops in the lenses of the eyes and progressively impairs vision. Changes in vision may also occur as a result of hemorrhages and the exudation of an opaque substance within the retina of the eye. In fact, discovery of such changes during a routine eye examination sometimes provides the necessary clue to the presence of diabetes and upon fuller diagnosis may help the doctor judge how far the condition has progressed.

Diabetes mellitus does not always follow a benign course beginning insidiously in adulthood or the middle years. The disease can also strike children and adolescents, beginning as early as age three or four, and in such cases it may pursue a far more explosive and devastating course. Discovery of the disease in a child may follow the abrupt and dramatic onset of extremely frequent and copious urination, constant hunger, and unquenchable thirst for a period of only a week or two before he reaches the state of diabetic coma; indeed, diabetes in children is often first discovered when the child suddenly and inexplicably goes into a profound coma. When this happens it creates a true medical emergency, for the child is literally at death's door, and unless the diabetic acidosis and coma can be swiftly reversed he may die before treatment can take effect. Most modern hospitals today stand prepared at all times to deal with this kind of emergency; an acidosis or diabetic kit containing all the necessary equipment is kept immediately at hand, and medical personnel are well trained in the necessary procedures. But it may be some time before aid reaches the victim, or before he can be brought to the hospital, and even under the best circumstances six or eight hours may elapse before the attack can be brought under control and the crisis passes. Thus this is a situation in which a few minutes can make the difference between life and death.

The severity of diabetes in children is so extreme compared to the disease in older people that for many year specialists have suspected that there are two distinct forms of the illness, a milder "adult type" and a far more severe and deadly "juvenile type." But so far it appears that the differences are quantitative rather than qualitative; when diabetes afflicts a child, it is apparently the result of a massive loss of the islet cells in the pancreas, whether due to a congenital abnormality or some other unknown factor, whereas in adults the islet cells "burn out" more slowly, or else insulin is perhaps produced in adequate quantity but is blocked or prohibited from doing its job properly by some kind of insulin-inhibiting mechanism. In any event, diabetes in a child causes the same degeneration of blood vessels and nerves, the same kidney damage and the same visual damage that occur in an adult diabetic, except that these changes progress much more rapidly and may shorten the life of the child in comparison to the relatively normal life span of the adult diabetic.

Before the discovery and isolation of insulin, there was no effective treatment for any case of diabetes, juvenile or adult. Children who developed the severe disease suffered a fulminating course that ended in diabetic coma and death. Adults with a milder form of the disease could often prevent severe complications by rigid attention to the diet, thus avoiding high concentrations of blood sugar, but they were seldom able to survive for more than five to ten years after the onset of the disease. Obviously the isolation of insulin from animal extracts in 1921 offered great hope that all diabetics might be returned to a relatively normal life, and insulin isolated from oxen, sheep, horses and swine had been pressed into use in the treatment of diabetes by the mid-1920s, long before the exact chemical structure of this complex hormone was known. It seemed reasonable to assume that if diabetes was due to underproduction of insulin in the victim's body, and if satisfactory replacement insulin could be derived from animal sources, then control of the disease should be possible just by having the diabetic take the right amount of insulin for his needs at the right times.

And in point of fact, this assumption was true. Insulin derived from animal sources *did* prove to be effective in treating diabetes in humans. But unfortunately this approach to treatment was not quite that simple. There was no effective way to achieve the extremely delicate feedback balance that would ordinarily keep just the right amount of insulin entering the blood stream at just the right times. Dosages of insulin from animal sources were difficult to standardize, and this replacement insulin could not be taken by mouth, since the hormone was a protein substance which was completely destroyed by the digestive enzymes. Thus it could be given only by hypodermic injection, and because of the frequency with which it had to be given—four or five times a day with the earlier insulin extracts—patients who were old enough to do so had to learn to administer it to themselves. Even today, now that standardized and longer-acting forms of insulin have been developed and only one or two doses a day are necessary for most diabetics, self-injection is still necessary, and it raises an additional problem: the amount to be used at each dosage time can be determined only by testing the urine for evidence of sugar and metabolic breakdown products such as acetone at regular intervals every day, another chore the patient has to learn to manage himself. And there is little margin for error because of another hazard that is ever present whenever insulin is being taken: the threat of inadvertent overdosage that can lead to *insulin shock*. This condition, also known as *hypoglycemic shock,* is a massive body reaction that can occur when an excessive amount of insulin in the blood stream causes the blood sugar level to drop dangerously low. The victim suddenly becomes pale and agitated, chilling and perspiring copiously, with pulse racing and blood pressure dropping; loss of consciousness often follows in a matter of minutes if the situation is not immediately recognized and treatment begun to restore the blood sugar level closer to normal. Indeed, in some diabetics insulin shock is a hazard as great as or greater than diabetes.

In spite of all these problems, the use of insulin in the treatment of diabetes has proved an enormous benefit to most victims of the disease. In older patients the disease often can still be treated primarily by careful diet regulation, with only a small amount of supplementary insulin each day to provide relatively "smooth" control. For those with more severe diabetes, a variety of different forms of insulin have been developed, and the physician can carefully match the kind and amount of insulin to the individual patient's needs. Most large hospitals have instituted "diabetic schools" in which newly diagnosed patients can be taught precisely how to master self-injection techniques, how to recognize the symptoms of insulin shock when they appear, and how to manage other important details in the control of the disease: diet, exercise, and the testing of urine for sugar and acetone, among other things. Urine testing has been made remarkably simple by the development of such special home-testing equipment as chemically sensitive test tapes that can be dipped into a urine sample to reveal the presence and relative amounts of sugar and acetone by easily observed color changes on the tapes. In the case of childhood diabetics, parents are taught how to care for their children, and even children seven or eight years old can often learn to handle the basic necessities of urine testing and insulin injection.

Most people with diabetes have been able, with careful instructions from their physicians and with additional help from such training programs, to master the day-to-day problems of insulin use and the overall control of the disease. Some, however, have special problems. Many juvenile diabetics, for example, tend to swing wildly from a wave of excessively high blood sugar one hour, owing to lack of enough insulin, to a sharp overdose of insulin an hour later, owing to massive utilization of the sugar. People, whether children or young adults, whose blood sugar levels show this kind of wild, unpredictable fluctuation are spoken of as "brittle" diabetics, and they present the most difficult problem in effective control because of the dual threats of diabetic coma and insulin shock. Fortunately, impending insulin shock can be forestalled, if it is recognized, by eating some candy or drinking sweetened orange juice in order to raise the level of blood sugar quickly the moment symptoms begin to appear. Those living closely with a brittle diabetic must also learn to recognize insulin shock; even if the victim has fallen unconscious, sugar can be administered by means of rubbing honey on the insides of his cheeks or under his tongue. Brittle diabetics in particular should carry identification indicating their condition so that proper help may be obtained if they are found unconscious. If insulin shock is profound enough to cause unconsciousness, the victim should always be taken to a hospital and seen by a doctor even if he "comes around" as a result of first-aid measures, since the occurrence of such a reaction may be a clue that his diabetes is not being controlled correctly or that some other problem has arisen that may require modification of his treatment program.

Other individual problems can arise in the control of the disease. A juvenile diabetic must learn to adjust to his condition and the lifelong need for careful observation, a properly balanced diet and the continual use of insulin and other medications; yet after years of enforced "slavery to an insulin syringe," children entering adolescence often become extremely rebellious, intentionally cheating on their diets or even refusing to continue treatment. Diabetes can be, of course, a severe emotional strain on both the victim and his parents, but rebellion, indifference, carelessness and other emotional overreactions do not alter the fact of the disease. They can, however, markedly affect its outcome; even two or three years during adolescence in which diabetes is poorly or incompletely controlled can result in partial blindness, for example, or fifteen to twenty years' worth of degenerative damage. Fortunately, once maturity is reached, juvenile diabetics usually undergo a renewed capacity for responsibility to their own health and return once more to the necessary treatment program.

Extremely old people with diabetes also tend to become "brittle," and the difficulty is compounded by the fact that with a certain degree of senility they tend to have trouble remembering what to eat, or what they have eaten, or whether they have taken their insulin or not. Ultimately these patients must either have some family member undertake responsibility for their medication and diet or be placed in some kind of nursing home situation where responsibility for their care can be taken out of their own hands.

Finally, certain conditions which pose little or no threat to the normal individual can become serious dangers to the person with diabetes, however mild it may be. The occurrence of infection anywhere in the body, for example, will frequently distort the control of diabetes completely, apparently because of the body's increased demand for energy necessary to fight off an infection. Special attention to personal hygiene is essential, and even minor cuts and abrasions must be treated properly and promptly with debridement, sterile dressings and sometimes even antibiotics to head off any possibility of infection. Vigilant dental care is necessary for the same reason. Particular attention must be paid to care of the feet; among the early degenerative changes brought about by diabetes is progressive atherosclerosis, and the feet—which have relatively poor circulation under the best of circumstances—are especially vulnerable to minor injuries which, among diabetics, can easily lead to a slow-moving, indolent gangrene in these extremities. Diabetics should wear well-fitted shoes and clean, absorbent socks at all times, with frequent changes if the feet perspire heavily. Activities that might lead to blistering of the feet should be avoided, and great care must be exercised in trimming toenails to avoid damage to surrounding tissues. Any foot injury, no matter how apparently mild, should be brought to a doctor's attention; scrupulous preventive care in this area can pay enormous dividends in terms of avoiding prolonged and crippling disability.

Other conditions may also present special hazards to diabetics. Any surgical procedure, for example, usually increases the patient's requirements for insulin very sharply until the period of physical insult is over; indeed, surgeons often seek to avoid any kind of operation that can possibly be by-passed, in the case of severe diabetics, because of the difficulty in controlling the disease during the operative and postoperative period and the increased risk of diabetic acidosis following the operation. Pregnancy is also particularly hazardous to a diabetic because of the additional physical strain placed on the mother's body. Even a mild diabetes tends to become more severe during the course of a pregnancy, with a much higher incidence of such complications as toxemia, high blood pressure, defective infants or miscarriages. In addition to the increased likelihood of congenital defects in babies of diabetic mothers, these babies are often unusually large and delicate, with edema accounting for an excessive birth weight. Although there is no evidence that there are abnormal levels of blood sugar in these babies, they are usually treated as premature regardless of their size. Because of the strong familial tendency to diabetes, children of known diabetic mothers should also be checked at regular intervals, particularly during episodes of infection, in order to detect any early appearance of sugar in the urine. What is more, the ravages of the disease upon the mother's body tend to be exaggerated during pregnancy. If a woman has severe diabetes of the juvenile type, she should be emphatically discouraged from undertaking a pregnancy at all, and even if the condition is mild, repeated pregnancies should be avoided.

Other conditions may be less threatening but still require careful attention. If a diabetic is obese, for example, weight reduction and carbohydrate control may prevent the condition from becoming more severe; in fact, many mild diabetics could actually control the disease by diet alone if they would only lose 15 or 20 pounds. In a diabetic child great care must be exercised to protect him against his own sweet tooth; control of a severe form of diabetes can be rendered almost impossible if the child is eating candy on the sly. Finally, alcoholic beverages are literally poison to all but the mildest diabetics, since they deliver quantities of carbohydrate to the blood stream and throw dietary and medical control completely out of balance.

Because of the many problems associated with the use of insulin in treating diabetes, researchers have sought for years to find a kind of insulin that could be taken by mouth rather than by injection, or for some other oral medication that could be substituted. In the 1950s several drugs were discovered which seemed to lower the blood sugar in diabetics. Certain of them are close relatives to the sulfonamide drugs in their chemical structure, although they have no antibiotic action, and all have proved most effective in treating mild to moderately severe diabetics, particularly those who develop the disease after the age of thirty. It is still not known precisely *how* these drugs lower blood sugar. The sulfatype agents appear to stimulate production of insulin in mild diabetics but have no effect on the blood sugar in a severe diabetic who has no natural insulin production at all; others of these drugs appear to potentiate the activity of whatever insulin is naturally manufactured, so that the individual with poor insulin function can more effectively utilize whatever insulin he has, while still others may enter into certain of the biochemical reactions in which carbohydrates are broken down into heat and energy.

Unfortunately, these oral medications have not proved to be the panacea for diabetics that was initially hoped. They do seem to help diabetics who develop their symptoms after the age of thirty and those who are controlling their diabetes, with difficulty, by diet alone. In fact, in many cases the oral medicine makes it possible for these relatively mild diabetics to discontinue the regular dosage of insulin or to greatly reduce the amount or frequency of administration. But in juvenile diabetics or in people with an especially "brittle" form of the disease these medicines are of little help. They are clearly not adequate substitutes for insulin, and there is still considerable question about whether they help prevent the degenerative changes seen in diabetics' blood vessels, kidneys or eyes.

These, of course, are long-term changes, and much more observation and data about the oral medicines must be gathered before a final judgment can be made. Meanwhile treatment of severe diabetes must still rest on careful regulation of the diet, the use of insulin, and special vigilance against both diabetic acidosis and insulin shock. Even at that, with blood sugar levels apparently well controlled for years, there is still a question about the efficacy of treatment of diabetes over the long term, and some authorities now believe that the degenerative changes of this disease progress at a certain accelerated rate regardless of how carefully the outward manifestations of the affliction are controlled. Clearly there is still much that is not known about this complex and commonplace disease. But research continues, and as knowledge of the biochemistry of the body increases, the time may yet come when even the most severe diabetics can be successfully and simply treated in order to live comparatively long and normal lives.

Hypoglycemia. Far less common than diabetes is another condition involving carbohydrate metabolism in the body and the function of the islet cells in the pancreas. It is a rather vague syndrome commonly known as hypoglycemia—simply, "abnormally low blood sugar." The condition tends to occur in attacks at times when the victim has gone without food for several hours. Symptoms include sweating, chilliness, pallor, headache and dizziness, an increase in heart rate and an odd sense of apprehension, all of which may be severe enough to cause unconsciousness. The victim may also frequently show emotional instability during an attack, sometimes quite a sharp change in personality, and become temporarily querulous and irritable. These changes can be marked enough to lead to an incorrect diagnosis of hyperemotionalism or psychoneurosis, but they do, in fact, stem from organic causes when the tissues and organs of the body are deprived of the necessary supply of blood sugar. Taken together, these are, of course, the typical symptoms of insulin shock, and hypoglycemia most commonly occurs in diabetics as a result of an overdosage of insulin or, occasionally, an overdosage of the oral antidiabetic medicines.

Hypoglycemia, however, is not always related to diabetes; a variety of other organic disorders can also cause an attack. For example, just as diabetes mellitus may in some cases arise because of tumors or inflammatory diseases of the pancreas that destroy the islet cells, hypoglycemia may be due to tumors of the islet cells that cause a proliferation or swelling of the Beta cells that manufacture insulin—a so-called functioning tumor which results in a marked increase in the production of insulin in the body. Hypoglycemia can also be the result of damage or disease to the liver which impairs that organ's metabolic processing of glucose. Overactivity of the islet cells can also be a secondary effect of

diseases of the adrenal cortex or of the pituitary, both endocrine glands which secrete hormones that enter into the "feedback" system that helps control the amount of insulin being manufactured. Although no specific "insulin-stimulating hormone" produced by the pituitary gland has yet been discovered, destructive diseases or lesions of the pituitary lead to a disruption of the carbohydrate metabolism in the body as reflected by episodes of hypoglycemia, possibly as a result of excess production of insulin or of excessive sensitivity to normal quantities of insulin, as well as evidence of other endocrine gland disfunctions. Finally, hypoglycemia may very rarely occur without any definitive cause whatever and in a few victims remains an annoying and unpredictable condition leading to intermittent distress all their lives.

Treatment of hypoglycemia obviously depends first on finding its cause, if possible. An acute attack, however, is treated by giving the victim dextrose or some other swiftly assimilable sugar by mouth; hospitals usually keep a "shock solution" of orange juice mixed with glucose on hand for emergency use in treating both diabetic and nondiabetic patients. When the attack is severe enough to cause unconsciousness, injections of adrenalin or a glucose solution can be used to rally the victim. If the victim knows of his condition, he usually carries some candy or other source of rapidly available sugar to swallow when the symptoms of an attack begin to appear. Little can be done in the way of first-aid treatment for the victim who loses consciousness other than summoning medical aid immediately, but if he is known to be vulnerable to hypoglycemia, rubbing the inside of his cheeks or the underside of his tongue with honey will introduce enough sugar into the circulation to help him rally from the attack. Although they can be very alarming, even severe attacks are seldom fatal, but both diabetics and nondiabetics who are vulnerable to this condition, as well as their families, should learn to recognize the symptoms and be prepared to deal with them.

In nondiabetics a careful and expert physical examination must be done to rule out tumors of the pancreas or disorders of the liver, adrenals or pituitary, and treatment planned accordingly. When no cause for the disorder can be found, careful attention to the diet to provide high-protein and high-fat foods in frequent feedings will often prevent attacks.

Perched like small caps on the upper pole of each kidney, the tiny adrenal glands have their own blood and nerve supply and function quite separately from the kidney. But for all their unimpressive size, they exercise a profound influence over the healthy functioning of the body because they produce a variety of different hormones: *epinephrine,* which is manufactured in the cluster of cells at the heart of the adrenal gland, the *adrenal medulla;* and a number of adrenocortical hormones, of which *cortisone* is perhaps the most familiar, which are manufactured in the cells of the thick outer layer or *adrenal cortex.* In general these two portions of the adrenal gland function separately, each doing its own job without much relation to the other, and both are stimulated and regulated by different hormones secreted by the pituitary gland. But it is obvious that any type of disease or destructive lesion of the adrenal gland can conceivably damage both the medulla and the cortex and disturb the overall production of adrenal hormones. Similarly, diseases or disorders of the pituitary can profoundly affect overall adrenal function. But there are also certain kinds of disease which affect only the cells of the adrenal medulla or the adrenal cortex.

Addison's Disease. One of the earliest of all endocrine gland disorders to be recognized and described as a disease entity was an odd and fatal condition characterized by progressive anemia, weakness, feebleness of the heart, gastrointestinal disturbances and a bronze-colored pigmentation of the skin, all associated with a disfunction of the adrenal glands in a report published by the English physician Thomas Addison in the year 1849. At that time Addison had no idea of the different functions of the adrenal medulla and the adrenal cortex, but today we know that the symptoms he first described are, in fact, the result of a disease of the

adrenal cortex and consequent underproduction of the adrenocortical hormones. In rare cases the condition, now known as adrenocortical insufficiency or Addison's disease, arises as a result of some kind of destructive lesion of one or both adrenals—tuberculosis, for example, or the development of cancer—but in most cases this insidious and slowly progressive disease occurs without any distinguishable cause. It can turn up in all age groups and is equally distributed between men and women. Its main manifestations are easy fatigue, weakness, and sometimes fainting under conditions in which the body's reserves are being taxed, as in the midst of a severe infection, or in times of injury or trauma. Other characteristics are weight loss, a tendency to become dehydrated, and unusually low blood pressure—one of the very few conditions in which low blood pressure is an element of illness or disorder. All these symptoms may occur either to a mild or to a marked degree, but however mild, the disease is truly dangerous and ultimately fatal if not discovered and treated.

The basic defect that leads to Addison's disease is destruction of the cortex of the adrenal glands with the result that insufficient cortisone and other adrenocortical hormones are produced. These complex hormones have a multitude of functions within the body, but perhaps their most important overall effect is to aid the body to adapt to, and thus often to survive, situations of stress, those situations which place a sudden drain upon the body's energies and capacities. During a severe infection, for example, the adrenocortical hormones help the body resist the onslaught of the invading organism. Similarly, they aid in resisting shock and other ill effects of trauma or physical injury, help the body get through the critical early stages of recovery after a surgical operation, and even enable the body to adapt to extremely hot weather by controlling the amount of salt that is lost by excessive sweating. The victim of Addison's disease, with a diminished amount of these stress-adaptation hormones, is unable to handle such "emergency situations" normally and may in fact respond to an acute infection, an injury, a surgical operation or even excessive sweating with a severe intensification of all the Addisonian symptoms—extreme weakness, profound shock, dangerously low blood pressure, heart failure or even kidney shutdown due to an impairment of circulation. This massive failure to adapt to stress in time of need and the extreme physical symptoms that result are spoken of as an *Addisonian* or *adrenal crisis,* and unless treated vigorously, it may be fatal.

One of the most dramatic and devastating examples of the desperate trouble the body can face because of an insufficiency of adrenocortical hormones is seen in fulminating cases of meningococcal meningitis (*see* p. 199). In this condition, hemorrhage into the adrenal glands destroys their function and brings on the sudden occurrence of profound shock which is rapidly fatal unless it is quickly diagnosed and replacement therapy started with one of the potent cortisone-like hormones. The victim may have had perfectly healthy adrenal glands until the invasion by the meningococcus organism occurred, but the profound shock that results is very like what happens to the body in an Addisonian crisis.

Until cortisone and other adrenocortical hormones were identified and isolated, the victim of Addison's disease lived on the razor's edge, vulnerable to dangerous crises any time his body was subjected to stress, and ultimately death occurred within five to seven years after the onset of symptoms. Then in 1934 the American chemist and physiologist Edward Calvin Kendall, who had isolated the active principle of thyroid hormone 20 years earlier, succeeded in isolating one of the adrenocortical hormones. Within two years eight more hormones in this family had been identified and today we know of more than thirty. In 1949, after years of study, the most well known of the adrenocortical hormones, cortisone, was successfully used in the treatment of rheumatoid arthritis and rheumatic fever. Today, in addition to naturally formed hormones extracted from the adrenal cortex of animals, a wide variety of very potent synthetic cortisone-like hormones have been developed, and they have totally revolutionized the treatment of Addison's disease, since it has become possible to supply them to those unable to manufacture adequate quantities themselves.

With the careful use of such replacement therapy, individuals who might otherwise have died in a few years from Addison's disease, after a prolonged and debilitating illness, are now able to maintain comparatively normal lives with little or no disability from their condition. In fact, John F. Kennedy was afflicted with Addison's disease long before his election to the Presidency, but was nevertheless able to undertake one of the most rigorous jobs in the world. However, successful treatment depends upon careful and continued medical supervision to adjust dosages of the replacement adrenocortical hormones, based upon the weight and changing physical condition of the patient and many other factors. Careful attention must also be paid to diet and other aspects of general health to prevent sudden changes in medication requirements. In short, Addison's disease today is controllable but not curable.

Adrenocortical Overactivity. Overactivity of the cells of the adrenal cortex with a consequent overproduction of cortisone and other adrenocortical hormones is extremely rare but can, on occasion, cause two main kinds of disorder. If such overactivity produces an excess of the so-called *androgenic hormones*—the male sex hormones which are manufactured in the adrenal cortex as well as in the gonads—the victim may develop a collection of symptoms known as the *adrenogenital syndrome.* These symptoms are manifested in various ways according to the age and sex of the victim, but in general they result in abnormal masculinization of both male and female. The male child may display premature development of the genitals along with other secondary sex characteristics such as deepening of the voice and early growth of facial and body hair. If the condition is present during the fetal life or early infancy of the female, a form of hermaphroditism may result, with an abnormal enlargement of the clitoris and the development of masculine traits. The older female child also begins to display masculine characteristics, and the adult female suffers a marked interruption of normal sexual function, together with masculinization of her appearance. Excessive production of other adrenocortical hormones can lead to *Cushing's syndrome,* the development of a characteristic kind of obesity, wasting of muscle tissue, retention of salt and water leading to marked edema, the onset of hypertension and in many cases the appearance of diabetes mellitus due to the interactivity between the adrenocortical hormones and the insulin-producing islet cells in the pancreas. Either or both of these conditions can usually be diagnosed by careful measurement of the quantity of adrenocortical breakdown products that are passed out in the urine; when excessive amounts of these hormones are released into the blood stream, excretion of their characteristic breakdown products is markedly elevated.

Treatment of both conditions depends upon discovery of the underlying disease, if possible. In many cases these adrenal overactivity disorders arise simply from enlargement of the cells in the adrenal cortex for reasons unknown, but occasionally a "functioning tumor" of the adrenal cortex may be responsible for the overproduction of hormones. In the latter case, surgical treatment of the tumor can bring a reversal of the manifestations of both conditions, but when no tumor is present, administration of quantities of cortisone-like hormones is often effective in counteracting the excessive natural hormone production and reversing its symptoms. This may sound much like fighting a fire by pouring on gasoline, but administration of these hormones in ample quantities tends to inhibit both the production of natural adrenocortical hormones and the formation of ACTH, the adrenocorticotrophic hormone manufactured by the pituitary that stimulates hormone production in the adrenals.

The chief problem in dealing with these diseases is to determine exactly where the fault lies; both the adrenogenital syndrome and Cushing's syndrome, for example, may well be a result of a tumor or hypertrophy of the adrenal cortex itself, but they may also be a result of a functioning tumor of the part of the pituitary gland that produces ACTH, thus stimulating adrenal overactivity. The complex interrelation of all of the glands of the endocrine system is essential to normal body function, but it also makes the practice of endocrinology one of the most complex and demanding of all medical specialties. Today, in fact, many physicians specially trained in endocrinology often subspecialize in the treatment of the diseases related to a particular gland.

Pheochromocytoma. By far the most common adrenal gland disease is a fascinating disorder that most laymen have never heard about. It is caused by the excessive production of epinephrine or adrenalin as a result of a functioning tumor of the adrenal medulla, known by the jaw-breaking medical name of pheochromocytoma (from the Greek, meaning "tumor of dark-colored cells"). This kind of tumor usually develops from cells in the center of the adrenal gland, and since the cells of the tumor produce adrenalin even faster than the normal cells, a steady or periodic outpouring of a large excess of adrenalin reaches the blood stream. According to medical definition, a pheochromocytoma is a benign tumor; that is, it does not tend to invade surrounding tissue or seed itself by way of the blood stream or the lymphatic system to distant organs. Thus it is not a cancer, but it stirs up quite enough trouble as it is, because its excess production of hormones causes a galloping hypertension (high blood pressure) which can prove to be extremely dangerous.

A few years ago pheochromocytoma was considered a very rare disease, and a highly infrequent cause of hypertension, but in recent years studies based on autopsies of thousands of patients who either died of high blood pressure or were known to be hypertensive have indicated that this benign tumor is far more common than previously thought. In fact, some pathologists today believe that as many as 15 percent of all persons who suffer some degree of hypertension have pheochromocytomas as a causative factor. If further studies substantiate this contention, the discovery may prove to be extremely important, simply because the hypertension caused by a pheochromocytoma is one form of the disorder which can be permanently and completely cured simply by surgical removal of the diseased adrenal gland.

It is for this reason that a person found to have elevated blood pressure is well advised to undergo a complete and thorough physical examination to try to pinpoint any identifiable cause. Hypertension caused by a pheochromocytoma usually begins gradually in much the same fashion as hypertension from any other cause, often starting in the third decade of life. In many people the hypertension is *persistent,* and the symptoms include recurring headaches, excessive perspiration, racing or palpitation of the heart and, frequently, a fine tremor of the hands. Further, these people are often thin and present the sort of nervous and jittery appearance that is also characteristic of hyperthyroidism, so that this cause for their symptoms must be ruled out. In older people who develop a pheochromocytoma, hypertension may occur in spasms or paroxysms lasting perhaps 15 to 30 minutes during which blood pressure spikes up to an abnormally high level, accompanied by severe headaches, sweating, pallor and tremor, all of which seem to resolve of their own accord in a brief period of time, only to recur later. Between these paroxysms the blood pressure may be relatively normal, and the disease can be missed altogether if the patient fails to mention the fact that he has strange, dizzy, jittery spells associated with rapid heartbeat, sweating and tremor.

Suspicion of this disease warrants certain special laboratory and clinical studies that help in the diagnosis. Twenty-four-hour urine examinations may reveal a high level of adrenalin breakdown products being excreted by the kidneys. In addition, there are certain drugs which counteract the effect of epinephrine and which, when administered as a test, cause a very sharp drop in blood pressure for a few moments in the person with a pheochromocytoma, but not in a normal person. Further, in patients who ordinarily have normal blood pressure with only periodic paroxysms of hypertension, it is possible to trigger a hypertensive episode using certain other drugs such as histamine. Surgical treatment is not without hazard, especially if the hypertension has been persistent, but in the vast majority of cases the tumor can be safely removed and the cause of the hypertension relieved.

Considering the large number of different hormones manufactured by the pituitary gland, its intimate relationship with the hypothalamus and thus with the nervous system, and its complex interrelationship with the other glands of the endocrine system, it is easy to see why any disease affecting the normal structure or function of this "master" gland will have far-reaching effects all over the body. Pituitary gland disorders are relatively uncommon, but when they do occur, they can be responsible for some of the most bizarre symptoms known to medical science. In general, these diseases are related either to *hyperfunction* (overproduction of hormones) or *hypofunction* (underproduction of hormones) of certain cells in the pituitary. Both of these abnormal and seemingly opposite conditions often stem, oddly enough, from the same cause: the growth of a pituitary tumor. If it is a functioning tumor, overproduction of hormones results, but if it is a nonfunctioning tumor, the normal cells of the pituitary are damaged or destroyed and underproduction is the result. The symptoms of each condition, of course, are dramatically different.

Two of the most important hormones produced in the anterior pituitary are the growth hormone, which is secreted by special cells called *acidophils,* and the adrenocorticotrophic hormone (ACTH) secreted by quite different cells known as *basophils.* A functioning tumor of the acidophils causes an excessive amount of growth hormone to pour into the blood stream, resulting in marked abnormalities in the physical growth of the body. If this overproduction of growth hormone occurs before the individual has reached physical maturity, it can cause continued proportionate growth of all of the long bones and other bones in the body. The result is known as *pituitary gigantism,* and victims have been known to attain a height of 8½ feet or more before excessive growth stops. If overproduction of the hormone begins after physical maturity has been reached, its effect is to stimulate overgrowth of certain parts of the skeleton still capable of increasing in size; there can be a gradual enlargement of the hands and feet, overgrowth of the bones of the skull over the eyes, and marked enlargement and protrusion of the jaw, all of which occur together with enlargement of the nose and a general thickening and coarsening of facial features. This condition is known as *acromegaly,* and the overall changes in features, sometimes described as gorilla-like, and the size and shape of the hands, are so striking that a diagnosis can sometimes be made at a single glance. Further careful examination often uncovers such additional symptoms as visual disturbances, headaches, loss of libido, and evidence of mental deterioration, while laboratory studies may reveal the presence of a secondary diabetes mellitus and/or hypertension. The treatment of both gigantism and acromegaly is based on either X-ray irradiation of the pituitary gland to slow down its secreting function or, if possible, surgical removal of the tumor. If the tumor is benign these conditions can often be arrested by one or the other of these approaches, although the overgrowth of bone cannot be reversed.

A functioning tumor of the basophilic cells in the anterior pituitary, on the other hand, causes an overproduction of the adrenocorticotrophic hormone (ACTH), which in turn stimulates the adrenal cortex to produce excessive amounts of the adrenocortical hormones and results in *Cushing's syndrome,* which is described above. Diseases due to underproduction of various pituitary hormones are even less common than those due to overproduction, but can arise as a result of congenital underactivity of the secreting cells, or when a nonfunctioning tumor destroys part of the gland, leading to a decreased production of growth hormone, ACTH or other pituitary hormones. If this underproduction is congenital there will be a proportionate arrest of the normal growth of all the bones of the body, which leads to the condition known as *pituitary dwarfism*—the "midget" who is well proportioned and of normal intelligence but diminutive in size, perhaps no more than three feet tall. This condition is completely unrelated to *achondroplasia,* a disease of skeletal formation, often hereditary, that results in dwarfism in

which the arms and legs are relatively shorter than the trunk, the hands and fingers are stubby, the skull is disproportionately large, and the bridge of the nose is depressed. The achondroplastic "dwarf" has a perfectly normal production of growth hormone and is not the victim of pituitary disease at all. (*See* p. 307.) Unfortunately there is no treatment for pituitary dwarfism. No one has yet succeeded in either isolating or synthesizing the growth hormone, so there is no way to supply it when it is missing, and animal extracts are not active in humans. Pituitary dwarfs tend to lead relatively normal lives in spite of their diminutive size, although in many cases the condition is accompanied by retarded sexual development.

Underproduction of other anterior pituitary hormones, particularly those manufactured in the basophilic cells, can lead to a variety of abnormalities, often because of a lack of the "trophic" hormones that would normally stimulate other endocrine glands to function. Thus damage to the anterior pituitary because of infection, cancer or hemorrhage may lead to such conditions as undescended testicles in a child or underdevelopment of the genitals in either male or female, conditions often associated with marked childhood obesity. This rare condition was described in 1901 by the Austrian neurologist Alfred Fröhlich, and is still known as *Fröhlich's syndrome.* Treatment depends upon discovering and treating the underlying pituitary gland lesion, but often victims of this condition can be aided by treatment aimed at supplying the hormones, such as androgens, which are not being formed due to lack of pituitary stimulation. Equally rare is *Simmond's disease,* the result of massive pituitary destruction due to hemorrhage or tumor, usually appearing in women and leading to atrophy of the genitals and breasts, cessation of menstruation, loss of thyroid and adrenal function and premature aging. Unusual as these conditions may be, they do occasionally occur, and any child who fails to show evidence of normal sexual maturation at the age of puberty (eleven to thirteen), particularly in association with obesity, or displays any change in normal libido or secondary sex characteristics should be examined by a doctor so that the possibility of abnormal pituitary function, among other things, can be investigated.

One final disease related to abnormal pituitary function, again a very rare condition, splendidly illustrates the often odd and indirect way in which certain hormones help regulate the function of the body. This disease is called *diabetes insipidus;* it has no connection whatever with diabetes mellitus, but is characterized by a progressively increasing excretion of huge quantities of extremely dilute but otherwise perfectly normal urine, combined with a constant excessive thirst. This condition may occur with no apparent cause whatever, but occasionally is a secondary result of cranial injury, meningitis infections or cerebral hemorrhage in the posterior pituitary area. Careful investigation shows that the urine does *not* contain measurable quantities of sugar, but the various "dehydration tests" indicate that the kidneys are virtually unable to concentrate urine.

What could cause a condition of this sort? Ordinarily a large quantity of water is filtered through the capillaries in the kidneys into the kidney tubules, carrying with it dissolved waste materials; then as this highly dilute urine is passed on along the kidney tubules, the cells of those tubes, under normal circumstances, reabsorb most of the water back into the blood stream while "closing the gate" to return of the dissolved wastes. Thus the final urine, moderate in amount, which is passed down the ureters into the bladder, contains a much higher concentration of dissolved waste materials than the fluid originally filtered by the kidneys. The action of the cells in the kidney tubules, however, is unusual for a membrane, in that the reabsorption of water is normally much more vigorous than could be accounted for by simple diffusion. These cells literally "pull" water back into the body, and this curious characteristic is directly related to the influence of the posterior pituitary hormone *vasopressin,* which acts as a so-called *antidiuretic hormone* (literally, a hormone that prevents the loss of water in the urine). When production of this hormone is impaired, the kidney's ability to recover extra water from urine is also impaired. In effect, kidney tubule cells are forced to stand by helplessly while enormous quantities of water are lost that would ordinarily be reabsorbed. When this occurs, the victim will pass huge quantities of urine (as much as 40 quarts a day in severe cases) and must, naturally, take in enough water each day to keep from becoming dehydrated. Even so, this disorder is accompanied by an extremely dry skin, with diminishment of normal sweating and salivation, and severe constipation because of reabsorption of water through the intestinal walls.

When this rare condition occurs, investigation may reveal a destructive tumor of the posterior pituitary, and surgical removal may be indicated. If the tumor cannot be removed, or if the condition is caused by some other unknown factor, symptomatic control of the massive urine production can often be achieved by the administration of an extract of the posterior pituitary. Additional help may also be obtained, oddly enough, by the use of certain drugs which ordinarily increase urine production and are thus known as *diuretics* but which, in the case of diabetes insipidus, act to decrease the loss of free water, reducing urine volume by as much as 50 percent.

Thus diseases and disorders of the pituitary, or any other gland in the endocrine system, include some of the oldest and most unusual conditions known to medical science. Fortunately most of the hormones formed by these glands have such pronounced effects upon the body that abnormal function comes to the attention of the victim early, and the chances of early diagnosis are very good. In addition, enough is now known about the various hormones and how they work that it is possible, with rare exceptions, to treat endocrine diseases effectively and return their victims to relatively normal healthy lives in many cases or, at least, to palliate distressing symptoms.

52. Diseases and Disorders of the Urinary System   713

53. Disorders of the Male Genital Organs   734

54. Disorders of the Female Genital System   745

Because the major organs of the urinary system are in the same location in the body as the organs of the male or female genital systems, and in some cases serve both systems in a dual role, it is common to discuss these systems together. Actually, they perform distinctly different functions. The urinary system not only serves to filter soluble waste materials from the blood by way of the kidneys and to dispose of these wastes in the urine, but it also helps the body maintain the proper internal balance of water and many other vital chemical substances. Proper function of the urinary system is as essential to life as are the functions of the heart or the lungs, and knowledge of how these organs do their job is necessary to the maintenance of good health. The genital or reproductive organs are not essential to life, but rather serve in the procreation of future generations. Further, they provide the physical mechanisms of reproduction in addition to influencing sexual behavior, one of the major aspects of human psychology. Both the urinary and the genital systems are subject to certain special disorders, but in many cases the damage these conditions cause can be minimized or even prevented by a clear understanding of the way these organ systems normally function and what steps can be taken to keep them free of disease.

Diseases and Disorders of the Urinary System

It is a common practice to discuss the urinary and genital or reproductive systems as if they were one unit, the so-called urogenital system whose organs and functions are somehow interconnected. Even more commonly, medical textbooks speak of the genitourinary (GU) system as if it were a single organ system with a single purpose. In terms of the anatomy or structure of the body, perhaps there is some justification for this; certainly the organs of the urinary system and those of both the male and female reproductive systems are located in close proximity. In the woman, for example, the urinary bladder is in contact with the lower end of the uterus and is vulnerable to various disorders as a result of stretching of tissue by the enlarging uterus during pregnancy or because of mechanical irritation during intercourse. But from the standpoint of function or purpose, the urinary and genital systems make strange bedfellows, for only one organ, the penis, which carries the male urethra from the urinary bladder to the outside, performs double duty both to evacuate urine and to deposit sperm-laden semen in the vagina of the woman during intercourse. The other organs of these two systems in both the male and the female perform sharply different and separate functions, operating quite independently of each other. Thus discussed in this chapter are only the diseases and disorders affecting the structure and function of the organs of urinary excretion—the kidneys, the ureters, the bladder and the urethra.

The Urinary System

The process of urination or micturition is certainly one of the most familiar of the body's functions, and under normal circumstances most people think no more about it than they do about breathing. Urination is, however, usually a voluntary process undertaken in habitual response to a gentle nervous stimulus. It may seem at first glance to be a very rudimentary process, and many people think of it with some degree of secrecy or shame. But it is, in fact, a complex and vital function, no less important to the health of the body than respiration. The frequency of urination and the amount and constituent ingredients of the urine itself are of extreme significance in diagnosing disorders not only of the urinary system but of other body functions as well. Thus the necessity of understanding just how the organs of the urinary system really work.

The urinary system and the kidneys in particular perform a much more complex function in the body than mere janitorial service. Of course, this function is important, too; potentially harmful waste materials, particularly nitrogenous wastes, produced as a result of the utilization of protein building materials in the cells and then dumped into the blood stream, must be removed from the body. It is these waste products, including ammonia and urea, which account for the pungent odor of urine.

713

But the kidneys do not serve simply as a collection point for these waste materials; they filter them out of the blood stream *selectively,* retaining many useful chemicals the body cannot do without so they may be reabsorbed into the blood stream. Thus the kidneys regulate the amount of several chemical substances retained in the body, conserving them for reabsorption when the body faces a shortage and unloading the excess when blood stream concentrations become too high.

The kidneys also serve to maintain a stable "internal environment" in the body by regulating its fluid content. The body's physiological functions could not take place without the fluid part of the circulating blood, or the lymph and tissue fluid that bathes every living cell. It is the kidneys that are largely responsible for the total amount of fluid retained within the body, conserving water when necessary by excreting only small quantities of highly concentrated urine, and unloading excess fluid when it accumulates in the tissues or the blood stream by releasing large quantities of very dilute urine.

Closely allied to this function is the conservation or excretion of sodium chloride, the major "salty" chemical in the body fluid which serves indirectly to regulate the amount of fluid conserved or lost by the body. When an excess quantity of salt is present in the blood stream, it tends to hold more water in the tissues, and will do so until the kidneys have excreted some of the excess, thus releasing unnecessary water and passing it in the urine. On the other hand, if the body is short of salt, the kidneys actively retain it until the body has accumulated the normal level of tissue fluid. This dynamic balancing act is accomplished by the kidneys working closely together with two other mechanisms that regulate the body's salt and water content: the loss of water from the lungs—every adult human being loses approximately a liter, or slightly more than a quart, of water from his body every 24 hours by exhalation—and the loss of water and salt from the sweat glands, which release another half-liter of body fluid a day in perspiration.

The kidneys also manage many other delicate balancing acts by means of their filtering func-

tion. They help maintain the precise level of acidity or alkalinity in the blood and tissue fluids, again balancing their activity with the action of the lungs, which reduce the body acidity by releasing carbon dioxide. The kidneys, however, excrete acidic ions when the acidity of the blood stream is too high, and alkaline ions when the alkalinity is above the normal neutral point. Further, they also control the amount of other saline chemicals retained by the body; known as *electrolytes,* these chemicals include magnesium, potassium, and chlorides, all vital to normal body function. Perhaps even more remarkable, the kidneys use a unique two-way filtering mechanism to prevent the escape of blood sugar or glucose into the urine. Under normal circumstances, dissolved glucose is actually filtered out of the blood stream in one part of the kidney and then actively pulled back into the blood stream in another part. The kidneys also act as a one-way filter, permitting water to be filtered out of the blood stream but blocking the passage of large protein molecules such as albumin, thus protecting the body from a steady drain of protein building materials. In short, the kidneys have an uncanny ability to "pick and choose." It is estimated that more than a quart of blood passes through the kidneys every minute, and from that the kidneys continually filter out those substances the body does not need and retain those that it does.

This essential function is accomplished by means of an intricate system of capillaries and collecting tubules which make up the main body of the kidneys themselves. These organs, located on either side of the vertebral column just below the level of the lowest rib in the back, are rather nondescript in appearance—small, reddish-brown bean-shaped structures, each about five inches high and two or three inches thick, which are enclosed in tough fibrous capsules and held in place behind and outside of the peritoneum by a network of connective tissue. The blood supply to the kidneys is provided by the *renal arteries* which branch from the abdominal aorta on either side; usually a single artery supplies each kidney, but occasionally a renal artery may divide so that the upper and lower portions of the kidney are supplied by separate branches.

Venous blood from the kidneys is returned to the abdominal vena cava by way of the *renal veins*. On either side the adrenal glands are perched on the upper curve of the kidneys like small triangular caps, but they have no anatomical connection with the kidneys except by proximity and have their own blood supply. (*See* Fig. 52–1.)

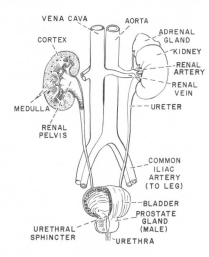

Figure 52–1.
The urinary system.

Within the body of the kidney the vital filtering process is carried out by multitudes of microscopic units known as *nephrons*. Each nephron consists of a tiny convoluted knot of capillary blood vessels, the so-called *glomerulus,* which receives blood from the renal artery and looks like a tiny tuft of twisted yarn under the microscope. Each glomerulus is enclosed in a microscopic *capsule* which leads to a long, looping *tubule;* glomerulus, capsule and tubule together make up the nephron unit. Ultimately the ends of tubules from thousands of nephrons cluster together to form pyramid-shaped structures called *papillae* which carry urine into a triangular collecting space known as the *kidney pelvis* at the inner, pinched-down margin of each kidney. Each kidney pelvis, in turn, drains into a narrow tube, the *ureter,* which extends downward to the urinary bladder.

The function of each nephron unit is a miracle of physiological engineering. The blood passing through the glomerular capillaries is under pressure, but cannot flow freely owing to the narrowness of the vessels. Thus quantities of water containing dissolved waste materials and body salts diffuse out of the glomerular capillaries into the capsules surrounding them, and thence into the tubules. Only the blood cells and larger protein molecules in the blood are too large to filter through the walls of the glomerular capillaries under normal circumstances. As this copious watery filtrate passes down the tubule, almost all the water is actively reabsorbed into the blood, along with certain of the dissolved chemicals—glucose, for example, or sodium ions and small blood protein molecules—as a result of the action of chemical catalysts or *enzymes* in the cells making up the tubule walls. Unwanted waste products, together with a small amount of water—perhaps a total of a quart and a half a

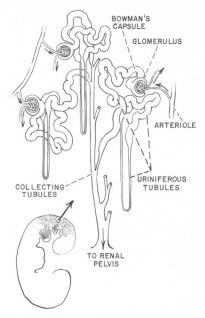

Figure 52–2.
Nephrons in the kidney.

day—remain in the tubules and pass on into the kidney pelvis as urine, which is then drained into the urinary bladder for disposal.

Not all the complex biochemical mechanisms

that help regulate this selective process of filtration and reabsorption of substances in the renal tubules are yet fully understood, but both the antidiuretic hormone produced by the posterior pituitary gland and various adrenocortical hormones are known to have important influence, especially on the rate at which salt and water are filtered. Whatever mechanisms are at work, the process is both selective and varied; materials such as potassium ions, sodium ions or bicarbonate ions, together with water enough to keep them in solution, may either be reabsorbed or be passed on for disposal in accordance with changing requirements of the body, while waste substances such as urea, phosphates, oxalates and creatinine are consistently filtered out of the blood and passed on in the urine.

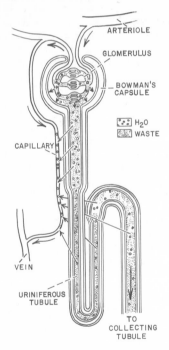

Figure 52–3.
Schematic diagram of filtration in a nephron.

Thus the kidneys are, in a sense, an important adjunct to the circulatory system—a sort of service station at which dissolved substances in the blood may be filtered out or retained as needed. But they have other important functions as well.

They play a part, not yet fully understood, in the production of red blood cells. In addition, they have a vital role in the regulation of blood pressure. Any time blood flow to the kidneys is impaired so that insufficient oxygen reaches the cells, a hormone known as *renin* is released by the kidneys. This substance triggers a biochemical chain reaction which causes small arteries and capillaries in other parts of the body to constrict, thus increasing the blood pressure and —at least theoretically—increasing blood flow to the kidneys. This mechanism also reflects the enormous amount of oxygen the kidneys require at all times to perform their task; the brain is the only organ in the body that requires more.

In comparison to the complex structure and function of the kidneys, the rest of the urinary system seems remarkably uncomplicated. The ureters are essentially drainage tubes, less than a quarter-inch in diameter, which extend from the kidney pelvis to the bladder on either side. Ordinarily these tubes, formed of smooth muscle tissue and lined on the inside with epithelium, function without any attention or conscious sensation, but whenever one becomes obstructed, squeezed, stretched or inflamed, special nerve endings create a sensation of pain, sometimes quite severe, which is felt in the low back and flank on the affected side, often radiating into the groin. This type and location of pain is so characteristic that its presence is an important diagnostic clue that the ureter is not functioning properly.

Finally, the ureters empty into the urinary bladder, a storage receptacle for urine situated low in the abdomen just beneath the pubic bone and in front of the uterus in the female. (*See* Fig. 54–1.) The bladder also is constructed of layers of smooth muscle and is sensitive to stretching; when accumulated urine fills the bladder to a certain point, the individual becomes aware of a characteristic, progressive discomfort until the bladder is emptied. Release of urine is normally initiated voluntarily anywhere from four to ten times a day, but once the sphincter muscle guarding the bladder exit is relaxed, the muscular walls of the bladder contract involuntarily, resulting in almost complete emptying. During urination the urine is passed from the bladder through another tube, the *urethra*, to the outside. The urethra is a very short tube in females, less than two inches long and passing directly under the pubic bone to the urinary orifice located just above the vaginal opening and just below the clitoris. In males, the urethra is much longer, passing directly through the *prostate gland* soon after leaving the bladder, and then through the length of the penis to the orifice at the tip. It is here, specifically, that a urinary tract structure does double duty as a reproductive organ; secretions from the prostate gland are emptied into the urethra, together with sperm stored in the adjacent *seminal vesicles,* to form the *semen* which is ejaculated from the penis under the force of rhythmic muscular contractions during the male sexual climax.

The amount of urine normally produced and voided in a 24-hour period will vary greatly, depending upon the general degree of hydration of the body, the environmental temperature, the amount of perspiration, the amount of fluid taken in, and many other factors. Some individuals habitually void more frequently than others but in smaller amounts. Others may have periods of excessive urine formation at one time or another because of the diuretic action of beverages such as coffee or beer. Doctors become alarmed if the total urinary output falls below 500 cc.'s (about a pint) in 24 hours, because it is often a sign of impaired kidney function. On the other hand, urination of more than 2 liters in a day may also indicate a disorder—diabetes mellitus, for example, or pituitary gland disease. In any event, the contents of the urine itself are an important gauge of general health; during a physical examination the specific gravity of urine is measured as a check on the kidney's normal, healthy ability to concentrate urine, and laboratory examinations are performed to detect the presence of any substances that urine does not normally contain.

Anything which influences or alters the structure or function of the delicate filtering system in the kidneys will obviously have an immediate effect on their efficiency in maintaining the body's internal environment. Certain drugs or chemicals—the caffeine in coffee, for example—can dilate the capillary tufts in the glomeruli, thus temporarily increasing the amount and speed with which water is filtered from the blood stream. This causes an increase in the amount of water passed as urine, and although the urine is more dilute than normal, there is usually no change in its normal chemical composition. Other drugs, including some widely used *diuretics* ("urine producers"), can cause a marked increase in the amount of urine produced, and in fact are used to draw excess water from the tissues and expel it in the urine.

Physical injury, diseases and disorders of the kidneys themselves can also have marked effects on their function. Swelling of kidney tissue as a result of infection or inflammation, for example, can block the normal flow of blood through the glomeruli and thus sharply reduce the amount of urine that can be formed. In addition, damage to the glomerular capillaries can occur as a result of certain inflammatory diseases, so that certain blood proteins—albumin, for example—can leak out of the blood vessels into the urine, something that never happens under normal conditions. Such damage can sometimes be so severe that whole red cells pass out in the urine as well. Thus the appearance of either red cells or albumin in a urine specimen is usually a signal that something has gone wrong with the basic function of the kidney, although bleeding from some source lower in the urinary tract—from the ureters or the bladder, for instance—can also be at fault. Narrowing or obstruction of the arteries and arterioles entering the kidneys can trigger the release of renin into the blood stream and cause a sharp elevation in blood pressure; and conversely, prolonged high blood pressure itself can lead to a narrowing and hardening of the arterioles entering the kidney. In certain individuals this becomes a vicious circle which can ultimately lead to a continuous, dangerous degree of hypertension and progressive impairment of kidney function as well. When one or another of these malign influences impairs the structure or function of the kidney, it can cause an increase in the blood stream of the nitrogenous wastes which cannot be effectively excreted any other way; and when these chemicals reach a certain elevation, a highly dangerous and often even fatal condition known as *uremia* ensues.

One characteristic of severe uremia, which illustrates the body's attempt to get rid of a useless breakdown product in some way, is the excretion of small amounts of urea in perspiration; the victim of exceptionally severe uremia is often found with a powdery rime of urea on his skin, the so-called uremic frost.

Thus normal, healthy function of the kidneys is absolutely vital to the general health. But other parts of the urinary system can also become involved in various diseases or disorders. Certain of these conditions—infection, for example, or the development of benign or malignant tumors—can occur in the ureters, the bladder or the urethra just as they can occur anywhere else in the body; other conditions, such as the formation and passing of stones, are more peculiar to the urinary system alone. What is more, certain characteristic signs and symptoms are generally associated with urinary tract disease: pain in the small of the back or the flank, pain and burning at urination, increased urinary frequency, increased nocturnal urination, or the passing of blood in the urine, to mention but a few. A physician performing a complete physical examination will be concerned at anything suggestive of urinary tract malfunction, and one important medical specialist, the *urologist,* is trained in the diagnosis and treatment of urinary tract diseases alone.

Kidney Calculi or "Stones"

One of the most familiar disorders of the kidneys is the development of calculi or "stones" —hard concretions of relatively insoluble chemicals, varying in size from very small to very large, which build up within the kidney pelvis. These stones can cause severe illness and agonizing pain when they make their way into the ureter either to lodge and obstruct the drainage of the kidney or to "pass" down into the urinary bladder or urethra. Less commonly, stones may also form in the bladder, where they occasionally reach a remarkable size and partially obstruct the outflow of urine, prevent complete emptying of the bladder, or contribute to chronic, refractory bladder infections.

How do kidney stones form? Obviously no solid material, as such, can be filtered out of the blood stream by the kidneys, but there are certain kinds of chemicals which can pass through the kidney's filters in small quantities, dissolved in water, and then later precipitate out as a solid. Some chemicals precipitate out when water is reabsorbed by the kidneys so that they become supersaturated in the urine in the kidney pelvis. Other substances may remain in solution in the slightly alkaline environment of the blood stream but precipitate out as solids in the usually slightly acidic urine; or conversely, substances that remain in solution in the blood stream may be precipitated out if the urine becomes more highly alkaline than normal. These substances, which include calcium carbonate, calcium oxalate, calcium triphosphate and pure urea, can collect over a period of time and build up layer by layer to form stones. Usually such concretions are passed down the ureters and into the urinary bladder as tiny hard granules. If so, they may then pass out with the urine without causing any symptoms whatever. Occasionally, however, they remain in the pelvis and sometimes become large enough to fill the entire interior collecting chamber of the kidney, forming a "cast" much as if the inside of the kidney had been filled with plaster of Paris. (*See* Fig. 52–4.)

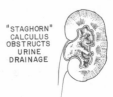

"STAGHORN" CALCULUS OBSTRUCTS URINE DRAINAGE

Figure 52–4.

The mere presence of such calculi in the kidney does not necessarily mean that symptoms of acute disease will develop; many people have been found to have huge kidney stones that have obviously taken years to develop but have never caused any symptoms. Trouble comes, however, when a stone or the fragment of a stone enters the ureter from a kidney and then wedges there or impacts before it reaches the bladder. Characteristically, this turn of events occurs without warning; it is recognized by the onset of excruciating pain centered in the small of the back on one side or the other and radiating down to the groin. The pain, which arises from stretching and abrasion of the smooth muscle lining the ureter, is typically spasmodic or "colicky" in nature, striking hard for a few minutes, easing off for a few minutes, and then striking again. So severe is the pain of this so-called *ureteral colic* that mild analgesics such as aspirin have no effect; often the patient requires stiff doses of a powerful narcotic to control pain until the stone is passed or until it is possible to remove it. Along with the pain, in most cases of ureteral colic the stone has scratched and scraped the tissue sufficiently to cause bleeding, and red blood cells appear in the urine. The combination of sudden excruciating pain, blood in the urine and accompanying symptoms of shock are usually sufficient to make the diagnosis. Similar symptoms may occur if a stone too large to enter the ureter nevertheless blocks the outlet from the kidney pelvis; in such a case, however, the pain is usually felt higher in the small of the back and remains more constant as a result of back pressure of urine in the kidney.

Very often even an acute kidney stone attack will clear up spontaneously with the passage of the stone into the bladder and thence out with the urine, a process that can sometimes be as painful as ureteral colic. As soon as such an attack is over and the victim has recovered, careful X-ray examination of the kidneys, ureters, bladder and urethra—and, in many cases, a cystoscopic examination of the interior of the bladder with a lighted tube—should be made to determine if more stones are present. They usually are, and future attacks can sometimes be avoided by attempting to dissolve the stones by special diet programs designed to acidify or alkalinize the urine, depending upon the substance making up the stones. In other cases surgical removal of a threatening kidney stone may be recommended, a decision usually made by a urologist.

Serious trouble can arise if a stone becomes and remains impacted in the kidney pelvis or ureter, for it can obstruct the drainage of urine and ultimately lead to back pressure of urine within the kidney and permanent destruction of kidney tissue. When a stone is impacted and cannot be dislodged by conservative means, it may be necessary for the urologist or surgeon, using a general anesthetic, to perform a cystoscopic examination, inserting a special lighted instrument into the bladder through the urethra and then threading a narrow probe up the ureter in order to locate the stone and mechanically remove it. Retrieval of the stone in this fashion is usually followed by immediate relief of symptoms and speedy healing of any damage that has been done. When this procedure is undertaken, however, X-rays are usually made at the time of surgery to detect the possible presence of other stones as well as to help evaluate any damage to the kidneys. A severely damaged kidney may ultimately have to be removed if the damage proves irreversible.

No one knows why one person forms kidney stones and another does not, but it is known that those who do form them tend to form them repeatedly. In terms of long-term prevention, the use of medicines to acidify or alkalinize the urine can often be helpful in preventing recurrence, but obviously the ideal is to prevent the formation of kidney stones in the first place. In some cases they form for inexplicable reasons, but there are a number of factors that can *predispose* a victim to the formation of kidney stones, and when the disorder is discovered, the doctor generally performs a thorough urinary tract examination in order to eliminate any such predisposing factors.

Perhaps most frequent of these factors is a chronic kidney infection or some urinary tract obstruction which causes poor drainage of urine, a condition known as *urinary stasis,* which gives dissolved minerals in the urine time and opportunity to precipitate out. A study of the kind of stones present may give the doctor a clue to an underlying cause for the disorder; stones made up of calcium compounds, for example, may result from excessive excretion of calcium in the urine as a result of a parathyroid gland disorder, or from prolonged treatment of a peptic ulcer with diets including quantities of calcium-rich milk or cream. Long periods of immobilization may also act as a predisposing factor, and patients who are bedridden or immobilized in casts, for example, should be turned frequently and take other such simple preventive measures as drinking an abundance of fluids. Physicians know other measures that can be taken to prevent the precipitation of various kinds of body chemicals in the urine, so it is important in the event of a kidney stone attack, even if it terminates of its own accord with the passage of the stone, that a doctor be consulted in an effort to prevent recurrence.

Infections of the Urinary System

Of the many disorders of the urinary tract, bacterial infections of one or both kidneys, the bladder or the prostate are probably the most common. Any of these can begin with an acute attack which may then progress to become a continuing, recurrent or chronic condition that may do severe damage to the kidneys. Infectious bacteria can reach the urinary tract via the blood stream any time an infection somewhere in the body releases them into the circulation. But most urinary tract infections are of the so-called ascending type, in which bacteria gain entry to the body from outside by way of the urethra.

Pyelitis and Pyelonephritis. Pyelitis is a bacterial infection of the kidney pelvis and collecting tubules, while pyelonephritis is an infection which involves both the pelvis and the basic filtering mechanism of the kidney, the nephron. Infection of any tissue tends to cause inflammation, swelling and engorgement with blood due to dilatation of the blood vessels in the area. The kidneys, however, are enveloped in a tight fibrous capsule which cannot stretch, and when they become infected and inflammation and swelling occur, the result is the onset of a very characteristic kind of pain. It is first felt as a dull nagging ache in the small of the back on one or both sides and then becomes progressively severe until virtually any pressure, motion or change of position may be excruciating. Usually the pain is localized in the back, but in some people it may radiate to the lower abdomen or groin as well. It is not colicky in nature but continuous. In addition to the pain, there is usually a marked elevation in temperature to 102° or 103° or even higher, with nausea and vomiting, general

malaise, headache, and frequently pain and burning on urination due to irritation of the bladder by infected urine. Very often the infection follows an acute course with spiking fevers and chills, and general toxicity sufficient to prostrate the victim. The urine may be scanty due to impairment of the kidney's filtering function by the infection, which also frequently imparts a very characteristic foul "dead mouse" odor to the urine. Dead white blood cells or pus, bacteria and occasionally red blood cells fill the urine; and the sediment in the urine may reveal fragments of cells from the kidney tubules destroyed by the infection.

Kidney infections of this type are not to be trifled with. Permanent damage can be done to the kidneys unless speedy treatment is instituted, and the infection may be severe enough to block off normal kidney function almost completely and cause a fatal uremia. It is important to secure an uncontaminated urine specimen for bacteriological culture before treatment begins, but when the causative bacteria has been identified treatment with antibiotics or sulfa drugs or both should be started at once and continued for a period of several days after the fever and pain have subsided and repeated urine specimens reveal no evidence of white cells or bacteria. Careful follow-up is also essential to see that the infection does not become chronic and remain smoldering in the kidneys, and to help alert the doctor to such serious complications as a kidney abscess. If the infection does become chronic, more and more kidney tissue may be destroyed, with resulting scarring and atrophy of the infected organ until it gradually becomes incapable of function at all. In long-term, untreated cases the damage and scarring can be so extensive that removal of the kidney becomes necessary.

It is possible for acute pyelitis or pyelonephritis to be caused by bacteria carried by the blood stream from some other purulent infection in the body—a boil or carbuncle in the skin, for example. Pyelitis, however, is more often an ascending infection, far more common in women than in men because the female urethra is only about one to one and a half inches long and provides easy access to the urinary tract for bacteria invading from the outside. Pregnant women are particularly prone to both pyelitis and infections of the bladder when the enlarging uterus presses on the ureters and partially obstructs the drainage of the kidneys. This is why the doctor caring for a pregnant woman checks her urine at regular intervals during the pregnancy. Pyelitis is also a frequent complication of labor and delivery, a miscarriage, a "D and C"—dilatation of the uterine cervix and curettement of the uterine cavity for diagnostic purposes or to interrupt a pregnancy—or some other gynecological disorder. Apart from these predisposing conditions, both pyelitis and pyelonephritis most commonly occur as a result of some other underlying factor, particularly the presence of an obstruction to the normal drainage of urine which permits invading bacteria to lodge and grow in the kidney or anywhere along the urinary tract, whether they are filtered from the blood stream by the kidneys or enter by way of the urethra. Obviously, if the underlying condition is not corrected, the infection can return repeatedly. Thus when an otherwise healthy person comes down with a kidney infection, a thorough examination of the urinary tract is necessary to look for possible obstructive lesions —kidney stones, for example, or enlargement of the prostate, which can obstruct the passage of urine through the urethra. In fact, a complete physical examination is also a necessary precaution because some other conditions, such as the presence of diabetes, an underlying tumor in the kidney, or an unrecognized tuberculosis of the kidney, can be predisposing factors in both kidney and other urinary tract infections.

One particulary dangerous form of kidney infection is caused by invasion of the kidney by tuberculosis bacilli with a resulting *tuberculous pyelonephritis*. In most cases this infection reaches the kidney via the blood stream from some other infectious source in the body, usually a tuberculosis of the lung. (*See* p. 212.) The infection develops slowly in the kidney, often with few or no symptoms until widespread damage has been done. Then at some point the chronic activity of the tubercle bacilli becomes suddenly acute; the victim becomes severely ill, with repeated episodes of high, spiking fever, night sweats, weight loss and ultimately the persistent appearance of blood in the urine. Diagnosis is made on the basis of the acute illness in a person with a history of pulmonary tuberculosis, from evidence of kidney damage found on special X-ray examinations, and by culture of the tubercle bacilli from the victim's urine. Once tuberculous pyelonephritis is diagnosed, the acute infection can be effectively quieted with the use of such antituberculosis drugs as streptomycin, isoniazid and para-amino benzoic acid (PABA), but all too often the organism is so firmly entrenched and has done such extensive irreparable damage that surgical removal of the infected kidney is necessary.

Cystitis. Acute cystitis, or infection of the bladder, may stem from the same variety of causes and predisposing factors that contribute to infections of the kidneys. It is, however, most often an infection of the ascending type, caused by a bacterial invasion through the urethra, and is particularly prevalent among women during pregnancy, although men are also affected. Like kidney infections, it may occur far more readily when there is some obstruction of the drainage of urine. The infecting organism is often a colon bacillus of some sort, but staphylococcus organisms are also often at fault.

Acute cystitis may begin abruptly or insidiously. In an acute attack the first symptoms may be a sudden marked increase in the frequency of urination, accompanied by a painful burning sensation when the urine is passed. Even though this sensation may be extreme, the victim of an acute bladder infection finds himself suffering an abrupt urge to urinate every few minutes but succeeds in passing only a small amount of urine. Frequently urethritis—infection of the urethra—accompanies the cystitis, which merely compounds the condition. In most cases the urine appears perfectly normal, but microscopic examination of a urine sample reveals great quantities of dead white blood cells or pus. Red cells are also often present as a result of the inflammation. The acute attack may be accompanied by a low-grade fever and a certain amount of general malaise, but more often the symptoms are quite localized. If the infection starts more slowly, the first symptom noted may simply be an increase in the nocturnal urge to urinate; the victim who normally sleeps the night through may find himself waking three or four times during the night to empty his bladder, a condition known as *nocturia*. This frequent urge may persist during the daytime as well, sometimes with no particular discomfort associated with urination—but *any change from normal* in the pattern of frequency of urination, day or night, whether or not accompanied by pain and distress, should be assumed to signal a bladder infection until proven otherwise, and a doctor should be consulted.

In very acute cases of cystitis the inflammation of the bladder lining may occasionally be so severe that blood-tinged or even frankly bloody urine is passed; laboratory examination of the urinary sediment can usually determine whether the bleeding is coming from the urinary bladder or from the kidneys. Even if there are no other urinary tract symptoms, blood appearing in the urine even in small amounts is an urgent danger signal. Its presence may indicate nothing more serious than an acute bacterial infection which can easily be cleared up, but it can also be a first warning of the development of a cancer in the urinary system, and it demands immediate and thorough investigation.

Most cases of acute cystitis can be very quickly and effectively treated with the use of modern antibiotic or chemotherapeutic drugs. Various of the highly soluble sulfa drugs, taken by mouth, are excreted in high concentration in the urine and reach the infected bladder this way in therapeutic quantities. In acute cases a physician may prescribe a broad-spectrum antibiotic in addition to or instead of a sulfa drug, if there is a history of sulfa sensitivity. Since these infections are so often caused by coliform organisms which are insensitive to penicillin, that drug is not ordinarily used unless a bacteriological culture of a urine sample has proved to be penicillin-sensitive. In addition to an antibacterial medication, if symptoms of severe frequency, urgency and *dysuria* (painful urination) are present, the doctor may prescribe one of a variety of medicines which, when excreted in the urine, act as surface anesthetics to alleviate these symptoms. Most common of these medicines are certain

aniline or other dyes which stain the urine a bright red-orange or pale blue-green color, and if the doctor neglects to mention this fact, his patient may be badly frightened. It is not difficult, however, to differentiate between the abnormal color of urine due to such medicines and the murky, rust-colored urine that indicates the presence of blood.

If an acute cystitis is neglected, or if treatment is not carried on long enough to eradicate it completely, the infection may become entrenched as a low-grade chronic inflammation; then it can persist for months or years with occasional acute flare-ups and may be extremely difficult to deal with. Patients themselves often contribute to the development of this problem when they stop taking medication the moment acute symptoms of cystitis subside, acting on the theory that they will then have some medicine left to use if the symptoms recur. This is, of course, a risky practice; as with any other prescription medicine, treatment for cystitis should be completed according to the doctor's directions to ensure eradication of the disorder.

When chronic cystitis does occur, effective treatment may require the use of a low dosage of sulfa medication for a prolonged period of time. Stubborn chronic infections of this sort may justify special X-ray studies or a cystoscopic examination of the bladder to determine if some obstructive lesion is helping prolong the infection. Occasionally in women who have borne a number of babies, cystitis is perpetuated by the presence of a *cystocele,* a condition in which the connective tissue supporting the bladder above the vagina has been stretched and scarred, allowing an outpouching of the bladder down against the vaginal vault to form a pocket or pouch which cannot be readily emptied of urine and thus provides a convenient place for infection to be harbored, or a *urethrocele,* in which a portion of the urethra has been stretched to form such a reservoir for urinary stasis. A thorough physical examination can reveal the presence of these conditions, and if conservative treatment does not clear up the infection the doctor may recommend surgical repair of the mechanical defects. If, in the female, there has been scarring of the urethral outlet to the bladder which interferes with passage of the urine, a simple series of urethral dilatations performed in the doctor's office under a mild local anesthetic may help relieve a long-chronic cystitis.

In males infection of the prostate gland or prostatic enlargement may be a factor in partially obstructing the urinary outlet; again, careful physical examination should reveal the presence of such a condition. (*See* p. 739.) Although prostatitis can and does occur from no distinguishable cause, it is very frequently a complication of gonorrhea, a venereal infection. (*See* p. 248.) In the male gonorrhea is initially a urethritis or infection of the urethra, which may then ascend to infect the prostate gland. When untreated, the initial symptoms—a painful purulent discharge from the penis which occurs from 24 hours to 5 days after sexual contact—may subside, but the infection can then be disseminated in the blood stream to appear in other parts of the body, particularly as gonorrheal arthritis or gonococcal infection of the knee joints.

In the female the gonococcus also causes a urethritis, but in addition the bacteria find lodging in the vaginal vault or in the glands inside the entrance of the vagina which normally produce lubricating mucus. The infection is significantly more difficult to eradicate in the female, and late complications may include an ascending gonococcal infection which reaches the Fallopian tubes and can lodge there to cause acute inflammatory disease of the pelvic organs or, as a chronic complication, the formation of abscesses obstructing the tubes, the reason why gonorrheal infection is so often incriminated as a cause of female sterility. Gonorrhea is a pernicious infection that requires thorough, prompt and persistent antibiotic treatment until all evidence of the infection is gone, with careful follow-up to be sure there is no recurrence.

The Twin Destroyers: Nephritis and Nephrosis

The gravest disorder of the urinary system is, of course, *renal failure;* that is, the loss of the kidney's capability to excrete nitrogenous waste material from the blood stream and conserve the body's water and electrolyte balance. Renal failure, whether complete or partial, swift or gradual, temporary or permanent, is not a disease in itself; rather it is the end result of a variety of other disorders of the urinary system or of a disease process elsewhere in the body that ultimately affects kidney function. But of the many conditions which may lead to renal failure, there are two groups or families of kidney disease that stand out above all the others. They are, first, a group of nonbacterial inflammatory diseases that primarily affect the glomeruli and thus are collectively called *glomerulonephritis;* and, second, another group of noninflammatory degenerative conditions which arise from unknown causes and primarily damage the cells in the collecting tubules. These latter disorders, spoken of collectively as *nephrosis,* lead to the so-called *nephrotic syndrome,* a highly characteristic cluster of signs and symptoms by which this type of disorder can be readily recognized.

Glomerulonephritis. In 1827 the famous British physician and physiologist Richard Bright first described the group of inflammatory disorders of the kidney that are still often referred to as Bright's disease, but are now generally called glomerulonephritis. Bright described this condition in terms of four symptoms associated with it, two of which are invariably present, and the other two present a great percentage of the time. The invariable symptoms are the appearance, either abruptly or insidiously, of quantities of both red blood cells and the blood protein albumin in the urine, neither of which is ever present under normal circumstances. In addition to these twin symptoms of *hematuria* and *albuminuria,* most victims develop some degree of water retention in the body, or *edema,* and most also develop an elevation of blood pressure or *hypertension* ranging from a very mild degree to a severe and malignant form of this abnormal condition.

Today we know that Bright's symptoms may sometimes occur in a number of different kidney disorders, but generally they appear as a result of a diffuse inflammatory change throughout both kidneys characterized by swelling and breakdown of the capillary walls in the kidney's glomeruli, followed by swelling of the interstitial tissue of the kidney and either a swift or slow impairment of the kidney's ability to produce normal urine and excrete the nitrogenous wastes piling up in the blood stream. Actually, glomerulonephritis usually occurs in one of two similar forms: as a sudden illness called *acute glomerulonephritis;* or else in a prolonged indolent form, known as *chronic glomerulonephritis,* that evolves slowly over a period of months or years or remains as a continuing chronic residual following an episode of the acute phase of the disease.

Today, after more than a century of careful study, we are still not entirely certain what causes this inflammatory condition. The kidneys are not infected by bacteria; but in the great majority of cases, acute glomerulonephritis appears, most commonly in children or young adults, a week or so after the onset of an acute streptococcal infection of the nose or throat, in much the same way that acute rheumatic fever appears following a completely separate and distinct streptococcus infection. And, as in acute rheumatic fever, acute glomerulonephritis seems to behave in many ways like an allergic reaction. Authorities today theorize that certain strains of streptococci have so-called *nephrotoxic* qualities; that is, they produce poisons which specifically attack kidney tissues and in some unknown way change or alter them so that they behave like "foreign" proteins. According to this theory, the body responds by making antigens against its own kidney cells, causing the damage and breakdown of blood vessels in the kidney and the inflammation that occurs at the same time.

At least 90 percent or more cases of glomerulonephritis begin as a severe and acute disease in which quantities of red blood cells and albumin appear in the urine some one to four weeks following an attack of streptococcal pharyngitis or tonsillitis. Simultaneously a puffy swelling appears in the cheeks and eyelids, sometimes followed by swelling of the feet or ankles. In some cases, there is an elevation of blood pressure, and the victim also suffers from headache, malaise, a sharp loss of appetite, and frequently a moderate amount of aching in the small of the back in the region of the kidneys. These symptoms may be so mild and transitory that they escape notice completely, and specialists strongly suspect that there are a great many very mild cases of acute glomerulonephritis that are never called to a doctor's attention, but rather clear up spontaneously after a day or two of minor symptoms with no residual aftereffects.

On the other hand, extreme cases can occur in which the kidney's capacity to produce urine is seriously impaired and the victim's urine output drops almost to nothing. There may also be marked hypertension, even to the point of convulsions, or such extreme edema and hypertension that the victim goes into acute congestive heart failure and may even die in the first few days of the illness. Victims of severe attacks may also develop blurring of vision owing to hypertensive hemorrhages from the arterioles in the retina or to increased intracranial pressure from hypertension and edema of the brain. There is always some degree of renal failure accompanying these symptoms; higher and higher levels of nitrogen are retained in the blood stream, and in some instances this condition is prolonged and severe enough that the victim develops uremia.

Unfortunately, even today there is little that can be done to treat acute glomerulonephritis effectively other than to treat the underlying cause: that is, to destroy any remnant of the streptococcus infection, first with high doses of antibiotics and then with continuing lower dosages to prevent a recurrence of the infection, and to relieve symptoms that may be present in order to help the patient "ride out" the acute course of the disease. Thus, as long as blood in the urine, edema or hypertension is present, the patient should be kept at rest in bed; the doctor will pay careful attention to the maintenance of proper balances of fluid and such substances as blood protein, potassium and sodium, reducing these sharply if kidney function is so impaired that the amount of urine is greatly diminished. Decreasing the salt in the diet, for example, helps reduce the amount of fluid retained in the body's tissues and also helps minimize or even prevent the development of hypertension. If there is severe kidney impairment, it may be necessary to reduce the amount of protein in the diet temporarily, since protein breakdown products will already have reached a high concentration in the patient's blood. The severity of the condition can change from day to day or hour to hour in any given individual, so a severe case is best treated in a hospital where good laboratory facilities are available and careful control of the patient's intake of fluid and food and output of urine can be maintained. Some physicians feel that the basic inflammatory process in the kidney is suppressed to some degree by the use of the cortisone-like hormones and they will prescribe these medications, although other authorities question their value or effectiveness.

In most cases of acute glomerulonephritis (some authorities say as high as 95 percent), the condition is self-limited, and the acute phase of renal failure begins to subside within a period of a few days to a few weeks, sometimes as quickly as within 24 to 48 hours, with simultaneous improvement of kidney function. Of those affected severely enough to require hospitalization, records indicate that more than 95 percent improve, with fatalities due to uremia, heart failure or the effects of hypertension or convulsions limited to perhaps 3 or 4 percent. Of those who survive the first acute period, the vast majority recover completely, although some trace of the illness, such as the continued pas-

sage of red blood cells or albumin in the urine, may persist for as long as two years. And among the approximately 90 percent of those who recover completely, virtually all proceed through life with no permanent damage to the kidneys and with no recurrence of the condition, even in the face of recurrent streptococcus infections. Some 8 to 10 percent, however, fail to recover completely; such persons enter the prolonged *chronic* phase of the disease in which there is measurable and progressive impairment of kidney function over a period of months or years, sometimes even decades, with occasional acute recurrences.

In the long run it is chronic glomerulonephritis which constitutes the real danger and tragedy of this disease, for its victims are often young people who must face a lifelong threat of death, sooner or later, due to renal failure. In some the downward course may be quickly progressive, extending only six to twelve months before the kidneys fail to such a degree that uremia or hypertension with heart failure proves fatal. Others may live almost indefinitely but must survive with only a fraction of their normal kidney function, which becomes progressively impaired until uremia ultimately ends in death.

Until about 20 years ago there was absolutely

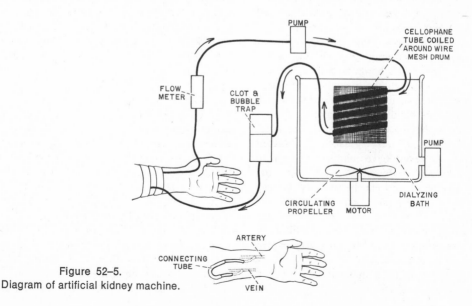

Figure 52–5.
Diagram of artificial kidney machine.

nothing that could be done for those with such severe glomerulonephritis that they died swiftly in the acute phase of the disease, or for those who developed the chronic disease and lived out a shortened life with the disorder continuously whittling away at their kidney function. There was no way to help the kidneys perform their function artificially, no way to repair a damaged kidney or improve its function. But modern medical research has recently made great strides in two different directions. First, physiologists and engineers working together have developed an effective *artificial kidney machine* through which a patient's blood can be circulated, waste material removed by a process known as *dialysis,* and the blood then returned to the patient's circulation. The first really practical kidney machine was developed in 1945 by the Dutch physician Willem J. Kolff, working under conditions of extreme handicap during the German occupation of the Netherlands in World War II. In 1947 Kolff's kidney machine, modified by the American surgeon-engineer Carl Walter, was successfully used to combat uremia in human patients at Peter Bent Brigham Hospital in Boston. Early kidney machines were used for only brief periods—to sustain a patient through the crisis of kidney failure during an attack of acute glomerulonephritis, for example—but as more machines were developed, victims of chronic and irreversible renal failure were also treated. Today, in such cases, the artificial kidney machine must be used approximately three times each week for 8 to 12 hours at a time. Until a few years ago, these kidney machines were large and clumsy, could be used only in hospitals with the assistance of highly skilled medical personnel, and could handle only a very limited number of patients at very great cost. Recent refinements, however, have made it possible to .build smaller but equally effective machines that are easy to operate and can be used by patients in their own homes, under continuing medical supervision.

Modern artificial kidney machines still have grave disadvantages. They are extremely expensive to own and operate, often well beyond the means of those who cannot survive without them, and even the machines owned by hospitals cannot begin to handle the large number of patients who require their use. It is still necessary for the patient whose kidneys have ceased to function to be "plugged in" to the machine, so to speak, for set periods of time two or three times a week without fail; the blood going through the machine must be treated with an anticlotting agent such as heparin, and frequent blood transfusions are necessary because the machine destroys a certain number of red cells every time it is used. Blood chemistry examinations must be performed regularly at least as often as once a week to check the efficacy of the treatment, and all these procedures add to the continuing yearly cost. Modern techniques have been perfected whereby permanent catheters are inserted into blood vessels in the patient's arm to be used for connection with the kidney machine, but that still does not solve the problem of the patient's utter dependency for his life on a machine which is subject to mechanical failure or may become useless because of power failure at a critical moment.

Thus at the same time that artificial kidney machines were being developed, surgeons began to experiment with transplanting a healthy kidney from a donor into the body of the patient suffering from complete and permanent renal failure. In a few cases in which the donor was an identical twin or close blood relation to the recipient, kidney transplants have proved to be remarkably successful, but in most other cases the body's rejection of the "foreign" organ has led to continuing trouble and ultimately to failure of the transplanted kidney. Experimentation continues, however, using not only human kidneys but also kidneys transplanted from higher primates such as chimpanzees. Research and experimentation also continue in an effort to find ways to overcome the body's "rejection reaction," and in some cases transplanted kidneys have remained in place and functioning for as long as two to three years before they were ultimately cast off by the body. But until a final answer to the problem of rejection is found, kidney transplants still remain a less than perfect solution which, like the use of artificial kidney machines, has comparatively limited applicability. These two approaches—the artificial kidney machine and kidney transplants—do save lives, but much research remains to be done before either can be widely, effectively and inexpensively used.

The Nephrotic Syndrome. Another common and potentially dangerous kidney disorder, similar in some ways to glomerulonephritis, is classified as the nephrotic syndrome because it is characterized by a group of related symptoms resulting from a defect in kidney function that can be caused by a large variety of different injuries or pathological processes. These symptoms include three marked changes from normal: first, the loss of large quantities of protein in the urine, not only albumin but other blood proteins as well; second, the resultant depletion of these blood proteins, particularly albumin, in the circulating blood; and third, the appearance of edema, a marked amount of fluid retention in the body, particularly in the ankles and legs. A fourth symptom—an elevation of the level of fatty lipid materials in the blood stream—is also present in a great many cases.

The nephrotic syndrome can take a variety of forms, depending on its cause. Unlike nephritis, it is not an inflammation and ordinarily involves the renal tubules rather than the renal blood supply. One form, fortunately quite rare, characteristically occurs in children between the ages of one and six, for reasons unknown, and many young victims spend the first few years of their lives suffering from massive edema and malfunctioning kidneys, sometimes to the point that death ensues. Very little is known about the cause of childhood nephrosis, and treatment of this form of the syndrome is a job for a pediatrician with wide experience in managing the disease. The disorder has a tendency to heal spontaneously in most cases if the sufferer can survive through months or years of the illness.

A number of victims of chronic glomerulonephritis develop the nephrotic syndrome together with other symptoms such as high blood pressure, but this group of symptoms also can appear in individuals who have no history of any kind of glomerulonephritis prior to the onset of the syndrome. The syndrome also commonly occurs in victims of severe diabetes mellitus which was uncontrolled at some time; in these cases the nephrotic syndrome apparently results from arteriosclerotic changes in the capillaries of the kidney, which often occur at a greatly accelerated rate in diabetics. Finally, some people develop the nephrotic syndrome as a result of allergic reactions to certain drugs or poisons.

Whatever the cause, the most striking feature of the nephrotic syndrome is the development of edema, often manifested as a puffiness around the eyes in the morning and the swelling of ankles at the end of the day, although the amount of swelling may vary greatly and its severity may fluctuate. Other symptoms include a loss of appetite and a tendency to nausea and sometimes diarrhea; these symptoms, added to the terrific drainage of blood proteins from the body into the urine through the malfunctioning kidneys, may lead to serious malnutrition, wasting of muscles and weight loss, in spite of the generalized retention of body fluid. Fatigue, weakness and depression may also be present.

Nephrosis in children has a reasonably favorable outlook for the majority of victims; approximately half will eventually heal spontaneously over a period of two to five years. Some die during this interval as a result of renal failure or an intercurrent infection which the body cannot fight effectively; perhaps a third who do not die eventually lose their edema but develop a persistent and progressive degree of renal failure that leads to fatal complications similar to those of chronic glomerulonephritis. In adults the course of the syndrome depends upon the underlying disease, but in the majority of cases the syndrome tends to persist and its victims eventually die of progressive kidney failure.

There is no very satisfactory specific treatment of the nephrotic syndrome. In some cases the use of cortisone or ACTH has been found helpful, and many patients may be maintained by intermittent treatment with these drugs over a long period of time. When helpful, they produce diuresis—that is, a pouring out of retained tissue fluid in the urine—but usually this effect is transitory and fluid retention recurs when the cortisone hormones are discontinued. Restriction of salt in the diet is helpful in reducing the amount of fluid retained in the tissues, and a diet rich in protein should be encouraged to help make up for the loss of protein in the urine. When renal failure is severe or continuing, the artificial kidney machine may be necessary to sustain life. Finally, treatment must include careful watchfulness for infections and vigorous treatment when they occur; in fact, infection is so common a problem in children with the nephrotic syndrome that many physicians recommend continuous prophylactic use of antibiotics as long as the disease is in an active stage.

A third form of kidney disorder, known as *preeclampsia* or "toxemia of pregnancy," has symptoms similar to both glomerulonephritis and the nephrotic syndrome and is directly related to the pregnancy; it is completely relieved in most cases by delivery of the child by either induced labor or Caesarean section. This type of kidney disease is discussed in more detail in connection with pregnancy and childbirth. (*See* p. 832.)

Acute Renal Failure

In glomerulonephritis and the nephrotic syndrome, the malfunction of the kidneys is a result of pathological changes in the glomeruli or in the tubules carrying urine into the kidney pelvis and the ureter. Both disorders can lead to prolonged or even permanent malfunction, but there are a number of conditions in which sudden, partial or complete failure of the kidneys to excrete water and the normal wastes and electrolytes appears on a temporary basis, as a result of injuries or temporary changes that occur in the body. For example, severe dehydration and salt loss due to excessive sweating without adequate replacement of water and salt, or due to hemorrhage, can reduce the amount of blood flowing to the kidneys and cause a reduction or even cessation of urine flow which may persist until water and salt are taken in again. If the blood supply to the kidneys is reduced for too long—a matter of six to twelve hours, usually—permanent damage to the kidney collecting tubules may occur; and when water loss is acute and prolonged, as in cases of summer diarrhea and vomiting in small children or in untreated cases of cholera, death may ensue from renal failure.

The onset of clinical shock associated with severe injuries, burns or overwhelming infections can also be followed by damage to the kidney tissue and sharply reduced urine output. This type of "renal shutdown" may persist for hours or even days after treatment of the shock has begun, and kidney failure is one of the major factors in the development of so-called irreversible shock; that is, shock that has reached such a profound state for so long that no amount of treatment can reverse it. Blood transfusion reactions can also cause injury to the kidneys when kidney tubules are plugged up with hemoglobin pigments released from hemolyzed red cells in the blood; the same sort of condition can occur from a crushing injury in which quantities of muscle tissue have been damaged, releasing hemoglobin or myoglobin (a pigment present in muscle cells) into the blood stream to plug the kidney. Finally, this type of acute renal failure can occur due to poisoning by such substances as mercury compounds or carbon tetrachloride, both of which directly damage the kidney tissue, or due to allergic reactions to drugs, particularly sulfonamides, which are excreted in the kidneys.

Acute renal failure is not ordinarily unheralded; rather, it occurs secondarily to other conditions. Its main symptom is the abrupt drop in the amount of urine passed over a 24-hour period from the normal minimum of about a pint a day to perhaps only a cup or less, often filled with tissue debris from the kidney. Treatment of the condition requires hospitalization and skillful medical management, since the amount of water, proteins and dissolved electrolytes taken in must be carefully balanced against the diminished urinary output. The otherwise healthy body can tolerate a marked degree of renal shutdown for a period of several days, even for a period of weeks in some cases, and still recover good excretory function; if the victim survives, the end of renal failure is usually marked by a sudden daily increase in the volume of urine up to one or two quarts a day. Fortunately, the conditions that bring about acute renal failure can usually be corrected or correct themselves given a little time. With the availability of the artificial kidney machine, it is now possible for the patient whose life is threatened by acute renal failure to have the benefit of dialysis long enough for kidney failure to be overcome and good function recovered. Thus a disorder which once was all too often fatal today can be effectively treated, particularly if the underlying cause of the kidney failure is diagnosed and treated promptly.

Other Urinary Tract Disorders

Congenital Defects. Like any other organ system, congenital structural defects occasionally affect the kidneys and can lead to functional disorders. Sometimes the structural abnormality has no significant effect; it is not unusual, for example, to find an individual who has one kidney lower than the other, a condition sometimes popularly known as a "floating" or "fallen" kidney, which has no effect whatever on kidney function unless the ureter is pinched off, causing back pressure. Other harmless anomalies include a bifid kidney (a kidney on one side apparently divided in half, with two separate urine-collecting tubes merging into a single urethra farther down) or even two kidneys on the same side. Such conditions are usually discovered in the course of physical examinations, and if kidney function is unimpaired there is no need for treatment. Occasionally, however, structural abnormality has more significance. Sometimes, for example, a defect in the structure of the renal artery going into the kidney, or its surrounding tissue, leads to a constriction which limits the amount of arterial blood to one kidney. This defect does not seem to have any ill effect upon the function of the kidneys, since the one normal kidney can easily handle blood filtration for the entire body; but as the victim begins to acquire mature growth, the increasing constriction of a renal artery may produce the effect of generalized severe high blood pressure. It is because of this abnormality, among other things, that X-rays of the kidneys and special renal function tests are commonly included in the complete physical examination of patients with high blood pressure, since surgical correction of the constricted portion of the artery may bring about a complete cure of the high blood pressure.

Polycystic disease of the kidneys is an uncommon hereditary condition in which much of the tissue of both kidneys is replaced by cysts. Thus the kidneys are incapable of functioning properly from birth on, and as the victim grows older the cysts gradually increase in size, progressively crowding out normal kidney function. Although people may live for some years before this condition is discovered, symptoms of progressive hypertension, blood in the urine or uremic poisoning begin to appear in adulthood, and the disorder may be fatal by middle age unless life can be maintained by the use of a kidney machine. This is a rare abnormality, but its victims are certainly among those who will profit when widespread and inexpensive means of "kidney substitution" finally become available.

Hydronephrosis. Any condition, whether an anatomical defect that leads to constriction of the ureter draining urine into the bladder, or an infection that obstructs drainage of a kidney, or an obstructing kidney stone or tumor, can lead to a backup of urine in the kidney, with a progressive increase in pressure and a limitation of the kidney's function. But because filtration of the blood in the kidneys does not depend purely on relative osmotic pressures, an obstructed kidney may continue making urine, which cannot adequately drain and stretches the kidney pelvis and then kidney tissue itself until back pressure actually begins destroying kidney function. This condition, known as hydronephrosis, is usually secondary to some other lesion in the urinary tract and is often discovered on X-rays which reveal an enlarged and poorly functioning kidney. The presence of any degree of hydronephrosis creates a situation in which bacterial infection in the kidney can flourish, and acute infection may do even further damage. If the obstruction is due to some sudden or acute cause, the patient suffers severe pain in the flank, much as in a case of acute pyelitis, but if the obstruction is caused by an aberrant blood vessel partially obstructing the ureter, or by a tumor or some other obstruction in the kidney, bladder or ureter, hydronephrosis may occur gradually and relatively silently over a period of time, sometimes causing severe kidney damage before the condition is discovered.

Treatment of hydronephrosis depends upon accurate and early diagnosis of the cause of obstruction, removal of the obstruction by whatever means necessary, and vigorous treatment of any infection present with antibiotics or sulfonamides. Once the acute situation is controlled, and sufficient time has passed for the injured kidney to resume its function, a variety of tests can be performed to assess the amount of lasting damage to kidney function.

Urinary Tract Injuries. Penetrating wounds, blows to the back, such as the infamous "kidney punch" in boxing, or crushing injuries or fractures of the pelvis can, of course, involve the kidneys, the ureters, the bladder or the urethra in mechanical damage or rupture. Diagnosing this condition is one of the physician's first concerns with an accident victim, and the first clue to such internal injuries is often the appearance of blood in the urine or the inability to pass urine. Modern diagnostic techniques are used to pinpoint the location and extent of the damage, and injuries of the urethra, bladder or ureter can usually be surgically repaired with excellent return of function. A ruptured or crushed kidney, however, is usually treated conservatively, unless it is obvious that a dangerous amount of bleeding is continuing. If an operation is necessary, the urologist will do his best to repair the kidney surgically, and will remove it only if there is no alternative and if he has been able to demonstrate that the opposite kidney is functioning adequately. Fortunately, the kidneys are among the vital organs which are paired in the body, and one healthy kidney can do the work of two if necessary, although life depends upon its continuing normal function.

Cancers and Other Tumors of the Urinary System. Like all other tissues and organs, the kidney, ureter, bladder and, more rarely, the urethra are vulnerable to the development of both benign and malignant tumors. Most tumors that arise in the kidney itself are malignant carcinomas, but a high proportion of them tend to become encapsulated and grow very slowly. When they erode into blood vessels in the highly vascular kidney, however, cancer cells may be spread widely throughout the body. One particularly notable cancer of the kidney, the so-called *Wilms's tumor,* is a malignant growth that often occurs in early childhood and may grow to a remarkable size before it is detected. It is usually an encapsulated cancer, however, and with exceedingly careful surgical removal so that the capsule is not broken and cancer cells seeded into the abdomen, cures can often be achieved. Most kidney cancers must be treated by surgical removal of the diseased organ. Because the kidney, like the liver and the lung, has a vast system of capillary blood vessels, one might expect that it would be a common site for the spread of cancer from other organs, but metastatic cancer in the kidney is actually comparatively uncommon.

Cancers originating in the ureters or the urethra are also relatively rare. The bladder, however, is a frequent site for the development of cancers. Even benign tumors arising in the inner lining of the bladder tend to invade bladder tissue and become cancerous unless they are diagnosed. When detected early, abnormal growths in the bladder can often be surgically excised, but when a cancer there is more advanced, the best treatment may be the implantation of radium or radon seeds in the tumor area to curb the growth with direct radiation, or the application of X-ray or cobalt radiation treatment.

As with other cancers, the key to successful treatment of urinary tract cancer lies in early diagnosis—and here nature is often cooperative. The cardinal symptom of tumors developing anywhere in the urinary system is the occurrence of blood in the urine, and this should never be ignored if it occurs. If more than the most microscopic amount of blood is present in urine, it becomes stained slightly brownish-red rather than the normal straw color, and turbid rather than clear; where there is a great deal of bleeding, the urine may well appear dark brown to dark red in color. On the other hand, early in the natural history of urinary tract tumors only microscopic amounts of red blood cells may be passed in the urine, quite invisible except by microscopic examination. Hence the importance of urinalysis as a part of routine physical examinations. Red cells are never present in the urine normally, but in the case of women, a certain amount of blood from menstrual flow can easily contaminate a urine specimen and confuse the issue of possible bleeding from the urinary tract. That is the reason that regular physical checkups and urinalysis are not usually performed until three or four days after the end of a menstrual period. In an emergency, an uncontaminated urine specimen can be removed from the bladder by means of a urethral catheter, but in most cases temporizing for a few days will not cause any irreparable harm.

In addition to blood in the urine, the development of urinary tract tumors can also cause dull aching pain in the back or low abdomen, loss of appetite, and fever. If the tumor is obstructing the drainage of urine into the bladder, it may cause back pressure in the kidney and hydronephrosis which is first detected because of pain and pressure in the back. Modern diagnostic techniques, including X-rays, cystoscopy and retrograde pyelograms are used to track down the presence of a tumor, its location and whether it is benign or malignant.

Blood in the urine, pain in the back and fever do not, however, necessarily mean the presence of a cancer. Acute cystitis (bladder infection), for example, may cause sufficient inflammation of the lining of the bladder that there is capillary bleeding into the urine. Blood may also appear during or following the passage of a kidney stone. Finally, perfectly benign tumors, such as small polyps or *papillomas* in the bladder may be the source of bleeding, and these may often be completely removed at the time of the cystoscopy. When a malignant tumor of the kidney, ureters or bladder is discovered, early treatment is, of course, vital, and must be planned according to the nature and location of the tumor.

Neurogenic Bladder. This is a disorder in which nervous control of the bladder has been impaired by injury or disease that has damaged the nerve roots in the lower spine, the spinal cord or the brain, with a consequent loss of voluntary or even reflex ability to empty the bladder. In these cases, the bladder empties only by means of involuntary dribbling of the overflow, a condition known as *incontinence,* or by application of direct pressure over the lower abdomen. In other cases in which there has been a complete transection or separation of the lower part of the spinal cord, the reflex arc between the urinary bladder and the transected portion of the cord may remain intact, and the victim develops an *automatic* or *reflex bladder.* In this condition, a person has no sensation of his bladder being full or of a desire to void, but when the bladder reaches its maximum capacity, it empties itself completely by reflex action with little or no warning. Efforts are made to "retrain" the bladder reflex so that the patient can have some warning that the bladder is about to empty, and those who have lost their reflex activity are taught a system of periodic voiding. In some cases "indwelling" or permanent catheters are inserted into the bladder, so that voiding can be controlled by unclamping the catheter or allowing it to drain into a urinal or a bag strapped to the leg. In such instances the catheter must be irrigated regularly with special sterile solutions to prevent clogging or possible infection. Neurogenic bladder is a condition that often complicates diseases of the spinal cord, brain or blood vessels in elderly patients, and incontinence poses difficult nursing problems. If the patient lives at home, however, some member of the family can be taught to manage relatively well, except in extreme cases when professional care may be necessary.

Detecting Urinary Tract Disorders

Often the first clue that something has gone awry somewhere in the urinary tract is the appearance of one or more of the major warning symptoms: increased frequency of urination, pain or burning with urination, an unusual sense of urgency to urinate, increased nocturnal urination, blood in the urine, or pain in the back, flank or pelvis. These are things physicians check for in the course of complete physical examinations, and patients should recognize that any change from normal in urinary function may be a signal of possible trouble that deserves prompt medical investigation.

Various laboratory and X-ray examinations are also useful adjuncts to diagnosis. The simple urinalysis is one of the easiest and least costly of all lab studies, but it can reveal the presence of sugar, albumin, crystals, bacteria, or red or white blood cells and other abnormal constituents in the urine, often in a matter of a few minutes. Urine specimens should be freshly voided into immaculately clean containers, preferably at the doctor's office unless the patient is instructed otherwise. If the urine is to be cultured for bacteria, the container must be sterilized and special collection techniques may be necessary to avoid possible contamination.

Blood chemistry examinations may also help focus on the nature and extent of urinary tract disease, primarily through the measurement of the level of nitrogenous waste such as urea or creatinine in the blood at the time of examination. The efficiency of kidney function may also be tested by remarkably simple "clearance" tests, in which carefully measured amounts of certain dyes or other rapidly excreted and easily measurable chemicals are injected into the blood stream, and then the total time necessary for the kidneys to completely clear them from the blood is clocked. If significant amounts of these substances remain longer than expected in the circulating blood, this is an indication, often quite accurate, of some impairment in the kidney's function.

X-rays of the kidney and urinary tract are, of course, invaluable aids in diagnosing disease and disorders of the urinary system, but they are by no means simple and routine as, for example, a chest X-ray is. Either one or both of two fairly complicated types of X-ray examination may be necessary to assess the condition of the kidneys, ureters and bladder. The simplest, both for the physician and the patient, is the *intravenous pyelogram* (IVP). Essentially this is a "clearance test" employing a special radio-opaque dye; that is, a substance that shows up in X-rays much the same as bone does as a "contrast medium." The dye selected is a foreign material which is normally filtered out of the blood by the kidneys and discarded in the urine in a matter of a very few minutes. Thus, after suitable preparation (a special diet to prevent for-

mation of gas or stool in the colon which might obscure the kidney region on X-ray, followed by an enema the morning of the examination), the radio-opaque dye is injected intravenously, usually into the patient's arm. Within a matter of ten minutes enough of the dye will have been gathered by the kidney from the blood stream to begin to show an X-ray shadow of the interior of the kidney on either side; and in successive film exposures at intervals up to an hour, the concentration of the dye in the urinary system will not only demonstrate the shape of the inside of the kidney, but will also provide some indication of the speed and efficiency with which each kidney handles the filtration of the dye. This procedure is extremely useful in determining kidney malfunction, evidence of infection, tumors, stones or other mechanical defects in the urinary system. Since the dye in the urine is carried down to the bladder, it also presents the opportunity to observe any abnormalities there, such as a tumor or obstruction of one of the ureters.

The main problem with an IVP is that at best a shadowy picture of the inside of the kidney is obtained, and frequently there are some areas that cannot definitely be considered either

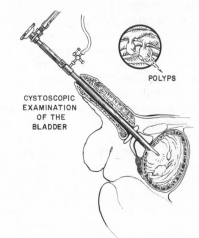

POLYPS

CYSTOSCOPIC EXAMINATION OF THE BLADDER

Figure 52–6.

normal or abnormal. When a finer definition of the inside of the kidneys is needed, or when some potentially serious symptom such as gross blood in the urine is being investigated, *retro-*

grade pyelograms may be necessary. For this procedure the patient is usually hospitalized overnight and a general anesthetic is used the following morning while the urologist or surgeon performs a *cystoscopy,* the insertion of a narrow lighted tube into the urethra in order to visualize directly the interior of the bladder. Then, with the aid of this instrument, the urologist threads tiny catheters up into the ureters from the bladder and injects a radio-opaque dye into the kidneys under slight pressure. Extremely sharp X-rays can then be taken and will often show very clearly lesions which appeared only equivocally on the IVP's. Needless to say, this procedure is more difficult, more uncomfortable and more costly to the patient than an IVP and IVP's will be used alone as a screening examination or selected first if there is a chance that they may provide sufficient information. If retrograde pyelograms are still necessary, however, they usually involve only a single overnight stay in the hospital. In addition to performance of retrograde pyelograms, cystoscopy is also an important technique for investigating possible urinary tract malignancies, for removing polyps or biopsy specimens from within the bladder, for crushing stones or for allowing direct medication or cauterization of lesions of the bladder or urethra. With such a variety of investigational techniques available, most urinary tract diseases and disorders can be detected early, but only if the victim seeks medical aid immediately when any irregularities of urination or other untoward urinary tract symptoms occur.

Disorders of the Male Genital Organs

With a few relatively minor exceptions, men and women can be afflicted with the same diseases and disorders of the urinary system, but when it comes to malfunctions of the genital or reproductive systems, there is, naturally enough, a wide divergence. Compared to the female, the structure and functions of the male genital organs are quite simple and uncomplicated. Disorders are rare, and those that do occur are often easy to diagnose and treat because the male genital apparatus is largely external. On the other hand, not only are the woman's genital organs primarily internal, but their structure and functions are considerably more complex; they are vulnerable to a wide variety of disorders that can often be difficult both to diagnose and to treat. In the long run, of course, normal, healthy genital function is of equal importance to both male and female. Its primary physiological purpose is reproduction of the species, but that purpose is served perhaps two or three times, perhaps only once, perhaps even never during the course of a lifetime. But aside from the process of reproduction, the functions of the genital organs have a profound influence on the overall health of mind and body, and they are, in turn, strongly affected by a complex of physical and psychological factors. Further, sexual intercourse is not solely a means of propagation; it is a unique form of physical and emotional communication between the sexes, of great importance not only to a relationship but to the individuals within it. No less than the body's

other organ systems, it is essential, then, to understand the structures and functions of the male and female genital systems and the variety of conditions that can lead to malfunction.

The Male Genital System

Both males and females have special glands or *gonads* specifically designed for the formation of the special reproductive or germ cells, the *sperm* in the male and the *ova* in the female. In the mature male the sperm are formed in the *testicles* or *testes,* twin glandular organs the size of pecans suspended between the legs in a pouch known as the *scrotum.* During a male baby's embryonic development, the testicles first arise from tissues within the abdomen; only about a month before birth do they normally descend down a natural canal into the scrotum. There they are supported in part by a thin sheath of muscle tissue which, when stimulated by cold or unexpected touch sensations, involuntarily draws the testicles up close to the groin. This arrangement in human males is a rather useless throwback to our more primitive evolutionary origins. In simpler animals such as the ground squirrel, sperm can be formed only during a periodic rutting season, when, in response to the female's *estrus* or period of receptiveness, the male's testicles are temporarily lowered into the scrotum; the cooler temperature there then stimulates sperm production. In humans, of course, there is no such season, and a healthy mature male develops sperm cells in quantity—up to many millions per day—over a period of five decades or more without any seasonal variation.

Sperm production in the human male is, however, controlled by a delicate balance of hormones produced not only by the testicles themselves but also by the adrenal cortex and the pituitary gland. (*See* p. 684.) The androgenic or male hormones testosterone and androsterone produced by the testicles, together with androgens from the adrenal cortex, are responsible for the maturation of the testicles at puberty and cause development of other male sex characteristics, while the so-called follicle-stimulating hormone (FSH) produced by the anterior pituitary acts upon special cells within the testicles to stimulate formation of sperm. These sperm-forming cells are found in the walls of miles upon miles of microscopically small, convoluted *seminiferous tubules* that make up the bulk of the substance of the testicles, and this process of sperm formation goes on more or less constantly from the time of puberty until the sixth or seventh decade of life or even longer, so that the male normally has a continuing supply of sperm throughout his adolescence and mature adult years.

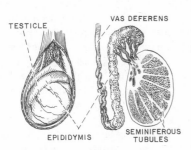

Figure 53–1.

Once manufactured, the sperm empty into a long twisted tubule, the *epididymis,* which partially covers the testicle (*see* Fig. 53–1) and then straightens out into a larger duct called the *vas deferens* which rises up out of the scrotum, into the abdomen, around the bladder, and down toward the urethra. It is the vas deferens, easily felt as a firm, cordlike tube in the upper part of

the scrotum, which is severed and tied off in the male sterility operation known as *vasectomy,* a procedure which effectively prevents sperm from reaching the urethra for expulsion.

Other structures contribute to the passage of sperm during ejaculation. At the base of the bladder two sacular structures, the *seminal vesicles,* produce a fluid which is carried by means of ducts which join the vas deferens near its entrance into the urethra to form the *ejaculatory duct.* Immediately adjacent and just below the bladder is a walnut-sized organ, the *prostate gland,* which actually surrounds a segment of the urethra; its function is to produce a sticky fluid which mixes with sperm and fluid from the seminal vesicles to form the *semen* in which sperm are carried out of the body through the penis during ejaculation. An extremely delicate chemical balance is maintained in the fluid portion of the semen which helps the sperm survive for a period of several hours following ejaculation, providing the semen remains at body temperature and is not permitted to dry.

MALE REPRODUCTIVE ORGANS

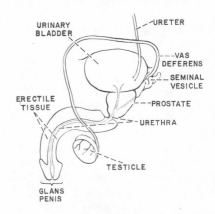

Figure 53–2.

The penis itself, a soft, flaccid tubelike organ some two to four inches long at rest, is equipped with both a rich blood supply and an intricate network of sensory nerves, particularly concentrated in a highly sensitive region around the head or *glans penis.* At birth the glans is covered by an elastic fold of skin known as the *prepuce* or *foreskin,* a bit of tissue which can be surgically removed by *circumcision* without interfering with sexual function (*see* p. 737). Both the main body or *shaft* of the penis and the glans are composed of *erectile tissue,* mostly a spongy network of blood vessels and elastic connective tissue. During sexual stimulation the arteries leading to the penis enlarge, while the veins draining blood from it constrict, so that the organ becomes stiff and erect, expanding in both length and circumference. An erection can occur as a result of mental as well as physical stimulation; indeed, during some phases of sleep penile erection occurs quite commonly in connection with dreams. When stimulation of the penis is increased, particularly by friction (as during sexual intercourse), an involuntary climax or *orgasm* is reached which triggers powerful contractions of the muscles at the base of the penis, as well as skeletal muscles of the back, legs, and arms. These genital contractions force some four or five cc.'s of semen containing as many as 500 million sperm out of the urethral opening or *meatus* at the tip of the erect penis in an ejaculation of remarkable force. At the same time, erection of the penis is also usually at its maximum, making deep penetration possible. Of course, sexual climax in the male is not necessarily dependent upon intercourse; it can also be induced by physical stimulation during masturbation and often occurs involuntarily in a nocturnal emission induced by dreams.

The sperm themselves are tiny oval-shaped cells equipped with long, whiplike tails which make them motile. Moving in a swarm, they are able to find their way from the upper end of the vagina into the interior of the uterus and even up the Fallopian tubes in order to permit fertilization of an ovum if one is available. At one time it was assumed that most sperm were superfluous, since only one was necessary for conception, but it is now believed that a multitude of sperm surrounding a ripe ovum are necessary to help break down a protective wall around the egg cell by means of enzyme action in order for any sperm to penetrate. Thus if fewer than 100 million sperm or more are present at any one ejaculation, fertilization is unlikely to occur—one of the possible causes of

relative infertility which can often be made to respond to treatment when it is detected. (*See* p. 741.)

A great deal has been made of the relationship between male sexual function and general health, and unfortunately much misinformation is still all too commonly accepted. The range of normal in male sex activity can vary from active intercourse as often as twice or more daily to as seldom as once a month or less, depending upon individual circumstances; neither extreme has either a salubrious or a damaging effect on the general health. Nor does masturbation have any known deleterious effects on the health so long as it does not become an exclusive, self-centered substitute for normal sexual relations. Excessive sexual activity may well be physically exhausting, especially if it is at the expense of sufficient sleep, and prolonged abstinence may well lead to a build-up of physical and emotional tensions— usually relieved, in part, by nocturnal emissions —but there is no level of sexual activity that is "necessary" to normal health. Under ideal circumstances, however, sexual relations are immensely gratifying and do contribute positively to the relaxation of muscular tension, restful sleep, peace of mind and a healthy renewal of energy for the day's work that lies ahead. What is more, despite the fact that sexual activity is accompanied by other temporary physiological changes—increased respiration, increased heart rate, increased perspiration and an elevation of blood pressure—there is little evidence that these changes can lead to physical harm except in individuals who already have severely impaired cardiovascular or respiratory function. But any question about the advisability of sexual activities in the face of illness or disability should be brought to a doctor's attention.

Congenital Anomalies and Structural Defects

Congenital abnormalities of the urinary and genital systems seem significantly more frequent than in any other organ system in the body, particularly in those organs in the male that the two systems share in common—the urethra and the penis. When these abnormalities do occur and are not corrected they can, of course, interfere with both urinary and genital functions. The urethra may, for example, open anywhere along the upper surface of the penis rather than at the lower side of the tip of the glans, a condition called *epispadias.* More common is the opposite condition, *hypospadias,* in which the urethral opening may occur anywhere along the underside of the penis or even, in some cases, in the region between the scrotum and the anus. The opening may be of normal size and shape, in spite of its abnormal location, or it may appear as a narrow open trench because of the incomplete formation of the urethra. Even when the location of the urethra is normal, running through the length of the penis to the tip, there may be a congenital stricture or narrowing of a segment of the urethra or constricting bands or valves within its walls obstructing the free flow of urine. In rare cases the urethra may not form at all or be present only as a solid band of tissue without any opening through it. Any of these structural abnormalities usually are observable at birth or very soon after, and they can and should be corrected surgically as soon as possible. Otherwise the afflicted child may come to associate pain and discomfort with his genitals and eventually become aware of his abnormality, which in addition to any impairment of function it may cause can also have profound psychological effects. If surgical correction is postponed until the child has reached the age of conscious awareness, genital defects, like any other visible abnormality, should be treated matter-of-factly, without undue emphasis or concern, and the child should be told exactly what the problem is and what can be done to correct it.

Another common abnormality is *phimosis,* a condition in which the prepuce or foreskin encloses the end of the penis so tightly that erection is impossible or extremely painful. Since urination is virtually always possible through an opening at the tip of the foreskin, this disorder sometimes escapes notice until puberty, but often is discovered in younger boys when bacteria become lodged between the prepuce and the glans and cause a painful and recurrent type of infection. Such infections usually respond well to vigorous antibiotic treatment, but subse-

quent *circumcision* (surgical removal of the foreskin) is advisable to prevent recurrence. For many centuries circumcision of male babies has been practiced as a religious rite in the Jewish and Islamic faiths, but most physicians today strongly recommend that *all* newborn male babies be circumcised immediately after birth, the time when this procedure is the easiest, least threatening and least painful. Not only does it correct any possible degree of phimosis that may be present and make it far easier to maintain ordinary personal hygiene and avoid bacterial infections, but it is now well established that carcinoma of the penis, which occasionally occurs at the base of the glans penis in uncircumcised males, is virtually nonexistent in those individuals circumcised from childhood.

Less amenable to surgical correction is a penis which is congenitally abnormally large or abnormally small, a condition that may become a concern at the time of puberty. Actually there is an extremely wide variation within the limits of normal in the size of this organ, and in most cases size has no effect whatever upon function. But a man may fear ridicule because of the small size of his penis or suffer totally unnecessary feelings of "unmanliness." For such persons the greatest help may well be the mature realization that true manliness has nothing to do with the physical size of the penis. Conversely, the man with an unusually large penis should recognize that the size of erection is not necessarily proportionate to the flaccid size of the organ and that most mature women are able to accommodate virtually any penile size without either injury or discomfort.

Undescended Testes (Cryptorchidism). If, by the time of birth, one or both of the testes have failed to descend from their place of origin within the abdominal cavity down into the scrotum, the condition is known as cryptorchidism. In some cases, especially when the condition is bilateral, it may be caused by a hormonal deficiency. In other cases, one testis may have partially descended but become trapped in the subcutaneous tissues of the groin. It is not uncommon for this condition in particular to go undiscovered for quite some time after the child's birth; and since one testis is in its normal location in the scrotum, the fact that the other one is missing may not be discovered until the child approaches puberty.

When the condition is found bilaterally, the testes can often be induced to descend by the administration of hormones, usually undertaken between the ages of five and seven. If this treatment is not effective, surgical correction may be recommended. The same holds true for one undescended testis, even though the other may have descended normally. A testis cannot develop its sperm-producing capacity within the abdomen or trapped in the groin, and if it is not brought down into the scrotum before the age of seven or so, it may be rendered permanently sterile. In addition, undescended testes are far more vulnerable to injury and trauma, and statistically more likely to develop abnormal cell growth or tumors. Their secretion of the vital sex hormones may also be impaired, retarding the development of the genitals and influencing the secondary sexual characteristics. Finally, an undescended testis is almost always accompanied by an *inguinal hernia,* a condition in which a loop of bowel from the abdomen bulges through or becomes trapped in a muscular defect created by the inguinal canal, the passageway through which the testis normally descends. (*See* p. 875.) Examination of the male infant's testes is, however, a routine part of the procedures of childbirth. If a defect is discovered, modern pediatric surgical techniques and anesthesia now make it possible to correct the defect.

Nonvenereal Infections and Inflammations

Both the male and female genital organs are particularly vulnerable to syphilis, gonorrhea and other venereal infections, as well as their seriously debilitating body-wide complications if these conditions are not diagnosed and thoroughly eradicated by treatment. (*See* p. 243.) But the genital organs are also vulnerable to certain types of infections or inflammations that are not specifically venereal; that is, not transmitted by sexual contact. In uncircumcised males, for example, the area at the base of the head of the penis underneath the foreskin is a common site of bacterial infection, particularly in those, children or adults, who do not keep that area clean. Antibiotic treatment is indicated, followed by circumcision to prevent recurrence when the foreskin is so tight that it cannot be stretched back over the head of the penis to permit thorough cleaning.

Another inflammatory condition, known as *acute epididymitis,* can arise, quite often without any apparent cause, to affect the tissues and cords from which the testes are suspended in the scrotum. The onset is often quite sudden, with the occurrence of pain, fever, chills, and acute swelling of the scrotum, sometimes to a remarkable degree. Prostate gland infection may or may not be present concurrently. Treatment consists of bed rest with scrotal support to relieve the pain of tension in the area, the application of ice packs, antibiotic therapy, anti-inflammatory enzymes and medication for pain as needed. This condition can often be frustrating to the patient because it can so thoroughly disable him from normal daily activity and may take a matter of some weeks before symptoms have regressed. Prompt medical attention and treatment offer the best prospect for a relatively short period of illness.

Acute orchitis, inflammation of the testes, may accompany acute epididymitis, or it may occur separately as a complication of some other systemic infection, most commonly mumps in adolescent or mature males. The complication seldom occurs, however, in males before puberty. Typically there is fever, pain and marked swelling of the testes, together with other clinical manifestations of the primary disease—in the case of mumps, pain and swelling of the salivary glands. Treatment of the primary disease, bed rest, scrotal support, the application of ice bags and medication for pain are helpful in combating the condition. Unfortunately, in some cases of mumps orchitis there is sufficient permanent damage to the structure of the testes that after recovery a period of testicular atrophy may occur, often resulting in complete sterility. Cases of infertility in a married couple can often be traced to the husband who has a grossly inadequate sperm count (or none at all) as a result of a case of mumps in adolescence or young adulthood.

A noninfectious source of acute pain and swelling in the testes is the condition of *torsion,* in which one of the testes becomes mechanically twisted on its pedicle and lodges that way in the layers of connective tissue within the scrotum. If the testis cannot be readily untwisted, or if the swelling caused by torsion holds the testis out of place, its blood supply may be seriously impaired. The pain of this condition can be prostrating, and the condition represents an acute surgical emergency, since any significant period of impaired circulation may result in permanent damage to the function of the testis or may even lead to gangrene. The surgeon's job is to correct the torsion and relieve the impaired blood supply as quickly as possible. Even more common is injury to the testes from a direct blow or other trauma. The testes are, of course, extremely sensitive to the slightest pressure, even that of crossing the legs the wrong way, and a severe blow may not only be agonizingly painful but may be followed by swelling and impairment of circulation to the injured gland. Thus proper protection is extremely important, particularly during any form of contact sport, with the use of an athletic supporter fitted to hold a protective metal cup.

Prostatitis. In men from young adulthood on, another type of genital tract infection that can cause varying degrees of disability is acute or chronic prostatitis, a bacterial infection of the prostate gland, through which the male urethra passes on its way from the bladder to the penis.

In some victims prostatitis may develop so slowly that there are no particular symptoms other than the presence of low-grade fever, a feeling of fatigue, a slight increase in frequency of urination, increased nocturnal urination, and a moderate degree of incomplete emptying of the bladder. Often, however, even in these slow-developing cases, active infection is discovered by the physician performing a rectal examination because pressure on the prostate gland reveals acute tenderness. In others the infection may occur quickly, with severe swelling in the prostate gland, pain which is often felt radiating into the testicles, chills, fever, and difficult urination. On examination the prostate may be exquisitely tender to pressure. Massage of an infected prostate gland via the rectum helps empty the gland of pus, which may be present in considerable quantity, and the resultant relief of pressure within the gland can greatly reduce the pain. Although prostate infection is usually considered a disease affecting old men, an acute prostatitis very frequently occurs in young men from twenty to thirty-five. In some cases the infection and ensuing pain may even require potent analgesic medicine.

Acute prostatitis requires immediate and vigorous wide-spectrum antibiotic treatment to avoid septicemia as a complication. Bed rest is advised, and three or four hot tub soaks or sitz baths per day will help relieve pain, establish drainage and improve circulation in the infected area. Again, inadequate treatment of the acute condition, or inadequate follow-up to make sure that the infection has been completely eradicated, can lead to a chronic prostatitis that may continue as a low-grade debilitating infection for years with occasional acute flare-ups. In addition, this kind of infection can cause strictures in the urethra which further obstruct passage of urine, and these may ultimately require surgical attention to reestablish a normal urethral passage. Since prostatitis may also develop as a result of venereal infection, particularly gonorrhea, pains should be taken to culture exudate from the infected prostate in order to identify any possible causative organism, so that more specific antibiotic treatment can be initiated as necessary.

Prostatism. Often confused with prostatitis because of considerable similarity of symptoms, yet quite a different condition, prostatism or *benign prostatic hypertrophy* is a gradual noninfectious and noncancerous enlargement of the prostate gland which often begins in men of middle age and continues into later years. This condition may be present without symptoms for decades, and when symptoms do start they may be subtle: minor difficulty starting the urinary stream, some degree of incomplete emptying, a tendency to drain a little urine after urination seems complete, and *nocturia,* the necessity to urinate two or three times or more at night. In some cases, however, prostatism becomes acute enough that the enlarging gland constricts the urethra passing through it, obstructing urinary outflow to a marked degree so that the victim becomes vulnerable to bladder or kidney infection because of the obstruction. Diagnosis is made from the history, and discovery of an evenly enlarged prostate gland on digital rectal examination. When prostatic hypertrophy is marked enough to cause urinary obstruction, surgical removal of the obstructing part of the gland may be necessary. Fortunately, a benign prostatic hypertrophy does not tend to become cancerous, and in many cases may require no specific treatment for prolonged periods.

Other Urinary Tract Infections. Far less commonly than in the case of prostatitis, urethral infections of any sort may also spread to the seminal vesicles and cause symptoms very similar to those of acute prostatitis. Diagnosis can often be established by the discovery of swollen, tender seminal vesicles on digital rectal examination, and treatment of the two conditions is essentially the same. Finally the prostate, the testes or other parts of the male genital system can become infected by tuberculosis, usually spread to this region via the blood stream from the lungs or by the urinary tract from a tuberculous kidney. Diagnosis is difficult, depending upon identification of the organism by means of smears and cultures prepared from a urethral discharge; tuberculous infections here, as in other regions, are often "silent" until well entrenched. Once diagnosed, vigorous treatment with the antituberculous drugs can prevent further spread and control or cure the infection.

Cancers and Other Tumors

Benign or malignant tumors of the male genitals are comparatively rare, and it is usually the patient who notices a swelling or a lump and calls the doctor's attention to it. *Carcinoma of the penis* first appears in the vicinity of the glans of an uncircumcised man as a small, painful sore which seems to resist healing. This condition is rare in age groups under forty or forty-five. Any sore on the genitals, however, should be called to a doctor's attention immediately, whatever the age of the patient, since the primary stage of a syphilis infection usually takes this form. Dis-

covered early, carcinoma of the penis can be treated with radium or other forms of radiation, but in advanced stages surgical excision may be necessary.

Occasionally a mass felt in the scrotum may turn out to be a benign disorder resulting from *embryonal rests;* that is, the survival after birth of certain of the formative tissues that were involved in the embryonic development of the genital organs but were not completely lost with the maturation of the baby. Simplest of these is a *hydrocele,* a small cystic collection of fluid in the scrotum which forms within a portion of the peritoneal pouch carried down into the scrotum with the testis as it descended from the abdomen. A *spermatocele* is a similar cystic pocket containing sperm which was pinched off from the connective tissue in the scrotum that came down with the testes. These conditions are not painful, but there is enough evidence that embryonic rests can develop into cancer that surgical removal of such cysts is usually recommended, and the surgery is relatively minor in nature. A similar cystic condition, known as *varicocele,* can be formed by varicosed veins developing within the scrotum. This abnormality is often associated with a dull aching in the scrotum and a constant feeling of heaviness or tension, but again the condition can easily be repaired by surgery.

Rare but relatively dangerous are true cancerous tumors which develop in the testis itself. Of the main kinds of cancer known, one called a *seminoma* is extremely sensitive to radiation, so that after surgical removal of the involved testis, radium therapy has a very good chance of killing any remaining tumor cells. Another kind, known as a *teratocarcinoma* or *teratoma,* requires more radical surgery supplemented by X-ray therapy. A third kind, one of the most malignant of all tumors, is the *chorioepithelioma,* which is similar to the highly malignant cancer that occasionally occurs in women from retained products of conception after a miscarriage. When it occurs, this tumor spreads so quickly that there is little that can be done for the patient.

When it comes to cancer, the male has a splendid advantage in the accessibility of his external genital organs to examination and his familiarity with their normal structure and function. Much is made about self-examination of a woman's breasts at regular intervals, but rarely do we hear a similar procedure suggested for men. Self-examination of the male genitals is, however, an excellent precautionary measure in addition, of course, to the commonsense fundamentals of cleanliness and hygiene. All male children should be taught these fundamentals, and any adolescent or adult male who notices a lesion of the penis or scrotum, or any other structural or functional abnormality of his genitals, should report the condition to a doctor without delay.

Of all cancers of the male reproductive system, by far the most common is *cancer of the prostate gland*. This disease is a major cause of death among males from the age of forty on, with the incidence increasing sharply in older age groups. An internal cancer that is not subject to discovery during self-examination, it first manifests itself as a small, hard lump of tissue in the prostate gland within easy access of the physician's examining finger. In most cases, however, cancer of the prostate is relatively slow-growing and tends to invade and spread in the gland itself before metastasizing to other parts of the body; therefore chances of a doctor's discovering it during appropriately spaced physical examinations are excellent. On the other hand, this cancer may be completely "silent" until it has progressed extensively. Early symptoms may include progressive difficulty urinating or emptying the bladder completely, or the appearance of traces of blood in the urine, but these manifestations do not always appear until too late—a major reason that men over the age of forty should have regular complete physical examinations, including rectal examinations, at least once each year. Once the disease has spread to other areas, such as to the bone of the pelvis or the spine, certain changes in the blood chemistry provide further diagnostic aid; the rise in the level of an enzyme known as acid phosphatase in the serum is, for example, indicative of cancer of the prostate. The diseased gland is surgically removed as early as possible, and surgery is followed by treatment with the female sex hormone estrogen, which appears to suppress the growth of this kind of tumor. Overall statistics indicate that cancer of the prostate is one of the cancers which is amenable to treatment if detected in its early stages, and with proper treatment the patient may enjoy many additional years of life. But there is no question that routine periodic physical examinations of all men over the age of forty would cut in half the number of deaths from cancer of the prostate and double the number of "five-year cures"; that is, five years of life after treatment with no sign of recurrence or metastasis of the tumor.

Disorders of Reproductive Function

The proper functioning of the genital or reproductive system in males is obviously not necessary to life in the same way, for example, that proper function of the circulatory or nervous system is, yet few things can cause more acute distress to a man at virtually any age than some malfunction of his reproductive organs. Even though the malfunction may be due to an organic illness or abnormality elsewhere in the body, it can still have profound psychological as well as physical effects. One such condition is *priapism,* an abnormally persistent erection of the penis which can become very painful and can so slow down the circulation of blood through that organ that blood clots or thrombi form in the engorged veins. Priapism can occur as a result of some disease or disorder of the nervous system which causes irritation of the nerve roots in the lower spine, or it may arise from some other irritating stimulus such as a stone in the bladder, urethral infection or prostatitis. Treatment is aimed first at diagnosis and control of the underlying cause of the abnormal erection, and the earlier this is done the less chance there is of thrombosis of the veins in the penis, followed by persistent enlargement and engorgement.

Male *infertility* or *sterility* is a much more complex and commonplace problem. It is defined, in general, as the inability to manufacture or ejaculate normal sperm in sufficient quantity to make conception possible, and it may be caused by a wide variety of conditions. Obviously, if one or both of the testes are nonfunctioning or only partially functioning, as a result of mumps orchitis or some other infection, congenital abnormality or physical injury, the sperm count may be low or completely absent. Certain endocrine gland disorders such as hypothyroidism may cause infertility, as well as the gradual decline in reproductive function that comes with advancing age. In some cases, the sperm cells themselves, while present in sufficient quantity, may be abnormally formed or abnormally inactive; in other cases, the quantity of ejaculate formed may be insufficient to carry the sperm to the desired destination. An obstruction of the seminal tract, as a result of an injury, a congenital abnormality, an infection and even a surgical procedure used to treat some other condition, can also block sperm production and ejaculation. Finally, there are many cases in which the insufficient manufacture or ejaculation of sperm cannot be traced to any known organic cause.

Infertility in the male does not necessarily interfere with sexual relations, but for the married couple who actively desire children, it is a matter of very serious concern. Male infertility is, of course, only one of any number of factors that can contribute to a barren marriage. Further, when it is discovered to exist, it need not necessarily be either a pathological or a permanent condition. But the first step in determining if it is a contributing factor is a microscopic examination of a semen sample. Granted only a single sperm is needed at the right place at the right time to fertilize the female ovum, but there is evidence that conception seldom occurs unless the total number of sperm ejaculated at the appropriate time to fertilize an available ovum is in the range of 130 to 160 million or more at the least. The motility of the sperm is also of significance; in normal men, 60 percent of the sperm should maintain vigorous motility after four hours at room temperature, and 25 percent should still be in motion after 24 hours. Most experts consider a sperm count as low as 20 million per cubic milliliter sufficient for fertility, but any number lower than that must be regarded as suspicious in cases of infertility.

Once a low or absent sperm count has been diagnosed, however, a careful physical examination and overall evaluation of the patient must be undertaken to investigate any underlying physical or psychological disorder that may account for it. It is recognized that such environmental factors as physical exhaustion, nutritional deficiencies, obesity, alcoholism or drug intoxication may well depress sperm count in a man. So also may excessively frequent sexual relations; abstinence of some 72 hours is necessary after an ejaculation to permit the build-up of sperm in the semen to its maximum possible count, and daily intercourse, for example, can effectively deplete the number of sperm present in any given ejaculation below the level that makes conception likely. Repeated ejaculations within an even shorter period may depress the sperm count still further each time, as well as deplete the quantity of prostatic fluid necessary to carry the sperm.

There was a time not long ago when infertility was widely, but quite unjustly, regarded as always the fault of the female, and men often stubbornly refused to put themselves to the test in any way. But a medical examination of a couple suffering from infertility should, of course, be a joint venture involving both the man and the woman; in fact, infertility in the male is often much easier to diagnose and is no less amenable to medical treatment and knowledgeable instruction than female infertility.

In many cases of relative male infertility, careful instruction of the couple to aid them better to identify the woman's period of vulnerability to conception immediately after ovulation can help them plan intercourse at the most advantageous time; abstinence from relations for from three to four days before that time may help ensure an adequate supply of sperm. Occasionally hormone therapy with thyroid extract may help increase the male sperm count; in other cases when the sperm count cannot be increased, *artificial insemination* of a woman with her husband's semen may help deliver a high enough concentration at the right time to be effective. Simultaneous use by the woman of certain hormones to help increase her susceptibility to conception—oddly enough, precisely the same hormones used in a different manner in "the Pill" to suppress ovulation (*see* p. 919)— often will supplement treatment of the relatively infertile male and lead to a desired pregnancy. Above all, approaching the problem as forthrightly as possible, with full communication among husband, wife and doctor, will at least provide an ideal climate in which to investigate the causes of male infertility and help overcome them.

Male impotence, the inability of the male to obtain or maintain an erection sufficient for sexual intercourse, is an entirely different condition and may pose problems of quite another sort. It may appear in one of two forms: either as an inability to obtain an erection at all (or for long enough for adequate sexual performance); or as a result of excessive excitability and premature ejaculation. In either case, both conception and satisfactory sexual relations are impossible, and impotence can be a serious concern not only to the man but to his wife as well. It is particularly insidious in that it is an emotionally self-reinforcing condition; that is, a failure to maintain an erection or a premature ejaculation on one occasion may engender discouragement, doubt and loss of self-confidence which, in themselves, may markedly affect adequate sexual performance later.

Any discussion of male impotence, to be useful, must define terms, simply because many cases of "impotence" that come to a doctor's attention are not truly impotence at all, but merely reflect the physiological norm for the man's age. Male children have erections as a result of external stimuli from the first days of infancy on, but it is not until puberty that an interest in sexual relations and release (libido) arises and ejaculation occurs due to masturbation or nocturnal emission. In most males the lifetime peak of potency and libido is reached sometime before the age of twenty and then is maintained well into the thirties with a gradual decline in the late thirties and early forties. Many men in their mid-forties become aware for the first time of a lessening of emotional or physical interest in sexual relations. Part of this, no doubt, is due to age and the decreasing amount of the male sex hormones the body manufactures, but often there are strong emotional factors involved as well. Sexual performance is inextricably linked to a man's concept of himself as a man, and with its gradual decline he may very well feel that not only is he growing old but he is becoming less "masculine." In an effort to prove to himself and others that this is not true, he may be drawn to young women, or simply to women different from his wife, often with a marked temporary increase in his sexual drive and performance. Also in early middle age, the circumstances of his life may have become thoroughly routine; he can never be young again and he resists growing old. Thus any change may seem desirable, and it is not without reason that the forties can be the "dangerous age" for many men. It is also at this age that many men exhibit an excessive concern with their potency, which in itself may affect their sexual performance. In their fifties and sixties, however, most men are able to adjust to their advancing age and declining physical prowess, and although sexual interest and potency are maintained by many even into the seventies, eighties and nineties, the level of interest is far less and far less compelling.

Thus potency varies with age and any number of other physical and psychological circumstances, and true male impotence must be considered to refer specifically to recurrent inability to perform sexually in view of these varying circumstances in each individual case. Frequency of intercourse must also be a factor in determining whether or not true impotence exists. An inability to perform sexually more often than usual, or after a longer interval than usual, need not necessarily be a sign of impotence, and impotence in the face of some aggravating circumstance—during or after a physically tiring illness, for example, or an emotionally exhausting experience—may be a frequent occurrence without signaling true impotence. The state of body and mind of both partners markedly influences sexual performance, and impotence is not uncommon during a period of some unresolved conflict between husband and wife. Only when occasional incidents of impotence recur frequently and consistently should the condition be considered abnormal and the advice of a doctor sought.

The first step in dealing with true impotence is a complete and thorough physical examination, for there are a wide variety of organic conditions that may be at the root of the trouble. The doctor checks specifically for evidence of any structural defects of the entire genital system and for evidence of any disease or disorder which may be influencing sexual function. He also searches for any evidence of malfunction in other endocrine gland systems, since diseases of the pituitary, the thyroid or the adrenals may well influence potency. Such conditions as diabetes mellitus, debilitating diseases of the liver or heart, excessive fatigue, alcoholism, drug dependence —any of these may have an influence on a man's potency. Occasionally a patient may have an idiosyncratic reaction to a particular drug or medicine; certain of the medicines used to combat nervous tension or depression, for example, sometimes cause a temporary loss of libido.

In the absence of a discernible organic disorder, a careful examination of all possible extenuating circumstances must be undertaken. Impotence due to premature ejaculation, for example, may be a result of relatively infrequent coitus or an excessive sensitivity of the penis that can be controlled with the use of a mild anesthetic ointment. On the other hand, it may also be purely emotional. Nervous tension, shyness or apprehension of failure may all contribute to both aspects of impotence and may sometimes be overcome with the use of a moderate amount of alcohol prior to sexual relations. Alcohol taken in small amounts may help lower inhibitions, but its excessive use retards sexual performance and is, in fact, often a major contributing cause of impotence. Above all, a frank and open discussion among husband, wife and doctor may be an important step in not only discovering the emotional factors that can inhibit normal sexual function, but in providing the knowledge, understanding and reassurance necessary to overcome them.

Many men are under the impression that impotence can be easily eliminated by the use of hormone shots, and it is true that medication with testosterone, the male sex hormone, can make up for modest underproduction of this hormone by the body and improve sexual performance. However, this drug is believed to be capable of stimulating the development of cancer of the prostate gland and is used only most sparingly and reluctantly. Other than this, however, virtually anything that is acceptable to both partners and works is valid, and often close communication, understanding and love between husband and wife are all that is necessary. In some cases, unfortunately, simple solutions cannot be found, and impotence can persist, often to the point of disruption of the marriage. In the absence of any evident organic disease, such a situation suggests the presence of deep-rooted emotional disturbances, and consultation with a psychiatrist may be in order. It is a very rare case indeed in which some help cannot be obtained by one or another of these approaches.

Certainly the normal, trouble-free function of the male genital system is as important to the individual's general health and emotional well-being as that of any other organ system, and while it is remarkably free of life-threatening diseases and disorders, even a minor misfunction can sometimes lead to a disproportionate degree of discomfort. Thus, like any other organ system, it deserves a certain amount of common-sense attention and hygienic care. Cleanliness is, of course, of primary importance. Experimentation and physical abuse of the genitalia should be avoided, and any sign of disfunction, however minor, should be reported to a physician promptly. Finally, it is well to remember that a doctor can often serve as a helpful consultant even in the absence of any symptoms or disorders. He can, for example, be an excellent source of sexual information in general and answer questions about genital function that so often trouble adolescent boys and even adult males. He should not, however, be expected to take on the responsibility for an adolescent's sexual education and behavior; that responsibility belongs to the parents. Nor is the family physician a substitute for a marriage counselor or a psychiatrist in dealing with grave marital or emotional problems. He can, however, help to the full extent of his medical knowledge and experience and, perhaps even more important, make an appropriate referral when he feels that a problem is out of his province.

Disorders of the Female Genital System

Of all aspects of illness and health care, there is probably no other area that has been written about at greater length than disorders of the female genital or reproductive system. Even so, there is still widespread misunderstanding or outright ignorance about its structure and its normal, as well as abnormal, function. There is less confusion about male reproductive function, perhaps because it is far less complex than the female and, of course, the male genital organs are largely external. In the female, however, the main reproductive organs—the ovaries, the Fallopian tubes, the uterus and the vagina, together with the various ligaments that hold them in place—are all internal, housed in the bowl-shaped and relatively protected area formed by the bones of the pelvis which come together at the pubis in front and join the sacrum at the base of the spine in the back. This "pelvic girdle" of bone forms the floor of the abdominal cavity, and the female genital organs or *pelvic organs* are thus, in one sense, located internally in the lower abdomen. Physicians distinguish, however, between the abdominal organs of the digestive tract above, which are completely enclosed within a slippery protective lining, the *peritoneum,* and the female genital organs of the pelvis which are outside and below the peritoneal space. This is not entirely an artificial distinction, because the peritoneum actually forms an effective barrier isolating pelvic organ disorders below the barrier from disorders of the digestive tract organs above. Even in a pregnancy, when the enlarging uterus presses up higher and higher into the abdominal area, it is

still considered to be in the pelvis. Indeed, the only direct communication between the peritoneal cavity above and the pelvic area below is at the point where the fimbriated or finger-like ends of the Fallopian tubes reach up in close contact with the ovaries. Here, at least theoretically, it is possible for invading bacteria, pus, menses or other materials present in the pelvis to make their way up the tubes and "spill out" into the abdominal space, a very important consideration in some disorders of the reproductive tract.

Most conditions of the female reproductive organs, however, are located in the pelvis, are characterized by symptoms in that region, and generally cause pain or distress due to irritation of the peritoneum only when the disorder is in the immediate region where the peritoneum covers the top of the pelvic organs. What is more, in the female the genital organs and the urinary tract organs, while in close proximity, are normally entirely separate, with no "sharing" of structures such as is the case in the male. The female urethra, for example, comes down from the bladder above but quite separate from the vagina, and although it emerges above the vagina in the genital crease, it has no direct internal connection with the reproductive organs. Thus there is somewhat less likelihood in the female of "mixing" infections of the genital tract and the urinary tract than in the male.

The Female Genital System

The process of reproduction in all but the most primitive living creatures requires the con-

745

tribution of both the male and the female of the species, but in human beings, as with other mammals, the female must carry the major share of the burden. Human egg cells or *ova* are produced in the female gonads, the ovaries— oval-shaped, peanut-sized glands that lie in the pelvis on either side of the uterus. Unlike the male gonads, which produce male germ cells or sperm by the millions more or less continuously, ovum production by the ovary is far more spar-

CROSS SECTION, FEMALE REPRODUCTIVE ORGANS

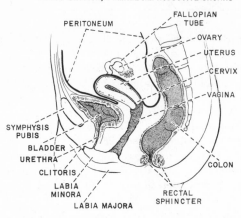

Figure 54–1.

ing. Only once every 28 days, on the average, does a rudimentary ovum mature in one of the ovaries, growing from a tiny nest of special cells known as a *follicle*. At the time of sexual maturation hundreds of thousands of immature follicles—potential ova—are present in each ovary, but ordinarily only one follicle matures at a time. As the ovum approaches maturity, a process that requires about 10 days, it grows to a size larger than any other cell in the human body, and with its surrounding follicular cells it actually forms a small blister-like growth on the surface of the ovary. Finally that blister ruptures and the ripened ovum is discharged—the process of *ovulation*. On rare occasions two or even more ova may ripen simultaneously; if two are fertilized, each with a different sperm, a twin pregnancy can occur, leading to the development of *fraternal* or *nonidentical twins*. Fraternal twins are born simultaneously, but have quite

individual hereditary patterns and thus resemble each other no more than children of the same parents born years apart; they may even be of different sexes. More rarely, a single fertilized ovum may break apart in the very earliest stages of embryonic growth and develop as two (or even more) separate babies with the same hereditary patterns. These babies then become *identical twins,* always of the same sex and of very similar form and feature.

To be fertilized, however, a ripened ovum must first come in contact with sperm from the male. Thus, when an ovum is discharged from an ovary it is not just released willy-nilly into the pelvic region. Each ovary is partially enveloped by the soft, finger-like ends of a *Fallopian tube* or *oviduct,* a narrow tube some 5½ inches long which extends up in a curve from the upper corner of the uterus, one on each side, to provide a channel to conduct the ripened ovum down into the internal cavity of the uterus. Each Fallopian tube is lined internally with tiny hair-like *cilia* which help sweep the ovum downward, a journey that takes approximately 48 hours. The uterus, for its part, provides a place for the fertilized ovum to lodge and grow. In its normal nonpregnant state the uterus is a pear-shaped organ some 4 inches high and 3 inches wide, located low down in the midline of the pelvis, where it is supported in place by fibrous ligaments which also help support the ovaries and Fallopian tubes. The walls of the uterus are formed of a special kind of interlaced muscle tissue which surrounds a central chamber or cavity. This internal cavity is lined with a soft, vascular tissue known as *endometrium* which is prepared by hormonal action following each ovulation to aid the implantation and growth of the ovum in the event that fertilization takes place. The lower end of the uterus, called the *cervix,* is attached to the upper end of the vagina, and the interior uterine cavity is connected to the vagina by means of a narrow *cervical canal*. Normally plugged with mucus, this canal can open sufficiently to permit the drainage of blood and degenerated endometrial cells from the interior of the uterus during menstruation, and it is ordinarily open enough to permit motile or moving sperm deposited in the vagina to find their way up into the uterine cavity and thence into the Fallopian tubes to make fertilization of an ovum possible. When a pregnancy develops, however, the uterine wall is capable of stretching to an amazing degree to accommodate the growing fetus until, after approximately nine months of fetal development, it

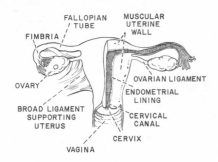

Figure 54–2.
Structure of the uterus and ovaries.

consists of a thin sac of muscle tissue rising well above the navel and pushing all the movable digestive organs aside. Thin as the muscular wall of the uterus may be at this time, the muscle itself is still remarkably powerful, and with the beginning of labor it begins contracting in rhythmic waves, forcing the baby down toward the birth canal while the cervical canal at the lower end thins and dilates to permit the baby to emerge.

At most times the *vagina* is merely a blind pouch or canal lined with mucous membrane which connects the cervical end of the uterus with the outside. But the vaginal walls are highly elastic, capable of stretching to receive the erect penis during sexual intercourse, and stretching still more at the time of labor to permit the birth of the baby. Prior to first intercourse the entry to the vagina is normally partially blocked by a thin crescent of mucous membrane, the *hymen* or "maidenhead," which is usually torn or stretched, with a minimum of discomfort and bleeding, by the penis during the initial copulation. The *external female genitalia* appear as a creaselike structure, the *vulva,* consisting of the entry to the vagina or *introitus;* two protective folds of tissue, the *labia majora* or outer folds

and the *labia minora* or inner folds, which ordinarily cover and protect the introitus; a small button-like structure located above the introitus (and above the urethral outlet) which is equipped with an extremely rich supply of sensory nerves, known as the *clitoris;* and two sets of mucus-secreting glands, the Skene's glands and the Bartholin's glands, which produce a slippery lubricating fluid during sexual arousal which greatly aids the insertion of the penis into the vagina. During sexual stimulation the labia, which are richly supplied with capillary blood vessels, become somewhat swollen and congested, while the clitoris becomes erect and extremely sensitive to touch; indeed, the entire genital region and the breasts and nipple tissue as well become highly responsive to tactile sensations. These sensations may intensify to the point of a pleasurable climactic nervous discharge or *orgasm,* more diffuse than in the male, accompanied by spasmodic contractions of the muscular walls of the uterus as well as by tightening of skeletal muscles all over the body. Contrary to popular belief, there is no discharge of fluid from the female during orgasm, nor does any sexual sensation arise from within the vagina itself. It is probable, however, that the uterine contractions during orgasm do tend to draw sperm that are deposited in the vagina up into the uterine cavity.

But the basic function of the female reproductive organs depends upon far more than sexual stimulation alone. Conception becomes possible only when sperm come in contact with a mature ovum that has been released by an ovary, and this occurs only at approximately 28-day intervals as a result of the interaction of certain powerful hormones produced both by the anterior pituitary gland and by the ovaries. (*See* p. 686.) For approximately ten to twelve days following the end of a normal menstrual period, the prime mover among these hormones is *estrogen* produced by the ovaries, the "female sex hormone" which is also responsible for feminine features and for such other secondary sex characteristics as breast development and the relatively scanty distribution of body hair found in women. During this interval following a menstrual period, estrogen stimulates the new development of the soft, vascular endometrial lining of the uterine cavity. At the same time a powerful hormone produced by the anterior pituitary gland, the so-called *follicle-stimulating hormone* (FSH), triggers one of the tiny nests of follicular cells in the ovary to begin forming a new ovum. Another pituitary hormone stimulates the final maturation of the ovum and its release from the ovary at the time of ovulation. Once ovulation has occurred and the new ovum has started its journey down the Fallopian tube, the nest of follicular cells from which it arose produces yet another hormone, *progesterone,* which further prepares the endometrial lining of the uterus to hold and nurture the ovum in the event that it is fertilized.

The passage of the mature ovum down the Fallopian tube takes approximately 48 hours, and it is during this time and this time alone that conception can occur. If sperm are deposited in the vagina during this interval, they can find their way up into the uterus or even higher into a Fallopian tube to meet and fertilize the ovum. Normally the ovum will make its way down into the uterine cavity even if it is fertilized in the tube and will then become lodged or *implanted* in the specially prepared endometrial lining, where it will begin to divide and grow. If by some mischance it becomes lodged in the tube instead, it will usually die, but on rare occasions it may implant there to become a *tubal* or *ectopic* ("out-of-place") *pregnancy,* a dangerous complication which, when it occurs, usually requires surgical intervention. (*See* p. 820.)

If conception occurs and the fertilized ovum becomes implanted, the level of progesterone produced in the ovary (and later by the special nurturing organ, the *placenta,* developed by the fetus) remains high, preventing menstrual flow when it would next be expected. Indeed, the first clue that a pregnancy exists is usually the failure to menstruate at the usual time. What is more, no further follicles are stimulated until the pregnancy is over, so that ovulation comes to a temporary halt. If, on the other hand, conception does *not* occur within about 48 hours, the ovum simply dies and disintegrates; the nest of follicular cells in the ovary from which it came shrinks up to form a tiny scar with no further hormone-forming activity, and the endometrial lining of the uterus, thus suddenly deprived of progesterone, begins to degenerate as the blood vessels supplying it constrict. Some ten days following ovulation shreds of this degenerated tissue lining, together with small quantities of blood, begin to drain from the uterus into the vagina, the onset of a normal menstrual period during which flow will persist from three to six days on the average. Then, once again, estrogen stimulates the preparation of a new endometrial lining in the uterus, FSH from the pituitary again triggers the maturation of another follicle in the ovary, and the whole female reproductive cycle begins again. Most authorities agree that there is no consistent physiological relationship between this hormonal cycle in the female and any waxing or waning of sexual desire, but there may well be a psychological relationship. For example, a woman who actively desires *not* to become pregnant may feel more free to engage in intercourse immediately before, during or after a normal menstrual period than at any other time because she knows that conception will be unlikely; and whereas people may avoid intercourse during the menstrual period as a matter of individual preference, there is no evidence whatever that sexual relations at such times are in any way harmful.

For all practical purposes, then, the occurrence of normal, regular menstrual flow is merely the end result of a chain of events, controlled and regulated by hormones, that began at the end of the previous menstrual period almost a month earlier; in a sense it is mute physiological evidence that a conception has not occurred and that another female reproductive cycle is about to begin. The first menstruation or *menarche* occurs when a girl begins to ovulate at the time of puberty between the ages of eleven and fourteen, and menstruation normally continues in recurring near-monthly cycles, except during pregnancies, until the age of forty-five to fifty, when pituitary and ovarian hormone production begins to fall off sharply. At this time, known as *menopause* or "change of life," both ovulation and menstruation become increasingly irregular and presently cease, bringing an end to the woman's ability to conceive. This, of course, is a perfectly natural phenomenon, but it is often accompanied by a variety of uncomfortable symptoms which may require intermittent or sometimes prolonged treatment.

What kinds of diseases and disorders commonly afflict the female reproductive organs? In addition to those normal physiological changes and possible disorders that may result from conception, pregnancy and delivery, which are discussed elsewhere (*see* p. 811), they generally fall into four main categories: disorders due to abnormal structure or development; infectious or inflammatory diseases; cancers, tumors and cysts; and finally, disorders of the female reproductive function itself.

Congenital Anomalies and Structural Defects

In the female certain minor structural abnormalities, if no less common than in the male, are often less frequently discovered simply because her genital organs are largely internal. Thus the woman is seldom bothered about whether her uterus is large or small, or whether her vagina is somewhat longer or shorter than normal. More serious anomalies are characteristically discovered either in childhood at some time prior to the age of puberty, when congenital defects or accidents of embryonic development become evident, or later in life after the childbearing years when a structural breakdown of the connective tissue in the pelvis often causes anatomical changes that require attention. True congenital malformations are relatively infrequent and often so minor that they pass unnoticed; still more infrequent are malformations which render normal sexual activity impossible without correction of the defect.

Certain abnormalities of the hymen or maidenhead, for example, may well require minor surgical intervention before normal intercourse is possible. Under normal circumstances this structure is a thin crescent of mucous membrane which partially occludes the entrance to the vagina, leaving enough room for drainage of menses or even for the use of tampons by older adolescent girls. It serves no known purpose and is usually ruptured during initial intercourse; its presence or absence, however, cannot be taken as a reliable indication of a girl's virginity, since in some cases intercourse is possible without disturbing the hymen, and in other individuals it may be accidentally ruptured prior to initial sex relations—as a result, for example, of horseback riding, tree climbing or some other vigorous athletic activity. Occasionally, however, the hymen will be *imperforate,* completely obstructing the vaginal entrance. Normal menstruation is impossible under these circumstances, and the uterus and vagina may form a large cystic mass filled with blood and serum if the condition is not discovered prior to puberty and the hymen incised and removed by a simple surgical procedure. More commonly it may be normal in size but abnormally thick, so that efforts to rupture it during intercourse are unsuccessful. In such cases a simple surgical incision can resolve the problem, preferably before intercourse is attempted—just one reason why every girl should have a thorough physical and pelvic examination at or about the time of puberty, and again in preparation for marriage.

Another congenital anomaly which occurs occasionally is the partial or total absence of the vagina. Once this condition has been discovered, however, there are a variety of ways to correct the defect by means of reconstructive surgery to permit the eventual assumption of normal sexual activity. In other cases, there may be either a complete double uterus or a bifid (divided) uterus, sometimes with the development of a double vagina and double cervix lying side by side. Often only one set of these organs is functional, and usually the woman can engage in perfectly normal sex relations, conceive, and even bear children without medical intervention, although in some cases reconstructive surgery may be necessary. Occasionally a malformation of the Fallopian tubes leads to an inability to conceive, and there are also abnormalities of the location or even the number of ovaries, sometimes with the total absence of one, or the presence of a third ovary. In such cases one or more of the ovaries may be abnormally formed and nonfunctioning. Such anomalies are generally of importance only in relation to the possibility of infertility, of abnormal pregnancies, or of a predisposition to infections in the tubes. In the absence of any problems nothing need be done, but corrective surgery may sometimes be necessary in an effort to restore normal reproductive function.

Another anomaly of reproductive structure and function, *hermaphrodism,* can, of course, afflict both the male and the female. True hermaphrodism, in which an individual has both functioning ovarian and functioning testicular tissue, is exceedingly rare, however; most instances of so-called double sex are in reality cases of pseudohermaphrodism or false hermaphrodism. These individuals generally have functioning glands or gonads of only one sex, together with part or all of the genital structures of that sex, but in addition they may also have undeveloped and inactive organs of the opposite sex. A female pseudohermaphrodite, for example, may have functioning ovaries but a vagina too small for normal intercourse and a markedly enlarged clitoris; a male pseudohermaphrodite may have functioning testes but a small penis and the external genitalia of a female. In cases of both hermaphrodism and pseudohermaphrodism, evidence of sex may be misleading at birth, and the infant is often cast in an inappropriate gender role; that is, the infant who appears to have a penis at birth is brought up as a boy, but at puberty he is subject to a baffling variety of hormonal influences as the physical and psychological characteristics of the opposite sex begin to predominate. When the condition is discovered, reconstructive surgery and hormone therapy, in some cases, may enable the individual to assume the most natural sex role, and psychiatric help is also useful in treating the condition. Very recently it has become possible to perform *chromosome typing* in order to determine the true sex of the individual as a further aid to correct treatment. It is one of the tragedies of our society that this disorder, as well as the doctors who have pioneered in its study and treatment, have been regarded with almost universal suspicion. Only recently have we come to realize that hermaphrodism in any form is a disorder no less deserving than other congenital abnormalities of the most knowledgeable and skillful treatment.

A structural defect that has also been the subject of a great deal of medical controversy is the abnormal placement of the uterus within the pelvis, a condition that is usually not discovered until young adulthood. Normally, the uterus is tipped forward almost horizontally in the pelvis with the neck or cervix extending slightly downward in the direction of the rectum and meeting the vagina at approximately a right angle. (*See* Fig. 54–3.) It is not unusual, however, for the

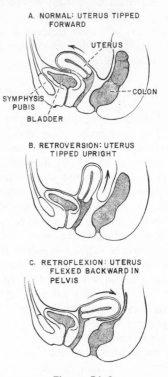

A. NORMAL: UTERUS TIPPED FORWARD

UTERUS

COLON

SYMPHYSIS PUBIS

BLADDER

B. RETROVERSION: UTERUS TIPPED UPRIGHT

C. RETROFLEXION: UTERUS FLEXED BACKWARD IN PELVIS

Figure 54–3.

uterus in some women to be *retroverted* or pushed back so that instead of lying horizontally at a slight downward angle it is stationed more or less vertically in the pelvis. Nor is it unusual for it even to be *retroflexed* or tipped backward so that the main body of the uterus is folded over the top of the cervix and presses against the lower colon.

Such so-called retrodisplacements of the uterus have been recognized for many years by obstetricians and gynecologists. In some cases they appear to be structural abnormalities present since puberty; in others they may occur later in life as a result of stretching of the ligaments supporting the uterus during one or more pregnancies. But even today there is no clear consensus among gynecologists about whether retrodisplacements actually mean anything in terms of illness. Often these conditions will be found in women who complain of more or less continuing pain or pressure in the pelvis, or who suffer from pain or discomfort during intercourse, or who are bothered by vague backaches or a variety of other symptoms, usually more pronounced at the approach of menstruation. Probably in many such cases the discovery of an abnormally placed uterus is purely coincidental and has nothing to do with the symptoms. On the other hand, many women with such complaints have been completely relieved of their symptoms by the test use of a *pessary,* a ring-like supporting device inserted and worn in the vagina to tip and hold the uterus in the normal position. In such cases, many gynecologists feel that surgical correction of the retrodisplacement, with the use of internal sutures to hold the uterus forward, is the best long-term solution. Retrodisplacement of the uterus has also been blamed in various cases for causing spontaneous miscarriages or for the inability of the woman to conceive. Again, even gynecologists cannot agree; some feel that surgical intervention is indicated, but certainly a search for other possible causes of frequent miscarriages or relative infertility should be made before surgery is undertaken.

Even among women with perfectly normal reproductive organs, there are many who suffer a certain amount of tissue breakdown in the course of their childbearing years which leads to various symptomatic structural defects later in life. Often these defects are directly related to the number of children the woman has borne; carrying and bearing a child inevitably causes a certain amount of stretching and relaxation of both muscle and connective tissue in the vagina and in the tissue surrounding the bladder above and the rectum below. This may lead to a weakening of these tissues during repeated pregnancies, so that the bladder begins to sag and bulge down against the roof of the vagina, forming the sort of pouch known as a *cystocele,* or a portion of the lower colon near the rectum bulges up through the floor of the vagina to form a pouch known as a *rectocele.* Up to a point, neither of these structural defects necessarily causes symptoms, but as time goes on, the woman with the cystocele has increasing difficulty fully emptying her bladder and becomes more susceptible than normal to bladder infections or cystitis. An even more distressing symptom which commonly occurs is stress incontinence—inadvertent loss of urine when coughing, sneezing, straining at stool or even, in severe cases, just with walking around or climbing stairs. At the same time, there may be the increasing problem of constipation, and often the woman with a rectocele finds that she must press down on the floor of the vagina with her fingers in order to have a satisfactory bowel movement.

When these defects are severe enough to become symptomatic, it is often advisable to have them repaired in a so-called *vaginal plastics operation,* in which the cystocele and rectocele (both usually occur together) are pushed back into normal position and held there by reconstructive repair of the roof and floor of the vagina, bringing muscle and connective tissue in from either side to prevent the outpouching. This is an elective operation performed at the patient's convenience and is a relatively satisfactory procedure for most women with this problem. After a period of convalescence of some six weeks, there is marked relief of symptoms and the patient can return to physical activities she had previously been forced to give up. In most instances surgery is permanently effective, but the aging process in connective tissue goes on, and there are occasional cases in which one or both defects may recur some years after the original repair. The decision to repeat reconstructive surgery at that time must be based on the severity of the symptoms as well as the age, general health and cardiovascular status of the patient.

Just as the muscle and soft tissue surrounding the vagina may become weakened and atrophied with age, the muscles and ligaments supporting the uterus may become stretched as a result of repeated pregnancies and allow the uterus to slide down or *prolapse* into the vagina, a condition that can be aggravated by chronic constipation which forces the woman to strain at stool. Occasionally the prolapse will become so severe that the cervical end of the uterus can be felt or even seen at the vaginal orifice. Depending upon the age of the patient and various other factors, a choice may be made for surgery to resuspend the uterus in its normal position through an abdominal incision or to perform a *hysterectomy* (removal of the uterus) either abdominally or by means of a vaginal procedure in which the uterus is brought down and removed through the vagina in order to spare the patient an abdominal incision.

There was a time not long ago when gynecologists were inclined to perform hysterectomies at the drop of a hat, regarding the uterus after childbearing age as a useless organ and a potential source of trouble. Today the criteria for this operation are somewhat more selective, as are the criteria for any pelvic operation approached by way of the abdomen. A doctor will usually seek other means to relieve the symptoms of any uterine disorder until he is thoroughly convinced that the trouble cannot be corrected except by surgery. Prophylactic hysterectomies, undertaken before any symptoms occur, are rarely recommended or performed.

Inflammation or Infection of the Genital Organs

The female reproductive organs are vulnerable to invasion by a variety of infectious organisms, both those which cause the venereal infections spread primarily by sexual contact and those which are contracted from the environment or result from an infection elsewhere in the body. Of the venereal infections, gonorrhea and syphilis are by far the most common, and potentially far more dangerous in women than in men because they are more difficult to diagnose. Untreated, both infections may be passed on repeatedly, afflict an unborn or newly delivered infant, cause infertility or sterility, and progress to involve the entire body in debilitating disease. (*See* p. 243.) Thus it is of the utmost importance to consult a doctor at the onset of any unusual symptoms of the genital area, or even in the absence of symptoms after a sexual contact that is regarded as suspicious.

In many cases, infections or inflammations of the genital area are not venereal at all. Any number of bacteria and parasitic organisms may attack the external skin surface of the genitals, as well as the interior surfaces of the vulva and vagina, causing irritation, swelling and sometimes unusual vaginal discharges. One of these, called *vulvovaginitis,* is an inflammation of both the vulva and the vagina, attended by acute itching of the external genitalia, pain and burning on urination, and a moderate amount of thin, milky discharge spoken of as *leukorrhea.* In many cases this is a superficial infection caused by one of the coliform bacteria, and it can be speedily and effectively treated using a vaginal antibiotic cream or gel. Frequently simple attention to personal hygiene and the use of a very mild vinegar douche (1 tablespoon of vinegar in a quart of warm water) will help restore the normally acid condition present in the vagina and will clear up such a bacterial infection.

More troublesome is a vaginitis (inflammation of the vagina) that is caused not by a bacteria but by a single-celled protozoan organism, the *Trichomonas vaginalis.* Symptoms again include persistent external genital itching and burning, occasionally painful urination and a leukorrheic vaginal discharge. The *Trichomonas* organism is easily identified in the course of an office visit to the doctor by microscopic examination of a vaginal swab, and it can be destroyed by use of one of a variety of medicated douches the doctor will prescribe, together with a special antitrichomonal medication known as Flagyl which is used simultaneously in vaginal suppositories and in pill form taken by mouth. This kind of vaginitis is frequently recurrent, and it is now recognized that the male may also harbor the *Trichomonas* organism by means of an asymptomatic infection and then reinfect the woman after she has stopped treatment. Thus in recurring cases of *Trichomonas* infection it is often wise for both husband and wife to be treated at the same time and to abstain from sexual relations for the week to ten days necessary to eradicate the organism.

A similar vaginitis quite as common as trichomonas infections is *monilia,* a fungus infection caused by *Candida albicans,* the same fungus organism that causes thrush in babies. (*See* p. 863.) This infection also causes severe itching and burning in the perineal region, as well as a whitish vaginal discharge. Once identified it is treated by cleansing douches and use of an antifungal agent known as nystatin in capsules taken by mouth as well as in vaginal suppository form. Monilia is particularly common as an overgrowth that occurs when the victim has been taking a broad-spectrum antibiotic for a prolonged period of time. Thus doctors often give nystatin simultaneously with the antibiotic as prophylaxis against monilia overgrowth.

Occasionally nonvenereal bacterial infections can invade the upper female reproductive tract and cause an acute inflammatory condition in the entire pelvis. Often this kind of *pelvic inflammatory disease* (PID) cannot be differentiated from a gonorrheal infection when it becomes acute, causing considerable pain in the pelvis, a spiking fever, chills, nausea and an elevated white blood count. The symptoms are such that the condition must also be carefully differentiated from an acute pyelitis (kidney infection) or even an acute appendicitis or diverticulitis. Treatment consists of rest, intensive treatment with antibiotics to destroy the invading organism, aspirin and analgesics as necessary to control pain and fever, and abstention from intercourse until the infection clears up. All too often women afflicted with this condition tend to stop treatment as soon as acute symptoms improve but before the infection is totally eradicated, which can lead to recurrent or chronic pelvic inflammatory disease and progressive damage to the reproductive organs.

Pelvic inflammatory disease is particularly a threat immediately after childbirth or after such surgery as a diagnostic dilatation and curette-

ment (D and C) of the uterus, when infectious organisms are more readily able to gain access to the uterus or tubes. It is for this reason that the doctor pays so much attention to regular measurements of temperature, frequent visits and examinations, and any sign of pain developing in the woman during these vulnerable periods. Often, in such cases, the first symptom of a pelvic infection is the presence of a peculiarly foul-smelling discharge. When this occurs there should be no hesitation or delay about contacting the doctor, since the length and severity of the illness can best be limited by early diagnosis and treatment.

Fortunately, in modern hospitals where every possible precaution against infection is taken during childbirth, *childbed fever* or *puerperal sepsis,* an acute and often fatal pelvic inflammatory disease contracted during delivery and usually caused by streptococcus or staphylococcus organisms, has become largely a thing of the past. (*See* p. 207.) But it remains a threat from another source—the illegal abortionist, or even from misguided attempts at self-abortion. Bacterial contamination is only one of the possibly fatal consequences that can result from such abortions, and when they occur they must be treated promptly and vigorously to save the victim's life. Social attitudes and laws regarding abortions are in the process of change, however, and one of the benefits that may be hoped for in the future is a sharp decline in the number of women who have recourse to illegal abortion.

Another disease of the female reproductive tract is bacterial infection of the Bartholin's and Skene's glands which lie near the outlet of the vagina and normally provide lubricating mucus during intercourse. Such an infection, if untreated, will form either infected abscesses or develop into sterile cysts. In both cases there is a hard, palpable and usually painful nodule that can be felt on either side of the vagina just within the introitus. Occasionally antibiotic treatment alone will help resolve these infections and surgery is not required, but in most cases incision and drainage of the abscess, followed either by excision of the infected gland or *marsupialization,* a surgical technique for keeping the infected gland permanently open until it can heal, is the best guarantee of prevention of further infection.

Finally, there is a type of infection which is usually relatively free of symptoms, but which is perhaps the most common of all inflammatory processes in the female reproductive tract, *acute or chronic cervicitis.* This is an inflammation of the lower end of the uterus, the cervix, and frequently the only symptom is a moderate amount of thin, watery vaginal discharge. In severe cases there may also be some spotting of blood between menstrual periods, one of the more common reasons the patient calls the doctor's attention to the condition.

The cervix can be examined visually by means of a *speculum,* and in cervicitis the surface of the epithelium covering the cervix is broken and there is some abrasion or erosion that sometimes involves the entire cervix, sometimes only one area. Frequently this area of inflammation tends to bleed readily when touched, which explains why women with the disorder occasionally find spotting the day following intercourse. Since the cervix is a sensory "dead area"—that is, it has no pain nerve endings—there is no pain. The physician is concerned about this condition because it often appears very much like the changes in the cervical epithelium seen in an early cancer. Thus he will take a Pap smear of the cervix for examination by a pathologist and will then prescribe a medicated douche or vaginal cream to be used for a period of a week or so. Assuming a "normal" report on the Pap smear, if the cervicitis does not clear up promptly, the doctor may stimulate healing by touching the eroded areas with an electrocautery, a completely painless office procedure. If the cervicitis is still refractory to healing, or too extensive, or if there is a recurring pattern of abnormal bleeding, a diagnostic D and C may be indicated, and the eroded part of the cervix can be surgically removed during this procedure. It is usually done to rule out the possibility of a cancer within the uterus and to provide more accurate study of the eroded portion of the cervix to be sure that there is no malignant change in the cells there. Healing following a D and C generally takes approximately six weeks to

two months, and special precautions against the development of infection must be taken.

Tumors, Cysts and Cancers of the Female Genital System

A great deal of publicity has been given to the importance of watchful vigilance on the part of every woman for any sign of reproductive tract tumors; and justly so, for the pelvic area is a frequent site for a variety of abnormal growths, and the most common of all reproductive tract cancers, carcinoma of the cervix, is one of the few kinds of human cancer which can easily be detected so early in its course, by appropriate diagnostic means, that it can actually be cured in a high percentage of cases.

Carcinoma of the Cervix. A slow-growing tumor, *carcinoma of the cervix* begins in the epithelial cells lining the neck of the uterus, and the earliest signs of the disease that can be detected are minor changes in the growth pattern, shape and staining qualities of a patch of these epithelial cells. At first there may be no visible change that the doctor can see on examining the cervix, but even at that very early stage, abnormal cells on the surface of the cervix can be discovered by means of the so-called Pap test or Pap smear, named after George N. Papanicolaou (1883–1962), the Greek-American physician and cytologist who was one of the researchers who developed the technique. Cells for microscopic pathological examination are removed by painlessly scraping the surface of the cervix during the course of a routine office examination. Cancerous cells can be detected in this way long before the growth becomes visible or any symptoms appear; hence the necessity of regular medical checkups, in which the Pap smear plays an important part.

Occasionally, when cervicitis or inflammation of the cervix is present, it is impossible to determine whether any abnormal changes in cell growth detected by the Pap smear are the result of inflammation or the beginning of a tumor; in such a case the cervicitis is usually treated and then the Pap smear repeated. If abnormal cells are still present, the physician or gynecologist then recommends a diagnostic dilatation and curettement (D and C) of the uterus, as he would with a markedly abnormal Pap smear in the first place. Abnormal cells on a Pap smear may indicate possible cancerous changes within the uterus, or in the cervical canal, as well as possible cancer of the cervix itself. The D and C permits a biopsy to be taken from the interior of the uterus as well as a biopsy of the cervical canal and the cervix proper. In this brief surgical procedure, usually done in a hospital with the patient under a general anesthesia, the gynecologist uses a series of metal dilators to open the cervical canal enough to insert a narrow instrument with a sharp loop or *curette* on the end into the uterus. He then scrapes the interior cavity of the uterus to obtain biopsy samples of the endometrium for pathological examination to be certain the abnormal cells in the Pap smear have not drained down from within the uterus. At the same time he excises the epithelial lining of the cervix, and this tissue is also examined by the pathologist. In its earliest stages, the abnormal cell growth of carcinoma of the cervix is diagnosed as *carcinoma in situ;* that is, cancerous changes all located in one small surface area without any evidence of invasion of deeper cell layers. In such a case, the pathologist can often determine by his examination that the entire area involved in abnormal growth has been removed. If the patient is a young woman who has not yet had a family, the doctor may encourage her to undertake a pregnancy as soon as possible, since the hormonal changes that occur in the course of a pregnancy seem to inhibit the development of early cervical cancer. Then once the pregnancy is over—or in the case of a woman beyond childbearing age—surgical removal of the uterus is usually recommended as a means of being as sure as possible that all remnants of the early cancer have been excised. The percentage of cures of early cervical cancer is very high—as many as 90 to 95 percent of all cases cured without recurrence.

In some cases, however, the diagnostic D and C reveals that the cervical cancer has reached a more advanced stage and deeper cell layers of the cervix have been invaded by tumor tissue. The degree of invasion varies, and in this more advanced stage, radium treatment is customary, since cancer of the cervix tends to be extremely sensitive to radiation and to recede with this kind of treatment. Thereafter, surgical excision of the uterus and all surrounding tissue often provides the best hope for cure, unless the spread is so great that the surgeon regards it as inoperable. In the latter case, palliative treatment with radiation often provides control for prolonged periods of time.

Fifty years ago carcinoma of the cervix was one of the most common and almost invariably fatal forms of cancer in women. Today, thanks to the special cell-staining technique of the Pap test, the discovery of an advanced cancer of the cervix is a completely preventable tragedy. The Pap test is not 100 percent accurate—gynecologists estimate that it fails to pick up an early cervical cancer about 15 percent of the time— but it is a simple procedure that requires only a pelvic examination, and is so inexpensive that it can, and should, be performed on every woman over the age of twenty at regular intervals. Carcinoma of the cervix may take as many as six or seven years to change from the very early *in situ* stage to a more advanced stage, so that even with 15 percent failure, there is an extraordinarily high probability that regular semiannual or annual Pap tests will reveal a cervical cancer in its early stages when it can be completely cured. Contrary to popular notions, cancer of the cervix is *not* influenced in any way by either the frequency or the vigor of intercourse, nor by the use of medications, douches, tampons, or any other physical manipulation. By undertaking a regular program of pelvic examinations and Pap tests, there is no reason why any woman today should let a cervical cancer go undetected beyond its earliest stages.

Uterine Myomata (Fibroids). Whereas carcinoma of the cervix is a malignant tumor, however slowly it may grow, another extremely common form of abnormal tissue growth, the so-called fibroid tumors which develop in the walls of the uterus, are almost always benign. These tumors are composed of fibrous tissue that begins growing in the muscular wall of the uterus for reasons unknown; they are characteristically multiple and frequently attain massive size. Fibroids have been removed that were as large as or larger than baseballs. When located in the middle of the uterine wall in the upper portion of the organ, fibroid tumors may be detected by the doctor during a pelvic examination as a marked enlargement of the uterus, in the absence of any other signs suggesting pregnancy. If the fibroids are located near the outside wall of the uterus, they may actually grow into a palpable mass that can be felt to the right or the left of the uterus; in other cases when fibroids grow near the central cavity of the uterus, they may come to fill the cavity and produce a pattern of abnormal menstrual bleeding, spotting after menstrual periods are over, or prolonged periods of scanty menses. Finally, as the fibroids grow larger, circulation of blood to the fibrous tissues may be impaired and some amount of cellular death occurs in the tumors themselves with resultant bleeding between menstrual periods. The enlarged uterus may also press against adjacent organs, particularly the bladder, causing pain and difficulty in urination.

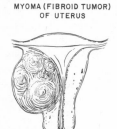

MYOMA (FIBROID TUMOR)
OF UTERUS

Figure 54–4.

Abnormal vaginal bleeding of any sort, whether a disturbance of the normal menstrual flow or bleeding between menstrual periods, is a cardinal sign that *something* is wrong with the normal genital functions that should be investigated without delay. This should be doubly emphasized in any woman of menopausal age or older, since the dangers of pelvic cancer become markedly greater with advancing age. Often when an abnormal bleeding pattern results from fibroids, the physician can diagnose the condition with reasonable accuracy just by pelvic examination. Nevertheless, when there is a history of abnormal vaginal bleeding, a diagnostic

D and C will be recommended to rule out some other source of the bleeding, such as a cancer of the interior of the uterus, before accepting fibroid tumors as the final diagnosis.

Treatment of fibroids depends upon the size, location and number of the tumors, the symptoms, if any, that they cause, and the age and childbearing history of the patient. The mere presence of fibroids is not, in itself, a reason for surgery unless they are rapidly increasing in size or causing symptoms such as painful pressure on the bladder or bowel or abnormal bleeding. Small fibroids do not necessarily interfere with conception or pregnancy, although they may, if located near the inner surface of the uterus, account for an occasional spontaneous miscarriage. If the fibroids are larger, they can definitely interfere with conception and pregnancy or produce an erratic pattern of menstrual bleeding that never settles down to normal, or they may simply take up so much space that it is wise to have them surgically removed. If the woman is of childbearing age and wishes to be capable of future pregnancies, the tumors can be removed from the uterine wall and the uterus reconstructed by suturing. When childbearing is no longer a consideration, however, a hysterectomy is often a better and more permanent way to resolve the problem. Other factors—a great deal of bleeding at menses, for example, or menstrual periods so prolonged that anemia gradually develops, or pain and pressure symptoms—may also militate for surgical intervention and correction. When a woman with known fibroids is pregnant and approaching term, many obstetricians favor performance of a Caesarean section for delivery of the baby, often planning a hysterectomy at some later date for treatment of the fibroids if this is indicated.

Cancers of the Uterus. These malignant tumors, which must be clearly differentiated from a slow-growing and accessible carcinoma of the cervix, arise in the interior of the uterus, often from the glandular tissue lining the uterine cavity, in which case they are called *cancer of the endometrium.* Other cancers occurring in this region are those highly malignant tumors that develop from retained fragments of embryonal material after a miscarriage, the *chorioepi-*

thelioma. Much more infrequently, a cancer may arise from muscle or fibrous tissue in the wall of the uterus, a type of tumor known as a *uterine sarcoma.*

In any of these cancers the first clue that something is wrong is usually the onset of intermenstrual vaginal bleeding; that is, bleeding or spotting that occurs sometime between the end of one menstrual period and the beginning of the next. In other cases, the bleeding may be at the time of menstruation, but with a change in the normal menstrual pattern such as more copious or prolonged bleeding than usual. For example, it is not uncommon for a woman to notice such a minor shift in pattern as the tendency to have spotting for two or three days after the bulk of menstrual flow has ceased. Whatever the abnormality, at the first evidence of abnormal bleeding a woman should see her doctor, for the best hope of successful treatment of a uterine cancer is early diagnosis and treatment.

The great majority of all cases of abnormal vaginal bleeding are not due to cancer at all, but to one of a multitude of perfectly benign disorders which can readily be diagnosed and differentiated from cancer. For example, the tissue lining the interior of the uterus may suffer *hyperplasia,* a benign overgrowth which often occurs late in the menstrual cycle when a conception has not taken place, and there can be bleeding or spotting from this overgrowth. Again, the glandular tissue lining the inside of the uterus can form *polyps* which, because of their poor blood supply, may tend to break down and bleed. Bleeding may be due to a benign cervicitis, which can be both diagnosed and treated with relative simplicity. And, in addition, there are a variety of changes that can occur in the ovaries and cause hormonal imbalances that lead to an abnormal bleeding pattern. Finally, benign tumors such as fibroids may be causing marked distortion of the normal menstrual pattern. Women beyond menopause, in whom menstruation has stopped, should be particularly alert to the onset of vaginal bleeding, even though the source of the bleeding in most cases is found to be perfectly benign. For example, fibroid tumors occur in as many as one-third of all women over the age of forty, and this is a very common cause of postmenopausal vaginal bleeding. Thus there is no reason for any woman to fear abnormal bleeding symptoms, but there is reason for concern. These symptoms must be investigated because occasionally cancer *is* at fault and early diagnosis offers the best opportunity for successful treatment.

When a uterine cancer is discovered, treatment will depend on the kind of cancer, as revealed by a biopsy of tissue taken during a D and C, the age of the patient, the length of the history of symptoms, and any evidence of metastasis that can be found. In most cases surgical removal of the uterus, often including removal of the tubes and ovaries as well, is the treatment chosen, but this type of surgery may often be preceded by radium or deep X-ray therapy to stop the growth and spread of the cancer. Surgery may also be followed by postoperative irradiation treatment in hopes of eradicating any spread of the tumor that might have occurred. In general, uterine cancers reach an advanced stage of development before such symptoms as abnormal bleeding appear, so a much lower percentage of cures and a higher percentage of ultimate fatalities result in spite of the most skillful treatment. However, treatment by means of surgery and/or irradiation may, even in advanced cases, prolong comfortable life by many months or years, and should be undertaken as soon as the presence of the disease is discovered.

Cysts and Tumors of the Ovaries. In the year 1809 in a small Kentucky village a young American physician named Ephraim McDowell performed the first successful abdominal operation in America—60 years before Lister's pioneering work on surgical asepsis and some decades before the first general anesthesia was available. Yet for all this, McDowell's patient survived the removal of a large ovarian tumor and safely recovered from the surgery.

The performance of that operation was a historical milestone in medicine, but the disorder leading to the surgery was well known even then. It has long been recognized that women's ovaries are particularly vulnerable to a variety of troublesome and often dangerous pathological changes. Among these changes are the development of inflammatory cysts of the ovaries, the development of cysts as a result of the normal ovarian function of producing and releasing ova, the growth of cystic (that is, large fluid-filled) tumors, and the development of a variety of ovarian cancers. Although each of these disorders arises from a different cause, they may all present much the same kind of symptoms and similar findings on physical examination; thus differentiation of a benign from a malignant disease is an extremely difficult diagnostic challenge even today.

Inflammatory cysts of the Fallopian tubes, the ovaries or both arise directly as a result of infection, and these balloon-like collections of serum, often mixed with pus or blood or both, may attain a size large enough to fill the lower abdomen. Inadequately treated gonorrheal infection is a major factor in the development of these cysts, as is bacterial contamination in the process of an illegal abortion. But infection introduced at the time of childbirth or during a diagnostic D and C or as a result of a nonspecific inflammatory disease can also be a factor. Such cysts may be relatively painless but can become so large that they press the other pelvic organs out of position, leading to a feeling of fullness or heaviness in the pelvis. What is more, normal ovarian function may be damaged or completely destroyed, on one side or both, and it is frequently a change in the menstrual pattern— cessation of menses, pain during menstrual periods or some abnormal bleeding pattern—that first brings the patient to the doctor.

Other kinds of cysts can produce much the same picture. Occasionally when a ripened ovum is released from a follicle in the ovary there may be a small amount of bleeding at the site of release, which can lead to the formation of a small to medium-sized *corpus luteum cyst* filled with clear or bloodstained serum. Multiple benign but space-taking *follicular cysts* may form in areas of the ovaries where ova have failed to ripen and then have degenerated while still immature. Often the formation of such cysts is associated with some disruption of the normal menstrual pattern, and when there has been an unusual amount of bleeding following the release of a mature ovum, the cyst may grow to the size of an egg and be quite easily detected by the physician on pelvic examination. Also a disorder called endometriosis (*see* below) can lead to the implantation of cells from the inner lining of the uterus on the surface of the ovary, and these implants may give rise to remarkably large cysts filled with quantities of clotted or degenerated blood.

Cystic tumors of the ovary are a different matter. These are true "new growths" which arise from cells in the stroma or supporting structure of the ovary, sometimes from immature islands or "rests" of embryonic tissue, sometimes from an overgrowth of different types of adult cell. Cystic tumors frequently become very large and fluid-filled, varying in size from the diameter of a baseball to the size of a small melon, and are usually associated with menstrual disturbances and/or pain with menstruation, or sometimes with the cessation of menstruation. It is now believed that most such cystic tumors— there are many different varieties classified according to the kind of cells from which they arise and the particular details of their pathology —begin as benign overgrowths of normal cells, but all too often the cells forming the walls of the cysts may undergo malignant or cancerous change sooner or later. Finally, there are outright cancers arising from ovarian tissue which may be cystic but which are often formed as solid cancerous growths.

The diagnosis of all of these abnormal growths depends upon many factors: the age of the patient, the pattern of symptoms, the history of previous pelvic disease or infection, and—most important of all—the performance of a careful and thorough pelvic examination at regular intervals, as well as at any time that abnormal menstrual symptoms occur. Inflammatory cysts, for example, may appear at any time, but are usually associated with a history of previous pelvic infection and are most common in women in the age group from the mid-twenties to mid-thirties. Cysts arising from hemorrhage in the ovary at the site where an ovum has been released are quite common among teen-age girls and young adult women, while cystic tumors can appear at any time from puberty on through the childbearing years, with the incidence of frank malignant tumors of the ovary increasing with age.

Whenever an ovarian cyst or tumor is discovered, surgical exploration and pathological identification of the nature of the lesion may be necessary. Since ovarian cysts are seldom cancerous in women under the age of thirty-five, the surgeon may temporize to see if a small cyst goes away spontaneously. In women over thirty-five the risk of possible cancer is too great, and surgical exploration is indicated, as it is at any age if the cyst is large. There are some kinds of benign cysts which completely disappear quite spontaneously; but others which may be benign at first may persist and then undergo malignant change. Thus the decision for surgery is often made not because the physician is sure that the tumor is dangerous, but because he cannot be certain that it is not malignant without examining the lesion at surgery and, if necessary, taking a biopsy for immediate pathological examination. Statistics indicate that approximately 15 percent of all ovarian tumors discovered on physical examination are malignant, while many others may sooner or later become malignant if not removed. When evidence of cancerous change is found during surgery it is often quite early in the course of development, and thus the chances for recovery are good. In treating ovarian cancer, however, just as in the treatment of cancer of the uterus, the best results are obtained not only by surgical excision of the tumor and surrounding areas, but also by the use of intensive X-ray irradiation following surgery. Irradiation before surgery may be indicated as well if the surgeon feels quite certain from his preoperative examination that a cancer is present—for example, if the mass in the vicinity of an ovary is hard and nodular and if there is a fixed thickening of fibrous tissue surrounding the area. With modern treatment methods approximately 60 percent of all women who are found to have malignant change in a cystic tumor of the ovary, or a frank cancer of the ovary, survive for five years or more after surgery. Even when the cancer cannot be completely removed, the patient may have a number of years of normal life before the disease becomes incapacitating. When a suspicious cyst or tumor of an ovary is found at surgery to be completely benign the surgeon will still seek to remove it, preserving the ovary unless the organ has been so severely damaged by pressure or scarring that it can no longer function to produce either ova or ovarian hormones. Since the ovaries are paired organs, a woman can still retain her reproductive capacity and normal hormone production even after one ovary has been surgically excised.

Endometriosis. One of the more common of all female pelvic disorders is a strange condition known as *endometriosis,* a form of abnormal tissue growth very much like, although not identical to, a tumor. In recent years endometriosis seems to be affecting more and more young women, and it was first associated with such a wide variety of signs and symptoms that gynecologists were at a loss to understand precisely what it was. For the most part, these symptoms included various kinds and degrees of pain felt in the pelvic region during the few days prior to menstruation and continuing into the menstrual period proper. In some cases pain would appear as a low backache; in others it would be felt in a localized area in the pelvis, aggravated by intercourse, bowel movements or pelvic examinations. There might also be an occasional failure to menstruate, even though the painful symptoms occurred on schedule, or menstruation would be scanty or irregular.

Gynecological surgeons in search of the source of these symptoms frequently discovered odd little nodules of tissue that could be felt upon pelvic examination, particularly in the small pocket known as the cul-de-sac between the neck of the uterus and the colon; and this condition was often associated with firm fibrous adhesions in an area where the uterus ordinarily is quite readily movable on examination. On surgical exploration these patients were found to have a multitude of small reddish-purple tumor-like growths scattered hither and yon on the outer surface of the ovaries, on the tubes, and most particularly on the back surface of the uterus, even studding the peritoneum to the rear of the abdomen. Microscopic examination of the nodules revealed that they were implants of tissue virtually identical to the tissue lining the interior of the uterus, the *endometrium,* which is filled with glands and engorged blood vessels after ovulation in preparation for a pregnancy. This material sloughs off when a pregnancy does not occur and makes up, together with blood, the substance of the menstrual flow. These "endometrial implants," however, were not within the uterus at all, but were found completely outside, as though endometrial tissue fragments had been released into the lower abdominal cavity where they implanted on the outer surface of various pelvic structures and began to grow.

How did these fragments of aberrant tissue get there? And why were the pain and distress they seemed to cause cyclical? By the early 1920s, investigators had found several different factors that were apparently related to the development of endometriosis. For example, a very high percentage of young women afflicted with this problem were found to have retroverted or retroflexed uteruses—far too high a percentage for this finding to be considered coincidental. Second, a great many of these same women had either difficulty or no success whatever in conceiving. Many of them also had symptoms of endometriosis that appeared after the performance of a procedure known as the Rubin test, in which radio-opaque dye had been forced into the Fallopian tubes under pressure in order to determine if there was a blockage of the tube preventing conception. And even among those women who contracted the condition without retrodisplacement of the uterus, a high percentage seemed to have intrauterine polyps or some degree of stricture of the cervical canal which tended to obstruct the normal escape of menstrual flow from the uterus during menses.

Today it is widely accepted that endometriosis occurs when, for one reason or another, normal menstrual flow is obstructed and back pressure tends to carry menstrual blood containing live tissue fragments and cells from the endometrial lining of the uterus up the tubes and out their fimbriated ends into the abdominal cavity in the vicinity of the ovaries. These cells, although nonmalignant, seem to have the capacity to implant themselves and grow on the surface of the ovaries, or on the peritoneal surface covering the back of the uterus and down into the cul-de-sac. The growth of such cells is not necessarily very impressive—perhaps a nodule of tissue half a centimeter across will form—but the tissue is the same as the endometrial tissue of the uterus and is responsive to the same hormone activity in the body. This means that following ovulation, endometrial "colonies" outside the uterus begin proliferating cells and glands just as the lining of the uterus does, as if anticipating the implantation of a pregnancy. When no pregnancy occurs, these bits of tissue, markedly swollen and located in areas where pain-sensitive nerves can be stretched, torn or pressed, cause the syndrome of pain which reaches its height at the beginning of the menstrual period. Once the hormonal balance changes so that menstrual flow begins, the endometrial implants slough off cells and blood to form small fluid-filled cystic bodies which then decline in size until the next menstrual period.

Later experimental studies have proved that the female hormones or estrogens definitely stimulate the growth and swelling of endometrial implants, while progesterone, the female hormone of pregnancy, tends to reduce the lesions in size. Thus the use of progesterone-containing hormones such as the Pill used for conception control, in larger doses, is often effective treatment. In selecting the choice treatment in a given case, however, the gynecologist considers a number of things. Endometriosis occurring in younger women may be relatively mild, with only minor symptoms, but the general rule is that the condition tends to get progressively worse when it starts in a young woman who has had no children and may, in fact, present a constant menace to the function of her ovaries or her ability to conceive. Thus the gynecologist is inclined to perform surgery to excise the endometrial implants that can be found and to suspend the uterus back in a normal position if it is retroflexed. In addition, diagnostic D and C's, Rubin tests and other surgical manipulations within the uterus are customarily postponed until after a menstrual period has ended to reduce the risk of forcing particles of endometrial tissue out through the tubes and into the abdomen. Finally, any strictures or obstructions of the cervix or mouth of the uterus that might cause retention and backflow of menses can be repaired preventively.

When a surgical approach is indicated, the amount of surgery performed must be decided on an individual basis. In the case of a young woman who has never been pregnant and wants to have children, the surgeon will usually do as little as necessary to provide relief of the symptoms, and then turn special attention to helping her conceive, since endometrial lesions tend to regress and remain subdued throughout a pregnancy. Similarly, they tend to atrophy and become subdued after menopause, and thus the age of the patient and individual plans for childbearing must enter into the decision for treatment. The woman of thirty-five or forty with severe endometriosis and no desire for further children may require total removal of the uterus to effect a cure. In such cases, however, removal of the ovaries is also essential to prevent recurrence, since large, painful endometrial implants may respond to the ovulation cycle even when the uterus has been removed.

Disorders of Menstruation

A large number of diseases and disorders of the female genital organs can interfere with a woman's reproductive capacity, and most of those conditions present pain in the pelvis, some disturbance of the menstrual pattern, or both, as symptoms. Indeed, the onset of a change in a woman's normal pattern of menstruation is often the first and major symptom that leads her to consult a doctor. Part of the doctor's job, however, is to determine what constitutes a variation from normal. For example *amenorrhea* (absence of menstrual flow) is, of course, quite normal before puberty and in some perfectly normal girls menstruation may not begin until the age of thirteen or fourteen, just as it may begin as early as the age of nine in others. Whenever menses begin, the first few periods may be scanty or grossly irregular before a more regular pattern becomes established. A doctor's examination is advisable if such irregularity continues for more than the first year of menstruation, but even

then there may be nothing wrong that will not correct itself with further physical maturation. Amenorrhea is also quite normal some time after the age of menopause, but the time may vary widely from individual to individual, and there may be a perfectly normal interval of irregular or scanty periods before menstruation finally ceases; thereafter, of course, it is the appearance of vaginal bleeding that is abnormal and a danger signal to the physician.

Between puberty and menopause, however, most women do establish a reasonably regular and predictable cyclic pattern of menstruation; even women whose periods remain "regularly irregular"—closer together than the average 28 days, for example, or further apart than average—can at least predict within a few days when a period should come due, and it is usually the woman herself who must provide the doctor with the criteria of what can be considered normal in her case. The complete absence or "missing" of an expected menstrual period may signal a variety of abnormal conditions. The onset of a pregnancy is by far the most common cause, but in the absence of pregnancy a broad range of physical or even psychological disorders may be at fault. Certainly if amenorrhea occurs between these age limits in the absence of a pregnancy, medical investigation is necessary to determine why.

Dysmenorrhea (difficult or painful menstruation, sometimes called *menorrhalgia*) is a different matter. Many women have some discomfort related to their menstrual periods—cramping, for example, headache or backache on the first day, and so forth—and this may be entirely within the range of normal. A change in the usual pattern, however, with totally new discomfort or a marked increase in the degree of discomfort, is suggestive of an abnormality or disorder of some sort and should receive a doctor's attention. The appearance of *menorrhagia* (excessive menstrual flow) again must be balanced against the normal pattern of the individual; some women have copious flow at each menstrual period while others have relatively little, and it is a change in the normal, expected pattern that suggests a disorder. Finally, *intermenstrual bleeding* of *any* sort is abnormal and deserves medical attention. In the presence of an early pregnancy it may signal an impending miscarriage; in the absence of a pregnancy it is symptomatic of some disorder that demands investigation.

Premenstrual Tension. Since time immemorial the interval just before and during menstruation has been popularly associated with a wide variety of irritating symptoms long regarded as "nervous" or "psychosomatic" in nature, and not entirely without reason. In many ancient cultures women were regarded as "unclean" during menstruation, and sexual relations were rigidly proscribed until menstrual flow ceased. More recently, but before reliable contraceptive techniques had become widely available, fear of an unwanted pregnancy could often cause a marked increase in nervous tension just prior to the time a menstrual period was expected. But today we know that a great many women suffer from a generally harmless but irritating physiological disturbance for a period of time ranging from three to seven or more days prior to the onset of menstruation—a condition marked by very real symptoms arising from real and treatable physical causes, but still rather deceptively known as premenstrual tension. Some time after ovulation, usually a few days prior to the beginning of menstruation, the woman finds herself increasingly nervous and irritable for no apparent reason, often given to outbursts of anger or fits of depression. Headaches ranging from very mild to severe are frequently part of the syndrome, and in many women the change in emotional tone is so great that "she acts like a different person," in the terms often used by husbands. For a long time this syndrome was thought to be almost purely psychosomatic and was erroneously thought to be due to worry about a possible pregnancy, or even a device for discouraging sexual advances. Oddly enough, this increasingly marked degree of tension would characteristically vanish completely a few hours after the onset of menses, seemingly corroborating the "fear of pregnancy" idea.

More careful and detailed study of the condition, however, has revealed another factor to be present: there is generalized fluid accumulation throughout the body, sometimes demonstrable as edema of the ankles, for example, during the few days prior to menstruation, and this accumulation is lost within 24 hours of the beginning of menses. Today most authorities regard premenstrual tension as primarily a physiological condition in which sodium ions are retained in the body, thus retaining fluids in the body as well, as a result of increased steroid hormone activity during the latter third of the menstrual cycle. It has even been suggested that the increase in nervous irritability and emotional instability could be due to a generalized edema of nervous tissue all over the body, including the brain. Armed with these ideas, physicians have found ways that this annoying condition can be helped.

In many cases all that is needed is aspirin for the relief of minor headache and a mild sedative, such as small doses of phenobarbital, during the last day or two before the period to counteract nervous irritability. In severe cases, a somewhat more prolonged preventive treatment is undertaken which involves administration of diuretic drugs for a week or more prior to the expected onset of menstruation, together with abstinence from salty foods, both measures designed to help dehydrate the body somewhat. Relatively small doses of a daytime sedative such as phenobarbital can also be used three or four times daily during the last three days before the period begins. This program usually relieves the headaches, nervousness and irritability quite significantly, but in some cases a tranquilizing drug may be recommended along with a sedative. Most cases of premenstrual tension can be prevented in this way, and those that are not can be dramatically reduced in severity.

In premenstrual tension there is, at least in theory, a plausible physiological relationship between the approach of menses and a certain degree of emotional tension. It is an all too popular misconception, however, that psychological factors can have a mysterious but powerful influence on the menstrual cycle to speed it up, delay it, and cause irregularities, pain or other menstrual disturbances. There is little if any scientific evidence to support this contention, but the converse may often be true. Women are understandably sensitive to any irregularity in menstrual function, and even the most minor variations from what is expected may engender seemingly exaggerated emotional responses. Most women learn to take occasional minor irregularities in stride, but any change from normal, however minor, should be discussed with a doctor if it is associated with significant emotional disturbance. A careful and thorough physical examination will help identify any potentially serious disorder, and at the very least will relieve both doctor and patient of unnecessary or continuing worry if all is found to be normal.

Menopausal Syndrome. The time of menopause is a time of far-reaching physical and emotional changes in the lives of most women, often affecting their husbands and families as much as themselves. These changes and the disturbances they engender are discussed in detail elsewhere. (*See* p. 933.) It is sufficient to note here that declining hormone production in the ovaries and anterior pituitary gland at some point between the ages of forty-five and fifty-five signals the end of ovulation and the beginning of certain distressing symptoms of physical as well as emotional change. Among the physical signs and symptoms of menopause the most notable are the onset of irregular and scanty periods of menstrual flow, followed presently by the complete cessation of menses; a tendency to water retention, as evidenced by swelling of the ankles and sometimes the fingers; and the experiencing of so-called hot flashes—sudden wavelike sensations of heat, flushing or tingling of the face and extremities, often physically uncomfortable and sometimes alarming in their intensity. Menopause is also commonly accompanied by unpredictable episodes of nervous irritability, occasional instability of emotional tone or mood, and a tendency to periods of intermittent anxiety and depression. Any or all of these symptoms may be suffered intensely for prolonged intervals by some women and few, if any, by others. All are a result of normal physiological changes taking place within the body, however, and even when severe can usually be ameliorated by appropriate medical treatment, most notably the intermittent administration of synthetic estrogens to relieve hot flashes and the use of diuretics and sedatives or tranquilizers as required, respectively, to encourage the release of retained body fluid and to provide temporary relief from nervous tension.

Disorders of Reproductive Function

A commonsense consideration of the mechanisms of ovulation and conception shows that any abnormality of the ovaries, tubes or uterus might impair normal reproductive function simply by preventing, in one way or another, the successful meeting of a viable sperm with a viable ovum. As in the male, a distinction is made between *true* or *absolute infertility,* in which the reproductive organs are permanently incapable of normal function, and *relative infertility,* in which some potentially correctable condition interferes with conception. True, infertility may result, for example, from surgical removal of the ovaries or uterus in treatment of a pelvic cancer, from destruction of the ovaries by a viral infection such as mumps, from some congenital or acquired condition which impairs the normal formation or maturation of the female reproductive organs or from surgical ligation of the tubes as a permanent means of conception control. In most cases, however, failure to conceive when a pregnancy is desired is the result of relative infertility caused by some undiscovered condition affecting either the male or the female which renders conception difficult or impossible unless the condition can be identified and corrected. Pelvic infection involving one or both tubes, for example, can completely obstruct the movement of an ovum down into the uterus. Fibroid tumors within the uterine cavity can also obstruct the passage of sperm and reduce the likelihood that a fertilized ovum will find a place to implant in the uterine wall in order to grow. Ovarian cysts or conditions such as endometriosis may interfere with ovulation and lead to relative infertility. Sometimes disorders of the thyroid or the adrenal cortex may cause hormonal disturbances that interfere with normal ovulation or menstruation until they are diagnosed and treated.

The investigation of relative infertility requires a careful search for any kind of underlying organic illness that might be interfering with conception. A semen analysis should always be done on the husband early in the investigation to spare the woman unnecessary investigative procedures if the cause of the infertility is an impairment in the husband's sperm production. Function of the thyroid gland should be evaluated, and the basal body temperature of the woman should be recorded for a period of several months to help pinpoint the frequency and time of ovulation. The basal temperature, taken first thing in the morning before arising, eating, drinking, or smoking, ordinarily remains very much the same each day throughout most of the month, but the temperature at the time of ovulation usually drops a few tenths of a degree below the normal baseline, and then 24 hours later rises abruptly to a few tenths of a degree above the baseline before settling down to normal again. Of course other things can interfere —the presence of an upper respiratory infection, for example—but in most women keeping a regular chart of morning basal temperatures will help establish the time of ovulation. Efforts to achieve a pregnancy can be timed accordingly, with sexual intercourse planned to coincide with ovulation after two or three days' abstinence prior to that time.

Once all the information possible has been gathered, treatment will be indicated by the findings. Congenital abnormalities sometimes can be corrected surgically, and other defects such as damaged tubes, ovarian cysts, retroversion of the uterus with endometriosis, and so forth can be treated. A low dosage of thyroid taken daily is often helpful in achieving a pregnancy even when the patient's basal metabolism rate is normal. In recent years many cases of relative infertility have been successfully treated with the same combination of hormones that are used, in a somewhat different manner, in the Pill to prevent ovulation. It has been found that when these potent hormones are used throughout two or three menstrual cycles and then abruptly withdrawn, there is a marked increase in the woman's tendency to ovulate and conceive following the withdrawal, and this procedure often helps when all else fails.

Finally, other factors that may be contribut-

ing to relative infertility must be considered. One such factor may be a degree of so-called *sexual frigidity*—the inability of the woman, for one reason or another, to respond normally to her husband's sexual advances. Frigidity in itself cannot directly interfere with conception, since conception depends upon union of a sperm with an ovum regardless of the woman's physical or emotional response to the sexual act. But frigidity from any cause can grossly interfere with the frequent, regular sexual relations that make conception more readily possible. In many cases frigidity in the female may be the result of pain during intercourse, a condition known as *dyspareunia,* arising from such causes as chronic pelvic infection, infection of the urethra or bladder, endometriosis or even an excessively restrictive repair of the vaginal introitus following the delivery of a child. In any such case the cause can be determined by physical examination and, if possible, corrected.

Frigidity due to emotional or psychological causes is far more frequent and may be far more difficult to deal with. Any number of factors can contribute to the condition: the woman's conscious or unconscious attitudes toward her husband or toward sex and marriage in general; unfortunate sexual experiences in childhood or adolescence; the husband's sexual performance, which for one reason or another may seem inept or repugnant; the conscious or unconscious fear of pregnancy, or even the converse, a desire for pregnancy so intense that a normal, relaxed and loving atmosphere for sexual relations is unattainable. In many cases consultation with a trusted family physician may help pinpoint such contributing factors and suggest an approach to improving the emotional climate and relieving the condition. Sometimes simple sex education for the wife or the husband or both may be all that is necessary to dispel misconceptions or temper unrealistic expectations; in more complex situations psychiatric consultation for one or both may be extremely helpful.

Success in detecting and dealing with disturbances of reproductive function, however, or with any disorder of the female genital tract, depends upon regular periodic physical examinations, combined with normal attention on the woman's part to maintain physical cleanliness and to detect and report any changes from the normal as early as possible. The vast majority of female genital disorders are either preventable or readily correctable, but a physician cannot work alone; the preservation and protection of the genital organs and normal reproductive function, perhaps more than with any other body function, must depend upon intelligent and knowledgeable cooperation between doctor and patient.

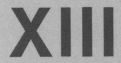
55. Emotional Conflict and Our Mental Defenses   769

56. Disorders of the Mind   778

In most human illnesses physicians and scientists have long recognized a basic principle of cause and effect. Familiar symptoms ordinarily arise from physical changes or alterations in the normal function of various organ systems—changes which can often be detected and identified by physical examination or chemical analysis. But for centuries one broad class of health disorders, the diseases of the mind, seemed to evade this cause-and-effect principle. No one could explain why these mysterious illnesses came about, nor could the most careful examination reveal any consistent differences in physical structure or biochemical function between the apparently well and the mentally ill. Thus it is hardly surprising that diseases of the mind were so long considered the most bewildering and frightening of all human disabilities. It was not until the late 1800s, with the studies of the great Austrian psychologist Sigmund Freud and others who followed him, that the doors were at last thrown open to the scientific investigation of mental illnessses; for the first time the possible emotional roots of these debilitating disorders were explored, and it became clear that many diseases of the mind could be prevented, treated, and even in some instances cured.

Today an understanding of mental illnesses depends on a basic understanding of how the normal functioning of the mind evolves from earliest childhood through successive stages of growth and maturity to adulthood. With such a background understanding we can then make sense of the broad major categories of mental illness, ranging from the often minor but still distressing psychoneurotic reactions to the grave and frequently dangerous mental derangements of the psychoses and, in a class by themselves, the many so-called "behavior disorders" with their own crippling effects on their victims and their close association with such disparate socio-medical disorders as chronic alcoholism, sexual deviation, or drug habituation and addiction. Only by recognizing the identifying characteristics of these disorders and understanding the fine line which so often divides the normal from the abnormal can the individual or his family recognize when to suspect the presence of mental illness and when to seek expert help in its care.

Emotional Conflict and Our Mental Defenses

Human beings are vulnerable to a multitude of physical injuries and diseases, disorders that involve some identifiable pathological change in the structure or the biochemistry of the body and result in a variety of symptoms. As prevalent as these diseases are, however, there is yet another kind of human illness, seemingly unrelated to any known structural or physiological changes, which occurs far more frequently and perhaps causes more human suffering than all the physical diseases put together. These disorders as a group are often spoken of as *mental illness,* but such a catchall term is far too general, because the disorders in this family range all the way from the mildest and most transitory episodes of depression through more chronic, persistent and disabling emotional disturbances to the extremely severe and often permanent mental illnesses. In addition this family of disorders also includes certain of the so-called psychosomatic or emotion-related illnesses which are often considered at least partially "mental" in origin yet which *do* involve identifiable structural or biochemical changes in the body.

A number of disorders affecting the brain and the nervous system, and thus capable of altering the normal function of the mind, are *not,* however, considered in the category of mental illness. These disorders include congenital defects in the formation of portions of the brain and nervous system, and certain congenital metabolic defects leading to mental retardation or impaired mental functions (*see* Part VI, "Patterns of Illness: The Nervous System"). Accidents and

injuries to the brain may also lead to mental impairment, as may such physical conditions as brain tumors (*see* p. 366), infections such as encephalitis or meningitis (*see* p. 199), or the so-called toxic brain syndromes resulting from damage to brain cells by various intoxicants or poisons (*see* p. 371). Many other identifiable disease processes, including the impairment of circulation to the brain that occurs in old age (*see* p. 367), may likewise affect the function of the mind but are nevertheless considered to be primarily physical rather than mental afflictions.

Primary mental illness—disorders or disturbances in the normal function of the mind in the absence of any identifiable physical disease— covers a wide area, and even today experts cannot entirely agree upon definitions and classifications. One major reason is the extreme difficulty in specifically distinguishing what is normal from what is abnormal, simply because every human being is unique in the way his mind works. Every human being also suffers to some extent from conscious or unconscious *emotional conflict,* a condition in which many of the mental illnesses are believed to be rooted, and seeks in one way or another to resolve these conflicts in certain recognizable patterns of behavior. Thus the distinction between normal and abnormal is often merely a matter of degree; equally often it may lie in the way other people—family, friends, physicians—interpret another person's behavior.

Despite such confusion, however, some general definitions are possible. The term *neurosis* or *psychoneurosis,* for example, is used to describe a primary mental disturbance ranging from the mild to the moderately severe, usually rooted in unconscious emotional conflict and characterized by abnormalities of thinking and behavior; the victim may suffer severe emotional discomfort, yet he remains in full intellectual contact with the real world around him and is capable of coping with it, albeit imperfectly. *Personality disorders* are more severe mental disturbances in which the victim suffers great difficulty in coping normally with either his own emotional conflicts or the real world around him and adopts unrealistic, antisocial and in many cases self-destructive behavioral patterns in order to survive. *Psychosomatic illness* is a form of mental disturbance in which unresolved emotional conflicts cause physical symptoms and even pathological changes in the body, by means not clearly understood, so that the mental disorder is largely manifested by physical illness. Finally, the term *psychosis* is used to describe particularly severe, profound and often prolonged mental disturbances in which normal mental defenses fall apart, the personality is severely crippled, and the victim loses contact with the real world, withdrawing into a private, internal world of fantasy, delusion and hallucination from which he may never entirely return.

Throughout history the social reaction to the most serious of the mental disorders, the psychoses, has been one of fright or revulsion or both. There is no question that many "madmen" have been born into or achieved positions of great importance in their societies and have, even in our own century, markedly altered the course of human events. But in most cases victims of severe mental illness in the past have been isolated and imprisoned, driven out of society or even killed. For centuries they were considered to be "possessed of devils"; their erratic behavior and their capacity to do violent damage to themselves or others was early recognized, and these "lunatics," so called because it was thought that Luna, the moon, exercised some evil effect upon their minds, were often the victims of brutal rites of exorcism, burned as witches or simply locked up in madhouses.

There they were starved, beaten, chained and treated with incredible cruelty; no attempt was made to help them in any way. Gradually, such persons came to be treated more humanely, but even so they were sometimes subjected to bizarre experiments to "bring them to their senses," and asylums were more like prisons than hospitals. It is only within the last hundred years, with the emergence of *psychiatry* as a medical specialty, that grave mental afflictions have been regarded as treatable illnesses.

Severe mental disorders account for only a relatively small segment of the total population suffering from mental disturbances of one degree or another. But the milder forms of emotional disturbance, the psychoneuroses, occur with the most widespread frequency. It has been estimated that of all the people who visit doctors' offices, approximately one-third are found to have no identifiable physical illness at all, while another one-third suffer from psychosomatic illnesses which are caused, precipitated or aggravated by emotional factors. In short, these disorders are far and away the most common form of human illness known.

Considering this, popular attitudes toward mental illness today are a little surprising. Victims of psychoses, or, to use the legal term, the insane, are still regarded by many with fear and apprehension; they are committed to public or private institutions where, it is assumed fatalistically, little or nothing can be done to help them, while patients who have, in fact, recovered from severe mental illness are looked upon with considerable curiosity and suspicion. Yet, in ironic contrast, the milder forms of mental disturbance are often considered to be quite fashionable. Forms of behavior once thought merely "eccentric" are now classified as "neurotic"; and the vocabulary of psychiatry and psychoanalysis, a popular form of treatment for psychoneuroses, permeates every cocktail party conversation. People take great pride in psychoanalyzing themselves and others, describing their psychosomatic ailments and discussing their compulsions and complexes, all too often with little or no knowledge of what these terms really mean. Perhaps more serious is the lack of understanding of the very fine line that can divide relatively innocuous neurotic behavior from a severe personality disorder or a crippling psychosis.

The medical science of psychiatry, in spite of the many advances it has made in recent years, is still in its infancy. Investigations of the human mind and the incredibly complex range of human behavior have barely begun. We still have only the dimmest ideas of how the brain functions to control thought and action, and of the distinctions between normal and abnormal behavior. Unlike the physical disorders of other organ systems, psychological disorders have so far defied any easy classification or cause-and-effect relationships. At one extreme, many researchers are convinced that some as yet undiscovered biochemical flaw lies at the root of the more severe mental illnesses, while at the other extreme a few prominent psychiatrists contend that the whole concept of "mental illness" is invalid and that true mental disease does not actually even exist. But despite such controversy, the extensive study of both normal and abnormal human behavior has revealed that certain distinctive patterns occur frequently enough to be considered prevalent and typical, and it is in the study of these distinctive behavioral patterns, as intricate and unpredictable as they are, that an understanding of the various forms of mental illness begins.

Anxiety

To understand what a "true" neurosis or psychoneurosis is, what it can do, how it can be treated, and how successful treatment may be, it is important to consider one of the most common of all emotional reactions—a reaction which virtually every human being harbors at one time or another and which is perfectly normal up to a point, but beyond that point becomes abnormal and destructive. This emotional reaction displays itself in many ways and has been called many things, but it is perhaps most familiar under its medical name: anxiety.

Many people are confused by the doctor's use of this term. In nonmedical usage it means simply "worry" or "concern" or even in some cases

"eagerness." But in medicine, the term has a very specific and limited meaning: anxiety is defined as a painful or apprehensive uneasiness of mind about some impending or anticipated ill fortune, and this emotional reaction often manifests itself in a variety of physical symptoms. In many cases, of course, it is based upon very real problems about which the individual is completely and consciously aware—the threat of losing a job, for example, or the quite natural degree of concern experienced when a husband, wife or child is ill. In such cases anxiety is chiefly characterized by worry, the process of turning a problem over and over in the mind in search of a solution or of anticipating a problem and trying to work out an advance plan of action. In these instances anxiety doubtless serves a useful purpose; it is, in a sense, a warning of danger which can engender enough painful distress and uneasiness of mind that the individual is driven to search for some constructive and satisfying solution to troublesome problems just to relieve the discomfort of the anxiety.

In other cases, however, anxiety may arise from external events also perceived quite consciously by the individual but over which he can exert no influence or control. In such a situation anxiety may be constant and is often manifested as fear or dread. A chronic or terminal illness, for example, can give rise to this kind of severe and prolonged anxiety. In such cases the anxiety may be fruitless; no amount of worry effects a solution, nor does continuing dread or fright, yet the anxiety may become painful enough that the mind must find some means or mechanism to relieve it. When the degree of anxiety is *appropriate* to the cause, it remains a normal emotional reaction no matter how painful it may be, but when anxiety becomes so extreme that it seems *inappropriate* to the cause, exaggerated beyond common reason or engendered by anticipated ills or external events that are unrealistic or blown out of proportion, the border line between normal and abnormal emotional distress may be crossed.

A far more common and disruptive form of emotional distress, sometimes impossible to recognize without medical or psychiatric help, is anxiety—often extreme—that arises as a result of unresolved emotional conflicts in an individual's mind of which he is not consciously aware at all, or else only vaguely or incompletely aware. The origin and nature of these hidden, internal emotional conflicts, "the mind at war with itself," so to speak, are still very poorly understood; we simply do not know enough about how the mind works to understand precisely why such hidden conflicts arise. However, they *do* arise, manifesting themselves in certain recognizable patterns so very often in so many people that they have become familiar to the physician or psychiatrist. Various possible explanations for these hidden conflicts have been proposed from time to time in the search for effective ways to deal with them. By far the most familiar explanation today, and by far the most useful in terms of understanding and treating hidden anxiety-producing conflicts, is contained in the theories of the great Viennese psychiatrist Sigmund Freud (1856–1939), and later modified and expanded to some extent by his co-workers and disciples.

Freud's theories about how the mind is constructed and how it functions have the unfortunate reputation of being too complicated for anyone but psychiatrists to understand; yet his basic ideas, in their simplest form, are remarkably sensible and easy to comprehend. We need to think of the mind and the personality as two quite separate, although closely related, entities, each of which has a specific structure. The *mind* is the element in an individual which functions in reaction to stimuli from the nerve cells of the brain, the nervous system and the sensory organs; it is the element which perceives and reacts to sensory stimuli, which feels, which thinks, which wills or desires, and—most important of all—reasons. Freud recognized that every human mind functions on two very distinct levels: the *conscious level,* of which the individual is completely aware, and the *unconscious level,* below the level of conscious awareness and beyond the reach of normal memory or recall.

Among the functions of the conscious mind are the reception of recognizable impressions of the outside world by means of the sensory organs, the control of voluntary movements and

the proper operation of higher intellectual faculties—for example, the ability to learn, to think, to remember, to act, to make decisions, and to perceive and react to pleasure and pain. The unconscious level of the mind, which Freud considered by far the larger and more important portion of the mind's structure, is the part that harbors our instincts, generates many of our desires, controls our habit patterns, and acts as a repository for memories which go all the way back to infancy—perhaps even to prenatal life—but which still exert a powerful influence on how we think and behave even though they may be "forgotten," filed away beyond the reach of conscious recall except under certain unusual circumstances. It is the unconscious level of the mind which remains oddly "alert" to stimuli while the conscious level of the mind is at rest, as during sleep, and our dreams are based upon unconscious information, often very strangely distorted or altered so that when we consciously remember them they seem to make no sense. Finally, the unconscious level of the mind often serves as a silent but potent auxiliary to the functioning of the conscious level of the mind in the process of thinking, frequently providing solutions to problems that conscious thought has not been able to resolve; and the unconscious level of the mind may also act to protect the conscious mind from painful, threatening or unacceptable memories simply by burying them away in the memory vault far beyond the reach of conscious recall. In short, the conscious and the unconscious portions of the mind are organized together to enable the individual to perceive and think, to act appropriately and to adapt successfully to every form of human experience.

What, then, do we mean when we speak of an individual's *personality?* Perhaps it is easiest to regard the personality as the totality of each and every human organism, including all the functions of the body and both the conscious and the unconscious mind. Every personality is unique, for it is the sum total of all the individual's physical and psychological traits and tendencies, as well as the distinctive patterns of thought, action and reaction that characterize his behavior. Thus the personality is an extremely complex entity, consisting of all the elements of human nature (those characteristics built into the individual at birth) and human nurture (those characteristics that are derived from learning and experience). It is the function of the mind to incorporate and utilize these various elements that are built into, or impressed upon, the individual; so, in a sense, the human personality is a direct result of the way in which the mind operates to achieve this complex task. Many authorities postulate that this essential mental function is largely determined, and thus the personality largely formed, by the time the individual is five or six years old. Others claim that the way in which the mind works, and the personality patterns that result, can change, or be changed, in later stages of the life cycle. But certainly both mind and personality are profoundly influenced throughout life by new information, new experiences and new environmental situations, and if fundamental change is not possible, the mind must be flexible enough to adapt to or "make peace" with these new circumstances. If it is not, the individual's overall personality will be affected. Thus when we speak of a "mental breakdown" or a "mental illness," we actually imply not merely some disturbance of the mind's function but rather a disturbance or disorder of the whole personality.

According to Freudian theory, the structure of the personality is divided into three parts, each identified by what it contributes to the whole personality, and all three coexisting in a sort of dynamic equilibrium, each balancing and modifying the function of the others. The first of these parts is made up of all the instinctual and unconscious drives and desires inherent in every human being, a collection of more or less primitive or uncivilized cravings for food, for sexual satisfaction, for mastery over others and over the environment—in short, those needs that can be considered basic to every animal organism. Freud referred to this part of the personality as the *id,* a part which is essential to survival and which makes urgent and continuing demands upon the individual, yet a part which, if allowed to dominate the personality, would result in extremely selfish and antisocial behavior and even, eventually, self-destruction.

In the human being, however, the avaricious

id does not go unchecked. A second part of the personality structure, Freud postulated, is made up of complicated controlling mechanisms impressed upon the individual by outside influences —by parents, by teachers, by society and by the environment, among other things—all of which act as a restraint upon the insistent demands of the id. These controls, consisting of all sorts of moral and social values, taboos, obligations, and above all, feelings about right and wrong, good and bad, proper and improper, have been hammered into the personality structure so early in life that, like the id, they are deeply embedded in the unconscious mind. Also like the id, this part of the personality makes insistent demands upon the individual, essential to some degree at least to his survival as a social being, but if allowed to dominate the personality, it, too, can be as self-destructive as an untrammeled id.

We have long known this second segment of the personality structure as the *conscience.* Freud used the term *superego,* but whatever it is called, it exerts a powerful influence over the instinctual drives and, indeed, over the whole personality. That influence may be either beneficial or harmful, for while the superego may hold in check some of the less desirable forms of sexual and social behavior, it may also impose such rigid and unrealistic standards that the individual feels he can never measure up, no matter how he behaves. The result is often a sort of silent self-punishment which is experienced as a feeling of *guilt.* Sometimes the individual is aware of these guilt feelings and understands perfectly well why they have arisen, but far more often the conflict between the id and the superego lies buried deep within the unconscious mind and the individual is not consciously aware either of guilt feelings or of the "unacceptable" behavior which generated them. What he may feel in circumstances of this sort is a vague uneasiness of mind, an apprehension or brooding fear—in short, anxiety.

But the structure of the personality is not complete with just the id and the superego. Indeed, these two parts of the personality structure together provide little individuality. Everyone's id is made up of approximately the same sort of instinctive desires and cravings, and everyone's superego, although derived from different sources, provides the same general restraining influence over the id. Individuality arises from the third part of the personality structure, that unique part which is consciously aware of the world outside and responsible for conscious thought, emotions and actions. It is from this highly unique, conscious and self-assertive segment of the personality—the part Freud called the *ego,* from the Latin word meaning "I"—that each individual derives his personal concept of reality, the sense of his own worth or self-esteem, and his singular identity as a human being distinctly different from all other human beings.

It is a major function of the ego to mediate the conflicting demands of the aggressive id and the repressive superego and thus devise patterns of thought and behavior that will satisfy the requirements of both in ways acceptable to the individual and to his external environment. Thus the ego is the powerful compromising influence which draws the entire personality structure into a unified and healthy whole. The ego is also charged with protecting the personality, especially from the painful and potentially self-destructive effects of guilt and anxiety. These feelings arise when an unresolved conflict exists between the id and the superego, or when parts or the whole of the personality is in conflict with the external environment, particularly with the social environment made up of other personalities. When these conflicts exist on the level of conscious awareness, the ego attempts to resolve them in appropriate patterns of thought and behavior, and if it is successful, the individual is said to be able to "adjust." But far more often these conflicts are unconscious, beyond the reach of any simple or logical resolution. In this case the ego may be driven to resort to a variety of devices and subterfuges, largely stemming from the unconscious mind, in an attempt to stave off the anxiety produced by hidden conflicts and thus shield or protect the personality.

The Sources of Emotional Conflict

Although much is still not clearly understood about the development of the mind and the personality, it is apparent that every human being from the beginning of life is inevitably confronted with challenges and conflicts, both external and internal, which must somehow be mastered or resolved if the personality is to grow, develop, and eventually mature. These conflicts are inherent in being human, and most authorities believe that they originate, and must be resolved, during certain particular times of life.

Infancy. Many of the internal conflicts which can result in damaging anxiety and guilt are thought to arise during the individual's earliest years. The newborn infant, for example, is utterly dependent upon others for the satisfaction of his needs for physical comfort, emotional security and mental stimulation. Just how these needs are met helps shape the infant's first awareness of himself, his relationship with others and his view of his environment, and deprivation of any of them may plant the seeds of incipient mental illness as infantile feelings of distrust or insecurity arise. Yet at the same time the infant's utterly selfish, urgent and continuous demands cannot be met forever. As he grows, more and more controls are placed over his behavior, and the result is an inescapable degree of conflict, some of which will inevitably remain locked up in the infant's budding personality, capable of influencing his later development.

Childhood. Additional conflicts, also inescapable, arise as the growing child begins to meet his first major challenges on the road to maturity—the search for individual identity, the struggle for mastery of his developing body and control over his environment, and the emergence of the all-important question of his own sexuality. If the infant's personality seems mostly composed of an all-demanding id, in childhood the developing superego imposes increasing restraints, many of them decidedly unwelcome. The child is unable to understand adult thinking processes and standards, yet he is constantly told what is right and wrong and forced to abide by what seem to him to be totally incomprehensible rules in such sensitive areas as toilet training, rivalry with brothers and sisters, and sexual experimentation. Above all, the child's evolving emotional relationships with his parents, among the most profound he will ever experience because they are so all-important to his life, give rise to inevitable conflicts as he passes from deep attachment first to the parent of one sex, then to the other. Parental overprotection or indifference during these shifting explorations can result in anxiety, guilt, shame, self-doubt and confusing combinations of opposing feelings; and from this period the child emerges with indelible early impressions regarding his own individuality, self-esteem and sexual orientation which will persist for the rest of his life.

Adolescence. If childhood is largely involved with the problem of the mastery of physical skills and the establishment of an individual and unique self-awareness, adolescence is concerned with mastery of intellectual skills and explorations into the world of adulthood. Adolescence is often regarded as a time of major crisis in which the individual seeks to throw off the mantle of parental control and become a person "in his own right." Maturing sexually, the adolescent is also faced with the disturbing challenge of developing healthy emotional relationships with individuals of the opposite sex outside the family, driven by demanding appetites, yet restrained by family values and impressions of right and wrong. In fact, virtually all of the challenges and conflicts of childhood are, in a very real sense, repeated on both the conscious and the unconscious levels during adolescence, but with the added urgency of imminent adulthood and adult responsibility looming around the corner. Often the success with which these conflicts and challenges were met in childhood determines how the adolescent fares in a similar quest for self-mastery, confidence, independence, identity and purpose.

Maturity. The child is the father of the man, and if the adolescent has weathered the emotional conflicts and storms that have come before, he will enjoy, in mature adulthood, handsome dividends in meaningful social relationships and the intimate relationship of marriage, in finding creative and purposeful work and in developing the capacity for responsible and confident parenthood—in short, a full range of expressions of a whole, mature personality on the physical, psychological and social levels, including the ability to meet new challenges and roll with whatever punches come along. But to the extent that old conflicts remain unresolved and influential, and to the extent that all the challenges of development, both physical and emotional, have not been fully met, the adult will be less than fully mature, and his personality less than fully equipped to deal with internal and external conflicts, regardless of the face he presents to the world. And to a certain extent at least—a condition shared by virtually everyone to some degree—it will be necessary for his ego to employ special devices to protect the personality from the recurring specter of anxiety, caused by these unresolved conflicts.

Defense Mechanisms

The protective devices used by the ego, sometimes remarkably elaborate, are very appropriately known as defense mechanisms. They are not easy to categorize, for they are complex and often put together by the individual in unique and unpredictable combinations. They are, in themselves, by no means abnormal; virtually everyone has recourse to them in his everyday behavior. And up to a point they are exceedingly useful, perhaps even necessary in coping with trying life situations. In an individual whose ego is strong and well developed, these defense mechanisms often succeed in resolving or at least compromising hidden emotional conflicts and allaying the guilt or anxiety they cause. But sometimes they are not so successful; the conflicts remain unresolved or recur, and then the defense mechanisms themselves must become a permanent part of the personality to help ward off the continuing threat of anxiety. In a sense, the ego in such cases is tricked or trapped into evolving patterns of thought and behavior that may markedly alter the personality or distort the individual's concept of reality. The degree to which defense mechanisms are successful varies from individual to individual and from situation to situation, of course; it is only when they are unsuccessful, break down or require further reinforcement by even more profound personality changes that they can be called abnormal and can lead to a baffling collection of symptoms or behavioral patterns which psychiatrists regard as neurotic or, when grossly exaggerated, even psychotic.

Just what are these defense mechanisms? Their technical names may not be familiar, but the patterns of behavior that result will be readily recognizable. Chief among the successful defenses are the various forms of *sublimation,* the relief of anxiety by directing energy and activity away from threatening or anxiety-producing desires and rechanneling them toward more socially acceptable goals—in effect substituting some "good" or "harmless" activity for some other activity considered "bad" or "harmful." The adolescent boy, for example, is "forbidden" or prevented, by his upbringing and his concepts of right and wrong, from relieving his sexual appetites by means of direct sexual contact, so he gains relief by rechanneling his sexual energies into more socially acceptable activities such as participation in vigorous competitive sports. Similarly, the adult who has strong aggressive feelings may find "acceptable" expression in the keenly competitive business world.

Projection is another very common device in which the individual seeks to escape self-blame and anxiety arising from his own "unacceptable" feelings by projecting or ascribing those feelings to someone else; a child, for example, who dislikes a teacher intensely but has been taught never to criticize an adult might say, "My teacher doesn't like me." The direct opposite device, known as *introjection,* occurs when the child, shamed by his classmates for liking the teacher, might declare, "I hate her," and actually behave in class as if he did.

Some defense mechanisms are directed more toward blocking off or concealing the cause of the anxiety—"getting rid of the evidence," so to speak—than at relieving it. Frequently unacceptable impulses or thoughts, at one time quite conscious, are thrust into the unconscious by a disapproving superego which tries to stamp out *all* unacceptable or disagreeable ideas. When the impulses are completely banished from consciousness so that they cannot be recalled like an ordinary memory, this unconscious process is called *repression.* When a threatening or unpleasant thought or experience is consciously

"forgotten," the process is known as *suppression* or "blocking"; often such thoughts or experiences seem to have been wiped out of the memory altogether until some later experience happens to call them forth and they are suddenly "remembered" as clearly as if they had just occurred. Certain other defense mechanisms are clearly devices to help the individual "make peace" with his hidden conflicts and the anxiety they produce; the man who is unconsciously striving for status and prestige in his job at any cost because of inner feelings of inadequacy or worthlessness may insist to himself and others—and actually believe—that his only motive for advancing himself so ruthlessly is his wish to provide for his wife and children, an example of a device known as *rationalization.* Still other defense mechanisms involve unconscious reactions against unacceptable impulses or feelings—"denying the facts," so to speak—and are known as *reaction formations.* One of the most familiar of these is *compensation,* as exemplified, for example, by the mother who unconsciously reacts against "unacceptable" feelings of anger and hostility toward a child by excessively "mothering" and overprotecting him. Similarly, a man may react against or deny unconscious feelings of inferiority by thinking of himself as a superior person, a device known as *reversal.* And feelings of shame or disgust associated with perfectly normal, acceptable adult sexual activities are common reaction formations against childhood interest in sex which were labeled "bad" or "dirty" at the time they first appeared.

These are only a few of the many defense mechanisms that have been recognized by psychiatrists as commonplace ways in which the ego seeks to protect the personality from the painful and destructive effects of anxiety and guilt engendered by deep-seated unconscious conflicts. Since everyone, no matter how emotionally mature, has some chinks in his emotional armor, the use of these unconscious mechanisms is the common lot of mankind. Whether they result in "normal" or "abnormal" patterns of behavior in any given individual is largely a matter of degree. At best, these mechanisms serve a useful purpose in helping the personality cope with both internal and external conflicts, inducing only slight distortions of reality and seldom requiring treatment. In some, however, the use of defense mechanisms may involve the substitution of certain "beyond the line" or abnormal patterns of behavior, sometimes quite bizarre in nature, as a means of burying or guarding against anxiety.

When this process of substituting a lesser ill for a greater—we might call it "faking out" the conscious mind—involves no loss of contact with the real world, no grave impairment of thinking or faultiness of judgment, we speak of the resulting emotional disturbance as a *psychoneurosis*. When thinking and judgment are impaired to the point that normal, socially acceptable patterns of behavior are impossible, or seem insufficiently rewarding, even though the individual still remains in contact with the real world, a more serious *personality disorder* is present. When the substitution of more accept-able behavioral patterns involves translation of the unresolved source of anxiety into actual physical symptoms, sometimes even into actual organic disease, we speak of the end result as a *psychosomatic illness*. And finally, when the internal conflicts are so destructive and the anxiety, guilt or fear so completely intolerable or so flagrantly threatening that they cannot be hidden or defended against without actual damage or disintegration of the structure of the personality to the point that the individual's ego can no longer distinguish accurately between the real and the unreal, the result is a massive crippling of the personality structure, together with a breakdown of the orderly function of the mind which is known as *psychosis*. Together these disorders constitute the four broad categories of mental illness, each characterized by particular symptoms, and each posing particular problems in diagnosis and treatment.

Disorders of the Mind

To see more clearly how psychoneurotic reactions arise, how they make people behave and why, we might consider the behavior of a man engaged in a very commonplace yet complex activity—driving an automobile. In essence, a car is simply a mechanical extension of the driver's body, responding to directions originating in the driver's mind, and the process of driving is primarily a conscious, voluntary act. But precisely *how* the driver operates his automobile depends heavily upon the structure of his personality. One part of his personality, corresponding to the id, has the instinctive desire to drive down the center of the road at 100 miles per hour, forcing everybody else off into the ditch. But this desire is restrained by another part of the personality, corresponding to the superego. The driver has been taught certain ideas of common courtesy, certain attitudes of "right" and "wrong"; he is aware of the possibility of an accident and further aware that there are laws imposed by society with regard to how a car may be driven, and policemen stationed here and there to enforce those laws. Thus, a third part of the driver's personality, corresponding to the ego, must find a happy medium between these two opposite influences that will satisfy each to a certain extent but, more important, will enable him to reach his destination safely.

Even when a compromise of this sort has been effected, however, the driver's personality must be concerned with other external dangers or threats—the special hazards of bad road conditions, for example, or the unpredictable actions of other drivers—and this concern quite naturally engenders a certain amount of anxiety. Some of these dangers are very real, and this kind of anxiety is probably good for the driver's safety. But in addition, certain internal threats and dangers, less apparent than obvious external hazards, may create even more anxiety in the driver's mind. The driver may be unsure of himself, for example, or uncertain of his ability to drive safely. To allay uncomfortable anxiety from these internal, often unconscious, sources, or to quiet feelings of guilt about driving at all in the face of such uncertainty, the driver's personality may resort to a variety of mental defense mechanisms which then markedly affect his behavior.

At one extreme, the driver may simply refuse to drive, saying, "I've tried and tried, but I just can't get the hang of it"—a form of denial in which he excuses himself from the responsibility altogether and thus finds a simple, if self-limiting, solution. Far more commonly, he continues to drive but quiets his anxiety with less direct defenses. He may, for example, tell himself, "It doesn't matter; everybody else is a rotten driver too," using the defense mechanism of projection. He may employ identification: "Listen, I'm just as good a driver as that guy who won the Indianapolis 500"; or displacement: "Talk about *me;* my wife is the worst driver in the world, and when I get home I'm going to tell her so." In most cases the use of such defense mechanisms is perfectly natural and normal; they amount to little more than minor and comforting unconscious tricks of the mind which succeed splendidly in quieting the driver's anxiety or guilt and protect his personality without seriously interfering with his overall behavior behind the wheel. In short, they work sufficiently well that the driver is at least able to get where he is going with reasonable safety, and they involve no significant disorder of the mind.

The Psychoneuroses

In some cases, however, these simple defense mechanisms do not work adequately. If the driver's personality is beset by internal anxieties and conflicts so severe that they cannot readily be quieted by simple defenses, he may then become vulnerable to a variety of more serious emotional reactions, often involving highly uncomfortable or disruptive physical symptoms. Such reactions, known as *psychoneurotic reactions* or psychoneuroses, frequently cross the dividing line from the normal to the abnormal. Usually arising from anxiety that is all out of proportion to any apparent cause, or from anxiety due to totally unconscious unresolved conflicts, these reactions often appear quite irrational and, when severe enough, can have very marked, even bizarre, effects upon the driver's behavior, whether he is driving his car or engaging in other activities.

Anxiety Reaction. Perhaps the most common of these psychoneuroses is known simply as an anxiety reaction. It is exemplified by the driver who becomes tense, nervous and fearful virtually any time he drives his car, even under the best of traffic conditions. If he drives for long, or if road conditions worsen, he suffers steadily mounting anxiety and tension; he grips the wheel, slows down, drives overcautiously and dreads each new encounter with another car. Ultimately his rising anxiety may culminate in a crisis, a so-called *anxiety panic state,* in which he perspires, his heart pounds, and he feels all the other physical manifestations of acute terror, massive indecision, even a sense of being "frozen" at the wheel, incapable of doing anything at all. Usually he can manage to control the car until he reaches his destination, but occasionally his panic may become so severe that he must pull off the road in order to "get hold of himself" before he can go on. He does not give up driving, however, apparently more willing to suffer acute discomfort each time he drives than to try to deal with his anxiety or the internal conflicts that cause it, even though his driving capability may be seriously impaired by the neurotic reaction. What is more, because driving itself is clearly not the cause of such irrational anxiety, the driver's anxiety reaction may well invade other aspects of his life, and he may suffer similar episodes of mounting anxiety and panic whenever a family, social or business encounter becomes even slightly difficult. Carried to an extreme, such unresolved and "free-floating" anxiety may ultimately impair his behavior in virtually everything he attempts to do.

Phobic Reaction. In another quite different form of psychoneurotic behavior, overwhelming anxiety arising from some unconscious conflict or forgotten and distorted past experience can create morbid, uncontrollable and totally irrational fears known as *phobias.* A phobic reaction results from an individual's unconscious attempt to deal with anxiety not by resolving its real cause, often long forgotten, but by avoiding some other sort of situation that, he thinks, triggers it. Thus a childhood terror of the dark, never resolved and completely erased from the adult driver's conscious memory, may come to the surface as a morbid fear of driving a car through tunnels. The victim of such a phobia may be an excellent driver in every other way, yet may find himself completely unable to take his car into a tunnel, perhaps driving miles out of his way in order to avoid such a situation. Such a morbid fear might seem preposterous to anyone riding with the driver; indeed, it may seem preposterous to the driver himself, yet his irrational fear or phobia may be completely out of his control.

Of course phobias, like other psychoneurotic reactions, are by no means confined solely to driving experiences. They may involve virtually anything in the world outside or within the mind itself. Among the most common are neurotic fears of certain kinds of diseases—cancer, for example, or a venereal disease. Others include the irrational and uncontrollable fear of being in a confined or crowded place, known as *claustrophobia;* the morbid fear of high places (*acrophobia*); or the fear of being alone in wide-open spaces (*agoraphobia*). Individuals may also develop morbid fears, always far out of proportion to any real danger, of certain kinds of insects, such as spiders or wasps; of animals such as dogs or cats; of dirty bathrooms; or of certain sounds or forms of language. Strange as it may seem, an individual may even develop a morbid and irrational fear of having a morbid and irrational fear, a condition known to psychiatrists as *phobophobia.* But whatever form the phobia may take, it is always merely a symbol of, or a substitute for, the hidden causative conflict, and it is with this substitute that the victim deals consciously, sometimes successfully avoiding the painful effects of anxiety if the phobia does not enter too importantly into his everyday activities.

Obsessive-Compulsive Reaction. A phobic reaction is an extreme form of displacement—unconsciously creating a substitute for the real anxiety-producing conflict and then quieting anxiety by avoiding the substitute as much as possible. Another form of displacement is the obsessive-compulsive reaction, in which the victim's mind again creates a substitute for the hidden conflict, and then proceeds to worry and suffer anxiety about the substitute rather than suffering the anxiety of the real causative conflict or attempting to resolve it. The automobile driver, for example, might become obsessively convinced that his right front tire is leaking, and he must stop to check the pressure every quarter of an hour or so. There is clearly a strong element of self-punishment in this form of neurotic reaction; even though he knows rationally that there is nothing wrong with the tire, the driver nevertheless feels *compelled* to perform the substitute act as a ritual to somehow atone for the insecurity at the root of the causative conflict. Like phobias, obsessive-compulsive reactions may be centered on virtually any life activity, sometimes affecting just a single action, sometimes involving the victim's entire manner of living. Compulsive hand-washing, for example, is commonly seen, in which the victim feels compelled to wash his hands 30 or 40 times a day, even though he realizes rationally that they could not possibly be that dirty. Compulsions may involve dressing in a certain ritualistic order or fashion every day, or suffering the urge to urinate every hour on the hour day and night, and if for some reason the ritual is interrupted or prevented, the victim may suffer unbearable anxiety. In some the reaction may take a much broader form, compelling the victim to do virtually everything meticulously and precisely, according to certain rigid, orderly patterns, from the moment he awakens to the moment he retires. Such obsessive-compulsive behavior can be a dreadful nuisance and can consume considerable time and energy, but like anxiety reactions and phobic reactions, in lesser degrees it is common enough to be considered normal. Even when it becomes abnormally excessive— that is, psychoneurotic—it is not necessarily incapacitating.

Depressive Reaction. Another common neurotic phenomenon, the depressive reaction, can be seriously incapacitating and dangerous as well. In this form of behavior, the victim punishes and torments *himself* rather than displacing his anxiety with a substitute that can be avoided or relieving it by means of compulsive, ritualistic behavior. The victim of a depressive reaction responds to his anxiety with a feeling of overwhelming depression and worthlessness; he is convinced of his inability to cope with certain aspects of his life, or indeed with anything at all. The automobile driver despondently admits to himself that he is a bad driver, whether he really is or not. He tells himself that he does not *deserve* to drive, that anybody would be a fool to trust him behind the wheel. He may complain about the traffic, or his eyesight, or his coordination, but in reality he feels that it is his own worthlessness that is to blame. Some victims of depressive reactions mask such feelings by feigning a sort of false or forced cheerfulness, perhaps even bravado; in other cases the victim becomes enveloped in an apparently impenetrable cloud of gloom, often marked by uncontrollable episodes of weeping or even thoughts of suicide. By means of valiant conscious or unconscious efforts the victim may fend off the persisting anxiety for a time, with apparent success, only to plunge without any outward warning into a prolonged period of anxiety panic or black depression during which he is completely incapable of doing anything at all for hours, days or even weeks, thus totally disrupting his normal pattern of life.

This kind of sudden and disruptive psychoneurotic crisis—with or without an associated anxiety panic state—which occurs after a long period of exhausting effort to "hold the fort" and keep things functioning normally is commonly described as a "nervous breakdown," an episode which may be relatively mild and transitory in some cases but may cause prolonged and persistent disability in others. It is certainly the most dangerous of the psychoneurotic reactions, not only because of the ever present possibility that the despondent victim may attempt to take his life, but because the deepening depression can, in some cases, cross the shadowy line from mere psychoneurosis into the more profound mental disorganization of psychosis. Again, as with other psychoneurotic reactions, occasional minor episodes of depression—"blue moods," so to speak—are normal and commonplace, but prolonged feelings of worthlessness or just "giving up" are not, and the seriousness of the mental disorder in such cases depends upon the depth, duration and appropriateness of the depression.

Dissociative Reaction. The dissociative reaction, far less common than other forms of neurotic behavior, is "giving up" of another sort. The automobile driver does not merely deny that he can drive; he denies that he is himself in various degrees of forgetfulness, "absentmindedness," amnesia or even, rarely, in the so-called split personality syndrome in which the victim acts, speaks and remembers as one person part of the time and as a totally different person at other times. In essence the driver may become a "new and different person," or at least a distorted version of the old person, when he gets behind the wheel. He may be able to drive perfectly well in this guise, but the condition is nevertheless incapacitating, since the victim forgets the facts of his real life or his disguise as he switches back and forth, even though he may behave quite normally in either state.

Conversion Reaction. One final form of psychoneurotic reaction to acute anxiety, also comparatively uncommon today, is conversion reaction, or conversion hysteria. In this form of behavior the individual facing a high level of anxiety, often involving physical threat, manages to change or "convert" the anxiety into the sudden onset of dramatic physical symptoms which make it impossible for him to continue the threatening activity. The automobile driver, in response to a particularly frightening experience on the road, suddenly goes blind, or his arm becomes paralyzed so that he cannot use it, even though there is nothing whatever organically wrong with his eyesight or his arm muscles and reflexes. The symptoms, however, seem perfectly real to the victim, and they serve a convenient purpose; now he cannot possibly drive, and the symptoms will often persist, or recur, until everyone including himself is fully convinced that expecting him to drive again under any circumstances would be foolhardy. In other forms of conversion reaction one or both legs may become paralyzed, or the victim may suddenly develop complete anesthesia of his hands and wrists up to the mid-forearm, or simply be overcome by a sudden overwhelming sleepiness when faced with a threatening situation. Such conversion reactions, obviously, are naïve and childlike in nature, yet the "secondary gain" they produce can be very significant, particularly when the symptoms effectively shield the victim from having to face the threat that triggers them.

Whatever form these psychoneurotic reactions may take, and however much they may seem, on the surface, to "help" the victim avoid the painful anxiety that arises from some unconscious conflict, they cannot ordinarily be considered beneficial. They may succeed in protecting the personality to some extent, but they do nothing to resolve the causative conflict. Further, they result in aberrant or distorted patterns of behavior that are an additional burden, and a source of additional anxiety, to the victim; and there is always the possibility that these psychoneurotic defenses may crumble and the personality may disintegrate, causing even more serious derangement of the mind. On balance, then, even mild psychoneurotic reactions are usually more damaging and crippling than they are useful, and the victim faces the choice of either finding some sort of effective treatment or else continuing a life seriously impaired by neurotic illness.

Treatment of the Psychoneuroses

Truly effective treatment of the various forms of psychoneurotic behavior can be exceedingly difficult. The first step, of course, is a thorough physical examination to rule out any active organic disease which may be causing some of the apparently neurotic symptoms or, more commonly, may be aggravating them. In many cases the victim of neurotic distress can find some relief simply by "talking out" his symptoms, fears, conscious anxieties and feelings of guilt with some trusted and knowledgeable adviser or counselor. Many people, including family physicians, priests, ministers, marriage counselors, psychologists, and social workers have had special training in such counseling, and although they are not equipped to undertake intensive therapy or treatment of profound psychoneurotic disturbances, they often can provide helpful guidance and reassurance to individuals suffering relatively minor or temporary neurotic reactions. Occasionally the mere assurance of a family doctor that no organic disease is present or reassurance from a qualified adviser that the victim is not "going insane" or "losing his mind" may be at least temporarily helpful—although this kind of relief is often quite short-lived, and the counselor may find himself having to repeat the same assurances over and over, often with increasing frequency. Even when the counselor can help the neurotic individual develop an understanding of the probable cause of his anxiety and distress by helping him recall long-forgotten and painful memories and feelings, his neurotic symptoms may not be relieved in the least, since a superficial or intellectualized "recognition" of the underlying causes often does nothing to decompress the overpowering emotional charge surrounding these memories. What is more, in cases in which the underlying

cause is (or was) extremely painful, threatening or emotionally distressing to the victim, he may unconsciously feel that the neurotic reaction and patterns of behavior, however troublesome, are really far safer and easier to live with than the buried and "forgotten" originating causes of the anxiety would be if they were suddenly brought to mind. Thus the individual suffering a psychoneurotic reaction may quite unconsciously struggle to avoid having it effectively treated, even though he protests that he really wants to cooperate in treatment. Or in some cases, one form of psychoneurotic reaction may disappear only to be replaced by another, possibly more damaging one. Finally, in the case of severe psychoneurotic reactions there is the danger that well-meaning but unskilled counseling may be unconsciously interpreted by the victim as such a threat to his defenses that it may inadvertently push him across the "defensive line" into a full-blown psychosis.

In short, counseling with a family doctor, minister or other "outsider" may be helpful in dealing with relatively minor or temporary psychoneurotic reactions, but such counseling is severely limited in scope, and can be dangerous unless the counselor is experienced enough to recognize when more specialized help is necessary. Most severe psychoneurotic reactions are far better treated by a psychiatrist, a physician specially trained in the diagnosis, understanding and treatment of neurotic and psychotic diseases, utilizing one or another form of *psychotherapy* to discover the root causes of the unconscious conflicts underlying the neurotic behavior of the victim. One particular type of psychotherapy, originally devised by Sigmund Freud and his followers, is known as *psychoanalysis,* often a lengthy, time-consuming and costly form of treatment since it seeks, by means of encouraging the neurotic patient to search out for himself, through free association, dream interpretation and other techniques, the emotionally loaded memories, experiences and traumas that have long been hidden in his unconscious mind. In a sense, the patient "relives" these experiences and, with the analyst's help, gains new insight into what actually happened and why, how he reacted at the time and how that reaction affects his present behavior. In theory, this insight enables the patient to deal directly with unconscious conflicts, thus relieving his anxiety and permitting him to control or alter neurotic patterns of behavior. There are several different "schools" of psychoanalysis, each adhering to certain analytic beliefs and techniques; further, it is a form of treatment so very difficult and demanding that even physicians trained in psychiatry must take special training in psychoanalysis. There are, in addition, many competent and qualified "lay analysts" who are not physicians, but who have studied psychology and then undertaken special training in psychoanalysis. Thus it is imperative that anyone considering this form of treatment investigate the credentials and qualifications of the analyst very carefully.

Over the years psychoanalysis, although helpful in some cases, has proved somewhat disappointing, partly because of highly unpredictable results (overall, only some 10 percent of the patients so treated are permanently freed of all neurotic reactions, although many more are greatly helped), and partly because of the time, effort and cost involved. Thus psychiatrists have sought quicker and more effective means of psychotherapy. The use of hypnotism to help alleviate neurotic symptoms and the use of drugs to open up the memory to painful experiences have both been tried, sometimes with great success, sometimes with less. In general, all these techniques fall into one of two broad categories. In *directive psychotherapy* the therapist actively interprets the patient's past and present neurotic reactions and frequently seeks to advise him and help him adjust to the circumstances of his life. In *nondirective psychotherapy* the therapist "takes a back seat," so to speak, urging the patient to seek out and interpret for himself the source of his neurotic conflicts, and then use this insight in regulating his behavior.

In recent years the use of various medications has considerably broadened the approach to treatment of psychoneuroses. Ordinary sedative medications are not particularly useful because they do nothing to help relieve anxiety or depression, but a number of drugs are now known that can provide a great degree of relief for both. They include the very gentle tranquilizing drugs such as meprobamate (also known by such trade names as Miltown and Equanil), the much more potent medications which appear to inhibit certain biochemical reactions in the brain and thus help relieve anxiety, whatever the cause, and certain other equally potent drugs which are particularly helpful in combating and relieving psychoneurotic depression. In general none of these drugs is ideal in all cases; although they have relieved many patients of anxiety, agitation or depression, sometimes quite dramatically, they are by no means a cure-all. Indeed, particularly deep degrees of depression with the ever attendant threat of suicide even today may require confinement in a neuropsychiatric hospital or the use of such heroic and distressing forms of therapy as convulsive shock treatment (*see* below). In all events, the use of *any* medication, to say nothing of shock therapy techniques, is the sole province of a qualified psychiatrist or, in the case of drug therapy alone, a physician with wide experience in the field of neurotic illness.

It is precisely because no single approach to treatment has yet proved, in itself, singularly successful in relieving the symptoms and distress of psychoneurotic reactions that new and different techniques are still being devised and explored. *Group therapy,* for example, has frequently been successful in relieving symptoms in a number of patients simultaneously, and it is particularly useful in situations in which patients with similar neurotic problems can meet and interact with one another, under a psychiatrist's guidance, to help "work out" their emotional conflicts. *Play therapy* is a nonverbal form of treatment which permits emotionally disturbed children to act out their unconscious angers, hostilities and frustrations in games with toys or dolls, thus enabling the psychiatrist to understand and help them. Even newer approaches to treatment such as encounter groups, consciousness-raising sessions and so-called sensitivity sessions are being explored by psychiatrists and laymen alike as possible avenues to understanding individual and group behavior, although to what degree these techniques will prove lastingly useful remains to be seen. It is an undeniable fact, however, that any form of treatment in unskilled or unscrupulous hands can be emotionally devastating. But it is important to emphasize that the help of properly qualified professionals can be obtained. It is folly for the victim of a neurosis to settle for a disturbed and crippled life when consultation with a physician or psychiatrist may provide precisely the help necessary for recovery, or for the family of the neurotic to allow him to ignore or deny his disability when professional care may enable him to understand and resolve his emotional conflicts.

Psychosomatic Disorders

Defense mechanisms and the psychoneurotic reactions are not the only defenses available to the personality. In many cases an alternative reaction pattern may develop in which the personality's defense against anxiety or guilt is expressed through physical symptoms—real and distressing—in various organs or tissues of the body, particularly those that are associated with the autonomic or "involuntary" nervous system. Known as a *psychosomatic disorder,* this kind of reaction differs greatly from the neurotic conversion reaction in that it actually affects the functions of the body, frequently producing structural changes which may even threaten life, and by the fact that the physical illness thus produced appears to have no particular direct relationship to the anxiety itself.

Many people have difficulty understanding how emotional disturbances alone can cause physical symptoms, even though they can accept as perfectly normal such commonplace psychosomatic reactions as the wave of faintness and nausea, sometimes even vomiting, that may overcome an individual after a sudden and frightening experience, or such a phenomenon as *blushing,* in which the emotional reaction to an embarrassing situation causes the blood vessels in the skin to dilate, resulting in a pink flush, usually of the face and neck. These, of course, are minor but familiar examples of the intricate and inseparable connections between the functions of the mind or *psyche* and those of the body or *soma*—connections that are maintained both by nervous system signals and by biochemical reactions, particularly those involving

hormones. In general, psychosomatic reactions are triggered by *stress,* which may arise from either external sources or internal conflicts or, most commonly, both; and the severity and duration of the psychosomatic reaction are often directly related to the severity and duration of the stress. Intense, prolonged, severe emotional stress, whether from external sources or from internal conflicts, can induce the mind to send out incorrect nervous or chemical signals, or correct signals to an excessive degree, leading to physical disfunction.

The psychosomatic disorders that can result are characterized, in most cases, by symptoms that primarily and persistently affect a single organ system or "target area." These physical symptoms can involve any part of the body, but certain tissues and organs are more frequently affected than others. For example, in many individuals the skin is affected, with the development of hives, itching, or even the sort of skin tissue breakdown known as eczema. In others the respiratory tract may be the "target area," with severe episodes of bronchial spasm or asthma, or a tendency to excessively rapid breathing. When the musculoskeletal system is the "target area" the victim may have chronic and recurrent backaches, muscle cramps, tension headaches or recurring episodes of stiff neck; when the genitourinary system is involved, there may be symptoms of menstrual disturbances, painful urination, urgency or episodes of urinary incontinence. Symptoms relative to the nervous system are often vague and ill defined—bizarre types of headaches that come and go, episodes of blurred vision, perhaps an inability to concentrate, or a tendency to become fatigued unreasonably soon, a pattern of insomnia or nervous intolerance to noise, or even mildly disturbing emotional overreactions. Some of the most dangerous, indeed life-threatening, psychosomatic disorders are those in which the target area involves either the heart and blood vessels or the gastrointestinal tract; in the former, there may be mild symptoms such as sudden episodes of rapid heartbeat or shortness of breath, troublesome symptoms such as migraine headaches, or dangerous disorders such as sustained hypertension. Any or all of these may involve very real and demonstrable structural or organic changes from the normal, but at the same time they are intimately related either to external stresses or to unresolved anxiety and emotional conflicts or both. Thus it is no more possible to develop the disorder without the emotional component being present than it is to treat the illness effectively and permanently without also searching out and relieving the underlying cause of anxiety or conflict, or relieving the external stress. The most vulnerable of all "target areas," however, is the gastrointestinal tract, and among the variety of gastrointestinal diseases which involve pathological change but which also involve a heavy overlay of anxiety or emotional conflict are peptic ulcer, chronic indigestion, ulcerative colitis, obesity due to continued compulsive overeating, or its direct opposite, anorexia nervosa, a condition in which the victim is compulsively unable to eat or to hold food down and will literally waste away and starve to death if some way of treating the neurotic basis of his illness cannot be promptly found. (Psychosomatic disorders of each of the various organ systems are discussed in greater detail in those chapters dealing with the other diseases and disorders of the system.)

In some ways psychosomatic disorders that result at least in part from deeply entrenched anxiety, guilt or emotional conflict seem easier to deal with than the sometimes bizarre and often incomprehensible psychoneurotic reactions. Excess acid production in the stomach can be counteracted by giving the patient antacids, and a bleeding peptic ulcer can be coaxed to heal by medical treatment or relieved by surgery, just as severe hypertension can be "controlled" by a variety of drugs acting on the part of the autonomic nervous system responsible for contraction or dilatation of the smaller blood vessels. The effects of external stress—the pressure of work or household responsibilities, for example—can often be counteracted by making a conscious effort to change the tension-ridden life style to some degree, to slow down, relax and provide for adequate recreation. But unless the more deep-seated internal psychological component of a psychosomatic disorder is effectively treated concurrently with its physical manifestations, the disease tends to recur or persist, all too

often in a pattern of progressive seriousness and disability.

If the psychological component of the psychosomatic disease is not too well entrenched or influential, a helpful form of treatment may simply be an honest discussion of the individual's problems, thoughts and emotions with his family doctor or some other trusted friend or adviser. Often, however, the individual refuses to acknowledge that any psychological or neurotic element exists, insisting upon concentrating all treatment efforts on relief of the physical symptoms; or he may be foolishly ashamed of "allowing his nerves to get out of hand," so to speak, and may thus tend to minimize the psychological component of his disorder. In the long run, however, recognition of the close interrelation between mind and body in every psychosomatic disorder is necessary before truly effective treatment is possible. Individuals in whom the symptoms of physical illness are particularly severe or potentially life-threatening should seek psychiatric treatment, if necessary, even after the apparently successful treatment of the physical illness, in order to help prevent recurrence.

Personality Disorders

Yet another group of crippling and often tragic disorders of the mind occupies a place in the dim gray area between the psychoneuroses and the psychoses. These conditions, generally classified as behavior or personality disorders, seem to result not from neurotic reactions designed to protect the personality from the pain of anxiety or guilt by repressing or disguising it in some way, as in the psychoneuroses, or from the disintegration of the personality structure, as in the psychotic states, but rather from some developmental defect, flaw or arrest in development of the personality. The victims of these disorders seem to behave quite rationally and normally up to a certain point, but then begin to reveal evidence of a "flawed" personality—not in neurotic distortions of reality or in psychotic disintegration, but rather in an inability to feel normal emotions, adhere to normally acceptable patterns of behavior or form normal relationships with others. Instead of finding ways to suppress or compensate for their unconscious feelings of anxiety, they *act out* these feelings in their everyday behavior, so that in a very real sense the manner in which they defend their personalities *becomes* their personalities.

The victim of a personality disorder may, in some cases, behave like an angry, unruly child, or depend heavily upon others for emotional support. Or he may manifest extremely antisocial reactions, or distorted or deviant patterns of sexual behavior, rather than a normal, mature heterosexual orientation. And in many personality disorders, the strong urge for self-punishment is manifested in such persistently self-destructive behavior as repetitive criminality, compulsive overeating, alcoholism or drug addiction.

As with other disorders of the mind, the degree of the disturbance is the key to how well or badly the victim can get along in society. If the degree is minor, the individual may manage to get by, sometimes very successfully, without seeking or requiring any form of treatment. In such cases there can be a real question whether or not the person is "sick" at all particularly if the disorder does not seriously interfere with his life or prove harmful to others. It is when the personality disorder is so extreme that the victim demonstrates real potential for harming himself or others that he must seek, or be compelled to seek, treatment. Even then, diagnosis of a personality disorder may be difficult, and the victim extremely resistant to treatment. Many victims of personality disorders are extremely clever and intelligent, capable of projecting a captivating, although fraudulent, charm when it suits their purposes. In general, however, they reveal their crippled personalities in three telltale ways: *they are unable to accept responsibility,* since they are unable to comprehend what responsibility means except in terms of looking out for themselves; *they are unable to learn from experience,* since they make the same antisocial or self-destructive mistakes over and over and over again; and *they are unable to love,* or indeed form any kind of healthy, balanced or constructive human relationship.

Personality disorders are classified in several different categories, although they seldom, if ever, occur in an uncomplicated form or unaccompanied by patterns of psychoneurotic behavior. Perhaps the simplest and most common of them is the *inadequate personality,* also known as the *passive-dependent personality*. The terms are particularly appropriate, for the victim of this disorder does seem to be completely inadequate, physically, mentally and emotionally. His behavior is generally indecisive, and he is unwilling or unable to assume responsibility for either himself or others. With childish helplessness, he clings to a parent, a sibling, a friend or a spouse, constantly demanding emotional support yet incapable of returning affection to any degree. Socially he is self-effacing and is usually incapable of any sustained work. He may be completely dependent and harmless, or he may give vent to his underlying anxiety by tormenting the very people on whom he depends. Many victims of this disorder simply pass through life unnoticed, while others may reveal their inadequacy and dependence by becoming drifters, alcoholics or drug addicts.

The *schizoid personality* is chiefly characterized by aloofness and indifference to others. Incapable of sustaining a normal social relationship, the schizoid simply withdraws, often priding himself on his independence and often capable of sustained, and even brilliant, creative work. He is usually regarded simply as a "loner," yet the schizoid may also become a recluse, reacting with extreme hostility and even violence to any intrusion upon his privacy. The person with a *paranoid personality* is also incapable of normal human relationships, yet unlike the indifferent schizoid, he is excessively preoccupied by what others think of him. Self-centered and suspicious, he may believe that he is the victim of continual persecution and always blames his own failures on others. Again the paranoid person may be regarded simply as eccentric by those around him, whether he withdraws and becomes a "whiner" or whether he insists upon his own superiority and acts out his hostility toward others. The person with a *cycloid personality* is the victim of unpredictable and inappropriate moods. Sometimes these moods fluctuate from elation to depression, but more often the personality is dominated by one or the other. Extreme energy, high spirits and impulsive actions may characterize the personality of the cycloid on one hand; on the other hand, he may be extremely serious, unhappy and depressed. In either case, the mood seems unrelated to the circumstances of the individual's life, yet there is little that can be done to alter it. In fact, all of these forms of personality disorder so dominate the individual that even if they are recognized as "illnesses," they are virtually impervious to treatment. They represent, in essence, a faulty adaptation of the mind so deeply entrenched that both the personality and the concept of reality are distorted. If the distortion is slight, victims of these disorders may get along very well, but there is always the threat that even this faulty adaptation may break down and the border line into psychosis may be crossed.

The *psychopathic personality* is characterized by a more extreme form of behavior in which the victim's personality is "frozen" into fixed patterns of aggressive, hostile and antisocial actions. Typically he can love no one and accept nothing, and he cannot or will not distinguish right from wrong or shoulder responsibility for his own acts. A great many psychopathic personalities manifest their disorder during childhood by incorrigible behavior and an apparent inability to control their aggressive and destructive instincts. They live in a vicious dog-eat-dog world of their own making; some become repeated runaways, and others remain at home but defy family and community values. In time they may be committed to detention homes and reformatories, later they graduate to petty crime and ultimately they live most of their lives in and out of penal institutions or neuropsychiatric hospitals. Again, most commonly, there is a self-destructive element to the behavior of these individuals; intelligent as they may be, they commit their antisocial acts with such apparent stupidity and disregard for self-preservation that it often seems they are *seeking* detention and punishment. Unfortunately, neither confinement, nor punishment, nor conventional forms of psychiatric treatment have proved particularly helpful in correcting these disorders; even today they

represent one of the mosh difficult therapeutic problems that psychiatrists have to deal with.

Sexual Deviation

Personality disorders do not necessarily lead to a direct confrontation or a violent clash between the victim and society. Indeed, certain very common forms of aberrant behavior are far more destructive to the victim than to the society in which he lives. Sexual deviation and the various patterns of behavior that characterize it are generally ascribed to some arrest or distortion of the individual's personality development during childhood or youth. Even psychiatrists cannot agree about the precise sort of trauma that may cause such an arrest in personality development, or whether, in fact, sexual deviation is an expression of a neurotic internal conflict. However, from infancy on through childhood and adolescence each individual passes through successive stages of psychosexual development. At certain points this development is mainly concerned with the anatomical sexual structure of the body—the child discovers that he is physically equipped as a male or female. At other points, development involves the discovery and exploration of pleasurable feelings related to the sex organs, whether male or female. At still other points, each individual develops strong emotional ties, first with the parent of one sex, then with the parent of the opposite sex, and invariably these emotional ties are related to similarities or differences in sexual structures as well as to pleasurable sexual sensations. In most individuals the end result of these developmental stages is the emergence of an adolescent personality aware of its precise sexual nature and with sexual impulses that are strongly *heterosexual;* that is, directed toward individuals of the opposite sex. Earlier and transitory *homosexual* attachments to parents or others of the same sex, perfectly normal at certain stages of development, have largely been "outgrown" or left behind; emotional attachments of love and affection remain, but sexual interest has moved on. Then, with the approach of adulthood, the dominating heterosexual impulses are confirmed and reinforced repeatedly, not only by sexual contacts with the other sex leading to courtship, marriage and mating, but also by the approval of these heterosexual impulses by the society in which the individual lives.

In many individuals, however, this pattern of heterosexual psychosexual development, regarded as normal in our society, is interrupted or arrested at some point. Any number of factors may cause such an interruption. One parent, for example, may be absent during critical stages in the child's development, or may be so emotionally weak or dominated by the other parent that the child cannot form the normal emotional attachment, leaving a "hole," so to speak, in the fabric of his development. Distressing or frightening incidents may occur, related directly or indirectly to sexuality, which may shame or terrify the developing child and in one degree or another distort the normal progress of his psychosexual development. Whatever the cause, one of the most common results of such arrested psychosexual development is the retention, as a part of the individual's personality, of unusually strong and still-powerful homosexual impulses into adolescence and adulthood.

Precisely how the individual's personality reacts to and deals with these impulses, often deeply buried in the unconscious, will determine the pattern of his sexual behavior. In most cases the individual suffers so much unconscious anxiety and guilt at harboring such feelings—which are, after all, widely condemned in our society— that he suppresses them forcibly, burying them so deeply that they never emerge into his conscious sexual behavior at all. The homosexual impulses remain *latent* or unexpressed, while the individual proceeds to live a heterosexual life as if denying that the homosexual impulses exist. Sometimes a single homosexual experience in childhood or adolescence may prove so threatening, terrifying or repugnant that the individual blocks the incident from his conscious memory and fights down feelings that might result in any further such experience. And in many cases such suppression works reasonably well, enabling the individual to live an "acceptable" heterosexual life without any outward evidence or awareness of personality distortion. The victim may often

"act out" this suppression to some degree or another, however. A man, for example, may compensate by engaging compulsively in outwardly "masculine" activities; he may react to real or imagined homosexual behavior in others with fierce condemnation, never recognizing how threatening to himself any hint of acceptance of such behavior might be; he may also harbor an uneasy, lifelong antipathy to women, his own heterosexual contacts notwithstanding, without ever realizing why. In general such minor distortions in his behavior are far less disruptive than acceptance of his homosexual impulses would be, even though he may spend his life in continual unconscious conflict with himself as a result.

Other individuals, rather than suppressing powerful homosexual impulses, recognize them and then act upon them, seeking to relieve their anxieties and impulses in *overt* or actual expressed homosexual contacts, even though such contacts, for social reasons, may be carefully concealed. Some may lead a virtual double life, striving to maintain a heterosexual façade, including marriage and parenthood, while engaging in homosexual activities in secret, either regularly or intermittently. Others openly or covertly eschew any sexual relationship with the opposite sex, in effect accepting and settling for homosexual relations alone. But whatever the pattern of his behavior, the overt homosexual is not only in direct conflict with the mores of a rigidly intolerant society, but in most cases is in grave conflict, conscious or unconscious, with himself as well.

Is overt homosexuality an illness? If so, can it be cured? There are as many answers to these perennial questions as there are homosexual individuals, and in each case the answer must depend upon the behavior of the individual and the consequences it has upon his life. Surely homosexual behavior is not normal according to the yardstick of our society; nor can it properly be considered a mere "variation of normal," as some militant homosexual groups would imply, for its roots lie in an abnormal, if not pathological, disturbance in the individual's psychosexual development. All this notwithstanding, there are multitudes of homosexual individuals who have found workable, tolerable and satisfying adjustments in homosexual relationships—individuals who probably live more "normal" lives under these circumstances, with fewer destructive anxieties and internal conflicts, than if they were to deny their feelings. Such homosexual adjustments may well be limiting or even self-damaging to the individual; they may result in a bleak and attenuated emotional life; but insofar as they are not personally or socially incapacitating they cannot arbitrarily be considered a manifestation of illness. On the other hand if the homosexual finds himself, as is often the case, in such intolerable conflict with himself or with society that his homosexuality does become incapacitating, then some form of psychotherapy may well provide an avenue of release or adaptation, if not cure. With powerful motivation on the part of the patient, and with skill and patience on the part of the psychiatrist, it is possible in many cases to identify and repair the rent in the fabric of the homosexual's personality, but each affected individual, in the long run, must decide for himself whether his condition is, for him, an illness and if so, whether it is worth it to embark on the long journey of counsel and possible cure.

Other forms of sexual deviation may arise when an individual's psychosexual development is arrested or distorted in such a way that full emotional and physical satisfaction cannot be achieved by the normal avenues of genital sexuality in sexual intercourse, so that some substitute or supplement to genital sexuality must be found. In *voyeurism,* for example, the victim may find his highest sexual satisfaction, culminating in orgasm, from watching others engaged in sexual activities, from window peeping, or from watching erotic peep shows or movies. The *exhibitionist* derives sexual satisfaction from exposing himself to others or from "performing" sexually while others are observing. In *sadism* the individual is sexually excited by the act of causing pain to others, while in *masochism* sexual arousal may depend upon the individual himself being painfully tormented. Other forms of sexual deviation include *nymphomania,* in which a woman seeks in vain to attain sexual fulfillment which her unconscious conflicts will not permit

by engaging in compulsive but meaningless sexual relations with a long succession of male partners, and *satyrism,* in which a man seeks repeatedly to confirm his masculinity, which he unconsciously questions, by means of a succession of meaningless sexual "conquests" of females. Perhaps most bizarre of all forms of sexual deviation is *fetishism,* in which the individual is unconsciously so gravely threatened by any direct sexual confrontation with another person, male or female, that his mind diverts his sexual interest to such inanimate objects as shoes or articles of clothing.

In the vast majority of cases such deviant impulses arising from arrest or distortion of the individual's psychosexual development are never translated into the overt patterns of a behavioral disorder. The impulses may be suppressed altogether or, more commonly, displaced or converted into more socially acceptable—or at least harmless—patterns of behavior. Thus the potential voyeur may relieve his impulses by reading erotic literature, collecting erotic photographs or telling off-color jokes; the exhibitionist may turn his energies to physical culture and body building; and sadistic or masochistic sexual impulses may be shifted from the sexual area altogether, with sadism translated into arrogant, sarcastic or cruel social treatment of others, and masochism acted out by inviting criticism from others or indulging in various forms of self-criticism or self-punishment. In other cases, however, the impulses are acted out in overt deviant sexual behavior, and again the line between satisfactory and essentially harmless adjustment and a true, potentially dangerous personality disorder may be a matter of degree. To the extent that the deviant behavior is crippling or harmful to the individual himself, or harmful to others, it may require active or even forceful restraint and psychiatric treatment. Any form of treatment, to be successful, must be aimed first at identifying the underlying flaws in the individual's personality, and then at aiding him to find socially acceptable avenues of release or adaptation. Unfortunately, however, successful treatment must also depend upon the patient's own motivation to be cured; overall results are by no means satisfactory, and in some cases individuals who threaten themselves or others with actual or potential harm on account of sexual deviation may require confinement in neuropsychiatric hospitals or correctional institutions until effective treatment can be accomplished.

Alcoholism

There is probably no other drug in history which has been used as long or as consistently in human societies as ethyl alcohol, a colorless aromatic liquid which is produced in the fermentation of sugars or starches by the action of microscopic plant organisms known as yeasts. Probably the earliest men were aware of the intoxicating qualities of fermenting berry juices or grains; certainly throughout recorded history man has been skillful in the production of wines and beers of low alcoholic content, and techniques for distilling brandies and other higher-concentration alcoholic beverages have been known at least since the 12th or 13th century A.D. At various times the drug has been used not only as an intoxicant, but also as a pain reliever or anesthetic, as a soporific, as an aphrodisiac, and as an adjunct to religious rituals and celebrations. In our modern society it is used, in some form or another, by the vast majority of the adult population. Thus it is hardly surprising that alcohol also plays an integral part in one of the most widespread and disabling of all human illnesses, chronic alcoholism.

In a very real sense alcohol is a drug of paradox, for it lends itself equally well to pleasant, relatively harmless use by many individuals and to dangerously destructive use by others. Because it can be absorbed directly into the blood stream from the stomach when used in modest quantities, its effects are felt very quickly, yet when used in large or undiluted quantities it can produce an intense chemical irritation of the stomach lining, leading to an acute gastritis and often followed by nausea and vomiting. In modest quantities it acts as a harmless appetite stimulant, yet in larger quantities it can dull or even destroy the appetite because, like a simple sugar, it can be utilized by the body for calories in place of food. In small quantities alcohol can act as a relaxant and tension reliever

by blunting the activity of the higher nerve centers in the cerebrum, temporarily easing social inhibitions and helping to quiet feelings of shyness, inferiority or inadequacy, effects that are often interpreted as "pleasantly stimulating" even though they actually result from depression of higher nervous system function; but in larger quantities it can cause a serious, although temporary, impairment of virtually all brain functions, inducing alcohol intoxication in which the drug interferes with vision, balance, muscle coordination and judgment, and ultimately culminates in a stuporous sleep until the body can rid itself of the drug through exhalation of alcohol vapor from the lungs and destruction of the drug by the liver. The residual effects of an occasional moderate overdose of alcohol may be no more serious, prolonged or disabling than the throbbing headache, nausea and general malaise of the "morning-after hangover," yet when the drug is used habitually in large quantities it can cause progressively serious and irreparable damage to the body and can ultimately lead to an early death.

The long-term physical damage that can result from habitual excessive use of alcohol arises in two quite different ways: direct damage to the central nervous system, particularly the brain; and indirect damage that occurs as a result of chronic malnutrition in the excessive drinker. Prolonged excessive drinking can cause physical destruction of brain cells and often may lead to such physical symptoms as recurrent episodes of violent trembling and shaking, sometimes accompanied by nightmarish hallucinations. This condition, which often occurs at the height of a prolonged period of excessive drinking, or when a bout of heavy drinking has suddenly been terminated, is known as *delirium tremens* or the "d.t.'s"—literally, a "trembling delirium." In other cases the brain damage may lead, over a period of time, to generalized mental deterioration in which the processes of thinking become slowed and muddled and physical coordination is permanently impaired; in extreme cases a form of dementia can evolve in which the victim is unable to manage even such simple basic activities as dressing, bathing or feeding himself without help. But secondary effects of excessive drinking, due to malnutrition, can be equally devastating. Because the habitual excessive drinker often has little appetite for food and ignores his own nutritional needs, he may lose weight, become anemic, and gradually develop symptoms of any of the vitamin-deficiency diseases. In particular, he may develop a painful *peripheral neuritis* affecting the hands, wrists, ankles or feet as a result of insufficient quantities of the B vitamins. Even more dangerous is the development of *cirrhosis of the liver* as a result of chronic protein starvation, in which liver cells are destroyed in increasing numbers and the liver then becomes scarred and finally atrophied in its attempt to repair the damage. Such a cirrhosis may also result from malnutrition due to other causes, but so many habitual excessive drinkers fall victim to the disease that it is commonly regarded as a condition primarily associated with overuse of alcohol.

The really tragic potential of alcohol, however, arises not merely from the physical effects of excessive drinking, but from the vast complex of chronic physical and emotional impairments that characterize the condition known as alcoholism. This term does not generally apply to the great majority of people who are moderate social drinkers using alcohol in small quantities on occasion as a relaxant, tension reliever or social lubricant; nor does it apply to most individuals who use larger amounts of alcohol daily at the "cocktail hour" as a habitual enjoyable ritual, or even to those who very occasionally overindulge to the point of marked intoxication. To these people, alcohol is an adjunct to their daily lives, not a necessity; in general they can control both the amount that they drink and the times and circumstances that they choose for drinking; they do not generally depend upon alcohol as an emotional crutch to enable them to face the problems of the day; and they can, in most cases, continue moderate use of alcohol over prolonged periods, even for years, without suffering any particular lasting physical or emotional damage.

Unfortunately, there are a large number of people who cannot exercise this kind of control over their use of alcohol. These are individuals who drink compulsively and cannot control

when or how much they drink. Further, they are usually individuals whose emotional development has been arrested or impoverished at some point in their lives, who feel inadequate to the everyday tasks of living, and who have depended heavily upon the emotional support of others during their early years, and ultimately come to depend upon alcohol as an emotional support. Often they are individuals who cannot accept responsibility for their own behavior, individuals who are perpetually seeking escape from the pain of their unconscious emotional conflicts and anxieties, or individuals who are unconsciously seeking to punish themselves, acting out the guilty feelings they harbor as a result of behavior long since buried in the past and consciously forgotten. Whatever the cause—and the causes vary widely—these are people who develop a powerful emotional dependence on alcohol, not a physical addiction but an emotional addiction so strong that they become powerless to control it. At the same time they develop a *tolerance* for alcohol, so that larger and larger quantities are required to produce the desired obliterative effect. Often they come to drink constantly during their waking hours; often they drink secretly, if those around them disapprove, or in solitude. As the alcoholism continues they become increasingly incapacitated, unable to perform their work adequately, losing their jobs, alienating those closest to them, rejecting any aid, watching their marriages deteriorate, while the progressive damage done by excessive alcohol whittles away at their physical health. The intervals they spend without the support of alcohol become nightmares; many are injured, even killed, by accidents that occur during periods of intoxication; many die of pneumonia or other conditions that arise from physical exposure. Many more spend their lives going "off the wagon" and then back on again, trying to bring their alcoholism under control, while still others live wasted lives, literally and figuratively drowning themselves in alcohol without ever really facing up to the fact that they are victims of a deadly and destructive illness.

Can alcoholism be cured? The answer must be extremely guarded, for this is one of the most resistant of all illnesses to effective treatment.

First it must be recognized and identified, and the chronic alcoholic himself is often the last to recognize or acknowledge that he is seriously ill. Recognition is all the more difficult considering that many individuals who are habitually heavy users of alcohol may, in fact, not be alcoholics because they lack the emotional dependency upon alcohol that marks the true alcoholic. Thus the mere amount of alcohol an individual consumes is not necessarily diagnostic of alcoholism, and indeed the line separating the heavy social drinker from the developing alcoholic may be all but indistinguishable even to physicians or psychiatrists. Certain clues may help identify the illness, however, or at least raise the level of suspicion. Solitary drinking is one such clue, for instance, since this is obviously the direct antithesis to "social" drinking. Morning drinking is rarely consistent with any normal life style, since even heavy social drinkers recognize that alcohol impairs their judgment and capacity to do their work effectively; the individual who must consistently "drink to get the day started" is almost certainly alcoholic. Increasingly frequent episodes of acute intoxication, and the occurrence of two- or three-day "benders," are far too common manifestations of alcoholism to be ignored. Similarly, the individual who becomes seriously upset or panicky when alcohol is not available at a time he is accustomed to drinking is clearly declaring his dependency upon alcohol. Perhaps most telling of all, however, is the individual's *inability to stop drinking when common sense and his own self-interest dictate that he should.* The person whose pattern of drinking is obviously threatening or impairing his normal, everyday performance, or his thinking capacities or judgment, yet who continues in that pattern all the same, is either alcoholic already or is rapidly on the road to chronic alcoholism.

Numerous methods of treatment have been used in attempting to deal with alcoholism. Few have proved outstandingly successful, largely because they have attempted to treat the symptom of the disorder—the drinking itself—without dealing with the underlying emotional causes of the dependency. For years simple withdrawal was the only avenue of approach known, and it still is used today, even though it fails far more

often than it succeeds. The alcoholic is hospitalized—often virtually imprisoned—in social treatment facilities or sanitoriums where alcohol is not available, and kept there until he has "dried out." Various facilities such as steam baths, massage and hydrotherapy tanks are used to help the alcoholic over the period of extreme nervous irritability or even delirium that may result from sudden withdrawal—more a manifestation of a psychological shock or a panic reaction than actual physical withdrawal symptoms—and a nourishing high-protein diet and various forms of social recreation are also provided. Such treatment is generally regarded as socially acceptable, but it is rarely permanently effective unless the victim himself recognizes his disability and vigorously desires to stop drinking. Combined with intensive psychotherapy, withdrawal treatment has a somewhat better chance of success, but again much depends upon the motivation of the victim; psychiatric therapy is generally wasted if the victim refuses to recognize the gravity of his problem and consciously or unconsciously resists treatment.

Another form of treatment involves the use of the drug Antabuse, a medication that has no discernible effect on the alcoholic as long as he abstains from alcohol, but which renders him violently ill with nausea, vomiting and excessive sweating whenever he takes even a small drink. Again, this treatment is successful in a small percentage of cases in which the victim genuinely wants to stop drinking, but more commonly fails because it never approaches the underlying psychological causes of the illness. Antabuse treatment may well help the alcoholic stop drinking for a brief time, but all too often the compulsive drinking pattern is resumed as soon as the medication is stopped.

Probably the most successful form of treatment available today is the group support and group psychotherapy practiced by the organization known as Alcoholics Anonymous (A.A.). This organization, with chapters in virtually every city or town in the country, is composed entirely of individuals who were once uncontrolled alcoholics but who have succeeded in achieving at least temporary control over their alcoholism, usually with the aid of other A.A.

members. The basic principle of the A.A. approach to treatment is that no one can understand the problem of an uncontrolled alcoholic better than someone who has been alcoholic, and that the act of helping other alcoholics end their drinking is the best form of reinforcement of the member's own resolve to stop drinking. The A.A. will not accept a candidate for membership until he is able to recognize and admit publicly to the group that he is an alcoholic who cannot help himself without aid; indeed, each A.A. member speaking at a group meeting or discussion will preface his remarks with the flat statement, "I am an alcoholic," although he may not have been drinking for years. According to the A.A., alcoholism is a permanent state, and the alcoholic will remain vulnerable to use of alcohol in any form or in any quantity as long as he lives; to the alcoholic there is no such thing as "controlled social drinking." Once an alcoholic can accept these premises and ask for help, other members of A.A. will rally to his aid, help him discuss the problems that may have led to his drinking, provide him with firm emotional support in his effort to stop, and finally enlist him in the "therapeutic" task of helping others.

Psychiatrists and physicians have criticized the work of A.A. on various grounds. It is an "amateur" organization, in effect administering group psychotherapy without the benefit of skilled psychiatric guidance, and there is undoubtedly some potential in such an organization for doing emotional harm to individuals as well as emotional good. Such criticism, however, misses the important point: that the A.A. program *works,* and works more effectively in treating and curing alcoholism than any other form of treatment known. Some A.A. members drop out and backslide; some succeed only after repeated attempts to conquer their alcoholism; but a great many others succeed on a permanent basis. There is no question that Alcoholics Anonymous deserves resounding credit for salvaging multitudes of lives that would have been totally wasted, or prematurely lost, without it. Certainly anyone who recognizes that he has a problem with alcohol, or anyone who recognizes alcoholism in a member of his family,

should be advised to contact the nearest chapter of Alcoholics Anonymous.

Despite the work of A.A., and despite other forms of treatment, chronic alcoholism remains a major health threat in our country today; by conservative estimate some 15 million people in the United States alone are alcoholic. Thus research continues to find more widely effective forms of treatment. In recent years behavioral psychologists have experimented with various means of conditioning alcoholics to avoid alcohol; group psychotherapy programs have been reinforced, for example, by administering mild but irritating electrical shocks to alcoholics every time they reach out for an alcoholic drink. It is still too early to evaluate such experimental programs, but *any* plausible approach to treatment deserves attention and hopeful support. Alcoholism is an insidious and pervasive health destroyer in our society, and it will remain a growing threat until predictably effective means of combating it are discovered.

Drug Abuse and Addiction

As little as 30 years ago the only notable "drug problem" in the United States, other than the problem of alcoholism, involved the physically addicting narcotic or so-called hard drugs, chiefly the derivatives of opium, including morphine and heroin, and the derivatives of coca leaves, most notably cocaine. Although there was an illicit traffic even then in these drugs, addiction most commonly occurred as a result of their use for pain control or local anesthetic, but the number of people affected was so small that addiction or drug abuse was then a relatively insignificant health problem. Today, however, abuse of these and a multitude of other drugs and chemical substances has become a massive health problem throughout the Western world. Most disturbing of all, the problem has primarily affected adolescents and young adults in ever increasing numbers, and most efforts to deal rationally with it are handicapped by a proliferation of false or distorted information and emotional overreactions that make calm and reasonable consideration impossible.

Any useful discussion of drug abuse or addiction must begin, then, with a simple classification of the *kinds* of drugs that constitute the problem, what the nature of their action may be, and what real dangers they pose to the user. For purposes of clarity the most commonly abused drugs today can be described in four major categories, even though the actions of many individual drugs may lap over into two or even more of these categories. They are the *stimulating drugs,* the *depressant drugs,* the "mind-altering" or *hallucinogenic drugs,* and the *physically addicting drugs,* also known as *narcotics.* Each category has its own characteristics and its own hazards.

The Stimulating Drugs. The major drugs in this category, also commonly known as pep pills, uppers, or speed, are the *amphetamines,* a group of potent cerebral and cardiovascular stimulants. The most familiar of these are amphetamine sulfate or Benzedrine, dextroamphetamine sulfate or Dexedrine, and methamphetamine; certain other cerebral stimulants also fall in this group, most notably products sold under the trade names of Ritalin and Preludin. All these drugs have a broad spectrum of effects: they are prescribed by physicians in small doses as antidepressants and mood-elevating agents because they tend to induce euphoria; they are widely used as adjuncts to weight reduction because they depress the appetite control centers of the brain; they elevate the blood pressure and increase the heart rate; and they induce a marked acceleration and stimulation of the thinking processes. When larger doses are taken, the individual becomes physically and mentally stimulated or "high," euphoric, overcome by restless energy, uninterested in food, and often sleepless for days on end. Large doses may also result in such prolonged supercharged physical and mental activity that the user is left physically exhausted when the drug effect wears off. Stimulant drugs are normally taken by mouth and are not physically addicting—that is, no physical craving for the drug occurs—but emotional habituation is commonplace, with the user coming to depend upon the physical and emotional lift provided by the drug and to dread the emotional "letdown" or depression that tends to

ensue when the drug effects wear off. Finally, the user develops a tolerance to these drugs, so that increasing doses are required to bring about the desired effects. The drugs are particularly dangerous when administered intravenously, since the full-blown effects then appear with shocklike impact, and the danger of an overdose is extreme. Even the most reckless drug experimenters acknowledge that "speed kills," and there is no question that inadvertent overdoses have led to death from cerebral hemorrhage, heart failure, or exhaustion and exposure.

The Depressant Drugs. The most commonly used depressant drugs are the barbiturates, frequently prescribed as sedatives, sleeping pills or adjuncts to light anesthesia. Sometimes called downers, reds or redbirds, yellows or blues (all taken from the color of the capsules in which they are most often dispensed), these drugs in normally prescribed doses depress the higher cerebral centers, slow down thinking processes, and induce a pleasantly drowsy readiness for sleep. In larger doses they can seriously depress the respiratory centers of the brain and induce marked mental dullness and confusion in some, or physical and emotional agitation in others. Depressant drugs are particularly dangerous when used in combination with the stimulant drugs to induce an agitated dementia, or when used in addition to alcohol; in fact, many deaths due to overdosage are the result of the use of barbiturates for sleep after a period of heavy drinking. The confused victim loses track of how many sleeping pills he has taken and swallows repeated and eventually lethal doses. Serious overdosage of the barbiturates leads to a stuporous coma in which respirations are so seriously depressed that the victim fails to exchange enough oxygen to sustain life. Treatment of an overdose must include pumping the stomach to remove any unabsorbed drug that may still remain, followed by administration of cerebral stimulants and inducing physical activity by walking the victim or moving his arms and legs to stimulate circulation and breathing until the absorbed drug can be removed from the blood stream via the kidneys or detoxified in the liver. Like the stimulant drugs, barbiturates do not cause a physical addiction but do lead to a marked psychological or emotional habituation when used for a protracted period. Physical tolerance also occurs, and when the drug is withdrawn after the body has become accustomed to high doses, severe emotional reactions, anxiety panic states or even convulsions may occur.

In some cases barbiturates are used much the same as alcohol, by passive-dependent individuals who seek escape from unconscious emotional conflicts, or use the drug as an emotional support to help them face the daily problems they feel unable to cope with alone. Others who live crushingly high-tension lives use them as a part of a vicious daily cycle of drug consumption, including amphetamines to get started in the morning, heavy use of alcohol throughout the day and evening, and barbiturates in heavy doses to "calm down" and get to sleep at night, followed the next day by more amphetamines to overcome the "hangover" from the barbiturates in order to get started again. As physical tolerance to such drugs builds up, these people may come to require staggering quantities of each in order to maintain the level of drug effect they seek, and thus subject their bodies to a physical and emotional pounding that no organism can long withstand. Unfortunately, there is also an increasing use of barbiturates, often in combination with various stimulant drugs, among young people solely for the euphoric "kicks" these drug combinations often provide, without consideration for the very real, perhaps mortal, threat of inadvertent overdosage that may occur at any time.

The Hallucinogenic or "Mind-Altering" Drugs. One of the most widespread areas of illicit drug use in recent years has involved a variety of drugs which bring about such striking temporary alterations in mental function or perception that their users describe them as "psychedelic," "mind-bending" or "consciousness-expanding." The most widely used of these substances, and by all odds the least dangerous, so far as is known, is *marijuana,* prepared from the dried leaves and flowers of the common hemp plant, *Cannabis sativa,* which still grows widely as a weed in many parts of the United States. This drug, also commonly known as pot, tea, grass, or weed, is ordinarily smoked, although its effects can also be obtained by eating it. However it is used, marijuana essentially induces a mild euphoria, a degree of physical relaxation, a diminishment of inhibitions and, in larger doses, a sort of drowsy intoxication. Such higher brain functions as judgment, concentration and short-memory retention are impaired; those affected by marijuana are often voluble, but have trouble following conversations or pursuing complex trains of thought. Some experience a distortion of time sense, so that time seems to move far more slowly—or more swiftly—than normal. Visual and aural perceptions are often keyed up, and the individual may feel he hears more when listening to music, or that he observes with a richer awareness than usual. Some experience an aphrodisiac effect; others feel that their emotional responses become more open and meaningful, while still others may withdraw. True hallucination is uncommon and apparently related to excessively heavy dosage or continued heavy use. On the other side of the coin, some experience panic reactions, feelings of terror, or outlandish and frightening nightmares with marijuana use, while others claim to feel no effect at all. In general the mental state or expectation of the user seems to influence the effect obtained from the drug. *Hashish,* a refined or concentrated marijuana product made from more potent strains of the hemp plant than are ordinarily found in North America, has a long history of use in the Middle East, North Africa and India, and has also appeared on the American scene in recent years. This form of the drug, also usually smoked, produces all the physiological effects of marijuana in exaggerated form, and its use results far more frequently in hallucinations, profound intoxication or mental disorganization than with plain marijuana.

Certain widely held views about marijuana are simply untrue. It is not a narcotic, despite the fact that it is defined as such under federal drug statutes; it causes no physical addiction, nor any physical tolerance. As an intoxicant, passive-dependent individuals may use it as a means of emotional support or escape and may develop a psychological dependence on the drug, but its use can be discontinued at any time with no physical effects. Although its use temporarily impairs judgment, it is not usually associated with bizarre or antisocial behavior; whereas the heavy drinker may feel impelled to go out and drive his car on public highways, endangering the lives of all who come near him, the marijuana user is more likely to spend the evening sitting on the living room floor in semitorpor listening to records. What is more, there is no convincing scientific evidence to support contentions that marijuana use is often a "stepping stone" to the use of more dangerous drugs such as the addicting narcotics. Heroin addicts may well often reveal a past history of marijuana use, but there is as yet no reason to believe that any but a few marginal marijuana users ultimately "escalate" their drug use to heroin.

This is not to say that marijuana is harmless, or that its use should be encouraged. The fact is that not enough is yet known about the long-term effects of marijuana use to support a scientific judgment about any possible deleterious effects it may have. Certainly many of the often-described "horrors of marijuana" are either gross distortions or outright falsehoods, and it is unfortunate that they have been presented to the public as true; and the very fact that the drug has been proscribed by law has made serious scientific investigation of its properties and effects extremely difficult until recent years. Much remains to be learned; many authorities suspect, although they cannot yet prove, that marijuana as it is used in this country is little more than a mild euphoriant and intoxicant that may well be less harmful to the body—and to society as a whole—than alcohol. It is also very possible that classification of marijuana as a dangerous narcotic in the eyes of the law, with mere possession of the drug treated as a felonious criminal offense punishable by years of imprisonment in many states, may well be far more harmful to our society than legalization and controlled sale would be, and a growing body of respected medical and legal opinion today has recommended that criminal sanctions be lifted and that use of the drug by mature individuals be legalized.

Even so, the frequent use of marijuana by young people during their preteens and adolescent years—among the most formative years of their lives—can only be deplored. Whatever else may be said, marijuana *is* an intoxicant; it *does* have distorting physiological effects on the function of the mind, and, if nothing else, it serves as an "attractive nuisance" to teen-agers who need all their wits about them while learning to deal with the tensions and trials of adolescence; indeed, there is nothing that can profit them less at this time in their lives than the employment of *any* drug-induced escape mechanism to interfere with their normal growth toward maturity. Unfortunately, marijuana use is widespread among young people today, and likely to become more so. Parents must realize that the great majority of adolescents will probably experiment with the drug at one time or another; "scare tactics" will not prevent this, nor will lectures or threatened punishments. Parents should adopt a balanced view toward such experimentation, taking pains to condemn the use of the drug without condemning the adolescent, and seeking primarily to discourage continuing use in every way possible. Certain clues will often alert parents when a teen-ager has moved beyond the point of mere experimentation; in many cases school work suddenly deteriorates, the teen-ager becomes secretive and reclusive in his behavior, uninterested in classes or extracurricular school activities, excessively sleepy at times when he ought to be well rested, or inclined to spend extraordinary amounts of unaccounted time away from home. None of these things necessarily indicates drug use, of course, but any of them should at least arouse parental suspicions and suggest careful but unobtrusive observation of the adolescent's behavior patterns. Providing him with unembellished factual data about the effects and dangers of *all* drugs may help discourage experimentation with those more dangerous than marijuana. When a problem of continuing use of marijuana, or experimental use of other drugs, does arise, parents should have no hesitation in confronting the adolescent, making it clear that continuing use will not be tolerated, and seeking professional help and guidance, beginning with a trusted family physician. Drug abuse is a problem today in virtually every community, and in many communities parents, physicians and other responsible citizens have joined forces to combat it, pooling both knowledge and experience in order to provide troubled families with support and guidance in dealing with drug abuse in their own homes.

Other hallucinogenic drugs have proved far more dangerous than marijuana, for a number of reasons. One of these is *lysergic acid diethylamide,* more commonly known as LSD or merely "acid," a colorless, tasteless chemical which is taken in capsule form by mouth or dissolved in water and used on sugar cubes or mixed into beverages. It is an extremely potent drug which can, even in tiny doses, produce a profound distortion of perception and mental functioning. Although its precise action on the mind is not yet understood, its use induces colorful and sometimes frightening visual, auditory and tactile hallucinations so intensely real to the user that he describes the drug experience quite accurately as "taking a trip" to a fantastic hallucinatory world. Time sense, color perception, virtually all the senses are distorted or intensified as the line between reality and fantasy is obscured, and some authorities believe that the drug temporarily induces a mental disorganization or dissociation disturbingly similar to that which occurs in the grave psychotic disorder known as schizophrenia. The LSD drug experience has been described by many as "awesome," "consciousness-expanding" or "mind-bending," but in many cases users of the drug find themselves suddenly and without warning suffering the nightmarish horrors and irrational, paralyzing terror of "bad trips"—and these may occur even in those who have used the drug many times before without apparent ill effects. What is more, whatever its chemical action on the brain, LSD use has in many cases triggered or precipitated true psychoses, and instances have been verified in which individuals who have apparently recovered from the effects of the drug some six to eight hours after a dose have later experienced spontaneous recurrence of the drug effects days or even weeks later without any repeated dosage.

There is much yet to be learned about what, precisely, LSD does, and controlled scientific research has been sorely hampered by the wide-spread and uncontrolled illicit use of the drug, but there can be no question that LSD presents a real and totally unpredictable hazard to the user. Although it causes no known physical addiction, its use can lead to mental and emotional trauma against which the victim may be totally defenseless; it has the potential to unhinge the most stable mind and presents a particular threat to any user who is already mentally unstable. In our present state of knowledge, the LSD user is literally gambling with his sanity, and there is no known way that the substance can be safely used.

Much the same holds true for certain other hallucinogens which have appeared from time to time on the illicit drug market in this country. *Mescaline* and *peyote,* derived from certain species of cacti found in Mexico and the southwestern United States, are intoxicating drugs which produce hallucinations of color and sound and ecstatic sensations similar to those produced by LSD; indeed, field tests have indicated that most underground products sold under these names in the United States are, in fact, LSD or are mixed with LSD. Other hallucinogens are derived from certain Mexican mushrooms and have probably been used for centuries in native religious rites. All present the same dangers; all are rightly classified as "dangerous drugs"; and all should be shunned by anyone who places any premium on the healthy function of his mind.

The Addictive Narcotics. Even the potential hazards presented by the hallucinogenic drugs cannot hold a candle to the life-wrecking capacities of the physically addictive narcotics—drugs which enter into the body's biochemical reactions in such a way as to produce a physical craving for repeated doses, or to produce physically and emotionally agonizing withdrawal symptoms when the drug is no longer available. One such drug is *cocaine,* an alkaloid derived from coca leaves, which was introduced to medical use in the early 1900s as a local or surface anesthesia, but which has since been largely abandoned in favor of less dangerous agents because of its powerful addicting properties. Far more commonly used, however, are various natural or synthetic derivatives of *opium,* an alkaloid-containing resin of the

Oriental opium poppy, including raw opium itself, purified products such as morphine, heroin and codeine, and such synthetic opiates as meperidine (trade name Demerol), dihydromorphinone (Dilaudid) or methadone (Dolophine). Raw opium has been smoked as a soporific, dream-inducing narcotic for many centuries in Oriental countries where opium addiction has been a more or less acceptable part of the culture. Many of the derivatives, especially morphine, codeine and the synthetic narcotics, have been prized in Western medicine as potent painkillers, and still have perfectly legitimate medical uses as such today, but heroin, the most violently and swiftly addictive drug of them all, has no legitimate medical use whatever and is produced today only to supply an ever growing illicit narcotics trade.

Addiction to one or another of these drugs generally arises in one of two ways. Despite the extreme caution with which they are prescribed by physicians and surgeons when needed to combat pain, some individuals become addicted quite innocently in the course of treatment of a prolonged painful illness or injury, or during the painful period of recovery from certain kinds of surgery. By far the majority of such so-called pain addicts have comparatively strong, well-structured personalities and have relatively little problem withdrawing from the narcotic once the pain is gone. Some, however, may remain addicted, particularly if there is some degree of continuing pain or if they are of the passive-dependent, anxious, inadequate and frightened personality type sometimes described by doctors as "the addictive personality," inclined to grasp and cling to any emotional support available, even the treacherous emotional support of a narcotic drug. Some such individuals, no longer able to obtain the addicting drug legitimately from their doctors, may begin making the rounds of doctors' offices, exaggerating the pain of their afflictions in order to obtain medication; others may turn to the underworld of drug sellers or "pushers."

Far more commonly, however, addiction to narcotics begins directly through foolish experimentation, an irresponsible search for "kicks," ordinary but imprudent curiosity, or social pressures in a drug-oriented underground culture. Although both cocaine and heroin are commonly used illicit drugs today (heroin use is far more widespread), the patterns of drug effect and drug addiction are similar for both. Heroin (diacetylmorphine) is a bitter-tasting white crystalline powder, usually mixed or "cut" with milk sugar before it reaches the addict. It can be used either by sniffing the powder into the nostrils for absorption through the mucous membrane or by mixing it with water and injecting it hypodermically into the subcutaneous tissues under the skin or directly into a vein.

This drug, known in the narcotics argot as junk, horse, H or smack, produces a drowsy stupor, a marked sense of euphoria and a feeling of soaring elation and calm self-confidence in which the user, for a while, feels equal to anything, capable of handling any task or solving any problem. Hunger is forgotten, sexual frustrations are forgotten, inadequacies vanish as the user feels himself master of his body and all the world about him. The drug's effects, which may last three to four hours, are usually terminated by sleep and a deep sense of depression upon awakening as the drug-induced illusions fall away. Repeated use of the drug will restore this illusive world, but very quickly a larger amount is needed to produce the desired effects, and the user finds the prospect of life without the ego-boosting effects of the drug to be more and more frightening. Physical addiction begins to develop with the second, third or fourth dose, perhaps even with the first if a large dosage is used, and very soon the addict is prompted to repeated dosage by the highly unpleasant physical symptoms of withdrawal that begin to appear: nausea, vomiting, abdominal pain, profuse sweating, violent tremors, a sense of pressure in the chest, even convulsions, all accompanied by a rising emotional state of panic and terror. Ultimately the addict comes to use ever increasing doses more to stave off the agony of withdrawal symptoms than for the primary euphoriant effect of the drug, which tends to become more and more blunted as time goes on. To the addict, obtaining enough of the drug to maintain himself becomes the most imperative thing in his life, and with his growing need he must pay whatever his supplier may demand. Confirmed addicts in our major cities may require two or three hundred dollars a day to support their habits, and many turn to selling the drug, entrapping others in the addiction, in order to fund their own addiction.

The physical effects of such drug use can be grave indeed. Quite aside from the addiction itself, the addict becomes indifferent to food, losing weight steadily and falling victim to protein starvation and vitamin deficiency diseases. His sexual drive diminishes, an inability to concentrate or perform adequately at his work frequently spells the end of any job he may hold, and the drug use acts as a shattering trauma to his nervous system. He is constantly vulnerable to contracting infectious hepatitis or septicemia from contaminated injection equipment, and since he has no way to determine the amount of drug actually contained in any given dose, he is always in danger of coma or death from inadvertent overdosage. Indeed, overdosage is perhaps the most common cause of early death among addicts, and it is probable that many overdosage deaths occur by deliberate intent of the drug supplier, who uses this means to get rid of addicts who are becoming troublesome. But the greatest tragedy of all is the pervasive social damage caused by widespread addiction, with children of high school or even grade school age being enticed into addiction by suppliers seeking to broaden their clientele and their profits.

No one knows precisely how widespread heroin addiction and other forms of narcotics addiction may be in this country today, but there is little question that the problem pervades virtually all of our major cities and many of our smaller towns as well. Many addicts are those who simply do not have the wit or the motivation to reject enticing overtures to narcotics use; many adolescents are trapped into addiction by their need to conform to the behavior of their peers or to "show off" before those they admire. Unfortunately, many others who become addicted are individuals with passive-dependent or otherwise crippled personalities, making them less able than most to face the agonies of withdrawal. And until very recently, the only approach to treatment of addiction was enforced withdrawal; addicts were imprisoned in narcotics wards of federal hospitals or in neuropsychiatric wards and held there for weeks or months until withdrawal was over. There was very little attempt at social or emotional rehabilitation, and virtually no effective psychiatric care available.

Today new approaches are being explored, in the face of the growing need. Addicts are regarded more as victims of illness than as criminals. Group therapy is being explored in institutional settings. Grass-roots "open door clinics" have been established in many communities, with "flying squads" of ex-addicts, doctors and other personnel ready to go to the aid of the addict who calls for help. One promising program of treatment involves the use of a milder narcotic, methadone, in regularly rationed daily doses, to help the heroin addict overcome the physical agony of withdrawal. Some have criticized such programs as "substituting one addiction for another," and to a degree this is true; but when used in combination with individual or group psychotherapy to aid the addict in rebuilding a shattered or crippled personality and in identifying and treating the unconscious conflicts and anxieties that have made him more vulnerable than others to addiction in the first place, the methadone program may well prove the best weapon available to combat hard narcotics addiction.

Fortunately, there is help and support available to addicts today, or to families of addicts. The first port of call, in the event of suspicion that someone in a family has become addicted, is the family physician. Not only can he help establish whether addiction is present or not, he can also recommend whatever treatment institutions or facilities are available in the community. Parents who suspect possible addiction in an adolescent in particular should not hesitate or delay in finding help; this is not the kind of problem that can be effectively handled alone, and delay in finding help may literally be fatal. In virtually every case not only physical but emotional problems are involved, and the victim all too often is helpless to help himself.

Other Drug Abuse. At least passing mention should be made of certain other forms of drug abuse that occasionally appear. Among pre-teen-agers and adolescents one of the most dangerous is *glue sniffing,* a term that is generally applied to the inhalation of intoxicating fumes not only from model airplane cements but from other aromatic solvents. Many of these substances contain carbon tetrachloride or other chlorinated hydrocarbons which can act as violent poisons to cells in the liver, leading to destruction and scarring of the liver and, ultimately, to death from cirrhosis and liver failure. Other such substances have caused even more sudden death from suffocation, respiratory collapse, renal failure or unknown causes. The use of any solvents, paints, model cements or glues should be carefully supervised by parents, and any untoward behavior on the part of a child using such substances should be reported to a physician or poison control center without delay.

Finally, it must be recognized that many drugs and medicines used for legitimate treatment of illness may have poisonous effects if taken in overdoses, or if used experimentally by children. Many of the tranquilizing drugs, for example, may be splendid therapeutic aids when used under a doctor's direction, but can be dangerous poisons if misused. With medications of every kind so readily available, children may take literally *any* drug without the least idea of what it may be or what effects it might have. Children should be taught a healthy respect for drugs from the earliest years on, and any medicines kept in the house should be stored in cabinets or drug safes that can be locked.

Psychosis: Most Dread Disease of All

The most severe forms of mental illness are those disorders in which the victim's internal conflicts are of such a grave magnitude and so adamantly unresolvable by any of the normal or neurotic reactions that the personality's best efforts at defense finally break down. The personality itself begins to disintegrate, with the functioning of the mind so totally distorted that the ego is unable to distinguish the real world from a dream world fabricated in the mind, and the victim becomes preoccupied with totally unreal or fantastic *delusions* (false beliefs) and *hallucinations* (false visual, auditory or other

sensory impressions). His intellectual and emotional perceptions and responses become so distorted or impaired that he slips into a nightmare world of phantom terrors, fear, agony and hopelessness. These disorders, known as *psychoses,* may sometimes result in behavior which appears, to the outside observer, to be cheerful, euphoric, "blissfully" childlike or "happily" withdrawn, but those who have recovered from these disorders, and the physicians who specialize in their treatment, describe the psychoses as the most dreadful of all human illnesses, a living hell of internal conflict and torment.

Schizophrenia. Of the different patterns psychotic disorders may take, schizophrenia is by far the most common, the most destructive, the most resistant to treatment, and the most likely to remain permanent or to recur episodically over long periods of time. Some 70 or 80 years ago this profound form of mental illness was called "dementia praecox" because it so commonly occurred in children, sometimes as young as age six or seven, and in adolescents and preadults; but the term has fallen into disuse because this disorder is not a true dementia in which there is irreparable damage to the mental functions, nor is the disease confined only to young people. It can first appear in either males or females at virtually any age from infancy through mature middle age, although it is comparatively rare for the first episode of the disease to occur after the age of forty. What is more, contrary to popular mythology, schizophrenia (which means, literally, "splitting of the mind") is not related to those rare and celebrated cases of "dual personality" in which the victim assumes one or more widely differing roles and may shift back and forth between them, an uncommon form of personality disorder. (*See* p. 781.) Rather, it is a disease that is mainly characterized by a progressive withdrawal from reality, a sort of massive "dropping out" of the individual from the people and the world around him, and a preoccupation with delusions and fantasies, all of which are manifested in often bizarre and incomprehensible patterns of behavior. The "splitting of the mind" refers to the profound dissociation of the individual from appropriate mental and emotional responses to his environment, and also implies the "splitting up" or disintegration of the normal personality structure.

Often the victim of schizophrenia is a person who has been limping along, psychologically speaking, on the border line of outright psychotic derailment for many years; frequently he may have been recognized as a "schizoid" or "schizophrenic-like" personality by a physician long before an outright psychosis develops. Some such people are extraordinarily timid, self-conscious, shy, sometimes highly suspicious, dissatisfied with themselves, easily hurt by comparatively innocuous slights, and socially withdrawn. Others merely appear to be rather dull, lifeless personalities, seldom stirred by emotion and inclined to be cold, uninterested or even calloused in their behavior toward others. In some cases the transition from a comparatively normal state into schizophrenia comes in the form of a very sharp *psychotic break* which may be triggered by a severe emotional shock, a sudden loss, illness, failure, or more recently, an unfortunate drug experience. More commonly, however, there is a somewhat more gradual prolonged and insidious change in mood, outlook and behavior which may occur over a period of weeks or months.

Typically the victim may seem to be increasingly preoccupied with his own thoughts, increasingly shiftless and lazy, at least to outward appearances, and often handles a normal day's work or normal social intercourse with increasing difficulty. In some cases he may appear taciturn, deeply withdrawn or unresponsive, ruminating at great length on an imaginary physical illness or on sexual topics. Or he may become increasingly suspicious and then begin to express feelings, quite without any apparent basis, that people are talking about him or laughing at him behind his back, trying to ostracize him from their company, or plotting among themselves to do him some grievous harm. The full-blown psychosis appears in a complete break with reality when the victim begins, for example, to talk to God about these feelings, or tears apart the refrigerator to find the hidden machine that observes his every action, or carries a loaded gun to shoot the "assailants" who are plotting against him, or to kill himself before they get him.

Schizophrenia is not really a simple disease entity; although it is characterized chiefly by withdrawal, it exists in a variety of forms and may result in many different kinds of abnormal patterns of thinking and behavior. Sometimes there are feelings of persecution, sometimes euphoria, sometimes depression. Frequently the victim becomes depersonalized; that is, he seems to be standing aside and watching his own actions and words from afar with little or no interest in or reaction to them. Delusions and hallucinations may be extremely vivid and sometimes seem more real than anything in the outside world. The victim may play with language, coining new words which are nonsense to anyone else but which he invests with grave significance, or he may create and inhabit a completely imaginary world. Strangely enough, however, there is usually no disturbance in consciousness, orientation or memory, and if the schizophrenic demonstrates any of these apparent impairments, it is almost invariably because some element of his personality derangement compels him to pretend that he is unconscious or cannot remember or does not know where he is. Even when he appears to be totally oblivious and unresponsive to anything around him, it has been demonstrated time and again that some part of his mind remains perfectly wide awake and alert and that he will remember distinctly everything that happens to him while he is in this state.

When schizophrenia is active and acute, any or all of these symptoms or behavioral patterns may be present, one at a time or all together; but certain patients often manifest one or another symptom in an exaggerated form so that specific types of schizophrenic behavior predominate. When withdrawal, lability of emotion, and diminishing interest in and response to the external world are present without any marked delusions or hallucinations, the psychosis may never be diagnosed and the victim may never seek medical help. He may become unable to work effectively, or may lose his job and withdraw deeper and deeper into himself and into bizarre but apparently harmless patterns of behavior so that family and friends may recognize that he is ill without understanding exactly how, or how gravely. Or he may simply wander off to lead a hand-to-mouth existence as a social derelict. In these circumstances, chances of schizophrenics such as these receiving effective help in terms of treatment are relatively small, even though they may eventually be hospitalized.

Schizophrenics who display other dominant patterns of behavior are often hospitalized much more quickly, for obvious reasons. One of the most common forms of the disease is *paranoid schizophrenia,* in which the victim has false ideas of being persecuted, threatened or harmed. These delusions have no basis in fact and are often totally illogical or even contradictory, yet the victim may act upon them as if they were completely real. Paranoid schizophrenia is regarded by psychiatrists as a particularly grave form of the disorder, more likely than any other form to become entrenched and permanent, far harder to deal with, and always fraught with the twin threats that the victim will become so terrified of his persecutors that he will attempt suicide or become so convinced that the world is plotting against him that he commits some violently antisocial act. Many of the tragic incidents in which a moody but otherwise apparently normal individual suddenly runs amok shooting people until he can be subdued are actually extreme manifestations of undiagnosed paranoid schizophrenia.

Another form of schizophrenia is characterized by more fragmentary fantasies and delusions, and the victim often shows a tendency to inappropriate laughter, inarticulate or incoherent babbling, sudden shifts from hilarity to weeping, childish behavior such as soiling or wetting the bed and an increasing silliness of response to external stimuli. Although victims of this so-called *hebephrenic schizophrenia* seem "happier" than other schizophrenics, they soon withdraw completely from contact with the real world or the people in it, and the disintegration of the personality is often more severe than in any other form of the disease.

Yet another form of the disease is *catatonic schizophrenia,* in which the victim retreats into a totally inattentive, completely preoccupied, and virtually stuporous state, sitting in the same place hour after hour without moving a muscle, sometimes not even blinking his eyes. Catatonic schizophrenics may remain in this weird and dreamlike state for days or weeks, rarely moving, apparently paying no attention to hunger or to offered food, sometimes even retaining urine or feces far beyond the limits of normal tolerance. Characteristically they hold their arms and legs in awkward positions for prolonged periods, or will allow someone to move a limb and then continue to hold it in that position. Occasionally victims may exhibit an "excited" phase of this manifestation of the disease and carry out extremely energetic but purposeless rituals of motion, sometimes to the point of exhaustion. But catatonic schizophrenia seems to be a form of the disease most likely to have periods of remission; that is, periods in which all the symptoms of the psychosis suddenly disappear and the individual returns to normal and may remain well for years.

Speaking generally, however, schizophrenia tends to be either a disease of steady progressive deterioration that requires lifelong confinement in a mental hospital or an illness that displays a pattern of intermittent acute recurrence interrupted from time to time with remissions. All forms of treatment of the disease are therefore aimed primarily at inducing and maintaining remissions, rather than attempting a "cure," although there are many reported cases of individuals with schizophrenic reactions which have cleared up under treatment and have never again recurred.

Schizophrenia is one of the most difficult of the mental disorders to treat effectively with psychoanalysis or other forms of psychotherapy, since it may require weeks or months of persistent work on the part of the psychiatrist just to establish contact with the patient. One of the earliest experimental uses made of the extremely potent hallucinogenic drug lysergic acid diethylamide (LSD) soon after its discovery was in the treatment of schizophrenics. It was perhaps the first time in medical history that treatment consisted of the *doctor* taking the medicine. This powerful drug was discovered to create a temporary hallucinogenic state or disturbance of the mind which seemed very similar to the mental disturbance of acute schizophrenia, and psychiatrists hoped that by taking the drug they would better understand their patients' delusional state and be able to establish more effective contact with them. Any kind of meaningful verbal communication is usually impossible with severe cases, however. Sometimes various forms of physical therapy are successful in establishing contact with a schizophrenic patient, in which case psychotherapy may prove effective; but this, too, is often a long and time-consuming process, particularly in the overcrowded and understaffed circumstances that all too often prevail in mental hospitals.

Thus other forms of treatment, quite severe from the viewpoint of the outside observer, have been used because they seem to be more successful in establishing contact with the patient, reversing the progress of the disease or inducing at least a temporary remission. One such form of treatment is *insulin shock therapy,* the administration of sufficient insulin to induce the patient to go into insulin shock and a hypoglycemic coma. Obviously this treatment can be handled only in a neuropsychiatric hospital where careful control can be maintained by experienced physicians over the amount of insulin the patient is given, the length of time he is allowed to remain in insulin shock, and the way he is brought out of it by the administration of adequate doses of glucose. However, insulin shock therapy is attended by so many dangers, including the possibility of physical damage due to convulsions, that it is now seldom used. *Electroshock therapy,* also less frequently used than previously, is another form of treatment in which the patient is rendered unconscious and convulsions are induced by carefully controlled electric shocks to the brain. The theory in both these forms of shock therapy is that, in the face of such a severe and "real" trauma, the patient's mind will rally to save his life. In some cases, this is exactly what seems to happen, but the remission may be only temporary, requiring additional shock treatment, although the patient often does recover to the degree that other forms of psychotherapy may be attempted. Electroshock therapy also has other drawbacks, not the least of which

are the terror felt by the patient and the threat of fractured vertebrae due to the violent convulsions caused by the electric shock. These dangers can be markedly diminished by the administration of muscle-relaxant drugs and a short-acting but effective anesthesia. The treatment is also generally accompanied by some degree of amnesia, which may last two or three months before clearing up, and if shock treatment is used too frequently there may be lasting impairment of memory. For these reasons, electroshock therapy must be carefully adapted to the individual patient's needs, and the decision to administer this form of treatment is never made lightly. Yet another form of treatment, involving surgical severing of certain nerve tracts in the brain, was once used in an effort to control maniacal and potentially dangerous activity on the part of schizophrenics, but most authorities today agree that such treatment, which tended to reduce the patient to a placid, vegetable-like condition, was worse than the disease, and such so-called *psychosurgery* has been largely abandoned.

Today far more reliance is placed on the techniques of *chemotherapy* or *psychopharmacology* in treating all forms of severe mental illness, sometimes in addition to, but often instead of, electroshock therapy. The use of various of the new "mind-affecting" medications, including tranquilizers and antianxiety or antidepression drugs, have gained widespread acceptance among psychiatrists, even though they seldom "cure" the patient, or even, for that matter, lead to remissions or recoveries any more frequently than other forms of treatment. The real value of these drugs in the treatment of schizophrenia or any of the other psychoses lies in the fact that they can relieve symptoms, particularly of anxiety, hyperactivity and often depression as well, to a sufficient extent that patients can leave the hospital, return safely to their homes and families, undertake their normal activities and, in many cases, remain, under medication, relatively free of alarming or antisocial symptoms for prolonged periods of time. Even if they must stay in the hospital, their behavior can be controlled, and they become more amenable to the various forms of psychotherapy. It still remains to be seen, however, whether these drugs, in the long run, will be helpful in permitting the victim of schizophrenia sufficient stability to enable him, over a period of time and with the continuing aid of psychotherapy, to reorganize and reestablish his shattered personality.

Paranoia. A psychotic disorder very similar to paranoid schizophrenia, yet markedly different from it in some ways, is the rare condition known as true paranoia in which the personality disorganization of the victim is limited to a persistent and consistent delusion, usually of persecution; sometimes delusions of grandeur are also present, but there may be little else in the way of overt evidence of mental breakdown. In the classical form of true paranoia, uncomplicated by any other kind of mental illness, a complete and complex behavioral system may be built up in a perfectly logical way based on just one single false or delusional belief, in sharp contrast to the variable delusions and inconsistent behavior of the paranoid schizophrenic. In essence, the victim loses contact with only one aspect of reality, but if the delusion of persecution is intense and pervasive, all of his intellectual and emotional reactions are affected by it. In severe cases, he may be driven to commit a violently antisocial act to "protect himself" or "get even," and feel perfectly justified in doing so.

In less severe cases, paranoia may exist in a highly systematized form, yet its victims may never be suspected of mental illness. They may simply withdraw to protect themselves and become recluses, or their continual and persistent suspicions may be regarded as merely "eccentric." Other more aggressive paranoiacs may seem perfectly normal to all outward appearances, but spend their lives complaining bitterly of their "persecutors" or enter into an endless succession of groundless lawsuits. Varying degrees of paranoia can accompany almost any other kind of mental disturbance, and in its mildest form it is classified simply as a personality disorder. But the line that divides a personality disorder and a full-blown psychosis is very fine, and regrettably, it is often only after the paranoiac has crossed that line and committed some

destructive or criminal act that the condition and the necessity for hospitalization and treatment are recognized. In its earlier and milder forms, paranoia may be amenable to the various techniques of therapeutic treatment, but in more severe cases the delusion is so firmly entrenched that the true paranoiac is virtually impossible to reach and recovery from the condition is extremely rare.

Manic-Depressive Psychosis. A third form of severe mental illness which, like schizophrenia, occurs most frequently between the ages of fifteen and thirty-five, is the manic-depressive psychosis, a condition characterized by unpredictable and exaggerated swings of mood back and forth between the highly excited, euphoric, irrepressibly enthusiastic heights of mania to the blackest depths of hopeless depression. Everyone may have "moods," of course, and feel bright and chipper one day and dull and blue the next. In the normal person such variations in mood are appropriate to the changing circumstances of his life, but if elation or depression, or more rarely an unpredictable fluctuation between the two, comes to dominate the personality, whatever the circumstances, the behavioral patterns that typify the so-called cycloid personality are established. Again, the line between the cycloid personality disorder and the true manic-depressive psychosis can be extremely fine. The cycloid may be generally elated or depressed, or subject to comparatively mild variations in mood, and still be able to lead a reasonably well-adjusted life. In the manic-depressive, however, contact with the real world is lost, and the mood, almost always of exaggerated length and intensity, takes over completely, dominating his every thought and action. In the manic phase of the illness the victim behaves with such frantic enthusiasm that no one can keep up with him. He may talk, criticize, argue endlessly, hopping from one idea to the next in bewildering succession. Often he is physically overactive, frenziedly busy, undertaking ambitious or impractical projects and then abruptly dropping them, singing, shouting to passers-by, making indecent proposals to people in the highest good humor, far too excited to eat, sleep or rest. These manic episodes may terminate in total physical exhaustion only to recur, and unless the victim is restrained, his rash and irresponsible behavior may lead to serious difficulties for his family and friends, and to the victim himself.

The other side of the coin, and the more frequent form of the illness, is the depressive stage, which may be mild, acute and short-lived, or abysmally black and prolonged. The victim undergoes a massive withdrawal; he may scarcely speak or move and is consumed by feelings of guilt and worthlessness. Deep depression is also a prominent feature of other forms of mental illness, particularly schizophrenia, but in the true depressive it is especially dangerous, for he is perfectly capable of acting on his feelings and taking his own life.

Individual cases of the manic-depressive psychosis vary; some may consist of single or recurring manic episodes with little depression, whereas others may be predominantly depressive. In either case, this form of mental illness is one which very often improves and disappears of its own accord, although it may recur, and is somewhat more amenable to treatment than schizophrenia. Untreated, a manic attack may last five or six months, and a depressive attack as long as a year or more. Tranquilizing drugs to control the excitement of the manic phase, and antidepressant drugs and central nervous system stimulants to terminate a spell of psychotic depression, have proved extremely effective in treatment. In especially severe cases, electroshock therapy may also be used in conjunction with medication, and extensive psychotherapy is usually essential to help the patient establish more realistic patterns of behavior. During the recovery phase from an episode of this psychosis, however, family members must be aware that the danger of suicide continues to exist, particularly as the psychotic symptoms seem to subside, and careful observation is necessary during convalescence.

Involutional Melancholia. One other form of psychotic disorder tends to occur in older people, from the late forties into the sixties, and is still known by the rather quaint, old-fashioned term "involutional melancholia." And that is exactly what the disease is: a psychotic state in which the individual's anxiety and agitation are characterized by an involution or "turning inward" of feelings, worries, or delusions combined with a pervading sense of helpless melancholy. This state in a woman may be triggered by menopause and the loss of her childbearing potential, sometimes interpreted by her as symbolic of the end of her worth and desirability; in a man it may be stimulated by the waning of physical and sexual vigor, and a sense that time is passing him by. In both, the disorder may begin with intermittent spells of weariness, pessimism, irritability, insomnia, and sometimes episodes of weeping unrelated to any specific cause. As the melancholy deepens, the victim becomes depressed, anxious, preoccupied with his health and obsessed with delusions of his worthlessness or his impending death, often expressing guilt feelings about early, and usually minor, indiscretions. Hallucinations may occur, often in the form of reproving or punishing voices, and there is often apprehension because of ideas of impending destruction. Depression can become the blackest imaginable, and there is no other psychotic disorder in which suicide is attempted so frequently or so seriously.

Ordinarily patients with involutional psychosis are best treated at a mental or neuropsychiatric hospital, not only because of the threat of suicide, but because of the need for constant observation to assure that they are eating properly and getting adequate sleep and exercise. For many years this psychosis was recognized as the one from which the highest percentages of victims might ultimately recover spontaneously; some 40 to 45 percent would finally emerge from their depression with nothing but supportive and protective care, although recovery might not occur for two or three years. When electroshock therapy was first introduced, it proved notably successful in speeding up recovery; as many as 80 or 90 percent of the victims of this disease were found to respond favorably to electroshock treatment and recover far more quickly than would otherwise have been expected. And this is still the treatment of choice if intensive drug therapy with the powerful antidepressant medications and central nervous system stimulants proves ineffective or inadequate in relieving the disorder.

Changing Attitudes Toward Mental Health

In many ways we know little more about the true nature of mental disorders than we did three hundred years ago, but at least in recent decades there has been a welcome and far too long delayed change in social attitudes toward mental illness. With the pioneering work of Freud, his contemporaries and his followers, and with the rise of modern psychiatry as an important medical specialty, we have become, if anything, too preoccupied with healthy and "normal" emotional reactions and relationships and "adjusting" those that seem unhealthy or abnormal. But at least the severe forms of mental illness are no longer swept under the rug, thanks to these social changes, and there is reason to hope that one day victims of mental disorders will be treated with the same solicitude and care as the victims of other illnesses.

One aspect of these changing attitudes is the widespread recognition that a healthy mind is just as important as a healthy body, and that it is just as appropriate—and important—to seek to prevent the ravages of external stress and internal conflict, whenever possible, as it is to protect the body from physical breakdown. Furthermore, people have come to recognize the extreme importance of the developmental stages of infancy and childhood, that seedbed of mental and emotional disorder, and the necessity of providing the child with the essentials for his emotional and intellectual growth and security as well as his physical growth and development, whether at home, in school or in his environment. People have also come to recognize what it means to be "human"—the simple fact that no one is ideally perfect or perfectly normal, and that everyone has emotions that require expression and, when they cause conflicts, resolution as well. Perhaps most important of all, people have come to recognize that having emotional problems does not necessarily imply mental illness. Emotional problems are the common lot of mankind, and they can be serious, breaking up marriages, disturbing families and causing unimaginable grief and pain. Seeking help for such problems, whether through the counsel of doctors, psychiatrists, priests or ministers, or through contact with social agencies, need not be considered an admission of mental disturbance. But some emotional problems can and do occasionally expand into more serious mental disorders, and when they do they must be recognized and treated.

When a disturbance arises in a child or adolescent, the parent must be responsible for recognizing that something is wrong and take steps to correct it. Sudden alterations in a child's behavior, apparent personality changes, tendencies to withdraw into silent noncommunication, or the appearance of extremes of rebelliousness may provide clues to possible trouble. Frequently the schools may be better able to recognize developing problems than parents; regular communication with a child's teachers is vastly important in assessing possible emotional disturbances. In adults, recognition of possible mental disorders must be their own responsibility, or that of spouses, other family members or friends. In elderly people, recognition again may depend upon relatives or children. But at whatever age, if suspicion of mental illness arises, it is essential that someone take action, and the *right* action. The advice of amateur analysts or well-meaning friends must be avoided, as well as the services of faddists and the mental-health quacks who proliferate in our society.

In many cases the place to start in seeking professional help is with the family doctor—but here one must be careful not to expect too much. Many physicians, preoccupied with the diagnosis and treatment of physical ills, are not widely experienced in treating severe mental disorders. In most cases, however, the family physician can at least recognize a mental disorder, help rule out the presence of any organic mental disfunction, and then arrange a proper referral with a psychiatrist, or with one of the mental health agencies, public or private, that stand ready to help. Many university health centers, for example, have facilities for testing and evaluating the mental performance of children, and the staff of such a center may include psychiatrists skilled in dealing with mental disorders in children, social workers experienced in child guidance, or psychologists who are trained in recognizing behavior disorders and equipped to measure a child's behavior against standards of normal and recommend programs of observation or corrective treatment. In addition, most large communities today have competent professionals skilled in marriage counseling, family therapy, occupational guidance and other specialties. Recently there has even been a proliferation of business, religious or social groups that get together for the purpose of discussing their problems and "letting off steam." But before joining any such group one should be certain that its activities are being guided by a competent professional in psychology, psychiatry, social work or behavioral counseling. It is just as ridiculous to allow inexperienced amateurs to tamper with the mind and emotions as it would be to let an amateur take out an appendix.

Far too many families faced with the suspicion that some member is the victim of a serious mental disturbance try to ignore it, temporize with it or seek to handle it themselves, often aggravating the illness and seriously upsetting their own lives as a result. No approach could be more foolish; and the more serious and disabling the disturbance, the more important it is to seek proper psychiatric advice. When commitment to an institution for psychiatric treatment is necessary, legal advice may be necessary as well. The decision to commit a mentally disturbed patient to an institution is a delicate one from which many families shrink. Certainly commitment proceedings can be abused, when, for example, a family simply wishes to get rid of an "incompetent" oldster or gain his power of attorney, but there are many cases in which commitment is not only best for the patient but often the only way that psychiatric help can be obtained. Abuse today is far less common than even a few decades ago; the insane *do* have rights that are recognized by psychiatrists and legal authorities alike. But when commitment is necessary, and undertaken only with the best advice and in the patient's best interests, there is no reason to draw back from it.

When the victim of a mental disturbance is institutionalized for treatment, either voluntarily or through commitment, this is by no means the end of the family's responsibility. When a choice of institution is possible, this should be carefully investigated. Then once the patient is hospitalized it is the family's responsibility to visit him as frequently as the psychiatrist thinks appropriate, keep check on his progress and prepare for the day when he may come home. When discharge is possible, it is well to remember that mental illnesses are no different from physical illnesses in that they may require very specialized forms of supportive treatment at home during convalescence, as well as care to prevent recurrence when that is possible. Continuing competent psychiatric counseling will help set any guidelines necessary for convalescence and later preventive home care. It is true that care of the mentally ill in this country is not all that could be desired; institutions are overcrowded and understaffed, and those who have been hospitalized for mental disturbance are still socially stigmatized. It is the concern of everyone that these inadequacies and injustices be corrected, but it should be the special concern of those who have encountered the frightening and disorganizing experience of mental illness in their own lives or families.

Unfortunately, for all of the study and work that has been done in regard to psychoneurotic and psychotic illnesses, there is still no consistently reliable treatment that can cure these conditions. We do not even completely understand what the relationship is between the mind, the personality and the body in these illnesses, nor where the "ultimate pathology" is to be found. In recent years more and more evidence has accumulated to suggest that there may be some chemical or biochemical basis for certain of the psychoses, particularly for schizophrenia. The fact that certain drugs such as LSD, mescaline, the amphetamines, even marijuana to a limited extent, can temporarily induce hallucinations and other symptoms uncomfortably similar to those seen in acute schizophrenic reactions has presented researchers with the tantalizing prospect that psychosis or even psychoneurosis may not necessarily occur solely as a result of psychological or emotional disturbances, but may have some chemical cause which, once identified, might be corrected and the disease cured. Could schizophrenia basically result from some genetic flaw in the biochemistry of the brain? Could it be, perhaps, a hereditary trait which predisposes certain individuals to the risk of personality disintegration under certain kinds of stress? We do not yet have the answers to these questions, but certainly the war against disease cannot be considered over until answers to the mysteries of mental illness have finally been found. In the meantime, we can at least feel confident that progress is being made, and that more victims of these diseases are ultimately able to return to their homes and some semblance of normal life than ever before in man's history.

XIV

THE TRYING TIMES OF LIFE

57. Progressing Through Pregnancy   811

58. The New Baby   850

59. The Childhood Years   867

60. Adolescence and How to Live with It   899

61. The Prime Years   909

62. The Hazards of Middle Age   926

63. Aging and Death   944

Until quite recently, physicians have usually been regarded as "healers," and the diagnosis and treatment of illness are certainly the primary functions of all the medical professions. But doctors today are vested with another equally important responsibility: the *prevention* of illness before it occurs. Disease prevention is not solely the doctor's responsibility, however; it must also depend on the active and continuing cooperation of the patient. Everyone has come to realize that this kind of doctor-patient cooperation is essential to a long and healthy life, but it is particularly important during certain "trying times" when the human body may be vulnerable to a number of unique health hazards. These hazards may never evolve into actual illness at all; they are, in general, simply part of the normal patterns of human life, starting with pregnancy when life begins and passing through successive stages of development in infancy, childhood, adolescence, maturity, middle and old age. During each of these stages certain physical and psychological problems may arise which are not precisely illnesses, but which can nevertheless be puzzling and possibly even a threat to continuing good health. In dealing with such problems the physician must rely not only on his professional skills but also on his understanding and personal concern for his patient. The patient, in turn, must have the knowledge and foresight to anticipate these problems and, in cooperation with the doctor, take the proper preventive measures. Then, and only then, can preventive health care at every age be truly effective.

Progressing Through Pregnancy

Of all the medical specialists, probably none has a more singularly satisfying group of patients than the obstetrician. They are, for the most part, healthy young women who have never been more physically fit—or happier—in their lives. Their condition is not an "illness" at all, even though minor discomforts and annoyances may occur during any pregnancy. Many women, for example, are uncomfortable with the breast engorgement and nipple enlargement that accompany pregnancy. Morning sickness is no delight for anyone, and as pregnancy advances, weight control and fluid retention frequently become nagging problems. That "pregnant look" may prove awkward for some, and inevitably, at term, there are the discomforts of labor and delivery. But all of these are a normal part of being pregnant, and while pregnancy makes exceptional demands, both physically and psychologically, most women are admirably equipped to handle them.

Why, then, are obstetricians or other experienced doctors needed to care for pregnancies? Simply because pregnancy can, on occasion, involve certain dangerous hazards which may arise swiftly with or without warning at any time along the way, and an experienced doctor must be ready to act immediately and knowledgeably to protect not only one life but two. Fortunately, these hazards are rare, and until the time of delivery, the doctor acts chiefly as a consultant and adviser. In his role as a watchful guardian, however, his best ally is obviously the patient herself and her knowledge of what will happen during her pregnancy, particularly what she should consider normal and what should be a cause for concern. Yet for all that has been written, many women know little of even the most fundamental aspects of pregnancy and childbirth. Worse yet, their heads filled with half-truths and the advice of well-meaning friends, many approach pregnancy and delivery with fear, and fear is the worst enemy of all.

Of course some degree of apprehension is inevitable as a woman faces her first pregnancy, but with knowledge and understanding, that apprehension almost always proves to be groundless. Modern medicine has made great strides in minimizing any discomfort and pain, as well as in diagnosing particular problems and preventing unexpected complications. But ultimately the successful progress of a pregnancy depends upon the woman herself, and the creation of a new life is surely one of the most wonderful and rewarding experiences a woman can have.

Pregnant or Not Pregnant?

Technically, a potential pregnancy begins the instant a living male sperm penetrates a mature, living female ovum to create a single "fertilized egg"—a momentary encounter called *conception*. This can, of course, occur only after *ovulation,* when the ovum manufactured in the female ovary is released and enters the long, narrow *Fallopian tube* to begin its passage down toward the cavity of the uterus. In most cases the meeting between sperm and ovum occurs in the

Fallopian tube, and after a brief interval the newly fertilized ovum then begins to divide and redivide, becoming an *embryo*. This potential pregnancy becomes a true, viable pregnancy within two to five days thereafter, when the growing embryo reaches the uterine cavity and lodges in the specially prepared lining of the uterus in the process called *implantation*.

By its very nature, the precise moment of conception cannot be determined. The sperm, normally deposited by the man in the woman's vagina during sexual intercourse, is highly motile and may remain alive for 24 hours or longer in the female reproductive tract. Thus chances for conception are very good as long after ovulation as a ripened ovum survives—a matter of 24 to 48 hours. Indeed, complete sexual union is not even necessary for conception to take place. Sperm are quite active enough to find their way into the vagina and travel upward following mere surface contact of the external genitalia.

The point is that conception takes place silently, without fanfare, perhaps many hours after sexual contact and with no immediately detectable physical or biochemical effects. Even the woman's fertile period—the two-day interval after ovulation has occurred—is often difficult to pin down exactly. Some women do have a distinct, measurable change in their basic body temperatures, a matter of a few tenths of a degree, at the time of ovulation, but for many even this is difficult to measure for certain, and most women are quite unable to guess, except within a span of days, just when they might be able to conceive. Thus, the beginning of a pregnancy is inevitably a *fait accompli* for a matter of days or even weeks before there is any way to determine for sure that it has in fact occurred.

And as silently as it begins, a pregnancy may also silently end. It is impossible to determine how many potential new pregnancies perish within the first brief hours after conception, before the fertilized ovum can become safely implanted in the uterus. Certainly a great many do. Fertilization may occur at a time when one germ cell or the other has already become too old or weak to sustain development. Even a healthy conception may fail to implant properly in the uterine lining, or some other condition may interfere with implantation or development. In any event, the fertilized egg—or even a tiny bundle of embryonic cells—may be expelled without a sign that new life ever flickered. But what about pregnancies that do survive and begin healthy new growth? Curiously enough, even these remain undetectable for a time. In most cases the first hint a woman has that she may be pregnant is the unexpected failure to menstruate at the usual time.

Pregnancy and Menses. The menstrual cycle is regulated by the female sex hormones—primarily *estrogen* and *progesterone*—which are produced and secreted into the woman's blood stream by the ovaries and adrenals under the influence of another hormone secreted by the pituitary, all "ductless" or *endocrine glands*. These hormones, acting in delicate balance, stimulate the growth and maturation of an ovum in one of the ovaries and then trigger ovulation. But the chain of events that culminates in the onset of menstrual flow actually begins much earlier. By the time of ovulation, the uterus, again in response to the action of the sex hormones, has developed a thick interior lining of epithelial tissue, rich in blood vessels and glands, to prepare a place for the ovum to implant and to grow if it should be fertilized. Usually, of course, this advance preparation is unnecessary; the ovum is not fertilized, and it subsequently deteriorates and is expelled. In such a case, the uterine lining begins to break down as its rich blood supply is curtailed by the action of the sex hormones. Presently, approximately 10 days after the "expected" conception fails to take place, fragments of the uterine lining, together with serum and some blood, are expelled in the normal menstrual flow. Then a few days later, again under the influence of the sex hormones, a new uterine lining begins to develop in preparation for the next ovulation and "expected" conception. (The role of the sex hormones in regulating menstruation and reproductive function is discussed in greater detail on p. 686 and p. 748.)

This menstrual cycle, with its succession of hormonal "triggers," is an orderly sequence which normally occurs over and over, from puberty through menopause, at regular intervals of 24 to 28 days. The cycle is broken when an ovum is fertilized and a pregnancy begins. Then, with the embryo implanted in the uterus, the uterine lining does not break down, and the next regular menstrual flow does not occur. Obviously, if every menstrual cycle were identical, and if a new pregnancy were the *only* thing that could disturb it and cause menses to cease, there would be no source of confusion. A missed period would be presumptive evidence of pregnancy, and a woman would need only to wait for the confirming evidence of the other physical changes that accompany the early stages of pregnancy.

But the fact is that every menstrual cycle is *not* identical among women in general or even in individual women. Some women are markedly irregular, with frequent delays in onset, while others may have periods beginning several days earlier than expected. Furthermore, conditions other than pregnancy can delay menstrual periods or cause them to be missed altogether. Thyroid gland disorders and other diseases, for instance, can lead to delayed periods with scanty flow, or even cause periods to be missed. Cysts, tumors or other disorders of the ovaries can also cause menstrual irregularity or even temporary cessation of menses. Even severe emotional upsets can occasionally have a disturbing effect on the menstrual cycle. Thus a missed menstrual period can be regarded only as "suggestive evidence" that a pregnancy has occurred, not as definite proof.

In many cases, of course, there is no need for positive early confirmation of pregnancy. A woman who has missed a menstrual period and thinks she is probably pregnant can assume that she is until proven otherwise and just wait expectantly for other physical signs—particularly morning sickness and breast engorgement—to confirm the assumption. But in other cases early confirmation of pregnancy may be highly desirable. A woman who has had previous early miscarriages should report any possibility of pregnancy to her doctor without delay, since special medication can be prescribed to help her body maintain a pregnancy. Other women may want their suspicions of pregnancy confirmed as soon as possible for purely social and personal reasons. For whatever reason, the prospect of having a baby can hardly be ignored, and a variety of laboratory and clinical tests have been devised to help confirm early pregnancy.

Hormone Withdrawal Tests. Since these tests are designed essentially to stimulate the onset of normal menstrual flow if a pregnancy is *not* present, they should perhaps be called "nonpregnancy tests." Simple to perform, inexpensive, and quite harmless to the embryo in the event that a pregnancy is present, these tests are widely employed because they afford reliable proof that a woman is *not* pregnant earlier than any other kind of test. Special hormone medications are given to the patient, either by injection or by mouth, for a period of some three days. At that point abrupt withdrawal of the medication will often trigger a delayed menstrual period. Since these hormones are those that normally regulate the menstrual cycle, their use in this fashion cannot harm a new pregnancy; if anything, they would help sustain it. Furthermore, the test can be performed within a few *days* of a missed menstrual period. If menstruation begins, of course, the question is settled: the woman is not pregnant. If menstruation is not stimulated, additional tests are necessary to definitely confirm pregnancy.

The Pregnant Urine Tests. These are true pregnancy tests, depending upon the appearance in a woman's body of certain special "hormones of pregnancy" which are produced *only* when a new pregnancy is present and well implanted. Such hormones first begin to appear very early, but are present in the woman's blood stream and excreted in her urine in measurable quantities only two to three weeks after conception—about a week after the first missed period. Until recently such laboratory animals as rabbits, mice or frogs were used in the performance of these pregnancy tests, but today simple and speedy test-tube measurements of the hormones of pregnancy, especially the one known as *chorionic gonadotrophin,* are usually performed and can identify a new pregnancy as early as within 10 days of a missed menstrual period if the period is missed because a pregnancy is present. These new testing methods are not only less costly than the old laboratory animal tests, but also avoid the "false positive" results that so frequently plagued the older testing methods.

Prenatal Care: The Doctor-Patient Team

Probably there is no other time in life when a close, cooperative doctor-patient relationship is more important than when a woman finally knows that she is unmistakably pregnant. Ideally, of course, a woman should consult a doctor *before* undertaking a pregnancy, in order to be as certain as possible that her health is in topnotch condition and to determine ahead of time if there are any factors that might make a pregnancy inadvisable. Certain conditions—for example, the presence of diabetes mellitus, a history of a recent German measles infection, a history of serious Rh problems with past pregnancies, a family history of hereditary diseases, even a history of distressing emotional or marital problems—might militate against a pregnancy or involve special circumstances that must be prepared for in advance. Once pregnancy has been confirmed, the watchful guidance of a physician is especially important during the early months when a variety of problems may arise. If the doctor who helped confirm the pregnancy customarily handles obstetrical cases, he may offer to undertake the prenatal care, or if not he may recommend a specialist who will.

Once an attending physician has been decided upon, the program of prenatal care begins in earnest. The first step is a careful and complete physical examination, with special attention to potential trouble spots—the breasts, the pelvic area including an examination of the positioning of the uterus, any previous medical or surgical history that might affect the pregnancy, a thorough history of all previous pregnancies and deliveries, and a review of the family history to detect any hereditary factors that might be important. As a part of this initial examination, blood tests and blood typing are done with special attention to the Rh factor of the mother (*see* p. 833) as well as a complete urine analysis. A blood test to determine immunity to rubella (German measles) is also done at this time, so special precautions can be taken

to protect the nonimmune patient. With this groundwork for prenatal care established, the physician then outlines the pattern of office visits he considers necessary throughout the rest of the pregnancy—usually at least one visit per month during the first six months, with increasingly frequent visits thereafter as the time for delivery approaches—and discusses those items that are chiefly the patient's responsibility. Most physicians, for example, advise careful attention to diet, with emphasis on protein and iron-rich foods in sufficient quantity to maintain both mother and fetus in good health without taking on excess calories or gaining excess weight, which can cause serious complications. If a woman is considering "natural childbirth," (*see* p. 839) she should let her doctor know at this point. In most cases the patient is advised to continue a normal pattern of work and exercise, as well as normal sex relations, until the terminal six or eight weeks of the pregnancy. Although very moderate use of tobacco, alcohol or coffee has no direct deleterious effect on a pregnancy, many doctors urge their pregnant patients to use the necessary self-discipline of the prenatal period as a golden opportunity to stop smoking permanently and to reduce any habitual use of alcohol or coffee to a bare minimum. What is more, any woman even contemplating pregnancy should avoid using *any* drugs not specifically prescribed by her physician. Finally, the attending doctor will make certain his patient understands the cardinal danger signs which must be called to his attention any time they appear: abdominal pain, vaginal bleeding or spotting, pain or burning upon urination, or any evidence of cramping, for example. Obviously, the whole purpose of setting forth a prenatal care program early in the pregnancy is to help ensure as normal and trouble-free a pregnancy as possible, as well as to anticipate any complications before they occur. Then, during later prenatal visits, the patient can be instructed in what to expect as the time of labor and delivery approaches. Many obstetricians today, recognizing that parenthood involves the father as well as the mother even though the mother carries the major prenatal burden, also make arrangements to consult with the father prior to delivery time, and some doctors even conduct classes or seminars for husbands and wives together, not only to explain what happens during a pregnancy, but also to help prepare prospective parents for the broader range of physical and emotional problems that may arise after the baby is born.

The Expected Date of Confinement

Once the fact of pregnancy has been positively established, the next and most obvious question is: When? The time the new baby is due to arrive is often called the "expected date of confinement" or EDC. It is important as a "target date," of course, but it should not be taken too literally. Unfortunately, a precise EDC can never be pinned down with accuracy. It is usually impossible to determine precisely when conception took place, and to further confuse the issue, some women carry a child a few days or even weeks longer than the "average" gestation period, while others may go into labor prematurely. Thus an EDC is merely an educated guess of the baby's arrival date, based upon an "average" term of pregnancy; but in most cases, on the average, the baby can be expected within a few days before or after the estimated date.

When a new pregnancy is confirmed, the expectant mother can use a simple rule of thumb to estimate the approximate due date—the same rule the doctor uses. Babies, on the average, require about 280 days of growth and development between the time of conception and the time of birth—approximately 9 calendar months or about 40 weeks. Since it is difficult to use an event that did *not* happen—a missed menstrual period—as a basis for measurement, the date of the beginning of the *last normal menstrual period* is determined, 10 months are added, and 14 days are then subtracted. The resulting date falls in the middle of a two-week period during which the baby will *probably* arrive—a simple calculation that is accurate at least 95 percent of the time.

This rule-of-thumb calculation works out well in most cases—but not always. Some women simply do not know when their last normal menstrual period was. Perhaps they do not remember, but in some cases a woman may have a certain amount of vaginal bleeding that resembles menstrual flow at period time during the first and even the second month after conception, with a new pregnancy well established. Ordinarily, when this "postconception spotting" occurs, it is very slight and has no significance; but in some women it can be heavy enough to be confused with a menstrual period, and thus upset due-date calculations. When this happens, or when the time of the last normal menstrual period cannot definitely be established, the doctor must reevaluate the expected date of confinement as the pregnancy progresses in light of other signs of the baby's growth and development.

The First Trimester

Once pregnancy has been established, doctors usually find it convenient to divide the gestation period into three trimesters, each approximately three months or 13 weeks long. Each of these periods is characterized by definite patterns in the growth and development of the baby, and by certain changes in the mother; each is also associated with certain distinctive problems, annoyances and potential hazards.

The development of the embryo during the first trimester is truly astounding; within an interval of just 13 weeks a single cell—the fertilized ovum—evolves into a miraculously complex new organism approximately 3½ inches long with recognizable legs, arms and human features, and with virtually all the organ systems already developed in miniature and rudimentary form. Within 24 hours after conception the fertilized ovum, usually still moving down the Fallopian tube to the uterus, divides first into two cells, then progressively into four, eight and sixteen to form a still-microscopic solid mass of cells by the end of approximately four days. Three days later these have multiplied still further, to form a sort of hollow, fluid-filled ball which has by then become firmly buried or implanted in the soft vascular tissue lining the interior of the uterus, with cells from that uterine lining growing over it to cover and protect it. By the end of approximately eleven days, another remarkable change has taken place in the tiny embryo: one group of large cells has developed into a cluster in the center of the fluid space—the future fetus itself—while other embryonic cells have begun to form an enclosing sac of membranes around it. In addition, a stalk of cells—the primitive *umbilical cord*—has formed leading from the new organism to a special pad of cells in contact with, but still separate from, the wall of the uterus—the rudimentary *placenta* through which the new baby will continue to absorb nutrients from the mother's blood stream until the actual moment of birth.

Thus, remarkably enough, within two weeks following conception the stage is set for the entire future development of the new baby. During subsequent weeks in the first trimester the cells of the embryo divide and differentiate, first into three layers that will form the nervous system and skin, the bones and muscle, and the gastrointestinal tract, respectively, and then into the

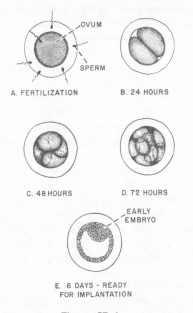

Figure 57–1.

rudimentary organs themselves, while the placenta and umbilical cord continue their development. By 4½ weeks the brain, jaw and heart have all begun to differentiate, and arm and leg

buds have formed; by the end of 8 weeks facial features have appeared, rudimentary arms and legs have formed, skeletal muscles and bones have begun their early development, and arteries

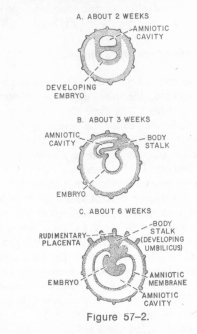

Figure 57–2.

and veins are differentiated. It is at this time that the new organism, still only 1½ inches long, leaves the embryonic stage of development and becomes a *fetus,* complete with recognizable human form and features. During the remaining five weeks of the first trimester the fetus continues to develop both in size, to a length of 3½ inches or so, and in refinement of virtually all its rudimentary organs.

During this first trimester of pregnancy a variety of changes also take place in the mother's body, some very marked, some so subtle as to be barely noticeable. Most of these changes are induced by the special hormones produced in the cells of the ovary after ovulation, and by the newly developed placenta—the bed of richly vascular tissue evolved from embryonic cells to provide the major physical point of contact between mother and baby during gestation. Many of these changes are of no serious medical concern; they are simply part of the process by which the mother's body prepares to feed and sustain the baby both before and after his birth. First of all, ovulation and menstruation cease, to resume only after the baby has been born. The mother's blood supply in-

THE EMBRYO AT 7 WEEKS

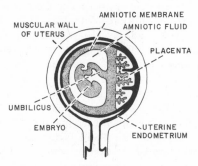

Figure 57–3.

creases as much as 20 percent during the first trimester in order to carry sufficient nutrients and oxygen to supply the baby as well as herself. The breasts normally enlarge during this period, as the milk-producing glands and ducts begin to develop in preparation for the beginning of lactation, even though actual milk secretion must await hormonal signals following delivery. The nipples also become larger, darker and more prominent, and the tiny glands around the base of the nipples become larger.

Other symptoms and signs of early pregnancy may be less noticeable. The mucous membrane of the vagina, for example, takes on a bluish color owing to increased arterial circulation in the pelvis and early impairment of drainage of venous blood from the area because of the increasing pressure of the enlarging uterus against the pelvic veins. At the same time there is often a colorless vaginal discharge resulting from increased vaginal secretions. Toward the end of the first trimester the mother will notice the first signs of abdominal enlargement and will also become aware of increased frequency of urination because of the pressure of the uterus on the bladder. Finally, many woman experience curious cravings for unusual foods, as transitory as they are peculiar, and may also be bothered by minor emotional disturbances, their moods swinging erratically from fits of exuberance to

mild depression and back at unpredictable intervals. None of these things has any alarming significance; they are a normal part of pregnancy. But another phenomenon of early pregnancy, equally normal, may become acutely annoying and require medication.

Morning Sickness. Strictly speaking, the term is inaccurate, because "morning sickness" does not necessarily occur only in the morning. Some women experience it only when retiring at night, while others may be bothered with it off and on all day. In most cases it is one of the earliest suggestive signs of pregnancy, most commonly occurs upon arising, and is often triggered by the smell of cooking food. Whenever it occurs, it is characterized by a wave of retching and vomiting which may begin with embarrassingly little warning. Some women notice morning sickness only once or twice, if at all, while others may experience it more or less daily from the second or third week of pregnancy through the end of the third month or early in the fourth. In perhaps 50 percent of all pregnancies it becomes irritating enough to require treatment.

The simplest means of control is to confine the morning meal to a cup of tea and a piece of dry toast, postponing heavier meals until later in the day. Many obstetricians seek preventive control by prescribing small doses of various effective *antiemetic medications* to be taken routinely during the vulnerable period. These preparations may not completely obliterate the symptoms, and may result in a bit of sleepiness as a side effect, but they will usually keep morning sickness under reasonable control until it finally disappears. The annoyance often vanishes so quietly that it is hardly noticed; the expectant mother awakens one morning and realizes that it has been a week or more since she was last bothered. And once gone, morning sickness is unlikely to recur.

In a very few cases the problem becomes more serious; simple measures do not control it, and the patient may suffer repeated episodes of vomiting, day after day, to the point of severe disability. Obviously, such a development is decidedly *not* normal, and the doctor should be consulted immediately. Sometimes conditions other than pregnancy can cause this so-called pernicious vomiting and must be diagnosed and corrected. A woman may develop a vicious circle of gastrointestinal irritation, so that all food intake must be stopped for a brief interval until the cycle can be broken. On rare occasions, pernicious vomiting may require a brief period of hospitalization and use of more potent medications for control. Even more rarely the vomiting may become so intractable that the obstetrician must consider termination of the pregnancy to protect the mother's life. Such extremes are most unusual and can normally be prevented by dealing vigorously with morning sickness the moment it becomes anything more than a minor annoyance.

The Hazard of Miscarriage. One of the most serious problems that can arise during the first trimester of pregnancy is the threat of miscarriage or, to use the medical term, *spontaneous abortion*. Ordinarily, when the embryo implants in the uterine lining, within a matter of weeks a special sustaining organ called the *placenta* is formed to carry nutrients and oxygen to the embryo from the mother's blood stream via the umbilical cord, and to return the new baby's waste products to the mother's blood stream for disposal. When delivery time comes, the placenta, by then a large and well-developed pad of spongy tissue and blood vessels, becomes detached from the interior of the uterus and is expelled as the "afterbirth."

The blood vessels of the placenta are not connected directly with the mother's, but instead simply lie side by side. Even so, once the embryo is firmly implanted, it is usually very secure and not easily dislodged or damaged. The widespread idea that a blow to the abdomen, or a sudden shock or fall, may cause a miscarriage is not generally valid; it would take a severe blow indeed to injure or dislodge a well-implanted pregnancy. But an embryo is not always well implanted, or it may fail to survive the first critical three months for other reasons. As a consequence, a surprising number of new pregnancies are lost during the first trimester.

There are some women, in fact, who seem to have great difficulty retaining any pregnancy at all, tending to miscarry again and again, through no fault of their own, a condition called *habitual*

abortion. Some anatomical irregularity of the mother may cause repeated miscarriages, or occasionally an endocrine disorder may be at fault, but in most cases there is no specific cause for this condition. In recent decades a number of new medicines have been developed which help support healthy pregnancies and tend to prevent spontaneous abortion. With their help, many women who had given up all hope of ever carrying a baby to term have succeeded, and these same medicines can be used to counteract a threatened miscarriage.

But miscarriage is not restricted to a few women afflicted with habitual abortion. It can happen to any woman, carrying any pregnancy, for no apparent reason. In fact, statistics show that one-third of all women who become pregnant have at least one *identified* spontaneous abortion at some time during their childbearing years. And this is a very conservative figure; since many spontaneous abortions must occur so early in the pregnancy that they are not even recognized as miscarriages, the experience is almost certainly more widespread than the statistics indicate.

Whatever the cause of a spontaneous abortion, it only rarely occurs suddenly or without advance warning. Usually the first symptom is the onset of cramping in the lower abdomen, often more annoying than painful. This may persist for several hours or even a day or two, intermittently, before the woman notices spotting of bright red blood from the vagina. Occasionally a brief episode of severe cramping is followed almost immediately by spotting, frank bleeding or the passage of fragments of tissue. When this occurs the doctor should be notified at once, and the tissue fragments carefully saved for his examination. In any case, the occurrence of even a small amount of vaginal bleeding must be regarded as a grave sign during the first trimester, and the doctor should be called at once, day or night. At this early stage of a *threatened abortion*, the embryo may yet be alive and healthy, and prompt treatment may help turn the tide. But the doctor also knows that if the miscarriage progresses, dangerous hemorrhage may follow. The more time he has to prepare for any exigency, the better.

The first step in combating a threatened abortion is absolute bed rest. It can be vital for the mother's protection as well as the baby's, since any physical activity, even an increase in heartbeat due to excitement or apprehension, can exaggerate the threat of losing the pregnancy. The doctor will usually prescribe a potent sedative to further curb physical activity and will examine his patient to determine, as accurately as possible, how far the threatened miscarriage has progressed. Up to a certain point, there is still a chance that the pregnancy may be saved; but once the cervix of the uterus begins to dilate, or bits of embryonic tissue are passed, a stage is reached called *inevitable abortion,* a point of no return beyond which the pregnancy is certain to be lost, no matter what is done. The kind of further treatment he will prescribe depends upon how far things have gone. If hemorrhaging occurs, he stands ready to deal with it with the use of medications or even surgery when necessary.

As little as fifteen years ago, the obstetrician treating a patient with a threatened abortion had to rely upon bed rest and sedation alone; there were no *active* steps he could take to help prevent the miscarriage. Recently, however, it has been discovered that the administration of large doses of certain hormones normally produced in a woman's body early in a pregnancy may help materially in preserving a healthy pregnancy when spontaneous abortion threatens. These medicines cannot turn the tide if the embryonic placenta has already begun to detach from the inner wall of the uterus. Nor can they help preserve a malformed or otherwise physically handicapped pregnancy. But administered properly and early enough, it is thought that they may save healthy pregnancies, at least in some cases.

When a threatened abortion is treated successfully, by rest, sedation and hormone medication, the cramping ceases, the spotting or bleeding stops, and the mother can go home after two or three days to a period of limited activity, then gradually move back to normal activity if there is no evidence of recurring symptoms. When the hormone medications have been successful in helping overcome the crisis, the doctor will usually prescribe their continuing use in diminishing doses for a prolonged period, perhaps even until the mother actually feels the baby's first movements in the fourth or fifth month, or until the baby's heartbeat is audible in the stethoscope. In fact, these medicines have been so successful in preserving pregnancies that many obstetricians prescribe them for patients with past histories of habitual abortion; therapeutic doses are administered from the moment a new pregnancy is definitely confirmed, often with gratifying results. Ironically, these same hormone medications were found to have another effect when used by nonpregnant women. Taken in small doses geared to a woman's normal menstrual cycle, they suppress ovulation temporarily for as long as they are administered, and today they form the basic ingredients of the well-known Pill used to prevent or control pregnancies, and to increase chances of conception after withdrawal of medication. (*See* p. 919.)

In many cases preventive and supportive measures are unable to avert a threatened miscarriage. The fetus may already be dead or may have some grave developmental defect or abnormality that is incompatible with its survival; the placenta may already have begun to separate from the uterine wall, or some other irremediable changes may have taken place. When this occurs, cramping and bleeding continue in severity until the fetus, together with its surrounding or "decidual" tissue, is finally expelled. Sometimes this expulsion is *complete;* there is a brief period of severe cramping, perhaps with copious bleeding, then the bleeding falls off sharply and the cramping subsides. The tissue that is passed is then examined by the hospital pathologist; although the cause of the miscarriage can rarely be determined in this way, it can be determined whether or not the expulsion was complete. If it was, the patient can be released from the hospital to spend a few days in bed at home. The doctor will check her for any evidence of fever, continued bleeding or infection during the next 48 hours, then allow her to resume normal activities within another 48 hours if all goes well. Ordinarily the uterine cervix, which dilates during expulsion, returns to normal within a month. Most obstetricians advise patients recovering from a miscarriage to abstain from sexual relations for about six weeks. The healing uterus is very vulnerable to infection during this interval, but regular menstrual periods can be expected to resume within two to three months, and a new pregnancy can then be undertaken without threat.

However, in many spontaneous abortions, expulsion is *incomplete* and fragments of tissue are retained within the uterus. In such cases there is often continuing, even profuse, bleeding and cramping which persists until all the decidual tissue is finally expelled, or until the obstetrician intervenes surgically to remove the retained fragments. This procedure, done in the operating room under general anesthesia, is called *dilatation and currettage* (D and C) and is much the same operation performed when a biopsy of tissue from within the uterus is required for diagnostic purposes. (*See* p. 754.) A D and C performed after an incomplete abortion is a very brief procedure, undertaken with the greatest delicacy and care; the cervix is usually already dilated, and retained decidual tissue is gently removed with forceps, followed by a momentary currettement (scraping) of the uterus. All tissue removed in this fashion is submitted to the hospital pathologist to determine, if possible, the cause of the miscarriage and to rule out cancer as a contributing factor. The chief advantage of treating an incomplete miscarriage with a D and C is that it puts an end to any threat of hemorrhagic bleeding, and recovery is usually rapid. The postoperative course is much the same as that following a complete miscarriage, although surgical intervention slightly increases the risk of infection. Again, sexual relations are countermanded for approximately six weeks, and normal menstrual periods resume within two to three months. Today obstetricians recognize that even a very early pregnancy terminated by abortion can give rise to later Rh factor problems, so the Rh-negative woman who suffers a spontaneous abortion is now usually immunized against Rh antibodies as soon as the pregnancy is ended.

There are many obstetricians who elect to perform a D and C almost categorically after any spontaneous abortion, whether it appears to have been complete or not. These doctors contend that rarely, if ever, is all decidual tissue expelled, a certain risk of continued hemorrhage remains as long as tissue is retained, and on rare occasions retained decidual tissue has been known to develop into a type of malignant tumor known as a *chorioepithelioma*. Thus, although all obstetricians do not agree, many consider a D and C after a spontaneous abortion to be a necessary extra measure of protection.

A miscarriage early in pregnancy is almost always a disappointing turn of events for the prospective parents. It is quite natural to wonder why it happened, what they did wrong, what could have been done to prevent it, and if it will happen again. The mother, in particular, may blame herself, but it is important to realize that feelings of guilt and self-doubt are virtually always groundless. No one knows why the majority of miscarriages occur, but there is ample evidence to show that a healthy pregnancy is remarkably tenacious. Rarely, if ever, do physical activities, sexual relations or emotional reactions disturb it in the slightest. Perhaps the embryo failed to implant properly, or the developing fetus may have been defective in some way. There may have been some disturbance in the mother's body, completely beyond her control—a feverish illness or an endocrine gland disorder, for example, or an undetected diabetic condition. Whatever the reason, it need not necessarily happen again. It is far more common for a single miscarriage to occur in the midst of several healthy, undisturbed pregnancies than to have a succession of miscarriages. In short, a spontaneous abortion may be the end of a pregnancy, but it is not the end of all pregnancies. The first concern after a miscarriage should be the mother's physical recovery, and the diagnosis and treatment of any known contributing cause. Then, without recriminations and with renewed confidence, there is time to begin again.

Misplaced Pregnancies. Another problem of the first trimester of pregnancy occurs only rarely—perhaps only once in every 275 cases—but if it does occur it constitutes a true emergency that requires immediate treatment. It is an *ectopic* or misplaced pregnancy, commonly known as a tubal pregnancy.

The mature ovum is usually met by a sperm and fertilized while it is still passing down the Fallopian tube leading from the ovary to the uterus. Ordinarily, the fertilized egg continues its downward course and implants in the lining of the uterus, but on occasion it may become lodged somewhere in the tube and proceed to grow there. This is more likely to occur when a woman's tubes have been scarred as a result of a pelvic infection, but it also may occur without any history of previous pelvic disorder. Even more rarely, the developing embryo may implant on the ovary itself, or even somewhere in the lower abdomen completely outside the uterus. However, the term "ectopic pregnancy" covers all such misplaced pregnancies, whether they occur in a tube or not.

At first there is no clue that anything unusual has happened. The woman's menstrual periods cease, she can have morning sickness as with any pregnancy, and her body undergoes the same physical and hormonal changes one would expect if the embryo were implanted normally within the uterus. Her body even tries to accommodate the misplaced pregnancy: blood vessels supplying the tube become enlarged, and a vascular placenta forms. But, of course, the tube cannot accommodate a pregnancy; there is not enough room to allow an embryo to grow for more than a few weeks. Ultimately the embryo dies and degenerates; the tube itself becomes inflamed, much like a diseased appendix, and finally ruptures into the abdomen, tearing the engorged blood vessels in the region and often leading to a sudden internal hemorrhage of massive proportions.

Fortunately, an ectopic pregnancy is often diagnosed before this grave state of affairs develops. Sometimes it is spotted during a routine prenatal examination. Sometimes the patient begins suffering from abdominal pain, at first mild and generalized, then severe, constant, and localized in the lower abdomen on one side or the other. Nausea and vomiting may accompany the pain, which is more severe and persistent than that of ordinary morning sickness, and may be recognized as characteristic of *peritoneal irritation*. The patient may also develop a low-grade fever and an elevated white blood count; in fact, the condition may greatly resemble early acute appendicitis, except that the pain can be centered on the wrong side.

When symptoms of this sort appear in a woman who knows she is pregnant, with no evidence of a kidney infection that might be a contributing cause, the doctor will be highly suspicious of an ectopic pregnancy and will probably initiate the only safe form of treatment: surgical exploration of the patient's abdomen to confirm the diagnosis and remove the ectopic pregnancy before it can reach the stage of rupture, or so-called laparoscopic examination of the interior of the abdomen, employing a lighted examining instrument on a long, narrow tube that can be passed through the abdominal wall in the operating room and sometimes make an open surgical exploration unnecessary. But often these symptoms appear before the patient knows for certain that she is pregnant. In this case the obstetrician may delay surgery long enough to confirm the pregnancy and to obtain surgical consultation, with the patient under close hospital observation. Occasionally a surgeon operating on a young woman for supposed acute appendicitis will discover an ectopic pregnancy instead. In any event, the occurrence of persistent localized abdominal pain, nausea and vomiting in a woman who may have an early pregnancy must always be regarded as a gravely serious situation until proven otherwise. If these symptoms are ignored, or if they are mistakenly considered just "one of those things" that goes along with a pregnancy, even when they appear as late as the third or fourth month, rupture and hemorrhage may result. With prompt surgical treatment, most victims of ruptured ectopic pregnancies can be saved, but they will usually suffer a longer convalescence than if the condition is discovered and treated before rupture occurs. In either event, treatment of an ectopic pregnancy usually necessitates removal of the involved tube and sometimes the adjacent ovary as well if it has been damaged by inflammation. So long as the other tube and ovary are normal and unaffected, however, the woman will still retain the capacity for ovulation, conception and normal carriage of future pregnancies.

Anemia. A far more common and less serious

problem of early pregnancy is the development of a characteristic form of anemia, a condition in which the content of normal red cells in the mother's blood stream is sharply decreased. One of the early changes that takes place in a woman's body during pregnancy is an increase in the rate that red blood cells are produced. Extra blood is needed, both to assure the baby's needs and to provide the mother with a margin of protection against the blood loss that normally occurs at delivery. Characteristically, the production of additional blood is always ahead of the need; new red blood cells are manufactured in abundance during the early months of pregnancy. But their normal manufacture depends upon a sufficient quantity of *hemoglobin,* the oxygen-carrying component in the red cells that, in turn, is limited by the amount of iron available in the mother's body. Without an extra supply of iron to meet the increased demand, the new red blood cells produced are very small and deficient in hemoglobin, and the patient develops a so-called iron-deficiency anemia.

If the mother's diet is adequate and well balanced, this form of anemia may not become serious, although there may be *some* degree of pallor and fatigue. Many women, however, actually find themselves becoming short of breath on exertion due to a decrease in their blood's oxygen-carrying capacity, and may feel so constantly tired that they have difficulty carrying out even the most basic daily activities. If this condition is allowed to continue without treatment, it can become a serious threat to both mother and baby during late pregnancy and at delivery.

The anemia of pregnancy usually cannot be prevented simply by increasing the iron content of the diet. Most obstetricians immediately start their newly pregnant patients on a special mineral preparation which contains extra iron and a generous supply of calcium and phosphorus to aid in the formation of the baby's bones and teeth. Unfortunately, many women neglect to fill their prescriptions, or they take their "pregnancy pills" only sparingly. True, a developing anemia can be easily diagnosed from the routine blood tests taken during prenatal visits, but prevention of this condition is much easier than cure. Once it has developed, it may persist throughout the pregnancy and complicate delivery.

Drugs and Infant Deformities. Aside from morning sickness, some degree of unusual emotional tension, and predictable vitamin and iron deficiencies, there are relatively few conditions that require any medications at all during pregnancy. Nevertheless, until quite recently, medications of various sorts, known to be perfectly safe under normal circumstances, were often routinely prescribed; no one gave much thought to the possibility that during pregnancy they might have tragic effects on an unborn baby. Then in the early 1960s the walls came tumbling down. A new drug called thalidomide, widely prescribed in Europe as a tranquilizer and sedative during pregnancy, was found to cause grotesque deformities in the arms and legs of thousands of newborn babies, an ordinarily rare condition known as *phocomelia.* As the thalidomide tragedy unfolded, other drugs were discovered to have more subtle effects on unborn babies. The tetracycline antibiotics, in widespread use for more than 15 years, were found to affect the development of the teeth, hair and nails of unborn babies when taken by expectant mothers. Doctors realized with horror that the damaging effects of many drugs, especially new and unfamiliar ones, might not be revealed for years after a baby was born, but that virtually any drug or medication taken by an expectant mother might cross into the infant's blood stream and pose a threat to normal development, especially if taken during the early months of pregnancy when the new baby's major organs are in the most rudimentary stages of formation.

Thus, doctors today are extremely cautious about prescribing *any* medicine to expectant mothers, with the exception of a very few that are known to be safe, unless there is no alternative. The drugs normally prescribed for morning sickness, nervous tension and iron deficiencies are known by long experience to be harmless to both mother and baby in normal dosages. If a woman is under treatment for some other medical condition when she becomes pregnant, her doctor may choose to withdraw the medicine during the first part of her pregnancy, if possible, in order to be on the safe side. If she develops some complicating condition during pregnancy, the doctor must prescribe medications with particular care. The woman, on her part, should feel perfectly free to query her doctor about any medications he may prescribe and must completely avoid self-medication of any sort—even headache tablets—without her doctor's express approval. Sulfa preparations and aspirin in particular should be avoided during the last 2 months of pregnancy. Thanks to a "high index of suspicion" on the part of both doctor and patient, the incidence of drug-induced damage to unborn babies has been sharply reduced in the last decade. But with the easy availability of so many pills and potions, continued vigilance is absolutely necessary.

German Measles (Rubella). The threat of drug-induced damage to an unborn baby can be minimized by the vigilance of both doctor and patient, but another similar threat is not so easy to control: the damage that can be done to the baby when an expectant mother contracts rubella, commonly known as German measles, during the first trimester of her pregnancy. (Rubella is discussed in greater detail on p. 180.) Why this particular virus infection, alone of all the "childhood rash" diseases, should affect an unborn child so seriously is not known, but there is no longer any question that it can severely disrupt the normal development of the fetus and cause such congenital abnormalities as cataracts, deafness, a wide variety of infant heart defects, or even mental retardation. Statistics show that if an expectant mother contracts the infection at any time during the first three months of her pregnancy, there is a 25 percent chance that her baby will have at least one serious structural defect, and up to a 90 percent chance of other minor defects.

What can be done to prevent this dreadful threat? Until the development of an effective, long-acting vaccine, the best possible prevention against inadvertent rubella infection during pregnancy was for a woman to contract the disease—and know she had it—before she became pregnant. One attack of rubella, even during early childhood, confers lasting immunity, so that reinfection during a later pregnancy

is highly unlikely. But the disease is not as infectious as red measles or chicken pox, for example, and many women reached childbearing age without ever having had it. To add to the confusion, some girls actually had rubella without ever developing the unmistakable rash or other symptoms to identify it. Thus, until recently, some medical authorities advocated deliberate exposure of female children to rubella to ensure that they would be safe from the infection later during pregnancy.

The new rubella vaccine, first widely used in the United States in 1969, completely changed the picture. This vaccine, which contains a live but *attenuated* or "weakened" rubella virus, can be administered safely to children at any time between the age of one year and the onset of puberty, and it stimulates the formation of antibodies against rubella so effectively that prolonged immunity against the infection is achieved. It is too early yet to know if the immunity engendered by the vaccine will prove to be permanent after a single inoculation, or whether booster shots will be recommended in the case of girls approaching the age of puberty; but in either case, a high degree of protection against rubella infection during pregnancy is at last possible.

Unfortunately, the rubella vaccine cannot be generally recommended for use by girls after puberty or for women of childbearing age because the virus in the vaccine, even though attenuated, may still linger in the body for weeks or months after the inoculation and could conceivably damage a fetus if a pregnancy should occur during this interval. Also unfortunately, there are still many women who have never been immunized either by an active rubella infection or by means of the vaccine, and who thus remain vulnerable to the disease early in pregnancy. Once the infection has occurred under these circumstances, the damage may be done and nothing can prevent it. In such cases, most physicians feel that therapeutic abortion is justified to prevent the birth of a possibly crippled child when the infection occurs during the first trimester of the pregnancy. If the infection occurs later, modern surgical techniques can correct many rubella deformities after the baby is born. Many other afflicted children, with the courage and loving support of their parents, have survived to live happy and productive lives in spite of their deformities. It is to be fervently hoped that widespread use of the rubella vaccine among schoolchildren during the next decade will drastically reduce the nationwide incidence of rubella and, with it, the number of cases in which such a difficult decision must be made.

The Second Trimester

Whereas the first trimester is marked by dramatic changes in the tiny embryo as it develops into a diminutive but unmistakably human fetus, the changes in the mother's body are mostly quiet, preparatory alterations which are often hardly noticeable. Although some potential hazards exist, that period is commonly notable for the *lack* of dramatic changes; with the exception of a few minor discomforts, it may hardly seem that the mother is pregnant at all. But during the second trimester, the situation reverses. The fetus, with its major developmental changes almost complete, spends its fourth, fifth and sixth months primarily in growing markedly in size, with gradual maturation of its organ systems; it is the mother who undergoes a wealth of obvious physical changes during this period. Fortunately for her, this middle trimester is probably the least hazardous period of her pregnancy; those problems that do arise are relatively minor in nature and can be minimized by preventive action.

From the fourth month on, the normal physical changes of pregnancy become increasingly evident in the mother. With the uterus steadily enlarging, the upper portion or *fundus* becomes palpable above the pubis by the end of the third month. A month later it can be felt as a firm mass in the lower abdomen about the size and shape of a large grapefruit. By the end of the fifth month the uterus reaches up to the navel. It continues to enlarge steadily until, at term, it seems to fill the whole abdomen. Also during this time characteristic pinkish *striae* or "stretch marks" often appear on the skin of the abdomen due to the action of hormones of pregnancy. Because of pressure of the uterus on other abdominal organs, most women notice a marked increase in urinary frequency after the third or fourth month, and constipation becomes a universal and chronic annoyance.

At the same time, other changes occur. At some point during the fifth month the doctor can hear the first faint sounds of the baby's heartbeat with his stethoscope, clearly distinguishable from the mother's pulse by its speed (120 to 140 beats per minute) and its odd mechanical sound, like the ticking of a watch under a pillow. About the same time the mother will notice faint fluttery sensations in her abdomen—the first tentative movements of the baby within the uterus. A week or two after this initial "quickening," the baby's movements will continue as a daily phenomenon, so regularly and unmistakably that one must be concerned if they are *absent* for more than a day or so at a time.

All these changes are natural and normal, observed with a sense of excitement and wonder by the mother, and with a certain degree of amusement by the father—until he actually feels the baby move under his hand or hears the faint but determined heartbeat in the doctor's stethoscope. This is often the time that it first dawns on prospective parents that a new life is really present; the pregnancy ceases to be an abstract medical condition and becomes, suddenly, a "person" with a life all its own. During this second trimester the expectant mother is usually scheduled to see her obstetrician at least once a month, but if a problem arises which seems to require investigation, she should never hesitate to call her doctor before her scheduled appointment.

Weight Control and Fluid Retention. Almost all expectant mothers have some trouble with weight control, partly because the unborn baby is increasing in size and partly because pregnant women tend to retain fluid in their tissues, particularly noticeable as swelling or *edema* of the ankles. In fact, for many women pregnancy seems to be one long battle with the bathroom scales. Is the battle really worth it? The fact is that excessive weight gain during pregnancy, even if it results only from fluid retention, does not *in itself* have any direct or specific ill effects on either mother or baby. Nevertheless, it is so frequently associated with potentially serious complications that the relationship, however indirect, cannot be ignored. Doctors know from long experience that the woman who loses control of her weight is usually the woman who will have trouble as pregnancy progresses, whereas the woman whose weight gain is well controlled usually has a trouble-free pregnancy, enjoys an uncomplicated delivery, and gives birth to a healthy child. It does not *always* happen that way, but it does often enough that most doctors are adamant about weight control.

Obviously a woman must expect to gain some weight during pregnancy. But how much is normal, and how much is excessive? The way to arrive at a reasonable figure is to calculate backward, adding up the *loss* of weight that might normally be expected at the termination of pregnancy. A full-term baby weighs, on average, 7½ pounds. The placenta and umbilical cord, delivered together as the "afterbirth," account for another 1½ pounds. The amniotic fluid surrounding the baby inside the uterus and lost during delivery weighs approximately 2 pounds. In addition, the uterus and breasts gain in size and weight during pregnancy, perhaps another 3½ pounds, and this, too, will ordinarily be lost once the baby has been delivered and nursing discontinued. Finally, there is a normal increase in the mother's total blood volume, and some additional fat deposited throughout her body, totaling perhaps another 7 or 8 pounds. All this adds up to approximately 20 to 22 pounds. Thus weight gain during pregnancy in excess of 20 pounds (slightly less in smaller, light-boned women, slightly more in larger women) must be considered excessive.

Twenty pounds may seem very generous, but mathematically it means only about 2½ pounds of "permissible" gain per month, often difficult to achieve. In the first trimester there is usually no problem holding weight gain to a total of 4 or 5 pounds, but during the second trimester there is often at least one month when weight seems to surge sharply, and the last three months can be the most difficult of all. Some women, of course, have no trouble. In fact, pregnancy can offer the perpetually thin woman a welcome chance to put on a little extra weight; it is the woman who is already overweight, or who has a tendency to gain weight easily, who may have the greatest difficulty. But pregnancy can be an excellent opportunity for the overweight woman to trim down even her prepregnant weight. She must exercise weight control anyway, and if she can hold her weight gain down to just 18 pounds, or even 15, she can emerge from the hospital with a bonus of "real" weight loss she might never have achieved otherwise.

Diet control is, of course, the most important step in preventing excess weight. Eliminate starches, pastries and desserts completely, and concentrate on lean meats, salads, vegetables, fresh fruits, and adequate amounts (a pint a day at least) of low-fat (2 percent) milk. Retention of fluid can be minimized by avoiding salty foods like ham, bacon, sausage, or potato chips, and by leaving the salt shaker off the table. The doctor can provide more specific recommendations for diet control. A mild diuretic or kidney-stimulating drug may also be prescribed, especially if water retention seems excessive, and later more potent diuretics are sometimes necessary if water retention becomes a more difficult problem.

In the long run, however, the key to sensible weight control is close cooperation between doctor and patient throughout the pregnancy. Continual vigilance and honesty are essential. Once excess weight has been gained through neglect or self-indulgence, it is extremely hard to lose again, and it can endanger the pregnancy. If a relentless weight gain occurs in spite of genuine efforts at control, it can be an early clue that more serious complications of the pregnancy are developing, and the doctor should be consulted immediately.

Urinary Tract Infections. From the first prenatal visit throughout the pregnancy, it is imperative to bring a morning urine specimen to every doctor's appointment. Most women comply with this request without knowing exactly why these specimens are necessary. Urine examinations are, of course, more than an obstetrical whimsy; they provide the doctor with an important means of guarding the expectant mother against two possible complications of midterm pregnancy, one of them only annoying, the other potentially dangerous.

One of the earliest discomforts of pregnancy is an increase in urinary frequency, together with a tendency to void considerably less urine each time. There is an obvious mechanical reason for this: the enlarging uterus lies behind and almost on top of the urinary bladder in the pelvis, and the increasing pressure on the bladder diminishes the amount of urine it can store. Later in the pregnancy when the uterus begins to fill the whole pelvis, it also exerts pressure on the ureters, the narrow tubes that lie along the back of the abdominal wall and drain urine from the kidneys to the bladder. This pressure never completely obstructs the passage of urine into the bladder, but it does cause partial obstruction, with some pooling of urine both in the kidney and in the bladder. And since urine is an excellent culture medium for certain kinds of bacterial growth, the woman in midterm becomes more vulnerable than usual to both kidney and bladder infections.

If such an infection does occur, it produces marked increase in urinary frequency, pain and burning on urination, an aching pain in the small of the back, and the appearance of quantities of pus cells in the urine. When only the bladder is involved there may be no fever, but with kidney infections spiking fevers may occur, often associated with chills. Fortunately, actual kidney infection is comparatively rare during pregnancy; most urinary tract infections during midterm pregnancy are simple *cystitis* or bladder infections.

Once detected, a urinary infection can be treated quickly and effectively, usually with certain highly soluble sulfa drugs. If an infection seems resistant to sulfa drugs, or if the patient is allergic to them, the broad-spectrum antibiotics can be substituted. Either way, these infections are almost invariably controllable and do no lasting harm, as long as they are detected and treated early. Once well entrenched, however, they can recur throughout the pregnancy and even later; hence the necessity for repeated urine examinations.

In addition, urine specimens are regularly checked for sugar—diabetes sometimes first appears during pregnancy—and, even more particularly, for protein. Ordinarily no protein is found in the urine, but when kidney function is impaired, as it is in *toxemia of pregnancy* (*see* p. 832), protein molecules from the patient's blood begin to leak through into the urine along with water and various chemical wastes. Protein in the urine causes no direct symptoms, and can be detected only in the laboratory by careful urine examination. When it appears, however, it can be the symptom of a developing complication which may become life-threatening to both mother and child if it is not promptly treated.

Varicose Veins. Another problem of the second trimester can also arise as a result of the pressure of the enlarging uterus in the pelvis, especially in a second or later pregnancy. In the fourth or fifth month the veins carrying blood from the legs, the pelvis and the genital and rectal areas are compressed by the uterus, and the blood tends to back up and pool in these areas. When it does, the thin-walled veins stretch and enlarge, and the tiny valves inside the veins, which help regulate the direction of blood flow, begin to break down. The result can be the development of *varices* or varicose veins; the dilated and twisted veins often become visible on the calves, thighs or vulva, and sometimes appear in the rectal area as painful, protruding *hemorrhoids.*

Not everyone develops varicosities during pregnancy. Heredity plays a part; in some families women practically never develop them, while in others they appear even without pregnancies. When they do develop, they may vary in severity from a mere unsightly nuisance to an extremely painful and continuing problem. Varicose veins and hemorrhoids that develop during pregnancy regress to some degree after delivery, but often some permanent damage is done; varicosities may become worse during subsequent pregnancies and may even become a chronic condition.

Many women simply suffer with varicose veins and hemorrhoids because they think that surgery is the only possible treatment. Sometimes it is, in severe cases that persist after delivery. But steps can be taken, when varicosities first begin to appear, to prevent or at least minimize their development. First and most obvious, the expectant mother should stay off her feet as much as possible if varicose veins begin to appear. Even when she must remain physically active, she should sit down with her feet elevated above the level of the hips for brief periods at frequent intervals—perhaps 5 minutes every hour—and lie down with hips and legs elevated for a longer period—perhaps 15 to 30 minutes—midmorning and midafternoon. This at least will relieve venous pressure regularly and prevent constant, unrelieved engorgement and stretching of the enlarged veins.

Most doctors recommend the continual use of elastic supportive hose, held up with a garter belt, or supportive panty-hose. Constrictive circular garters should never be worn; there is no more certain way to *guarantee* development of varicose veins during a pregnancy. If elastic hose of the proper size cannot be found to provide firm but not tight support, ordinary 3-inch elastic bandages can be worn during the day when the expectant mother is on her feet; they should be anchored well around the bridge of the foot; wrapped in spiral fashion up the leg and secured with safety pins and a garter belt. Such wrappings may not be very attractive, but they can perform miracles in relieving the aching and leg cramps that so often attend varicose veins.

If severe varicosities begin to develop in spite of these measures, the doctor may recommend custom-made elastic stockings. They are more expensive than standard elastic hose, but they fit perfectly and apply scientifically calibrated pressure designed both to control discomfort from varicose veins and to prevent them from getting any worse.

Hemorrhoids and Constipation. Hemorrhoids present a more difficult problem, since there is no effective way to apply pressure to varicosed rectal veins. In most cases the hemorrhoids of pregnancy are merely annoying and tend to regress and disappear after delivery. Symptoms, which may include pain, bleeding, itching, or even protrusion of the hemorrhoids, are seriously aggravated by another perennial problem of pregnancy, chronic constipation. If constipation can be controlled, serious discomfort from

hemorrhoids can usually be avoided, but controlling constipation is not always easy.

Decreased bowel activity due to pressure of the uterus on the lower segment of the colon is commonplace in pregnancy, particularly in the second and third trimesters. Constipation in itself is no particular health hazard, yet it can be aggravating to the expectant mother. Dietary measures are an important step in relieving the condition. Doctors recommend quantities of fluids daily, including fresh fruit juice, some form of bulk in the diet, such as bran cereals or whole wheat bread, and free use of the mildly cathartic fruits such as prunes, figs or raisins. When this, combined with regular, unhurried bowel habits, does not do the trick, the obstetrician may prescribe an artificial bulking agent such as Metamucil, a powdery vegetable product which has no nutritional value but absorbs many times its volume in water and as it passes through the intestine forms a soft, bulky stool. Habitual use of chemical laxatives such as milk of magnesia or mineral oil should be avoided, but their *occasional* use on the doctor's recommendation can also help bring relief. If hemorrhoids are irritated by constipated stools, avoid straining to evacuate, and consult with the doctor about a safe, nonhabituating stool softener.

Multiple Pregnancies. Although it can hardly be considered a "complication" of pregnancy in the medical sense, the discovery of a multiple pregnancy during the second trimester can pose special problems. Twinning, the most common form of multiple pregnancy, occurs on an average of about once every 86 pregnancies, but in families with a history of twins on one or both sides, hereditary factors may increase the odds considerably. Twin pregnancies can arise in two ways. *Identical twins* develop when a single fertilized ovum in its earliest stages of cell division separates into two different clumps of cells, each of which then develops into a fetus. In such a case, the two developing babies share the same basic hereditary material, are always of the same sex, and appear closely alike in features and body structures. They also develop within the same membranous sac in the uterus, and at delivery the obstetrician can often determine at once that twins are identical by examination of the afterbirth membranes. *Fraternal twins* develop when two separate ova are produced and fertilized at the same time, and then both implant and grow. In such cases each twin has separate and different hereditary material; the sexes may be different, the physical features as different as those of single siblings, and each child develops within its own separate set of membranes within the uterus.

Multiple pregnancies involving triplets, quadruplets, quintuplets or even sextuplets do occur, although only rarely. Again, when early and repeated cleavage and separation of parts of a single fertilized ovum result in triple or higher-multiple pregnancies, the babies are identical, whereas babies developing from the fertilization of multiple ova at the same time are not. Until recently quadruplet and higher-multiple pregnancies occurred very rarely, but today an increase in multiple pregnancies has been related to the use of certain medications used to stimulate conception among women suffering from relative infertility.

Because twin pregnancies and deliveries are more difficult for the mother and place special demands on the obstetrician, it is important to detect twinning as early as possible. From the fifth month on, the doctor automatically checks the possibility of twins during each prenatal visit, whether he mentions it or not. The things that might make the expectant mother suspicious of twins—seemingly overrapid enlargement of the abdomen, excessive weight gain, or apparent overactivity of the "babies"—seldom have any significance; twin pregnancies often keep themselves well hidden and are usually detected only by careful prenatal examination.

What does the doctor look for? First, for truly abnormal enlargement of the uterus itself. Especially in a second pregnancy the doctor is usually able to feel the baby's head, rump and back within the uterus; if the baby feels too small for the size of the uterus, he will be suspicious and sometimes can palpate two heads and two buttocks. But the most convincing clue aside from X-ray evidence is the detection of two distinct sets of fetal heart tones with the stethoscope, distinguishable because one baby's heart rate is measurably slower than the other's.

Once a multiple pregnancy is discovered, both the parents and the doctor have an opportunity to make the necessary preparations. A woman with a twin pregnancy usually goes into labor somewhat prematurely; the labor may be longer and more difficult for mother and doctor alike, and the babies, usually smaller than average, may also require special attention. With modern obstetrical skills and facilities available almost everywhere in the country, the potential hazards of a twin pregnancy are only slightly greater than those of a single pregnancy and delivery. Even in cases in which three or more babies must be delivered, foreknowledge and advance preparation can reduce the risks involved to a bare minimum.

Premature Labor and Midterm Miscarriages. Statistically, the greatest proportion of miscarriages occurs during the first trimester of pregnancy. During the second trimester, when the new baby begins to move and fetal heart tones can be distinguished, that potential hazard is much diminished, but miscarriages and stillbirths sometimes do occur at this time, and a certain number of babies may be endangered or lost because of premature labor.

Why would a baby die *in utero* at this late stage? Sometimes a physical defect is present to which the baby finally succumbs. Sometimes the mother has an underlying illness—diabetes, for example—which can lead to the death of the baby at midterm. *Erythroblastosis fetalis,* a condition caused by Rh factor incompatibility between mother and child, can also cause the baby's death *(see* below). Other unusual circumstances may have less direct influence: malnutrition of the mother, illnesses such as high blood pressure or syphilis, and the presence of fibroid tumors in the uterus. Even the mother's age can be a factor; stillbirths are far more common among women in their late thirties or early forties than among younger women.

Whatever the cause, the distress of a baby *in utero* will usually be heralded by one of two symptoms: the baby may inexplicably stop moving, or the mother may begin cramping and spotting. In either event, the doctor should be notified at once. Fetal distress may trigger premature labor, and if the baby is born alive it can sometimes be saved. More often the baby is still-born, but the same care and precautions are necessary to protect the mother against hazards of hemorrhage and infection.

Premature labor is usually over quickly once contractions begin. If labor does not begin immediately, however, the doctor may induce contractions, using the same medicines that are employed to induce labor at term. But even if a period of waiting is necessary after the death of a fetus for the uterus to begin contracting to empty itself, there is no cause for alarm, nor any particular danger to the mother. Ultimately the lost pregnancy is always expelled, whether speeded up by medical means or not.

The situation is quite different when the baby appears to be alive and premature labor begins unexpectedly during the fourth, fifth or sixth month. Sometimes this occurs as a result of premature partial separation of the placenta or because of placenta previa, two complications that appear more commonly in the third trimester (see below). Occasionally premature labor is triggered by a physical trauma of some kind—an automobile accident, for example, or a bad fall. Even more rarely, it can result from a severe emotional shock. Most often, however, there is no identifiable explanation. Nor is there any reason to forgo normal physical activities, sports or sexual relations during this part of the pregnancy. In fact, no modern obstetrical authority regards restriction of these activities as either necessary or desirable.

When premature labor does occur, the first sign is usually the onset of rhythmic cramping contractions of the uterus. Frequently the membranous sac enclosing the fetus within the uterus in a watery bed of *amniotic fluid* will rupture spontaneously, with drainage of the fluid from the vagina. If either of these things occurs, the doctor should be notified as soon as possible. Occasionally medications can be used to quiet the contractions, if there is no sign of bleeding and the baby seems to be in no distress. Nor does rupture of membranes necessarily mean that premature labor will always begin. In many cases, however, rupture of membranes and uterine contractions are followed by vaginal bleeding, weakening of the baby's heart tones,

dilatation of the uterine cervix and, within a few hours, labor and delivery of a premature baby—sometimes stillborn, but sometimes very much alive.

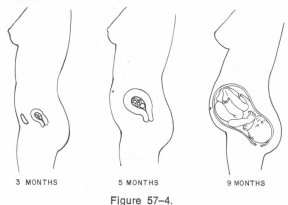

3 MONTHS   5 MONTHS   9 MONTHS

Figure 57–4.

The fate of the baby, if it is living when labor begins, depends heavily upon how premature the labor is, how large the baby is, and what sort of premature baby care is available. Babies weighing as little as 14 or 15 ounces at birth have been saved and have become thriving normal children, thanks to skillful nursing care and modern facilities; but most extremely small "premies" are either stillborn or survive only momentarily after birth. Every pound, indeed every ounce, can make a vital difference. If the baby weighs as much as 2 pounds, he has at least a fighting chance; perhaps 10 percent of such tiny premature infants survive. A premature baby weighing 3 pounds or more has a better than 90 percent chance of survival. Fortunately, when a premature baby survives its initial fight for life, its development in infancy and childhood is usually unaffected by its early arrival. Once the fight is won, it is won.

The Third Trimester

In many cases the most common "problem" facing a mother in the third trimester of her pregnancy is boredom. During this final period the fetus continues to grow and mature in preparation for delivery, but for the mother, it may be a time when she becomes thoroughly weary of being pregnant. By the twenty-sixth week the uterus is large enough to make the mother physically awkward and limit many of her activities, including sports participation and sexual relations, which become increasingly difficult and uncomfortable as term approaches. This is also a time when many minor annoyances—urinary frequency and constipation in particular—may seem interminable. During this period the breasts become markedly enlarged and heavy, and a special supportive bra is recommended. Inevitable discomfort and feelings of awkwardness can also be minimized by the use of loose fitting clothing or special "maternity clothes," flat-heeled supportive shoes and—if necessary on occasion—the use of a maternity corset.

The increasing pressure of the baby in the pelvis also causes a whole new series of perfectly normal but annoying discomforts. Low backaches are commonplace at this time, as are a variety of aches and pains in the hips and pelvis. In preparation for the baby's birth, there is a softening and relaxation of the cartilage and tendon binding segments of the pelvis together, so that these bones can separate slightly to allow the baby to pass more readily at delivery. As a result, the mother may experience twinges and feelings of weakness in the area of the pelvis, low back and hips, which, toward the end of term, can become almost continuous. Women complain frequently that they "can't get comfortable" or "can't stand up and can't sit down." A little aspirin may give partial relief, but the only real "cure" for these aches and pains is delivery.

Obviously, rest and relaxation are essential, and it is wise to limit physical activities as well. Some form of mild exercise is usually beneficial, but strenuous sports should be eliminated, and sexual relations, tub baths and swimming are usually forbidden during the last six or eight weeks. At this time, the uterine outlet begins to stretch and open, and there is a real threat of infection being introduced through the vagina as a result of such activities. Vaginal douching should be avoided for the same reason, unless specifically ordered by the doctor. Finally, traveling more than a few miles away from home is inadvisable. Even though the estimated date of confinement may be as many as six or eight weeks away, it is only an estimate, and labor can begin several days or even weeks sooner than expected.

But long as the third trimester may seem, the day of delivery is not far off, and the expectant parents—mother *and* father—should be well prepared in advance. Most obstetricians are associated with a particular hospital, but there should be frank discussion between patient and doctor about the kind of arrangements available and preferred by the mother-to-be. There should also be a clear understanding in advance of the approximate length of confinement the doctor normally advises, the total hospital costs the parents should expect, and whether the labor and delivery are covered by hospitalization insurance or not. In addition, parents should know in advance the costs of nursery care for the baby, and whether "rooming-in" facilities are available (*see* below). Then, by the seventh month, the expectant parents should visit the hospital, introduce themselves and make advance arrangements for admission when the time comes.

Preparations at home are also important. The purchase of baby clothes can often be postponed until the baby is ready to come home, but arrangements should be made in advance for a crib, feeding equipment, diapers or diaper service and other essentials. Often the obstetrician or his office nurse can be extremely helpful in suggesting specific items that will be necessary. Finally, the expectant mother should prepare a "hospital suitcase" at home, ready for use at a moment's notice, containing certain minimum necessities: cosmetics and toilet articles, a bathrobe and bed jacket, slippers and pajama tops, a couple of nursing bras, some note paper and a book or two. Store the suitcase in a convenient place, and when the time comes remember where it is.

During this last third of the pregnancy, doctor's appointments will be more frequent than before, at first every two weeks, then weekly. The reason is simple: at this time there are a few problems that may arise and require swift action. These "late complications of pregnancy" are not exactly commonplace, but neither are they rare. They are usually accompanied by clear-cut signs or symptoms; one is sudden vaginal bleeding, and another is sudden and inexplicable weight gain and fluid retention, often with ankle swelling. In either case, these symptoms require immediate medical attention.

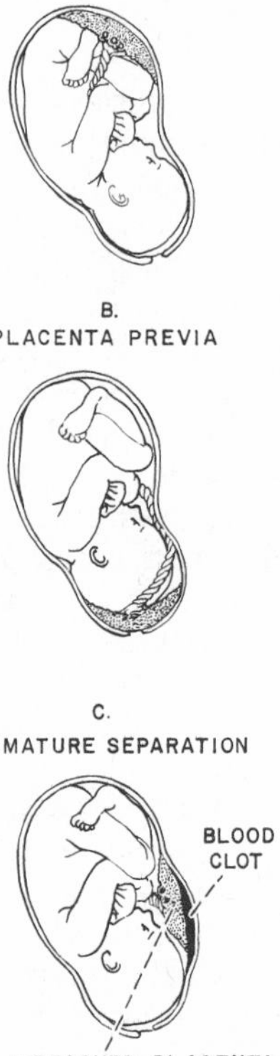

A.
NORMAL IMPLANTATION

B.
PLACENTA PREVIA

C.
PREMATURE SEPARATION

BLOOD
CLOT

DETACHED PLACENTA

Figure 57–5.

Placenta Previa and Abruptio Placentae. These relatively uncommon complications occur perhaps once every two hundred pregnancies, but historically they have been notorious as major causes of maternal and infant mortality. Today, thanks to early diagnosis, modern hospital facilities and obstetrical skill, maternal death rates have been reduced sharply, and even a high percentage of the affected babies can now be saved.

Placenta previa, the Latin term meaning "placenta first," describes one of these complications perfectly. Ordinarily a pregnancy is implanted high up on the interior wall of the uterus, and the placenta develops either beside the baby or above it, well away from the lower uterine opening. Occasionally, however, implantation is low in the uterus, and part of the placenta grows *across* the outlet through which the baby must ultimately be delivered.

There may be no hint of this condition early in the pregnancy; but in the last trimester the cervix or neck of the uterus begins to soften and stretch, and the opening begins to dilate somewhat. If the placenta lies across the cervical opening, part of its attachment is torn, leading to vaginal bleeding, either intermittent or steady. This kind of bleeding is quite different from the slight discharge of blood-streaked mucus which normally appears just as labor begins. There may be just spotting, or a more copious flow, but *any* frank vaginal bleeding at this stage of the pregnancy should be reported to the doctor immediately, day or night. It is *never* normal. When the doctor suspects placenta previa, careful observation in the hospital is necessary. If the bleeding is not too severe, he may have special X-rays taken to help establish exactly where in the uterus the placenta is located. If only a small edge lies over the cervical exit, he may be able to induce labor when the baby is mature and proceed with a normal vaginal delivery of a slightly premature baby. When the whole cervical orifice is covered by placenta, however, a surgical delivery by Caesarean section is mandatory.

Today the main threat of placenta previa to the mother is severe hemorrhage; the threat to the baby is loss of its oxygen supply before it can be delivered. With modern techniques of blood transfusion, swift surgical intervention when necessary, and skillful premature care for the baby, both these threats can usually be averted.

The other cause of vaginal bleeding late in a pregnancy is *abruptio placentae;* that is, premature separation of a portion of a normally implanted placenta from the wall of the uterus. When the separation is minor, affecting just the edge of the placenta, the bleeding may stop spontaneously and the separated edge may heal and scar. More frequently, blood gathers under the placenta, forming a *hematoma* or clot which then forces greater separation. The result is increased maternal bleeding and increasing fetal distress as the baby's oxygen supply is progressively impaired.

As in placenta previa, the first clue to premature separation of the placenta is the onset of vaginal bleeding some time during the third trimester, often accompanied by cramping pain. Again, careful hospital observation is imperative from the onset of symptoms, so that a Caesarean section can be performed at any moment if necessary. Since this complication, like placenta previa, usually occurs late in the pregnancy when the baby's development is almost complete, chances of a happy outcome are good if the doctor is notified at the first suspicious sign. Although no one knows why either of these complications occurs, both are more common among older expectant mothers, and placental abruption in particular seems to occur most frequently in women with underlying hypertension (high blood pressure). For this reason, among others, a growing number of obstetricians urge their patients to have babies before the age of thirty-five. Over that age the risk of complications with a first or subsequent new pregnancy materially increases.

Toxemia of Pregnancy. High blood pressure plays a very dramatic role in another more common complication of late pregnancy known as *preeclampsia* or, more familiarly, toxemia of pregnancy. The first symptoms of this condition may make their appearance late in the second or early in the third trimester, but it develops gradually, and if diagnosed soon after onset, it can be very effectively treated and controlled.

The primary signs of early toxemia are a sudden excessive gain in weight, progressive elevation of blood pressure and the appearance of protein in the urine. Originally toxemia, which is derived from Greek words meaning "poison in the blood," was believed to stem from some poisonous or "toxic" substance produced by the pregnancy. No such poison has ever been identified, but in certain women, for reasons unknown, pregnancy does seem to cause a progressive impairment of kidney function very similar to that seen in the acute kidney inflammation known as nephritis. Salt and water are retained in the body tissues instead of being excreted nor-

mally. Protein appears in the urine because of a breakdown in the kidneys' filtering capacity, and the blood pressure rises, owing to widespread impairment of normal circulation through the kidneys. If undetected or untreated, toxemia can lead to a puffy swelling of the ankles and cheeks, headaches and blurring of vision; ultimately the blood pressure can climb to dangerous levels, and convulsions may ensue, the condition known as *eclampsia*. If this condition is uncontrolled, death of both mother and baby can result.

Toxemia today seldom reaches these extremes; the early symptoms are almost always detected by routine weight, blood pressure and urine checks in the obstetrician's office, treatment is begun, and the dangerous crisis of eclampsia is averted. The condition goes away completely as soon as the baby is delivered, except for a residual hypertension in a small percentage of cases. But with vigorous treatment, preeclampsia can be prevented from progressing as delivery time is awaited.

In most cases restriction of dietary salt intake, the use of diuretic medicines to stimulate salt and water excretion by the kidneys, and the use of mild antihypertensive drugs are effective, and the expectant mother can safely carry her baby to term and a normal delivery. But toxemia tends to become progressively more severe, and progressively more difficult to control, as term approaches. Occasionally the condition gets out of hand during the last month, in spite of careful control measures, and delivery must be speeded up by inducing labor or a Caesarean section must be performed. Toxemia does not impair the baby in any way as long as the convulsive crisis of eclampsia is prevented; he simply begins "life on the outside" a few days or weeks earlier than expected. After delivery the mother experiences a sudden diuresis of the water retained in her body, and there is a dramatic fall of blood pressure to normal ranges in most cases. Occasionally some degree of hypertension remains as a permanent aftereffect, however, and any woman who has suffered toxemia in one pregnancy can expect a more severe recurrence in another pregnancy. Thus anyone with a history of previous toxemia should notify the doctor as soon as she becomes pregnant again.

Erythroblastosis or "Rh Disease." One peculiar complication of pregnancy which may first manifest itself during the last trimester is a result of a so-called Rh blood factor incompatibility between the expectant mother and the baby she is carrying. Technically, this condition, known as erythroblastosis fetalis or "Rh disease," is an affliction of the baby, not the mother, but it begins to develop before delivery and can sometimes cause miscarriages or stillbirths. Furthermore, although it cannot always be positively diagnosed before birth, it can usually be *anticipated,* an important consideration, since successful treatment can depend upon advance preparation, and the baby's chances for recovery are often greatly enhanced by inducing labor a bit before full term.

What is Rh disease and how does it come about? By far the greatest majority of people of every race are born with an inheritable factor in their blood, similar but not identical to the familiar A-B blood grouping factors. It is called the Rh factor because it was first discovered in 1939 in rhesus monkeys, but no one knows what purpose it serves or why it is absent in a small percentage of people. We do know that when a woman without the factor, classified medically as Rh-negative, has Rh-positive blood introduced into her body at any time, either by a transfusion of Rh-positive blood or during a previous pregnancy by a baby whose blood contained the Rh factor, permanent antibodies form in her blood stream to "protect" her against the Rh factor just as if it were a dangerous virus. These anti-Rh antibodies ordinarily do no harm, but they persist for decades in any Rh-negative person who has once become "sensitized." Thus, when an Rh-negative woman who has been sensitized by an Rh-positive transfusion or an Rh-positive pregnancy again becomes pregnant with an Rh-positive baby, her body treats the baby's Rh factor as a "foreign invader" and begins to form more and more anti-Rh antibodies.

In many cases only a few anti-Rh antibodies are formed, and no harm is done. But in some women there is a terrific overreaction. Antibodies pile up in the blood stream, cross over into the baby's circulation and begin destroying or "hemolyzing" the baby's red blood cells. In addi-

tion to causing an anemia in the baby, the hemoglobin pigment released from the red cells may have a severe poisonous effect on certain vital groups of cells in the baby's brain, causing permanent brain damage or even death. In severe cases this damage may begin relatively early in the pregnancy, leading to spontaneous abortion or a midterm stillbirth. But more often the dam-

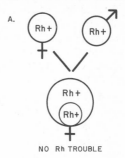

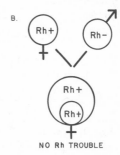

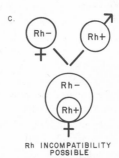

Figure 57–6.

age begins only at term, or immediately after the baby is born.

Since the cause of Rh disease was discovered, much has been learned about its mechanism and treatment. When a baby is conceived by two Rh-positive parents, by far the most usual case, there is no possible threat. The same is true if both parents happen to be Rh-negative, or if the mother is Rh-positive and the father Rh-negative. Only when the mother is Rh-negative and the father Rh-positive can trouble arise, and even then it occurs in less than 10 percent of cases. All the same, a pregnant woman's Rh factor is now always checked as part of the initial obstetric examination. If she is Rh-positive, there is nothing to worry about. If she is Rh-negative, the father's Rh factor will also be checked. If he is Rh-positive—and especially if he carries two genes for the positive factor—the mother's blood must be checked at regular intervals throughout the pregnancy for evidence of an increasing amount or *titer* of anti-Rh antibodies. Ordinarily the titer will remain low throughout the pregnancy, even if the baby is Rh-positive and the mother was previously sensitized. In a few cases, however, it will begin to climb, and both doctor and patient must be prepared for the possibility of Rh disease in the baby sooner or later. This preparation can take two forms. If the mother's anti-Rh titer is increasing rapidly, the doctor may seek to induce labor between the thirty-sixth and thirty-eighth weeks, but not earlier, since premature babies seem to tolerate later treatment very poorly. Even a Caesarean section may be justified if the titer is climbing ominously high. On the other hand, if the titer is not alarmingly high, the obstetrician may wait for normal delivery of the baby, but be prepared in advance for immediate, vigorous treatment if the newborn baby shows any evidence of Rh disease.

If, after birth, the baby becomes anemic or develops the jaundice characteristic of the disease, an *exchange tranfusion* must be performed. In this procedure the baby's blood containing the deadly antibodies is withdrawn a small amount at a time through the umbilical vein and replaced by freshly donated Rh-positive blood. In extreme cases as many as three or four exchange transfusions may be necessary before the baby's blood is completely flushed free of the damaging antibodies. But thanks to increasing skill in performing this life-saving procedure, as many as 75 percent of live-born babies with Rh disease can be saved before death or brain damage takes place.

Modern research has recently found a way in which the disease may soon be prevented completely, if steps are taken early enough. A new vaccine, recently introduced, can block the formation of anti-Rh antibodies if given to an Rh-negative mother at the time of delivery of her first Rh-positive baby. If given thereafter following each subsequent delivery the vaccine will, in effect, prevent the mother from ever becoming sensitized to the Rh factor, at least as a result of prior pregnancies. Today use of this vaccine is becoming a routine part of the obstetrical care of any pregnant Rh-negative woman, and it promises to become an effective weapon in preventing Rh disease in future generations of babies. For the Rh-negative woman who is already sensitized, however, this new vaccine will be of no help. The damage has already been done, but adequate forewarning and preparation usually prevent the condition from being fatal to the baby.

The Approach of Labor. Whatever individual differences there may be between pregnancies, and whatever complications may arise, pregnant women usually agree that the last month is the longest, and the last weeks seem interminable. It is impossible to know just when labor will begin; all the expectant parent can do is wait. During this interval the doctor can judge the mother's progress to some degree during weekly office examinations. By that time she will have become accustomed to the coming and going of rhythmic "contractions"—tightening or cramping of the uterus—associated with sensations of pressure and discomfort in the pelvis. Actually, these rhythmic contractions occur constantly throughout the last trimester of pregnancy or even longer; they are often so mild that most women fail to notice them. But they accomplish an important purpose: the gradual stretching and thinning of the lower end of the uterus so that the cervix can dilate readily when labor finally begins in earnest.

Often the onset of true labor is gradual, no more than a strengthening of these "mild" uterine contractions and an increase in their frequency until they become quite intense at regular intervals of 10 to 15 minutes. Characteristically, the pattern of labor contractions is like the breaking of waves on the beach; there is a steady build-up with increasing pressure and discomfort for a period of 60 seconds or so, followed by an abrupt relaxation in which pressure and discomfort are relieved completely. This pattern obtains even at the climax of labor when contractions occur one after another only a half-minute apart. Until the very end, the mother can always count on at least a momentary breather, free of discomfort, between contractions.

Frequently the beginning of labor contractions is heralded by the rupture of the membranes surrounding the baby in the uterus, and there is the sudden passage of a considerable quantity of fluid which has a characteristic musty, soapy smell. When this occurs prior to the onset of uncomfortable contractions, it usually signals that serious labor will commence within the next 24 hours, and probably much sooner; if it does not the doctor will usually seek to induce labor to avoid the threat of infection, or even consider a Caesarean delivery. The popular superstition that premature rupture of membranes will lead to a difficult, "dry" labor with deleterious effects to both mother and baby is, of course, completely unfounded; the production of amniotic fluid progresses continuously, so there is really no such thing as a "dry" labor. But infection is an increasing threat the longer the interval between rupture of the membranes and the onset of labor.

Many women think their membranes have ruptured when, in fact, they have not. Sometimes just a pocket or "bubble" of membrane ruptures, leaving the main membrane sac intact. More often, a particularly vigorous prelabor contraction presses the baby's head against the bladder, causing an involuntary loss of urine that is mistaken for amniotic fluid. In any event, premature rupture of membranes is no cause for alarm as long as the doctor knows about it when it happens. If he feels that the interval between the rupture and the onset of labor is too long, and his examination convinces him that the mother is "ready" at any minute, he may use

medicines to stimulate contractions; but unless he particularly favors induction of labor, he will probably be content to wait for nature to take its course.

However long the wait, sooner or later labor begins. For some this event looms up as a frightening and painful experience; for others, it is the triumphant climax of the pregnancy, a few brief hours which seem to epitomize the miracle of birth. It is, however, a universally accepted fact that the mother's attitude toward labor and delivery in a large measure determines how much trouble—or lack of it—she will have. If she is frightened and fights childbirth every step of the way, it will almost surely be an ordeal. No one can pretend that labor is "fun"; of course there will be discomfort, even moderately severe distress and some pain for a time, no matter what medicines the doctor uses to help. But if it is accepted and understood as a completely normal process, and if the mother approaches it with confidence in both herself and her doctor, she will almost invariably come through with flying colors.

Labor and Delivery

By modern standards the ways in which labor and delivery were handled even as little as 75 years ago seem unbelievably crude. At the turn of this century home deliveries were far more common than hospital deliveries, and the mother was often attended by a "midwife" rather than a doctor. Pain control, such as it was, depended entirely on opiates and barbiturates, drugs sometimes responsible for depressing the newborn baby beyond resuscitation. Ether and chloroform were the only anesthetics, and antiseptic techniques were still a novelty. It is hardly any wonder that the death of the mother or the baby in childbirth was accepted as commonplace. Today things are quite different in practically every respect. The overwhelming majority of all deliveries now occur in modern hospitals, with experienced nurses assisting the obstetrician and with facilities at hand to deal with virtually any complication that may arise. Safe and effective medicines are available to relieve apprehension and pain, and to promote the muscle relaxation that helps shorten the duration of labor. A wide variety of safe anesthetics exists for the safe delivery of the baby, including some that permit the mother herself to participate in the delivery. Obstetrical instruments and techniques allow the obstetrician to control the progress of the delivery and to protect the baby from birth injuries which once were so common. And the benefits of this modern-day revolution in obstetrics are clearly reflected in medical statistics: today the death of a mother in childbirth is a medical rarity, and the death of a baby almost equally rare.

In part this dramatic change has come about as a result of more open and honest communication between the expectant mother and her doctor. Today a pregnant woman is no longer "confined," and labor and delivery are no longer discussed in hushed and mysterious whispers. The obstetrician insists that his patient be fully informed, and the expectant mother has every right to know just how her doctor will conduct her labor and delivery. Only with this kind of advance information can the expectant mother make the preparations necessary for labor and know what to do when it begins; and with knowledge, self-confidence and trust, chances are the delivery itself will proceed without a hitch.

Preparation for Labor. Most women have ample notice that the onset of labor is imminent. Of course, some start regular, business-like contractions without warning at 2 o'clock in the morning and deliver their baby three hours later, but this is the exceptional case. Far more often, mild, wavelike contractions come and go for days and weeks before labor begins in earnest. Sometimes they can be quite uncomfortable, but they can often be ameliorated or even stopped simply by changing position—rolling over in bed, getting up and walking around, sitting down or standing up. Many women, particularly during a first pregnancy, may be convinced that these preparations for labor are the "real thing" only to have them stop completely for a few hours or even days before starting again.

Episodes of "prelabor" contractions can be aggravating, particularly when they recur day after day for weeks, but the doctor can evaluate their significance during the next scheduled office visit. The onset of real labor involves more than just uterine contractions and pressure; certain physical changes must occur before the expectant mother is "ready" for the contractions to proceed into active labor, and the doctor can identify these changes by means of simple digital vaginal examinations. Before active labor can begin, for example, the baby's presenting part— usually the head—must be "engaged" or wedged more or less firmly into the upper end of the birth canal. The doctor can palpate the uterine cervix, and if the examining finger can push the baby's head up and free with gentle pressure, the head is not engaged and imminent active labor is unlikely. Also, the uterine cervix, which dilates to permit the baby to pass down the birth canal, must have thinned or *effaced* and dilatation of the cervix must have begun before labor can start in earnest. There is nothing that can be done to hurry this normal progression of events; prelabor contractions are a necessary preparation for delivery. And if they are repeated and prolonged, when active labor begins it will probably be briefer and easier as a result.

False Labor. Occasionally an episode of prelabor contractions may be unusually intense and prolonged, accompanied by several other signs— the passage of some blood-tinged mucus, for example, or even the rupture of membranes— convincing everyone that labor has begun. Then, inexplicably, the contractions stop completely, or the expectant mother may have reached the hospital and the contractions may continue for hours before it becomes evident it was a false alarm.

False alarms occur frequently during a first pregnancy, and the doctor often encourages the mother to stay home and wait a while even if she really is in active labor. First labors characteristically start slowly and sometimes require as many as 12 to 24 hours to really begin in earnest. During a second, third or fourth pregnancy, however, these false alarms cannot be ignored, for there may be no way to distinguish them from true labor that can, and often does, begin precipitously. If the expectant mother reaches the hospital only to discover that it was, in fact, a false alarm, the doctor may decide to induce active labor if he feels the mother is ready. In any case, false labor is common; it is no one's fault, and in the long run it is better to go to the hospital than risk being unprepared for the onset of true labor.

Induction of Labor. Inducing labor means exactly what the term implies: coaxing or inducing labor to begin before its natural onset with the use of various labor-stimulating drugs. The most popular of these drugs is *oxytocin,* a hormone product of the pituitary gland which ordinarily stimulates normal labor by causing the muscular walls of the uterus to contract and relax in rhythmic fashion when pregnancy is at term. A commercial preparation of this hormone known as Pitocin can be administered in small individual doses by injection or by a continuous, carefully regulated intravenous infusion. When the baby's presenting part is engaged in the birth canal and when the cervix is adequately effaced and dilatation already begun, this artificial stimulation of uterine contractions is often enough to trigger natural labor, which in most cases will then take over and continue through delivery. The medication may be slowed down or stopped as normal labor takes over, but sometimes it is necessary to continue its use right through delivery if contractions dissipate when medication is stopped.

Contrary to popular notions, the obstetrician cannot arbitrarily decide to induce labor any time he chooses. If the timing is wrong, it can lead to a long and exhausting false labor, on one hand, or a precipitous and overviolent labor and delivery on the other. Some obstetricians favor induction because they feel it gives them a certain advantage in controlling the time and circumstances of labor and delivery. Others regard induction as tampering with a natural process which may subject patients to an unnecessary risk. Obviously it is not a technique that should be used simply because the mother, or the doctor, is impatient for labor to begin. Rather it should be reserved for those cases in which there is a valid medical or obstetrical reason for it— when a potential Rh factor problem exists, for example, or when toxemia may be a complicating factor, or when the mother has a past history

of precipitous labors with deliveries before she can get to the hospital. Even then it will never be attempted until certain criteria are fulfilled: the baby's presenting part must be engaged, the cervix thinned and effaced, dilatation started and the membranes ruptured.

The Progress of Labor. Ultimately, labor begins in earnest, whether naturally or by induction. Mild, intermittent contractions become regular, frequent and intense. There is some vaginal discharge of mucus, perhaps tinged with blood, and the membranes may rupture spontaneously with a copious discharge of watery fluid. Pressure increases in the lower pelvis, and the contractions become quite uncomfortable or downright painful. Most doctors instruct their patients to go to the hospital when their contractions occur at a specified interval and last for a specified period of time. They often arrive earlier than necessary, especially if it is a first pregnancy, but certainly if contractions become intense, painful and regular—five to seven minutes apart by the clock, not by guesswork—the time has come to notify the doctor and leave for the hospital.

Once the woman is admitted to the hospital, the progress of labor will be confirmed either by the doctor or by a member of the obstetrical staff, probably both. The routine usually includes an enema and the so-called perineal prep (shaving and surgical cleaning of the genito-anal region) and, if delivery is not already imminent, the administration of a mild tranquilizer or sedative. Apprehension is, of course, quite normal under the circumstances, and as contractions become intense, there is an almost irresistible tendency to tighten up muscles, which can thwart the effectiveness of labor. A mild tranquilizer or sedative can help relieve tension and make it easier to relax and let the contractions come with less discomfort. Other forms of "tranquilizers" can also help immensely at this point. Today most hospitals approve of the husband staying with his wife at least through the early stages of labor and often through the delivery, if the necessary preparations have been made in advance. There is probably no greater reassurance for the expectant mother, but only if the father knows what to expect and is not himself so tense and anxious that he communicates his anxiety to the mother.

Labor may be long or short, relatively hard or relatively easy, depending upon individual circumstances. But contractions, however painful they may be at their peak, are not continuous; when one contraction fades, there is a brief breathing spell before the next one begins. Bit by bit the baby is being eased down the birth canal, and the doctor will determine his progress with periodic examinations. If the expectant mother has not elected natural childbirth, she will be given analgesic (pain-relieving) medicines to take the edge off truly painful contractions, and here in particular her attitude and preparation are immensely important. The woman who is knowledgeable and relaxed may well do splendidly with no more than a single dose of a relatively mild analgesic such as Demerol to ease her labor until delivery begins. The woman who is frightened, tense and fighting all the way may require far more massive medication and may actually obtain far less relief from it. As a result, she may remain confused and tense throughout labor and ultimately deliver a heavily drugged baby. Whatever the length of the labor, however, progressive physical changes detectable by the doctor's examinations—particularly the degree of cervical dilatation and the progress of the baby's presenting part down the birth canal—will signal when the time has come for the mother to be moved from the labor room to the delivery room.

Anesthesia and Childbirth. Anesthesia is often a major concern in the mind of the expectant mother as she approaches delivery. Not many decades ago the anesthetic used most frequently was ether or chloroform, administered to "knock out" the mother at the moment of delivery. Today, fortunately, a wide choice of far safer childbirth anesthetics is available. Some still render the mother unconscious, although more safely than before, but many leave her conscious and actively able to assist in the delivery with a minimum of discomfort. If the mother has not decided to deliver "naturally," the choice of anesthesia usually rests with the doctor and may depend upon the personnel and facilities available in the hospital. The expectant mother's desires and preferences deserve prime consideration when a choice is available, but in general the doctor selects the anesthetic he considers the safest and most effective in each individual case.

Today several types of obstetrical anesthesia are widely used, each with particular advantages and disadvantages for both the mother and the baby. *Inhalation anesthetics* induce unconsciousness and total muscle relaxation in the mother, thus stopping pain; but they also stop labor contractions and thus cannot be employed until labor has reached a point that the delivery no longer requires the mother's assistance. What is more, the baby itself is often sleepy and sluggish from the anesthetic, some of which is inevitably absorbed from the mother's blood stream. Inhalation anesthetics can be safely administered in experienced hands, but their obvious disadvantages have led to a search for alternatives that enable the mother to remain awake and have little or no depressive effect on the baby.

One alternative is the use of *local anesthetics,* in which Novocaine-like medicines are injected to block or numb the nerves carrying pain sensations from the birth canal and the vaginal outlet. The *pudendal block,* applied just prior to delivery, is the most widely used local anesthetic in obstetrics, and in skilled hands it can be quite effective. Its disadvantage lies in the fact that it must be injected at precisely the right moment in precisely the right spot, and because no two women have exactly the same anatomy, it frequently fails to "take" adequately.

For this reason less localized *spinal anesthetics* are more frequently used, particularly a low spinal or "saddle block" anesthetic, so called because it blocks only the nerves supplying the "saddle" area that includes the lower pelvis, the rectal and genital areas and thighs. It is a true spinal anesthetic injected into the spinal canal well below the level of the spinal cord itself, and it has a number of advantages. It can be given very quickly as delivery time approaches, bringing complete pain relief within a minute or so. It leaves the mother completely awake and alert, able to assist with contractions by bearing down without pain or discomfort, and it has no depressing effect whatever on the baby.

But "saddle block" anesthesia has disadvantages as well. Because it tends to slow down or stop uterine contractions, it cannot be employed until late in labor when the baby is very near the point of delivery. Even then the uterus may have to be stimulated with Pitocin injections to complete the labor. Like any spinal anesthetic, it also often causes a temporary but troublesome drop in blood pressure immediately after administration, and about one out of ten women suffers a postanesthesia headache which may vary from mild to quite severe and last from a few hours to several days. More serious residual aftereffects such as paralysis, meningitis or permanent recurring headaches are virtually nonexistent. In fact, statistically, spinal anesthetics are among the safest and most reliable known when properly administered. Even so, many obstetricians, and their patients, prefer an alternative form of *subspinal* or *caudal anesthetic* when the hospital can provide the services of a skilled anesthesiologist.

Unlike the saddle block, the caudal is not a true spinal anesthetic at all. The anesthetic agent is introduced into an area at the base of the spine below and outside the spinal canal, where it can affect the nerves leading to the pelvic, genital and rectal areas only after they have left the spinal canal. The nerves controlling uterine contractions are not affected; thus it can be administered much earlier in labor than any other anesthetic. However, it tends to wear off fairly quickly, so it must be replenished from time to time. Usually this problem is overcome by threading a fine plastic catheter into the caudal canal at the base of the spine at the time of the initial injection and then leaving it in place during the rest of labor so that small quantities of anesthetic can be injected periodically as needed. This requires the continual attendance of an anesthesiologist, sometimes for a period of several hours, but the result is early relief from the pain of labor, effective muscle relaxation so that contractions can accomplish more in less time, and a mother who is awake, comfortable and able to contribute to the delivery.

Unfortunately, the bony caudal canal through which the anesthetic must be administered is extremely tiny and difficult to locate in some women; in others, the anesthetic is either only partially effective or does not "take" at all and hence cannot always be relied upon. There is also a certain incidence of "postspinal" headaches associated with a caudal anesthetic, even though it is not really a spinal anesthetic at all. Thus there is no one "perfect" obstetrical anesthetic, and the doctor must choose the one he feels more reliable and appropriate to the particular circumstances of the delivery. The search continues for the ideal anesthetic technique, but meanwhile labor and delivery cannot be expected to be completely painless, although they are far more comfortable and infinitely safer, both for mother and for child, than even a few decades ago.

The Pros and Cons of Natural Childbirth. It was partly in reaction to some of the very real hazards of obstetrics in the early decades of this century that the concept of natural childbirth appeared, first championed by the English obstetrician Grantley Dick Read and later modified and perpetuated by a variety of English, French and American obstetricians and clinics. The term "natural childbirth," however, seems unfortunate, not only because it implies that anything else is somehow "unnatural," but also because women have quite different emotional reactions to it. To some it evokes an image of an immensely enriching "back to nature" delivery without "stupefying" drugs or the use of surgical instruments; to others it suggests panting and suffering through labor and delivery completely unassisted. Neither concept comes even remotely close to what natural childbirth really means.

Read's contentions, briefly summarized, are that fear, apprehension, and the tendency to "fight" uterine contractions by tensing muscles are the chief sources of pain and difficulty during labor. By eliminating that fear through the knowledge of what to expect, and by preparing for labor with exercises in relaxation, muscle control and breathing, the discomfort can be reduced to a point that it can be easily and happily tolerated. Further, the brief period of real pain at the time of actual delivery can be made tolerable by yielding to the instinctive urge to expel the baby, and, by being awake and actively participating in the birth of her child, the mother experiences a sense of great psychological satisfaction that can be obtained no other way.

All of these contentions have a good deal of demonstrable validity. Fear and apprehension unquestionably *do* intensify the pain and difficulty of labor. Knowledge and advance preparations for labor *do* relieve both apprehension and physical distress. And certainly participating in the birth of a baby seems to be more gratifying to many women than being drugged into a stupor throughout labor and then rendered totally unconscious during delivery. But with modern obstetrical techniques and medicines, all of these benefits are available to a woman whether she follows a natural childbirth regimen or not. Why, then, go to all that trouble?

There is only one valid answer to this question: *because the woman wants to.* Not because her doctor thinks she should or should not; not because it is "fashionable"; not because of some imaginary benefits for the baby; above all, not because she elects it in a moment of enthusiasm and then feels trapped into sticking with her decision; but only because she sincerely desires to participate as fully as possible in the natural physical and emotional experience of having her baby without blunting or dulling her senses any more than is absolutely necessary, and is willing to work hard and tolerate a certain amount of discomfort in order to achieve it.

For the woman with this kind of motivation, a natural childbirth regimen may be the best possible decision. She must recognize, however, that it is not all that "natural"; preparing herself both physically and emotionally requires diligence and hard work. Her doctor must be willing to work with her, and doctors sincerely interested in natural childbirth are hard to find. She must also have the active support and encouragement of her husband. And, finally, she must realize that *no one* can predict in advance the amount of tension and discomfort she may experience in labor, no matter how carefully she has prepared; nor can anyone guarantee a completely trouble-free delivery. The decision to use medications *must* rest with the doctor; no matter how experienced and knowledgeable the mother, only the doctor can evaluate the progress of her labor and delivery. Even the most ardent medical

champions of natural childbirth use medications without hesitation when they are necessary.

Perhaps the most serious drawback to natural childbirth is the "fear of failure." Many women make the mistake of regarding it as an end in itself, a challenge that *they* must meet, rather than as a means to a comfortable and safe delivery. Thus they may be afraid to change their minds when the time comes, adding to the fear and apprehension they may already have about childbirth rather than lessening it. Or they may suffer quite unnecessarily with a grim determination that actually complicates labor and delivery. If they do change their minds, or if medications do become necessary, they may feel that they "couldn't take it," that they have somehow "failed" themselves and their babies, and suffer pointlessly from guilt and self-reproach. Some women even overreact emotionally to their success with natural childbirth, almost as if it were more important to pass that test than to have a baby.

Obviously these attitudes are antithetical to the real purpose of natural childbirth, which is, quite simply, to aid in a generally easier and speedier labor and delivery, whether or not some medications become necessary. For many women natural childbirth offers very little that cannot be obtained equally well with modern obstetrical techniques. But for the woman with sound motivation, careful preparation and real support from her doctor, it can be a beneficial and rewarding experience.

Terminal Labor and Delivery. Whether medications and anesthetics are used or not, the final result of labor is always the same, as long as no major complications arise. The tempo and intensity of the contractions begin to increase, further thinning and dilating the uterine cervix and forcing the baby down the birth canal a bit at a time, until finally a point is reached that delivery is possible.

During the baby's passage down the birth canal, most women experience an irresistible urge to work with their contractions, "bearing down" by adding the force of abdominal contractions to the strength of uterine contractions and speeding the progress of their labor. This is especially true when a saddle block anesthesia

has rendered "bearing down" relatively painless. In the case of a first delivery, as much
as an hour or two, perhaps even more, may
elapse from the time when the cervix is com-

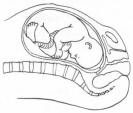

A. BEFORE LABOR

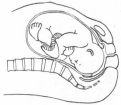

B. CERVIX DILATED, HEAD
ENGAGED

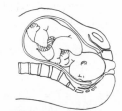

C. HEAD IN BIRTH CANAL
READY FOR DELIVERY

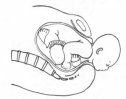

D. HEAD DELIVERED

Figure 57–7.

pletely dilated to the time when the baby's
head has moved far enough down the birth canal
for the scalp to be visible at the vaginal outlet,
and this interval of "hard labor" cannot generally be hurried. During subsequent deliveries
the walls of the birth canal, already stretched by
one delivery, are more flaccid and offer less

resistance to the baby, so that this stage of labor
is often much briefer.

In most cases the baby enters the birth canal
head first, with the head serving to stretch and
dilate the muscle and connective tissue of the
birth canal as it goes. It might seem that this
normal head presentation is "doing things the
hard way," and that a breech or feet-first presentation would be much easier on both mother
and baby by stretching the birth canal gradually.
In fact, quite the opposite is true. At term the
baby's widest cross-sectional diameter is through
his head, the next through his shoulders, and the
third through his narrow hips. The rounded,
somewhat moldable head serves as a wedge that
can do a far better job of dilating and stretching
the birth canal than the shoulders or the hips.
Furthermore, once the head has dilated the birth
canal, there is ample room behind it for the
umbilical cord to follow without suffering compression, and a good supply of blood can be
maintained up to the moment that the placenta
detaches after the delivery. Finally, once the
head has been delivered, delivery of shoulders,
hips and legs usually follows quickly, but if the
rest of the delivery is slightly delayed, at least an
airway has been established and the baby can
begin his own breathing movements. It is true,
however, that in its progress down the birth
canal the baby's head is "molded" or elongated
to a certain degree due to the pressure on his
skull, which is quite flexible and not yet firmly
joined together. When the mother first sees her
baby this elongation might seem quite extreme,
but it does the baby no harm and his head will
resume its normal shape within a few hours after
birth.

The last barrier to delivery of the baby's head
is the thick muscular floor of the perineum
which lies between the vaginal opening and the
anus. In a *spontaneous delivery* (that is, a delivery unassisted by forceps) considerable time
may be required for the baby's head to stretch
this thick, resistant layer of soft tissue sufficiently to make its way through. Since both
uterine contractions and "bearing down" become
most forceful at this point, it was once common
for this last barrier of tissue to be torn by the
baby's head in the process of delivery after a

prolonged period of pushing and stretching. Today, if necessary, the obstetrician usually makes a small surgical incision through the perineum to enlarge the vaginal opening, a procedure known as an *episiotomy,* in order to shorten the ordeal for both the baby and the mother. The mother is anesthetized and the procedure is performed just as the baby's head begins to emerge. It creates a clean surgical wound which can easily be repaired after delivery and heals quickly, certainly preferable to a ragged tear which may be far more difficult to repair properly. Once an episiotomy has been performed, the baby's head can be delivered with relative ease, followed quickly by delivery of the shoulders and arms and then the hips and legs. After such long preparation, actual delivery may seem almost anticlimactic. If the mother is awake under a saddle block or caudal anesthesia, however, she will know it has happened when she hears the infant's first indignant wail, and will have her first look at her new baby just a few moments later.

The Modern Use of Forceps. In any discussion of labor and delivery the question of obstetrical forceps invariably arises. Some doctors, it is said, "always" use forceps for their deliveries; others seem to condemn the practice. Why this difference of attitude? And which view is correct?

Obstetrical forceps are deceptively fierce-looking instruments, but essentially they are simply a pair of broad, curved metal plates with handles that articulate at a pivot point. The

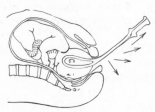

Figure 57–8.
Forceps delivery.

curved plates are so fashioned that they can be eased into the lower end of the birth canal, one at a time, to fit snugly about the baby's head. The handles of the forceps are then engaged,

and gentle traction can be applied to ease the baby's head out of the birth canal.

Forceps were first invented in the early 1600s to be used in emergencies when it was necessary literally to extract a baby, dead or alive, from the birth canal. Many women to this day equate the use of forceps with dire emergencies, and not entirely without cause. Forceps are still used to assist and hasten a difficult delivery, sometimes under emergency conditions in which the life of the baby might be lost without them. But today they are far more commonly used not just in emergencies, but as an added safety precaution in perfectly normal deliveries. The doctor may choose to use them *prophylactically* to shorten the terminal stage of labor, to protect the baby's head from a prolonged interval of pushing and pounding against resisting muscle tissue before it can be delivered, and to provide the baby with a protective sheath or "helmet" at the moment of delivery. Not all doctors use forceps routinely in this fashion; some still prefer to wait for a spontaneous delivery. But most obstetricians see little virtue in *not* using forceps, and feel that in most deliveries the advantages to mother and baby far outweigh the extremely remote risk of causing the baby even minor injury when they are properly applied.

After Delivery. Once the baby is delivered, the doctor and assisting personnel must quickly turn their attention to two patients, rather than just one. The baby's umbilical cord is clamped and cut, later to be cut shorter and firmly tied in the nursery. If the baby is not already squalling, and thus breathing, the doctor will stimulate it until it begins. The baby is then wiped to remove mucous secretions and the waxy coat of *vernix* on the skin that helped lubricate the delivery. Dilute silver nitrate drops are instilled in his eyes as a routine protection against gonorrheal infection. Then, before the baby leaves the delivery room the doctor makes a brief but thorough examination to be sure he is physically sound. In recent years pediatricians have come to realize that a variety of disorders which appear in infancy or childhood can frequently be anticipated on the basis of observations made by the obstetrician at the time of birth. The doctor checks the baby's degree of alertness and activity, the length of time that elapses before he breathes spontaneously, his color at birth, the presence or absence of infantile reflexes, and a number of other conditions. These observations are later evaluated against a so-called Apgar rating scale named for Dr. Virginia Apgar, a pediatrician who devised it as a means of prognosticating certain threatening disorders of infancy and childhood as early as possible and, conceivably, helping to ameliorate or even prevent them. The baby's Apgar rating is now customarily entered as statistical data in the hospital chart of the delivery. In this way a permanent record exists of the doctor's on-the-spot impressions of the baby's overall condition at birth. Such an examination takes only a few minutes after the delivery, but widespread use of the Apgar rating scale has already made it possible to anticipate, and sometimes to prevent, certain childhood disorders which might otherwise have progressed undetected for weeks or even months. Once this examination has been completed, the baby is carefully identified and then assigned to an assistant who keeps a close watch to see that he remains pink and responsive when he is taken from the delivery room to the nursery.

After delivery, the mother's uterine contractions continue as before, since the placenta still remains inside the uterus. However, separation of the placenta usually occurs a few minutes later—rarely longer than an hour after the baby's birth—and it is expelled as the *afterbirth*. There is always a certain amount of bleeding during the separation and delivery of the placenta, but once it has been expelled the continuing contractions of the uterine muscle tighten the uterus down into a firm ball low in the pelvis so that further bleeding is naturally controlled. In addition the doctor may administer Ergotrate, a drug that helps keep the uterus firmly contracted for the first few postdelivery hours. He may also prescribe small doses of Pitocin if the uterus still tends to relax enough to permit significant bleeding. He repairs the episiotomy incision immediately after delivery while the anesthetic is still in effect and examines the placenta carefully to see that it has been completely expelled. Even if only a fragment of placental tissue remains, it can cause later complications. Then, after a period of observation to be sure everything is stable, the new mother returns to her room for the postdelivery recovery period.

Complications of Labor and Delivery

Childbirth, in the great majority of cases, is a relatively uncomplicated process, but labor and delivery do not always follow the normal pattern. This, of course, is the main reason why there is an obstetrician in attendance. With his special knowledge and experience he can spot trouble in advance, where possible, and move swiftly to protect the mother and the baby when complications do occur. Some of these complications are extremely rare, but others occur frequently enough that expectant mothers should at least know what they are and what they may mean.

Breech Presentations. One of the most common *foreseeable* complications of labor is a persisting breech presentation of the baby when labor begins. No one knows why some babies enter the birth canal in this feet-first or buttocks-first position, but they do, and they often defy all the doctor's attempts to turn them around in the uterus by manual manipulation from the outside before labor begins. The position of the placenta or the length of the cord may have something to do with it, but whatever the cause, persistent breech presentations occur in about 3 to 4 percent of all labors, and some women tend to have recurrent breech presentations, perhaps as a result of some subtle difference in their pelvic anatomy.

In most cases a breech labor begins and progresses much the same as if the baby had entered the birth canal head down. The trouble arises at the time of delivery. The lower part of the baby's body is too small to dilate the birth canal enough to permit a speedy, spontaneous delivery of the head. If the body has been delivered but not the head, the baby is imperiled, since delay at this point may permit the placenta to detach, cutting off the necessary oxygen supply. When that happens, the baby can suffer acute oxygen lack, or even suffocate, if the head is not delivered immediately.

In most cases, the possibility of a breech presentation has been established before labor begins, so that a breech baby seldom comes as a surprise. Further, the techniques for speedy delivery of a breech baby's head have been known for centuries, and the doctor is fully prepared to handle this problem, either delivering the head manually or using special forceps developed for the purpose. Even so, there is a slightly higher mortality rate, overall, among breech babies than among babies that present head first, and the threat of damage or death to a breech baby is sharply higher than average if it is the

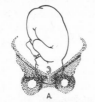

A.
VERTEX PRESENTATION
(HEAD DOWN)
MOST COMMON

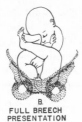

B.
FULL BREECH
PRESENTATION

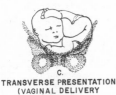

C.
TRANSVERSE PRESENTATION
(VAGINAL DELIVERY
IMPOSSIBLE)

Figure 57–9.

mother's first labor. This is particularly true if the mother has a small, narrow pelvis and the baby is comparatively large.

In fact, the danger to the baby is great enough,

in the case of breech presentation in a first pregnancy, that most obstetricians will be prepared to do a Caesarean section if a trial of labor fails. If the labor progresses well without complications, the doctor will proceed with a vaginal breech delivery; but if, in his judgment, some problem threatens as the labor proceeds, he will not hesitate to perform a Caesarean.

Other Malpresentations. A persisting breech presentation, while not exactly the rule, occurs often enough that it cannot really be considered abnormal. But other malpresentations, which occur far less frequently, are truly abnormal and sometimes arise solely by chance or because of some structural peculiarity of the mother's pelvis.

A *transverse presentation* occurs when the baby lies crosswise in the pelvis at the time labor begins. In such a position the baby cannot enter the birth canal at all, even though the membranes rupture and labor contractions become intense. *Arm* or *shoulder presentations* are more complicated variations of a transverse presentation; the baby's shoulder may be wedged into the birth canal, or an arm may be extruded. In either case, normal progress of labor is impossible. In a *face presentation* the baby's neck is somehow flexed so that the head enters the birth canal face first, a situation in which the baby's head may become firmly wedged and make vaginal delivery difficult.

As with a breech presentation, the doctor usually has advance warning before labor begins that a malpresentation may occur. Even when it occurs unexpectedly he can feel the presenting part in the birth canal and make the necessary preparations. X-rays will help confirm the diagnosis, and a Caesarean section will be undertaken without delay. Most obstetricians feel that this procedure is far safer than attempts at *internal version;* that is, reaching up into the uterus to turn the baby around and make vaginal delivery possible.

Disproportion. Another common mechanical cause for *dystocia* (difficult labor) is the presence of a marked disproportion between the diameter of the baby's head and the diameter of the birth canal somewhere along its length. Surprisingly, such a disproportion can rarely be diagnosed on the basis of the size of the woman or the baby; many small women have delivered eight- or nine-pound babies after a perfectly normal, uncomplicated labor. Occasionally, however, the bony structure of a woman's pelvis is narrowed or *contracted* just enough, regardless of her size, that the baby's head becomes lodged in the birth canal and fails to progress downward in spite of active labor. This situation can be further aggravated if the baby's head happens to engage in the occiput posterior position (with the face upward) rather than in the occiput anterior position (face downward) as is the normal case.

If the disproportion is slight, it may result in nothing more than a more prolonged and difficult labor than normal. If it is more marked, a Caesarean section must be performed. Usually the doctor will suspect a contracted pelvis from the time of his first physical examination. If he is in doubt, he will order special X-rays during the final month of pregnancy to permit actual measurement of the baby's head in comparison to the mother's pelvic outlet. Then, if disproportion is evident, a Caesarean section will be planned in advance. Even if an unexpected disproportion becomes evident only after labor has begun, the doctor will be prepared to perform a Caesarean if it proves necessary in order to avoid dangerously prolonged and fruitless labor.

Uterine Inertia. Another comparatively common complication of labor, uterine inertia occurs when the contractions of labor are too feeble, too short, or too infrequent to move the baby down the birth canal for delivery. It often complicates delivery in older women, or when labor has been so prolonged that the uterus has simply become "tired out." Uterine inertia is usually treated differently depending upon whether it is *primary* (that is, when contractions have been weak from the very beginning of labor) or *secondary* (when contractions diminish after a prolonged interval of active labor). In primary inertia, the problem is often resolved by the administration of small doses of Pitocin to intensify and prolong the contractions. In secondary inertia or "uterine exhaustion" after a long period of hard labor, the doctor may administer a sedative in order to quiet the contractions still

further temporarily, and allow the patient to sleep. In most cases strong contractions will return again after a few hours' rest.

The obstetrician uses certain well-established criteria in deciding when to intervene in a prolonged labor. Any sign of distress on the part of the baby—weakening or slowing of the fetal heartbeat, for example—is an indication for an immediate Caesarean section if vaginal delivery cannot be accomplished swiftly. He may also decide on a Caesarean section if more conservative treatment of uterine inertia does not produce prompt results. Further, after an episode of uterine inertia, the doctor is particularly alert for evidence of abnormal bleeding following delivery which may be caused by the failure of the uterus to contract adequately. Medications and transfusions, if necessary, can be used to counteract this complication.

Other Emergency Complications. Most of the common complications of labor and delivery are foreseeable and can be dealt with as a matter of obstetrical routine. But there are a few, less common but more hazardous, that can occur unexpectedly, often with no prior warning, and require swift emergency action.

Placenta previa and *abruptio placentae,* both of which may occur during the third trimester of pregnancy (*see* p. 831), can also first appear at the beginning of labor, heralded by the onset of copious bleeding. The doctor must then decide whether an immediate Caesarean section is indicated or whether to proceed with a vaginal delivery. *Rupture of the uterus* is a rare complication which may occur in women who have had a previous Caesarean section, or in multiparous women when labor is being induced. When it happens, swift surgical intervention becomes necessary. A similar emergency arises when a loop of umbilical cord *prolapses* or slips down from the uterus into the birth canal ahead of the baby's presenting part. There is always threat of this complication when membranes rupture early and there is room for the umbilical cord to slip into the birth canal before the baby's head is firmly engaged. When the head does engage, it presses against the cord and may cut off the baby's oxygen supply. This complication can usually be averted, if the problem is recognized early enough, by an emergency Caesarean section.

Caesarean Section. Named for the way in which it was believed that Julius Caesar was brought into the world, a Caesarean section is a surgical procedure used to remove a baby from the uterus by making an incision through the abdomen. Julius Caesar perhaps to the contrary, the procedure was not employed to deliver a living mother of a living child until the 1500s, and it was not until the late nineteenth century, with the dramatic improvement in all forms of surgical techniques, that the operation was considered reasonably safe. Today, thanks to effective anesthetics and the use of antibiotics and blood transfusions when necessary, the procedure is remarkably safe, offers the baby almost as good a chance for survival as a normal vaginal delivery, and provides an ideal means to save the mother from the hazards of complicated labor.

A Caesarean section is performed primarily in cases of malpresentation and disproportion. It is also usually performed in treatment of placenta previa or abruptio placentae, when immediate delivery is necessary to prevent dangerous hemorrhage, and when severe toxemia or childbirth convulsions threaten to complicate vaginal delivery. In addition, most obstetricians plan a Caesarean section when a woman has already had a previous Caesarean.

As a major surgical procedure, a Caesarean section is, of course, not quite as safe for the mother as an uncomplicated vaginal delivery. And there is the minor drawback of a somewhat longer post-partum (i.e., after delivery) recovery for the mother, since the abdominal wound must heal. A longer-term disadvantage, however, must always be weighed; once the wall of the uterus has been opened for a Caesarean section, it heals with a scar, and that scar will remain as a "weak spot" for the rest of the woman's childbearing life. In any subsequent pregnancy, there is always the possibility that this "weak spot" will tear in the course of labor and possibly even rupture. Bearing this in mind, the obstetrician caring for a woman who has had a previous Caesarean section may feel committed to perform another section to deliver each subsequent baby. This "once a Caesarean, always a Cae-

sarean" attitude is not a hard and fast rule, however; if the mother is a young woman in good health who has already had a normal vaginal delivery before her first Caesarean section, her doctor may elect a "trial of labor" with a subsequent pregnancy. But in practice, more than half the Caesarean sections performed today are "repeats," and in probably as many as 9 out of 10 women who have had an initial Caesarean, the procedure will be repeated with subsequent pregnancies, simply as a precaution.

The use of the Caesarean section has led to a steady decrease in mortality rates for both mother and baby in hospital deliveries, even in the face of the most serious emergency. Equally important, however, is the use of other modern obstetrical techniques, and the skill, experience and concern of the obstetrician as well as the other members of the specially trained obstetrical team.

The Post-Partum Period

There was a time not long ago when a woman's hospital confinement after delivery was always at least a full week and often even longer. But times have changed, perhaps because labor and delivery are not quite the "ordeal" they once were, thanks to modern obstetrical practices. Whatever the reason, most modern-day mothers are up and moving about the day after delivery and are permitted to go home with their new babies approximately two days later.

In the hours immediately after delivery, however, the doctor and the obstetrical nurses are very alert for any sign of certain early post-partum threats to the mother that may occur. The twin specters of *post-partum hemorrhage* and the clinical *shock* that may result from it must be guarded against. Sometimes delivery itself is accompanied by a greater than normal blood loss, but even when the normal and average 500 cc.'s or less of blood loss are not immediately exceeded, continuing bleeding from the uterus or into the soft tissues of the perineum may occasionally occur. Thus the mother's pulse rate and blood pressure are carefully monitored during the first 24 post-partum hours, and the doctor is prepared to order blood transfusions if necessary to cope with any problem. A third major post-partum hazard, uterine infection, although quite rare today because of modern aseptic techniques used during delivery, still does occasionally occur, manifested by a sudden spiking fever and abdominal pain arising at some time on the second or third post-partum day. Such infections, usually caused by strep or staph organisms, once ran a swift and often fatal course, so that *puerperal sepsis* or "childbed fever" was a dreaded complication. Today early diagnosis and speedy treatment with antibiotics on the first suspicion of infection can virtually always control such infections before they become well entrenched.

Certain other post-partum physical changes are perfectly normal and to be expected. During approximately three days following delivery, the woman's uterus *involutes* or shrinks in size, sometimes with accompanying crampy "after-pains" similar to but milder than labor contractions; by the time she leaves the hospital the top of the uterus will have receded almost to the level of the pubic bone again, and it reverts to normal size by the end of approximately three weeks. During this interval there is a normal discharge from the vagina, first bloody, then becoming milky white, known as *lochia,* a normal result of the healing process going on within the uterus where the placenta was attached. Normally the lochia has little or no odor; but should a foul or putrid odor begin to appear, this can be an early indication of infection and should be called to the attention of the doctor or nursing staff without delay.

Finally, normal changes take place in the breasts after delivery. If the mother has elected not to nurse, the doctor prescribes hormone medications which will suppress lactation, and the breasts will remain soft and gradually revert to normal size within a few weeks. If the mother is to nurse, hormonal changes in her body are triggered by the delivery of the child and placenta; within about 48 hours, the breasts engorge with milk. At this point, when the baby is put to breast, only a watery fluid known as *colostrum* emerges from the nipple—the same discharge noticed by many women during the last two months or so of pregnancy—but within another 24 hours in most cases an abundant supply of mother's milk will begin to emerge at each nursing.

Once the baby has been taken home, it is well to have some help with household chores for the first few days so that the mother has ample time for rest and for getting used to the new arrival. She should have plenty of nourishing food and fluids during this period and should report any unexpected symptoms—pain and burning with urination, for example, a sign of possible bladder infection—to her doctor. Tub baths must still be avoided, as well as sexual intercourse, until the doctor feels that all risk of introducing uterine infection is past, usually a period of about six weeks. At about that same time if he is a family doctor, he ordinarily performs a careful office examination of both mother and baby, and will discuss such questions as resumption of ovulation and menstruation, which usually occurs within three to four months following delivery, the diet controls that should be continued, and restoration of the feminine figure to prepregnancy proportions, aided and speeded up by exercises the mother should do on a daily basis to strengthen stretched and sagging abdominal muscles. If the baby is delivered by an obstetrician, care of the baby will be referred to a pediatrician or general practitioner.

Of course, if the baby was delivered by Caesarean section there is less risk of hemorrhage, shock or infection in the immediate post-partum period. Recovery is somewhat slower than following a vaginal delivery, since an abdominal wound must heal, but other aspects of the post-partum period are similar.

To Nurse or Not to Nurse. Probably no other single question related to childbirth has been discussed more widely, or more emotionally, than this one, both pro and con. As a result, a great many women have been thoroughly confused or misled. Some who really want to nurse their babies feel ashamed to say so, or fear they will not be able to, while others who really do not want to nurse feel somehow obliged to go through the motions. Doctors have often added to the confusion by taking an adamant stand on one side of the question or the other. But in the long run it is a decision that should be left to the mother herself and no one else.

There are, of course, some situations in which the mother is unable to nurse her new baby, perhaps because of her own physical condition or an insufficient production of milk, and in these cases the doctor's advice must be followed. But by far the greatest majority of healthy young mothers *can* successfully nurse their babies if they have the patience to learn how and are willing to put up with a certain amount of discomfort and inconvenience. The size of the breasts makes little difference; a woman with small breasts may have to nurse the baby on both sides at each feeding, but her total milk production will usually be quite adequate. Nervous tension and emotional factors, however, play an important role. Thus the most important consideration is whether or not the mother *really* wants to nurse. Like the decision for natural childbirth, the decision to nurse must be made willingly, sincerely and knowledgeably.

Nursing a new baby causes no damage or disproportion of the breasts, and it does offer certain advantages. Mother's milk is economical and available, and bottles, nipples and formulas are necessary only for occasional supplemental feedings. But the nursing mother must take special care of herself and her breasts, and obviously she must be "on call" day and night. Overall, however, nursing does not provide any particular physical benefits to either the mother or the baby, and, conversely, it does no particular harm *not* to nurse. The proper formula is just as good as mother's milk. As for any psychological benefits, they are largely a matter of personal conviction. Babies must be held and handled with warmth, love and intimate physical contact, and nursing can be a part of that intimacy, but the same closeness can also be achieved without nursing. Many people feel strongly that nursing does add to the relationship, but again that is something that only the mother can decide.

The widespread notion that the nursing mother will not menstruate is not at all true. Nursing seems to have no relationship to the onset of menses, which usually begins three to four months after delivery whether the mother is nursing or not. It *is* true that nursing mothers, *on the average,* remain somewhat less likely to conceive again while nursing, at least during the first twelve months after the baby is born. Beyond that point there is no significant difference. Obviously, then, the couple who wishes to avoid conception during the first several months after the birth of a new baby cannot count on nursing to prevent another pregnancy. With these pertinent facts, and with careful consideration of her own feelings, the decision to nurse must be left up to the mother. If she decides in favor of it, she can, of course, count on her doctor's help and advice. (The actual techniques and problems of nursing are discussed in detail on p. 853.)

Rooming In. This is a maternity practice, encouraged in some hospitals, whereby mother and baby remain together in the same room from shortly after delivery on, rather than keeping the baby sequestered in a separate nursery except for occasional brief visits to the mother during the day. The objective of rooming in is, of course, to allow mother and baby to get used to each other while they are still in the hospital. In addition, it is argued that the close, attentive care provided by the mother while rooming in is better for the baby psychologically than dispassionate care in a hospital nursery. If all hospitals had unlimited facilities for rooming in, and ample nursing personnel to supervise and teach in such a program, rooming in would doubtless provide many advantages that the ordinary nursery-oriented maternity ward cannot provide. However, most hospitals do not have these facilities.

If an expectant mother wants her baby to room in, she should make plans to go to a hospital where the service is offered. A young mother may be very eager to have her first baby within arm's length at all times. On the other hand, a woman who already has four children at home and has been looking forward to a couple of days of rest in the hospital after her delivery may emphatically *not* want rooming in. In hospitals where rooming in is available, the mother should be allowed to choose it or not as she wishes.

Circumcision. Here again it is a matter for the

parents to decide whether they wish to have a boy baby circumcised or not. But in this case, medical opinion is pertinent and leans heavily toward the affirmative. In terms of cleanliness and personal hygiene throughout life, as well as a measure to prevent possible infection, chronic irritation and even cancer, circumcision in infancy is usually recommended. Certainly if circumcision is to be performed at all, it is far simpler and less trying for the newborn baby than for the older child, adolescent or adult. The operation is a simple one, and contrary to widespread popular belief, removing the foreskin has no significant effect on the child's eventual sexual sensitivity or capability. However, medical arguments aside, if the parents do not want their baby circumcised, the doctor should respect their wishes.

Baby Makes Three

Especially in the case of a young couple, the appearance of a new baby inevitably alters their lives. The long waiting is over, and suddenly there he is. Much has been written about the profound emotional effects the arrival of the first baby has on both the mother and the father and about the change in their relationship and the problems that may follow. One problem, to state it quite simply, is the father who, no matter how much he wants and loves the new baby, may feel rejected or simply left out because the mother seems to concentrate a disproportionate amount of time, attention and affection on the baby. If a couple has a healthy and loving relationship, the advent of a new baby will, of course, strengthen rather than weaken it. But the fact remains that the baby *does* require excessive attention, time, love and care, and it is usually up to the mother to provide them. The days when the young couple could remain completely absorbed in themselves are over. Where once there were two, baby now makes three.

Most young parents accept this fact readily

and sensibly. After all, the baby is an important new member of the family. But he is not the *only* member of the family or even, necessarily, the most important member. Both mother and father also count, with their own needs for love, affection, communication, privacy and intimacy. Thus time should be planned for the mother and father to be by themselves occasionally, just as time should be set aside to be completely devoted to the baby. Young mothers soon come to feel cooped up, totally at the mercy of the baby, if they do not have some time to themselves. The father can help by sharing the work of caring for the baby and even taking over completely on occasion to give the mother a "breather." But simply taking turns is not the answer; just as mothers tend to feel restricted, young husbands come to feel ignored and left out unless they have *some* privacy with their wives.

Honest recognition that these problems exist is usually the first step in their resolution. Within two or three weeks after the baby is home, new parents should make an effort to find a reliable baby-sitter with whom they can confidently leave him for a few hours at a time. Then they should deliberately plan time as a couple, away from the baby perhaps as often as one evening a week, to spend with their friends or by themselves. New parents need these times to regain their balance as individuals and to reaffirm their relations.

If there is another child in the family, he should, of course, be included in the excitement and joy that a new baby brings; and he should be encouraged to share in some of the work, too. Time must be set aside by his parents, separately and together, to spend exclusively with him so that he will not feel left out. Perhaps most important of all is the realization that *every* member of the family counts equally. The family does not exist until a new baby arrives on the scene, and right then and there is the time to establish the patterns of love and care that will keep it together for many years to come.

The New Baby

During the first few days after she has given birth, most of the mother's time will be spent in resting and regaining her strength, and in getting acquainted with her baby. For new mothers, it is a time of revelation; but even for experienced mothers, it is doubtful that the sense of wonder at being able to see, hold and communicate with a newly born human being ever completely disappears. The baby is an individual from the moment he is born, and that individuality is expressed in a multitude of ways in the early days and weeks of his life. This is often a period of anxiety for the mother, too; no matter how many other babies she may have had, a new baby poses new problems, new questions and even new worries.

Any baby's first year is the most important in his life, barring none. He grows faster, learns more and develops more rapidly during the first twelve months than at any other time. It is also the time when the burden of responsibility on the parents is heaviest; the baby is more vulnerable to illness during his first year than during any comparable period in his life. Thanks to modern medical advances, the hazards that once threatened the lives and health of infants have been significantly reduced. But obviously the goal of a modern baby care program is to *prevent* trouble before it begins in order to give the baby the best possible start in life.

An important part of any preventive program is, of course, for the baby's parents, and for his mother in particular, to be fully informed about what to expect in the first weeks and months of

the new baby's life. Baby care is by no means "instinctive"; it requires a high degree of knowledge and experience to recognize not only those signs and symptoms that indicate a potential health problem, but also those patterns of behavior that are perfectly normal and should cause no concern. It would be impossible here to discuss every aspect of baby care in minute detail; whole books have been devoted to this topic alone, and expectant parents should ask the doctor, early in the pregnancy, to recommend those that he thinks are appropriate. No two babies are exactly alike; nor, for that matter, are any two mothers. Further, helpless and dependent as babies are, they are not as breakable as one might think. They are, in fact, remarkably sturdy little creatures—and they can communicate in their own way. With this in mind, with knowledge of the important, practical and up-to-date facts of baby care, and with love, patience and understanding, the new mother is well on her way to becoming a good mother.

Planning for Baby Care

When most women plan ahead for baby care, they think of baby clothing, bedding, diapers and all the other paraphernalia of the nursery. But the most important advance plan, which must be made before mother and baby leave the hospital, is an arrangement with a doctor to set up a routine program of baby care. The advice of relatives and friends is all right in its place, but it is no substitute for professional health care. The new mother may wish to go to her family doctor or to the doctor who supervised her pregnancy and delivery. She may prefer to consult a specialist in baby care, the *pediatrician,* or a child care clinic may be more convenient. Whatever her choice, it is of the utmost importance to "monitor" the first crucial weeks and months of the new baby's life.

Every doctor or clinic will have a different schedule which the new mother is asked to follow, but invariably it involves visits with the baby at certain intervals. Often the first checkup will be at approximately three weeks of age (unless of course the baby needs medical attention before then), with another checkup when the baby is six weeks old. Subsequently most pediatricians recommend protective shots beginning at about the third month, including immunizations against whooping cough, diphtheria, tetanus, polio, and later smallpox, rubella and red measles. The length of these visits is often very short, but they provide an opportunity for a brief but careful examination of the baby, and an opportunity to discuss the baby's growth and development with the doctor. They also provide the opportunity to make an excellent friend who can be enormously helpful. Most pediatricians have the invaluable assistance of an office nurse who has a wealth of experience and knowledge. A good pediatric nurse can answer a multitude of questions, thus making calls to the doctor unnecessary, and at the same time she knows when a particular problem should be brought to the doctor's attention.

It is most important to establish an open and honest relationship with the doctor who is caring for the baby, particularly in the matter of house calls and emergencies. Emergency situations can and do arise, and if the doctor does not make house calls, or if the child care clinic is open only during certain hours of the day, the mother should know well in advance whom to call or where to go to seek help. The doctor may be available day or night, or he may suggest an alternate physician who will take his calls if he is not available. He will also provide the names and telephone numbers of his own hospital or a convenient emergency facility that can be used to locate him or where the baby can be taken for emergency care. All of these names and numbers should, of course, be kept close at hand, and anyone taking care of the baby in the parents' absence should be carefully instructed in how to use them.

Perhaps more difficult is the question of determining just when a true emergency exists. New parents in particular often overreact in some situations and, in essence, create the emergency themselves, which can then lead to unnecessary worry, inconvenience and expense. With knowledge and experience this problem usually resolves itself, but the new mother should discuss quite frankly with her doctor just when she should, and should not, call. The doctor, in turn, should see to it that the mother is fully informed about those symptoms and conditions that do signal an emergency and those that do not.

In the long run, of course, it is better to be safe than sorry, and telephone calls in the middle of the night have long been a part of medical practice. A mother should not be afraid to "bother" her doctor, but at the same time she should be prepared to follow his advice. In deciding what to do, the doctor relies heavily on his personal knowledge of the baby and his assessment of the parents' ability to describe the situation accurately and to handle it. He may come immediately, or he may ask the parents to call back at regular intervals to keep him posted on the situation. He may feel that it is not an emergency at all, and arrange to call or visit at some later time or ask to see the baby in his office. On the other hand, he may ask the parents to take the baby immediately to a hospital emergency room. The parents should not be unnecessarily alarmed by this; in some cases, it may be easier for the doctor to reach the hospital than the home, and even if a true emergency does not exist, he may prefer to examine the baby and, if necessary, begin treatment under ideal medical conditions.

Obviously, then, it is essential to establish an atmosphere of open communication and confidence between the parents of a new baby and their doctor. He must depend upon their knowledge and common sense, and they must trust his professional experience and judgment. Further, the pediatrician, his nurse or some other child care professional is the best and most reliable source of information about the daily routines and procedures of caring for the new baby. Special precautions must be taken, particularly at first, in just how the baby should be handled —and who should be allowed to handle him. A new baby is not a toy, and the dangers of infection and carelessness are always present. In dealing with relatives and friends, and with older children in the family, the parents must first rely on their own judgment, but if some particular problem arises, they should not hesitate to ask the doctor's advice. The pediatrician's role is chiefly a preventive one. He is concerned with the baby not only when he is sick; his concern is with the normal, healthy growth and development of the baby throughout the early years of his life.

Babies Behave Like Babies

One of the wonders of motherhood is observing how incredibly individualistic even a very tiny baby is; yet at the same time all babies share certain physical characteristics and certain aspects of behavior in common. At the time of birth all the baby's bones are soft, and many have not yet become completely calcified. In addition, the large saucer-like bones of the skull have not completely formed, nor have they joined firmly together. Thus the baby has a noticeable "soft spot" just above his forehead, known as a *fontanelle,* and another smaller and firmer one where his head joins his neck at the back. These fontanelles will presently close as the skull bones grow together during the first year; in the meantime they are covered with tough fibrous tissue, so that injury is most unlikely. Babies' heads are always disproportionately large and heavy during infancy, and they display other physical stigmata: a receding jaw, a bulging belly, bowlegs and a thick layer of "baby fat." Babies often have blue eyes at first, but in many the eye color changes during the first six months to assume other colors.

As for characteristic behavior, all babies sneeze, yawn, belch, suck, have hiccups, pass gas, cough and cry. They may occasionally look cross-eyed, especially before they are able to focus their eyes on a bright object and "track" it; that is, follow its motion back and forth in front of them, an ability which does not begin to develop until the third month. Newborn babies sometimes appear deaf for the first few days or weeks because they do not respond to sounds by turning their heads the way older children or adults do, but they hear quite well enough to start and cry at sudden sharp noises very close to them. Most aspects of a baby's behavior have a logical and natural purpose. For example, sneezing is the only way in which he can clean mucus, lint or milk curds from his nose. Hiccups are little spasms of the diaphragm which have no grave significance; they can often be stopped by a few swallows of warm water. Coughing is the baby's way of clearing his throat, and the random, sometimes frantic physical movements of his arms and legs are a natural means of exploring the functions of his body and discovering things in the world around him.

Similarly, crying is his way of saying, "I'm hungry," "I'm wet," "I'm thirsty," "I want to turn over," "I'm too hot," "I'm too cold," "I have a stomach ache," or "I am bored." To one unaccustomed to a baby's behavior and personality, all this crying sounds exactly the same— noisy. But gradually the new mother will be able to distinguish between different *kinds* of crying, each with its particular volume, persistence, timbre—and meaning. A "hungry" cry sounds quite different from a "something hurts" cry, and each of these differs from a "things are pretty dull around here, let's get them stirred up" cry or an angry "if somebody doesn't pay attention pretty soon I'm going to have a tantrum" cry.

Early in the game the new mother tends instinctively to respond any time the baby cries, and the baby learns this lesson with uncanny swiftness. Naturally when there is a valid reason for crying, such a response is appropriate. But many mothers assume that there is a remediable cause for every crying spell, and become thoroughly upset, or even annoyed, when they have attended to all conceivable needs and the baby persists in crying. For these mothers, it is well to remember that crying does not necessarily mean that something is wrong, nor does it do the baby any harm. Even a perfectly satisfied and comfortable baby may cry for a little while each day, and if nothing else it ensures full expansion of his lungs. But if he cries for no remediable reason, or if it sounds like a fretful "nobody's paying any attention to me" kind of cry, there is no reason for the mother to be concerned or feel that she is doing something wrong. Let the baby go ahead and cry, with perhaps only an occasional reassurance that she is close by and will be there when he really needs her.

Finally, the baby sleeps a great deal during his first few months—sometimes so much that inexperienced mothers wonder if something is wrong. At first he may do little else but sleep and eat, but after a few weeks even a baby does not want to sleep *all* the time. Like anyone else, he gets rested, and then starts looking around to see what is going on. Within a couple of months most babies pick a definite period in the course of the day for a stretch of wakefulness between feedings. This is an ideal period for the baby's play time. During this interval, perhaps lasting from one-half hour to an hour and a half, remove the baby from his crib and permit him to kick freely on a bed or warm floor. If the baby will cooperate, the play hour can be scheduled before the late afternoon or early evening feeding, when the father is also home to enjoy it.

Bit by bit the baby's sleep and wakefulness will fall into a pattern, with a longer and longer wakeful period during each 24-hour span and, in most cases, a long sleep period some time during the day or night. Obviously it is to the parents' benefit if the long wakeful period occurs during the day and the long sleep period during the night. Often these two periods of the day can gradually be "developed" by encouraging the baby to be wakeful during daylight hours, and then offering him a full feeding when it is time for everyone to go to sleep. If the baby is not cooperative and, for example, begins to take his long sleep during the afternoon, it is possible to gradually work this sleep period around the clock a half-hour at a time simply by extending the wakeful period that precedes it a half-hour every day or two. In this way, eventually the baby's long sleep period can be made to coincide with his parents' sleeping hours. This kind of

"manipulation," within reasonable limits, is perfectly safe, and can spell the difference between several sleepless months for the parents and a comfortable spell of sleep at night. Other than this, however, it is usually wise to tamper with the baby's own feeding and sleeping schedule as little as possible. No baby yet has been known to starve when he is fed on a "demand" basis, and it is, of course, ridiculous to wake a baby in the middle of his long sleep period and give him a bottle just because the clock says that it is time for a feeding.

Breast Feeding

Feeding is one of the baby's first thoroughly pleasurable experiences, and his first love for his mother arises primarily from the feeding situation. Both mother and baby should be comfortable during feeding times, with the baby held in the mother's lap with his head slightly raised and resting in the bend of her elbow. Whether breast feeding or bottle feeding, hold the baby comfortably close, for it is physical contact and cuddling that supplies the vital emotional needs of this almost totally helpless creature at the same time that he is enjoying the pleasure of sucking, swallowing and satisfying his hunger.

If the mother has elected to breast feed the baby, her breasts and nipples should be washed once a day with soap and water. Then before each feeding, the breast should be rinsed with plain water and dried thoroughly. The nipple should be guided into the baby's mouth, and at the same time, the breast must be kept from pressing against the baby's nose so that it will not interfere with his breathing. Occasionally the baby must be encouraged to nurse; if his cheek nearest the breast is gently stroked, he will usually turn his head to hunt for the nipple. At other times, particularly if a relatively short time has passed since a very full feeding, he may simply be uninterested in nursing; there is nothing wrong with this, and he should be allowed the simple prerogative of choice.

All babies are born with a strong sucking reflex, but sometimes it may take a while to learn how to breast feed. As much as several days or even a week may elapse before mother and baby become accustomed to nursing and the baby is satisfied from the breast. During this early interval, if he still seems hungry after a nursing period, it is perfectly appropriate to supplement his breast feeding with an ounce or two of prepared formula in a nursing bottle. In most cases, however, the physiology of milk production in a woman's breast responds to the natural stimuli that occur during nursing; a breast that is completely emptied by nursing will be stimulated to produce more milk, while a breast that is only half-emptied will gradually tend to produce less milk. In this way the baby gets almost precisely the right amount of milk at each nursing, and the mother suffers little discomfort from breast distention owing to excessive milk production.

One great advantage of breast feeding is its flexibility and naturalness. There are no rules about when and how much, no anxiety about making sure that the baby gets at least two ounces but not a drop more. The baby may nurse from both breasts at each feeding if this seems to be his natural pattern. Ten minutes at each breast is usually long enough to empty the breasts temporarily, but mothers nursing their babies do not ordinarily set a kitchen timer. If for some reason the process must be speeded up, the baby may well be taken care of with a five- or ten-minute feeding, since he consumes about three-fourths of the milk in the breast in the first two or three minutes if he is hungry. On the other hand, breast feeding can also be extended if the baby is hungry and there is no great pressure on the mother's time. Nor are there any rules that say both breasts must be used; if preferred, and if the milk supply is ample, only one breast need be used at a feeding. Many mothers often allow their babies to feed at only one breast at a time in order to give the other breast a rest period, a procedure which helps prevent the soreness of the nipples that occasionally occurs when a baby is a particularly active nurser.

Breast feeding, however, does create certain problems that do not arise with bottle feeding. After the first couple of weeks, the mother's body responds quite emphatically to whatever nursing pattern has been established. Thus if circumstances make it necessary to delay nursing the baby for half an hour or even longer, or if the mother is absent for the usual nursing period, she may well find that her breasts fill, become distended and, in some cases, become quite painful. This problem can easily be relieved by purchasing a breast pump, a small, inexpensive, horn-shaped glass tube and receptacle with a suction bulb at one end. In a matter of a few moments enough milk can be withdrawn from the distended breasts, when circumstances demand, to relieve discomfort and help maintain the normal pattern of milk production. If the baby regularly needs a supplemental bottle feeding after nursing to fill him up, it is perfectly permissible to store breast milk obtained with a breast pump in a sterile bottle in the refrigerator at least until the next feeding. But mother's milk should not be used if it has been stored in excess of six or eight hours, even with refrigeration, and it should *never* be stored without refrigeration. Otherwise, the milk should be discarded.

Some babies need supplemental bottle feeding regularly, some need it occasionally, and some need it not at all. The mother must use her own judgment, bearing in mind that the baby may enjoy a period of fifteen or twenty minutes of sucking even when most of the milk has been emptied from the breast. A great deal can be learned simply by watching the baby closely, for he is enormously eloquent in his actions. A baby who nurses as if he had been deliberately starved for a week may well, after ten minutes or so, suddenly become massively indifferent to the whole idea, perhaps spitting out the nipple, allowing milk to dribble down his chin and grinning toothlessly. Or he may just go to sleep, only to wake up and wail vigorously the moment he is put down, and then pretend to nurse a few seconds before he falls asleep again. As a rule of thumb, virtually any pattern of nursing behavior is perfectly healthy as long as the baby does not remain too fretful too long, or show signs of discomfort or distress.

Many women are vaguely disturbed about breast feeding because they quite naturally associate the breasts with sexuality. Indeed, some women are even more distressed because they occasionally find themselves sexually aroused by the baby's nursing. But considered honestly and realistically, such feelings are not only perfectly normal, but appropriate. The breasts are richly endowed with sensory nerve endings and as erogenous zones play an important part in female sexuality, both in the act of intercourse and in the process of breast feeding. Thus nothing could be more natural than experiencing a sense of excitement, pleasure and satisfaction when nursing a baby, particularly when the circumstances of pregnancy have caused a period of abstention from sexual intercourse. If this or some other problem associated with breast feeding does trouble the mother, however, bottle feeding her baby is a perfectly satisfactory substitute.

Bottle Feeding and Formulas

The decision to nurse the baby by breast or by bottle is, of course, the mother's; and it should be made *before* the baby is born. (*See* p. 847.) If the mother elects to breast feed her baby, and if for some reason it does not work—an insufficient supply of milk, for example, or physical discomfort—there is no reason for feelings of guilt or inadequacy. Bottle feeding gives the baby all the nourishment he needs and still provides the opportunity for holding and cuddling. It does require, however, additional routine preparations.

There is a wide variety of baby bottles available on the market today, ranging from glass or plastic containers that can be washed, sterilized and reused, all the way to plastic holders equipped with presterilized disposable liners that can be filled with formula, placed in a holder, and then discarded after use. These disposable liners are also supposed to prevent air from entering the bottle during feeding, thus minimizing the need for "burping" the baby. In general, disposable feeding equipment, while certainly time-saving and convenient, is quite expensive in comparison with reusable bottles. If economy is a consideration, a dozen or so reusable glass or plastic bottles are a better investment; if speed and convenience are more important, the disposable variety may be a good choice in spite of the cost. In either case, the pediatrician or his nurse will be glad to offer recommendations.

When feeding the baby with a bottle, be seated comfortably and hold the baby with his head supported by the crook of the elbow and upper arm. Then tilt the bottle so that the neck and the nipple are always filled with formula. This helps the baby get formula instead of sucking and swallowing air. Most bottles, except for the collapsible and disposable type, and nipples are equipped with an automatic valve that permits air to enter the bottle as the formula is sucked out. Obviously, if the baby does not waste energy sucking and swallowing air he will get formula; in addition, swallowed air in his stomach may give him a false sense of being full, or may make him very uncomfortable.

An ample supply of nipples maintained in good condition—new enough to be firm as well as pliable, with the holes free from gummy residue—is important. Nipples deteriorate very considerably upon repeated boiling, and may become too soft for satisfactory use. Remember that the baby has a strong, natural desire to suck and will keep sucking on nipples even after they have collapsed, so take the nipple out of his mouth occasionally during the feeding. This will make it easier for him to suck, and will also let him rest a bit.

Never prop a bottle up and leave the baby to feed himself. The bottle can easily slip into the wrong position. Remember also that the baby needs the security and pleasure of being held at feeding time. Busy as the mother may be, this is an ideal time for her and baby to relax and enjoy each other, and no mother is too busy to devote a twenty-minute period every three to six hours to the pleasant game of feeding. The mother should be careful, however, to find a place to sit while either bottle feeding or nursing the baby in which she will remain relatively alert and able to observe any trouble the baby may be having. Particularly during nighttime feedings when the mother is wakened out of a sound sleep by the baby's hunger signal, it is tempting to sit propped up in bed dozing while the baby feeds. This procedure can be dangerous; it is all too easy for a dozing mother to fall asleep and inadvertently roll over on the baby. For nighttime feedings, at least, use a firm straight-back chair, just uncomfortable enough to discourage dozing off and falling asleep.

Whether the baby is bottle or breast fed, it is usually necessary to help him get rid of swallowed air, inevitably taken in during feedings, by means of "burping" or "bubbling" him. The most common way to burp the baby is to hold him upright over the shoulder and pat or rub his back very gently until he lets the air go. Or he may be placed on the mother's lap and leaned forward until he burps. Don't be alarmed if he spits up a little when he burps; this is perfectly normal until the baby's stomach gets used to handling food.

It is not always necessary to interrupt a feeding to burp the baby, but it should be done after each feeding at least. Of course, sometimes a baby may not burp because he does not need to. Don't try to force him, or panic if he does not burp. Finally, some babies swallow air when they cry or sleep, so it is a good idea to give the baby an opportunity to burp before feeding as well as afterward.

Much has been said on both sides of the still-raging controversy between "regulated" feeding times and a "demand" schedule in which the baby is allowed to eat when he is hungry. Most authorities today agree that the latter is by far the most satisfactory. A baby fed on "demand" will develop his own individual hunger schedule, which may extend from three to five hours between feedings. New babies usually "demand" to be fed every three hours, but may often go four or five hours between feedings once or more each day, or occasionally may need to be fed as little as two hours after a previous feeding. At least during the first two or three months most babies tend to go off to sleep immediately after each feeding; if they occasionally wake up and cry less than two hours after a feeding, they are probably not hungry. However, if it occurs consistently, it may be a clue that the amount or the richness of the formula may be insufficient.

The amount of formula the baby takes will vary from feeding to feeding. Sometimes a baby, just like anyone else, may not be hungry, and there is no way, of course, to make him want to eat. Most babies feed for fifteen to twenty minutes; occasionally they will take all of the bottle, and occasionally they will not. Don't worry about this; it is perfectly normal. As the baby grows and gains weight, he needs more formula, diluted with less water. When he begins to take all of his bottle quite regularly and sometimes cries for more, it may be time to increase the amount of his daily formula.

Naturally, babies have a steady and normal loss of water from their bodies, some of it lost as urine, some as perspiration, and some exhaled from the lungs during breathing. It is advisable to offer the baby lukewarm boiled water in a nursing bottle once or twice daily, preferably not within an hour of the next feeding. Some babies do not like water and may refuse to take it, but it is a good idea to offer it, especially during warm weather when the baby may perspire more than usual. Sometimes a small amount of corn syrup added to the water—perhaps half a teaspoonful in a four-ounce bottle—will encourage the baby who does not like water to take some. Alternatively, diluted orange juice, as soon as the doctor approves, may be offered instead of water.

After the baby has been fed and burped, put him in his bed. Placing him on his stomach will help expel any additional air bubbles that may still remain. It is also a good idea to rinse bottles and nipples with cool water immediately after feeding in order to remove milk before it forms a film. Squeeze water through the holes of the nipples to rinse them. This simple technique will make later washing with soap and water much easier.

It is important, of course, that the formula, the containers and other equipment used to feed the baby are as germ-free as possible. It is usually easier to prepare the formula separately and pour it immediately into already sterilized containers. A good way of sterilizing feeding equipment is called the "simple boiling" or "aseptic" method. The articles needed for this procedure are as follows:

A covered saucepan for boiling water for the baby's formula and drinking water; also used for warming bottles of formula before use.

Covered one-pint Mason jars for storing sterilized nipples and bottle caps.

A large, deep, covered kettle for sterilizing bottles, nipples, bottle caps and utensils. A sterilizing rack fitted into the kettle makes it easier to remove the contents.

Nursing bottles and caps. Between eight and twelve are usually enough unless the disposable bottle-bags are used. If they are, be sure to have two or three extra plastic holders in case they are accidentally broken.

A dozen or more nipples.

A quart, heat-resistant measuring pitcher calibrated in ounces.

Utensils: a long-handled spoon for stirring formula; tongs for handling hot bottles, nipples and caps; a funnel, a can opener, a bottle brush and a nipple brush.

Bottles, nipples and all utensils are customarily cleaned after each use, and then sterilized by submerging them in boiling water and boiling them actively for twenty minutes. After bottles and nipples have cooled, nipples may be inverted and the bottles capped with sterile screw caps for storage in the refrigerator or in a clean, covered container, to await future use.

The precise preparation of the formula itself will, of course, depend upon the doctor's instructions. Most formulas for very small babies are first prepared with approximately 12 parts of homogenized milk diluted with 15 parts of boiled water. Later this ratio is made richer, with more milk per unit of water. Whether the formula is prepared for bottle feeding or as a supplement to breast feeding as needed during the day, it should be made fresh every day and must be kept fresh, clean and sterile. Make enough at one time to last for a day, and then divide it into approximately the number of sterile bottles needed for the day. Some doctors enrich the formula somewhat by the addition of either corn syrup or simple sugar, but this is not necessary unless the physician specifically prescribes it. If for any reason the baby has difficulty with the formula that has been prescribed, don't hesitate to telephone the doctor and ask him to adjust the formula.

When filling bottles needed for the day's feedings, put nipples and caps on the bottles, taking care not to touch any part of the nipple that goes into the baby's mouth. Just before a feeding, remove a bottle from the refrigerator and warm it in a pan of hot (not boiling) water for a few minutes or use a bottle warmer. Do not touch the part of the nipple that goes into the baby's mouth. Test the temperature of the formula by shaking a few drops onto the inside of the wrist. It should feel warm but not hot.

Nipple holes should be the right size to help the baby suck easily. When the holes are the right size, warm formula should drip as rapidly as possible without forming a stream. If nipple holes are too small, the baby may grow tired of sucking before he gets all the formula he needs, whereas if they are too large he will get too much formula too fast and may not have enough sucking to satisfy. There is no way to make nipple holes smaller; large nipple holes indicate that the nipple is worn out and should be thrown away. If the holes are too small, they can be enlarged by heating a needle point red hot and then pushing it through the hole quickly. If the nipple holes become gummy, place the nipples in a pan of water, add a pinch of salt, and boil for a few minutes. Even when nipples are carefully washed and sterilized, a small residue of dried milk can form in the holes. If the holes still seem gummy after this treatment, discard them.

Finally, as a supplement to either breast feeding or bottle feeding, the doctor may recommend giving the baby vitamin drops after he is a week old or so. There are numerous good preparations for infant diet supplements, most of which include vitamins A, C and D, with vitamin B complex added when the baby is perhaps six months old. Ask the doctor if he has a particular preference; then shop to find the best price, since vitamin drops are often recommended for use all through the child's early years. Initial dosages will be very small, but when the baby's growth warrants it, the doctor will increase the amount. When giving vitamin drops, point the opening of the dropper toward the cheek inside the baby's mouth so that the drops do not fall too far back in his throat. A good time to give these vitamin drops, which are not particularly tasty, is immediately before a feeding so that the taste will be replaced by the taste of formula.

Solid Foods

There is no set rule about solid foods; every pediatrician has his own recommendations, and of course they should be followed. There is actually no need to force solid foods on the baby too soon; he will survive splendidly just on formula for the first three or four months. But many pediatricians believe that starting solid foods earlier not only helps the baby's gastro-intestinal tract accommodate to its future digestive role, but also provides a certain amount of bulk, in addition to nourishment, so that such large quantities of formula will not be necessary. Most babies can be started on solid foods at least toward the end of the first month, and sooner if the doctor recommends it. Often the solid food first recommended is a small quantity of rice, oat or barley cereal each day, perhaps a tablespoon-ful mixed with formula in a semifluid consis-tency. Use a small spoon to feed a baby, and remember it will take him a while to learn how to use his tongue and lips to help him swallow solid food. Next, many pediatricians will recommend approximately a tablespoonful of strained pear or applesauce per day added to the cereal; later, strained vegetables and meats will be added. The occasion of the baby's three-week checkup with the doctor provides a good opportunity to dis-cuss feeding of solid foods.

As to choice of solid foods, when the time comes, ready-prepared, jarred baby foods are so abundant in the markets, and so well advertised, that many young mothers today assume that no other kind of solid food will do. Unfortunately, this is a very expensive assumption, since the cost of these foods is significantly higher than the cost of the same foods prepared at home. True, it is more trouble, and special precautions must be taken in preparation to make sure the food is as germ-free as possible, but there is no significant difference, nutritionally or otherwise, between ready-prepared foods in a jar and the same foods cooked and strained at home. The convenience may be worth the additional cost, but in families where every penny counts, invest-ing in a V-shaped vegetable strainer and a wooden pestle can save a great deal of money during the time the baby must eat soft and strained foods.

Certain foods are deliberately withheld from the baby's diet until after the first six months or so. For example, strained meats are usually not added until the baby is used to strained vegetables or fruits and his digestive tract can tolerate the rougher consistency of strained meats. Wheat-containing cereals are also often withheld until the baby is six months old, as is egg yolk. Doctors who recommend this kind of caution do so because these are foods that are known frequently to be allergenic. In the first few months of life the baby is not able to cope as well with allergenic foods, if he should become sensitized to them, as he is when he is a bit older. In addition to these commonly allergenic foods, the baby may develop allergic reactions to almost any food, and any food which seems consistently to cause a rash or a colic attack following feedings should be with-drawn until the doctor can be consulted. (*See* p. 864.)

Bathing the Baby

Bathing the baby daily is important not only from the standpoint of hygiene but because chemicals in the urine and materials in the stool can be quite irritating to his very tender skin. In addition, bathing is a time of fun for both parent and baby. Most babies enjoy their baths im-mensely, and it is often there that they first begin to "respond like human beings," laughing and playing, splashing and having a fine time.

At most obstetrical hospitals there are nursing personnel in the maternity ward or nursery who will be glad to show the new mother how babies should be bathed, and any questions or problems can be referred to the pediatrician or his nurse. It is well to establish as soon as possible a fairly regular time for bathing the baby. The room should be warm with no drafts, and bathing sup-plies should be kept together to save steps. Until the navel (and circumcision) has healed, wash the baby by sponging; after healing, a tub or bathinette can be used. Only a small amount of lukewarm water (*never* hot) is needed.

Face: Wash with plain water and soft cloth, using no soap.

Eyes: Use cotton dipped in cool boiled water.

Nose and ears: Cleanse *only* the outer areas with a moist (not wet) cotton-tipped applicator. Do not attempt to cleanse inside either the ears or the nose. Babies will sneeze mucus out of their noses without any aid, and the excretion of wax in their ear canals encourages a natural self-cleansing process which needs to be aided only by cleaning the exterior of the ear canal daily. If a baby's ear seems to be plugged full of wax, or if some foreign object gets into his ears or nose, contact your doctor. *Don't try to remove it yourself.*

Mouth: No cleansing is necessary under ordinary circumstances. If a baby spits up, there is ordinarily no cleansing necessary afterward other than to offer a little water or orange juice. It is wise, however, to check the inside of the baby's mouth from time to time when he is crying, and ideally just before a feeding, to be on the lookout for the little white patches on the inside of the cheeks or on the gums which signal the common condition known as *thrush*. (*See* p. 863.) Tooth brushing should be started as soon as the child can manage it.

Head: During the daily bath, wash the baby's head with plain water and a soft cloth, but without using soap, in order to minimize the chance of getting soap into his eyes. Then once a week the head should be lathered gently with a mild soap, working the lather from front to back and keeping a Kleenex handy to catch soapy water drips before they get into the baby's eyes. Cleanse the soft spots well, and be sure to rinse the baby's scalp thoroughly.

Body: Use any mild soap. Be sure to wash in the creases. Rinse these folds well and be sure to get them thoroughly dry to avoid chafing and rashes. Pay particular attention to the genital and anal areas.

The baby may need a certain amount of skin protection between his daily baths. Natural substances such as cornstarch to powder areas that tend to chafe, or pure olive oil where indicated to soften the skin, are safest. Avoid perfumed baby oils and medicated powders or skin ointments unless specifically recommended by the doctor. The baby's skin is extremely delicate, and any of these products may be more irritating than helpful, even though they are prepared with the utmost care and with use for infants in mind. If the baby has areas of persistent chafing, or any other skin problem, consult the doctor.

Don't leave the baby alone in the bath even for one second. If the telephone rings, take the baby out of the bath, roll him in a blanket and carry him to the telephone, or else ignore it. The same goes for the doorbell. Even in the small amount of water in the baby's bath there may be enough buoyancy or slipperiness for the baby to turn over by himself and drown.

Don't bathe the baby close to a stove or a radiator. It can easily be too hot for his tender skin, and burns or a skin irritation may result. Similarly, *don't add hot water to the bath while the baby is in the tub.* His skin is not able to tolerate water that might merely be uncomfortably warm to you.

Keep the baby clean between baths; it will help prevent skin irritations and keep him tidy and "sweet." It is common for a flaky material known as *cradle cap* to form on the baby's scalp. It is not a sign of anything gravely wrong, but it can be a nuisance unless it is regularly removed. This is best done by applying Vaseline to the scalp in the evening once or twice a week and then rubbing it off with a soft towel the next morning. Ideally this should be done regularly so that cradle cap does not tend to cake and crust.

The baby's umbilical cord stump may not drop off for several days after he has been taken home. Keep the stump clean and dry, and do not tamper with it. If there is any sticking or oozing, carefully apply rubbing alcohol with a cotton applicator to help dry the sticky area. After the stump falls off there may be a few drops of blood, but this is no cause for worry. Also the baby may develop a small quantity of red moist granulation tissue, the so-called proud flesh, at the site where the stump dropped off. If so, it will usually dry, crust into a scab, and fall off without special attention. If it does not, the doctor at the three-week visit can speed healing by touching the area with a silver nitrate applicator, a painless form of chemical cautery.

When a baby is circumcised in infancy, there

may be a minimal amount of swelling, but not much, and there should be no bleeding. Commonly the physician performing the circumcision will wrap a strip of Vaseline-soaked gauze around the baby's penis and suggest that the mother leave it there until it dries and falls off. If there seems to be swelling, bleeding or irritation, call the doctor for advice. A sore area in a healing circumcision can often be relieved by the use of sterile Vaseline, but any manipulation of this small surgical wound should be done only on a doctor's instructions.

Diapers and More Diapers

A constant and inescapable headache in the care of babies is the need to change diapers whenever the baby is wet or soiled, and to keep a supply of diapers in good condition. Some babies may have a bowel movement after each feeding, at first, while many others may have only one or two a day from the start. Some babies go as long as 48 hours and are still within range of normal. Most babies strain when they have a stool, and some make a grand production of it, turning red in the face and puffing and grunting fiercely. Unless the stool is hard and pellet-like, this is perfectly natural. If stools are excessively watery or contain mucus, phone the doctor for advice. Similarly, if stools seem to be too hard and cause the baby difficulty in eliminating them, ask the doctor's advice. Laxatives are rarely if ever needed by a baby, and can be downright dangerous. *Never give a baby a laxative of any kind without checking with the doctor first.* As for urination, new babies may urinate small amounts as frequently as every hour at first, but soon settle in a pattern of bladder emptying at three- to six-hour intervals, usually during sleep periods or along with bowel movements.

It is well to change the baby's diaper as soon as possible after each bowel movement or wetting, at least within reason. Always be sure that the baby is dry when he is put to sleep, but there is no need to check him at ten-minute intervals during sleep to determine if he is wet. Otherwise diapers should be changed routinely as soon as it is noticed that they are soiled. Wash the diaper area clean with a soft cloth, soap and water,

rinse with warm water and then pat dry with a clean soft cloth. The use of a simple dusting powder such as cornstarch may help keep the baby's skin from chafing during warm weather.

Sometimes a baby's skin becomes irritated by contact with urine and a "diaper rash" develops. It is worthwhile noting, however, that all skin rashes on a baby are not necessarily diaper rash. Many babies have rashes that come and go without much rhyme or reason. Some of them may result from transitory allergies to certain foods, or from contact with some kind of clothing or bedding material. Any rash that persists or gets worse should be reported to the doctor, including a diaper rash. If it becomes severe, the doctor may prescribe specific treatment to help clear it up; in addition, it is often helpful to allow the baby with a severe diaper rash to sleep completely unclothed and exposed to air for part of the day, using a pad of diapers under him in bed without wrapping him up.

Most expectant mothers have a good supply of diapers given to them at baby showers. They are usually made of a loose-woven cotton material which can be laundered many times and reused. Soiled diapers should be rinsed in a freshly flushed toilet and then soaked in a covered pail of water kept in the bathroom for this purpose. If they are washed in an automatic machine, normal washing procedures with either soap or detergent should be followed, with an additional rinse if the machine permits. If a nonautomatic washing machine and soap are used, the diapers should be rinsed three times, and one-half cup of vinegar should be added to the last rinse. If a detergent is used the vinegar may not be necessary, but very thorough rinsing is a must.

Cut any way, the cleaning of diapers is one of the least attractive parts of caring for a baby, so it is not surprising that alternatives have been devised. One is the use of disposable diapers, absorbent paper material intended to be discarded after use. Unfortunately, most disposable diapers are made with a sheet of moisture-repellent material on the outside, so that, in essence, the baby is wearing plastic pants. They are also more expensive than cloth diapers, and they can be a real disposal problem; they cannot be flushed down the toilet and they add greatly to the volume of waste disposal in the household. Occasionally, they may be handy for travel, but in general they are not recommended. In fact, plastic or rubber pants of any kind, whether they are used over a cloth or a paper diaper, are not recommended. The vast majority of cases of diaper rash can be traced directly to the use of plastic or rubber pants. They may stay dry on the outside, but everything else inside, including the baby, stays wet. Even before the diaper is soiled, they cut off any contact of air with the covered area almost completely. Some mothers insist on the "convenience" of these pants, but the only excuse for using them, and then only occasionally, is when the baby is taken for a visit where an accident might be embarrassing.

A better alternative, in areas where it is available, is the use of a regular diaper service, a "baby's laundry" that delivers a fresh supply of diapers once or twice a week and takes soiled diapers back to be washed. Although this service, too, is more expensive than washing diapers at home, it is often provided at remarkably low cost and represents an enormous economy in the mother's time and energy if nothing else. Most services handle diapers properly and they are perfectly safe to use, but it would not hurt to check with the doctor or his office nurse to make sure of a firm's reputation before engaging it.

Babies Love Comfort

Perhaps more than anyone else, a baby is a lover of comfort, and he has no qualms about letting the world know the moment he becomes the least bit uncomfortable. This is hardly surprising, considering he spent the first nine months of his prenatal life cradled in the warm protected comfort of his mother's womb. Once he arrives in the "outside" world, however, he must have his comforts supplied by others, particularly the mother, until he is old enough to begin learning to take care of himself.

It is desirable, although not absolutely necessary, that the baby have a room to himself. This is not only for the baby's benefit; the mother needs some privacy, too, and some escape from the demanding presence of the baby. Inexperienced mothers frequently worry that if the baby is not immediately at hand they may not wake up if he cries; but fortunately, nature works in strangely logical ways, and the mother of a newborn baby seems to be equipped with a "third ear" that can catch her baby's cry, however feeble, anywhere in the house and bring her to instant wakefulness. Oddly enough, when studies were done to verify this seemingly magical capability, it was found that it is quite specific: a woman sleeping in a room adjacent to several babies would awaken instantly when her own baby cried, yet sleep blissfully through the cries of all the other babies.

Try to keep an even, comfortable temperature in the baby's room throughout the day or night. It is not necessary to heat the house up like an oven just because there is a new baby; the infant will adapt to whatever house temperature is normally comfortable for you. On hot days, be sure that there is some ventilation. On cold days, check the baby occasionally to see that he is covered enough to be warm.

A new baby can be expected to do a lot of sleeping, perhaps as much as 75 to 80 percent of each 24-hour day. Most babies prefer to sleep on their stomachs with their heads turned to one side, as soon as they are old enough to lift their heads. A very new baby should be allowed to sleep on his side; but put him down on a different side after each feeding. It can be dangerous to place a baby on his back to sleep because in this position, if he spits up some food, it is all too easy to breathe irritating stomach contents into his bronchial tree. Don't be overly alarmed, however, if he turns himself over during sleep. Some babies are extremely active in their sleep and simply will not stay put no matter what position they start out in. Mothers of babies who develop a habit of sleeping in the same position are sometimes upset because the baby's head seems to flatten on one side or his hair thins out in that area. But there is no reason for concern as long as the baby is getting the proper diet including supplementary vitamins. As soon as he grows older he will begin changing position in his sleep, and any distortion of his head will quickly correct itself.

As for preparing the baby's bed, bear in mind that pillows of *any* kind are a concession to the comfort of adults. The baby will sleep splendidly without a pillow unless he is taught to use it, and a pillow poses a real threat of possible suffocation. The mattress should be firm and flat, and should be protected by a waterproof cover. Next comes the soft baby sheet and one or two cotton blankets. Use only the lightest of bedclothes on top of the baby, keeping him in a room that is adequately warm rather than piling on blankets and comforters. Loose-weave cotton blankets will do as good a job of insulating as heavy down comforters, with the additional advantage that if the baby gets tangled up in the bedclothes, he can breathe through a light cotton blanket. If he is very active in his sleep, and tends to pull blankets up around his neck, it is wise to secure the blanket at the middle of the bottom of the bed and on two sides with safety pins. Don't wrap the baby up in a blanket, because this interferes with his freedom to kick.

The new baby does not require any more, and probably less, clothing than an adult, so take care not to overclothe or overcover him. Clothing should be loose and not too long to allow him complete freedom of movement. Dress him according to the temperature. Some babies develop allergies to certain fabrics, so watch for rashes in clothing-contact areas. As much as possible, make the baby a "cotton baby," using only cotton clothing and bedding that touches his skin, since cotton practically never causes allergic reactions. Bedding or clothing of wool, fur or feathers in direct contact with the skin is to be avoided until the child is two or three.

Ordinarily the baby's life pattern is centered on the indoors, but whenever the weather is pleasant it is a good rule to take him out from time to time. Babies born in the summer may be taken out in pleasant weather when they are only a week or so old. If a baby is born during the other seasons, he should be kept indoors for three or four weeks unless the weather is particularly balmy. Remember, however, that a baby's skin is exceptionally vulnerable to sunburn, and he should not be left for any length of time in the bright sun.

The new baby is clumsy, uncoordinated and physically weak at first, unable even to support his own head. When he is held, the mother should cradle him so that his head is always supported. Older children in the family often want to hold the baby, but they tend to be both careless and awkward about it; probably it is best to allow them only to "help" the mother hold the baby until he is older and stronger. Remember that there is no necessity, at this early stage, for any attempt at disciplining or training the baby, just love and enjoy him—*both* father and mother—and remember that he is a person in his own right. As such, he may not conform to what baby care books say, or to how some other baby in the neighborhood may be developing, but this is no matter for worry. The range of normal development in new babies is remarkably wide.

Watching the Danger Signals

Hopefully the new baby will enjoy exuberant good health from the first week of life onward, and it will be relatively seldom that he falls ill. Occasionally he may be cross, or his stomach may be upset, but these conditions are usually transitory and require little more than patience and love. There are, however, a number of illnesses to which babies are vulnerable, particularly upper respiratory and other infections. Obviously, commonsense precautions must be taken to protect the baby from colds and other everyday hazards, and if he does come down with a cold, the doctor should be consulted. Never give a baby even the mildest medication without the doctor's express approval.

The more serious illnesses to which the baby in particular is vulnerable are discussed in detail in the following chapter, but in addition an occasional emergency may arise that demands quick and knowledgeable action. As the baby grows older and begins to crawl and then to walk, he gets into everything, and he will swallow anything. A fall that might have caused a fracture should, of course, be brought to the doctor's attention, as well as any other physical injury, particularly burns. If the baby swallows pins or buttons or any other object that might cause internal injury, the doctor should also be called. Perhaps the most common emergency occurs when the baby swallows harmful medicines or poisonous substances. Such dangerous poisons as automatic dishwasher compound, strong detergents and other powerful household cleaners should be stored in a place inaccessible to young children. Similarly, any medicines, particularly aspirin, should be kept *locked in a cabinet* with the key well hidden. There are on the market small "wall safes" for medications equipped with combination locks that can be opened quickly by an adult but are safe from a baby's curiosity. The local druggist probably sells these lockers, or knows where they can be purchased. Finally, parents, or anyone entrusted with the care of the baby or any child, should be thoroughly familiar with the emergency procedures necessary in dealing with burns (*see* p. 119) and ingestion of poisons (*see* p. 116).

Fortunately, infant babies do not become ill very often, but when they do, diagnosis and treatment is a job for the doctor, and it goes without saying that the earlier he is called the more quickly and effectively the illness can be treated. *Any of the following signs of illness should be reported to the doctor at once: a fever of 101° or more taken by rectum; vomiting— not just "spitting up"—or refusal of food several times in a row; excessive crying; listlessness or excessive sleepiness; loose, running bowels, particularly if the stool is mixed with mucus and has a foul odor; or any unusual rash.* Any such signs may not necessarily have a serious cause, but the symptoms are suggestive enough of possible trouble that the doctor should know about them without delay.

Certain minor disorders occur so commonly among new babies that it is tempting to speak of them as "well-baby illnesses." Some of these deserve special note here, not because they are terribly threatening to the baby's health, ordinarily, but because they often alarm the new mother who has never encountered them before, and because any of them may become threatening to the baby if they are not promptly dealt with.

Colds and Upper Respiratory Infections. Babies are as vulnerable to these infections as are older children or adults, and are consider-

ably less capable of taking care of annoying symptoms by themselves. Most colds in infants appear first as runny noses, with or without a mild degree of fever; later, coughing develops as a prominent symptom. Sometimes vomiting or spitting up will follow a spell of coughing. Upper respiratory infections are discussed in more detail elsewhere (*see* p. 470), but mothers should be particularly wary that such infections in a baby do not continue without checking with the doctor. Babies cannot blow their noses, so the mother must clean away draining mucus when babies have a cold. A small rubber nasal suction bulb, available at the baby supply counter of any drugstore, can be a real help in clearing runny noses. Care should be taken that the baby sleeps on his stomach when he has a cold, since this will prevent drainage of mucus down into his chest. Temperature should be checked with a rectal thermometer after each sleep period. But perhaps the best clue to possible trouble is the *sound* of the baby's cough. A loose, moist cough is common in the presence of a cold, but a tight, dry cough, a wheezy cough or a harsh, croupy bark should be called to the doctor's attention at once, since active antibiotic treatment and careful observation of the baby may be indicated.

Thrush. This common fungus infection in babies, more annoying than dangerous in most cases, is caused by the growth of the fungus *Candida albicans* and usually first appears as white patches on the mucous membrane lining the baby's mouth. These patches can be distinguished from flecks of curdled milk because they do not dislodge easily with a moistened Q-Tip. Once discovered, the condition is usually easily treated with simple medication that the doctor will prescribe, but on occasion it can be irritating to the baby and may, under certain circumstances, tend to spread. Thrush may occur at any time, but is much more of a danger when a baby has been given a broad-spectrum antibiotic for a period of several days in treatment of an infection. Many of these antibiotics kill the normal bacterial flora living in the baby's intestine, or reduce the concentration of bacteria to a point that *Candida albicans* spores in the intestine are able to take root and overgrow the remaining bacteria. When this occurs, sometimes the patches of fungus are passed in stools and can be observed around the anus when changing the baby's diaper. The doctor is alert to this problem, and will usually take pains not to prescribe antibiotics for more than three or four days at a stretch unless absolutely necessary. Even a severe overgrowth of *Candida albicans,* however, can usually be cleared up quickly with the proper medicines.

Colic. Practically every baby regurgitates or spits up small quantities of food from time to time, often an annoyance for the mother but with little significance as far as the baby's health is concerned. In most cases holding the baby upright after a feeding and allowing him to "burp" or expel the bubbles of swallowed air he has taken with his food will minimize this kind of regurgitation. Some babies, however, actually appear to have pain in the abdomen after feedings, sometimes so regularly that they will begin crying within ten or fifteen minutes following each and every feeding, no matter how large or small. This pain is often accompanied by some degree of abdominal swelling and tenseness, and represents a form of cramping or spasm of the smooth muscle of the baby's gastrointestinal tract which is commonly known as colic.

No one knows the cause of infantile colic; in all probability it is a symptom that can arise from a wide variety of different causes. Some colic undoubtedly results from food allergies. Or it may arise from feedings that are too large and too infrequent for the baby to handle well, in which case the condition can be relieved by shortening the interval between feedings and feeding the baby less at a time. Most babies develop at least one interval between feedings that becomes longer and longer, but then appear voracious when feeding time comes again. A baby fighting frantically to take in as much of a feeding as possible in the least possible time might quite understandably have gastrointestinal cramps as a result. In addition, a baby who is rushed through a feeding may have colic as a result of rapid eating combined with nervous tension.

In most cases colic occurs only infrequently, and nothing needs to be done about it. In a child that seems to have this difficulty regularly, vari-

ous medications can often be of help. The doctor may prescribe a very small dose of one of the antispasmodic medicines to be given in drop form a few minutes before feeding to help overcome a tendency to intestinal cramping; in other cases a few drops of elixir of phenobarbital given either alone or in combination with an antispasmodic may help relieve tension if given a half-hour or so before feeding. Dosages of such medicines may seem to the mother to be ridiculously small, but babies themselves are small and often extremely sensitive to medicines; never give more than the doctor orders. Fortunately, even babies who have frequent or regular colic tend to outgrow it within the first month or two of life unless it persists as a result of food allergies.

Food Allergies. Although not as commonplace as many mothers think, food allergies nevertheless do occur in some babies. There are certain foods which are allergenic to many babies and which can cause continuing and repeated trouble if their use is continued, particularly if they are given to a baby very early in his life before he has had a chance to build up antibodies against the offending allergen. One such food, wheat, is so commonly allergenic that most pediatricians postpone the introduction of wheat cereals into the baby's diet until he is six months old or more, substituting rice or barley cereals that tend to cause less trouble. Egg yolk is another allergenic food which occasionally causes a baby great distress when it is introduced. Any sign of trouble that consistently follows feedings of egg should be a signal to the mother to discontinue eggs until she can discuss the problem with the doctor.

A third allergenic food, and a particularly annoying one, is cow's milk; many babies with persistent severe colic are relieved of the problem almost immediately as soon as cow's milk is eliminated from the diet. Allergies to mother's milk, on the other hand, are extremely uncommon, although not unheard of. Indeed, cow's milk is so often an offender that a variety of substitutes, usually formulas manufactured from soybeans and perfectly satisfactory for the baby's nutritional needs, have been developed. Mothers should remember that soybean milk tastes different from regular milk, and the baby may object to it at first if it is necessary to make the change, but most babies soon adapt. This is not entirely a panacea, because a certain number of babies prove just as allergic to soy products as to milk. In the rare cases when a baby is severely allergic to both, it is sometimes necessary to have recourse to such things as goat's milk; but a mother should never make this decision on her own. The pediatrician may well prefer first to attempt to suppress the baby's allergic responses by means of antihistamines or other medicines, a procedure that is often more satisfactory and much less expensive than putting the baby on a goat's milk formula for a period of months.

Basically the best solution to a food allergy problem is to avoid the offending food, if it can be identified. This does not necessarily mean that the child will have to avoid that food for the rest of his life; food allergies are often eventually "outgrown." When a baby does have an allergy, it may be wise to avoid the food that seems to be causing it for a period of a year or so, but then to try it again, particularly if it is as commonplace and important a food as milk.

Colic and gastrointestinal symptoms are the more common signs of food allergy, but this is not the only way the body may signal its distress at taking in an allergenic food. In some cases, for example, a food allergy may manifest itself by an outbreak of a rough, red and scaling rash, often very angry-looking, which most commonly appears on the backs of the knees and the inner creases of the elbows, but which may also appear on the scalp, the face or other parts of the body as well. This so-called *infantile eczema* may come and go and give so little trouble that no treatment is necessary, but in some cases it can be an extremely aggravating and itchy condition, particularly dangerous to the baby because infection can be introduced by scratching. On occasion a baby may become so badly covered with eczematous rash and secondary skin infection that such extreme measures as hospitalization and expert nursing care may be necessary to overcome it. Any such rash, however minor, should be called to the doctor's attention; in a great many cases the rash is found to be an allergic manifestation which can

best be controlled by identifying the offending food and removing it temporarily from the baby's diet. Infantile eczema can be an extremely long-term and difficult condition to treat, but careful attention to the doctor's orders for medication is necessary until the rash is relieved in order to avoid the threat of secondary infection.

Prickly Heat. A less difficult skin problem in babies, most common in the summertime, prickly heat or "red-pepper" rash results from plugging up and irritation of the sweat glands in the baby's skin; it is mildly irritating and may cause itching if severe. The easiest way to avoid prickly heat—or deal with it when it occurs—is to dry the baby carefully after a lukewarm bath, and then place the crib in a cool area free of drafts and let the baby go without clothing or covers when the weather is warm. The use of body oils or baby powders should be avoided, as they may contribute to the plugging of the sweat glands. If the rash persists or grows worse, the doctor should be consulted.

Infantile Diarrhea. Another disturbance that occurs most commonly in the summertime is infantile diarrhea. All babies will occasionally have loose, runny bowel movements for no identifiable reason, but with repeated watery stools the baby can become seriously dehydrated in a very short while, even within the course of a single day. This is particularly true if a bacterial or viral intestinal infection is present. For this reason, any episode of recurrent diarrhea should be reported to the doctor. Often the problem can be relieved with the use of a simple stool-firming medicine such as a suspension of kaolin and pectin, but medicines of this kind, or any other kind, should never be given to a baby without the doctor's express permission.

Every doctor caring for babies has his own preferences of medicines and nursing care supplies that he would like the mother to have on hand, and his instructions should be carefully followed. Most doctors recommend that the mother have a rectal thermometer at home, together with Vaseline for lubricating the tip before it is used, and rubbing alcohol for cleansing it after use. Unless instructed otherwise by the doctor, the mother should have plain unscented talc as a drying powder for the baby's skin and plain olive oil to protect the skin from drying or chapping. Follow the doctor's orders explicitly regarding any medicines to be kept in the home, and scrupulously avoid using any medicines that he does not recommend.

Bringing Up the Baby

From the moment a new baby comes home from the hospital, observation of his normal growth and development will be a joy that can be shared by every member of the family. Babies are fascinating creatures to watch for signs of progress, change, and the almost day-by-day emergence of a recognizable personality. Different babies develop at different rates, of course, and parents should not be alarmed if their baby fails to reach a certain bench mark of development at precisely the "right" time, but on the average babies do generally achieve certain developmental goals at fairly predictable times. The newborn baby at first is a comparatively limp, expressionless individual who seems constantly to be either crying, feeding or sleeping; but within the first four to six weeks he begins to smile, however fleetingly, when he is happy and within three months laughs freely in response to pleasant stimuli. During this interval he also begins to vocalize, "talking" or cooing to himself or in response to others. By the end of three months many babies have achieved the ability to lift and control their heads; control of hand movements comes at about four months, and the ability to roll over between five and six months of age. Then a much stronger, more self-reliant baby begins all manner of physical activities; his "baby fat" disappearing, and his muscles stronger, the seven- or eight-month baby attempts to sit up and then crawl, and at the same time develops a firm and purposeful grasp upon objects. Some babies crawl only briefly, graduating immediately to the more sophisticated skills of pulling themselves up and walking about with support; others develop consummate skill in crawling anywhere and everywhere with incredible speed, and abandon this form of locomotion only to go directly to unsupported walking at some point between nine and fourteen months.

As fascinating and enjoyable as the new baby's progress is, keeping up with him can be a lot of hard work. Perhaps unavoidably, the major burdens fall upon the mother, but other members of the family should be encouraged to help out whenever possible. Ideally, older children in the family should be aware of the mother's pregnancy and what it means from the time it obviously begins to show, and everyone can help in some way to get ready for the newcomer. When he does arrive, it is also advisable to find some area of responsibility that each child can take in caring for the baby; even a small child can help in some way, and nothing can be more important to engendering a feeling of family unity, mutual love, care and responsibility.

The Childhood Years

Newborn babies are incredibly resilient creatures, by no means the fragile and delicate things many new mothers assume them to be. They are natively equipped to raise a howl—literally—when hungry, wet, in pain, tired or irritable, and the speed with which they learn through their sensory perceptions, the sheer volume of data they absorb in the first few months of life, and the staggering capacity for adaptation that they demonstrate should all be powerfully reassuring factors to the inexperienced mother. Perhaps even more reassuring is the fact that a baby does not remain a baby for very long. The helpless little creature who was brought home from the hospital is suddenly crawling and then walking, talking, eating, playing, learning to coordinate his movements, and growing like a weed. In short, he has become a child.

Problems of Normal Growth and Development

It is hardly possible here to enter into a detailed discussion of all aspects of a child's normal growth and development. Whole books have been written on this subject, and a new mother would be well advised to ask the doctor caring for her baby to recommend the book or books he considers most helpful, and then read them carefully. Truly knowledgeable attention to a child's health care, however, including certain serious problems that may arise, demands some awareness of what is normal and what is not. Thus it is appropriate to consider briefly some of the highlights of normal growth and development that can be expected during the childhood years.

Physical Growth and Development. One naturally expects a healthy baby to grow, but many mothers are surprised to learn that children generally grow in spurts, with "leveling-off" periods in between, rather than in a steady fashion. Between birth and the age of three there is swift and steady growth; most babies in America at least double their birth weight in the first four to five months, and treble it by their first birthday. During the second year, growth and weight gain continue; there is a noticeable loss of "baby fat" at this time that is more than balanced by the growth and development of muscle tissue as the child becomes not only heavier but stronger. By the age of three the rate of growth begins to diminish, although it does not normally stop, and it continues to increase much more slowly through the age of nine or ten. Then, with the approach of puberty, there is another spurt, often quite dramatic, as the child develops an adult-sized body. In many children this abrupt spurt in height and weight again levels off at about the age of fourteen, followed by much slower growth to final mature height and weight; in others the adolescent growth spurt is stretched out and proceeds more slowly but also more steadily throughout the years of puberty and adolescence.

If the child's rate of growth slows down during the "leveling-off" period between the age of three and ten, however, maturation of his body continues at an accelerated rate. Both the nervous system and the musculature mature, so that the physical clumsiness and incoordination so common to children between the ages of three and six gradually disappear. Bone growth is particularly important during this period; babies' bones are only partially formed and calcified at the time of birth, but continue to form, calcify and grow at a steady rate until the age of nine or ten, as long as the child has a well-balanced diet including plenty of protein, vitamins (particularly vitamins C and D) and sufficient milk to supply the necessary calcium for bone formation. Even when the child's bones become calcified, however, they remain comparatively soft and flexible until the age of puberty, so that the tumbles and falls that are so commonly taken during childhood do not often result in fractures. Fractures do occur, however, and any injury followed by persisting pain, or one which causes a child to "guard" or avoid the use of a limb, deserves medical attention.

Various factors can impede the normal pattern of growth during this slow but steady growth period from the age of three to ten. *Malnutrition* is one such factor; and it may be present, even when the family has ample resources to provide enough food, because of poor *choice* of food. (Proper nutrition for the child is discussed in more detail on p. 887.) *Periods of illness* can also hinder normal growth, and many cases of apparent growth retardation are found, upon investigation, to be directly related to an interval in which the child had recurrent colds or ear and other respiratory infections. Impairment of normal growth as a result of some *endocrine gland disfunction* is far less common, but can occur and must be considered if no other cause can be identified. Finally, there are many cases in which a child's individual growth pattern may be perfectly normal, for him, yet seems slower or faster than normal in comparison to other children. Like adults, children can vary in body type and form, and the child who has inherited short, thick bones and a stocky, muscular body type will develop differently from a narrow-boned, wiry child. For this reason, many pediatricians favor the use of a comparative growth graph or grid by means of which they can compare a given child's rate of growth and development over a period of months or years with the patterns of growth shown by multitudes of other children. Such comparisons are particularly helpful in identifying an unusual *change* in a child's individual growth pattern that may appear at some time during childhood, signaling the doctor that something may be wrong and directing his attention to a search for possible causes.

But the normal development of a child from his first birthday on involves much more than a mere increase in height and weight. As evidences of increasing physical maturity appear, the child also develops an increasing capacity to control his body in certain important ways. He learns to crawl and then walk during his first year, and in the second year he moves on to more sophisticated activities—crawling and then walking up and down stairs, climbing on furniture, tricycle riding and so forth. The eruption of teeth follows a steady course; the lower and then the upper central incisors appear at approximately the age of six and nine months respectively, the lateral incisors at about one year; the canines and first molars erupt during the second year, and the second molars early in the third year. Even with these deciduous teeth the child is able to masticate food, and the transition from prepared baby foods to table foods can usually be accomplished at about the time of the child's second birthday, since by then his digestive apparatus is also ready for the change. At the age of six to seven the deciduous incisors are lost, to be replaced with the first permanent incisors, and from that point on to puberty children are steadily losing deciduous teeth and bringing forth permanent ones. Dental observation of the child should begin at least with the appearance of the deciduous molars, since the development of caries even in the "baby teeth" can be a threat to health. (Dentition and dental care are discussed in more detail on p. 415.)

Other changes occur simultaneously. With development of the nervous system, the child's need for sleep diminishes; by the age of two he will be awake much of the day, with a two-hour nap period in the afternoon. Most children continue to require a daytime nap until school age is attained, and an early bedtime in the evening is especially important once a child is unable to nap because of school activities. Lack of adequate sleep can make a child cranky and irritable, impede school achievement, and reduce natural resistance to infection, and parents must monitor TV-watching and other activities that children may find more tempting than an early bedtime. In addition, maturation of the nervous system is demonstrated by increasing capability and coordination of motor skills. During the period from two to five years the child learns to run, jump and climb; ability to cut or slice food or hammer nails remains crude until the age of six. By the end of the first eighteen months the average child will be able to speak at least a few intelligible words; subsequent development of speech varies widely from child to child, but by the age of six most children have a comprehensive working vocabulary of more than 2,500 words and can understand the meaning of many more when they are used in a familiar context. During this same interval the child usually accomplishes control of bowel and bladder functions, learns to feed himself with very little spilling, learns to dress himself except for tying knots—in short, he develops the groundwork for many important skills of daily living.

Teaching a child bowel and bladder control is often much less of a problem than parents expect. During the second year, most children develop a natural rhythm for bowel movements, and often signal their need with facial expressions that the mother can recognize. By placing the child on a training chair at such times and making this a pleasant part of the child's routine, bowel control can frequently be achieved by the child's second birthday. A start can also be made at bladder control during waking hours; subsequently, by offering the child the opportunity for toilet urination just before and immediately after each sleeping period, bladder control may be established by the age of three. Individual children may vary widely from such a pattern, however, and the mother is well advised to "let the matter ride" for an interval without any pressure if early attempts at toilet training prove unsuccessful. Most parents today recognize that positive reinforcement of successful attempts at either bowel or bladder control is far more use-

ful than punishing a failure by expressing anger or exasperation or withholding promised rewards. As long as toilet training is a generally pleasant, tension-free process in which success is rewarded by approval and failure is ignored, the child will move in the direction of control as quickly as he can; it is only when the training period is filled with anxiety, fear of failure and fear of rejection because of failure that the child's emotional development can be harmed and his ability to master control of these bodily functions impaired.

Even when control is established, children have occasional lapses, particularly in the area of bladder control, and no issue should be made of this; in fact, occasional nocturnal bed-wetting or *enuresis* very commonly continues, with decreasing frequency, up to or beyond school age. If at that time it continues as the rule rather than the exception, consultation with the doctor is in order. Occasionally an organic cause for enuresis is discovered—a minor but persistent bladder infection, for example—but in most cases continuing enuresis can be controlled by such simple measures as restricting the child's fluid intake during afternoon and evening hours, or the use of a mild sedative or tranquilizer to help relieve emotional tension connected with bed-wetting until the child can develop the habit of awakening enough to go to the bathroom at night when necessary.

From the age of five or six on to the beginning of adolescence there is a marked shift in the direction of the child's development. Whereas earlier his time, thoughts and energies were devoted almost exclusively to his own needs, learning to do things for himself alone, the child now enters a period of socializing with other children and learning the give and take of interpersonal relations both with brothers and sisters and with those outside the home. Many complex or delicate muscular skills, so hard to master earlier, come easily now; the child can dress himself, tie his own shoes, bathe himself, cut up his own food, entertain himself and undertake responsibility for keeping his own room tidy, recognize the wishes and rights of others, and participate in group activities. He becomes interested in people—and things—outside his immediate home and begins the long process of learning acceptable social behavior. Learning to read is often a source of great pride to a child, and of gratification as well, not only because of the "world of books" it opens up to him but because of the increased sense of independence and control that reading permits him. As he acquires a vocabulary, his ability to learn increases, as well as his capacity to obey and to recognize the difference between acceptable and unacceptable social behavior.

Emotional Growth and Development. These early years are not only a time of physical growth and the development of muscular capabilities, but of emotional growth and development as well. During the first five or six years of life children are almost inevitably egocentric; they are primarily concerned with their own immediate wants and needs, and depend heavily upon their parents or others in the family to provide for physical needs as well as to supply affection, protection and restraint. Competition with brothers or sisters for the parents' attention and love is intense and natural at this time, and it is pointless to expect small children to resolve this so-called *sibling rivalry* in an "adult" or "grown-up" fashion. Parents must set the ground rules and then enforce them with as little restraint as possible, and should be neither surprised nor perturbed to find children treating each other like savages. By the age of five or six, however, most children are capable of learning more "civilized" or socially acceptable ways of behaving toward others, and begin to discover that such heretofore alien concepts as sharing, patience, cooperation and pleasant socialization with others can often provide more gratification than single-minded egocentricity. As the child develops more confidence in his own ability to cope with his environment, and feels increasing security in his parents' love and support, his demands on others become less imperious, and as he is taught the limits of acceptable behavior by example and experience in dealing with others, a self-restraining superego emerges as an integral part of his personality.

This does not mean that a child suddenly becomes an angel at the age of six, or completely sheds his egocentricity. There will still be outbursts of selfishness, aggressiveness or outright hostility directed toward parents, brothers and sisters, teachers or friends outside the home. As long as these emotional storms are not positively injurious to himself or others, it is better to accept them matter-of-factly as a part of the child's normal emotional development than to force the child to hide or repress them. The child who is never permitted to express his anger or frustration, and thus to decompress harmlessly these potentially dangerous emotions, is likely to remain constantly angry and, ultimately, to express his anger in more devious and destructive ways. Most children, allowed reasonably free expression of their feelings, learn from experience that antisocial behavior does not work well; gentle reminders of this fact by the parents, with firm restraint where necessary but without reprisals, are far more helpful to the child's emotional growth than threats, physical punishment or emotional rejection. In addition, many common childhood activities offer the child an outlet for pent-up aggressive and hostile feelings. Competitive games and outdoor sports, for example, provide the child with both socially acceptable and emotionally satisfying release for these feelings, while team play teaches the advantages of cooperation, sharing and helping one another.

Few children, however, pass through this period of emotional development without at least transitory problems of one sort or another. Faced with a huge and bewildering world outside the family, as well as with changing relationships within the family, all children suffer some degree of anxiety, insecurity or guilt, and many express these feelings by way of various minor behavioral aberrations. Unconscious feelings of anxiety and insecurity, for example, may lead to such tenacious habits as thumb-sucking or nail-biting in some children. Others may maintain an excessive fondness for a favored stuffed animal or a special blanket, especially at bedtime, long after the need for such "islands of security" is ordinarily past. Many children develop morbid fears of darkness or thunderstorms as an expression of unconscious anxiety, while others have periodic bad dreams or nightmares. Recurrent bed-wetting after bladder control has been established is often a disguised expression of anger, hostility or a thwarted desire for more independence; the child may be, in effect, telling the parents: You can make me do other things I don't want to do, but you can't do anything about this; *I'm* in control here. In other cases temper tantrums may be employed as a thinly disguised, childlike attempt to assert control over the parents by frightening, embarrassing or tormenting them. This, however, is not the only possible reason for this particular behavioral problem; in some cases a temper tantrum may be the child's covert cry for more attention, while in still other instances the child may simply be following the example set for him by parents who may themselves use temper tantrums, in one form or another, to tyrannize their families or to get their own way.

Behavioral aberrations such as these are very commonplace among children of early school age who are caught between the desire to retain the comfortable security of the parental love and attention they demanded, and received, as infants and the equally powerful desire to become independent and "grown up" in the enticing and exciting, yet still frightening and confusing, world of give-and-take relationships with parents, siblings, or people outside the family. In most cases such behavioral disturbances are short-lived, and when parents feel that some form of control is necessary it is important that they recognize that the unacceptable behavior is merely a symptom of underlying emotional conflicts. Thus they must seek to help the child overcome the emotional problem, to express his anger or hostility in constructive ways and to increase his sense of security and self-confidence, rather than attacking the misbehavior as if it were the whole problem. When such behavioral aberrations seem persistent, appear to be growing worse rather than better, or seem to be interfering seriously with the child's emotional development, professional advice should be sought regarding specific steps that may be both painless and successful in correcting the problem. Such "old-fashioned" remedies as punishing the child for his temper tantrums, shaming him for bed-wetting, or painting his fingers with iodine to combat nail-biting are usually not only unsuccessful but may actually increase the underlying emotional problem rather than diminish it.

This is by no means to say that parents should assume an attitude of uncontrolled permissiveness during these important years in a child's emotional development. While it is discouraging to a child to surround him with an endless succession of unnecessary rules and restrictions, it is obvious that behavior that might be harmful to himself or others must be gently but firmly controlled. Harsh physical punishment is rarely if ever justified (*see* p. 896), but occasional punishment involving temporary loss of privileges or brief periods of restriction from enjoyable activities, when directly related to a given example of unacceptable behavior and instituted immediately, can help encourage the child to think twice before repeating the act at some later time. A child certainly needs continuing love and affection from his parents, and these should never be withheld as punishment, but an attitude of bland parental carte blanche in the face of antisocial or potentially self-injurious behavior is far more likely to be harmful to the child than helpful. For one thing, the child may interpret such permissiveness as indifference, and find himself faced with the appalling prospect that perhaps his parents just do not care how he behaves. Perhaps even more pertinent, the child actually *needs* reasonable, consistent limits set upon his behavior as a major means of discovering precisely what the expanding world around him will or will not tolerate. Thus parents who permissively draw back or refuse to set such limits fail the child in an extremely vital area. Even the small child can readily recognize that enforcement of limits need not mean rejection; parents can make clear the important distinction that they may dislike certain things the child does, yet still love the child. Without such reasonable limits set for him, the child will flounder; with such limits set and enforced, he can develop confidence in himself and learn the difficult art of socially acceptable behavior at the same time.

Perhaps most important of all to a child's normal, healthy emotional growth and development is the overall emotional atmosphere of the home, and many of the problems children may suffer are directly related to unfortunate and often quite unconscious attitudes and practices of the parents. The love and affection every child needs must be extended equally to all the children in the family, not just a favored one or two. When discipline is necessary, it must be consistent, so that every child in the family recognizes what the limits are. All too often parents, responding to their own unconscious needs, may lose sight of this basic need for equity and consistency in their relationship with their children; one child may be overindulged or "spoiled," to the hindrance of his normal emotional growth, while another may be subtly rejected, held at arm's length, so to speak, by one parent or another. Parents often make such unconscious mistakes as seeking to live vicariously through a child—placing demands and expectations upon him that are beyond his capacities or alien to his real interests—or constantly denigrating a child by repeatedly comparing him unfavorably to others. Such unconscious attitudes can be identified and controlled only if the parents are clearly aware that they may exist, and parents must remain constantly alert to signs of their appearance, difficult as this may be.

This problem often appears in relation to one particularly important aspect of the child's development, the area of sexuality. From the very beginning the child, like human beings of any age, is a sexual creature, and a vital part of his normal emotional development is his growing awareness of his sexual identity. Even during infancy the child discovers pleasurable sensations related to the genital region; virtually all children between the ages of one and six indulge in a certain amount of harmless and perfectly normal genital manipulation, and most continue this episodically to the age of puberty and beyond. By the age of six most children develop a natural curiosity about sex and become aware of structural differences between brothers and sisters, and between parents and children. Unfortunately, many parents communicate their own fears, uncertainties, inhibitions and restrictive attitudes toward sex to their children at precisely the time when the child should be learning frank, matter-of-fact acceptance of sexual differences. Again, the only way parents can avoid the communication of potentially damaging sexual attitudes is to recognize the problem and be prepared to respond to the child's natural curiosities with openness and understanding, answering questions factually and truthfully when they arise, but keeping the answers within the child's capacity to comprehend.

This need not be as difficult as it sometimes seems. A child of three years is perfectly aware that he has two arms, one nose, two ears and numerous toes on each foot; the same child is equally aware of the presence of a penis or vulva, as the case may be, and that these are parts of his body, too. Soon the child becomes aware that other living things reproduce and can accept with equanimity that the genital organs, aside from their connection with excretory functions, also provide him with the future means of reproduction. Before the age of seven or eight the child's sexual training can be confined to learning the correct names for the parts of his body and to simple, factual answers to sexually related questions. Obviously there is no point in belaboring a child of seven with a graphic, blow-by-blow description of sexual intercourse when he asks where babies come from; a simple statement that the father plants a seed inside the mother's body and that after the seed has grown into a small new human being, it makes its way through a natural passage to the outside world so that the mother can take care of it, a process known as "being born," will be quite sufficient to answer the question. Later, of course, the child will require more detailed and explicit information, but free, unembarrassed and matter-of-fact discussions of sexual matters, when appropriate, as a normal part of a child's upbringing, will pave the way for equally unembarrassed discussion later when the need for more detailed information becomes imminent. And while many parents may not find this easy, its importance can scarcely be overemphasized.

Indeed, parents soon discover that the entire process of child upbringing—or, more accurately, escorting the child through his early, developing years—is no easy matter; it is possibly the most difficult task parents may ever be faced with, and a task for which there is little formal training other than experience. Yet with the exercise of patience, concern and effort, most parents find themselves equal to the challenge, and are ultimately rewarded a thousand-fold when the child emerges as a physically and emotionally hardy, well-balanced, fascinating and unique individual, well prepared for the final journey through puberty and adolescence toward adulthood.

In many ways nature is on the side of the parents. For most children, these early years are a period of exuberant good health. Minor accidents and injuries are common, as are upper respiratory infections, ear infections, the familiar "childhood rash" diseases and certain more serious infectious disorders. (These disorders are discussed in detail in Part IV, "Patterns of Illness: The Infectious Diseases.") Fortunately, however, many of the diseases that once took a terrible toll among children can now be effectively treated by the use of the various antibiotics, or completely prevented by immunizations. One of the most essential aspects of child care is, of course, a careful and complete immunization program. The doctor will prescribe the schedule of immunizations he feels most advisable for each child. (*See* table for

a typical schedule of childhood immunizations recommended by many physicians.) Some shots can begin as early as three months, others can be safely postponed until a later age, and still others must be given in series extending over several months or even years. Thus it is of the utmost importance not only that immunization series be started at the proper time, but also that they be continued and *completed;* half an immunization is little better than no immunization at all. Parents should also keep a careful record of the immunizations given each child and put it with their other important papers. It can prove invaluable in case of an emergency, a move to another community, for school records and for travel abroad.

In spite of the widespread use of the "miracle" drugs and immunizations, there are still a number of conditions or disorders to which infants and children are vulnerable. Some of these may be congenital—that is, present at birth due to some hereditary or developmental defect; others may be the result of some external or environmental factor. Many of these disorders are particularly tragic because their victims are helpless and innocent children. Within the last half-century, pediatric medicine and surgery have

Routine Immunizations

Age	Procedure	Remarks
3 months	Diphtheria-tetanus-pertussis (DPT) #1 Trivalent oral polio vaccine (TOPV) #1	By injection—basic & vital By mouth—basic and vital
4 months	DPT #2	By injection
6 months	DPT #3 (completes basic series) TOPV #2	By injection By mouth
8 months	TOPV #3 (completes basic series)	By mouth
12 months	Measles virus vaccine, live Mumps virus vaccine, live Rubella virus vaccine, live	All by injection. May have combined measles-mumps-rubella vaccine in one dose, or may be given separately one month apart
18 months	DPT booster #1 TOPV booster #1	By injection By mouth
	Tuberculosis skin test	Any time after 12 months
5 years	DPT booster #2 TOPV booster #2	By injection By mouth Both given pre-kindergarten

Special Immunizations

Age	Procedure	Remarks
12 months on	Smallpox vaccination	*No longer a routine immunization in U.S.A.* Administered prior to foreign travel to endemic areas, or on the recommendation of a physician closely acquainted with child's individual needs and circumstances. Revaccination when necessary every 3 to 6 years
6 years on	Diphtheria-tetanus (DT) (adult type)	Follow-up booster for earlier DPT; booster every 10 years
As needed	Typhoid-paratyphoid	Prior to travel to Mexico, So. Europe, Middle East, other endemic areas. Advisable prior to any foreign travel, 3 injections 1-2 months apart
As needed	Yellow fever vaccine	Prior to travel to tropical endemic areas. Single shot, booster every 10 years
As needed	Cholera, plague	As recommended by physician or Public Health Service prior to foreign travel
As needed	Measles, immune globulin	Administered to susceptible (i.e. non-immunized) exposed child to prevent or modify measles after exposure. Effectiveness depends on how soon after exposure the globulin is given. Protection falls off rapidly (6 weeks)
As needed	(Hepatitis) immune serum globulin	Administered to child or adult exposed to infectious hepatitis (close contact) to prevent or modify infection. Should be given as soon as possible after close exposure. Protection falls off rapidly (6 weeks)

IMPORTANT NOTES:

1. Ordinarily only well children should receive immunizations, but minor infections such as common colds are not contraindications.

2. Interruption of the immunization schedule does not interfere with final immunity and does not necessitate starting the series over again, regardless of interval elapsed. Consult with doctor at once regarding lapsed immunization schedule.

made enormous strides in correcting, combating and even curing many disorders that were once almost invariably fatal or completely debilitating. Nevertheless, it is important for every parent to know what these conditions are, even though many of them are comparatively rare, in order to detect their symptoms as early as possible and to take steps essential for treatment.

Structural Defects Present at Birth

Among the most unfortunate human afflictions are structural defects caused by some genetic or developmental flaw that are present at birth and may afflict the newborn baby throughout his life. Most of these defects can be quite readily identified by the physician either at or very shortly following the time of birth in a routine but thorough physical examination. The examination may take so little time that the mother is unaware that it has been performed, but the physician's findings—including any suspicions of abnormality—are noted immediately on the hospital birth record. Most doctors today assess the baby's general condition at birth according to the so-called *Apgar rating* (*see* p. 843), a convenient means of detecting both obvious and subtle clues to any possible birth defects or abnormalities, particularly in the baby's respiratory, circulatory and nervous systems. An Apgar rating of 12, for example, indicates that all systems are functioning normally, as far as the doctor can observe, with no immediate evidence of trouble, while a lower Apgar rating suggests that some defect or abnormality requiring further careful investigation may exist. The advantages of such an examination are obvious. If a life-threatening defect is detected, treatment must begin at once to save the baby; and even if no obvious defect is found, the baby with a low Apgar rating can be watched with special care, further examinations and diagnostic studies can be performed, and any indicated treatment begun at the earliest possible time.

Cleft Palate and/or Harelip. These anatomical defects, which often occur together, result from an incomplete joining of the bony plate separating the mouth from the nasal passages during the baby's gestation. The defect may appear in all degrees of severity from a tiny harelip on one side to a bilateral harelip and cleft palate on either side. The name "harelip" is deceptive in that the upper lip defect does not occur in the center but on one side or the other, or both. In rare cases the defect in the hard palate may involve both sides and be so gross that virtually no palate separates the mouth and the nasal passages. Whatever the degree, this condition is not immediately threatening to the baby's life; but left untreated, it inevitably results in a disfiguring external defect of the lip, feeding and eating difficulties, and later, speech defects. Today, however, virtually all degrees of cleft palate and harelip are surgically correctable, in one or several successive stages. An infant born with this defect should be seen in consultation by a pediatric surgeon soon after birth, so that repair of the defect can be planned on an orderly basis as soon as the child has reached an age and size that permit it.

Cryptorchidism and/or Congenital Inguinal Hernias. Another common anatomical defect in male babies is the failure of one or both testicles to descend from the area in the lower abdomen where they are formed during gestation down the so-called inguinal canal into the scrotum.

Any time one or both testicles fail to descend, there is an area of weakness in the muscles and tissues of the abdominal wall in the region of the inguinal canal which permits the abdominal contents to bulge down through the defect to form a *hernia.* Sometimes a congenital hernia may be present even when the testicle has descended, owing to the failure of the inguinal canal to close up properly before birth. In any of these events, surgical intervention is necessary to bring the undescended testicle down into the scrotum, a procedure that can be done without damage to the normal functioning of the testicle, and to repair the hernia defect in the groin. Surgery is ordinarily performed as soon after the baby is about three months old as possible, since at that time it poses the least possible threat. It is wise not to postpone this procedure chiefly for two reasons: first, because the continued presence of the defect can lead to entrapment or incarceration of a loop of bowel in the hernia, causing an acute surgical emergency; and second, because an undescended testicle which is left too long in its internal location may atrophy and fail to function when it is finally lowered, or it may degenerate and become cancerous.

Female babies may have congenital inguinal hernias, too, although less commonly than males. Diagnosis of the hernia is often extremely difficult when a baby is newborn, particularly in females or in males when the testicles have descended normally. Further, there is reason to believe that they occur more frequently than was once thought, but may often actually heal themselves before they are detected. In any event, when a hernia requiring surgical correction is diagnosed on one side, the surgeon frequently discovers and repairs a similar defect on the opposite side during the course of surgery. When done at the proper time, the operation is well tolerated and the condition tends to recur only rarely. The baby is often permitted to return home within a day or two of the operation, with provisions made for follow-up in a clinic or doctor's office.

Umbilical Hernia. Perhaps the most common physical defect found in a baby at or immediately following birth, an umbilical hernia is caused by a weakness in the abdominal wall in the area of the umbilical opening or navel which permits a bulge or "bubble" of tissue to protrude through the opening, and may be especially marked when the baby is crying or straining. In a newborn baby who has just dropped the stump of the umbilical cord, a slight bulging defect is not at all uncommon, and many physicians believe that it will close spontaneously in a short period of time. However, nine times out of ten it can be treated quite satisfactorily by the simple expedient of *taping;* that is, pinching together two folds of skin on either side of the navel and holding them in place with a band of elastic adhesive. Taping for a period of two to three weeks often permits a minor umbilical hernia defect to heal and close without any further treatment.

When it persists, or is too large to close spontaneously, or seems to be growing larger, surgical treatment is indicated. The procedure is usually well tolerated and is rarely associated with any further complications if it is performed at the proper time and the baby is in good general health and in no distress from the hernia itself. Even without surgical repair, most umbilical hernias sooner or later close by themselves, but there is always the danger that a loop of bowel may become trapped or incarcerated in the defect, thus creating an acute and dangerous surgical emergency. As infrequently as this occurs, most pediatricians recommend elective repair of an umbilical hernia as soon as it is definitely established that the defect is not going to close quickly with the aid of more conservative measures.

Tongue-Tie. This extremely common anatomical defect can become a serious problem only if it is not detected and corrected early in a baby's life. Tongue-tie is caused by nothing more than a thin membrane of tissue that extends from the midline of the under surface of the tongue down to the floor of the mouth, restricting the free movement of the tongue. The defect may be so minor that it is virtually undetectable, or it may actually bind the tongue quite closely to the floor of the mouth. In infancy it causes little difficulty, since it does not interfere with crying, and usually restricts the baby's sucking ability only slightly. If left uncorrected, however,

the thin membrane may become thicker and can result in a significant speech impediment when the child begins to learn to talk. Physicians today regularly check newborn babies for this defect, and at that time the condition can be corrected simply and quite painlessly by lifting the baby's tongue with a special slotted instrument to stretch the membrane and snipping it with a pair of scissors. There is rarely more than a very small amount of bleeding, and healing is so rapid that evidence of surgical intervention is virtually impossible to detect within 48 hours. Even if the condition is not diagnosed until a child has grown to be two or three years old, the restricting bit of tissue can usually be cut in a simple procedure in the doctor's examining room with the use of local anesthesia. The incision heals quickly with no visible aftereffects.

Circulatory Defects. In addition to the several less serious and easily corrected birth defects described above, there are a number of other congenital anatomical flaws which are far more grave, usually because they impair some vital function and must be detected and repaired quickly, or at least as quickly as the baby's health warrants, to protect him from serious consequences or even death. Among these abnormalities are the various congenital heart defects which impair the proper function of the heart, affect the overall circulation of the blood, and thus may prevent tissues and organs from receiving the necessary supply of oxygen. The most familiar result of these defects is the so-called blue baby, who may exhibit the symptoms of oxygen starvation from the moment of birth. These and other circulatory abnormalities are discussed in detail elsewhere. (*See* p. 542.) Many of them were once considered "lost causes," but today with modern methods of diagnosis and treatment they are often readily amenable to surgical repair during childhood or, if necessary, even during infancy.

Gastrointestinal Defects. Structural abnormalities of the organs of the gastrointestinal tract can also pose a grave threat to the newborn baby. One of the most serious of these is a *tracheoesophageal fistula,* a condition in which the trachea and the esophagus fail to develop into two completely separate tubes. Instead there is an opening between them at some point, so that whenever the baby attempts to take food, it can be drawn into the lungs, causing choking and aspiration pneumonia. The defect is usually identified within a few hours of the baby's birth, frequently during the first attempt to feed him anything by mouth. The diagnosis can often be confirmed when the doctor attempts to pass a nasal catheter down into the baby's stomach; when this leads to intractable choking and coughing, it strongly suggests that the catheter has been diverted from the esophagus into the trachea through an opening or fistula. Since feeding by mouth may be impossible, the discovery of this defect is the signal for immediate emergency surgical correction. In some cases the condition may prove uncorrectable; there may be complete absence or *atresia* of the lower half of the esophagus, for example, or the necessary surgery may be so radical that the baby fails to survive the operation. But today, with the techniques, experience and skill of the modern pediatric surgeon, this grave defect can often be successfully repaired.

Other malformations of the gastrointestinal tract may be more difficult to diagnose, but still require early surgical correction. Damage to the fetus from known or unknown causes during the formation of this organ system may lead to atresia of either the small or the large intestine, thus preventing the passage of food materials, or the lower end of the colon may end in a blind pouch without an external opening, a condition known as *imperforate anus*. In most cases such malformations, once diagnosed, can be corrected surgically with good prospects for recovery. Other obstructive phenomena in the intestine are *Hirschsprung's disease* or *megacolon* (*see* p. 622) and *meconium ileus,* a condition in which the greenish-black material known as meconium normally found in the newborn infant's small and large intestine is markedly more sticky and viscid than usual and actually forms an obstructive plug somewhere along the length of the bowel. When discovered, surgical correction of the obstruction itself, together with any related structural abnormality of the bowel, is usually possible. Unfortunately, however, meconium ileus is very often related to a more serious

underlying disorder, an inherited glandular disease known as *cystic fibrosis* which may continue to threaten the health of the child. (*See* p. 893.)

Finally, one of the most common and dramatic gastrointestinal congenital defects may not indicate its presence until the infant is two to three weeks old, and on occasion may not appear symptomatic until the age of three or four months or more. This condition is *pyloric stenosis,* a marked narrowing and thickening of the pylorus, the valvelike sphincter muscle which guards the lower end of the stomach and relaxes intermittently to allow food to pass into the duodenum. No one knows what causes the disorder, and the obstruction may be as much a result of spasm of the muscle as of physical enlargement and thickening. In either case, however, the affected child has difficulty feeding and spits up excessively from the very first, and later develops a pattern of progressively more violent "projectile" vomiting a few minutes after each feeding. This symptom is often accompanied by constipation, sometimes by decreased urinary output, and a failure of the baby to gain weight, sometimes even a weight loss. All babies tend to lose some weight immediately after birth, but once the trend has been reversed with regular feedings, any further loss of weight is usually due to a failure to take in and hold adequate nourishment for one reason or another. In pyloric stenosis the severity of the obstruction depends on the degree of enlargement of the muscle and the amount of spasm present. In some cases the enlarged pylorus can actually be felt in the baby's abdomen as a hard lump the size and shape of a small olive. Diagnosis can usually be confirmed by X-ray examinations.

A conservative medical program to treat pyloric stenosis is in order at first. Small amounts of a mild sedative in combination with an antispasmodic medication are given to the baby a short while before each feeding, followed by frequent relatively small feedings of breast milk, prepared milk or cereal. When this simple approach is insufficient to relax the spasm of the pylorus and permit normal nutrition, or in cases in which the symptoms seem to grow progressively worse in spite of treatment, a surgical procedure is used to incise the hypertrophied pyloric muscle. With modern infant anesthesia this procedure offers an excellent chance for recovery from what could be a prolonged period of poor nutrition, or even a fatal form of obstruction of the infant's gastrointestinal tract.

Nervous System Defects. A fortunately rare congenital defect occurs in the internal chambers of the infant's brain when the cerebrospinal fluid generated there cannot properly drain through the passageways that normally carry it down along the spinal cord to bathe this great nerve trunk. The result may be *infantile hydrocephalus,* a condition in which cerebrospinal fluid is trapped in the ventricles of the brain. As more and more fluid is formed without any means of drainage, its increasing volume causes a progressive enlargement of the infant's head and a progressive loss of brain function due to destruction of brain tissue. For centuries infantile hydrocephalus, which manifests itself within a few days following the baby's birth, was a hopelessly incurable condition. Since the late 1930s and early 1940s, however, a variety of neurosurgical techniques have been developed to drain excess cerebrospinal fluid artificially. None of these approaches has been entirely satisfactory, but some offer temporary relief for at least a few years, and research and experiments continue to find more effective and possibly even permanent forms of treatment.

All forms of hydrocephalus are not necessarily congenital. The condition may, for example, arise as an aftermath of an attack of meningitis in which exudate from the infection, or scarring during the healing process, may narrow or obliterate the passages that drain cerebrospinal fluid. Occasionally the condition, whether congenital or acquired, appears to correct itself, and when the internal pressure of the fluid is not too great, it is not necessarily associated with brain damage or mental impairment. For the most part, however, the disorder is ultimately incurable because even the best medical and surgical techniques used to combat it are still only partially effective.

Other Physical and Metabolic Defects. Virtually every organ system is vulnerable to congenital malformations of various kinds which may cause later disability or even a threat to life. An abnormality in the development of the fetus may result in incomplete closure of the vertebral column, which permits an outpouching of tissue containing cerebrospinal fluid anywhere along the spine. The outpouching is called a *meningocele* or *myelocele,* and the condition is known as *spina bifida.* A meningocele or a myelocele is almost always associated with partial or complete paralysis of the limbs and often with hydrocephalus as well, but in some cases a malformed vertebral column does not result in neurological changes. If this occurs, the condition may never be identified until adulthood or middle age, at which time such an "occult" spina bifida malformation may sometimes be associated with weakness in the low back.

Other rare forms of congenital abnormalities are atresia of one or both of the ureters leading from the kidney to the urinary bladder which prevents normal urination; *arteriovenous fistulas* which connect an artery and vein and permit the passage of arterial blood directly into the vein; *craniostenosis,* a condition in which the bones of the infant's skull become firmly fixed and joined too soon after birth so that subsequent growth of the brain causes a sometimes marked deformity of the front and rear of the skull; *clubfoot,* which occurs when one or both of the infant's feet are either malformed or twisted out of normal alignment due to the position of the fetus in the womb; a malformation of the middle or inner ear which results in impaired hearing or deafness; and even an obstruction or incomplete formation of the lacrimal ducts that normally carry tears from the eye down into the nasal pharynx for disposal, so that the baby displays excessive tearing from birth on. Many of these conditions, when discovered early, are amenable to surgical correction, and continuing research into the causes, treatment and possible prevention of birth defects holds out the hope that fewer and fewer children will be afflicted with these conditions in future years.

Phenylketonuria (PKU). Congenital abnormalities are not always confined to structural or anatomical faults; occasionally a baby is born with a flaw in his body's biochemistry or metabolism, or some genetic defect may cause an obvious or hidden disability. For example, throughout recorded medical history there has been a certain very small number of newborn babies who, while they appear perfectly normal at birth, seem to undergo a mysteriously steady and progressive deterioration of brain function and intellect, which evolves into a degree of mental impairment equivalent to idiocy by the age of five or so. There appeared to be no known cause, nor any consistent history of injury or other untoward occurrence that might have resulted in brain damage. Only recently was it found that these afflicted children, from the very first week of their lives, consistently excrete abnormal amounts of a normal chemical breakdown product known as *phenylpyruvic acid* in their urine. Ultimately it was discovered that their mental deterioration was directly related to a biochemical or metabolic flaw which made it impossible for the victim properly to utilize a chemical substance known as *phenylalanine,* one of 22 amino acids present in protein. No one knows exactly why an excessive blood level of phenylalanine in an infant's body causes brain damage of this nature, but fortunately the defect can be discovered within the first month of the baby's life, before mental retardation has set in, by means of a simple and now routine form of urine examination. The mental degeneration can be prevented if the condition, now called *phenylketonuria* or PKU, is discovered early enough, by careful measures designed to reduce the amount of phenylalanine in the baby's diet to zero. So treated, the child with phenylketonuria, once he reaches the age of seven or eight, can resume a normal diet without any untoward effects.

Mongolism. While many inborn defects are insidious and difficult to diagnose, one form of mental deficiency makes itself known very early, usually at the time of birth, by the very appearance of the afflicted baby. This defect is known as *Down's syndrome* (*see* p. 376) or mongolism, so called because an abnormal fold of the upper eyelid and other facial features were thought to give the afflicted child an Oriental appearance. Other stigmata are the presence of an abnormal flaccidity of musculature in general, together with a very slow pattern of growth, an extraordinary vulnerability to upper respiratory infections, and mental retardation, with the child seldom progressing beyond a mental age of five or six.

For a long time the cause of mongolism was a complete mystery. There was no discernible hereditary pattern; the condition could appear once without warning in a given family, but with no other occurrences in the same family. However, the likelihood of mongolism did seem to correlate with the age of the mother; that is, a high proportion of mongol children were found to be born of women who were in their late thirties or early forties, late in their childbearing years.

The specific cause of the disorder is still unknown, but recent discoveries reveal that mongoloid children consistently have certain specific abnormalities in the pattern of the chromosomes in their cells, the protein material in the cell which determines all aspects of the body's structure and function. Since mongols rarely reach adulthood even today, and since they seldom mature sexually, the defective chromosomes are not known to be handed down to succeeding generations. Thus mongolism is caused by some genetic defect, but it is not known whether the defect occurs because of the influence of drugs or medicines the pregnant mother may have taken, because of the aging of the ovum or the sperm, that entered into the victim's conception, or because of some other factor. There is some hope, however, that a more detailed knowledge of the genetic structure of human cells and increasing skill in manipulating chromosomal patterns may one day lead to therapeutic measures that will offer relief to mongol children.

For the present there is no fixed rule of thumb to guide the parents of a mongol child; much depends upon the emotional makeup of the parents as well as their family situation. In a family in which such a child can be loved and well cared for even in the presence of normal siblings, his life may perhaps be far happier than in an institution, as these children usually are docile and amiable with little tendency toward ill nature or destructiveness. On the other hand, if the parents find themselves unable to develop a loving relationship with the child, or if his presence generally upsets the balance of family life, institutionalization may well be the wisest and kindest approach. Certainly such a decision should be made only after the parents have reviewed all the possibilities and discussed their individual situation not only with a concerned family physician or pediatrician but also with other professionals who are acquainted with the institutional care of mental defectives and trained in the care of mongoloid children.

Many parents feel that a mongoloid child is somehow "their fault," which is, of course, untrue. Equally unfortunate is the fear that another pregnancy may result in the birth of a child with a similar defect. With this particular condition, however, parents can be assured that the likelihood of a second mongoloid child is so extremely small as to be negligible, if the mother is still a young woman. Women beyond the age of thirty-seven or thirty-eight who have given birth to a mongoloid child might well be advised not to undertake future pregnancies. When late pregnancies do occur, a newly developed technique known as *amniocentesis*—withdrawing a sample of amniotic fluid from the uterus early in the pregnancy—may soon make detection of mongolism possible early enough that the defective pregnancy may be interrupted if the parents so desire.

Muscular Dystrophy. A congenital disorder affecting children which has been the subject of intensive research in recent years is known by the family name of muscular dystrophy, a term which means "abnormal or difficult behavior of the muscles." (*See* p. 288.) Although several different forms of muscular dystrophy are known, all have one feature in common: a progressive decrease in muscle size and tone in children, with increasing weakness and degeneration of muscle fibers in many areas of the body. No one knows the exact cause of this disorder; authorities suspect that some inheritable metabolic defect is the underlying cause, but just what that defect is has not yet been discovered. Symptoms often first appear when the child starts walking, and muscle weakness and resulting skeletal deformities such as *scoliosis* (curving or twisting of the spine), or muscle contractures progress until the child, in severe cases, becomes confined to a wheelchair or is

bedridden. Until quite recently there was no cure for muscular dystrophy, and little else but simple supportive treatment as long as the child survived. However, the Muscular Dystrophy Association has succeeded in raising funds to make intensive study of this disorder of children possible. There is still no specific drug therapy for the disease, but with a better understanding of the nature of the illness a great deal can now be accomplished in terms of physical therapy to aid the afflicted child by means of muscle-strengthening exercises, and by employment of muscle braces or even corrective surgical measures to prevent deformity and crippling. In the meantime, any family into which a child is born with this disease should be made clearly aware of the hereditary nature of the affliction in order to help discourage passing it on to future generations.

Environmental Illnesses

Quite apart from inborn or congenital defects, babies are vulnerable to a number of environmental illnesses during their early months which may then affect their lives permanently. *Congenital syphilis,* for example, can result from active infection of the fetus during gestation by syphilis organisms present in the mother's body if the disease is active, and this prebirth infection can cause severe structural abnormalities. Bony destruction of the bridge of the nose is one of the stigmata of this disease, as are malformations of the teeth and severe brain damage. Another disease acquired by babies which once caused great distress was an extremely virulent eye infection, *gonorrheal conjunctivitis,* contracted in the process of birth when the mother had active gonorrhea, and capable of destroying the sight of afflicted babies. This problem is still such a threat that it is now routine practice to instill drops of dilute silver nitrate solution into all newborn babies' eyes at birth to prevent any possible gonorrheal eye infection before it can take hold. (*See* p. 243 for a more detailed discussion of these venereal infections.)

Another acquired disease affecting the eyes of infants has had a singular history. For at least thirty or forty years this rare disease was known to cause a dense opaque membrane to form across the eye and in back of the lens as a result of hemorrhage within the retina, followed by detachment of the retina from the back of the eye, causing permanent blindness. Surgical removal of the membrane did not restore sight, since the membrane was formed as a result of irreparable damage to the retina itself. This condition, known as *retrolental fibroplasia,* first appeared when babies were approximately a week old, and completely eluded the efforts of pediatricians to identify any possible cause. Further, beginning in the 1940s there appeared to be a marked increase in the incidence of this disease, and it was discovered that it occurred most commonly in relatively small or premature babies, although some large, full-term babies also developed the condition. The only common denominator seemed to be that virtually all victims were babies with a history of respiratory difficulty shortly after birth.

This realization led to intensive study of the condition, but when the true cause of the disease was discovered, it came as a complete surprise: retrolental fibroplasia occurred only in babies, premature or otherwise, who had spent moderate to prolonged periods of time immediately after birth in an incubator or rockette which was supplied with a high concentration of oxygen to help them overcome respiratory difficulties. Subsequent studies showed that any baby subjected to a concentration of therapeutic oxygen higher than 14 percent for longer than a few hours was in danger of developing this disease. Of course, rich oxygen therapy has been discontinued, and the disease, once a major cause of blindness in the newborn, has completely ceased to occur.

One of the most vital transitions the newborn infant must make between life within the womb and life outside is the commencement of breathing motions and the aeration and inflation of the lungs. Needless to say, any condition which interferes with respiration during this period poses a grave threat to the baby's survival. Almost invariably the newborn infant's nose and throat are filled with a certain amount of tenacious mucus at the time of birth, and one of the first things the physician does after delivery,

prior to clamping and cutting the cord, is to use a suction device to clear away this mucus. The stimulus to begin breathing is related both to changes in pressure on the baby's body outside the womb and to the effects of anoxia as a result of clamping the cord and/or detachment of the placenta. In most babies all that is required is a mild irritating stimulus such as a slap on the back or a snap on the feet to cause crying, an action which automatically helps inflate the lungs. If the baby is somewhat torpid due to medications given to the mother, or otherwise breathing and crying only feebly, use of a rockette or other mechanical device for tilting the baby's body first slightly head downward and then slightly head upward helps maintain respirations in a regular sequence.

One type of respiratory disorder, however, sometimes eludes everything the doctor can do to prevent it. This condition, known as *hyaline membrane disease,* is marked by the onset of respiratory distress which begins a few hours after the baby's birth and grows progressively worse; air exchange in the lungs gradually diminishes and the baby must struggle harder and harder to breathe. It is now believed that this disorder is the result of inhalation of amniotic fluid by the baby at some time before birth, possibly because of respiratory movements initiated by partial obstruction of the cord. A collection of waxy *vernix* (the slippery material that "lubricates" the baby's body as it passes down the birth canal), cells from the skin, hair, and meconium thus gain entrance into the baby's large air tubes prior to birth. It is thought that this material is subsequently drawn into the smaller bronchioles to form a tenacious "membrane" which prevents normal air exchange. To date there is no known way to relieve or treat this condition other than to supply a relatively rich mixture of oxygen, and in some babies the disorder is so severe that it causes oxygen starvation and death by suffocation. In other cases, however, the baby's body, bit by bit, begins to tear down and absorb the "membrane," so that if he survives the first two or three days his breathing becomes progressively easier and ultimately he may recover with no residual aftereffects.

Another comparatively rare condition affecting the newborn baby's nervous system is the occurrence of intracranial bleeding as a result of the trauma of birth. Such bleeding, which can result in the formation of *subdural hematomas* —blood clots outside the baby's brain but enclosed within the meningeal membranes covering the brain—may produce little or no evidence of abnormality at first, but during the first few months of life it can lead to increasingly marked evidence of intracranial pressure. This occurs because the blood cells in the hematoma, upon breaking down, release electrolytes and other chemicals into the hematoma in higher concentration than outside, and the resulting osmotic pressure tends to draw more and more fluid into the area of the hematoma as if in an effort to dilute these chemicals to the same concentrations found in other body fluids. Fortunately, pediatric neurosurgery has, in recent decades, developed effective techniques for diagnosing subdural hematomas, and great relief can be obtained before any permanent brain damage occurs, in many cases, by means of surgical removal of the hematomas.

Cerebral Palsy

Of all the illnesses that can afflict infants and growing children, perhaps none is more tragic than a group of nervous system diseases in which damage occurs to one or more of those areas of the brain that regulate muscular activity, resulting in a type of disorder of the motor function of the body commonly known as cerebral palsy or CP. Cerebral palsy is not a single disease entity like measles or diabetes; rather, it is a kind of disorder that can range from the very mild to the extremely severe, arising from a variety of different causes and resulting in several different sorts of muscular disfunction depending on what area of the brain is damaged. In the majority of cases, however, the specific cause for the condition cannot be readily identified. One of the most frequent identifiable causes is the occurrence of some kind of brain injury to the baby as a result of a long and difficult labor or a traumatic delivery, but many children who later prove to have symptoms of cerebral palsy have no record of difficult labor or delivery, and even in those

that do there is little correlation between the severity of their symptoms and the degree of trauma noted at delivery. Another cause of these symptoms is the occurrence of Rh factor disease or *erythroblastosis fetalis* (*see* p. 833) which progresses to the point where the nuclei of certain brain cells are damaged by the time the baby is delivered. Still other cases can be traced to episodes late in the pregnancy, during labor or shortly after delivery, involving cerebral oxygen starvation or anoxia—for example, the baby whose head has compressed the umbilical cord so that he is starved for oxygen during the duration of labor, or the baby who for other reasons has weak and feeble respirations–and considerable respiratory distress early in life.

Whatever the cause, the symptoms of cerebral palsy are quite characteristic, although in very mild cases they may be subtle enough to escape notice for months or years. In some cases certain affected muscles of the extremities or trunk are abnormally rigid or *spastic,* sometimes to such a degree that normal walking or other muscular functions are nearly impossible. In other cases the victim may suffer from a continuous and uncontrollable slow, writhing movement of the limbs, jaw, neck or trunk, a condition doctors know as *athetosis* or *athetoid* (i.e., wormlike) *tremor.* Still others may suffer such severe muscular incoordination that they lurch and stumble as they walk, a condition known as *ataxia.* Which condition predominates depends upon which brain centers have been injured; in some cases all three may be present. Some children are so severely afflicted that they are unable to speak or swallow without enormous difficulty and may require considerable time and effort to accomplish even the simplest muscular tasks, if they can attempt them at all. A large proportion of children with severe cerebral palsy (as high as 70 percent, according to some authorities) have some degree of mental deficiency as well as their deficiency in muscle control, but far too many who have perfectly normal or above-average intelligence are mistakenly assumed to be mentally deficient because of their appearance, their inability to speak clearly or quickly, and their inability to control involuntary muscular movements. Many victims of the disease also suffer from convulsions which, if controllable at all, are treated by the use of massive doses of depressant medications sufficient to make the brightest mind react with exaggerated dullness. All in all, the child with a significant degree of cerebral palsy faces a lifetime of severe disability.

There is no way to cure the disease, to repair the damage done to brain and nervous tissue, or even to ameliorate the amount of muscular disorganization the victim suffers. Half a century ago, little was done to help afflicted children; they were usually sequestered at home, a source of shame and embarrassment to their families. Often the parents felt guilty, assuming that they were somehow at fault, although virtually everything that is known about cerebral palsy today indicates otherwise; only rarely can one actually find any incident in the course of the pregnancy or any preventable act on the part of the mother in the course of labor and delivery that might be directly or indirectly related to the occurrence of cerebral palsy. But equally false is the widespread attitude that nothing can be done to help the cerebral palsied child.

Treatment today is primarily designed to ameliorate the discomfort and disability of the child. In some cases the use of simple prosthetic braces will help support muscles and overcome awkward abnormalities of muscular movement. Patient and long-term training programs in the hands of experienced workers often result in significant physical rehabilitation, muscle reeducation, and marked improvement in speech—all important for the patient in order to lead as nearly normal a life as possible. Equally important are the efforts made to liberate the mind that is trapped in the crippled body and to help the patient utilize his full intellectual capacity. All cerebral palsy victims should have the benefit of thorough intelligence and psychological testing which will not only help reveal their true mental capacity, but will also help identify emotional disturbances which might interfere with either physical or intellectual training. Once reliable baselines have been established, skillful teaching programs can help the patient realize his fullest physical and mental potential.

Finally, it should be pointed out that a great

number of cases of cerebral palsy may never be detected at all simply because the telltale symptoms are absent. Many children with mild or "occult" cases of this disease may simply appear to be somewhat slow to speak or move, and, frustrated in their attempts to keep up with others of their own age, they become discouraged and fail to make any effort at all. Far from being dull-witted, however, they are often extremely bright. Here again, the importance of careful physical and neurological examinations, followed by psychological and intelligence testing, cannot be overemphasized. If the disease can be identified, the proper tutoring and training can make all the difference, physically, intellectually and psychologically, in the lives of these children. Cerebral palsy is no longer a shameful secret. Research continues today, not only to find out more about its causes and possible prevention, but also to learn more effective ways to help its victims lead full and fruitful lives in spite of disabilities which might seem at first to be insurmountable.

Convulsive Disorders

Another form of neurological disturbance which most often occurs in childhood is a group of so-called convulsive disorders, more commonly known as *epilepsy* or "epileptic fits." And like cerebral palsy, these disorders are surrounded by myths and misunderstandings.

Just what is a convulsion? This phenomenon or symptom, sometimes called a "seizure," a "fit," or a "spell," is a disturbance of the electrical conducting mechanisms of the brain, or more accurately, a disturbance of the way nerve impulses are transmitted in the brain and nervous system, which can result in several different kinds of dramatic and often frightening physical reactions. The most common form of convulsion, the so-called *grand mal seizure,* is similar in many ways to an electrical storm which suddenly appears on a summer day, rages violently for a short period and then dissipates. In a grand mal seizure, something happens in some portion of the brain—although what that "something" may be is often unknown—which sets up a focus of abnormal nerve messages, revealed on an electroencephalograph as a sudden electrical discharge, and then spreads to other parts of the brain. The physical result of this "brainstorm" is immediate and striking: the victim may let out an inadvertent cry and then abruptly lose consciousness and fall. Almost instantly the massive electrical discharge leads to a violent stiffening of virtually all the muscles in the body, with legs and arms becoming rigid, the back arched and the head thrown back and the jaws clamped; then, from this position of rigidity, the victim begins rhythmic jerking motions of the arms, legs and trunk muscles which gather in speed and violence to such a degree that he may do severe physical harm to himself. Like a great tidal wave of nervous energy the entire seizure may last no longer than 30 or 45 seconds, and rarely longer than a minute or two before the rhythmic jerking motions subside, the muscles relax, and the convulsion is over. There may also be an involuntary emptying of the bladder or the colon during the seizure. In some cases, once the muscles relax the victim may experience complete "nervous exhaustion" or fall into a deep sleep for a period of time, or he may immediately regain consciousness but be confused, frightened and uncertain of his whereabouts for a matter of minutes or even hours following the episode.

Sometimes a different form of seizure may occur which seems to start in one focal point or area. Rather than losing consciousness abruptly, for example, the victim may notice a twitching of a finger or thumb which then progressively extends into rhythmic jerking of the entire arm before the seizure passes or sometimes evolves into a full-blown grand mal episode. This kind of convulsion, spoken of as a *Jacksonian seizure* from the man who first described it as a separate form of convulsion, is most commonly associated with some specific and identifiable area of brain damage such as a scar due to injury of the brain, a brain tumor, or an area of injury due to trauma.

There are other forms of convulsions as well, more subtle, but nevertheless resulting from an abnormal neuroelectrical discharge in the brain. The second most common form is called a *petit mal seizure,* so named because it is much less

violent and far briefer than the grand mal episode. The victim, most commonly a child, has periodic brief lapses of consciousness without loss of muscular control; typically he may suddenly stop what he is doing and remain "frozen" for a matter of two or three seconds, then resume his activities as if nothing had happened. Sometimes he drops what he is carrying during this interval, but he is never aware that anything has happened. The so-called *psychomotor seizure* is very similar to the petit mal lapse of consciousness, except that it may last for a matter of several minutes during which the victim moves about, appears disoriented, perhaps mutters unintelligibly and seems totally unable to understand anything that is said to him. There have been cases of psychomotor seizures in which the victim wanders away and then regains conscious awareness in some totally different place, yet he is unable to remember how he got there.

A grand mal seizure in particular is often followed by a period of exhaustion, confusion and bewilderment, but there may be no such period following a petit mal attack, and a victim may have as many as fifteen, twenty or more such seizures in the course of a day without any loss of consciousness except during the brief intervals of the attacks. In extremely severe convulsive disorders, however, the victim may reach a point where he has repeated grand mal seizures one after another with little or no rest in between. This condition, much like one prolonged grand mal seizure, is known as *status epilepticus,* and should always be called immediately to medical attention, since vigorous treatment is necessary to halt the succession of seizures as quickly as possible before death from total exhaustion occurs.

While each individual case is different, there are certain things which are commonly associated with all convulsive seizures. One of the most peculiar is the feeling experienced by many victims of recurrent grand mal seizures just prior to an attack, an indescribable feeling spoken of as an *aura,* that sometimes warns the victim that a seizure is about to begin. Further, there are some victims who have seizures only as a result of a specific sensory trigger; a bright light, for example, or the odor of cooking bacon, or a particular tone or sound may invariably cause a seizure if medication is not taken to prevent it.

Convulsive seizures have been traced to a great variety of causes. One very commonplace cause, particularly in children, is the presence of a high fever, usually as a result of infection. The cause and treatment of these so-called *febrile convulsions* differ markedly from other convulsive disorders and are discussed in detail elsewhere. (*See* p. 151.) A far more frequent cause is damage to the brain from such infections as meningitis or encephalitis, often called "brain fever." In some cases these infections leave a permanent residual tendency to seizures of one type or another. Still other convulsions are caused by known injury to the brain as a result of trauma to the head in automobile accidents, brain injury at birth or anoxia sufficient to cause damage to the brain. Brain tumors, whether slow-growing and benign growths which damage brain cells by their excessive pressure, or malignant growths which actually invade and destroy normal brain tissue, can also cause convulsions. In addition, they can occur as a result of various kinds of poisoning or toxicity, particularly in cases of uncontrolled toxemia of pregnancy; they are often a feature of severe hypertension when high blood pressure is accompanied by water retention and edema of the brain.

These known causes, however, account for only a small portion, perhaps as little as 15 or 20 percent, of all convulsive disorders. In the vast majority of cases there is no specific cause, disease or precipitating condition that is known to account for the onset of convulsive episodes. Thus the victims of recurring convulsions that cannot be traced to specific causes are said to suffer from *idiopathic epilepsy*. True, in the great majority of such cases electroencephalograph measurements of the brain demonstrate the presence of abnormal electrical activity even when the patient is not having a convulsion, and in many cases a location or focus in the brain which seems to trigger convulsive seizures can also be identified. Thus many authorities argue that *some* form of injury or malformation of the brain is at the root of the trouble, whether it can be identified or not, but unfortunately identify-ing the area which seems to trigger convulsions does not lead to successful treatment. In fact, any form of neurosurgical operation on the brain for any reason may ultimately lead to the formation of a scar which may later become a focus of convulsive seizures.

Are convulsive seizures dangerous in themselves? They often are. In the case of grand mal seizures, the victim's loss of consciousness, combined with loss of muscular control and violent jerking movements of the body, can easily lead to severe physical injury. Unlike individuals who suffer from "fainting attacks" or even "hysterical convulsions"—that is, pseudoconvulsions that sometimes accompany psychoneurotic behavior either intentionally or unintentionally—the true epileptic does not choose a comfortable place to fall. The fall itself may lead to fractured bones, or he may severely bite his tongue if it becomes trapped between his clenched teeth. Injury to flailing extremities is not uncommon, and in some cases convulsions are accompanied by severe enough muscular rigidity in the back that crushing fractures of the lumbar vertebrae occasionally occur. In addition, among victims who have frequent grand mal convulsions without adequate control or preventive medication, there is often a steady deterioration of brain function. It is not known whether this deterioration is a result of convulsions or whether the convulsions arise because of some condition that causes degeneration of the brain, but in either case neurologists uniformly believe it to be of great importance to do everything possible to suppress or prevent convulsive episodes, not only to make life easier for the victim, but also in the hope that progressive brain damage and deterioration can be prevented.

Although it may be impossible to pin down the precise cause of a convulsive disorder, or to cure it even if the cause is known, it is often possible to suppress convulsions completely, or at least to diminish the frequency and severity of attacks by the use of various medications. By far the most familiar of these is a simple barbiturate, phenobarbital, administered either as white tablets taken by mouth or in an alcohol suspension known as an *elixir*. Phenobarbital is the chemical base from which a wide variety of sedatives and hypnotic (sleep-inducing) drugs have been derived, ranging from amobarbital (Amytal), which acts very swiftly to induce sleep and is often used as an aid to anesthesia, to secobarbital (Seconal) or pentobarbital (Nembutal), which react much more slowly and smoothly and have a longer period of effect. Phenobarbital itself has long been used for daytime sedation to provide rest and partial relief from worry, anxiety and stress, but when used in sufficient dosages, it is also successful in reducing the frequency and severity of grand mal seizures and is equally useful in treating psychomotor seizures and the dangerous status epilepticus. Phenobarbital alone, however, has one unfortunate side effect: quite large doses are often necessary to suppress convulsions, and while the patient under treatment may be free of convulsive episodes, he may also suffer continuing drowsiness and grogginess. This is particularly a disadvantage with children when the sedative side effect may interfere with school work or even normal play.

The development of an alternative drug, sodium diphenylhydantoin (Dilantin), has proved a great boon in the control of grand mal seizures. Today in most cases Dilantin is the medication of choice in treating this kind of epilepsy, although the drug also has sedative side effects and may cause the gums to become overgrown and puffy. However, side effects of either Dilantin or phenobarbital can often be overcome by using the two drugs in combination, with smaller doses of each. Dosages are carefully regulated by the physician, as the amounts of either or both of the drugs necessary may vary widely in individual cases.

For petit mal seizures, certain other drugs, particularly ethosuximide and trimethadione, are particularly useful in reducing the number of seizures per day. In resistant cases, or in cases of allergic reaction to these drugs, other alternatives have at least some value in control of the condition. All of the drugs used for convulsion control, however, tend to be toxic in a high dosage, particularly when taken for prolonged periods of time, as is often the case in epilepsy, and are also allergenic in nature, causing skin rashes, photophobia (light sensitivity) and

blurred vision. Any such reactions, or any other curiosity that comes to the notice of the patient, should be called to the doctor's attention without delay, and regular blood tests are necessary to guard against the possibility of anemia and bone marrow depression which occasionally occur with these medicines.

The best that can be said about these anticonvulsant medications is that they are very helpful, but not exactly a panacea. Authorities estimate that with adequate treatment grand mal seizures can be controlled in about 50 percent of cases, and their frequency can be markedly reduced in an additional 35 percent. The remaining 15 percent whose seizures cannot be controlled are often those with severe brain damage or with such progressive degeneration of the brain that the tendency to convulse increases beyond the controlling capability of the drugs. In petit mal seizures only about one-third are completely controllable with drugs, and the frequency of these brief seizures is reduced in another one-third of the cases. Psychomotor attacks are controlled in even fewer cases, but can be reduced in frequency in about one-half of all cases.

Convulsive disorders are, of course, a very frightening phenomenon, both to their victims and to those who witness them. It is perhaps for this reason that epileptics have been stigmatized by society for so many centuries. Considered dangerous, insane or feeble-minded, they were often ostracized or locked up in asylums. Today we are certainly better informed about the true nature of these disorders, but unfortunately the stigma still exists. It is particularly tragic when the victim is a child who may be completely normal in every other way, yet his teachers and playmates treat him as a "special case," eying him with apprehension and excluding him from everyday activities. Parents often seek to hide the affliction in their child, or consider him an invalid. Adult epileptics are subject to the same suspicion and "overprotection," and are often barred from employment for fear that a seizure on the job may cause some damage or harm, or simply social embarrassment.

Obviously attitudes such as these are extremely unfair and may cause irreparable psychological damage. Certain restrictions on the activities of those who suffer convulsive disorders are, of course, rational and necessary. Anyone vulnerable to seizures that cannot be fully and completely controlled with medication should not drive or be employed on jobs that depend upon total alertness and concentration. Even when convulsions *are* adequately controlled, any side effects caused by the medications must also be taken into consideration. This does not mean, however, that epileptics cannot lead full and productive lives. They can, and history shows that many epileptics have been men of remarkable achievement.

A child with a convulsive disorder well controlled by medication can usually progress in his school work and social activities without hindrance; only rarely are special teaching or social facilities necessary. Naturally, dealing with a long-term convulsive disorder can be a burden on the parents as well as on the child. They must see that the child takes his medication at the proper time, and is observed at suitable intervals by his doctor. They must also realize that conditions may change, and that medication effective in controlling convulsions may become inadequate, or conversely that the child may eventually require less and less medication.

It is also important for the family of an epileptic to be thoroughly familiar with the first-aid measures that must be taken to aid the victim of a seizure. A grand mal seizure cannot be stopped, but the victim should be rolled over on his side to allow his mouth to drain, restricting clothing should be loosened, and by the use of gentle restraint and padding, he can be prevented from harming himself. Some soft but firm object should, if possible, be inserted between the victim's teeth to prevent clenching of the jaws and biting of the tongue. Little can be done to aid the victims of attacks of lesser severity other than to prevent them from wandering off in a state of bewilderment and confusion, but if the victim has repeated attacks or falls into a deep sleep after a seizure, medical aid should be summoned as quickly as possible.

Finally, the epileptic must be accepted by both his family and society in general as a person with a special problem, to be sure, but not a cripple or a misfit. The condition should be regarded and discussed with complete honesty like any other medical problem. If the illness is accepted calmly and realistically, the epileptic can look forward, in most cases, to a long and useful life.

Disorders of Nutrition

Virtually everyone is aware of the vital connection between good nutrition and normal growth, development and maintenance of a healthy human body. We are a diet-conscious society and speak knowingly of proteins, carbohydrates, fats and the important part played by vitamins and minerals in our everyday diets. Considering this, it may seem ridiculous to discuss nutritional deficiency as a source of disease or disorder, at least in this country. Yet the fact is that nutritional deficiencies can cause trouble, and that deficiency diseases, varying from the relatively minor to the truly dangerous, are by no means rare, both among those who may make the wrong choice of foods and those who may have no choice. Children are often the victims of these diseases, but good nutrition is essential at every age and must be a lifelong concern. Such concern, however, must obviously be based on knowledge of what food substances are essential, why they are important and what happens when insufficient amounts are taken in with the daily diet.

Water. While it may seem odd to discuss water as an "essential food substance," the fact is that the body needs water in sufficient quantities more urgently than almost any other chemical substance. An individual may be able to survive for weeks, perhaps months, with little or no food, utilizing food substances already stored in the body, but he is in serious trouble if deprived of water for as little as 48 hours, and even 24 hours or less without water under tropical or desert conditions may be fatal. Water, the necessary solvent for all the chemical reactions in the body, and a major component of every living cell, is constantly being lost each day, some by way of the urine, some by perspiration and some exhaled as water vapor from the lungs with breathing. An adult male may lose as much as two and a half quarts of water or more each day in ordinary sedentary activities, and as much as five quarts or more can be lost in active work in a hot climate. Children lose proportionately less, of course, but the loss is just as steady. And since the body has no capacity to store extra water against future needs, the water lost each day must be replaced each day.

The major threat to the body when lost water is not replaced is *dehydration;* fluid from the circulating blood and from all the cells is leached out, often very swiftly when some disorder such as continuing diarrhea, or diarrhea accompanied by vomiting, forces more rapid water loss than normal. In children dehydration from such causes may occur within a few hours after the onset of diarrhea, and for this reason *any* continuing diarrhea or vomiting in a child must be promptly reported to the doctor. In either adults or children when water loss cannot be replaced by drinking water (i.e., when vomiting is present, or when the individual is unconscious and cannot be given water by mouth), fluid can be replaced either by means of intravenous infusion or by way of a nasogastric tube inserted into the stomach.

Carbohydrates. This essential group of foods, which includes all sugars and starches, is the body's major source of energy. These foods are called carbohydrates because they are basically chemical compounds of carbon, hydrogen and oxygen, and can be broken down during digestion into simple sugars, primarily *glucose,* which can be utilized for heat and energy within all the cells of the body. In addition, some of the carbohydrates taken in the diet are converted in the liver to a more complex form of sugar known as *glycogen,* which can be stored in the liver cells and elsewhere in the body for later reconversion into sugar. Thus a certain amount of carbohydrate storage is possible. Even greater excesses may be used by the body to manufacture molecules of fat for storage in the adipose tissues. Such foods as sugar, honey, potatoes, rice, corn meal, wheat flour, kidney beans, plantains, bananas and many other sweet fruits, as well as ethyl alcohol, are rich sources of carbohydrate; since many of these are also the least costly foods the world over, carbohydrate deficiency is most uncommon except in areas where people are subsisting on starvation diets. In many parts of the world, however, including our own country, there are many people in poverty who live almost exclusively on inexpensive carbohydrates, and thus suffer dietary deficiencies of other vital food substances.

Protein. Protein is the major body-building food for man, and indeed for virtually every member of the animal and plant kingdoms. Protein molecules are built up in an incredible variety of forms from various alignments or arrangements of nitrogen-containing molecular fragments known as *amino acids,* derived from the digestion of protein-containing food materials in the diet. For many centuries the chemical structure of protein, or even of amino acids, remained a mystery because efforts to break protein down into constituent chemical parts destroyed both the protein and its constituents. Today, however, we know that all proteins in the human body are constructed of various arrangements of a mere 22 amino acids, all of which are important to the healthy growth and maintenance of body tissues, and most of which are essential to life. The cell walls in tissues all over the body are composed of protein, for instance, as well as the genetic material within each cell. Muscle tissue is composed almost entirely of protein. The hemoglobin in red cells is an iron-containing protein material, and many of the hormones are basically protein in nature. Perhaps most important of all, multitudes of *enzymes*—the chemical catalysts that enable life-sustaining biochemical reactions to occur throughout the body—are proteins.

Important as proteins may be, chronic protein deficiency is one of the most widespread of all nutritional disorders throughout the world today. Virtually all of the protein-rich foods— lean meats, fish, shellfish, eggs, cheese and milk —are comparatively costly and either unavailable or beyond the means of multitudes of people, particularly in underdeveloped countries. Babies suffer especially when they are weaned from breast milk. And while it is true that many vegetables, beans, rice, corn meal and wheat contain *some* protein, diets utilizing these foods as staples without additional protein-rich foods seldom provide enough protein, and starchy foods such as plantains that are the staple diet of many people in tropical countries contain virtually no protein at all.

The results of chronic protein starvation are subtle but pervasive. Lack of dietary protein leads to poor physical growth and development, lowered resistance to infection, impaired nervous system development and diminished utilization of intellectual capacity. Lack of one particular amino acid known as *choline* results in damage to liver cells, ultimately leading to cirrhosis. In populations suffering from chronic protein starvation the average life expectancy is often less than half what it is in countries where protein is widely available. Thus any well-balanced diet must be based upon sufficient protein from meat, eggs or milk supplied each day and supplemented by carbohydrate supplied by fresh fruits, vegetables and cereal foods. Finally, a balanced diet requires daily supplies of three other vital food materials: fats, minerals and vitamins.

Fats. Basically, fats in the diet supply the body with two things: first, a concentrated supply of calories for production of heat and energy in the body cells; and second, a means of storage of excess calories for the body to use when the daily intake is diminished for one reason or another. Fats are taken in the diet in the form of meat fats, vegetable and cooking oils, naturally fat-rich vegetable products such as nuts, coconut, avocados or olives, and butter fat from milk, cream, cheese and butter. Fats account for the desirable flavoring of many cooked foods—a fat-free diet tends to be rather tasteless and unpalatable—and supplies the body with a surprisingly rich source of calories, since fats contain more than twice the calories, weight for weight, as are contained in either protein or carbohydrate. The body needs fat not only as a nutritional supplement but also for the biochemical synthesis of a number of fatty materials known as *lipids*. Some of these lipids enter into the formation of cholesterol and various of the cholesterol-like hormones, including the adrenocortical hormones and the sex hormones; others, formed in combination with phosphorus, become *phospholipids* which make up the fatty myelin sheaths that cover nerve fibers in many parts of the body and aid in the transmission of nerve signals. Unlike other food materials, the body has a remarkable capacity to synthesize fats and lipids from other food materials even when dietary intake of fats is very low; thus, overeating of any kind of food will ultimately result in the deposition of the excess over and above daily needs as fat globules in the adipose tissues. Similarly, when faced with relative starvation due to lack of food intake, the body can draw upon these fat stores for heat and energy. So long as the diet contains enough protein, the body will *selectively* utilize stored fat to supply needed energy, so that the individual seeking to lose weight by dieting will lose stored fat first as long as dietary protein is supplied in sufficient quantity—doubtless the source of the erroneous idea that "protein burns up fat" in a reducing diet. It is true, however, that the body can manage without dietary fat far better and longer than it can manage with a deficiency of any of the other vital foods. In a child's diet, however, it is important that all the basic food materials, including adequate fat as well as protein and carbohydrate, be supplied. During the early years this need is splendidly supplied by milk, which contains butterfat, and later by fats normally found in meats and vegetables as well.

In recent years much has been written about potential health dangers from eating certain kinds of fats. Biochemists distinguish between *saturated* and *unsaturated* fats; the former are fats in which certain carbon atoms in the fat molecule are already completely chemically bonded to oxygen or hydrogen or other carbon atoms, and thus these fats differ in physical and chemical properties from others in which certain carbon atoms remain free for chemical bonding with other atoms. As a practical rule of thumb, saturated fats are those, usually from animal sources, which remain hard or congeal at normal room temperatures, while unsaturated fats tend to remain liquid at room temperatures. Virtually all natural animal and vegetable fats are actually mixtures of saturated and unsaturated fats, but some natural fats such as peanut oil or vegetable oils contain a preponderance of unsaturated fats, and some manufactured margarines, cooking oils or shortenings are made up almost entirely of unsaturated fats and are thus termed *polyunsaturated*. Interest in this distinguishing feature of fats was aroused in the 1950s and 1960s when medical researchers began to suspect that saturated fats might be major offenders in forming the fatty deposits on the inner lining of coronary and other arteries, thought to be the precursors of the atheromatous plaques so characteristically present in arteriosclerosis. It was hoped that by reducing the amounts of saturated fats taken in the diet, individuals could slow the development of arteriosclerosis, or even prevent it. Most authorities still agree that the use of polyunsaturated fats is preferable to saturated fats in the diet, but the relationship of saturated dietary fats to heart or circulatory system disease is no longer thought to be quite so direct. These disorders are now known to progress and worsen even when the individual eats no saturated fats at all, and it is believed that the body will synthesize the offending fatty materials, at least to some degree, no matter what fats are eaten. It is still recognized, of course, that high-fat diets do contribute to obesity, and reduction of daily intake of fats is still an important part of any reducing diet.

Minerals. In addition to the three major food materials discussed above, the body also needs varying amounts of a number of nonnutritive minerals for normal growth, development and health maintenance. Calcium and phosphorus are vital to the formation and maintenance of normal bone, and calcium is needed for normal muscle function as well; a lack of dietary calcium, for example, will cause the body to draw calcium from the bone, and too low a calcium level in the blood can cause a type of convulsive muscle cramping known as *tetany*. Potassium is a vital mineral constituent in all the cells in the body, and plays an important role, among other things, in normal regulation of the heart rate. Sodium chloride—ordinary salt—is necessary to maintain the normal fluid pressures inside and outside the cells in all the tissues; an excess of sodium will cause the retention of water in the body as edema fluid, while the loss of sodium through excessive sweating or excessive urinary excretion can lead to dehydration, heat exhaus-

tion or an excessive viscosity or thickness of the blood due to loss of body water along with the salt. Iron must be supplied in the diet to aid in the formation of hemoglobin, and inadequate dietary supplies of iron can lead to *iron-deficiency anemia*. (*See* p. 515.) Small amounts of iodine are required as a vital constituent of the thyroid hormone thyroxin, and a lack leads to a form of thyroid gland enlargement known as *goiter*. (*See* p. 690.) Finally, trace amounts of other minerals, including magnesium, copper, manganese and fluoride salts, are important to the normal maintenance of a wide variety of biochemical reactions. Ordinarily, necessary minerals are taken in with the normal diet without special attention, but deficiencies can occur under certain circumstances. Many women, for example, suffer from iron deficiency during early pregnancy when their blood supply must be swiftly increased to take care of the growing baby. Calcium must be supplemented during pregnancy, along with iron and vitamins, to help provide calcium for the baby's cartilage and bone formation. For many years it has been customary for manufacturers to add trace amounts of iodine to table salt to combat iodine deficiency and goiter in areas where the diet has little natural supply of iodine from seafood or shellfish, the richest dietary sources available.

Vitamins. Vitamins are particular chemical substances, differing widely in their structures, which enter into the body's metabolism in a variety of ways. We speak of "the vitamins" as a close-knit family of substances, but they are actually quite independent and unrelated to each other. Some, like vitamin D, are highly complex chemicals while others, like vitamin C (ascorbic acid), are much simpler substances. The best source of most of these substances is from natural foods, since both plants and animals require them in their metabolism, too, but they can also be manufactured synthetically and taken as food supplements if necessary. More than a dozen different vitamins are known to exist, and although the specific function of some of them in human metabolism is not yet fully understood, it is well known that a lack or an inadequate supply of the more familiar vitamins can cause the temporary symptoms, or even the permanent disabilities, that characterize deficiency diseases.

Vitamin A deficiency is most frequently connected with visual disturbances, particularly night blindness, or poor visual adaptation in dim light, and most commonly occurs in this country not as a dietary deficiency but as a complication of various disorders of fat absorption in the bowel. (*See* p. 893.) Vitamin A is essential to the formation of the visual pigments in the retina, and is contained in nature in the yellow-colored pigment known as carotene which is found in abundance in yellow and green leafy vegetables and animal livers. Carrots, milk, butter, eggs, and liver are excellent sources of supply. A dietary deficiency of vitamin A is far less common in this country than in the Orient, parts of Africa, Mexico and India, where it is believed to be the most frequent cause of blindness in children. A severe deficiency, however, can also affect the condition of the skin and leave the victim more vulnerable to bronchial infections and infections of the conjunctiva or lining of the eye. Today vitamin A is artificially added to milk, butter and margarine, and in this form, in addition to eating a balanced diet, most children can be assured of a more than adequate supply.

Deficiencies of the family of B vitamins known as the "B complex" are even more uncommon in this country, turning up only occasionally in very low-income groups where diets are composed largely of refined carbohydrates, in alcoholics whose intake of all foods may be chronically inadequate, and in those who indulge in various dietary fads. Deficiencies of the B vitamins can result in two clearly distinguishable diseases—pellagra and beriberi. *Pellagra* is a disorder due to deficiency of niacin or nicotinic acid, one of the B complex vitamins, and is characterized by soreness of the mouth and tongue, cracking of the lips at the corners, sometimes diarrhea, nausea and vomiting, and in prolonged and severe cases, nervous system degeneration and chronic inflammatory skin rashes. These symptoms are reversible by the use of therapeutic dosages of nicotinic acid, if the disease is diagnosed early enough, but there is always the possibility of recurrence without a varied diet of meat, fish, cereals, eggs, milk and fresh fruits and vegetables.

Beriberi is caused by a deficiency of vitamin B_1, or thiamine, and is notoriously common in parts of the world where polished rice is the major food grain. The husks of rice are rich in vitamin B_1, but it is completely lost when the rice is polished and the husks discarded. Thus the disease can be avoided in these areas simply by eating unpolished rice. Beriberi causes a number of changes in both the nervous system and the heart muscle, with degeneration of the sensory nerve endings and thus disturbances in the senses of touch, temperature and vibration. There is also degeneration of motor nerves controlling movements of the fingers, arms, toes or legs, and when the heart is affected, enlargement, a rapid heartbeat, and eventually congestive heart failure may result. All these changes, if discovered early in the disorder, are completely reversible with vitamin therapy and an adequate and varied diet, although complete recovery may take a long period of time.

A deficiency of vitamin B_2, riboflavin, is also rarely seen in this country but may result when the diet consists mainly of potatoes, corn and rice. Its symptoms include inflammation of the mouth, tongue, nose and eyes, impaired vision and an increased oiliness of the skin of the face. Again the disease can be prevented, or its early symptoms reversed by an adequate and varied diet. Vitamin B_{12} and folic acid are essential to the body in the manufacture of red blood cells. A deficiency of these substances is most often caused by the body's inability to absorb them into the blood stream, although they may exist in adequate quantities in the diet. *Pernicious anemia* (*see* p. 516) and *sprue* (*see* p. 628) are two diseases which occur among both children and adults as a result of this condition, and they can be cured by vitamin supplements and treatment of the absorptive disorder.

Scurvy is a disease caused by a deficiency of vitamin C or ascorbic acid. In children the most striking manifestations of scurvy are changes in the bones which cause pain on motion, and a tendency to capillary hemorrhages under the skin, in the mouth and around the teeth. As long as the mother's diet is adequate, breast milk provides ample protection against scurvy in infants, but cow's milk, especially pasteurized cow's milk, is much lower in ascorbic acid content. Fresh citrus juices, notably fresh orange juice, are the best natural source of ascorbic acid, and other fresh fruits and vegetables contain quantities of it as well. Because vitamin C is destroyed by prolonged heating, heat-processed (pasteurized) or evaporated milk tends to be low in this vital substance, whereas fresh fruits and fresh vegetables, either uncooked or very lightly cooked, retain their ascorbic acid and help meet the daily necessary supply.

The symptoms of scurvy usually bring the victim to medical attention, and the disease is quite easily diagnosed from characteristic changes in the growth areas of the long bones, easily distinguished by X-rays of the knees or wrists. The disease is treated first by administration of ascorbic acid in pure chemical form, followed by an improved diet and multiple vitamin supplements containing vitamin C. Once scurvy is treated, abnormal bone growth reverts to normal, and permanent deformities are extremely rare.

Rickets due to a deficiency of vitamin D is often associated with scurvy because the disease also affects the growth and development of bone, particularly the deposition of calcium and phosphorus. Vitamin D controls the supply of these bone-forming minerals, and when inadequate vitamin D is present, especially during a period of rapid bone growth such as childhood, the disease can appear insidiously. Most of the changes occur at the place where cartilage covering the joints meets the shaft of the long bones, and one of the most common signs of the disease is deformity of the skull noticed in children from three to six months of age. Beading of the ribs can occur at the place where the cartilage joins the bony part of the ribs to form a line of swellings down either side of the chest, sometimes so striking that it has been given the name "rachitic rosary." Deformities of the long bones also occur, with bending of the bones and swelling at the joints. In addition, the muscles of the afflicted child tend to be small, flabby and poorly developed, so that children with rickets are often unable to sit erect, stand or walk at the usual age, and this condition is suspected in cases of children who do not walk until long after the expected time.

Fortunately one of the best of all supplies of vitamin D is perfectly natural: the body actually manufactures this vitamin in the skin upon exposure to ultraviolet radiation from the sun. For this reason the disorder is less common among children living in sunny climates than among those in gray northern latitudes, although those with dark or deeply tanned complexions do not derive as much benefit from the sun's rays. Children were once forced to choke down quantities of cod liver oil because of its high vitamin D content, but today a more pleasant source of the vitamin is available. Although milk is not naturally rich in the vitamin, it has become customary in the United States to "enrich" pasteurized milk by the addition of synthetic vitamin D, so that the child who receives an adequate amount of enriched milk (from a pint to a quart a day, depending upon size and age) will not suffer from rickets. Once again, the condition is easy to diagnose from the appearance of bones in X-rays, and occasionally it is discovered incidentally when X-rays are being taken for other purposes. There was a time in history when both scurvy and rickets took thousands of children's lives every year, and today they are still the major deficiency diseases suffered by children, but the remedy or prevention for both is widely recognized and easily and inexpensively provided.

Vitamin K is a less familiar vitamin, but an extremely important one because it is essential for the production in the liver of prothrombin, a substance necessary to the normal blood-clotting mechanism. Some vitamin K is derived from the diet, but most of the body's requirement is synthesized by the bacteria which normally inhabit the colon, and the aid of bile salts in the colon are required in order for the vitamin to be absorbed into the blood stream. Since newborn babies' colons are sterile, they have a natural vitamin K deficiency for the first three to five days after birth, and thus have a tendency to slow blood clotting until colon bacilli find their way into the lower gastrointestinal tract. For this reason doctors usually postpone simple surgery such as circumcision until after the baby is five days old. Later in life vitamin K deficiency may develop when sulfa drugs or antibiotics used to treat bacterial infections also destroy the normal colon bacilli, or when obstructive liver, gall bladder or bile duct disease prevents bile from reaching the colon. When detected, the resulting bleeding tendency today can be treated easily with small doses of synthetic vitamin K, so that deficiency problems seldom arise.

What about excessive amounts of vitamins? When the existence of vitamins was first discovered, it was thought that since they are necessary to normal growth and maintenance, one could not take too many of them. Today we know that excessive amounts of certain vitamins, particularly vitamins A and D, may actually be harmful and cause toxic reactions. In the proper amounts they are essential, particularly in infancy and childhood, and during pregnancy, but even though they are readily available in a bewildering variety of preparations and combinations, it is wise to rely on a doctor's advice for their use. Above all, attention to a well-balanced diet based on a physician's directions, supplemented by such vitamin preparations as he prescribes, is the best possible assurance that a child will receive adequate nutrition and avoid any deficiency problems.

Disorders of Intestinal Absorption in Children

Proper nutrition depends not only upon an adequate supply of vitamins and minerals in the diet, or even upon adequate quantities of protein, carbohydrate and fat, but also upon proper digestion, absorption and assimilation of these foodstuffs by the body. Within the past three or four decades a certain group of disorders, somewhat similar in nature but not identical, have been discovered to occur quite commonly in children, disorders of digestion or absorption of food materials and vitamins from the intestinal tract which have been found to account for certain long-unexplained patterns of illness, and in some cases chronic disease and death. There are two major members of this class of disease—*celiac syndrome* (sometimes called *celiac disease*), a chronic and recurring disorder of digestion and absorption which may retard the child's physical and emotional growth but which tends to disappear as the child grows older; and a disease known as *cystic fibrosis* (sometimes called *fibrocystic disease of the pancreas* or *mucoviscidosis*), a hereditary or familial disease in which inadequate quantities of digestive enzymes produced in the pancreas of the child, together with disturbances in glandular secretions elsewhere in the body, particularly in the bronchial tree, so severely impair the growth and development of the child that death may occur any time during childhood or, at best, early adulthood.

The cause of neither of these disorders is fully understood; even in cystic fibrosis, which is known to be a chromosome-borne hereditary disorder, investigators have not identified what causes the chromosomal change in the first place, nor have they identified which of the chromosomes is at fault. Of the two conditions, celiac syndrome tends to appear later, usually not until the baby is six months old or so, and then begins with the onset of persistent diarrhea following an episode of upper respiratory infection. Exactly what the relationship is between the infectious process in the body and the triggering of the baby's intestines' inability to absorb certain nutriments has not been determined. Once triggered, however, the diarrhea tends to persist, with the production of frequent loose, bulky and foul-smelling stools which, upon laboratory examination, are found to contain large amounts of undigested or unassimilated starches and fats from the diet. Even though the triggering respiratory infection may clear up quickly under antibiotic treatment, the attacks of diarrhea and malabsorption of nutriments may persist for weeks or months, compounded by a drop in the child's appetite, a dwindling of normal fat storage within his body, gradual weakening of muscle tissue, and a marked increase in irritability. In a typical case the physician sees a child showing evidence of severe malnutrition, severe vitamin deficiency and emotional misery all at once.

In most cases of celiac syndrome left untreated, the diarrhea gradually subsides after a few weeks or months, and the child once again begins to gain weight and develop strength, only to be struck by a recurrent episode again triggered by an upper respiratory infection. These recurrent attacks can appear and reappear cyclically throughout childhood, gradually becoming less severe as the child grows older. But fortunately there are some measures that can help cut down on the length of recurrences, lengthen the interval between them and generally help the child over the trying periods. Early attention and vigorous treatment of any and all identified infections is the first step, and both the number and the duration of the recurrences of diarrhea can be markedly reduced by preventing infections. Second, it has been found that the presence of a type of protein material known as *gluten,* found in such common grain foods as wheat, rye or oats, is deleterious, so that special diets completely free of gluten and including simple, easily digested sugars such as those in corn syrup, honey and ripe bananas help reduce the severity and duration of acute episodes. At the same time general nutrition can be enhanced by making the diet high in protein from lean meats, cheese, or egg white and fruits and vegetables, together with high doses of multivitamin preparations, especially of vitamins A and D and the B complex vitamins, all of which are poorly absorbed in the presence of the disease. Since anemia sometimes results from these episodes, such anemia-preventive medicines as folic acid and vitamin B_{12} are also added. This kind of regimen has been found to be extremely helpful in dealing with celiac syndrome when it arises, but treatment should be carefully monitored by a physician who has had experience in treating this disease. Complete recovery may require as long as one or two years to accomplish, but the disease does tend to clear up sooner or later. In severe relapses children may lose so much water in diarrhea that they require hospitalization and intravenous feeding, but in the long run the prognosis is good providing that adequate treatment is available.

Outwardly similar as it may seem to celiac syndrome, cystic fibrosis is a far more serious disease when it occurs. This disease also attacks children during infancy, often beginning within the first three months of life; and as in celiac disease one feature of cystic fibrosis is the production of extremely large, bulky frequent stools which are particularly foul-smelling because of the high content of undigested fat and protein they contain. Also as in celiac disease, as much as 50 percent of the total amount of foods taken in, including carbohydrates, fats and proteins, is lost in the stool. But the cause is basically different. Whereas in celiac disease the disturbance seems to be a disorder of absorption of digested foodstuffs from the intestine, cystic fibrosis is a result of marked diminution or absence of virtually all the digestive enzymes that are normally made by the pancreas. Indeed, cystic fibrosis is a multiple-system disease in which the secretory glands of the pancreas, the mucus-secreting glands of the respiratory system, and the sweat glands in the skin are all greatly impaired, leading to severe digestive insufficiency with consequent nutritional and vitamin deficiencies, chronic respiratory infections, and a marked susceptibility to heat prostration because of improper function of sweat glands. The prognosis for cystic fibrosis is also far more grave than for celiac disease, since many of its victims die in infancy, many more die in early childhood, and only a relatively few even today survive through adolescence into young adulthood.

The first hint of the presence of cystic fibrosis in a child may come very soon after his birth with the discovery of the presence of a type of small-intestinal obstruction known as *meconium ileus.* (*See* p. 877.) Normally the newborn child's intestinal tract is filled with a soft, black sticky material known as meconium which is ordinarily passed per rectum within the first 24 to 48 hours after birth, certainly as soon as the child begins taking feedings. In many children afflicted with cystic fibrosis, however, the disease process has already begun during fetal life, and excessively thick and sticky mucous secretions in the intestine, including sticky secretions from the pancreas or bile ducts or both, are mixed with the meconium to form a semisolid, putty-like plug which completely obstructs the lower end of the small intestine or ileum. Thus the baby reveals a syndrome of intestinal obstruction, often within minutes or hours after birth, and certainly as soon as feedings begin, complete with distention of the bowel above the obstruction, vomiting of feedings and obvious pain. Although on rare occasions meconium ileus can be resolved with conservative medical treatment to dislodge the bowel obstruction, in most cases a surgical emergency exists and the plugged section of ileum must be surgically removed. With modern anesthetics and pediatric surgical techniques, this procedure today has a far lower rate of mortality than was once the case, but those infants who recover from the surgery almost invariably develop other symptoms indicating that cystic fibrosis is the basic disease process.

These symptoms are primarily related to the respiratory and digestive tracts. Sticky respiratory tract secretions apparently plug up medium-sized bronchial tubes and make the infant far more prone than normal to respiratory infections, particularly bronchitis or pneumonia, with large areas of both lungs often involved in differing degrees. As in any obstructive bronchial disease, the alveolar air sacs that make up the substance of the lung tend to become distended or emphysematous, and chronic bronchial infection gradually dilates and destroys the muscular walls of the bronchi so that sacular pockets of infection, known as *bronchiectasis,* form along the track of the bronchial tubes. If the child survives to late childhood or adolescence, chronic sinus and middle ear infections also become part of the picture. At the same time marked malnutrition due to poor absorption of nutrients and vitamins from the intestine interferes with the child's growth, development and resistance to infection. Finally, excessive amounts of salt and other electrolytes are lost in perspiration, and thus the child is excessively vulnerable to heat prostration whenever the weather is extremely warm or whenever he has a fever.

In severe cases the main problem of diagnosis is distinguishing cystic fibrosis from the less threatening celiac syndrome. Evidence of severe respiratory tract infection on chest X-ray and signs of insufficient pancreatic digestive juice formation—determined by examining specimens of the stool and by securing samples of digestive juices from the duodenum, where pancreatic secretions should be present in large quantity— are both strongly suggestive of cystic fibrosis. In addition, a special laboratory procedure in which the child is induced to perspire heavily so the sweat can be analyzed is also a good diagnostic aid; the child with cystic fibrosis will have extraordinary elevations of sodium and chloride ions in his sweat. A chemical analysis of hair and fingernail clippings reveals high concentrations of both sodium and potassium in children with cystic fibrosis, sometimes as much as three times more than normal. A positive family history further confirms the suspected diagnosis, although the disease cannot be ruled out simply because no one knows of anyone else in the family who had it. The untimely death of an infant in the family from bronchitis or pneumonia must be regarded with suspicion, since not uncommonly children with cystic fibrosis die before the diagnosis is ever made.

A great deal about the nature, diagnosis and treatment of cystic fibrosis is still unknown or only poorly understood, but with modern treatment, its prognosis is at least somewhat brighter than before. In general, therapy consists first of vigorous antibiotic treatment of bronchial infections or pneumonia, followed by the long-term use of broad-spectrum antibiotics prophylactically to help prevent further infection. The sticky mucous secretions characteristic of the disease in the lungs and bronchi may be liquefied by means of such expectorant medicines as potassium iodide or glyceryl guaiacolate, used in conjunction with drugs to dilate the bronchi so that sticky secretions can better be expelled by coughing. At the same time adequate replacement of the missing enzymes from the pancreas, given either as powder or as tablets with each meal, helps the child digest and absorb more of the food he takes in. Fortunately children with this disease usually have a healthy or excessively good appetite, and are able to take in the quantities of food, sometimes from 25 to 50 percent more than the normal diet, necessary to obtain adequate nutriments, especially proteins, that will permit growth and development to progress.

Various complications of the disease may require surgical correction—the removal of nasal polyps, for example, or resection of parts of the lung damaged by bronchiectasis or emphysema. By maintaining a closely regulated program of treatment, including careful education of the parents about the nature of the disease and the importance of avoiding complications, there is reason to hope that cystic fibrosis will respond to treatment more and more frequently, and that the number of patients diagnosed in early childhood who actually reach adulthood will begin to exceed the present statistical limit of 10 percent.

Other Causes of Illness or Death in Children

There are certain kinds of cancer that afflict children, sometimes very young children, the most notorious of which is *lymphatic leukemia,* a far more common, swift and deadly killer in childhood than in later age groups. (The various kinds of leukemia are discussed in detail on p. 523.) Another form of childhood cancer is the so-called *Wilms's tumor* which develops in the kidney and arises from malignant changes in foci or "rests" of very primitive cells remaining in the kidney after its development is complete. This cancer, most commonly discovered within the first year of a baby's life, may be rapidly fatal, but surgical removal of these growths can be successful if diagnosis is made early enough. Other malignant growths afflicting children include *retinoblastoma,* which can develop in the retina of the eye, one of the most virulent of all known cancers.

Children are also subject to certain benign tumors which do not commonly appear in older age groups, particularly *hemangiomas,* growths of capillary blood vessels which often occur on the surface of the skin and appear as raised, mottled, reddish or reddish-purple lumps that occasionally enlarge sharply during the child's early months. These tumors, which are almost always benign, are usually discovered early because of their unusual appearance and may either be removed surgically or be destroyed by more conservative methods such as freezing with

dry ice, depending upon the size and the physician's preference, in those cases in which they do not gradually diminish in size and disappear spontaneously. Small hemangiomas which are frequently found at birth and commonly persist without any evidence of growth, particularly in the region of the back of the neck, are commonly known as "birthmarks" and have no pathological significance. On rare occasions a hemangioma may involve a large blotchy area of otherwise normal skin on the face, neck or elsewhere on the body, forming an area of dark bluish-red discoloration sometimes called a "port wine stain." Such a mark, while unpleasant cosmetically, does not tend to grow or become malignant, and may involve too large an area for effective treatment. These tumors are discussed in more detail elsewhere. (*See* p. 400.)

Another all too frequent cause of illness and death in infancy and childhood is not a disease process at all but the result of the *"battered child syndrome."* Although this term has come into use only within the last few years, and only within that time has become clearly identified with willful mistreatment of children either by siblings or by adult members of the family, the tragic phenomenon has, without doubt, occurred throughout history. In earlier decades doctors were familiar enough with the symptoms: a small child brought in for medical treatment, or even dead on arrival at a hospital, with multiple bruises and black-and-blue marks all over his body, sometimes fractured bones, damaged teeth, or burns, all ascribed to an "accidental" fall or other injury. The physicians seeing these children may have suspected that the injuries were the result of some form of "punishment" or simply physical abuse, but they were often restrained from reporting it to the authorities because of the lack of positive proof, or the threat of reprisal or litigation.

Today, however, the problem is finally out in the open, along with the other more readily recognizable forms of child abuse like neglect, desertion and abandonment. Extensive studies of unexplained and repeated injuries among children have outlined the medical means by which the battered child syndrome can be detected and have strengthened the proof necessary to support prosecution. Thus physicians are more and more alert to the telltale symptoms of the condition, and are now protected in most states by laws designed to encourage, or even require, the reporting of suspicious injuries to the proper authorities without putting the doctor in legal jeopardy. Social agencies, with the necessary legal authorization, also stand ready to remove the child from the custody of the abusive adult, and where possible to help the adult deal with the severe emotional or behavioral disturbance that is usually at the root of the problem.

Occasionally a child may be the victim of an injury inflicted by a parent not as a result of cruelty, drunkenness, or an emotional disturbance, but because the parent in punishing the child failed to realize his own strength, or perhaps because he momentarily lost his temper. Accidents like these, however, are seldom repeated, and the remorseful adult makes no effort to conceal his guilt. But every parent must realize that children's bodies are small and fragile, and that all but the mildest forms of physical punishment can cause serious injury. Some authorities regard any kind of physical punishment of a child as anathema and recommend instead withdrawal of privileges, social approbation, appeals to reason and other forms of "intellectual" discipline. Others contend that these forms of punishment are less comprehensible to a child, and that making him feel ashamed or guilty is far more cruel than mild corporal punishment on the spot, directly related to the misdeed, if possible, followed by permitting the matter to drop. Certainly the vast majority of parents do, in fact, use some form of physical punishment at least occasionally in training and disciplining their children. But certain kinds of physical punishment should *never* be used under any circumstances. For example, blows to the head, however "restrained," can inadvertently result in concussion and/or intracranial hemorrhage, or conceivably even fracture of the neck. Beatings with hands, belt or hairbrush can bruise or lacerate the skin and even fracture limbs, as can any form of bondage. The problem of discipline is certainly a difficult one, particularly with a rambunctious and unthinking child, but it makes little sense to

inflict pain in the hope of preventing misbehavior. If physical punishment is used, it should be extremely light and brief. Far more important, whatever the form of punishment, is to try to make the child understand what he has done wrong, why it is wrong, and why he must not do it again. And, of course, it is preferable that the child knows what constitutes wrongdoing *before* the misdeed has been committed. Parents whose standards of behavior are unnecessarily restrictive, or who continually make threats that they do not, or cannot, carry out, merely invite disobedience. In every case, punishment should be administered for the child's benefit, not the parents', and any form of discipline must be carried out with fairness, consistency, understanding and love.

Finally, there is one source of mortality among babies that occurs often enough that in recent years a great deal of research has been applied in hopes of controlling it. It is the so-called *sudden death syndrome,* the quick and apparently mysterious death of a child, usually within the first six months to a year of his life. Each year thousands of infants do indeed die suddenly for reasons that are never clearly understood. Sudden death may occur during what appears to be an otherwise benign illness; or it may occur with *no* apparent explanation. Yet, incredibly, for emotional reasons, these deaths are frequently never explored by such means as a post-mortem examination in an attempt to determine the cause. And even when post-mortem and other examinations are performed, all too often no really convincing explanation can be found.

Until recent decades, grave suspicion often rested unjustly upon the child's parents in the event of such a tragic occurrence. But intensive research has revealed a number of hitherto unsuspected causes for sudden death in infancy and early childhood. Leading among them are abnormalities attendant upon premature birth, often merely the aspiration of food or mucus into the respiratory tree which results in suffocation when the child is too immature or premature to have a well-developed cough reflex or the strength to expel such foreign material from the bronchial tree. Equally common are hemorrhages within the baby's head, either as a result of very difficult or prolonged labor or as a direct result of trauma at delivery, which can then lead to respiratory failure owing to unsuspected brain damage. Again, undetected and unsuspected malformations of the brain, heart, lungs, kidneys or other organ systems frequently lead to sudden death. Occasionally death occurs when a child has been subjected to excessive heat to which the immature temperature control mechanisms of his body are unable to adapt. Finally, it has been found that in some infants a fulminating and fatal infection—meningococcal meningitis, for example, or diphtheria—may run its course without producing the characteristic symptoms, sometimes even without the presence of a detectable fever. Occasionally such infections can be established only by obtaining a blood culture in which the bacteria are demonstrated, or by means of microscopic examination at autopsy.

The sudden death syndrome is not a frequent occurrence, but when it does happen it not only is tragic for the child but can be gravely traumatic for the parents, who often blame themselves for some act of omission or commission. The fact is, however, that in almost every case there is virtually nothing the parents could have done that would have altered the outcome. Nevertheless, it is exceedingly important for the sake of the parents' own equilibrium and emotional health that every possible step be taken to help identify the cause of death if possible. Parents are urged to permit post-mortem examination even in circumstances in which legal requirements do not demand it. When a probable cause of death can be established, the parents should confront it honestly and realistically with their family doctor so that any question of culpability can be firmly eliminated, and

so that the remainder of the parents' lives need not be spent under the pointless and destructive shadow of guilt.

In discussing the wide variety of disorders and diseases that can affect infants and children, it is all too easy to convey the impression that they live continuously on the brink of disaster. Obviously this is not true; a great majority of children get through these early years without any kind of serious illness. Certainly parents should be alert to the possibility of illness striking their child, and certainly a sensible program of preventive medical care should be a regular part of every child's early years. But children should not be smothered with overprotection; they must be allowed freedom to grow and explore—and freedom always involves certain risks. Trouble should not be ignored, but neither should it be borrowed.

A happy medium can be achieved with a close rapport between the parents of a child and the physician or clinic overseeing the child's health care. Visits may become fewer and farther apart as the child grows older, but they should never be completely eliminated or viewed as necessary only in emergencies. A child, like an adult, requires periodic health checkups. These visits serve an important dual purpose: they provide an opportunity for the parents to raise questions about the child's development and behavior and learn those commonsense rules that are necessary if they are to assume their share of responsibility in caring for the child, both in sickness and in health; and they provide the doctor an opportunity to keep abreast of the child's growth and development and thus be in a better position to advise the parents and treat swiftly and effectively any illness that might arise.

Adolescence and How to Live with It

With the exception of minor infections and injuries, and perhaps visual or dental problems that need corrective treatment, the late childhood years usually require little in the way of medical care. What is more, this period of exceptionally good health extends through the age of adolescence and physical maturation and, for the most part, right on into young adulthood. It is not at all uncommon for a boy or girl to go all the way from the age of seven or eight to the age of twenty-five without once darkening a doctor's door. In a way this is unfortunate, not because good health during these years is the rule rather than the exception, but rather because the young person tends to lose contact with the family doctor at a time when maintaining a line of communication, however frail, with some familiar and respected, yet impartial or "outside," adult can be of enormous value both to him and to his parents.

The fact is that the interval from late childhood through adolescence and early maturity, while largely free of physical illness, is nevertheless an extremely awkward, distressing and conflict-torn time of life. It is a time when young people are subjected to some of the most difficult emotional stresses that they will ever encounter without, in many cases, the intellectual and emotional experience necessary to handle them. It is a time when they have to adjust to startling physical and psychological changes largely by experimentation and through the painful process of trial and error. It is a time when many of the basic urges that motivate all mature human

beings—the search for identity, the need for physical independence, and the desires for self-determination, direct sexual expression, and adult respect and responsibility—make their first appearance. The adolescent no longer wants to be treated like a child, but he is reluctant to leave the security, dependence and irresponsibility of childhood behind. Yet when he tries to behave like an adult, he may run into direct conflict with his parents' values and with community customs and standards. On one hand he is told to "grow up," and on the other that he is "growing up too fast." No wonder adolescence is one of the most trying times of life.

In recent years it appears that there has been a marked increase in the separation or alienation of young people from their parents and from the conventional values, rules and prohibitions of adult society. A generation gap, surely, but today that gap seems wider than ever before. Today's parents who remember their adolescent years can find nothing comparable in their own experience. They did not smoke marijuana, listen to deafening and incomprehensible music, experiment with sex at the age of thirteen, grow beards and long hair, dress in rags and patches, and become actively involved in social and political causes. They criticized their parents, but they did not preach to them; they rebelled in small ways, but they did not revolt. The world has changed drastically in the last few years, and nowhere are those changes more evident than among the younger generation. Yet when it comes to the period of adolescence itself, there are those who say things have not really changed all that much. The music is different, but the theme is the same; styles may vary from generation to generation, but the substance remains. Adolescence is the bridge between childhood and maturity, and it can be crossed in a variety of ways. There is no way to get around it, and problems and conflicts are almost inevitable.

The fact remains, however, that many of these problems, and the intensity of the conflict, could be eased, or even by-passed, if both the older and the younger generations paused at some point to consider just what adolescence really is. In essence, it is that brief span of perhaps five or six years during which the child becomes an adult, physically, psychologically and socially. The physical changes of puberty come first, while intellectual and emotional maturity are slower to develop. A lot of ground must be covered, and it is very rocky ground, for all these changes proceed by fits and starts and are often reflected in completely unpredictable patterns of behavior. As trying as this transitional period may seem to parents, it is even more difficult for the teen-ager, and the need for parental love, patience, support and understanding is never greater.

The Problem of Puberty

Puberty can be defined simply as the process of sexual maturation, and it may begin as early as age nine (on rare occasions even earlier) or may be delayed as long as age fourteen or fifteen. These extremes are the exception, however; in general, puberty in males begins by age eleven and a half or twelve, and in girls often slightly earlier, perhaps by age eleven. The changes that accompany puberty do not occur overnight, however; whatever the age they begin, they occur gradually and continue over a period ranging from two to five years.

There is no mistaking these changes when they begin, because they are emotional and social as well as physical. Prior to puberty there is a period of segregation of the sexes, but without any particular sexual content. Boys tend to favor each other's company in their activities and in general regard girls with teasing or scorn.

Girls tend toward close friendships with other girls and quite seriously believe that they dislike boys. Even so, this prepubertal period is also characterized by a certain amount of curiosity about the sexual structure of the opposite sex, either clandestinely when concealment has always been the rule at home, or more openly when the family has not made an issue of sexual differences and where casual nudity, at appropriate times and places, has been permitted. In all probability it makes little difference, since boys and girls usually satisfy their curiosity one way or another regardless of family attitudes, and it is the wise parent who accepts this fact philosophically and takes great care to react to this basically "nonsexual" exploration with as little anxiety or fuss as possible. To subject the child to feelings of shame and guilt or fears of punishment for a perfectly natural curiosity may cause irreparable psychological damage.

With the onset of puberty, however, boys and girls begin to display a pronounced and obviously sexual interest in each other. Puberty itself is marked by three striking changes, all occurring more or less simultaneously: the growth and development of the sexual organs, an acceleration of overall physical growth, and the appearance of the so-called *secondary sex characteristics*. In the male there is a marked enlargement of the penis and testes, the appearance of pubic and axillary hair (and, somewhat later, facial hair); an enlargement of the larynx which causes the voice to "crack" and finally drop to a lower register; generalized muscular development and an increase in stature, sometimes as much as four or five inches in a single year; the development of a ravenous appetite; the rather sudden appearance of an overwhelming degree of body odor; and, frequently, the occurrence of unpredictable erections along with the ability to ejaculate either by masturbation or stimulated by sexual fantasies.

In the female the most striking and obvious change at the time of puberty is the onset of menstruation. Even today there are girls so ill prepared for the sudden appearance of vaginal bleeding that they are both frightened and embarrassed by it, reactions that are all the more unfortunate considering that they are unnecessary. By the time a girl is nine, she is old enough to understand that changes related to her sex may be expected, and she can be introduced to the idea that she will sooner or later begin menstruating by casual and matter-of-fact discussions, perhaps related to her mother's menstruation. One simple means of broaching such a discussion could be the purchase of a sanitary belt and pads for the girl, to be kept in her dresser in anticipation of the onset of menses. The mother should point out that menstrual flow may be minimal or irregular during the first year or so, and the girl can be forewarned that early menstrual periods may be heralded by some degree of crampy abdominal discomfort; she can also be forewarned that she may be unable to participate in certain activities, such as swimming, during menstrual periods. Care should be taken, however, not to overemphasize these negative aspects. The amount of discomfort and disability related to menstruation is to a large degree determined by the girl's mental attitudes and expectations, and the child who is taught that menstruation is a painful, distressing experience may find it to be just that. Thus it is important that the mother present menstruation as a normal part of growing up, an encouraging sign that the girl is becoming a woman, rather than as a "curse."

Other changes in the female at the time of puberty are somewhat more subtle. Pubic and axillary hair appear, and there is the beginning of breast development, sometimes quite suddenly. Increase in stature is not so marked as in the male, but the pelvis broadens and there is the appearance of a normal padding of fat in a female distribution throughout the body. There is also an increase in emotional lability or changeability which may or may not correspond with menstrual periods; like the boy, the girl has a new awareness of her own sexuality, and she, too, may masturbate.

In both sexes puberty is marked with increasing oiliness and porosity of the skin with accompanying acne. (*See* p. 393.) Increased oiliness of the hair is also common, and pubertal children should be encouraged to establish patterns of careful personal hygiene, including frequent shampooing. This is a time when showering is often preferred to tub bathing, a perfectly acceptable change so long as bathing in the shower is done thoroughly. The appetite increases at this time, and there is a real threat of obesity in some teen-agers, a condition that can be highly threatening to the young person's self-image, the idealized picture of himself that he develops and carries throughout adolescence. Usually this self-image is so strong that teen-agers will willingly work at taming acne and maintaining cleanliness and personal hygiene, as long as parents do not make such an overriding issue of it that the teen-ager takes it as a point of rebellion. Finally, parents should at least unobtrusively observe the physical changes that occur in order to be aware of any real abnormality—puberty delayed beyond the normal expected age limits, for example, excessive weight gain or abnormalities in the development of secondary sex characteristics that might suggest some hormonal disfunction. Any question of possible abnormality should be called to a doctor's attention, but this should be done, if it is necessary, without any undue fuss or emphasis that might alarm the teen-ager unnecessarily.

Puberty is accompanied by emotional and psychological changes that are often even more marked than the physical changes. In both sexes there are sudden "crushes" or infatuations with others (often somewhat older) of the opposite sex. These episodes tend to worry parents considerably, perhaps because of the unexpected *intensity* of emotion in such relationships; yet such liaisons are, in fact, a natural and useful step toward a healthy polarization of the sexes, and will usually take care of themselves with little more than concerned interest on the part of the parents. Sometimes more disturbing are similar infatuations that may occur with older members of the same sex, more commonly among girls than boys. Parents often fear that such relationships signify emerging homosexuality and overreact to them, when in fact they usually represent nothing more than the teen-ager's exploration of mature emotional relationships on the relatively "safe ground" of the same sex in preparation for moving into the comparatively unknown—and slightly frightening—region of heterosexual relationships. If such an infatuation seems to persist more than a few months, or if the pattern seems to repeat itself, parents should certainly seek the advice of a trusted family counselor such as the family physician, but in most cases such liaisons are short-lived and comfortably terminated by the teen-ager's own initiative.

Other psychological changes are very marked during puberty and early adolescence. In boys these often take the form of exaggerated rebelliousness, rejecting or challenging of parental authority, and increased aggressiveness or even hostility toward siblings, parents, teachers, school authorities, or the world in general. In addition adolescent boys tend to display secretiveness, an increased desire for privacy, recklessness, sloppiness of dress or manners, and often an imperiousness of demands that can be highly irritating to those around them. Many of these patterns of behavior represent nothing more grave than the sense of insecurity and isolation that the boy feels at this time. There must, of course, be some degree of control exercised by the parents over such moods and attitudes, but parents must also learn not to accept these manifestations entirely at face value. The boy who rages violently and noisily against the limitations placed upon his actions one minute will—quite literally—forget his rage ten minutes later and, paradoxically, assume that his parents have forgotten it also. Girls, in general, are likely to be somewhat more passive, obedient and tractable, but they too can exhibit rebelliousness and secretive behavior, and may be far more moody and emotionally changeable than boys. Both sexes begin to "run with the pack," seeking approval of their peer group rather than their parents. They usually devise styles of dress and language all their own; they may display extremes of self-consciousness and sensitivity; and they continually participate in sexual jousting and experimentation, endure "crushes," go "steady" with a different partner every month, engage in hero worship, take up moral or political causes, and struggle constantly to come to terms with their own sexuality and libido—all manifestations of a harrowing emotional search to find out who they are, and where and to whom they belong.

Parents often feel totally left out of this struggle—and to a large extent they should be, for this is an interval when adolescents must come to terms with their developing maturity at their own pace and in their own ways. It is not a time for parents to abdicate, however, because limits must be set on behavior, and mature guidance must be imposed, where necessary, even when it is not specifically sought. Parents should be particularly alert for behavioral patterns that may signal real trouble. Such grossly abnormal behavior as exaggerated withdrawal from social situations, continuing hostility toward brothers and sisters, or marked underachievement at school may suggest the emergence of a serious psychological maladjustment or even a mental disorder, and such patterns should be discussed with a family doctor, a child guidance specialist or a psychiatrist. Parents must be aware that problems of drug experimentation or even addiction may appear at this time, and should be alert at least to the possibility of behavioral patterns that may signal the emergence of homosexual tendencies, delinquency, or other patterns of antisocial or self-destructive behavior. In most families such gross maladjustments are the exception rather than the rule, and parents can reasonably expect their teen-aged children to adhere, at least basically, to their own standards of honesty and civilized behavior, but exceptions can occur in any family, and can often be prevented by early detection and wise parental guidance, aided where necessary by professional counsel.

For many parents, however, commonsense understanding of certain perfectly normal phenomena that characterize adolescence can relieve a vast amount of unnecessary worry and conflict. Some of these phenomena have to do with the child's sexual development, some with his social development, but all are of significant importance.

Masturbation. There are few concerns more sensitive to both parents and adolescents—or more shrouded with misinformation and needless distress—than masturbation, the stimulation of the genitals to orgasm, usually without a partner, by manipulation, friction or any other means short of sexual intercourse. Even though no other sexual activity is more universally practiced, masturbation has been openly condemned since the very beginning of our culture, and even today is still widely regarded (if not spoken of) as "the solitary vice." And reinforcing these attitudes are any number of perfectly ridiculous beliefs that masturbation causes blindness or insanity, pimples or a "coarse skin," or even enlargement of the genitals or premature loss of libido—all frightening ideas, and all entirely without any basis in truth. But perhaps the most destructive of all these myths is the moralistic contention that masturbation somehow is shameful, dirty, corrupt and perverted.

Where, in all these fictions, are the facts? First, there is the fact that masturbation in our culture is practiced by *virtually everyone* at some time during his or her sexual development and, even later, during sexual maturity. Second, masturbation is utterly harmless, both physically and psychologically, as long as it does not result in actual abuse of the genitals and is not arbitrarily associated with fear, shame and guilt. Granted that the practice of masturbation in adulthood to the exclusion of sexual relations with a consenting partner is a pity and may very well represent a form of neurotic behavior, but it is still harmless, and masturbation is a symptom of the neurosis, not the cause.

In point of fact, masturbation has some very positive and beneficial qualities. Aside from being a simple and undemanding source of physical pleasure, it can provide adolescents with a safe, unthreatening means of discovering their bodies' natural, healthy capabilities for sexual pleasure in private and at their own pace. It can also provide safe and private means for exploring both the normal and the less normal modes of sexuality by means of fantasy; for example, the sexual aspects of sadism, masochism, homosexuality, sodomy or incest can be sampled and found wanting (or at least uninteresting) through masturbatory fantasies without the need or the desire for further experimentation. Above all, masturbation can provide a safe and harmless release for sexual pressures which, by reason of age, conviction or social taboos, cannot find acceptable expression through the more direct avenue of sexual intercourse. In this same re-

gard, the necking or petting that is indulged in as a substitute (rather than a prelude) for intercourse is a normal and healthy attempt to satisfy urgent needs for intimacy and to find a safe outlet for sexual tensions without yet moving into the no man's land of full sexual contact.

Obviously any change in social attitude toward masturbation must depend upon the parents' understanding and realistic acceptance of a normal human practice. Of course there are limits to what is acceptable and what is not; an adolescent should not be permitted to engage in masturbation any time, any place or in any company. Masturbation is only a small part of a whole complex of often confusing and unpredictable patterns of adolescent sexual behavior, and the parents who realize this and who can discuss it with their children are well on their way to easing their own apprehensions and giving their children the understanding and support they need in this difficult area. No particular issue need be made of it, other than to suggest discretion and moderation. Even if parents cannot manage this degree of frankness in an open discussion with their children, they can at least keep their prejudices to themselves and stop perpetuating false and destructive ideas. Adolescents have enough troublesome problems and conflicts to deal with without the added burden of shame and guilt about masturbation. Parents who can pass it off as a normal and not terribly important part of growing up will do their children a favor without parallel.

The Problems of Sex Education

Surely one of the most difficult problems facing both parents and their children during the adolescent years is the question of sex education. Today's youth gather information about sex from a variety of different sources: from discussion with friends, from books, pictures and movies, from school programs on sex education, and lastly—in too few cases—from their parents. Some of these sources are perfectly reliable and valid, but in the absence of accurate information the sexual naïveté and even ignorance of teen-agers can be truly appalling and potentially tragic. All too often it is the parents' fault, especially when they have met every question about sex from childhood on with tight-lipped silence or stern disapproval, forcing their children to rely on the fancies and folklore of their contemporaries. But the children themselves may also be at fault, because as they grow older it is all too common for them to assume cockily that they know it all and that there is nothing they need to be taught. Yet the recent staggering increase in teen-age pregnancies and abortions, not to mention the resurgence of venereal disease among that age group in almost epidemic proportions, offers sad evidence to the contrary.

Obviously sex education is the only answer, and it must begin in the home. But many parents fail to recognize two very important facts: first, that we all are essentially sexual beings, and that sexual curiosity and experimentation begin at a very early age; and second, that sexual behavior and attitudes are *not* somehow instinctive and intuitive; they are learned—usually from the parents themselves. Even those parents who have never uttered the word "sex," or those who are obviously mistrustful or apprehensive about their own and their children's sexuality, set an example in the home to which their children will almost inevitably conform, or against which they will ultimately rebel. To complicate the problem even further, sex education in the home is not merely a question of supplying the right facts. Sex is much more than physical know-how; to be fully healthy and mutually rewarding and constructive, it must exist in an atmosphere of love, tenderness and consideration, and this example, too, is set by the parents whether sex is openly discussed in the home or not. How much better, then, for parents to assume this inescapable responsibility willingly and knowledgeably.

Yet many parents do not really know just where to start. They may (very wisely) have agreed to meet awkward questions from their children with casual frankness, yet when the questions turn up, without fanfare in the middle of dinner, the tendency is, in a wave of embarrassment, to pass them off with a "Let's not talk about that now," which the child interprets, with considerable insight, to mean: "Let's not talk about that, period." And when circumstances are right for private discussion, it may seem too

premeditated or artificial, embarrassing to both parent and child. Yet if a sympathetic rapport is not established between parent and child when he first begins to ask questions about sex, he will not come back for help and information when he grows older. Thus the best parents can do is to wait for clues. It is ridiculous, of course, to bombard a child with information that he cannot yet understand, but if a question *must* be postponed, it should not be postponed indefinitely. *Any* expression of interest or curiosity from a child, *any* question or confusion about social customs such as dating or "going steady" that seems to worry an adolescent, can provide an opening for frank discussion of sexual feelings and behavior. Parents are sometimes astonished about how much their teen-aged children already know, but they should never assume that some other person or agency has done their job for them; it is first and foremost their own responsibility. This does not mean that they should oppose sex education in the schools. Far from it. These programs can, and should, serve as an important adjunct to their instruction, particularly in the areas of the physiology of sex and the dangers of venereal disease. (*See* p. 243.) But books and lectures cannot convey two equally important aspects of sex education: the wisdom that comes only from experience, and a framework of personal values and social standards that must govern all forms of sexual expression. These can come only from the parents, not in angry recriminations and repressive prohibitions after the fact, but in frank and sympathetic discussions before a problem arises, and not in moralistic pronouncements, but in words and deeds that provide tangible, firsthand evidence of the validity of moral standards.

Many parents, in the light of today's relaxing moral standards, feel embarrassed or challenged if they express any opinions at all, fearing that they will appear hopelessly "square" in the eyes of their children. Yet it is vitally important, precisely because of changing standards, that parents communicate directly to their children these aspects of behavior that they consider right and wrong, acceptable or unacceptable, and an attitude of honesty and personal conviction in matters of sex can serve to good advantage.

Open discussion also provides parents with the opportunity to make clear *why* they feel that certain standards of sexual behavior are necessary. Teen-age friendships, dating and "going steady" are normal, necessary adjuncts to emotional development—but limits must be set. Teenagers can understand clearly that such sexual experiments as necking or petting, while acceptable to a point, can easily get out of hand. They can understand that their emotions and developing sexual urges can easily escape from control, and that certain prohibitions are necessary simply to protect them from their own behavior until they gain more experience in controlling themselves. Teen-agers can be taught sufficient respect for themselves and their bodies that they will resist the dangerous temptations of promiscuous behavior or premature intercourse, not because parents forbid it but because the images they have developed of themselves forbid it. Discussions of birth control, venereal disease, and the hazards of sexual experimentation can be effective only if they are presented within the framework of meaningful moral standards. Obviously, honest discussion and realistic restrictions on the teen-ager's behavior *before* trouble occurs are preferable—but mistakes are often made, and help and support from the parents at such times, free from useless and painful recriminations, may determine whether a mistake sets a pattern and permanently scars a life, or whether it becomes an episode from which the teen-ager may hopefully learn or even profit. Parents cannot successfully maintain an image of omniscience during this period, but they can understand that their children are human, too.

The Problem of Authority

Paradoxically, no matter how often they complain about "old-fashioned," "silly" and "pointless" parental rules and regulations, not only in regard to sex but in other areas as well, adolescents actually need and actively seek an authority to establish just and reasonable guidelines for their behavior. In fact, to an adolescent, there is no abandonment more complete than that of parents who react with total permissiveness, which is not far from indifference, or who avoid or neglect setting acceptable and consistent standards of behavior.

This is not something that an adolescent is likely to admit, or even to be consciously aware of. Indeed, as far as his conscious behavior is concerned, the main thrust of virtually everything he does is in the direction of questioning authority and throwing off dependence on his family in an attempt to establish his own identity and independence. Yet he is not quite ready to trust himself as an authority; teen-age boys as well as girls want desperately to "belong," and they conform slavishly to the styles of dress and behavior of their adolescent contemporaries. Peer group approval is no substitute, however, for parental authority, and most teen-agers know it. For their part, parents must recognize that this kind of conformity is necessary to the teen-ager; but freedom is not synonymous with license, nor independence with irresponsibility.

In essence, teen-agers want to enjoy adult privileges, or at least their interpretation of those privileges, without accepting adult responsibility for them and without yet possessing the mature judgment necessary to choose wisely among a bewildering variety of alternatives. Although they like to feel that they could be self-sufficient if necessary, they rely upon being fed, clothed and sheltered by their families, they count on using their allowances or money they have earned for luxuries or pleasures, not necessities, and above all, although unconsciously, they depend heavily on the love, concern, interest, help and protection of their parents, in the background, perhaps, but there when they are needed.

The adolescent years are packed with problems and difficult decisions for the teen-ager, boy or girl. Not only must adolescents adjust to new feelings about themselves and others, they must also begin to make choices about how, and with whom, they would like to spend the rest of their lives. Naturally they resent having these decisions made for them and rammed down their throats by parents who do not trust them or who are determined that their own needs and ambitions, not their children's, are to be served. Equally unfortunate are those parents who relinquish their authority completely. They often force their children into more and more extreme forms of rebellious behavior in an attempt to see just when their parents will begin to care. The children are left with no standards by which to measure parental acceptance and approval, which is extremely important to them, and they are compelled to make all the crucial decisions, often the wrong decisions, completely on their own.

Clearly, the solution to the problem of authority rests in compromise, not only in the realm of establishing realistic, consistent and just standards of personal behavior, but also in setting forth equally realistic expectations for both the present and the future, not for the parents' benefit, but for the teen-ager's. Parents must also be prepared to have even the most flexible guidelines tested by the energetic, ingenious teen-ager who, given an inch, will invariably try to take a mile. But parental authority is not an absolute; if it is truly effective, it will diminish as the teen-ager demonstrates his ability to assume responsibility for himself. Parents who never learn to trust their children usually have their worst fears realized. Teen-agers complain, often with validity, that they are never "given a chance" to prove their increased maturity or improved judgment, that some foolish transgression at the age of thirteen is still being "held against them" at the age of sixteen. Certainly the teen-ager must be given the benefit of the doubt; of course, he will make mistakes, but making the wrong decision, and learning to accept the responsibility for it, is an important lesson in growing up. The emphasis of parental authority, however, should not be exclusively on the mistakes, nor should the teen-ager be compelled to demonstrate daily how grown-up he is. All too many parents tend to punish transgressions, however minor, with much fuss and fanfare while virtually ignoring evidence of good judgment or maturity on the grounds that "it was the least they could expect." This sort of negative approach can be extremely discouraging to the adolescent. A far more positive and constructive approach is to acknowledge and reward mature and responsible behavior generously, and confine punishment and restriction of privileges to specific transgressions. Whatever the restriction, however, the teen-ager

should know about it in advance, and understand the reasons for it; and when it is administered fairly, and in the spirit of helpfulness rather than retribution, the teen-ager will continue to respect parental authority and try to live up to his parents' expectations. Applying a single standard to their own as well as to their children's behavior is probably as vital as anything else in maintaining the adolescent's respect. All too many parents expect their children to admit their misjudgments, acknowledge their failures and recognize their foolish decisions, yet adamantly refuse to do so themselves when occasions warrant. Parental authority cannot survive the merest suspicion of hypocrisy. Parents who demand that their children "do as we say, not as we do" are fighting a losing battle.

There is no easy solution to the problem of authority; obviously every situation is unique. A certain amount of conflict between parent and teen-ager is inevitable, but certain commonsense things can greatly reduce its magnitude. For example, parents can easily dispense with a multitude of petty and essentially pointless restrictions. Bizarre eating habits can be a source of almost endless bickering, but there has never yet been a teen-ager who has starved to death or even suffered serious malnutrition as a result of going without breakfast or lunch, snacking in midafternoon, gorging at dinnertime and raiding the refrigerator at bedtime. Similarly, there should be no needless restrictions on how teen-agers dress and wear their hair. The often bizarre styles of the younger generation are conceived in part as an attempt to establish individuality, which is important to a teen-ager, and in part simply to get a rise out of the adults. Viewed in this light they can be seen merely as the passing fancies that they usually are. Many other pointless restrictions can be eased on the grounds—expressed specifically in those terms—that the teen-ager is old enough to decide these things for himself. Indeed, expressing and demonstrating confidence in the teen-ager's attempts to mature is more useful than a thousand meaningless limitations. Granting adult privileges before they have been asked for can relieve a teen-ager of the feeling that he must constantly fight for every inch. But letting him know that responsible and mature behavior is expected in really important matters, and then rewarding it with a further extension of privilege, will help maintain his own security as well as provide him with meaningful goals. Finally, and above all else, keeping the lines of communication open is absolutely essential, for this constitutes a special problem in itself.

The Problem of Communication

There is an odd idea harbored by both parents and adolescents that the problem of communication as it is reflected today in the mistrust and misunderstanding that characterizes the much-publicized "generation gap" is something completely new and different. Nothing could be further from the truth. Generation gaps have existed for centuries, probably since the concept of the family first took form, but each new gap seems somehow wider than before. Parents forget that they once challenged their own parents' authority; they forget, confronted by a difficult teen-ager, how difficult they must have been at that age. Differences of thought, opinion and behavior are almost inevitable between generations simply because time does not stand still, and there can be no progress without change. True, today's changes seem more rapid and far-reaching than ever before. The ideas and beliefs, the standards of sexual and social behavior, the aspirations and goals that played such an important part in the older generation's upbringing have been challenged and even cast off by their sons and daughters. Naturally this is alarming to most parents; it can even be worrisome if their sons and daughters share their beliefs and goals but choose to express or pursue them in their own way. Paradoxically, parents have devoted years of love and care to give their children the education and freedom that will enable them to choose their own course through life, and then they object when their children exercise that privilege.

This is not to say that parents are always wrong, and their children always right. Far from it. Both sides of the generation gap are capable of making very serious mistakes, no matter how well intentioned. And perhaps the most serious is neglecting, or even cutting, the lines of communication that must exist in every family. It usually happens gradually, and usually both sides are to blame; the teen-ager feels his parents just do not "understand," and the parents feel that their son or daughter "simply will not listen to reason." Both are probably right, but that does not relieve either of the responsibility to *try* to listen and to understand. Ideally an atmosphere of love, trust and mutual respect should be built up between the generations from childhood on that will keep the lines of communication open. But even under ideal circumstances, adolescence is a particularly trying time. Although it is perhaps inevitable that parents and children will go their separate ways, there is no need for sullen silences, hostility, anger or displays of brute authority. They merely aggravate what might have been a minor difference of opinion into a major rebellion or even a complete break when communication is no longer possible, and both parents and teen-agers find themselves in a frightening situation that neither wants or can handle.

It is largely up to the parents to keep the lines of communication open in the family. They should have greater wisdom, experience and understanding—and if they can recall, they went through adolescence themselves once. It is all new to the teen-ager, and usually he begins to spend less and less time with his family at that age, preferring instead the company and activities of his own friends. That is why it is imperative that parents take every opportunity their children provide, and provide opportunities themselves, to exchange ideas and opinions, or simply to "keep in touch." There is no reason why dinner table conversations should be confined to "Don't gobble your food" or "Pass the butter, please." Too many parents and children only really talk when some problem arises, and by then it is often too late for calm and rational conversation. Frank and open discussion on a wide variety of topics keeps the lines of communication open, and lets each side know just where the other stands. Of course special problems will always arise, but then the teen-ager will not be afraid to express his views and come to his parents for help and advice. And the parents who really know how their teen-age sons or daughters feel, what is important to them and why, can provide the support, understanding and advice that they need.

In the long run, successful communication makes compromise possible, and the secret of safe passage through the stormy years of adolescence, more than anything else, is a willingness and ability to compromise, to find some middle ground upon which both parent and adolescent can agree, at least temporarily, even if it is only to "agree to disagree." Parents are often pleasantly surprised by their teen-aged children, who have no trouble communicating with their peers,

even if their language is somewhat unusual. The ill-mannered and lazy boy or girl suddenly becomes a model of decorum and industry as soon as he or she leaves the house. Both parents and children have many sides to their personalities, and communication is the only way they can be explored and appreciated. Inevitably, the family situation is charged with emotion, particularly during adolescence, but that emotion need not be destructive. In fact, with meaningful communication and compromise, family ties will survive, and when the journey through adolescence is over, the generations can come together again as mature adults.

The Prime Years

After successfully navigating the shoals of adolescence, the average young man or woman enters a prolonged period of life which can be almost completely free of serious health problems. We often speak of this period as "the prime years," and the term is singularly appropriate, for during young adulthood, the body is strong and fully mature, yet still youthful, and as long as reasonable attention is paid to health care, there are relatively few illnesses that pose serious threats. The insecurities, uncertainties and identity crises of adolescence have also been left behind, replaced by a sense of physical and emotional well-being, a sense of security in one's identity as a capable and mature adult, and a sense of confidence in one's healthy capacity to meet and overcome the challenges of life.

The prime years are not, however, all sunshine and light. With maturity comes the necessity to accept responsibility, not only for oneself, but as a husband or wife, as a parent in the family unit, and as a useful member of society as a whole. The choices that confront young adults, the decisions that they may make, are certainly as momentous and far-reaching as any they will ever face. They must decide what they will do for a living, where and how they will live, and, above all, with whom. Sexual maturity can pose a problem in itself, both within and outside the confines of marriage, and with marriage come the difficult problems of learning to live with a husband or wife, and the equally difficult decisions related to bringing children into the world. All too often these important decisions seem almost accidental, or are made

selfishly or impetuously without full awareness of their consequences. The fault usually lies in the fact that while the young adult may be physically mature, emotional and intellectual maturity come only with added years of learning and experience. With intelligence and foresight, however, the young adult can expect a full measure of health and happiness during the prime years and, at the same time, lay the groundwork for a long and rewarding lifetime.

Physical and Sexual Maturation

Physical and sexual maturity come at different times for different people; there is no set schedule, nor do men and women follow precisely the same developmental track. For both sexes full physical growth may be achieved anywhere from the age of fourteen or fifteen on to the early twenties, with the age of eighteen as a median. Even beyond this young men will continue to develop musculature up to a peak level in the early twenties. Although sexual maturity is technically achieved during puberty, between ages eleven and fourteen, young males are generally more capable of fertilizing an ovum in these early pubertal years than females are capable of becoming pregnant. While it is possible for a girl to conceive at the time of her first ovulation, a regular pattern of mature ovulation is not usually established until some years later. Breast development and other secondary sex characteristics may not reach the maximum until age sixteen, and in most young women the libido, or sex drive, and the capacity to enjoy sexual relations and achieve orgasm develop rather slowly and steadily from that age on to a peak in the mid-thirties. The young man's sex drive is generally more intense and more urgent in his middle and late teens, reaching a peak in the early twenties and then leveling off and beginning to taper gradually from that point on, although he is unlikely to become aware of any lessening of active sex interest until he reaches his forties or fifties.

Sexual maturity, however, involves a great deal more than physical capabilities; it inevitably gives rise to the difficult problems surrounding mature and responsible sexual behavior. Every young adult, male or female, must ultimately decide for himself how he will behave as a person, what standards he will adhere to, what he considers morally right or wrong, acceptable or inacceptable. It is not appropriate here to enter into the many complex factors upon which such decisions are based. It is worth mentioning, however, that the changes in social attitudes and acceptable patterns of behavior about which we read so frequently today, the wave of social and sexual permissiveness which seems to prevail and which some gloomily contend marks a new age of moral degeneracy in our society, may in fact be far more apparent than real. Beyond question there is more openness about premarital sexual experimentation among young people, for example, than was the case a generation ago. Certainly connubial arrangements made outside of marriage seem to be more frequent than ever before, and even more socially acceptable. And certainly there is a new sense of freedom from at least one of the deterrents to premarital sexual relations—the fear of pregnancy—as a result of the availability of highly reliable means of contraception. But whether all of these new trends really add up to a significant change in the way young people actually conduct their lives is seriously open to question. Among a minority of young people, undoubtedly, the "new morality" is very real. But many sociologists, physicians and psychologists doubt that any widespread change has taken place at all. True, all forms of sexual behavior are more openly and knowledgeably discussed among the young; for many sex is no longer a dirty word and sexual behavior no

longer a guilty secret. This, surely, is an important change, but the standards that govern responsible sexual behavior have not changed significantly, and with knowledge and understanding, young people may very well be better equipped than ever before to make the right decisions about their own behavior.

It is not difficult to define sexual behavior in the abstract. Among other things, it is the necessary means of ensuring the reproduction of the species, a completely normal human activity, a way to release physical and psychological tensions, and a source of intense pleasure and satisfaction. It is far more difficult, however, to define precisely what mature, responsible or even "healthy" sexual behavior involves. Inevitably, any such definition will be clouded by age-old social attitudes, legal limitations and personal prejudices. These considerations aside for the moment, many authorities have come to agree that the *motivation* behind sexual behavior is of primary importance. Responsible sexual behavior is motivated by feelings of love, tenderness, respect and consideration. Irresponsible and immature sexual behavior is motivated by feelings of anxiety, insecurity, hostility and the need for psychological reassurance or simple physical release. In short, responsible sexual behavior is a shared experience in which physical and emotional pleasure is both given and received. Obviously, then, if it is indiscriminate, promiscuous or selfish, it becomes little more than an unhealthy and often damaging neurotic compulsion.

Sex has always been the biological basis of male-female relationships, whether inside or outside of marriage, and it is perhaps hard to believe that the concept of "love" as the major criterion by which the selection of a sexual or a marital partner should be made is a comparatively recent one in human society. For centuries in most cultures (and in a great many even today), marriage was a practical business arrangement, worked out by those older and supposedly wiser than the participants, in which sexual availability was merely part of the bargain. Of course, in our modern Western society love includes mutual sexual attraction; in fàct, that is where it may begin in a relationship, and when sexual attraction starts to subside that is where the relationship may end. But love implies much more than sex; it involves the complete sharing not only of a bed but of every other aspect of daily living. It implies mutual trust and respect, shared beliefs and ideals, ambitions and goals. It also implies companionship; few people are capable of going through life completely on their own and even fewer desire to. A truly loving relationship must make room for two quite separate and individual identities; yet at the same time its participants must be able to achieve much more together than they could alone.

It has often been said that sex is easy; it is love that is so difficult. If there is a drawback to the increasing sexual sophistication among teenagers and young adults today, to relaxing moral standards and to the availability of effective contraceptives, it is the threat that sexual relations may come to be regarded as little more than a casual social activity. No idea could be more dangerous or further from the truth. Quite the contrary; sex is possibly the single most socially and emotionally loaded activity in which a human being can engage. Although it can be a continuing source of pleasure and fulfillment in a relationship, it can also be the source of inordinate pain and frustration. Irresponsible sexual behavior can have destructive long-range consequences not only in terms of creating an unwanted pregnancy, forcing a marriage where love does not exist or driving a woman to the extreme of abortion, but also—perhaps even worse—in terms of bringing an unwanted and unloved child into the world. Even if every precaution is taken to prevent conception, sex is still a powerful binding force between a man and a woman, and sex without love can have profound psychological consequences on both partners, sometimes permanently affecting their attitude toward themselves and their ability to trust and love others.

In short, *sex matters* whatever the changing social and moral circumstances, and no young adult can be said to be truly mature until he or she has come to understand this, has learned to check potentially destructive sexual impulses and channel them into more constructive outlets, and

can enter into and sustain a complete human relationship, not merely a sexual one.

These criteria apply equally, of course, to adults of every age, but for the young adult to whom both sex and human relationships may be quite new, and whose sexual drives are extremely intense, the problem of responsible sexual behavior can be very difficult indeed. Young people often ask, "How can we tell we're in love if we don't have sex?" and, unfortunately, there is no easy answer. Ideally, sex and love should be inseparable, but often one may precede the other; inevitably there will be some experimentation, and some mistakes. The real danger, however, is not in premarital intercourse per se—that is a decision that can be made only by the individuals most involved—but in considering sex selfishly as an end in itself, or as a casual social encounter, an obligation, a game, or even a weapon to influence the course of a relationship. The adolescent or young adult who enters into a sexual relationship for "kicks," or because "everyone else does it," or even because he or she is "swept away" by physical attraction, all too often discovers eventually that momentary sexual satisfaction can in no way measure up to the satisfactions of a complete human relationship.

Sexual intercourse is the most intimate form of human contact, and it cannot be considered lightly. In this regard, the sexual knowledge and awareness that seem to characterize today's younger generation can offer an unparalleled advantage. With the veils of secrecy, shame and ignorance lifted, a young couple can, and should, discuss their feelings about sex openly and frankly between themselves, and they can, and should be able to, ask their parents and trusted friends for their help and advice. Then, even though the decision must ultimately be their own, they can make it with their eyes wide open, fully aware of both the joys and the responsibilities that a mature sexual relationship entails.

Marriage

It is axiomatic that all marriages, even the most manifestly successful, have problems; the difference between one marriage and another lies not in the occurrence of problems but in their magnitude and the way they are handled. Nor are marital problems always necessarily a bad thing. Much as one may dislike storms, the dullest thing about a tropical paradise is the unremitting good weather. There are, however, some kinds of storms that are never desirable, and there are marital problems that can be profoundly disruptive or even fatal to a viable marriage relationship. Fortunately, certain of these problems can be anticipated, and in many cases the best time to detect and deal with them is *before,* not after, marriage.

The Decision to Marry. Although connubial relationships between young people outside of marriage are by no means uncommon today and are undertaken much more openly than they were a generation ago, often as a prelude to marriage, the formalization of marriage still involves physical, emotional, legal and material commitments that can be side-stepped in extramarital living arrangements. And whereas divorce is also by no means uncommon in our society, breaking up a marriage based on all these commitments is an exceedingly painful experience for both parties and, all too often, for the children they may have. Thus the decision to marry is one of the most profoundly important choices that young adults are ever called upon to make.

Among the many factors to be considered in making such a decision, the matter of age is of enormous importance. Statistics indicate beyond doubt that early marriages, undertaken in the late teens or very early twenties, before both partners are emotionally and intellectually mature, are by far the least likely to survive. All too often the very young couple, while physically mature, are still psychologically insecure, uncertain of their individual identities and goals, still basically selfish in their attitudes, and poorly equipped, as yet, to meet the mature demands and responsibilities of marriage. Such marriages are often based upon an emotional dependence that becomes a restrictive rather than a binding force as the couple begin to "grow apart," each developing and maturing along separate paths, discovering divergent interests and evolving

differing values—all aspects of normal emotional growth which should ideally be accomplished before marriage if it is to become a stable, permanently enriching relationship. Early marriages are also troubled by such material considerations as economic insecurity, disruption of the education of one or both partners, or immature attitudes toward the realities of living together. Above all, the mark of immaturity is clear in the frequency with which early-married couples rush into parenthood, with little consideration of the long-term responsibilities that raising a family entails.

Indeed, most of the major considerations that are basic to a wise decision for marriage are related to the question of emotional maturity. Sexual attraction is, of course, one important factor—but the couple should be mature enough to recognize that sexual attraction is not the same as love, and can prove to be a weak foundation for marriage if the relationship has no other supports. Ideally the marriage decision should be postponed until both partners are capable of considering the many other factors that are certain to be equally important, if not more so. One such factor is psychological compatibility—not merely the ability to "get along" together when the marriage is new, but the ability to provide mutual support, care and companionship during the many years ahead. Ideally, both partners should also share compatible attitudes, ideals, ambitions and goals in marriage, particularly parental goals, since there is scarcely any other area in which mature mutual understanding between prospective marriage partners is more important. Other considerations should include compatibility of religious, racial and cultural backgrounds, family attitudes toward the marriage, and sufficient financial security to make a marriage economically feasible. Above all, neither partner should allow external pressures to force a decision that he or she is not ready to make. The circumstances surrounding any marriage are perhaps never completely ideal, but both partners must be mature enough to make a realistic assessment of the problems that may arise, and with sincere and loving commitment be willing to work together toward their successful resolution.

Once the decision for marriage has been made, a thorough premarital physical examination for each of the prospective partners is very much to be desired. Most states require that premarital blood tests be done on both partners to rule out any possibility of untreated syphilis, a particularly important precaution because an unsuspected infection in the mother, or one transmitted to her before a pregnancy, can be passed on to the baby when a pregnancy occurs. But the premarital physical examination can and should have a broader purpose. It provides one means of ensuring that both partners are bringing healthy bodies to the marriage, and that no undetected disease or hereditary illness exists. If the examination of the woman reveals that the hymen might interfere with successful sexual relations, there is the opportunity to incise this membrane partially occluding the vagina, if the woman wishes, in a simple and painless procedure that can be done with a local anesthesia in the doctor's office. Finally, such an examination provides both the man and the woman an opportunity to discuss with their doctor such matters as sexual activities, personal hygiene and conception control, and to establish an avenue of professional counsel that can be invaluable when questions or problems surrounding physical or emotional adjustment or contemplated parenthood may arise.

Sexual Compatibility. Considering all that has been written about human sexuality in recent years, it is perhaps surprising how frequently sexual incompatibility emerges, even today, as a difficult and sometimes devastating physical and psychological problem in marriage. Any number of excellent and authoritative books are available which deal with the structure and function of the sex organs, the nature and means of sexual arousal and the techniques of sexual intercourse; the young couple contemplating marriage should ask their doctor to recommend the books that he considers particularly suitable and informative, no matter how sophisticated they consider themselves to be. The reason is simple: many of the problems of sexual adjustment that occur in marriage from the wedding night on actually result from little more than ignorance or misconceptions that lead the newly married couple

to expect too much too soon from their sexual relationship. It is amazing how many young people are prepared to explore and develop other aspects of their relationship slowly and patiently over a period of years, yet expect to achieve an ideal sexual adjustment overnight, and then are disappointed, puzzled, angry, frightened or distressed when this does not occur.

Such expectations, of course, are unrealistic. Sexual responses are just as complicated as any other form of human behavior, perhaps even more so, for an intimate sexual relationship involves two quite different people, each with his own needs, hopes, fantasies and expectations, and each with his own misconceptions, inhibitions, preferences and prejudices. All these personal factors must be patiently explored over a period of time before mutual satisfaction can be achieved. What is more, the distinct physical and psychological differences between men and women tend to make this process of mutual discovery and exploration more difficult at first, although more enriching in the long run. In the male sexual arousal is characteristically more swift and urgent than in the female, and at the same time more swiftly and completely relieved. In the female arousal is slower and more diffuse, as is her sexual release, both often dependent upon an atmosphere and feelings of confidence, intimacy and affection. In males the intensity of sexual arousal also tends to peak at an earlier age than in females; the woman's full capacity for sexual response may not be reached until she is in her early thirties. In practical terms, these and other differences between the sexes mean that mutually gratifying sexual behavior is by no means intuitive or instantaneous; it is a *learned response* that takes time, patience and understanding to achieve.

Many of the problems of sexual compatibility that come to a doctor's attention are due quite simply to a lack of understanding, or to impatience or selfishness on the part of one partner or the other. How frequently should a couple have intercourse? What positions are the most suitable? Which sexual preferences and practices are "normal" and which "abnormal" or "perverted"? Authorities of half a century ago, reflecting the restrictive moralistic attitudes and value judgments of their time, offered absolute answers to such questions; authorities today recognize that they can be answered only by the marital partners themselves. For example, it is known that there are no harmful health effects associated with *any* frequency of intercourse as long as it reflects the mutual desires and needs of both partners; harm can occur when one partner habitually inflicts his or her desires on the other, against the other's wishes or feelings—in short, when sexual invitation becomes a demand. The same may be said for decisions about techniques and practices; whatever is mutually gratifying to both partners can be considered "normal" for that couple, whereas any practice which is unpleasant to either partner must be considered "abnormal"—or at least unacceptable—for that couple. Unfortunately, such antediluvian concepts as the man's "right" to sexual satisfaction any time he wishes, or the woman's "duty" to make herself available whether she is interested at the moment or not, still crop up in our sexually enlightened society. Obviously such outmoded beliefs are the very antithesis of a sexual relationship that is equally rewarding to both partners, a vital component of any lasting marriage and a necessary emotional preparation for parenthood.

The important point is that sexual compatibility can almost always be achieved given such qualities in both partners as mutual love and concern, an ability to understand and communicate, and the patience and willingness to try. When incompatibility does appear, it can almost always be corrected given these same qualities, although in some cases professional guidance may be necessary to help a couple understand and resolve their problems. A trusted family doctor may be able to provide such help, and when incompatibility has deep-seated emotional roots, psychiatric consultation may be advisable. Religious advisers or qualified and experienced marriage counselors may also be called upon to help. The time to seek help, however, is when sexual problems first appear, rather than later when incompatibility has become firmly entrenched and deep, perhaps unhealable, wounds have been inflicted. In particular, such seriously disruptive sexual problems as male impotence or

female frigidity require professional assistance as early as possible. These problems are discussed in more detail elsewhere. (*See* p. 743 and p. 784.)

Psychological Compatibility. Both partners must make a profound emotional investment in marriage. Thus psychological compatibility is no less essential than sexual compatibility; and while this, too, may take patience, love and understanding, it can be achieved only through shared interests, communication and companionship. The old attitudes of male dominance and female inferiority or submissiveness in marriage are truly antiquated; both partners in a marriage must have equal opportunity to express themselves fully and to contribute to the direction of the relationship, just as both must share equally in the responsibility of making the marriage work.

Certain specific problems can prove very hazardous to this kind of shared relationship. And surely the greatest of these is infidelity. The concept of mutual faithfulness still lies at the heart of any marital or even nonmarital relationship, and infidelity by either partner is still the single most destructive act that can be undertaken. Second to infidelity, trouble with money is perhaps the most common marriage-wrecker; only by completely open discussion and mutual agreement on financial priorities can this threat be avoided. Any budget must, of course, be both realistic and flexible, and managing the budget must be a fully shared responsibility. Other hazards—problems with in-laws, for example, or the deadening effect of taking each other for granted, or even the problem of sheer boredom as a marriage seems to settle into dull routine—can again be avoided, or minimized, only by keeping the channels of communication open, discussing problems when they first appear, and periodically reassessing mutual desires and goals. Problems of psychological incompatibility can often be resolved by the couple themselves, but again professional counsel may be helpful, provided by a family doctor, a psychiatrist, a marriage counselor or even, in some cases, a mature nonprofessional friend. Whatever approach is used, however, the first and major step toward safeguarding a marriage from these commonplace hazards is an alert awareness on the part of both partners that such threats are very real, and a communicated and shared determination not to allow them to become divisive or corrosive influences on the marriage.

Parenthood

Children are, of course, an important concomitant to marriage, not merely from the standpoint of preservation of the species, but primarily in our society in terms of the personal fulfillment that childbearing and child rearing represent to the parents. The profound desire to have children is an integral part of human nature, and society at large heartily approves—to such an extent, in fact, that a couple who have been married for several years and have not had children are generally regarded with sympathy, or thought to be extremely selfish. Perhaps it is this unspoken social pressure that helps explain why so many young couples feel impelled to begin their families so early. The decision to have children is surely one of the most important that a couple of any age can make; it involves not only deciding when to start a family, but also how large that family will be and the interval that elapses between children. Yet all too often these decisions seem to be matters of pure chance or accident, usually the result of impetuousness, ignorance or carelessness. Pregnancies are sometimes even undertaken in a misguided attempt to satisfy some neurotic need of one or both parents, or in an equally unfortunate attempt to shore up a troubled marriage.

Obviously the baby who is unexpected or unwanted has a great deal against him from the start. But just what considerations should enter into the important decision to have children? First and foremost, the young couple must realize that children cannot help but be a mixed blessing. The first child, and each additional child thereafter, will profoundly alter the living pattern of the parents. Not only does each child represent an additional financial responsibility for a period of up to twenty years or longer, but far more significantly, each child represents a new, separate and distinct physical and emo-

tional responsibility that the parents must undertake and share, a responsibility which the vast majority of young couples must face as rank amateurs. It simply does not make sense to undertake such a responsibility until both partners in the marriage are fully prepared to do so.

Second, young couples who are mature enough to undertake the responsibility of children should also be mature enough to recognize that children in a family do not resolve problems. Rather, they *create* them. If the child is sincerely wanted, his arrival carefully planned, and his parents capable and willing to provide the love and affection he needs, the problems he will create will not be insuperable—but there will be problems, added on to whatever problems may already exist in the marriage relationship. Above all, it must be recognized that children are not possessions, or weapons, or mere reflections of the parents' egos; they are individuals in their own right. To use children as foils in marital jousting, consciously or unconsciously, is unthinkable.

The decision to raise a family is uniquely important to the mother, particularly the working mother. Fathers in our culture are generally excused from the time-consuming burdens of infant and child care, but recently we have come to recognize that combining marriage and motherhood with work outside the home may be not only an economic necessity in many families but also a source of psychological satisfaction for the wife. Much has been written in recent years about the "trapped housewife" and "momism," all true to a certain extent. But as yet our society is not well organized to accommodate the working mother; competent domestic help is a rarity, and adequate day care centers for preschool-age children are the exception rather than the rule. Thus the mother must realize that rearing children can indeed be an "interruption," perhaps lasting for years when one child follows another in rapid succession, and the husband must realize that fatherhood involves much more than simply paying the bills. If his wife works, or even if she does not, he must assume his share of domestic and child-rearing responsibilities.

Fortunately, few parents today are unaware of these considerations, and with the information and guidance available in the areas of family planning and conception control, there is no rational reason why parenthood ever need be undertaken prematurely or unintentionally. The first step, of course, in successful family planning is the use of an effective means of conception control. (*See* below.) Various public or private agencies or the family doctor should be consulted for reliable information in this area even before marriage. Most couples have no difficulty conceiving when the time comes, but such a problem can arise from any number of physical or psychological causes; again, honest and open consultation between both husband and wife and a trusted family doctor is an important first step in their successful resolution. (*See* p. 742.) And certainly before undertaking a first pregnancy, a young wife in particular should consult her doctor to detect, and prevent if possible, any factors that might complicate pregnancy and delivery.

Once a family has begun, serious forethought and mature consideration should also be given to the spacing and number of further children. Spacing is usually a matter of convenience, a decision that can be made in the best interests of the parents and the other children in the family; but the ultimate number of children is often a reflection of personal preference. Although large families have become increasingly rare in this country, there is no specific reason why a couple should not have numerous children if that is their sincere, mutual wish and if they are capable, both financially and emotionally, of handling them. Prospective parents should recognize, however, that there is little advantage per se in having a large family, whereas there are identifiable disadvantages, not the least of which is the very real concern about the population explosion. Rather than contribute to that, many young parents desiring a large family today limit their own children to one or two, and then add to their families by adoption, thus fulfilling both their own and society's needs. Adoption is also a happy solution for those couples who are unable to have children of their own, and there are any

number of private and public agencies that specialize in this valuable and humane service.

As carefully as a family may be planned, there is one thing that cannot yet be controlled: the sex of the child. Parental prejudices or preferences for one sex or another are most unfortunate, and may be particularly damaging to the child, but it is perhaps natural that many parents want both a boy and a girl, or after one or two children of the same sex would like at least one of the other. There has been considerable research into the matter of predetermining the sex of children, and some evidence has been unearthed to indicate that the odds that a child will be one sex or the other may be altered according to the time after ovulation that the conception takes place. Children conceived within the first few hours after ovulation, for example, are thought to be somewhat more likely to be male, while those conceived during the second 24 hours after ovulation are thought more likely to be female. This theory has even been used (tentatively) by some gynecologists in counseling their patients in an attempt to improve the chances of a male or female conception according to the patient's desire. But even if the precise time of ovulation in a given woman could be accurately determined—by no means a reliable proposition—it must be recognized that only a *slight shift of the probabilities* is possible in either direction, providing the theory in the long run proves true. In short, there is today *no* way to predetermine the sex of a child at the time of conception, nor is there any reason to expect this millennium to come at any time in the foreseeable future. Thus, again, adoption provides the only solution if the sex of the children in a family is a concern.

Finally, it should be said that the family, whatever its size and whatever the sex of its children, is the basic unit in our society, and although the so-called nuclear family has recently come in for a barrage of criticism, it will probably endure for years to come. The patterns of love, security and responsibility that are first experienced in the family setting are crucial to the emotional development of the child, and will have a telling influence both on his abilities to establish a family of his own when the time comes and on his abilities as an individual in his own right and as a responsible member of his society. In short, the family is surely the most important human environment, whatever the other social circumstances, and it is largely up to the parents to provide and sustain that environment. An awesome responsibility, true, but there is no reason for the mature young couple to be intimidated by it. The family is as old as human history, and becoming a parent, in spite of the problems, is one of the most natural and rewarding of all human experiences.

Control of Conception

For many centuries, the control of conception —both preventing it when it was not desired and aiding it when it was—has constituted one of society's most perplexing problems. It was, and still is, a problem of far greater dimensions than merely preventing the birth of unwanted children. In some cases, childbirth can seriously endanger the life of the mother and must be prevented on valid medical grounds; in other cases, there are equally valid medical reasons for helping a woman conceive who has not been able to do so naturally. We have also come to realize that controlling conception and the principles of planned parenthood offer innumerable advantages in a family in which too many children too soon may impose intolerable economic and emotional burdens. Further, the concept of birth control in the family unit has expanded to include the broader concept of population control in human society as a whole. Many of the world's most serious economic and social problems, not only in poorer and less developed countries, but also in those comparatively more affluent and advanced, can be traced directly to overpopulation, and the threat increases with every year. Thus the control of conception is both a very personal concern and a social problem of the greatest magnitude. Today, thanks to concerted and cooperative scientific research, we at last have the means at our disposal to solve this multifaceted problem.

Formerly, the only truly effective means of conception control, however unrealistic, was abstinence. A variety of mechanical deterrents have also been used for many years, but the only "natural" alternative to abstinence as a means of preventing conception is the so-called *rhythm method,* which depends upon an understanding of the female ovulation cycle and the capacity of both male and female to abstain from sexual relations during those times in the female cycle when the woman is vulnerable to conception. Ovulation occurs, in general, roughly halfway between the end of one menstrual period and the beginning of the next, and the time of ovulation can often be identified quite accurately by a change in the woman's basal temperature. To establish this basal temperature, which may vary with the individual, the woman takes her temperature with an ordinary fever thermometer upon first awakening in the morning, before getting up and moving around. The results are then recorded for a period of several weeks, and in most cases a slight rise in the basal temperature of from .4 to .6 of a degree indicates the time of ovulation. A few days following ovulation, the temperature again falls to the basal level. The woman is vulnerable to conception only during a period of approximately 48 hours from the time she has ovulated in any given cycle. Thus, abstaining from intercourse during the right 48-hour period will prevent an unwanted pregnancy.

The problem, of course, is to identify the right 48 hours, and the woman who chooses this method of conception control should consult her doctor for specific and detailed instructions. The change in basal temperature at the time of ovulation is a remarkably accurate indicator, providing the change is significant and uniform, and providing the woman goes to the continuing trouble of charting her basal temperatures. Unfortunately, in many women the change is relatively minor, a matter of .2 of a degree or so, and thus difficult to identify for certain; in others there may be just enough day-to-day variation in basal temperature for other reasons to make the time of ovulation impossible to pinpoint. Finally, many women grow weary of what seems to be a tedious and unnatural ritual and begin guessing instead of measuring, and that is the end of *that* method of conception control.

The only alternative to the measurement of basal temperature is to utilize the knowledge that in most women ovulation occurs at a precise time between the end of one menstrual period and the beginning of the next. However, this time may vary in the same woman as much as several days from one cycle to the next, and even when it is precise, it must be *measured backward* from the beginning of a new menstrual cycle, since menstruation occurs as a result of hormonal changes that arise after ovulation has taken place and the ovum has not been fertilized. In short, this method of calculation, more often employed than measuring changes in basal temperature among women who subscribe to the rhythm method, may require abstention from sexual relations for as much as a week to ten days during the interval from the end of one period to the beginning of the next in order to be certain of avoiding conception.

Considering the fact that many men and women are reluctant to engage, or opposed to engaging, in sexual intercourse while a woman is actually menstruating (a time which is, in fact, the "safest" period of all, as far as conception control is concerned), it is easy to see that the rhythm method can become highly intrusive and restrictive of natural patterns of sexual behavior. Sexual needs and impulses do not follow a calendar, and for this reason alone the rhythm method is often totally ineffective. One of the major joys of sexuality lies in its spontaneity and the freedom of either partner to invite intercourse when the time seems right, and to enjoy it without fear or tension. This is precisely the quality of sexuality that the rhythm method can destroy, perhaps even affecting the marital relationship itself. Apart from abstinence, it is surely the most difficult and demanding of the various means of conception control for both partners. Those who subscribe to it, by reason of their moral convictions or religious beliefs, must be able to cope with this consideration, and must realize that even with the most careful and con-

scientious adherence, the rhythm method can never be completely reliable.

Other means of conception control have both their advantages and their disadvantages, but one in particular can be completely discounted. *Coitus interruptus,* the practice of male withdrawal just prior to orgasm and ejaculation, is not only difficult but also manifestly ineffective as a means of avoiding conception, since secretions emitted from the penis during foreplay and intense sexual arousal carry multitudes of live sperm into the vagina even prior to ejaculation. Spermicidal jellies or foams, or spermicidal chemicals introduced into the vagina in the form of *suppositories,* may have some contraceptive use, but none of these chemicals effectively penetrates the cervix, the precise area where most sperm emitted with ejaculation are ordinarily deposited, usually with considerable force and pressure. Similarly, any form of vaginal *douche* after intercourse, while regarded as a desirable hygienic measure by many women, cannot be relied upon as a means of contraception. The use by the male of a protective sheath, called a *prophylactic* or *condom,* worn over the penis and usually made of rubber or some other impermeable material, can be considerably more effective in preventing sperm from entering the vagina during intercourse. In fact, the condom is widely used both as a contraceptive method and as protection against venereal disease, but here again it is not completely successful in either role. Condoms can break, slip or come off during sexual activity, they can be unpleasant to the female, and they may also dull sexual sensations for the male.

Most authorities agree that the ideal mechanical contraceptive is some type of barrier device worn by the female to obstruct the entry of sperm into the uterus. Such a device can be either permanently placed or temporarily inserted at some time prior to intercourse; it should remain in place at least for a time afterward; it can be handled with relatively little mess or bother, and has no effect whatever on the woman's sexual sensations and responses. The *diaphragm* fulfills all of these criteria at least reasonably well and, when used in combination with a spermicidal jelly, can be highly effective (as much as 97 percent) in preventing conception. The diaphragm is a simple dome of soft rubber supported by a flexible metal ring which, when properly inserted into the vagina, completely covers the mouth of the uterus. Initially, it should be fitted under the supervision of a physician, since women vary considerably in size; if it is too small it may be ineffective, and if it is too large it may be uncomfortable. Properly fitted and inserted, a diaphragm should not be felt by the woman at all, even in the midst of vigorous intercourse. After intercourse it should be left in place for a minimum of five to six hours (overnight is fine) and then removed only after thorough douching with warm water. However, a diaphragm can break and should be carefully inspected for imperfections before use, or if improperly inserted it can dislodge during intercourse. Thus, it, too, cannot be considered 100 percent effective.

Perhaps more effective, and far less troublesome for many women, is the use of an *intrauterine device* (IUD) or "coil," one of a variety of small, shaped bits of plastic or other inert material which can be inserted by the doctor into the cervical entrance to the uterus and then, in most cases, left there as a "permanent" contraceptive. Gynecologists are still not entirely sure whether IUD's work as effectively as they do because they impede the passage of sperm into the uterus, or because they prevent implantation of a fertilized ovum, or both, but it is known that these devices are extremely effective in preventing conception and may often be left in place for months or years, if desired, since, when properly placed, they do not usually come out, nor do they interfere with menstruation or sexual enjoyment. An IUD must, however, be inserted and subsequently checked for position by an experienced physician. It can be removed any time that a pregnancy is desired and then reinserted after childbirth until another pregnancy is desired. Insertion and removal are relatively painless procedures for most women, although some may find both insertion and retention quite uncomfortable. In these rare cases, of course, its use is impractical. IUD's are relatively new, and have been tested and used widely for only a few years. Much is still to be learned about their long-term effectiveness and safety; physicians are particularly watchful to be certain that there is no increased incidence of cervical inflammation or cancer in women using the device. But to date no evidence of such problems has appeared, and for many women the IUD has proved to be an ideal means of conception control.

Even more effective than any of these mechanical devices, and by far the handiest and simplest means of contraception, is the use of *the Pill,* one of any number of special hormone medications which, when taken orally on a regular basis by a woman, prevent conception by the most direct method of all, by preventing ovulation. All varieties of these medications work on the same basic principle: they contain the pregnancy-sustaining hormone progesterone or other hormones with progesterone-like effects; taken at the time that a follicle would normally begin to mature in the ovary, these hormones successfully block this maturation process just as progesterone would block it if a pregnancy were present, and thus prevent ovulation. When used intermittently, or in some cases continually—in very low doses, however—these hormones do not prevent menstruation; they merely create *anovulatory* (i.e., "ovulation-free") menstrual cycles so that conception is prevented while they are being used. If the medication is taken faithfully in the prescribed manner, it has proved to be virtually 100 percent foolproof; in fact, its record has been so impressive that many gynecologists regard an unexpected pregnancy in a woman who is taking the Pill as de facto evidence that she has not been taking the medicine as directed.

Unfortunately, some women suffer from troublesome side effects. These hormones tend to promote fluid retention in the tissues, for example, and occasionally a woman will be troubled by menstrual irregularities, intermittent bleeding and spotting before a menstrual period is due, and similar problems. Furthermore, there is some evidence, not yet fully established but too significant to ignore, that the use of certain of the contraceptive hormone preparations may render some women more than usually prone to such serious health threats as the development of blood clots in the veins or persisting kidney disfunction. Again, these medications are relatively new, and a long-range evaluation of their overall effects is not yet possible. However, this is no reason to abandon the Pill as a highly effective and desirable contraceptive method, nor should it cause undue concern to the woman who is using it. But obviously the Pill must be prescribed judiciously under the watchful attention of a physician, and the user must be alert to possible side effects, report them immediately to her doctor if they occur, and be fully prepared to abandon the medication in the event of any suspicious symptoms. Further, the woman who has just begun taking the Pill should be aware that it is not instantly effective; most physicians recommend that other contraceptive methods be used concurrently for at least a month after the Pill has been started and preferably for two full cycles before it can be relied upon. And anyone using the Pill with the serious intent of controlling conception must recognize that its effectiveness depends *entirely* upon absolutely faithful adherence to the prescribed dosage schedule. The woman who forgets her medication from time to time and then takes two or three pills at once to "catch up," or uses the Pill only sporadically or intermittently, is not only subjecting her body to the possible ill effects of uncontrolled hormonal meddling; she is also fooling herself. Such women should simply forget the Pill entirely and utilize one of the mechanical contraceptive devices.

It has often been said that the truly ideal contraceptive would be a harmless medication which could be taken by the male to interrupt sperm production temporarily, a reversible effect that would disappear within a brief time after the medicine was discontinued. So far this medication exists only in the realm of probability, but very active research is being conducted along precisely these lines, and the near future may well provide a breakthrough. In addition, research is progressing in search of effective contraception medications that might be taken by the woman on a once-a-month basis, or even a Pill that might be taken after intercourse and

still prevent pregnancy. Some authorities predict that such contraceptive medications may be ready for initial clinical testing in the very near future. Certainly if they prove both safe and reliable, they will introduce a whole new approach to modern conception control.

Of course the most completely effective, and final, answer to the problem of contraception is surgical: actually tying and cutting the Fallopian tubes of the female, a procedure known as *tubal ligation*, or cutting and tying the vas deferens, the tube in the male that carries the sperm from the testicles into the urethra, an operation known as *vasectomy*. Many physicians in the past have regarded these operations as mutilatory, destructive and permanent procedures which can have quite unpredictable physical and psychological aftereffects. Indeed, many hospitals have forbidden these procedures in their operating rooms, and of course they are abhorrent to the religious convictions of many doctors and patients as well.

In recent years, however, probably in part due to concern about the overpopulation problem, a more enlightened approach has been taken to these procedures. Today many gynecologists argue that a woman in her mid-thirties who has already borne two or more children, has a stable marriage and, with her husband's consent, does not wish to bear any more children under any circumstances, should at least be considered as a candidate for tubal ligation. The operation is a safe and simple one, and can be performed at any time, although the ideal time is a day or two after the delivery of a baby, when the uterus is still enlarged and the Fallopian tubes are more accessible to the surgical knife through a small abdominal incision. In the case of a man, vasectomy is even more readily performed at virtually any time, but many physicians who consider tubal ligations in a female acceptable under certain circumstances frequently reject vasectomy for their male patients on the grounds that the procedure may be psychologically damaging. It is a difficult contention to support with any kind of objective evidence, however, and this argument against vasectomy may be more emotional than scientific. In any case, the attitudes of both the medical profession and many men and women toward these procedures are in the process of change.

Nevertheless, changing attitudes and opinions aside, there remains one unalterable fact: both these procedures are permanent and cannot be reversed once performed. True, there are rare cases in which Fallopian tubes or the vas deferens have been reconstructed after an operation and made functional again, but the likelihood of success is far too small to count on. What is more, there is no way to foresee the future, and a procedure which may seem to be a perfectly rational step might later prove to be a tragic mistake—in the event of a remarriage, for example, or the death of one or more children in the family. For many these may seem remote eventualities, but in every case, these permanent procedures should be undertaken only after the most careful deliberation between husband and wife, thoughtful consultation with a trusted medical adviser, and in full awareness of all possible consequences. Certainly it is also advisable that temporary and reversible means of conception control be given most serious consideration first.

Abortion

Until quite recently performing an *elective abortion*—that is, purposely destroying a healthy, viable pregnancy without urgent medical indication—was anathema in our society, rigidly prohibited by law in virtually every state in the land. So-called *therapeutic abortion* was sometimes legally permitted in those rare instances when continuation of a pregnancy presented an indisputable threat to the health or life of the mother, but these criteria were rigidly interpreted in most communities. In many areas the law required the unanimous agreement of three or more physicians, including specialists in obstetrics and gynecology, in any case before an abortion was considered therapeutically justified, and even then many hospitals refused to permit such procedures in their operating rooms. As a consequence, women who were determined to terminate their pregnancies but could not meet the therapeutic criteria were forced into the hands of illegal abortionists at home or abroad, or were even driven to such dangerous extremes as attempting self-abortion. The results were often appalling; multitudes of women died of hemorrhage or infection at the hands of inept, illegal abortionists, and many more suffered permanent damage to their genital organs and perhaps even more pervasive psychological damage.

In recent years the whole question of elective abortion has become a matter for nationwide debate, and many state and local governments have made far-ranging changes in their abortion laws. In some areas laws have been altered to make abortions legal, when performed by qualified physicians under acceptable hospital conditions up to a specified point in the pregnancy, entirely at the option of the woman or couple involved; elsewhere medicolegal criteria for therapeutic abortion have been broadened to such a degree that even the possible threat of emotional harm to the woman on account of the pregnancy may be construed as "medical" justification for abortion. Thus legal elective abortions are now being performed by qualified physicians in many of the hospitals in a number of our states, with the strong likelihood that whatever restrictive laws remain will ultimately be relaxed.

The mere passage of more liberal laws, however, has not by any means provided solutions to the ethical and moral problems involved in elective abortion. Abortion is still adamantly proscribed by many religious, ethical and humanitarian leaders who argue that a new human life has begun, either at the moment of conception or at least by the time the fertilized ovum has become implanted in the uterus, and that any willful interference with that new life is tantamount to legalized murder. Those holding this view point out that the various available techniques for conception control provide the woman, or the couple, ample means to prevent conception if they so desire, but that there can be no justification for purposefully extinguishing a new life once it has been conceived. On the other hand, those favoring the legalization of abortion on a basis of maternal or parental option argue just as adamantly that a conception does not become a distinguishable human life until the fetus has developed sentience, certainly not before a brain and nervous system have developed, and until that point has been reached it is the mother, not the fetus, who deserves primary consideration. Proponents of this view also contend that every woman has an inalienable human right to control over her own body, and should not be forced by any law to carry to term a pregnancy, or bear years of responsibility for a baby, which she does not want.

Both views, of course, have certain merits. Moral considerations aside, many physicians take a third view: that in the past women who were determined to have abortions for whatever reason very often obtained them one way or another, often at grave risk to their health or even their lives, and that it is better to make abortion legally available under safe medical conditions than to encourage by default the dangerous practice of criminal abortion. When performed under carefully controlled medical conditions, abortions pose relatively little threat to the mother. The earlier an abortion is performed following conception and implantation of the fetus, the lower the risk; medical authorities agree that an abortion attempted after the third month of the pregnancy poses an unacceptable risk to the mother because of the grave threat of uncontrollable hemorrhage. When performed before the end of the third month, however, abortion can readily be accomplished by means of a D and C (see p. 754), in which the uterine cervix is dilated under a general anesthesia and the fetus dislodged from the interior lining of the uterus by curettement or scraping. Alternatively, the abortion can be performed with even less risk of uterine hemorrhage by dilating the uterus and introducing a suction device into the uterus to dislodge the fetus without direct instrumentation. Such procedures require only a few moments of time and a brief anesthesia, and can usually be accomplished with no more difficulty or long-term physical effects than a D and C performed, say, for the diagnosis of abnormal uterine bleeding. Properly performed, the abortion necessitates no more than a few days' convalescence at the most, and does not have any deleterious effect on the woman's ability to conceive later if she so desires.

No one, however, can make the moral decision for or against abortion in any given case except the woman herself, or the couple involved. Certainly medical advice should be obtained as soon in a pregnancy as any question of a possible abortion arises. Some physicians vigorously oppose elective abortion on the basis of their personal religious or ethical convictions, while others support the opposing view with equal vigor; but no one concerned with the problem should hesitate to ask for professional medical advice. Unfortunately, relaxation of abortion laws has not yet done away with illegal abortionists, who continue in practice largely because women are embarrassed to discuss the possibility of abortion with their family doctors. Such hesitancy is ridiculous today, and no woman should consider subjecting herself to the perils of an illegal abortion under the misguided notion that it will somehow be "easier" or "less trouble." Finally, there are both religious and social agencies, some favoring elective abortion and some opposing it, which stand ready to help the woman with an unwanted pregnancy, and any physician, regardless of his personal views, can provide references.

In short, elective abortion is readily available in this country today for any woman who emphatically wishes to terminate an unwanted pregnancy, but the moral and ethical decision to have an abortion must rest squarely in the hands of the woman herself. If an abortion is performed before the end of the third month of pregnancy, in most cases it poses little threat to the physical health of the mother, but no one can predict the long-term psychological effects that may accrue. If an abortion is likely to constitute a lifelong source of self-recrimination, regret or guilt, it should certainly be avoided; many agencies exist to help place an unwanted child for adoption if the mother decides to carry the pregnancy to term. Finally, it is irresponsible folly to rely upon elective abortion as an alternative to contraception when so many excellent and reliable methods of conception control are available. In the long run it is far better to take the minimal pains necessary to prevent a conception from occurring in the first place than to be faced later with the moral dilemma that elective abortion may entail.

Physical Illness During the Prime Years

For most people the prime years are remarkably free from illness aside from the common run of minor upper respiratory infections, influenza, or everyday injuries. A few serious or continuing illnesses, however, often make their appearance among this age group, and ironically, although many of them can be cured or controlled with the proper diagnosis and treatment, some can also be completely avoided with common sense and knowledgeable action.

Peptic ulcer disease, for example, is typically an illness that begins in young adulthood, often concurrently with undertaking the many responsibilities of marriage and parenthood. In some cases, undoubtedly, the emotional stresses of an unhappy marriage can contribute to the onset of this illness; in others, the tension of a competitive job and the pressures of growing financial responsibilities play a part. Whatever the cause, it is foolish to temporize with the symptoms of this condition or the emotional factors that aggravate it. Early diagnosis and treatment of both its physical and its psychological components are imperative. (*See* p. 648.)

Hypertension is another major illness which typically makes its appearance during young adulthood, often in a very mild and labile form, but with the potential for becoming permanently entrenched unless adequately treated. Again, the emotional tensions of these years of life doubtless contribute heavily to the development, in particular, of so-called benign essential hypertension. The condition can, however, be easily detected in a routine office examination, both its physical and psychological causes assessed, and its symptoms prevented or controlled effectively. (*See* p. 582.)

Still another commonplace distress of young adulthood related to emotional tensions is the occurrence of *migraine headaches,* particularly among women. Enough is known today about the behavior of these headaches that their symptoms can be combated and the condition at least

controlled. (*See* p. 338.) Similarly, although more related to biochemical changes than emotional stress, young adulthood for many young women is punctuated by episodes, sometimes infrequent and sometimes with monthly regularity, of so-called *premenstrual tension,* characterized by nervous irritability, emotional lability and fluid retention, all of which occur during the five or six days prior to the onset of menstruation. For many generations this unpleasant syndrome was widely believed to be an emotional concomitant to menstruation, but more recent evidence has shown that the condition involves very real physiological changes, and its distressing symptoms can be markedly alleviated, if not prevented completely, by the proper medications. (*See* p. 762.)

The prime years can also be afflicted by a variety of episodic, or even chronic, *allergies.* In some cases they may be a continuation of allergies suffered during childhood—asthma, for example, triggered by contact with specific allergens or by some emotional conflict. In other cases, brand-new allergies make their appearance, most commonly in the form of either skin reactions or the so-called nasal allergies. However, the diagnosis and treatment of allergies is a definite medical specialty, and with the proper testing and the use of medications, their symptoms can usually be prevented or effectively controlled. (*See* p. 387.)

Finally, three broad categories of health hazards often have their origins in the years of young adulthood, arising either due to *habit* or simply because of *neglect.* In the first category are those habits which, although perhaps not apparently or immediately hazardous to health, nevertheless lay the groundwork for serious trouble in the years ahead. For example, the habit of overindulgence in rich and fattening foods can lead to a lifelong struggle with obesity. Obesity begins insidiously with the gain of a few pounds at a time. At first the gain is hardly noticeable and is well tolerated by the body, particularly the energetic and youthful body, but then energy begins to diminish, the metabolism begins to slow down, and obesity becomes an established fact. When that happens, it poses much more than a problem of appearance; obesity is a contributing cause of many serious, and possibly even fatal, illnesses. Obviously the ideal time to establish sane and controlled eating habits to prevent obesity is *before* it has become entrenched. The alternative is to spend later decades attempting, usually unsuccessfully, to keep weight under control. (*See* p. 927.)

It is also during the prime years that the habit of overindulgence in alcohol begins to take hold. In some cases, the habit may evolve into acute alcoholism, one of the most destructive and life-shattering diseases known to man, which, once identified, requires the most skilled and tenacious medical and psychiatric treatment. (*See* p. 790.) More often, however, indulgence in alcohol never quite reaches the extreme physical and social abuses of pathological alcoholism; rather, it becomes an entrenched day-by-day dependence whose ill effects are more subtle yet no less destructive: the steady, excessive intake of relatively useless calories, again leading to chronic borderline obesity; the chronic taxing of such organs as the liver and the heart; and above all, the chronic impairment of both physical and mental functions owing to the insidious influence of this cerebrodepressive drug.

The numbers of young people who fall victim to this habit are legion; in this country they number in the millions. They are not alcoholics in the true sense, but neither are they merely "social drinkers." If they share a common characteristic, it is their vehement denial that their drinking is a problem. It is, in fact, much more than that; it must be regarded as a serious long-term health hazard. Obviously the best way to avoid this hazard is in the realization that the excessive use of alcohol constitutes a very real threat. Candid self-evaluation and reasonable self-discipline is the next step. It may not be necessary to give up alcohol completely, but some degree of control should be established by setting strict limits upon its daily use to confine the pattern of drinking to a harmless level.

Finally, tobacco smoking is a pernicious habit which, once entrenched, can be exceedingly difficult to break, particularly for the "heavy" smoker. The physical hazards of heavy cigarette smoking—the continuing burden and damage to the heart, and the massively increased vulner-

ability to carcinoma of the lung, to mention only the most serious—have recently received wide publicity. It is not scare propaganda by any means. Because of the complex nature of these illnesses, and the complex nature of the effects of cigarette smoking on the body, it has been extremely difficult to prove a direct cause-and-effect relationship between smoking and heart disease or lung cancer, and the task of unequivocally establishing that proof still continues, but there are few medical authorities who seriously question that the causative relationship exists. The best way to stop smoking is, of course, not to start; but for those who did start, and who continue to smoke, the time to stop is *now*. (*See* p. 590.)

All three of these destructive habits can be very difficult to break because of the powerful emotional factors that contribute to them. Yet with determination and will power it can be done; ultimately it is up to the individual. It is also up to the individual to prevent those illnesses that result from simple neglect of routine health care during the prime years. These illnesses can be just as tragically unnecessary, and their prevention is not a matter of will power at all. It is just a matter of common sense. A prime example is neglect of routine preventive dental care. Dental care is lavished upon children in our society, and when they grow up, they lavish it on *their* children, but not on themselves. This kind of neglect usually comes to an end in some acute dental crisis, and by that time the damage has been done. Everyone is aware of the necessity of routine dental checkups, if only to have the teeth professionally cleaned. Neglect of even this simple and painless procedure can, in later years, result in teeth damaged beyond reasonable hope of repair, the need for extractions, costly bridgework and the replacement of once strong and healthy natural teeth with artificial dentures. Jokes and stories to the contrary, a visit to the dentist is hardly an agonizing ordeal. The slight pain and inconvenience of routine preventive dental care are more than outweighed by its long-range benefits.

Neglect of foot care is equally common. Wearing ill-fitting shoes or high heels in defiance of both anatomy and common sense can result in calluses, corns, bunions, muscular aches and pains, impaired circulation, fallen arches and even actual deformities. (*See* p. 322.) The feet are probably the most consistently mistreated parts of the entire body, and their mistreatment can easily cause years of chronic pain or permanent disability. Obviously, comfort and proper support, not vanity or stylishness, are the first principles of preventive foot care.

Abuse of the eyes is somewhat less common, but there are many who resist wearing glasses, even though it is perfectly apparent that they are necessary. An annual checkup of eye function is simply a matter of common sense, both for those who already wear glasses and those who may need them in the future. The eyes are not changeless; like every other organ in the body they are vulnerable to the effects of wear and tear and aging. With proper care, these effects can be minimized and corrected. Abuse of the hearing can also be a problem, particularly in an age of ever increasing "noise pollution" and among a younger generation who seem to prefer music played at almost deafening volume. No one yet is certain of the long-range effects of excessive noise on hearing capacity, but the fact remains that impaired hearing, which may stem from a variety of causes, first becomes evident to the victim, and it is up to him to do something about it. Again hearing problems can, in most cases, be minimized or corrected, and refusing to admit that the problem exists, because of vanity or any other reason, can lead to years of partial, and quite unnecessary, impairment and even more serious damage.

It is probably one of life's greatest ironies that the years which are normally most free of physical illness—the prime of young adulthood—are also the years when preventive health care, at the least expense in time, trouble and money, is generally ignored. Attention during these years to regular programs of preventive health care not only can save money and time in the long run, but ultimately it can prolong life and provide greater assurance that the later years can be enjoyed with a minimum of preventable physical disabilities. Indeed, it is during these years of young adulthood that conscientious health care is most important. Young couples with growing children are responsible for the health of their families, which includes not only the children but themselves as well. A major step in fulfilling that responsibility is the investigation of the health facilities in whatever community the family lives, and the establishment of good cooperative relationships with doctors, dentists and other health care specialists who can not only provide help in emergencies but also supervise programs of preventive health care for every member of the family. But ultimately it is up to the young couple themselves to establish good health habits in their children by setting the example of practicing good health habits themselves.

62

The Hazards of Middle Age

People approaching their middle years—the forties, fifties and early sixties—are often beset with a perplexing mixture of feelings. Many enter "middle age" with an ominous sense of foreboding, frustration or loss, a sense that life is passing them by. Youthful ambitions and dreams, still unrealized, may begin to seem forever unattainable. The long struggle for material security may change into a worried struggle to hold on to what has already been secured. The frustrations of a dull and routine life are compounded by the knowledge that it is probably too late to change. And for many, there is the looming specter of poor health, for this is the time when body tissues and organ systems begin to break down even among those who have never suffered ill health in their lives.

On the other hand, there are those who take a more mellow view of middle age. For many it is an opportunity to look back with satisfaction on realized dreams and accomplished goals, to relax to some degree and begin to enjoy the fruits of earlier labors. There are also the satisfactions of success, of a position of importance and respect in the community, of the wisdom that comes from experience and the opportunity to exercise leadership. Others find deep satisfaction in their families, and in children old enough now to start families of their own. Those who maintain that "life begins at forty" are at least partially correct; it is certainly a time when a *different sort* of life begins to evolve, not always necessarily a better life, perhaps, but a life with a very different complexion.

Whatever one's view of middle age, there is probably no other time when good health is more vitally important. Inevitably, perfectly natural changes—both physical and psychological—begin to take place during the middle years, few of which can be prevented or ignored. Physically we begin to slow down; we tend to require more sleep, or at least more rest; we no longer enjoy quite the boundless energy of early years, and often find that it takes more time to accomplish less. Among women the beginning of *menopause,* the cessation of regular menstrual periods and the concurrent loss of the ability to bear children, is accompanied by physiological changes, and often emotional changes as well. In many men the sexual appetite begins to flag, however subtly, yet among many women freedom from the risk of pregnancy has an opposite psychological effect, with an increase in sexual interest and vigor.

For the most part these changes are natural and normal concomitants of the process of aging and have no relationship to ill health. Other changes and certain specific hazards, however, are very much related to health, particularly the increasing vulnerability to certain kinds of illness. A great many things can be done to avoid these hazards and illnesses. Obviously, a program of preventive health care, begun and followed in earlier years and continued through middle age, will pay the greatest dividends. If such a preventive program has been neglected, it is imperative that it begin immediately. There is certainly no reason for an excessive preoccupation with the minor aches and pains that are a normal part of middle age, but an awareness of those symptoms and conditions that can very easily evolve into serious illness is an important part of maintaining optimum health. Now, more than ever before, regular physical examinations and dental checkups are necessary at more frequent intervals; beyond the age of forty both men and women should have preventive medical and dental checkups at least every six months. It is also imperative that unusual symptoms of any kind be checked out with a physician *when they occur;* nothing can be more foolish than to ignore such symptoms, or write them off as "part of growing old." The middle years are a time for extraordinary vigilance to avoid or minimize certain hazards that all too frequently begin to appear.

The Hazard of Obesity

There is no question that the most common and overriding health hazard of the middle years, the one condition that does more than any other to predispose the breakdown of good health, is obesity. Excessive weight is by no means exclusively a problem of middle age. There are those who are harmfully, even dangerously, obese all their lives. But it is during the middle years that obesity commonly begins to afflict even those who have never before had a weight problem. Almost overnight, it seems, they find themselves becoming paunchy, their weight slowly creeps up, their clothing ceases to fit, the fat appears first in pads and then in rolls, and they are completely bewildered by this phenomenon when, as far as they can see, there has been no significant change in their life habits. Those who have had to control their weight periodically during more youthful days, and have always been able to do so with relative ease, suddenly find weight control much more difficult. The diets and weight loss programs that always worked before seem ineffective, and they cannot understand why.

There are, of course, several very good reasons why. First, *physical activity begins to decline.* Men and women who have always led comparatively sedentary lives tend to become even more sedentary. More active individuals who once enjoyed competitive sports and exercise begin to pass them up in favor of less strenuous activities. With a diminution in physical exercise, calories that were formerly burned off in this fashion are no longer used, but rather stored and gradually contribute to a growing layer of fat.

Concurrent with the decline of physical activity, *the body's overall metabolism also begins to slow down.* Although the thyroid gland, the powerful governor of the body's biochemical reactions, may show no measurable sign of flagging, body chemistry becomes infinitesimally more sluggish, less adaptable to extraordinary demands and changes. Other hormonal influences on metabolism—the action of the adrenocortical and sex hormones, for example—also diminish somewhat, affecting the overall chemical activity of the body. This slowing down is natural, even desirable, but unless it is accompanied by a reduction in the number of calories that are consumed each day, there will be further storage in the body of unused food materials as fat.

A third reason for the "creeping obesity" of middle age lies in *a subtle change in eating and drinking habits* that commonly occurs at this time. As other interests and pleasures diminish, many people—quite unconsciously—often depend more and more upon the satisfactions of food and drink. The "good eater" becomes a gourmet, and the social drinker, with more time on his hands, has two or three cocktails instead of one, and spends a Sunday afternoon in front of the television drinking beer. Then, too, in middle age there is often less concern about personal appearance; many people grow weary of the self-discipline necessary to keep their weight down. An extra helping or another drink is worth it, even if it does mean a few extra pounds. There is nothing wrong with good food and drink, of course. In fact, they are among life's greatest pleasures—in moderation. But alcohol is one of the most concentrated forms of calories a human being can consume, and rich foods often contain more calories than solid nutritional value. Self-indulgence in either or both, whatever their momentary satisfactions, can mean years of the discomforts and dangers of overweight.

Many people rationalize that increasing weight in middle age is "natural," like wrinkles and gray hair, and that little can be done about it. Some even claim that creeping obesity is really not as serious as it is made out to be. The truth is, however, that obesity is far from "natural," and in the middle years it is every bit as dangerous as, if not more dangerous than, during any other time of life simply because it becomes increasingly difficult to control. Obviously, an extra burden of weight is an extra load for the heart to carry, a heart that may already be slowing down. Obesity and increased blood pressure go hand in hand, and this is a time of life when hypertension can be lethal. Obesity and improper nourishment magnify and accelerate the process of arteriosclerosis, which tends to become widespread enough at this time of life without these predisposing factors. Muscles, bones, joints—in fact, virtually every organ system in the body, many of which may already be strained to a point of beginning disfunction—are burdened and impaired by excessive weight. There is no other condition more fiendishly capable of causing or compounding ill health.

Fortunately, many people are conscious of the problem of obesity. Weight control has become a popular health fad, possibly the only generally beneficial health fad the world has ever known. Multitudes of ingenious weight reduction schemes have been widely publicized and avidly read, including such curiosities as "the drinking man's diet," "the expense account diet" and "the grapefruit diet." Some are based on perfectly sound medical and physiological principles; others are pure nonsense. The very fact that new and ever more ingenious weight reduction programs continue to appear and sweep the best-seller lists suggests that somehow an ideal solution to this problem has not been found.

The basic fallacy of these programs, of course, is that almost without exception they seek to accomplish the impossible. They imply that obesity can be controlled without any particular effort or sacrifice, or if some self-control is necessary, it can be exercised for a few days or weeks and then back to the cream sauce and brandy nightcaps. In short, they imply that it is possible to eat one's cake and have it too, and that, unfortunately, *never* works, particularly in middle age when the natural adaptability of youth has flagged and when what might once have been a temporary annoyance has become a chronic and doggedly refractory condition. Obesity *can* be controlled, but it cannot be done without effort and sacrifice, nor can it be done in a few days. It cannot really be done effectively with a diet of specific foods, but only with the aid of certain prescribed attitudes toward eating. And yet, in their simplest form, the basic principles of successful weight control are fundamental and can be successfully applied by anyone who seriously recognizes obesity as a threat to his health.

The single most fundamental principle is self-evident: excessive weight can be lost only if the total amount of food taken in is consistently held slightly lower than the total amount of food actually used by the body. Once an ideal weight has been attained, the only way to keep it at a stable level is to make sure that the total amount of food taken in each day is *consistently and precisely the same* as the total amount of food actually used by the body each day. Notice that calories have not been mentioned. A *calorie* is simply a measurement of the amount of heat or energy contained in foods and released in the process of metabolism. If this heat or energy is not released or expended by the body, the foods are converted into and stored in the body as fat. Although different kinds of food have different caloric content and calories can offer a convenient means of measuring the total amount of food taken in, an elaborate calorie-measuring ritual is unnecessary as far as this basic principle is concerned. Every person has his own built-in measuring device: if you eat more food than you use, your weight begins to increase; if you eat less food than you use, your weight begins to decrease; if you balance your food intake with your food expenditure, your weight remains stable.

But how to accomplish this kind of control? Crash diets, in which the amount of food taken in is reduced to starvation levels for a brief period of time, are a hazardous affair. Such diets throw an extraordinary burden on the heart, create an abnormal situation in the gastrointestinal tract and bring about convulsive changes in the body's metabolic processes, any one of which may precipitate serious health problems. They may also lead to dangerous nutritional deficiencies. It is true that certain skilled doctors have, on occasion, tackled a case of gross obesity with a "crash diet" program: hospitalizing the patient and providing sufficient water for his survival but otherwise literally starving him in order to bring about swift weight reduction. Startling successes have been reported under such programs, but the patients have been selected from among those whose excessive obesity posed an immediate threat to their health, and the programs have been conducted under the most carefully controlled hospital circumstances. With the ordinary person this is not possible. Even more to the point, a crash diet suffers from one built-in flaw: no one can live with it for more than a short time. It does nothing to alter the basic eating and living habits which led to obesity in the first place. Thus, although weight may indeed be lost, it is almost invariably gained right back again the moment the program is over.

Indeed, the only practical and effective way to permanent weight control through the balance of intake and expenditure of food must lie in the realization that obesity is going to be a continuing, refractory and frustrating hazard that can be dealt with *only* by making certain permanent changes in daily eating habits—changes which can be pursued during a period of weight loss, but which can also be lived with on a *long-term* basis.

What sort of changes? The answer can be found in a brief review of the characteristics of certain foods. The great majority of people in America, and particularly those suffering from obesity, depend upon carbohydrate foods for a large portion of their daily caloric intake. These foods include not only the sugars (sweet desserts, cookies, pastries) but the basic starchy foods (bread, potatoes, rice, noodles, macaroni, spaghetti or other pastas). These foods provide calories for sustenance, they are among the cheapest foods available, and although they are of less nutritional value than certain other foods,

they are filling. The problem is that it is virtually impossible to control the amount of these foods that one eats. And those who depend upon starchy foods almost invariably tend to overeat.

By contrast, the protein-rich foods—the lean meats, eggs, fish and seafood, and cheeses—all contain the same number of calories as the carbohydrates, per unit of weight, yet they have the capacity to satisfy hunger and leave one feeling "full" after eating much smaller quantities. These protein-rich foods also have greater nutritional value, but unfortunately, they are much more costly, weight for weight, than the starches. Even so, they must form the solid core of any weight reduction program.

Fats are treacherous, for they contain more than twice the number of calories, weight for weight, than proteins and carbohydrates. Used in very modest amounts, fats or fatty foods improve the palatability of meals immensely. But used for cooking, as in deep-fat or pan frying, they add enormous quantities of calories to the diet without adding anything substantial to nutrition or the fulfillment of hunger.

Certain other foods have special desirable qualities in terms of weight control. Lettuce, celery, tomatoes and onions all have remarkably low caloric content, yet are not only tasty in salads but provide a filling bulk to the diet. Some starchy vegetables (sweet potatoes, rutabagas, beans or peas) contain as much starch as the starchy staples mentioned above, whereas other vegetables (members of the cabbage or cauliflower family, for example) are relatively low in calories and still provide satisfying bulk.

With these broad food categories in mind, it is easy to see the *sort* of diet which can be both satisfying to hunger and taste and at the same time avoid the dietary excesses that make weight control all but impossible. For example, although it may seem like heresy, most Americans could survive splendidly if they never ate another potato, slice of bread, dish of rice or bowl of spaghetti in their lives. These foods are often part of every major meal purely by habit. They do not need to be. A diet in which eggs are substituted for breakfast cereals, clear soups and chicken or tuna fish salad *without* the bread are substituted for thick luncheon sandwiches, and lean broiled meat, poultry or fish and a simple green salad flavored with a small amount of dressing and perhaps varied with a nonstarchy vegetable for dinner can supply all the nutritional needs of the body and provide varied and satisfying daily fare. When weight must be lost, a certain "attrition" can be practiced. Desserts, for example, can be eliminated. The quantity of milk one normally drinks can simply be cut in half. Alcoholic beverages can be confined to one drink a day, and the total amount consumed reduced by one-half. Wine with dinner can be eliminated during the weight-reducing period, or reserved for special occasions. The "second helping" habit can be dispensed with; it is almost invariably nothing *but* a habit, and every meal can be served in a single helping, eliminating the temptation to overindulge with seconds. We expect this at restaurants; why not at home? If something in addition to these measures is necessary to secure more rapid weight loss, simply reduce the *total amount* of food eaten at each meal by one-third.

Such a simple, fundamental program can be instituted by anyone, and it will work. Furthermore, it will help establish new and permanent eating habits that will carry the hard-earned rewards of a weight reduction period over to the everyday diet, making the maintenance of a stable weight at acceptable levels far more easily attainable. In establishing such a program, of course, certain goals should be set: an "ideal weight," a lower weight limit below which it is not necessary to go, and an upper weight limit which signals the need to apply the simple "attrition" measures discussed above. In most people, there will usually be a generous ten- to fifteen-pound spread between the lower limit and the upper limit, and this is the range within which everyone should try to remain, a range well below the level of chronic obesity. But everyone should be prepared to review his eating habits and readjust his "normal" and "attrition" diet programs as time passes and the need arises. A program that works well at the age of forty may be overindulgent by the age of fifty. The results can always be checked on the bathroom scales; if weight begins to climb, the program must be tightened down.

But just how does one determine his ideal weight in the first place, or select the upper and lower weight limits that should be observed in such a program? The first step is a frank discussion of the whole problem of excessive weight with a qualified physician. In fact, *no* weight-reducing program should be started without at least initial consultation with a doctor. Quite aside from establishing reasonable and realizable weight limits, the doctor can protect the overweight individual from potential harm by first checking out any possible physical reason for the obesity. Further, he can help the patient pinpoint particular habits that contribute to weight gain and then set guidelines for a weight reduction program tailored to his individual needs. Again it must be emphasized that sane weight reduction depends upon reducing the quantity, not the quality, of foods that are eaten, and any reducing diet must meet the body's nutritional requirements with a variety of healthful, nutritious foods—another area in which a doctor's guidance can be of great value. Finally, the question of exercise (*see* below) is also essential in weight control, and a doctor's guidance is particularly important in planning an exercise program that will aid weight reduction without throwing a dangerous physical strain on the body.

Unfortunately, there are cases in which a combination of reason, common sense and professional advice does not accomplish the weight reduction that is necessary; what then? In such refractory cases, it may be necessary to probe more deeply into the causes of obesity and the patient's inability to control it. Often there are underlying emotional reasons for overeating; indeed, in some individuals eating becomes a neurotic compulsion, a means of satisfying unconscious needs and desires, or of reacting to unconscious anxieties, fears or guilt feelings. In such instances, the professional advice of a doctor or a psychiatrist may help deal with these emotional problems and control the compulsion to overeat.

Many other cases of weight reduction failure, however, result simply from sagging will power. Fortunately, there are some medical aids that can sometimes be used safely and effectively to help overcome this problem. Most familiar are the "diet pills" that are often prescribed for their direct effect on the appetite control centers of the brain, medicines which act physiologically to make the patient feel less hungry. Most of these medicines, however, contain amphetamines, a family of drugs which do tend to blunt the appetite, but which may be thoroughly dangerous if overused or abused. Even in commonly prescribed doses the amphetamines act as potent heart, blood pressure and cerebral stimulants, often causing a distressing amount of physical hyperactivity, an inability to concentrate, a thoroughly illusory sense of euphoria and well-being, and a tendency to insomnia; higher doses merely exaggerate these effects. What is more, these drugs tend to be habituating; the body often develops a tolerance for them so that increasing doses are necessary to maintain the same effects, and when they are withdrawn after a period of use, an exceedingly distressing period of emotional depression may ensue. Thus, while these drugs undoubtedly have a useful role to play in weight control in some cases, their use should be carefully prescribed and controlled by the doctor. Certain other prescription drugs have appetite-controlling effects similar to amphetamines but without as many undesirable side effects. But whenever drugs of any kind are used for weight control, it is well to remember that at best they serve only as a crutch, and a very unreliable one if the will power necessary to maintain a weight-control program is lacking.

Finally, various organizations—both commercial and nonprofit—exist to help the overweight individual reduce. One should be wary of commercial weight-reducing salons or special diet products which advertise miraculous success, and at least consult a doctor before committing time and money to such programs. One voluntary organization, however, known as Weight Watchers, Incorporated, has established a good record for helping people who have had difficulty maintaining other weight-reducing programs. This organization, which operates on much the same principle as Alcoholics Anonymous, and has chapters in many communities, uses the positive reinforcement of fellowship, open recognition of the danger of excessive

weight, and mutual assistance and encouragement among members as a potent force to help the overweight person gain control of his weight problem. And indeed, more stress upon the positive benefits of losing weight, and less upon the dangers of continuing obesity, makes very good sense. Most obese individuals are both physically and psychologically uncomfortable—sometimes desperately so, whether they wish to admit it or not. Maintaining the proper weight takes a tremendous load off the heart and the respiratory system as well as relieving the musculoskeletal system of an excessive burden. Those who succeed in losing weight are rewarded by easier breathing, better physical condition, remarkably improved physical appearance, an ability to participate in many pleasurable activities that are difficult or impossible for the obese, and the ability to enjoy stylish clothing and a freedom of motion previously denied them. And because virtually everyone knows that weight control is not easy, the successful weight-reducer can also enjoy the hearty admiration of those around him even as he enjoys the prospect of better health, greater physical comfort, greater longevity and increased energy levels. Those who have succeeded bear happy witness that the rewards are worth the struggle.

Overexertion and Exercise

Most overweight people are at least aware of their obesity; it can rarely be said to sneak up on them. But another common hazard of the middle years, physical overexertion, often does.

It is perfectly natural for those in their middle years to have a well-established range of physical activities that put certain regular demands upon the body, whether at work or during leisure hours. It is also natural to expect to have certain physical reserves—excess energy or "demand capacity" that can be called upon under extraordinary circumstances. This, after all, is part of the makeup of the human body. Indeed, an awareness of and confidence in this built-in reserve, conscious or unconscious, is an important part of everyone's sense of well-being. The middle-aged man usually prefers to walk, for example, but he knows that he can run if he really has to. It may also be natural, if somewhat naïve, to assume that this physical reserve always remains the same. The truth is, however, that with advancing years physical capacities dwindle sharply; the underlying structure of the body simply cannot retain the strength and resilience it possessed in the prime years of the twenties and thirties. Those who assume that it does often find themselves in serious trouble when they attempt to call on physical reserves which are no longer there. The result of this kind of overexertion is frequently painful or even dangerous to health. Occasionally it can prove disastrous.

Obviously, this health hazard can be minimized by the realization that overexertion is a threat, and by the common sense to avoid it. Yet all too often people in their middle years attempt physical activities well beyond their capacities, or engage in some form of recreation or exercise that simply no longer makes sense. Shoveling snow, for example, is a perfectly normal activity for a young man, but it can be fraught with danger in later years. In fact, this single form of overexertion precipitates countless heart attacks every year. Other strenuous activities may take their tolls in less drastic but still painful ways. A middle-aged housewife who has spent two or three frantic weeks on a community project may suddenly collapse, physically unable to continue. The man who hardly lifts a finger all year round tramps ten miles through the woods on the opening day of hunting season, and is virtually paralyzed for the next three weeks with muscle stiffness. Another man tries pushing his stalled automobile to get it started one morning and discovers to his chagrin that in the exertion he has broken three ribs. And quite aside from the physical toll overexertion can take, it can also result in extreme fatigue, exhaustion, nervous tension and irritability.

Clearly, any kind of overexertion throws an excessive and hazardous burden on the body, and common sense should be enough to warn against it. For many, however, it is not quite that simple; it is painful to admit that one no longer has the physical capacities or reserves of previous years, particularly for those who have always derived considerable satisfaction from vigorous physical activity. Yet there is nothing quite so ridiculous or potentially damaging, both to the body and to the ego, as trying unsuccessfully to act like a college athlete when those days have gone forever. Typically, this kind of self-deception is practiced in two forms. First, there is the individual, man or woman, who believes he really could measure up to his former physical prowess, if he wanted to; but since he does not want to, he ends up doing nothing at all. And second, there is the individual who has to prove it, to himself or others, and ends up flat on his back. There is a big difference between overexertion and no exertion whatever, but they are similar in that both can pose a serious threat to the health. That threat can be avoided in only one way—a compromise between these two extremes in a *carefully controlled program of regular physical exercise*.

It is entirely possible to counteract the loss of physical reserves and to maintain a high level of physical conditioning by means of a sane, practical exercise program. And it is not only possible but essential to help counteract the ill effects of complete physical inactivity in the same way, for lack of adequate exercise can be as hazardous to people of middle age as overexertion. One result of inadequate exercise at this time of life is the development of obesity, discussed in detail on p. 927. But even more specific hazards may result. The respiratory reserves, for example, tend to diminish if the full natural breathing capacity is never taxed by moderate degrees of physical exercise. Muscles become flabby and incapable of producing the reserve that may be demanded by a sudden emergency. The appetite can become sluggish and the digestive tract less capable of handling desirable variations in the diet. Perhaps worst of all, cardiovascular function may be severely impaired by inactivity, with an increasing probability of trouble due to atherosclerosis, coronary artery disease or hypertension, all conditions that frequently come to a serious head during the middle years.

No program of exercise can be expected to recapture the strength and stamina of youth, but it can minimize the hazards of inactivity, contribute to overall physical and mental alertness and provide an accurate and useful awareness of just what the body can, and cannot, be called upon to do. But what kind of exercise program is desirable? This may vary greatly, depending upon the individual's own needs. Any exercise program should begin with a visit to a doctor for a careful professional assessment of the kind and amount of exercise that will be most useful in an individual case, together with careful consideration of the kind or amount of exercise that might be dangerous because of the individual's current physical condition. A truly effective exercise program will call forth physical reserves a little at a time, and then help maintain them at a level appropriate to the individual's age and physical condition. For some a gymnasium workout two or three times a week or a regular schedule of swimming, handball or tennis may provide a pleasant and practical form of physical conditioning. For others bicycle riding or an exercise bicycle in the basement may be the best answer. Many medical authorities feel that a regular program of jogging, begun cautiously after consultation with a physician in order to determine safe and sensible limits, can provide the best overall form of exercise for both men and women, since jogging not only exercises muscles but generates healthful extension of the cardiovascular and respiratory systems as well. For still others, weekend hiking or stream fishing regularly throughout the year will do the job. Even walking can be a beneficial form of exercise, so much the better if it is done on the golf course.

The most important thing, however, is not so much the kind of exercise as the amount, undertaken on a regular and continuing basis. Exercise fads or crash exercise programs, like similar diet programs, should be avoided, since they may in themselves constitute one of the most hazardous forms of overexertion. Any exercise program which is boring or inconvenient is not likely to endure for more than a few weeks at best, and as a long-term aid to health exercise should be an enjoyable part of everyday life for many years. Whatever the form of exercise, it should be undertaken slowly and gradually to build up the body in progressive and hopefully permanent stages, and in moderation to avoid the hazards of overexertion even when the body

seems to be in comparatively good shape. Without question a regular and carefully controlled program of exercise can markedly slow down the decline of physical strength and stamina which comes with advancing age, and provide a sense of physical fitness and well-being that cannot be attained in any other way.

The Menopausal Syndrome

From the time of puberty through the age of about forty-five, regular monthly ovulation and a subsequent periodic menstrual flow when pregnancy does not occur is part of the natural living pattern of women. This cycle of ovulation and menses is controlled by the balanced production and interaction of a variety of sex hormones manufactured in the ovaries, the adrenals, the pituitary and elsewhere. (*See* p. 763.) The time eventually comes, however, when ovulation and menstruation cease, and the woman's ability to conceive and bear children comes to an end. This period of physical and often emotional change is known as *menopause*. It is as natural as it is inevitable, and yet it is often a trying and even traumatic time of life.

In some women menopause may begin as early as the age of forty; in others it may be delayed until the early fifties; the vast majority of women, however, become menopausal in the five-year period between forty-five and fifty. Further, ovulation and menstruation do not suddenly stop; rather they decline gradually and sometimes erratically over a period of months or even years. Popular myth to the contrary, by far the overwhelming majority pass through this period with little or no trouble. But for some the distress is very real indeed and enduring enough to require medical attention. In general, menopausal distress, when it occurs, involves a combination of disquieting physical symptoms, an interval or recurrent intervals of intense nervous irritability, and a certain degree of emotional lability or changeability, all of which seem to be beyond conscious control. Any of these manifestations may occur singly or in combination, but fortunately all of them can be effectively prevented or treated.

What brings about these changes at menopause? Strange to say, no one knows for certain, nor does anyone know why one woman passes through this period without any significant distress while another may suffer inordinately. Certainly an alteration in the balance of sex hormones plays an important part. One of the most common physical symptoms of menopause is a sudden wavelike sensation of heat, flushing or tingling in the face and extremities, the so-called hot flashes, which are both physically uncomfortable and sometimes alarming in their intensity. For years gynecologists, reasoning that the end of ovulation is intimately associated with a sharp reduction in the natural supply of the sex hormone estrogen, have successfully treated hot flashes with injections of estrogen or with estrogen-containing medicines administered orally. Similarly, another common physical symptom during menopause is periodic episodes of water retention, as evidenced by puffiness or swelling of the ankles, combined with an increased degree of nervous irritability—symptoms very similar to those noted by many younger women during the few days prior to the onset of the menstrual period and sometimes referred to as "premenstrual tension." (*See* p. 762.) The sex hormones as a group have the capacity to cause the body to retain fluid, and it seems clear that the changing balance of various of these hormones at menopause accounts for these symptoms, which often can be relieved with the administration of a simple diuretic and the temporary reduction of the amount of salt taken with the diet.

The nervous and emotional manifestations of menopause, when severe enough to cause distress, can be more difficult to deal with. Psychiatrists have proposed a number of theories to account for some of these emotional disturbances. It has been suggested, for example, that women are unconsciously frightened by the incontrovertible physical evidence that they have lost the capacity to conceive and bear children; that they fear this lack of fertility will diminish their husbands' affection for them, on one hand, or that they will be unable to respond to their sexual demands on the other. Certainly it cannot be denied that sexual function and emotional behavior are intimately related throughout life,

and that menopause represents a profound change from the "normal" that has prevailed for thirty years or more. It is hardly surprising that a woman under these circumstances might feel some distress, or even a profound sense of emotional insecurity, perhaps aggravated by the realization that time is running out and that youth and physical beauty are fading. She may also feel that her children, approaching maturity themselves, no longer need her, and that her marriage has become a dull routine, rather than the loving supportive relationship of earlier years. Her husband may be preoccupied with his activities, and because this is the time when men, too, become concerned about their own fading youth and sexual potency, she may fear that he will be tempted to look elsewhere for reassurance, love, or just a break in the routine, if he has not already done so. And indeed, this actually happens often enough to lend some substance to such fears.

There is certainly no one who can provide more concrete help in combating such distressing emotional reactions than the husband himself, although it is unlikely that it will occur to him naturally to do so. For one thing, he is not undergoing the physical changes that bring such thoughts into focus in a woman's mind; for another, he may well have physical and psychological problems of his own that his wife fails to understand. But often with the intercession of a knowledgeable and trusted medical adviser, a husband can recognize the very great need that may exist for his emotional support, understanding and patience during this difficult period. At the same time, his participation may help him realize that time is changing him, too, and with that shared understanding both husband and wife can reinforce their own relationship and face together the emotional problems that are an inevitable part of approaching middle age.

There is also an ever growing armamentarium of medications that can help with the emotional distresses of menopause when they occur. One of the many tranquilizing drugs can help restore emotional balance and counteract irrational worries and baseless fears. Tranquilizers are frequently overused and often abused in our society, but when prescribed carefully and taken in moderation for specific purposes, they can be a very real help.

Fortunately, menopause even at its worst does not last forever; the woman who is severely tried by physical symptoms or emotional reactions usually finds that they subside spontaneously within a few months once a new hormonal balance has been established. What is more, there are certain positive aspects to menopause that deserve mention. Although ovulation and menstruation come to an end, the enjoyment of sexual relations need not; indeed, with the possible complication of pregnancy finally removed, a great many women experience a significant revival of sexual interest and an increased pleasure in the act. Neither does menopause necessarily signal the end of physical attractiveness; if a woman begins to "fall apart" at that age, it is probably the fault of negligence rather than of menopause. Sensible eating and drinking habits and adequate exercise are just as important for the woman of middle years as for the man. Further, although menopause does indeed signal a "change of life," the nature of the change is largely up to the woman herself; many women, free from the cyclic inconvenience of menstruation and frequently less burdened, at this time of life, with domestic responsibilities, are able to undertake outside activities and even full-time careers with much satisfaction and notable success. Certain commonsense precautions are in order, however. Although menopause does not automatically bring with it the threat of cancer, careful and regular self-examination of the breasts (see p. 450), prompt investigation of any sign of postmenopausal bleeding (see p. 939), and regular medical examinations including Pap tests to detect any sign of early cancer of the cervix are essential not only to continuing good health during the menopausal years, but to continuing peace of mind as well.

The Hazard of Depressive Reactions

In recent years physicians have become increasingly aware of a type of destructive emotional state that afflicts a great many people in their middle and later years, a condition that often goes totally unrecognized. This emotional hazard is known as the depressive reaction, or simply *depression*. It is characterized not merely by the "blues" which are an entirely normal emotional reaction that may occur from time to time at any point in life, but rather by a pervading sense of helpless gloom, a mixture of frustration and grief that can, on occasion, become so profound that the victim is virtually immobilized. Often the depression is accompanied by a looming sense of insecurity, a feeling of worthlessness and a loss of self-esteem. The victim may feel that life is totally meaningless and display a lack of interest in the events and activities that were once important to him, even cutting himself off from his family and friends. This reaction can affect both men and women, but often it is masked or disguised. In some, it may manifest itself primarily as an increasing degree of anxiety and worry, sometimes based upon real concerns, but more often irrational or unconscious apprehensions. At other times it may take the form of increasing ill temper and irritability. In its most profound form it can become a full-blown state of psychotic withdrawal which is still known today as involutional melancholia. (*See* p. 805.)

Depressive reactions, even when not that severe, can be extremely painful to the victim as well as to his family. They can also be profoundly disorganizing to an otherwise stable and comfortable life. Because they can lead to inattention or indifference to other aspects of health care, they can also precipitate physical illness and undo the value of years of preventive medicine. Occasionally, and often quite shockingly, they can result in suicide. Diagnosis of this condition, or its true depth, is very difficult at first, but individuals who are subject to periods of depression tend to establish a pattern of behavior that becomes clearly recognizable to doctor, family and patient alike once it has been identified.

Until recently there was little help for milder states of depression other than waiting for them to pass; the tranquilizing drugs, while sometimes helpful in relieving the anxiety that accompanies these reactions, seldom relieved the depression itself. Sometimes the mood-ameliorating drugs—

Ritalin (methylphenidate), for example, or the amphetamines—in moderate dosages could help turn a depression, but such drugs carried side effects which often made them dangerous for people in this age group. Profound and continuing degrees of depression were sometimes treated, often quite successfully, with electroshock therapy. (*See* p. 803.) In recent decades, however, a new family of drugs, often described as "psychic energizers," have appeared on the scene and hold forth real hope for the treatment and relief of depressive reactions without the potential dangers of shock therapy. Exactly what these drugs do in terms of physiology or biochemistry is not yet clearly understood; in use, they seem gradually to alleviate the depression while at the same time slowly stimulating or energizing the mental functions of the patient, enabling him to return to his normal life and activities free from pointless anxiety and worry. Often these medications must be used for prolonged periods and sometimes in high dosages; they do not work in a matter of a few minutes or hours like aspirin, but rather have a cumulative effect over days and weeks. Much has yet to be learned about their use, and they must still be considered potent and dangerous drugs, to be taken only under the prescription and careful supervision of a physician. But if their promise holds good, they may well provide a reliable, safe and much-needed answer to one of the most perplexing and frustrating health hazards that can afflict those in their middle years.

The Hazard of Cancer

Middle age, with its inevitable decline in physical function, is the time of life when virtually everyone becomes increasingly vulnerable to a variety of degenerative diseases and disorders. Perhaps the most prevalent, and certainly the most dreaded, of these diseases is cancer, and it ranks with arteriosclerosis, hypertension and old age itself as one of the greatest enemies of human life, an enemy that even today, after decades of the most intensive and highly specialized medical research, has not yet been conquered. Giant strides have been made in the diagnosis and treatment of cancer, but as yet there is no way to prevent it.

The fact is, however, that in individual cases even the most skilled and knowledgeable physician is, by himself, virtually helpless in combating malignant disease. He must depend more heavily upon each patient's knowledge, common sense and cooperation in dealing with cancer than in any other kind of disorder; in no other situation is a truly cooperative relationship between doctor and patient more important. But for all that has been written about this disorder, a shocking number of people are still ignorant of the most basic facts about cancer. This ignorance is tragic enough when early danger signs are disregarded or go unrecognized, but it is even more tragic when they are recognized and yet the patient is so frightened of cancer that he postpones medical attention to the point that effective treatment is no longer possible.

It has been said repeatedly, but it cannot be emphasized too much—*cancer can be cured and even totally eradicated, never to recur, in a great many cases if treatment is started early enough.* In many other cases not quite so fortunate, cancer can be treated so effectively that its victims may enjoy as many as five, ten or even more years of comfortable and productive life before final recurrence of the disease. Indeed, there are cancers once regarded as "terminal illnesses" which now, thanks to modern methods of treatment, are regarded more as "chronic diseases" with which the victim can live for years that would otherwise be lost to him. Finally, even in advanced cases, diagnosis and treatment can alleviate symptoms, help control pain, and permit the victim to live out his remaining weeks or months in relative comfort.

Virtually every organ and tissue in the human body is vulnerable to cancerous growth. The cancers that affect specific organ systems are discussed in detail in those chapters dealing with the other diseases and disorders of that system. But here it is important to describe cancer not as a single disease, but as a class or family of diseases, along with certain general characteristics that all cancers have in common, the signs and symptoms they cause and the modern techniques of diagnosis and treatment. It cannot be denied that cancer can be one of the most painful and destructive of all human illnesses, but nothing is accomplished by speaking of it in hushed whispers or refusing to admit that it exists. On the contrary, a knowledge of just what cancer is, and an honest awareness of the hazard it may pose, especially in the middle and later years, is an important first step in combating this disease.

What Is Cancer? Under normal conditions the various tissues of the body exhibit a predictable pattern of growth at various times in the individual's life. In the newly conceived embryo the fertilized ovum at first merely divides and then redivides, doubling its number of cells with each division but with all the "daughter cells" essentially identical to the "parent cells" from which they came. Doctors speak of these early embryonic cells as *undifferentiated* because none of them at first shows any tendency to develop into special kinds of tissue. Later, certain cells become *differentiated;* that is, they begin to take on the characteristics and functions of nerve, liver, bone or muscle cells, and thereafter these differentiated cells are responsible for the further growth and development of the special tissues and organ systems of which they are a part. At the time of birth virtually all of these specialized tissues and organ systems have been differentiated, but there is, of course, a long period of further growth; thus the final stages of differentiation of some tissues may be delayed for several years. The tissues of the ovary and the testis, for example, do not differentiate in the mature form capable of producing ova or spermatozoa until puberty. Others, such as the brain cells, are fully differentiated at birth and merely increase in size and length, with no capacity to regenerate or develop new cells when old ones have been destroyed. In most tissues, however, once mature growth is reached, there is a slow and steady turnover of cells as old ones die and new ones regenerate to take their place. This orderly process is carefully controlled by the genetic material contained in each cell and ordinarily there is neither too much nor too little growth and regeneration at any time.

Occasionally, however, for reasons as yet not clearly understood, certain cells in a body tissue break away from the orderly and controlled pattern of normal growth and begin reduplicating themselves at a far greater rate of speed. This accelerated and uncontrolled cell growth often becomes detectable as an enlargement or swelling within the organ or tissue and is thus called a *tumor* from the Latin word meaning "to swell." More accurately, when a mass of new tissue of this sort persists and grows independently of its surrounding structures and has no apparent physiological use to the body, it is called a *neoplasm,* which simply means "new growth."

In many cases neoplasms are composed entirely of cells very similar in nature to the original tissue cells from which they grew, and they tend to remain clustered in the localized area of the tissue where their growth took place. Although they may take up space and have harmful effects on the body by stretching or exerting pressure on surrounding tissues, these new growths do not have any tendency to spread or *metastasize* by invading surrounding tissues or by seeding more distant tissues. Rather, they remain localized in the area in which they grew and separate from the tissues around them. Neoplasms of this sort are called *benign* tumors. This term does not necessarily mean that they do no harm, but it does indicate that whatever harm they do is a result of localized pressure in other organs or tissues in the area where they grow. Once discovered and identified, benign tumors in most cases can be surgically excised and thus permanently removed. Examples of simple benign tumors include moles on the skin, polyps in the nasal passages, and ordinary warts, all relatively harmless. But one type of benign tumor which is extremely dangerous is a *meningioma,* a benign tumor that grows from the cells of the meningeal tissue stretched over the brain within the skull. Although such tumors are technically "benign" and merely grow larger without sending cells out to invade surrounding brain tissue, they can nevertheless be life-threatening simply because they take up space within a confined area and the pressure exerted by their increasing size can often destroy delicate brain tissue.

Other neoplasms have sharply different characteristics. Some, for example, grow far more rapidly than the cells of a benign tumor, and often lose all similarity to the cells from which they arose. This kind of tumor is tissue growth gone wild, completely free from the elements that control normal tissue growth. The cells of these tumors soon tend to invade surrounding tissue, destroying healthy cells and in some cases growing so swiftly that they outgrow their own blood supply and tissue dies at the center of the tumor. In addition, they tend to lose the normal capacity of cells to stick together, and individual cells can break off from the tumor and be carried in the blood stream or lymphatics, like seeds in the wind, to distant parts of the body, where they implant and begin growing just like the original tumor. Tumors of this wildly uncontrolled, invasive and spreading type are called *malignant,* and they make up the group of grave disorders known as *cancer.* The place where a malignant neoplasm first begins its growth is spoken of as the *primary lesion;* the multiple neoplasms that result from the spread of cancerous cells to distant parts of the body are called *secondary* or *metastatic lesions.* The difference between a primary and a secondary malignancy, from the medical standpoint, is very simple: before a malignancy has grown to the point of metastasizing, detection of the primary site of growth and surgical removal of the malignancy can effect a cure; once the cancer has begun seeding to distant parts, surgical treatment is usually either useless or of very limited value, and the best that can be done is to attempt to restrict the growth of the seeded lesions to keep them from impairing vital functions until such time as their growth becomes uncontrollable.

There is no way to determine just when a primary cancer begins its metastatic spread, but certain types of malignancy show individual characteristics of growth which doctors know well. Certain cancers of the skin, and cancer of the cervix or mouth of the uterus, characteristically grow slowly, can often be detected early because they occur in areas accessible to examination, and therefore offer excellent chances for complete cure. Other malignant neoplasms tend to seed so very soon after their primary growth

has started that the fatal moment of metastasis has almost always already occurred by the time the primary lesion is detected. Still other cancers are difficult to detect in their early stages because they affect deep-seated organs not readily examined, and may have no early symptoms related to them at all. Thus by the time they have grown to the point that symptoms occur, metastasis has already taken place and the chance of cure when diagnosis is finally made is usually very poor.

Finally, there are certain kinds of tumors, originally benign, which may become malignant and begin to invade surrounding tissue at some point after a period of benign growth. Tumors known to follow this pattern are called "precancerous," and since there is no way to tell at what point the benign tumor changes into a malignant growth, these particular tumors must always be treated as if they were malignant until proven otherwise. An example of this kind of precancerous tumor is the rectal polyp, which grows in the mucous membrane of the lower end of the colon. The vast majority of rectal polyps discovered during routine physical examinations prove to be completely benign when removed and examined by the pathologist. Occasionally, however, the pathologist's microscope will reveal malignant change within the tissue of the polyp with evidence of spread to surrounding tissues. At this stage, these precancerous tumors can be completely removed; left to themselves, they would become true cancers of the rectum and ultimately could seed cancerous growths in other parts of the body.

Cancerous tumors can develop from virtually any kind of tissue or any organ in the body, and are sometimes classified and named according to the type of tissue or organ in which they originate. Thus malignant tumors which develop from the skin or mucous membranes of the body are often called *epithelial carcinomas* or *squamous cell carcinomas,* while malignant tumors developing from connective tissue, bone or muscle are called *sarcomas,* and those which develop from glandular or secreting tissue in the body are called *adenocarcinomas.* Among adenocarcinomas, physicians sometimes make a further distinction between *functioning tumors,* in which the cancerous tissue continues to produce the secretions of the precursor gland, often in such quantity as to cause symptoms in itself, and *nonfunctioning tumors,* in which the wild cell growth has lost the ability to secrete. Obviously, this distinction can be particularly important in the case of cancers of such vital hormone-secreting organs as the various endocrine glands. In general, however, all these distinctions are more important to the doctor seeking to determine the ideal form of treatment than they are to the patient, who must be primarily concerned with the harm any cancer can do, its symptoms and how it can be detected early enough to make possible a cure.

What exactly do cancerous tumors do that is bad for the body, and how can they ultimately take life? Answers to these questions depend upon the kind of cancer and its characteristic pattern of growth. Early in their development cancers may appear to do no harm at all, but as the primary lesion begins to invade surrounding tissue massive cell destruction may occur. Similarly, wherever a secondary lesion implants and begins to grow, it destroys tissue and impairs the function of the invaded organ. Finally, a malignant growth anywhere in the body may erode through major or minor blood vessels, leading to hemorrhages which may, in themselves, be massive enough to be fatal. Any of these changes may bring pain, progressive loss of normal body functions and ultimately death. But even in the absence of such acute complications, growth of a cancer has other widespread and generalized debilitative effects. Often the body becomes toxic, a persisting fever occurs, and such symptoms as nausea, vomiting or loss of appetite appear. A marked weight loss begins, and the victim becomes unable to eat even when he knows his body is wasting away. Meanwhile the burgeoning growth of the cancer drains whatever energy remains until ultimately the victim may die from sheer exhaustion or starvation.

What Are the Symptoms of Cancer? Under certain circumstances cancer can produce virtually *any* symptom. But over the years certain particular symptoms have so frequently been associated with the early development of cancer that they serve as potential warning signs that

must not be ignored. It is important to bear in mind that other conditions may also cause these symptoms, and thus their discovery does not necessarily mean cancer. But their appearance should be regarded as a red danger flag, and their cause should be determined as quickly as possible. If the symptoms prove to be due to cancer, chances are that it is in the early stages of development and something can be done about it; if they are *not* due to cancer, their cause can usually be corrected and the mind relieved of worry. Among the most notable of these symptoms are the following:

Persistent hoarseness. This symptom may frequently result from perfectly benign causes, but it may also be an early clue to the development of cancer of the larynx.

Difficulty in swallowing. This symptom often appears early in the development of cancer of the throat or esophagus.

A lump in the breast or discharge from a nipple. Either or both of these symptoms may be an early sign of carcinoma of the breast, one of the most common of all cancers among women, and one, if detected and treated early in its development, that can be completely cured. In the vast majority of cases, breast cancer is first discovered by the woman herself performing a routine breast self-examination. Every woman should perform this self-examination carefully and regularly and lose no time in reporting any abnormality to her doctor. (*See* p. 450.)

A persistent cough. Many people shrug off this symptom as "smoker's hack," but it can be an early symptom of cancer of the lung. Smokers in particular should be alert to any increase in the frequency of coughing, and should have a chest X-ray taken at least every six months. Cancer of the lung is notorious for spreading beyond control before its earliest symptoms appear; thus even nonsmokers should have chest X-rays taken at least once a year.

Any abnormal bleeding. A doctor should be consulted at the first appearance of abnormal bleeding. Blood coughed up from the lungs or bronchial tubes, usually bright red in color, may signal lung or bronchial cancer. Vomited blood is usually a black grainy material resembling coffee grounds, and may indicate bleeding from a cancer of the stomach. The passing of red blood per rectum suggests a bleeding source far down in the colon, whereas passing a sticky black material resembling tar signals bleeding from some place higher up; either symptom may indicate cancer of the gastrointestinal tract. Any abnormal vaginal bleeding which appears between menstrual periods or which occurs after menopause should be investigated immediately. There are many gynecologic sources of abnormal vaginal bleeding other than cancer, just as some other condition may cause any form of abnormal bleeding, but again there is no sense taking a chance.

Any changes in a mole or pigmented area on the skin. Any increase in size or change in color may indicate that a benign mole has become a malignant tumor.

Unexplained fever. An occasional transitory episode of low-grade unexplained fever may arise from a dozen benign causes and is no reason for alarm. But a fever which persists without explanation, or which recurs, should be investigated. A persisting or recurring fever of unknown origin is frequently a clue to a hidden or "occult" infection, but it may also occur with certain kinds of cancer.

Unexplained weight loss. It is a rare person who loses weight under normal circumstances unless he is dieting. Thus any unexplained weight loss should be investigated, as it can be a clue to the development of cancer.

Any sore that does not heal. A lesion anywhere on the body that seems to resist healing for an abnormal length of time should be examined by a doctor without delay, as it may be a sign of early cancer.

How Is Cancer Diagnosed? The first step in diagnosing cancer is, of course, a complete physical examination. A careful evaluation of symptoms and other physical findings will often rule out the possibility of cancer, but when the possibility remains, certain laboratory tests are particularly helpful in making the diagnosis. Liver function tests, for example, can reveal patterns of malfunction that may indicate the presence of cancer. Certain enzyme systems in the body characteristically go awry in the presence of specific forms of cancer, and this can be detected by blood tests. Rarely does a doctor make a diagnosis on the basis of an abnormal laboratory test alone, but laboratory facilities can often aid in pinpointing cancer or help rule it out.

Perhaps the most important diagnostic technique lies in X-ray examinations. Lung cancers, for example, are often first suspected when an abnormal shadow is found on a chest X-ray. Gastrointestinal cancers or primary or secondary cancers of bone can often be seen in diagnostic X-rays. What is more, radiologists have recently developed new X-ray examination techniques to help in the detection of certain cancers. In the past few years *X-ray mammography,* a special technique for examination of the female breast, has proved to be of great value in helping the physician judge whether a lump in a woman's breast is likely to prove benign or malignant. Similar new techniques are continually being explored and perfected.

In many cases physical examination, laboratory tests and X-rays are sufficient to confirm the presence of cancer, but at times a diagnosis still cannot be made with certainty. It is in cases of this sort that *surgical biopsy* of a suspicious lesion becomes necessary; a portion of the tissue in question is excised surgically and then examined by a pathologist. In certain instances the biopsy may be done as a separate preliminary procedure, with the decision for further surgical exploration postponed until the pathologist can examine the suspicious tissue. Thus a surgeon who encounters an abnormal shadow on a chest X-ray, which he suspects might be carcinoma of the lung, may perform a *scalene node biopsy;* the small lymph glands in the neck just above the collarbone are removed surgically and examined for any evidence of the spread of cancer, since lung cancers most frequently first seed the lymph nodes in the chest and neck before spreading elsewhere.

In other cases, however, when it is considered dangerous to delay surgical excision if the biopsy shows cancer, a so-called frozen section biopsy can be performed while the patient remains in the operating room. For example, when a woman has a lump in her breast which is suspicious of cancer, it is customary for the surgeon to remove the lump itself, together with a small amount of surrounding breast tissue, and have the pathologist perform a frozen section examination of the mass then and there. The procedure involves freezing a segment of the biopsied tissue with compressed carbon dioxide, then making microscopically thin slices of the tissue and staining them for immediate examination, a procedure that can be performed in a matter of 15 or 20 minutes. If the pathologist determines that the lesion is benign, the surgeon then simply closes the small biopsy wound. But if he finds evidence of malignancy, the surgeon proceeds to do a widespread excision of the diseased breast and underlying tissue in hopes of removing all the adjacent areas to which the cancer might already have spread. The development of such biopsy techniques has been one of the great surgical steps forward in dealing with cancer, and frozen sections are often helpful in establishing (or ruling out) the diagnosis of cancer in many parts of the body.

How Is Cancer Treated? Benign tumors are normally either excised if their presence is troublesome or if they are known sometimes to be precancerous, or else left alone, depending upon the tumor and the physician's judgment. Malignant tumors, however, must be destroyed, together with any secondary tumors that have seeded from the primary, if cure is to be obtained. In most cases surgical excision of the cancer is the treatment of choice, particularly if the cancer is believed to be early in its development, and if there is as yet no detectable evidence of its having spread to adjacent or distant tissues. If the excision succeeds in removing all of the cancer down to the last trace, that cancer will be cured. Another cancer may conceivably develop in some other part of the body, but the original one will not recur. Unfortunately, it is often impossible to be absolutely *certain* that a given cancer has been completely removed before any of its cells have metastasized to distant areas. This means that periodic reexamination of the patient is necessary to detect any possible recurrence. Thus, rather than claiming absolute cure, physicians normally speak of "five-year cures" or "ten-year cures," which indicates that after excision there has been no evidence of

recurrence for five or ten years respectively. There are recorded cases, however, in which previous cancers have recurred as long as fifteen or twenty years after the original surgery; but in general the patient who has achieved a "five-year cure" has a very good chance of escaping recurrence, and a "ten-year cure" patient has an even better chance.

In some kinds of cancer that are known to be particularly sensitive to radiation, X-ray therapy or radium or radon therapy may be used either before surgery to reduce the size of the cancer or after surgery in hopes of destroying any seeded cancer cells that the surgeon could not detect. Since the first discovery of radioactivity in the late 1890s, it has been known that various forms of radiation in sufficient dosages could destroy living tissue, and it was soon found that the abnormal cells present in many cancers were much more vulnerable to radiation damage or destruction than healthy tissue cells. Thus radiologists sought to impair the growth of cancers, or even destroy them, by applying just enough radiation to the region of the tumor to damage the sick cells while leaving surrounding healthy tissue unharmed. Today radiation therapy is still one of the most swiftly growing fields of medicine as new techniques for the treatment of cancer are explored. For example, most major hospitals now have radioactive cobalt therapy equipment which permits an extremely intense irradiation of a small portion of the body containing a cancer with less damage to surrounding tissues than was possible with other radiation techniques. When the cancer is discovered to have invaded some vital organ so that excision might in itself prove fatal, or when the cancer's spread is found to be so wide that it is impossible to excise all of it surgically, and removing just a part of it would not benefit the patient, the cancer is considered to be *inoperable* and radiation therapy is often used as an alternative to radical surgery. Usually this treatment is palliative rather than curative because only a very few kinds of cancer are completely destroyed by radiation at dosage levels the patient can tolerate. Nevertheless, skillful radiation therapy may well cause temporary regression of the size of a cancer and may curb its wild growth for an indefinite period of time, thus offering the patient months or years of life before the disease again begins its inevitable march.

Finally, a great number of chemotherapeutic agents, potent drugs, usually quite toxic or poisonous, which damage or destroy cancerous cells more readily than the surrounding healthy tissue, have been used as a means of slowing down the growth of certain kinds of cancer. Leukemia, for example, can often be controlled by the use of certain of these toxic chemicals, at least for a while. Often these drugs are reserved by the physician until after surgical treatment in order to have them ready to use in the event of any sign of recurrence. In other cases they may be used concurrently, either with surgery or with radiation therapy, if the cancer is such that the doctor believes that every major weapon available should be used at once in hopes of obtaining a cure or prolonged palliation. In addition to these toxic chemicals, there are forms of cancers whose growth can be severely inhibited by certain natural or synthetic hormones. Cancer of the prostate gland in the male, for example, is often markedly retarded by administering female sex hormones or estrogens. On the other hand, male sex hormones or androgens are sometimes of value in combating recurrences of breast cancer in females after surgery.

As for the prognosis, the anticipated end result of cancer treatment, many different things must be taken into account. The chances for a cure, of course, are always better when a cancer is discovered early. The odds for cure are also much greater when thorough surgical excision is possible and when no evidence of spread to surrounding or distant tissues can be found. In some patients there may be a marked and prolonged beneficial response first to surgery, then to radiation therapy, and then later to chemotherapy or hormone therapy, with resultant control over the disease for years even when cure is not possible. But in other cases of virtually identical cancer, the patient may pursue a steady, rapid downhill course, failing to respond even slightly to any kind of treatment. No one knows why this happens in one patient and not in another.

In summary, every form of cancer has its own peculiar characteristics which may make the outlook more or less favorable for cure or long survival. And in spite of the concentrated efforts of researchers all over the world, the disease still remains a dangerous and unpredictable medical mystery. But researchers have by no means given up. One day, perhaps even soon, a cure for cancer—or a group of cures for different kinds of cancer—will be discovered. The underlying cause of most cancers is still unknown, and a great many causative factors have been implicated; but in recent years there has been increasing evidence that viruses may play a critical role. It is known, for example, that viruses enter cells in various tissues, and often have the capacity to alter the genetic makeup of the host cells, making them behave in ways that they are not normally programmed to do. Since it appears that cancers arise as a result of some change in the genetic makeup of certain cells which alters the natural controls over the rate and amount of growth of those cells, it is not surprising that researchers have long been suspicious of viruses as at least one causative agent in cancer. Certain viruses have even been clearly identified with specific cancers in animals, and researchers today are hot on the trail of viruses that may be causative in human cancers as well. Precisely which viruses no one yet knows, nor do we know how or why they are acquired by some people and not others, or how people could be protected against them. It is certain, however, that if specific viruses are indeed found to be important causative agents, then at some time vaccination against them may offer widespread protection against cancer. Meanwhile, every possible avenue to prevention, treatment and cure is being explored in an immense, world-wide research program, and whether vaccination becomes possible or not, it is entirely possible that in the years ahead "magic bullets" will be discovered to control or destroy cancerous growths, and that we will learn enough about the effects of this disease on the body that laboratory examinations can be devised to make early detection far easier than it is today. Until then, the best protection an individual has against this disease is not fear or panic, but watchful concern and immediate action any time the symptoms suspicious of cancer are encountered.

Other Health Hazards in Middle Age

Cancer is unquestionably a major hazard to health during the middle years, but it is not by any means the only disease process that threatens at this time in life. Arteriosclerotic heart disease, for example, often first begins to manifest itself at this time, and these are the years when coronary thrombosis first strikes its victims, when hypertension can become severe and debilitating, when gall bladder disease, kidney disease and a multitude of other "physical breakdown" diseases can begin to appear.

There was a time when the most that could be done was to sit quietly and wait for these or other diseases to manifest themselves with symptoms, and then struggle as best one could, often against serious odds, to accomplish cure. Today we are no longer so helpless. Indeed, it is precisely because modern medical techniques have made early discovery of these diseases of the middle years, including cancer, possible and thus massively improved the chances of cure that the whole concept of preventive medical care is so vitally important. In earlier years health care is often neglected with impunity. In the middle years such neglect can be suicidal. The only rational protection against the hazards of cancer and other degenerative diseases is to be thoroughly knowledgeable of their signs and symptoms and alert to their appearance; to make full use of the laboratory facilities and diagnostic X-ray techniques that are available; and to provide the family physician with the opportunity to perform periodic and thorough physical examinations in order to detect the early development of any illnesses at a time when control or even cure is possible.

This does not mean that the middle-aged man or woman must live in the doctor's office. But it does mean that symptoms, even relatively minor symptoms, must not be shrugged off. A persistent cough, persisting hoarseness, difficulty in swallowing, digestive distress or abdominal pain, sores that do not readily heal, changes in moles on the skin, coughing or vomiting blood or the passage of blood per rectum, abnormal vaginal bleeding, pain or distress upon urination, shortness of breath, persisting headaches, recurring fevers, night sweats, weight loss or loss of appetite—all these are symptoms that may have no significance at all, but any one of them can also be a vital clue to the presence of a disorder that must be dealt with promptly. The rewards of such diligence—of such ordinary, commonsense attention—can be very great indeed. Not merely additional years but additional decades of comfortable and productive life may be achieved. Middle age can, and should, be among the healthiest and happiest years of life, but good health can never be taken for granted; during the middle years it becomes more precious with every passing day.

Aging and Death

One of the most dramatic indications of the improving quality and efficiency of health care in the United States since the beginning of this century is the almost incredible increase in the life expectancy of the average citizen; that is, the number of years a newborn baby can be expected to live as of the time of his birth. In the year 1900 the average life expectancy of newborn babies in this country was estimated at 47.3 years—46.3 years for males, 48.3 years for females. In 1970, the most recent year for which these statistical estimates are available, the average life expectancy had increased to 67.1 years for the male, 74.6 for the female. These figures reflect a long-recognized fact: the average life expectancy of females has always been somewhat higher than that of males, and the difference increases with the increasing average age of the population. They also reflect a less readily apparent fact; if the figures are broken down between the white and nonwhite population, the average life expectancy of white males and females is between six and eight years longer than that for nonwhites—a clear indication that the average nonwhite family, often living in conditions of urban or rural poverty, does not have the amount or the quality of health care that is available to the average white family. Even so, increased medical knowledge and the greater availability of medical care have had a profound impact upon the overall life expectancy of the population, and there is no question that a great majority of those who live out longer lives do so in far better health and with

far greater freedom from illness than ever before. Certainly this represents the achievement of a major goal in preventive health care.

Success in one area, however, often creates problems in another, and the significant increase in the average life expectancy in this country is no exception. It has brought with it an equally significant increase in the total number of aging and aged men and women among the population, and this change in itself has created both social and health care problems of the greatest magnitude. At the beginning of the century truly aged people were comparatively uncommon. A great number of people died during their middle years while still actively involved in their working lives. In an average family perhaps one of the four grandparents might survive to be sixty-five, seventy or older; and by and large, the aged continued to live with one or another of their children, making up a natural and accepted part of the family circle. When illness struck, it was ordinarily handled like any other illness in the family; the elderly patient was cared for at home, if possible, or the children or grandchildren met the cost of medical care if the patient had no economic resources of his own. This was the normal pattern of life, and very few families gave serious consideration to any other.

Today that pattern has changed markedly. Now it is only seldom, except among families living in very poor circumstances, that the elderly take up residence with their children and grandchildren. Often it is a matter of personal preference: the elderly do not want to be a "burden" to their children, if they have the means to avoid it, nor do they want to give up their independence. Further, more and more of the aged continue to enjoy relatively good health, and thanks to the benefits of Social Security, Medicare and tax relief for those over sixty-five, many are able, at least in large part, to take care of their own needs. They may choose to continue to maintain their own households, often living near but no longer with their families. Among the more affluent there has been a massive movement to take up residence in retirement communities—homes or apartments designed specifically to meet the needs of relatively healthy aging people, often including medical and hospital services to deal with the minor health problems that occur with increasing frequency. The usual age for retirement in this country is sixty-five, and at that age men and women are by no means necessarily "old." Many are interested in exploring new activities and making new friends among people their own age, and retirement communities can offer these opportunities. In fact, the mass migration of retired people to the parts of the country with pleasant year-round climates has resulted in remarkable population shifts in such areas as southern California, Arizona, New Mexico and Florida. There has also been an increasing emphasis on housing for the aged, usually for those with more limited means, in urban apartment complexes, and although these projects have been criticized as a form of segregation, they can offer the elderly an opportunity to maintain their independence and take part in group interests and activities.

Many, however, are not able to do this. They may be reluctant to move from old friends and familiar neighborhoods, or they may not be able to afford it. The extremely aged, even though they may be in good health relative to their advancing years, nevertheless often need the kind of care and attention that only family and friends can provide, but their families may be unable to take on that responsibility, either for personal or for financial reasons. What is more, when illness does strike the aged, it is less likely to terminate abruptly in death than in decades gone by. The expenses of treatment can be enormous, or the condition may become chronic and require the kind of specialized care that the family cannot provide. To meet the needs of the elderly suffering from long-term chronic illness, multitudes of nursing homes have been established which provide professional medical supervision and care that is generally far less costly than hospitalization. Even so, they, too, can be expensive, and the decision to go to a nursing home, whether it is made by the elderly patient or his family, is a very difficult one. And finally, there is the problem of death itself. Whatever the other circumstances of life, the old person, and his family, must eventually come to terms with this ultimate enemy.

The social problems created by an ever increasing aged population are many and complex. These people are, in a very real sense, segregated from the more youthful world, often cut off from useful employment and even from social contacts with younger generations. They need adequate housing and the means to maintain independence and activity as long as possible, not in "geriatric ghettos" but as useful members of society. Ways must be found to utilize the wisdom, experience and abilities of the aged which, as history has repeatedly shown, can be remarkable indeed. Medical care for the aged is another problem; it must be provided at prices the elderly can afford, and some means must be found to meet the medical needs, often largely untended today, that lie in the gray area between reasonably good health on one hand, and illness requiring hospitalization or nursing home care on the other. In short, the concept of preventive health care must be expanded to include the needs of the aging as well as the young and the middle aged. Low-cost outpatient clinics emphasizing preventive health care could provide an enormously beneficial service, and they do so in those communities where they have been established. The medical field of *geriatrics* deals exclusively with the health care problems of the aged; the work of specialists in this field, known as *geriatrists,* has become increasingly important today and may well produce useful answers to the question of how good health can best be maintained during the declining years.

No lasting solutions to the social and medical

problems of aging can possibly be found, however, without the active cooperation and participation of the segment of the population that can help the most: the elderly themselves. Every aging individual faces unique and specific problems, and they can be solved successfully only by seeking to identify them in advance and then preparing and planning to meet them when they arise. Many of the physical and emotional problems of retirement, for example, could be avoided by advance planning. Problems of health maintenance could be minimized by knowledge of those changes that are normal in the process of aging and those that may signal more serious illness. Regular medical checkups are, of course, essential, as are thoughtful advance plans in case failing health requires hospitalization or nursing home care. Commonsense precautions and careful preparations, with the help of family and friends as well as the advice of a trusted medical consultant, are the only effective ways to deal with the problems of growing old. Today more than ever before, the elderly can look forward to many years of a relatively comfortable and healthy life. But the realization of that goal is to a great extent up to the individual.

A Healthy and Happy Retirement

There are few events that can have greater impact, for better or for worse, than retirement from an active job or career and the often abrupt change to a more leisurely and usually less structured way of life. In theory, such a change is viewed as a "reward": after years of hard work it is at last time to relax and enjoy the many activities that were once difficult or impossible. In fact, however, retirement proves to be a bitter disappointment for many—usually because they have not prepared themselves for it in advance.

Of course there are some people who never formally retire at all. Many self-employed business or professional men and women continue the pursuit of their lifework until the time they die. Others accept emeritus positions, contributing their services as consultants and reducing their activities only as they individually elect to

do so. These people, however, are the exception rather than the rule; in general, retirement is mandatory in this country, frequently forced at an age when the individual is not yet ready to cease work. Indeed, mandatory retirement often bears little relationship to the individual's continuing ability to contribute; it is simply viewed as a necessary business policy.

Whatever else it may be, retirement can hardly be welcomed if it is regarded—and accepted—only as being "put out to pasture." Everyone, young or old, needs to feel he is doing something useful and constructive. Everyone needs to feel needed; everyone needs to have his hours or days filled with relevant activity. To the aging individual, these are necessities to continuing emotional health, and to continuing physical health as well; in a very real sense a healthy body requires a happy mind, and all too many emotionally unfulfilled retirees spend increasing amounts of time brooding about their physical ailments and infirmities to the point that, like a self-fulfilling prophecy, their health indeed begins to break down.

Fortunately, the very fact that retirement is so often mandatory at a given age provides an opportunity for careful advance planning that can pay remarkable dividends in making the retirement years as fulfilling as earlier years in life. Assuming reasonably sound health, each individual can decide in advance whether he or she is willing and ready to retire completely, or whether other kinds of work can be sought. If the decision is to continue working, time and effort should be spent preparing for the new position; if formal employment is to be ended, time and thought must be directed to outlining the shape that retirement life is to take. Pleasure is important, of course, but so is continuing productive activity; many elderly people welcome retirement, for example, as an opportunity to expand their time and interest in useful social activities, on either a paid or a volunteer basis. Hobbies once limited to occasional leisure hours can be a source of continuing enjoyment and even profit. A part of the year can also be devoted to travel; in these days of mobile homes and campers, many couples, frustrated for years in their desire to travel, find in retirement the opportunity to realize their dreams both economically and enjoyably.

Obviously, financial planning is equally important if the elderly are to have the freedom to put their new leisure time to good use. Usually the financial base in retirement is more narrow than during full employment, and plans must be made to use funds that are available with every possible economy. Maintaining a large house, for example, may be an economic burden as well as hard work. Planning for future security must include not only the necessary living expenses but also the means to enjoy the pleasurable "extras" and, of great importance, the ability to meet unexpected medical costs. In general, financial plans should be primarily directed toward *freedom from worry,* insofar as possible, and toward setting a living scale that will be both practical and enjoyable now and in the years to come.

At the same time, retirement planning should take social and emotional needs into consideration. Provision should be made to maintain close ties with old friends and family, but new friends and new social activities should also be sought out as a spur to intellectual stimulation. In particular, the elderly person should make every effort to keep in touch with the young by not only taking an interest in the lives of his children and grandchildren, but also by participating in neighborhood and community activities and organizations. The effort will be repaid many times over in terms of richer, more interesting and varied lives for both the elderly and the young.

Finally, planning for retirement is predicated upon continuing good health, and rational steps must be taken to ensure that good health is maintained, insofar as possible. A program of preventive health care that is important at any time of life is all the more important during the declining years. Special attention must be paid to such health concerns as proper nutrition and adequate amounts of rest and exercise. Elderly people tend to eat less, and often become bored with cooking and dining, yet their nutritional needs remain basically the same as in earlier years and must be properly fulfilled. Many older people sleep less at night than they once did, but require additional rest at other times of the day.

And exercise, while necessary, can be scaled down according to the individual's physical capacities. In addition, regular medical examinations are essential to help discover any potential health hazards. Many older people draw back from medical checkups out of fear that something truly serious may come to light, but this attitude makes even less sense during the later years in life than it does earlier. Serious diseases and disorders may well occur in old age, but many can be cured provided they are detected early enough that irremediable damage has not yet occurred.

The fact that many of the health hazards of old age require surgical intervention also frightens many elderly people, yet there has never before been a time when surgery could be performed more successfully and with less distress and briefer convalescence than today, thanks to the enormous strides made in recent years both in surgical techniques and in anesthesia. Increasing health hazards are an inevitable part of the picture during the later years of life, and both planning for the care of health problems when they occur and increased vigilance against symptoms and conditions that may signal serious illness are essentials to a healthy and happy retirement.

The Physical Process of Aging

An important part of maintaining good health during the later years necessarily involves an understanding of those physical changes that are normal at this time of life and those that should be a cause for concern. No one knows precisely why the process of aging occurs, but certain changes begin as early as the third or fourth decade of life, and others appear at progressively later stages. These alterations in normal structure and function of the body with increasing age involve all of the organ systems, and in addition to those illnesses that may pose a threat at any time of life, certain kinds of disorders present particular hazards during the declining years.

Infectious Diseases. Although there are no infectious diseases which strike elderly people exclusively, there are certain kinds of infections which are more dangerous to the elderly because of changes that occur in the normal process of aging. Older people are less physically active than the young, of course, and have fewer energy reserves with which to fight off infections. Life is more sedentary, and nutrition is often poorer as well. Consequently even minor infections, such as head colds or other upper respiratory illnesses, tend to be more severe in the elderly. Viral infections in particular take a heavier toll among old people; they may drag on for weeks at a time and are more likely to be complicated by secondary bacterial infection. This is especially true of the various head cold and influenza viruses; winter flu is particularly dangerous to the elderly because it tends to be more severe, to cause more general debility, and to leave the victim more vulnerable to secondary bronchitis or pneumonia. For this reason, most physicians urge their older patients to have "flu shots"—influenza vaccinations—at the beginning of each winter season, and "cold shots" may also be helpful in minimizing the risk of head colds. It is also wise for the aging to seek medical attention at once any time an infection strikes. By careful attention to treatment, and by the use of broad-spectrum antibiotics to fend off possible bacterial infections that may come on the heels of viral infections, the risk of this kind of difficult infection can be substantially reduced.

Urinary tract infections can also be especially trying to older people. In males, hypertrophy or enlargement of the prostate gland often prevents complete emptying of the urinary bladder, leaving a reservoir of urine in the bladder to act as a medium for the growth of bacteria. In women a similar condition can occur owing to the breakdown of tissue supporting the bladder above the vagina, which permits an outpouching of the bladder known as a cystocele to form. Finally, *diverticuli* of the bladder—small outpouchings due to a breakdown in the muscular wall of the bladder, or *polyps* obstructing the bladder outlet, may afflict either men or women. Again, while these changes are not uncommon as a part of the aging process, the risk of continuing urinary tract infection can be minimized by early investigation of any urinary tract symptoms that

may appear, including increased urinary frequency, increased nocturia (nighttime urination), or any evidence of pain or burning associated with urination.

In short, the lowering of resistance and the increased vulnerability of the elderly to infections of any kind can be offset by increased vigilance and early medical consultation and treatment of any infections that may appear.

The Musculoskeletal System. Many changes occur in this organ system as a result of the normal process of aging. With advancing age the bones become increasingly brittle; in addition, calcium is gradually withdrawn from the bone, even when dietary supplies of calcium are adequate, resulting in a generalized thinning of the bone substance which is known as *osteoporosis*. Usually this does not become evident upon X-ray examination until the sixth or seventh decade of life, but the process probably begins in middle age. The cartilage covering the ends of articulating bones becomes gradually thinner than normal, while the ligamentous binding of the joints becomes less elastic, and the joint space becomes narrowed. These changes, which occur over a period of years, may cause no symptoms other than occasional episodes of joint pain, usually associated with episodes of overuse of the joint, but in some the changes progress to the degree that *osteoarthritis* becomes an increasingly disabling annoyance. The features of this condition and its treatment are discussed in detail elsewhere. (*See* p. 317.)

Another normal aging phenomenon is the gradual degeneration and narrowing of the cartilage pads that lie between the vertebrae, combined with an increasing degree of osteoarthritic overgrowth or "spurring" of the bodies of the vertebrae. As a result, elderly people actually tend to lose stature, and their spines become more rigid and immobile than before. Although these changes need not cause any specific symptoms, they do impair the speed and agility of motion, cause difficulty in turning the head or twisting the body, and contribute to a "slowing down" of physical activity. In addition, the body's ability to heal broken bones is markedly impaired with advancing age, so that fractures are a particular hazard to the elderly.

This hazard can be reduced by certain common-sense steps the older person may take. Wherever possible, living on a single floor of a house is easier—and less risky—than living in a house where stair climbing is necessary. When stairs in the home are unavoidable, special lift devices can be installed so that the strain of stair climbing not only on the musculoskeletal system but on the heart and respiratory systems as well may be reduced. Older women should substitute sensible flat-heeled shoes for the high-heeled variety. All older people should dispense with such common household hazards to stability as loose rugs, slippery floors, raised carpet edges or other nuisances, and must take particular care to avoid icy porch steps or sidewalks in the winter. Installation of metal handrails on the wall alongside the bathtub can help make it possible for elderly people to avoid potentially disastrous falls in the bath. Finally, the use of a cane as an additional support when walking need not be restricted only to those who cannot walk without one. Although many people indignantly regard the use of a cane as a concession to old age, the fact remains that a cane can provide a remarkable degree of additional support, and use of a cane as soon as one becomes aware of decreasing agility can prevent disabling and dangerous fractures.

In addition to skeletal changes, there is also a certain degree of muscle atrophy that occurs as part of the aging process, resulting in less physical strength and stability of motion than in earlier years. To a large degree, however, this change is a result of declining overall physical activity, and healthy muscle tone and strength can be maintained, even into very old age, with the aid of a program of regular physical exercise. Even when more vigorous forms of exercise from earlier years must be abandoned, a reasonable exercise program can and should be continued. Any such program should, however, be reviewed regularly by a physician and modified periodically, as necessary, to see that the form and amount of exercise is realistically within the person's physical capabilities, and to avoid the threat of overextension.

Many elderly people escape serious musculoskeletal problems for many years but still suffer intermittently from minor but annoying forms of distress: aching muscles, recurring episodes of bursitis, periodic low back pain, even a waxing and waning of discomfort from mildly arthritic joints. Victims of this sort of annoyance often chalk it up to "rheumatism" or just "growing old" and assume that nothing can be done about it. There are many medications available today, however, beginning with plain aspirin and including a whole spectrum of "safe and sane" analgesic and anti-inflammatory drugs, that can be used from time to time, as needed, to combat this form of distress. The time of a regular physical examination offers an ideal opportunity to discuss this kind of problem with the doctor and initiate a simple but effective treatment regimen which, in many cases, can virtually eradicate the "minor annoyance" type of aches and pains so often associated with aging.

The Nervous System. Changes in the nervous system as a result of the aging process are often more subtle than those occurring in the musculoskeletal system, and vary much more from individual to individual. A great many people suffer no noticeable nervous system deterioration at all for many years. Others may experience a gradual slowing down of mental activity, a slight but progressive impairment of reflexes, occasional difficulty following conversation or periodic difficulty selecting words or formulating answers. Some notice occasional memory lapses, often in relation to unimportant matters. Quite commonly there is diminishment of the senses of smell and taste, and hearing loss frequently occurs. In addition, changes in certain nerve centers and nerve circuits in the brain as a result of aging may lead to the development of such symptoms as tremors of the hands or head as well as changes in sleep patterns—insomnia at night, for example, together with a tendency to doze off from time to time during the day.

In general, however, changes in nerve tissue itself due to aging are comparatively minor; the major symptoms associated with impairment of brain or nervous system function among the elderly stem primarily from the impairment of other organ systems which causes secondary nervous system disfunction. For example, the development of bony projections or spurs on the vertebrae in the areas where the spinal nerves emerge, a result of developing osteoarthritis, may cause pressures on those nerves and lead to the intermittent aching in the limbs known as *neuralgia,* a common complaint of older people. A greater threat is the progressive impairment of blood circulation to the brain owing to arteriosclerosis of the cerebral blood vessels. In such a condition, great numbers of brain cells can be destroyed as a result of continuing long-term oxygen starvation, leading to the progressive widespread impairment of brain function associated with *senility,* including severe memory lapses, marked impairment of the speed and quality of mentation, and a progressive degree of "childishness" that often occurs as the higher brain centers are slowly damaged. In other cases a more dramatic kind of change may occur when an arteriosclerotic cerebral artery or arteriole is suddenly blocked by a blood clot or thrombus, causing a so-called *cerebrovascular accident* or *stroke.* A stroke may impair higher mental functions, interfere with sensory perception, and even lead to partial or complete paralysis of one or more limbs if the motor nerve centers of the brain are affected. Such serious disorders as progressive senility and cerebrovascular accidents are discussed in more detail elsewhere. (*See* p. 367 and p. 360.) The important point to be made here is that prevention of such disorders, insofar as it is possible, must depend upon preventive care of the cardiovascular system more than of the nervous system.

In short, most changes in the nervous system due to aging result from changes or disorders in other organ systems, emphasizing once again that the proper function of the body as a whole depends upon the proper function of all of its parts. In any regular physical examination, particularly among the aged, a careful assessment of nervous system function is essential, so that the doctor can detect any progressive change, however minor. He can then search out changes in other organ systems that may be contributing and take the necessary preventive or treatment measures as soon as they are indicated. In this regard, because nervous system changes are often less than obvious, and because symptoms are so often subjective—that is, more noticeable to the patient himself than to anyone else—the doctor must depend upon the patient's calling his attention to any changes that have been noticed, however minor or insignificant they may seem. Preventive measures may include things as diverse as modification of the diet to increase the intake of proteins, vitamins and minerals, medications to help improve cerebral circulation, mild sedatives to help overcome nervous irritability or the annoyance of insomnia, or gentle cerebral stimulants to help elderly patients feel more "perky" during their waking hours. Thus, although some degree of nervous system loss may be expected as an aspect of aging, much can be done to enable the aging individual to continue using his mind and nervous system to the highest degree of efficiency possible.

The Cutaneous System. Many of the most obvious—and to some, the most distressing—changes resulting from the normal aging process occur in the cutaneous system, in part because the skin, hair, teeth and nails are all on display, so to speak, for the world to see. With advancing years much of the fatty tissue underlying the skin is absorbed, while the elastic connective tissue fibers become stretched. As a result, the skin loses much of its turgor and wrinkling begins, a process that continues progressively throughout the remainder of life. In addition, because of progressive impairment of capillary circulation, the skin becomes thinner, smoother and shinier than in earlier years. In many people, especially those with fair complexions, large irregular pigmented areas known as *liver spots* may appear, particularly in the skin of the hands, arms and other exposed areas. Circulatory impairment also accounts in part for a progressive degree of thinning of the hair, not only on the scalp, but on other areas of the body as well, and the hair remaining becomes thinner and more brittle. Graying due to loss of pigment in the hair often starts as early as the second or third decade of life, but in most people becomes marked only in middle age or later. Male pattern baldness, discussed elsewhere (*see* p. 410), often proceeds at an accelerated rate, and although few aging women experience balding to the degree that it appears in males, general thinning of hair in females is often quite marked in the ages from sixty on.

For the most part such skin and hair changes are not only normal in aging people, but are also irremediable, and although many women seek to slow or mask these changes with the use of cosmetics or even such cosmetic surgery as "face-lifting" procedures, whatever improvement that is achieved tends to be only temporary. In the long run careful attention to adequate nutrition and commonsense hygienic care of the skin is of more value in holding skin changes to a minimum than the application of cosmetics, ointments, hormone creams or other expensive—and essentially useless—preparations. Acceptance of the inevitable changes as they come about is an important part of "growing old gracefully." In fact, the elderly person who keeps his body in trim and his mind active has a beauty and dignity all his own.

The loss of teeth and the need for dentures is by no means exclusively a problem of aging—poor dental care may result in the loss of teeth even during young adulthood—but many elderly people suffer needless anguish trying to avoid the necessity of dentures by making do with decaying, broken or missing teeth to the point that they are no longer able to masticate their food properly. Many such people condemn themselves to a progressively narrow range of foods that they can eat, substituting unappetizing or unpalatable soft or ground foods rather than taking the steps necessary to be fitted with adequate dentures. Eating becomes a chore rather than a pleasure, meals become irregular and nutritionally inadequate, and the overall result is a steady deterioration of eating habits that can, in many cases, lead to a degree of malnutrition verging upon starvation. Even more tragic are those elderly people still trying to use dentures fitted decades before which have become so ill-fitting, uncomfortable or unsightly that they are essentially useless. Obviously the best way to prevent this state of affairs is the maintenance of a lifelong program of preventive and corrective dental care; but even when this has not been done, proper dental attention undertaken later in life to preserve sound teeth when possible, or to provide attractive, comfortable and well-fitting dentures, need involve only modest expense and can pay handsome dividends in terms of comfort, appearance, good nutrition and continuing good health.

The normal process of aging can also, of course, affect the structure and function of such special sensory organs as the eyes, the nose or the ears. Little can be done to overcome the natural loss of the sense of smell that occurs with aging as a result of deterioration of the olfactory nerve endings in the nose; but this is fortunately the least important of all the senses, and the one most easily done without. The most striking natural change in vision that may begin any time from middle age on is impairment of accommodation—the ability to adjust quickly from close vision to distant vision and back. This occurs because the crystalline lenses in the eyes become gradually stenosed or hardened. Impairment of circulation to the retina may also lead to some decrease in visual acuity. Thus many aging people find it necessary to wear glasses for the first time in their lives, while those who have used glasses during earlier years often need adjustments. Because vision is perhaps the most precious of all our sensory contacts with the world around us, it is particularly important that elderly people have regular eye examinations as frequently as necessary to keep abreast of changes or deterioration in vision. Among other things, such examinations will enable the doctor to detect such potentially serious eye disorders as *glaucoma* (*see* p. 430), a condition that is reversible if discovered early enough, but which can cause blindness if treatment is not undertaken, or the development of *cataracts* (*see* p. 430), a clouding of the normally transparent lenses of the eyes that can cause progressively poorer visual acuity. There is no way that the development of cataracts can be slowed or prevented, but in cases in which vision is severely impaired they can be surgically removed, a comparatively simple procedure in the hands of an experienced ophthalmologist, and visual acuity restored by means of specially prepared corrective lenses.

A certain amount of hearing loss is also a normal part of the aging process, but the amount and nature of the loss may differ greatly from individual to individual. Often the loss is so slowly and subtly progressive that family members or friends recognize it before the victim does. At one time little could be done to correct hearing loss, but today a multitude of miniaturized and unobtrusive hearing devices are available that can restore hearing in most cases as long as the auditory nerve remains intact and functioning. In other cases hearing loss is due to the deterioration of the tiny bones or *ossicles* in the middle ear, a condition known as *otosclerosis,* and improvement in hearing can be achieved by a simple but delicate surgical procedure in which the normal vibratory motion of the ossicles is restored. Ideally, any degree of hearing loss should be assessed by a physician as soon as it is suspected. Most large communities also have speech and hearing centers where the kind and amount of hearing loss can be analyzed, and the patient can be referred for corrective treatment or fitted for a suitable hearing aid. Most authorities, however, emphasize that the best results are achieved if corrective treatment is undertaken early, before hearing is severely impaired—in short, as soon as any significant hearing loss is detected.

Respiratory System. There are surprisingly few changes in the structure of the respiratory tract organs as a result of aging per se, and most disorders of respiratory function that occur with advancing years arise from the impaired function of other organ systems, particularly the cardiovascular system, or else as a result of permanent damage to the lungs or bronchial tubes from diseases or disorders that arose earlier in life. Because elderly people tend to be more sedentary and limited in the amount of physical activity possible, they also tend to more shallow respirations, moving much less air in and out of the lungs with each breath. This not only reduces the individual's *vital capacity*—an indirect measure of the amount of fresh oxygen available for oxygenation of the blood with each breath—but it also leaves portions of the lungs underinflated, leading to the collection of mucous secretions in the smaller bronchial

tubes; the individual is thus more vulnerable to bronchial infections or pneumonia than in earlier years. In addition, the vertebral column, affected by some degree of spinal arthritis, is often bent forward and fixed so that the individual is more stooped or "hunched over" than normal, further crowding lung tissue and making full inflation of the lungs more difficult. As long as the elderly person remains physically active, with sufficient regular exercise to keep the lungs well inflated, this limitation of breathing space is of minor consequence and there is little threat from pulmonary stasis or incomplete respiratory filling; but if an illness should render the victim bedridden or otherwise immobile for long periods of time, this becomes a very real threat and special provision must be made to ensure enough movement in bed, together with forced respiration, to counteract the danger. It is for this reason that such an accident as the fracture of a hip is so much more dangerous to an older person than to someone younger; not only does the bone heal more slowly, but if the victim must be immobilized for prolonged periods, he is also in grave danger of troublesome or even fatal pulmonary infection. This explains why surgeons treating fractured bones in elderly patients are inclined to surgical pinning or fixing of the fractures in order to get the patient out of bed and moving as quickly as possible—not because of trouble with the fracture, but because of the danger of respiratory tract complications.

Other forms of respiratory impairment can, of course, result from damage to the lungs or bronchial tubes from earlier disease. A long-standing bronchial obstructive disease due to chronic bronchitis, heavy cigarette smoking or bronchiectasis can lead to *pulmonary emphysema,* a stretching of the air pockets in the lungs which can take its greatest toll in respiratory impairment during the victim's declining years. But even in the face of these conditions, discussed in detail elsewhere (*see* p. 494), much can be done under a doctor's guidance to minimize respiratory distress and to achieve the most efficient pulmonary function possible under the circumstances. The use of bronchial dilating medications, taken either by mouth or by means of an aerosol spray, plus a regular program of bronchial drainage—the so-called bronchial toilet—to clear secretions from the chest and help keep respiratory passages open, can materially improve impaired breathing even in older patients who have sustained extensive respiratory tract damage from the past. Such a program can also help the older patient suffering from fibrosis or scarring of lung tissue due to long-term hypertension—again, a matter of getting the most respiratory function possible even in the face of a degree of irreparable pulmonary damage. Finally, pulmonary congestion resulting from the collection of fluid in the lungs can arise as part of the syndrome of *congestive heart failure.* (*See* p. 580.) This condition can bring about sudden and frightening respiratory distress, including abrupt episodes of severe shortness of breath, but when heart failure is identified as a factor in respiratory impairment, marked improvement of breathing capacity can be achieved by effective treatment of the heart failure.

The Cardiovascular System. Perhaps the most far-reaching changes that occur in the process of aging involve the structure and function of the cardiovascular system, reflected by impaired heart function, progressive damage to the arteries and arterioles, or both. The heart is a faithful and tireless servant throughout life, but with advancing age it tends to weaken and enlarge, functioning less efficiently and markedly less capable of compensating for any extra demand placed upon it. At the same time the burden upon the heart is slowly but steadily increased as a result of changes in the structure of the arteries and arterioles. Even in the absence of any disease process, the arteries become more rigid and less elastic with advancing age, leading to an increase in the arterial blood pressure, less capacity for the vessels to expand with the force of the heartbeat, and—ultimately—a greater load on the heart as it works to force blood through these less resilient vessels. Virtually everyone suffers some degree of progressive *arteriosclerosis* sooner or later, and with advancing age the arteries become even more rigid. When arteriosclerosis is advanced, it may also seriously impair the circulation of blood to the heart itself, further impairing the heart's

capacity to keep up with the work load thrust upon it. Finally, even a comparatively minor degree of *hypertension* in earlier years tends to become more marked with advancing age; rather than increasing and decreasing in a labile or changeable fashion, the hypertension becomes fixed and unchangeable, further overburdening the heart.

Both arteriosclerosis and hypertension, discussed in detail elsewhere (*see* p. 592 and p. 582), thus become serious health threats during the declining years, even if earlier manifestations of these so-called degenerative disorders have not been severe. Arteriosclerosis can affect the arteries of the kidneys, leading to impairment of renal function; it can affect the cerebral arteries, resulting in strokes, progressive senility or senile dementia (*see* p. 367 for more detailed discussions of these conditions), or it can affect the heart itself, resulting in coronary artery disease, angina pectoris or coronary thrombosis (*see* p. 600). Long-term hypertension can result in chronic overtaxing of the heart, impairment of kidney function, chronic fibrosis or scarring of tissue in the lungs surrounding the pulmonary arterioles, or even cerebral hemorrhage. (*See* p. 582.)

In view of all the cardiovascular complications that *can* occur, it is both surprising and encouraging to consider the number of people who suffer comparatively little from these long-term disabilities, even in advanced old age. What is more, risk can be minimized even at this point by adherence to a reasonable and commonsense program of preventive health care. A morbid preoccupation with cardiovascular system function is unnecessary, but care can be taken to avoid situations that might place an excessive physical burden on the heart. At the same time, attention should be paid to regular daily exercise to keep the cardiovascular system in tone and trim. The diet should include adequate amounts of protein, vegetables, salads and fruits, with fatty foods, starches and rich pastries held to a minimum. Obesity merely increases the burden the heart must carry; a stable weight should be maintained. Ample rest is necessary. Many older people are extremely sensitive to cold, owing to the general impairment of circulation that is a normal part of aging, so the house should be kept warm, and vigorous outdoor exercise in cold weather, a notorious strain on the cardiovascular system, should be carefully avoided. Finally, any symptoms suggesting heart or circulatory impairment, including progressive shortness of breath upon exertion or during the night, heart palpitations or episodes of rapid heartbeat, or any form of chest pain should be checked out with a doctor without delay. As with so many other conditions, impairment of cardiovascular function can often be counteracted, or at least well controlled, as long as it is discovered early and treatment begun before the heart is irreversibly overtaxed.

The Gastrointestinal System. A variety of distressing gastrointestinal symptoms is so commonly associated with advancing age that many elderly people accept such ailments as inevitable, even though much can be done to relieve them. Symptoms including a sense of bloating after meals, excessive belching, sometimes with regurgitation, acid indigestion, abdominal distention, excessive gas formation, specific food intolerances or recurrent constipation do indeed occur more frequently with advancing age. In part, they are a result of changes associated with aging alone. In many elderly people there is a diminishment of acid gastric secretions and progressive impairment of gall bladder function; production of alkaline digestive juices by the pancreas may also be reduced. Certain items of the diet—onions, cabbage and fatty or greasy foods in particular—are poorly digested and frequently associated with bloating, belching and gas formation. Many aging people develop individual idiosyncrasies to other foods which, however unexplainable, cause real digestive distress. Often intolerance may develop to highly spiced foods or foods containing irritating fibers or excessive roughage. Digestion and elimination may be further impaired by such extraneous factors as inadequate mastication, possibly because of poorly fitting dentures, sluggish intestinal motility related to overall physical inactivity, or long-established dependence upon laxatives to improve bowel function.

Although such symptoms as these do not signal any grave gastrointestinal disorder, they can be extremely uncomfortable and annoying, particularly when they follow a recurrent pattern. Often they can be controlled simply by attention to careful mastication of food and elimination of foods that seem consistently to cause distress. In some cases indigestion and bloating can be relieved by the use of a mild antacid medication after meals; in other cases, tablets containing bile salts or supplementary digestive enzymes are extremely helpful, while much of the discomfort of bloating and gas formation can often be counteracted with the use of a mild antispasmodic, sometimes combined with a sedative, when excess intestinal motility and cramping occur. Any program of medication should be prescribed by a physician after a careful examination to be as certain as possible that no serious underlying gastrointestinal disorder is at the root of the trouble. Other commonsense measures, such as taking smaller but more frequent meals or ensuring that meals are taken in pleasant surroundings in the absence of tension or nervous irritation, can further help maintain gastrointestinal function at the highest possible level of efficiency. Sometimes remarkable relief can be obtained by gradually learning to dispense with laxatives which may be acting as a long-term gastrointestinal irritant.

Certain symptoms, of course, can signal more serious digestive tract trouble, and should be called to a doctor's attention without delay. Recurrent vomiting, persisting or recurring abdominal pain, intermittent diarrhea and constipation, or the passing of blood as a black semisolid coffee-ground material in vomitus, as frank red blood in feces, or as sticky, tarry-black stools require prompt medical investigation to rule out the possibility of potentially dangerous illness, or to ensure speedy diagnosis and treatment if some serious disorder is present.

The Urinary and Genital Systems. Ordinarily, kidney function continues unimpaired by aging unless kidney damage has been sustained as a result of some earlier or continuing disorder— kidney infection, for example, or kidney damage resulting from hypertension, arteriosclerosis or diabetes. However, aging people often are more vulnerable to various lower urinary tract disorders and infections. The symptoms of these disorders may include incomplete emptying of the bladder, some increase in nocturnal urination, a marked increase in urinary frequency, and pain and burning during urination. Even the mildest of these symptoms should be checked by a physician to determine whether they are within normal limits or a sign of more serious trouble.

There is no set age at which sexual activity must be terminated; many couples maintain some degree of regular sexual activity into their late seventies or early eighties, whereas others may prefer much more intermittent sexual contact. In elderly women the decline in the natural production of female sex hormones brings about a gradual atrophy or shrinkage of the mucous membrane lining the vagina, and this combined with a natural diminishment of the production of lubricating mucus may render sexual intercourse uncomfortable or even painful, but often this change in vaginal tissue can be slowed by the local administration of small amounts of estrogen in the form of vaginal creams or suppositories. As aging progresses in the male there is a slow atrophy of the testicles, with concomitant decrease in sperm formation, and a decrease in the natural production of male sex hormones results in a gradual decrease both in interest in sexual intercourse and in the capacity to obtain or maintain erection. Periodically there are cases reported of men in their eighties or beyond who have impregnated younger women, but at best they represent the extreme outer limits of normal. Temporary reversal of these natural changes associated with aging is possible with the administration of supplementary quantities of sex hormones, but this practice is condemned by most physicians today because of the risk that estrogen administered to an aging woman may stimulate the development of breast cancer, while testosterone administered to elderly males has been associated with an increased incidence of carcinoma of the prostate. Thus most authorities recommend letting well enough alone, and the vast majority of aging people, both male and female, are able to make perfectly comfortable physical and psychological adjustments to the gradual decline in their sexual capacity

Growing numbers of elderly people today enjoy years of continuing good health that might have been impossible only a few decades ago. All are not so fortunate, however. Old age has always been, and still remains, the time of life when acute illness may strike suddenly and without warning, and also the time when many of the degenerative diseases begin to take their inevitable toll. Although a number of disorders that appear in later years can be effectively treated and even cured, there are many others that come to stay as prolonged chronic illnesses that require continuing medical treatment and nursing care, and even then may ultimately terminate with death. Acute and transitory episodes of illness may often be successfully treated at home, or may require only a brief period of hospital care before home convalescence is possible. But in cases involving such serious disorders as severe, chronic or recurrent heart disease, severe hypertension with progressive kidney failure, cerebrovascular accidents or strokes, inoperable or recurrent cancers, or progressive senility arising from cerebral arteriosclerosis—to name only a few of the most common chronic illnesses of the later years—brief hospitalization may not be enough to meet the need, and long-term plans must be made to provide for whatever degree of continuing medical and custodial care is necessary.

Precisely how this can best be accomplished is a decision that must depend upon the type of care that is required and the individual family situation. When the elderly patient is mentally unimpaired and needs only concerned observation and immediate help in the event of a change for the worse rather than continuous nursing, home care may be the best and by far the least costly solution to the problem, and the solution most often preferred by the patient himself. In many cases the patient's spouse can provide the necessary care, with as little change as possible in their normal living arrangements. In other cases one of the patient's children can provide the necessary care and family support in a spirit of kindness and love. If an elderly patient can be cared for in the home without gravely disrupting family activities and living habits, it can provide both grown children and grandchildren an opportunity for a close and rewarding relationship that might not otherwise be possible in these days of far-flung and highly mobile family life. When the elderly patient has left the hospital after treatment for a prolonged illness but still requires considerable medical attention, a growing number of hospitals have home nursing care programs that can provide the necessary medical aid and supervision at a fraction of the cost of continuing hospitalization. Or the patient's family may be able to manage his care by themselves, with the proper instruction in whatever nursing procedures are necessary, and with occasional home or office visits with the doctor in charge of the case. A private nurse when necessary or periodic visits by a visiting nurse, a program maintained in most major communities, can also be of great help. Specific problems and techniques of home nursing care are discussed in greater detail elsewhere (*see* p. 157); here it is enough merely to emphasize that care of the chronically ill elderly patient is often possible in the home, that various forms of help are available to families seeking to provide such care, and that often the patient is more content and comfortable under these circumstances.

On the other hand, the family must also weigh realistically the possible deleterious or destructive elements that may be introduced into the pattern of family life in attempting to care for an elderly patient in the home. There are certainly cases in which a mentally confused, senile, overly demanding, pain-ridden or completely helpless patient cannot reasonably be treated at home, particularly if it is already overcrowded, or if there are several small children. It can be wrong to permit such a patient to dominate and disorganize normal family life; and it may be equally unwise, when the patient needs rest and tranquillity more than anything else, to subject him to the turmoil of noise and activity so common in homes filled with busy parents and exuberant children. Although it is a judgment

that each family must make for itself, the needs of the younger family members should probably take precedence under ordinary circumstances; an obligation that might seriously threaten the maintenance of a stable, productive and healthy family life should not be undertaken if that threat is more than minimal. Nor is it usually a good solution for a family to try to "hang on" in anticipation of the imminent death of the patient; although some chronic illnesses do end abruptly in a sudden terminal change for the worse, many others may drag on for months and years.

The medical decisions concerning the elderly patient's care must obviously be made by the attending doctor; if full hospitalization is unnecessary, no one is better qualified to recommend the kind of nursing care that would be best suited to the patient's needs. Such an adviser can, among other things, also suggest ways the family can better adapt to the care of an elderly patient at home with the least amount of family disorganization and dissension. If that is not possible, many nursing homes of high quality and with excellent facilities can provide the necessary care. The decision for nursing home care cannot be made hastily, however. Economic considerations as well as the personal preference of both the patient and the family must be carefully weighed. Equally necessary is a thorough investigation of the nursing homes available, and here, too, a doctor's advice and recommendations can be invaluable.

There was a time not long ago when many families felt guilty even considering such a decision; it often seemed tantamount to deserting a member of the family or "sending him away to die." But when a family is torn between their love and responsibility for an elderly patient and the equally pressing needs of other family members, it may well be the better part of compassion to find a living situation for the elderly patient that will satisfy his own particular health and custodial needs without imposing an intolerable burden on the rest of the family. Certainly maintaining him in a well-staffed and well-equipped nursing home need not amount to "desertion" unless the family elects to make it so. These facilities can be found in most communities close enough to home that visits are possible at regular intervals. Family holidays and special events can be enjoyed together, and the elderly patient who might ultimately come to be resented as an onerous full-time burden can often, in fact, become a far more welcome member of the family.

The Right to a Dignified Death

Obviously no one can predict when death will come. No rules apply; actual events often totally confound the most informed medical predictions. The individual who appears at the age of seventy-five to be hale and hearty and in abundant good health may develop acute heart failure and die with bewildering suddenness, while another individual suffering chronic liver failure, chronic high blood pressure, chronic heart disease and recurring cancer all combined may survive crisis after crisis and still live on. The days when a doctor gave a patient "six months to live" are virtually gone forever; most doctors have more sense than to make such predictions. Still and all, the likelihood of impending death poses certain problems for the doctor, for the elderly person, and for the family—problems for which there are no clear-cut solutions but which deserve thoughtful consideration.

One constantly recurring question is whether or not an individual known to be suffering from a grave and eventually terminal illness should be told about his condition. Every doctor has his own personal feelings about this question, some adamantly inclined one way or the other. If there is a consensus among physicians today, however, it would probably be a somewhat cautiously qualified yes: in most cases it is probably not only morally right but also, in the long run, better for the patient's own well-being to know the true state of his health.

Certainly there are cases in which this might not apply. Every practicing physician has encountered patients who, when faced with the truth about their physical condition, even when the outcome was not entirely certain, have simply given up, "withdrawn from life," and entered into a state of physical and emotional collapse that has quite unnecessarily precipitated the end.

A patient's "fighting spirit" and his "will to live" can often play a vital role in turning the tide against even the gravest of illnesses. If from his personal knowledge of the patient the doctor feels that the truth may have an adverse effect, he may well decide to tell a responsible family member, but withhold it, at least temporarily, from the patient himself. On the other hand, every doctor has encountered patients who have repeatedly signaled in subtle or obvious ways that they simply do not want to know the truth. In most such cases there is little question that the patient is aware or at least deeply suspicious of the true nature of his condition, yet has made a decision, consciously or unconsciously, to ignore or deny it as long as possible. Here again the physician must decide, based upon his personal knowledge of the patient, whether the truth will be beneficial or harmful in the long run. Obviously every case is different, and the decision does not rest solely with the doctor; it must be considered both by the physician and by some responsible person close to the patient, either a family member or a trusted friend. Occasionally, too, a decision in the opposite direction must be made; there are cases in which the dying patient does not want his family or friends to know, or cases in which the doctor may feel that telling the family the truth may cause such an unfortunate emotional reaction that the patient will be adversely affected. In each case the doctor must do what he thinks will be of the greatest benefit first to the patient and then to the family. There is no excuse, however, for a doctor to temporize or avoid frank discussion with the patient or a family member or both in the face of a grave and almost certainly terminal illness; the truth must be told, since it will become obvious sooner or later anyway, although great discretion must be exercised in deciding how, to whom, and even when the revelation is made.

By and large most patients want to be told the truth, and should be given the opportunity to set their affairs in order and to make their own peaceful accommodation with the inevitable. The one thing that no physician or family member has a right to do, however, is to destroy the patient's hope when any reasonable hope exists.

If there is even a slender chance that recovery may be possible, it is up to the doctor and the family to preserve the patient's hope; and when there is really no hope whatever, the doctor, family and friends must do everything in their power to reassure the patient that everything that can be done is being done, and then provide as much help and emotional support as is possible for whatever time is left.

But just as the patient in most cases has the right to be told of the true nature of his illness, so also should he have the right to a dignified death. Modern medicine can perform virtual miracles in supporting, maintaining and sustaining life; advanced medical techniques have, in fact, made it possible for many people with illnesses once considered extremely grave or even terminal to turn the corner and recover. Nevertheless, there are all too many times, in dealing with truly terminal illnesses, particularly among the aged, when the physician and hospital staff, in their zeal to preserve and sustain life as long as possible, utilize these techniques simply as a matter of routine without regard to the patient or the inevitable outcome of his illness. Thus lives have been prolonged simply because they *could* be prolonged when it certainly would have been far better to allow a terminal illness to take its normal course. In some cases families have literally been impoverished by the costs of prolonging life far, far beyond the limits of good medical judgment and compassionate care in situations that were clearly and inevitably hopeless. And in all too many such cases death becomes a long, drawn-out ordeal for both the patient and his family.

There is no question that moral considerations enter into this problem. There are physicians who argue that to yield to death while anything can still be done to postpone it is to betray their moral and professional injunction to preserve life. There are those who fear that if the one extreme is not pursued, the other extreme—giving up hope too soon or the irresponsible or arbitrary application of euthanasia—is necessarily bound to follow. Whatever the medical or moral arguments, however, there are certain steps that can and should be taken when such a problem arises. There should, of course, be close and frank consultation between the physician and the family when a decision to permit death appears imminent. Such consultation should, when appropriate, include the participation of the patient's or family's religious counselors. From the physician's standpoint, consultation with other physicians whose knowledge and judgment he respects can and should also be undertaken. Such simple and sensible procedures as these can, in most if not all cases, aid in finding both a medically and a morally acceptable course to follow.

XV

OUR MODERN MEDICAL RESOURCES

64. The Medical History and Physical Examination   961

65. Laboratory Tests, X-Rays and Other Diagnostic Aids   968

66. The Doctor's Training   983

67. The Many Kinds of Doctors   991

68. Our Modern Hospitals and Auxiliary Medical Services   1001

69. Medical Costs and How to Meet Them   1011

A great number of people are involved in the business of modern health care: doctors, nurses, laboratory technicians, aides, hospital administrators, therapists, pharmacists and many more. The work of medicine is done in a variety of facilities: doctors' offices, medical clinics, private or public hospitals, outpatient departments, emergency rooms and even mobile medical units. Because these professional services and facilities exist in such bewildering variety, many people are not aware of all these medical resources that are available to them, or are perhaps somewhat intimidated by the "mysteries" of diagnosis and treatment or the complexities and costs of professional medical care. The fact is, however, that there is nothing mysterious or frightening about modern medical care. Its goal is quite simply the prevention and cure of human disease, and that goal is unattainable without the understanding, confidence and cooperation of the patient himself. Thus it is up to every individual, even if he never becomes a patient, to be fully informed about the modern medical resources available to him and his family in order to use them to their best advantage.

The Medical History and Physical Examination

As little as a hundred years ago, most people regarded a doctor's services as an unwelcome necessity, to be sought out only in cases of dire emergency. Hospitalization was even more unwelcome; it could mean pain, inconvenience and a prolonged convalescence if the illness were not fatal, but all too often hospitals were places where people went to die. Fortunately these attitudes have changed, in large part because the medical profession and our modern medical facilities have themselves changed. Treating and curing illness is still an important part of the doctor's job, but equally important, and a far better use of his knowledge and skill, is the prevention of illness. Hospitals, too, now play both a diagnostic and a preventive role, and with the facilities available today, many illnesses can be nipped in the bud before massive damage and debilitation occur. Even in the case of serious injury or illness, hospitalization is not the ordeal it once was, and successful treatment and rapid recovery are the rule rather than the exception.

Under these circumstances, there is no reason to be apprehensive about consulting a doctor. In fact, frank and regular consultations with a medical adviser are essential if he is to perform his job effectively. It is a serious mistake to assume that the medical professions can perform miracles when a patient neglects his own health or postpones seeking the proper medical care. These "miracles" are invariably the result of knowledge, skill and hard work, and they can be achieved only with the active participation of the patient himself, preferably *before* illness strikes.

It is, of course, up to the patient to select his own physician or medical facility; professional ethics prevent doctors from soliciting patients. Once that selection has been made, the process of diagnosis can begin; but no matter what the complaint, the doctor must first *see* the patient, *hear* him describe his symptoms, and *examine* him carefully. In other words, for all the progress that has been made in medical practice, the modern doctor must begin his diagnosis in exactly the same way his predecessors did, on the basis of what the patient tells him (the medical history) and what he himself can detect (the physical examination). True, diagnostic aids and techniques have become very sophisticated, but they are still only aids, and must take second place. The first step is a one-to-one consultation between doctor and patient; the patient must be prepared to give frank and accurate answers to the doctor's questions about his past and present medical history, and cooperate fully in the performance of the physical examination. There is nothing difficult or demanding about these initial diagnostic procedures, but they are so important in the prevention and treatment of illness, both to the doctor and to the patient, that it is appropriate here to describe them in detail.

The Medical History

When you first consult a doctor, he will, of course, assume that you are bothered by symptoms or signs that do not seem normal, and he will ask you to state succinctly just what is disturbing you. Thus his first inquiry will be about your *chief complaint*. This may be crystal clear—"I hit my thumb with a hammer and it hurts"—or it may be very vague—"I just don't feel well, somehow." Obviously this chief or presenting complaint is a necessary "opening move" in any careful medical consultation.

Once the chief complaint has been stated, the doctor's next step is to elicit a detailed *history of the present illness*. When and how did the initial symptoms begin, and what has happened since you first noticed them? What other symptoms seem to be associated? What did you do about the symptoms? What medicine have you taken? Here the important thing is a narrative account of all the aspects of the chief complaint, preferably expressed in your own words; the doctor may say very little other than to prompt you with an occasional question. He knows that the words the patient himself uses to describe a pain, an ache or a feeling of pressure may provide the vital clue to the cause of the symptom—and he must avoid putting words in the patient's mouth. Once you have finished, the doctor will have particular and pointed questions to ask, for he will already be sorting out in his mind a number of possible diagnoses, and now must begin to narrow the field, ruling out some suspicions, perhaps confirming others. Many things may be related to your symptoms, whether you recognize any relationship or not: your eating habits, the kind of work you do, the amount of emotional tension you feel, your normal pattern of waking and sleeping, and so forth. Sometimes this kind of direct questioning is embarrassing to the patient, or seems irrelevant, but the doctor knows from experience how often the clues to a diagnosis may be hidden in everyday aspects of the patient's life that he might never think to mention.

With the chief complaint defined as well as possible, the doctor will next inquire about your *past medical history,* especially if you are new to him as a patient. A past illness does not *necessarily* have anything to do with a current complaint, but often there is a direct relationship. Obviously, the doctor needs to know of illnesses that might have had lasting effects on your health—rheumatic fever, for example, or tuber-

culosis; he also wants to know the details of any previous surgery. But more important, the doctor knows he will ultimately be treating a person, not just an illness, and the better informed he is about that person's medical background, the better the job he can do. If your past medical history is particularly lengthy or complicated, he may ask your authorization to contact doctors who previously treated you, and to ask for a transfer of records.

Further, your *family history* and *social history* may provide additional clues and invaluable background knowledge. Many illnesses, if not frankly hereditary, nevertheless show distinct patterns of *family predisposition*. Diabetes is one example in which a family history of the disease may be very significant. Other illnesses with a strong family predisposition include hypertension (high blood pressure), certain kinds of heart disease and cancer. As for social history, knowing about your home and family surroundings, the kind of work you do and the conditions under which you work, and your social habits and activities not only helps the doctor see you as a three-dimensional human being but also helps him establish realistic guidelines for the treatment and handling of your illness.

As a final step in taking your medical history, the doctor will throw out a sort of medical dragnet in the hope of picking up other relevant information about your health that may have been missed. In a so-called *review of systems* he will ask questions related to the general health and function of each organ system—the digestive system, the nervous system, and so forth. This is a search not only for clues to the diagnosis of your chief or presenting complaint but for indications of any other kind of illness or disorder that may also be present. Often the questions make little sense to the patient, but each one is keyed to reveal a particular class of disorder if such a disorder is present. Essentially, the review of systems is an extra precaution the doctor takes to be sure that in concentrating on a patient's chief complaint he does not neglect some other perhaps hidden disorder.

Complicated as a medical history may sound, an experienced doctor can usually accomplish it very thoroughly in the course of half an hour or less. Throughout his medical training he has gained skill and proficiency in interviewing patients, and by the time his training is over, the technique of taking a history is so thoroughly mastered that he is unlikely to miss much when he is treating patients of his own.

The Physical Examination

The medical history is only the first step toward arriving at a diagnosis. By the time it is complete the doctor will have narrowed his mental list of possible diagnoses down to the few that seem most probable—his so-called *differential diagnosis*. He may even have arrived at a single "most likely" diagnosis on the basis of the history alone. But a patient's medical history is, after all, only a *subjective* description of his symptoms and may be very difficult to evaluate accurately. What one patient may describe as an agonizing pain, another might mention only as a minor annoyance. Thus the doctor will try to corroborate his tentative diagnosis by finding demonstrable signs of the illness or disorder, physical changes from the normal, by means of a *physical examination*.

Strictly speaking, the doctor begins his physical examination the moment you walk in the door, for his eye has been trained to pick up very subtle peculiarities or deviations from the normal any time he sees a patient. Quite unobtrusively he makes mental notes of the patient's skin color or complexion, any puffiness of the cheeks, a tremor of the hands, a stammer, a hoarseness of voice—any one of a dozen characteristics that may be revealed during the course of the medical history. This sort of "overall inspection" may, in fact, prove the most revealing part of the physical examination because it can tell your doctor a great many things of which you may not be aware.

The physical examination proper is designed to examine all parts of the body briefly but thoroughly for any physical signs of illness. It takes place in more or less the following order:

The Skin. Throughout the examination the doctor observes the skin for any abnormality. The general skin tone and the health of the hair and scalp are important indications of general health; so is any collection of fluid in the tissue underlying the skin, a condition known as edema. Scars, growths, lumps or any other peculiarities will catch the doctor's practiced eye even though they might be missed by an untrained person. When he presses the skin over the shinbone with his thumb, for instance, he is looking for the telltale "pitting" or depression that would indicate the presence of edema.

Ears, Nose and Throat. In examining the ear, the doctor uses a lighted magnifying instrument called an *otoscope;* through the funnel-shaped *speculum* of the otoscope he can see the ear canal and the eardrum itself. A foreign body lodged in the ear canal, or a wax plug that may be interfering with your hearing, will be plainly evident; so will the reddening or bulging of the eardrum that indicates a middle-ear infection. The inside of the nose may be examined with the same instrument, using another kind of speculum to spread the nostrils. Usually the mouth and throat are examined with an ordinary flashlight and a wooden blade to depress the back of the tongue and permit a clear view of the throat, the tonsil beds and the palate. He will also examine the tongue, and although he is not a dentist, he will look for evidence of gum disease or tooth decay as well.

The Eye. In examining the eye, the physician has one of the most extraordinary opportunities in the whole physical examination. The external examination with a flashlight is simple enough, but with a small magnifying instrument known as an *ophthalmoscope* the doctor can also observe the interior of the eye, particularly the retina that lines the inside of the back of the eyeball. This is the only place in the body where both veins and arteries can actually be directly observed, for these tiny vessels lie exposed on the surface of the retina. In the presence of longstanding hypertension or arteriosclerosis, characteristic and recognizable changes can be observed in these blood vessels, suggesting the same disorder in other vessels throughout the body. Other illnesses may also announce their presence in the examination of the retina; diabetes, for example, is not only associated with increased arteriosclerosis, but may in severe cases show a typical kind of exudate collected on the retina. To the patient an examination of the interior of the eye is simple and painless, but to the doctor it is an invaluable diagnostic procedure.

Thyroid, Lymph Glands and Vascular System. After completing the eye, ear, nose and throat examinations, the doctor will proceed down the body, beginning with an examination of the thyroid gland. This organ, wrapped around the front of the windpipe just below the Adam's apple, can be examined best with the doctor standing behind the patient and feeling the throat with his fingertips as the patient swallows. Normally the thyroid is smooth and soft to the touch, but with practice the doctor soon learns to detect an enlargement of the gland (sometimes called a goiter) or the presence of any irregularity or nodule. In case any such abnormality is noted, further laboratory examinations are necessary to help identify the nature of the enlargement or growth.

Also in the neck, under the jaw and behind the ears, are a number of lymph glands—patches of tissue that form at the juncture of lymph channels. These glands, among other things, form lymphocytes, one of the kinds of white blood cells that help the body fight off infection. Ordinarily lymph glands are too small and soft to be detected at all, but when infection is present in the region, these glands become swollen and tender and provide an important clue that something is awry. Swollen lymph glands in the neck, for example, often indicate infection in the throat or ears. The doctor will also check for lymph gland swelling just above the collarbone, under the arms and in the groin.

At the same time, he will check what can be observed about the condition of the vascular system of arteries and veins all over the body. We normally think of taking the pulse at the wrist, but the doctor will also check pulses in your feet to be sure there is no evidence that some condition is impairing the circulation to the lower extremities. The doctor will also measure and record your blood pressure, or have his office nurse do it. He is looking, of course, for any evidence of hypertension—an abnormal elevation of blood pressure—but at the same time he recognizes that factors other than disease may push your blood pressure above normal. Nervous tension alone may elevate your blood pressure when you first enter the doctor's office; thus, if the initial measurement is a little high, the doctor may check it again later when you are more relaxed. If you are curious or worried about your blood pressure, ask your doctor what your reading is and what it means. Most doctors nowadays are perfectly willing to tell their patients what their blood pressure reading is, and inform them whether it is normal or not.

Along with pulse and blood pressure, the doctor (or his nurse) will also check your temperature with a fever thermometer and measure your respiration rate. In fact these three simple measurements—temperature, pulse and respiration, or "TPR"—are such an important reflection of your life processes and are so helpful in detecting illness and following its progress that doctors traditionally speak of them as "the vital signs." Blood pressure measurement is often included in this designation as well.

Examination of the Heart and Lungs. To examine the lungs the doctor must rely on indirect methods: *observation* of the expansion and contraction of your rib cage as you breathe, *percussion* of your chest with his finger, and *auscultation*—actually listening to the sound of your breathing with the aid of a *stethoscope*. Unlikely as it may seem, he can learn a surprising amount in a very short time using these simple examining techniques. When he observes limited chest expansion, for example, he will suspect that the patient may have chronic emphysema, actually moving very little air in and out of the lungs with each breath. By thumping or "percussing" the chest with his finger as he listens, he can detect sounds that may indicate a solid growth of some sort in the lung itself, or a collection of fluid in the chest cavity. Finally, with the stethoscope the doctor can hear a wide variety of squeaks, squawks and wheezes as you breathe which may signify collections of mucus in the lungs, partial obstruction of the smaller air tubes, or a dozen other things, depending upon the particular nature of the sound.

Many people erroneously assume that the stethoscope must contain some special kind of sound-amplifying device, but in fact it is really nothing more than a pair of hollow tubes connected to earpieces at one end and to a hollow bell or diaphragm at the other. The faint sounds you make when you breathe are magnified by this instrument much as your voice is magnified by a megaphone.

Precisely the same sort of indirect methods are used to examine the heart, and here—as in the examination of the lungs—the doctor's skill and experience interpreting faint differences in sound are extremely important. By percussion of the patient's chest with his finger he can outline the approximate size of the heart and determine whether it is enlarged or not. With the stethoscope he can hear the cycle of "heart tones" arising from the opening and closing of the heart valves and from the surge of blood moving through the heart and into the great arteries leading from it. He may listen to these heart tones from several different areas on the chest wall, since certain of these characteristic sounds are transmitted more clearly to one part of the chest than another. Thus the sound of the mitral valve closing can best be heard high up in the chest to the left of the breastbone, while the aortic valve sounds are more clearly audible in an area to the right of the breastbone.

Normal heart tones are heard as a steady, rhythmic *lub-dup, lub-dup, lub-dup,* slowing down or speeding up slightly with the cycle of respirations. But various heart disorders can cause marked changes in these sounds or their rhythm. When a patient is in heart failure his heart rate may be very fast, with the heart tones taking on a sound similar to that of rapid hoofbeats—a so-called gallop rhythm. Certain disorders of the heart valves may cause a variety of abnormal or extra heart tones known as "murmurs" to become audible. Some heart murmurs have no grave significance at all; some perfectly healthy children, for example, will have audible heart murmurs at one time or another, usually most marked during periods of rapid growth. These innocent or "functional" murmurs generally vanish by the time of late adolescence. But other murmurs never occur innocently, and may be so very characteristic of specific heart disorders that the doctor can make an accurate diagnosis the moment he hears them. One such

murmur, characteristic of a damaged mitral valve, suggests to the doctor that the patient has probably had severe rheumatic fever at some time in his life, with permanent damage to his heart valves, even though the patient himself may not remember the illness.

Finally, the stethoscope may reveal another kind of disorder in the course of the heart and lung examination: a coarse, scratchy *friction rub* that can occur when the delicate membranes lining the heart or lungs have become infected or inflamed. A friction rub produced by rubbing of the pleural membrane lining the lungs and the inside of the chest cavity will be heard each time a breath is taken, while the scratchy sound arising from an inflamed heart lining or pericardium will recur with each heartbeat.

Actually, it takes considerably longer to describe the heart and lung examination in words than to perform it in the doctor's office. But assessment of these organs in a physical examination *is* limited at best, and your doctor may need other kinds of studies—a chest X-ray, for example, or an electrocardiogram—to help him in his evaluation. With the aid of all these techniques together, however, he can gain a remarkably accurate impression of the condition of these vital organs.

Examination of the Abdomen. Again, direct examination of the abdominal organs is impossible, but at least these vital organs are not confined in a rigid cage of bone as the heart and lungs are. With the patient lying flat on his back, the doctor can use the tips of his fingers to press and probe, seeking first to feel various organs or masses that are palpable, and second to localize the region from which pain arises, if abdominal pain is present. The edge of the liver can often be felt, just below the rib cage on the right, when the patient takes a deep breath. The spleen is normally too small and soft to be palpable, tucked up high in the upper left corner of the abdomen under the rib cage, but in the case of certain diseases it becomes enlarged and firm and can readily be felt. Organs such as the stomach, the pancreas, the gall bladder and the intestines are not normally palpable, but by probing all four quadrants of the abdomen with his fingers the doctor can search for masses that should not ordinarily be there. If a patient's severe abdominal pain arises from an acute gall bladder attack, for example, the doctor may be able to feel the swollen, painful gall bladder protruding below the edge of the liver. Occasionally he may find totally unsuspected conditions as well. A woman, for instance, may have developed a completely painless cyst of an ovary which is so large it can be palpated during an abdominal examination. Finally, the doctor will check for any evidence of a hernia or "rupture"—a potentially dangerous condition in which part of the abdominal contents (usually a loop of intestine) has pushed through a weak spot in the abdominal wall into the groin.

Examination of the Genitalia. In male patients this is a simple, straightforward procedure by which the doctor can determine in a matter of a moment or so any abnormality of the penis, scrotum or testicles. In women, whose major genital organs are located internally in the lower abdomen or pelvis, the procedure is necessarily more complicated, and can be somewhat embarrassing until one recognizes that the pelvic examination is as much a matter of routine to the doctor as an examination of the ears or throat.

A pelvic examination involves two steps, after the external genitalia have been inspected for abnormalities. First the vagina and the cervix (the lower end of the uterus) are examined directly with the aid of a vaginal *speculum*—an instrument inserted into the vagina to hold the vaginal walls apart so that the cervix can be seen. This type of examination can be performed without pain or difficulty on most girls or women beyond the age of puberty; a special narrow speculum is used when the vaginal opening is still partly obstructed by the hymen. In women over twenty the doctor may take this opportunity to transfer some of the surface cells from the cervix onto a glass slide, to be stained and examined later by a pathologist for any sign of cancer cells. This is a so-called Pap smear and is most valuable for the early detection of cancer of the cervix at a stage when it is completely curable; the same technique can be used to detect cancer in cells taken from many other parts of the body as well.

In the second part of the female pelvic examination, the physician palpates the internal genital organs directly by placing one hand on the lower abdomen and inserting fingers of the other hand into the vagina. By means of this *bimanual examination* he can actually determine the size of the uterus, as well as the size and location of the tubes and ovaries, with surprising accuracy. He can also detect any abnormal growth, cysts or other anatomical variations that may exist. In adolescent girls the usual bimanual examination is often omitted because of the hymen, but much of the same information can often be obtained by means of a digital rectal examination.

The Rectal and Proctoscopic Examination. Like the examination of the cervix, the doctor's examination of the rectum and the lower few inches of the colon is primarily designed to detect cancer. Cancer occurs quite commonly in this region, but it often can be detected very early by means of this admittedly awkward procedure. The rectal examination is simple, accomplished by the doctor with a gloved finger; such conditions as hemorrhoids or rectal fissures are detected this way, and in a male patient the prostate gland is examined at the same time for any abnormalities. The proctoscopic procedure, in which the lower segment of the colon is examined by direct vision, is more complicated. For this the patient must first have a cleansing enema, either at home or in the doctor's office. Thereafter, the doctor inserts a *proctoscope*—a narrow hollow tube bearing a light in the end—through the anal orifice and examines the lower six to eight inches of colon, where some 90 percent of all cancers of this region begin. Awkward and uncomfortable as this examination may be, it is the best possible way to spot a beginning cancer of the rectum or colon while it is still curable, and should be a part of any complete physical examination of patients thirty-five years of age or older.

The Neurological Examination. As a final step in your physical examination, the doctor will make a survey to assess the function of your nervous system. Obviously direct examination of the brain, the spinal cord and the vast network of motor and sensory nerves in the human body is impossible; the best the doctor can do is to check various *reflexes* and conduct a series of simple screening tests to demonstrate how the nervous system is working, watching carefully for any abnormal results that might indicate some malfunction.

Thus, in a matter of a few moments he can check out the function of the twelve *cranial nerves* providing for vision, hearing, eye movements, control of the tongue and swallowing, motion of the facial muscles and so forth. Next he will test the deep *tendon reflexes* in the forearms, below the kneecaps and in the Achilles' tendon in the heel. Since coordination of muscle activity is part of the job of the nervous system, he will test your sense of balance, asking you to stand on one foot, with your eyes open first, then closed. If something in your medical history has suggested some possible abnormality of the nervous system, he will conduct an even more rigorous nervous system examination, or may even refer you to a *neurologist*—a specialist in nervous system diseases—for more detailed examination. (*See* p. 992.)

Other Aspects of the Physical Examination. The various procedures described above make up the bulk of a complete physical examination; but your doctor, rigorously trained as an acute observer, will notice many other things as he proceeds through the examination. For example, he will check for any sign of jaundice—a yellow coloring of the skin—and for any abnormal odor on your breath that might provide a subtle clue to the presence of diabetes, liver disease or kidney failure. He will examine your legs for evidence of varicose veins, note the quantity and texture of your hair, and observe your skin for any sign of tiny capillary hemorrhages or unusual bruising. In a really thorough physical examination your vision and hearing should also be checked, and if you are over forty a special eye examination should be performed to detect the early onset of such eye diseases as glaucoma, one of the most common causes of blindness in later life.

If you are a woman, regardless of your age, your doctor will carefully examine your breasts for any abnormal lumps or masses. If you have never learned the simple technique of regular monthly breast self-examination, here is your golden opportunity to learn how. (*See* p. 450.)

Finally, as part of his examination, your doctor will order certain laboratory and X-ray studies if he feels that they will help him evaluate your health status, or help him confirm or rule out various tentative diagnostic impressions. These special aids to diagnosis are discussed in detail in the following chapter.

Timing Your Physical Examination. A complete physical examination is, of course, unnecessary every time you visit your doctor's office. Such an exam would be superfluous if you are merely seeking relief from a head cold or some other minor complaint, and in that case the doctor would probably confine his examination to the region that is immediately affected. If you are a new patient, however, or present more than a casual complaint, he will ask you to plan time for a complete examination as soon as possible, and you should insist on it. Such an examination will require more of the doctor's time, and will involve more expense than a cursory office checkup, but it is of vital importance that it be done; no doctor can hope to provide good medical care "flying blind."

Indeed, more and more people today realize that the *prevention* of illness, through regular physical examinations, is far less costly and painful in the long run than treatment and cure once illness has struck. In fact, complete physical examinations undertaken at regular intervals will ensure that your doctor remains completely familiar with the condition of your health—and with you as a person—at all times. Thus he can turn his efforts toward *helping you maintain optimum good health* year after year. Discuss with your doctor the interval that makes the most sense for *you,* and then stick to the program you agree upon. In general, such preventive examinations are most useful if they are performed when you are feeling *well,* rather than *ill;* that way your doctor can best regard your health picture as a whole without being preoccupied with some acute problem that requires immediate and concentrated attention.

65

Laboratory Tests, X-Rays and Other Diagnostic Aids

In recent years science fiction stories have painted rather alarming pictures of the "automated medical care" we may all receive a few decades in the future. According to these stories, patients will go not to a doctor but to a huge diagnostic computer, where they will provide their medical histories by filling out punch cards; samples of blood, urine and other materials will be taken automatically; robot arms will poke and probe, vital signs will be registered on tape, X-rays will be taken, heartbeats measured, and other studies done as patients move along through the machine like cars on an assembly line. Finally, diagnoses and treatment recommendations will be printed on read-out sheets and thrust into the patients' hands as they emerge at the other end, without human contact with a single live physician.

A fantastic idea? Not entirely. Certain types of diagnostic aids have already been automated, and a trip through a modern diagnostic clinic often has certain aspects of an assembly line about it. But at least in the foreseeable future, good medical care will continue to depend, as it always has in the past and still does today, on a close human relationship between doctor and patient.

The basic core of such medical care is the complete medical history and physical examination described in the previous chapter. With nothing else but these to go on, a well-trained and experienced doctor can diagnose the great majority of common health problems, and chances are good that he will miss very little.

Even so, he will also use a variety of diagnostic aids to help him either confirm or rule out various tentative diagnoses or to help spot certain disorders which may not be readily apparent upon physical examination and may not yet be causing any discernible signs and symptoms. Among these diagnostic aids is a multitude of *laboratory tests* designed to provide information about the functions of the body; a variety of *X-ray examinations* which allow him to see portions of the body which would otherwise be inaccessible to study; and a number of *special diagnostic studies* such as bacteriological cultures, antibiotic sensitivity tests, blood-typing and cross-matching procedures, or electrocardiographic examinations, all designed to provide vitally useful data for the doctor to add to what he has already been able to learn about his patient.

Laboratory Studies

Every modern medical office has access to an up-to-date, well-equipped clinical laboratory to which samples of blood, urine and other specimens can be sent for examination, and the lab technician who performs or oversees these special tests is in many ways the doctor's good right arm. With the literally hundreds of different laboratory studies that have been perfected, it may seem that everything requires some kind of test. In practice, however, the doctor will order only a few basic laboratory studies as a routine part of a physical examination. Other lab tests will be performed only if something in the patient's medical history or physical examination suggests that more information is needed in a particular area, and many other tests are done only rarely, in the face of specific indications.

Most laboratory studies fall into two general categories: the *microscopic examination* of various tissues or fluids from the body, and the *chemical analysis* of body fluids to detect any abnormal biochemical changes. Two of the most basic laboratory studies, the *complete blood count* and the *routine urine analysis,* actually involve a little of both. These two studies provide so much useful information about body functions that they are always a part of a complete physical examination, and indeed may be performed as part of any office visit.

The Complete Blood Count. This examination actually involves half a dozen separate tests. Among other things, the number of red cells (*erythrocytes*) and the number of white cells (*leucocytes*) in a tiny diluted sample of blood are counted under the microscope, and the results compared to known normals. The red cell count, together with a measurement of the amount of oxygen-carrying hemoglobin in the cells, and the ratio of red cells to serum in a centrifuged specimen of blood, will reveal whether anemia is present or not, and can even indicate to the doctor whether the anemia is caused by deficient iron in the diet or stems from other causes. As for the white cell count, an increased number of these cells usually indicates an active bacterial infection somewhere in the body, while an abnormally low white cell count is often suggestive of virus infection. More information is gained when a specially stained blood smear is examined under the microscope, and the various kinds of white cells present are enumerated in a so-called *differential* white cell count. In the presence of bacterial infections, white cells called *granulocytes* and *monocytes,* formed in the bone marrow, usually predominate; in virus infections, *lymphocytes* formed in the lymph glands tend to be more numerous. This differential white cell count can provide other useful diagnostic clues as well. For example, a number of oddly shaped lymphocytes of a very distinctive type may be found in the blood

in the presence of infectious mononucleosis, a common viral infection of adolescence and young adulthood. Similarly, the appearance of large numbers of incompletely formed or "immature" white cells in a differential smear may be an early but unmistakable indication of leukemia, appearing long before any other symptoms have occurred.

Another part of a complete blood count is a measurement of the speed with which red cells settle to the bottom of a tube of blood that has been mixed with an anticoagulant to prevent it from clotting—the so-called *erythrocyte sedimentation rate.* Ordinarily the red cells will settle out relatively slowly, but in the presence of debilitating illnesses such as rheumatic fever, or in longstanding infections, the rate of sedimentation is much faster. Although this is not a specific diagnostic test to identify any single disorder, it can provide the doctor with a vital clue that some hidden disorder may be present.

The Routine Urine Analysis. This test also involves microscopic examination of urine sediment and a chemical analysis of the urine itself. Normally the urine contains no solid matter other than a few harmless crystals of excreted wastes. In case of kidney or bladder infections, however, white blood cells may be seen under the microscope, and in certain other kidney disorders red blood cells or fragments of kidney tissue appear in the sediment. Chemical analysis may reveal the presence of *albumin,* a blood protein that appears in the urine only in abnormal situations, or traces of *sugar,* often the earliest clue to the presence of diabetes mellitus. Finally, the doctor can tell if the kidneys are doing an adequate job of concentrating urine by a simple measurement of its specific gravity.

The Blood-Clotting Test. Another familiar lab test is the measurement of *bleeding time* and *clotting time* of the blood, most commonly performed when a child is about to be subjected to surgery such as a tonsillectomy. The bleeding time is simply the length of time a person continues to bleed from a minor wound, usually a needle prick of the finger or the ear lobe. Bleeding ordinarily will stop in a matter of two or three minutes, but under abnormal conditions, such as in the presence of hemophilia, it may continue for hours or even days. The clotting time, usually measured simultaneously, is the time it takes blood removed from the body in a glass capillary tube to show the first evidence of a sticky clot. If either of these measurements suggests any disorder of the blood-clotting mechanism, other special tests can be done to help pinpoint the exact nature of the disorder.

Blood Chemistries. In addition to the routine tests that are part of a physical examination, a number of other studies known as blood chemistries are often performed, either as screening tests to reveal early evidence of such disorders as diabetes or kidney disease or as special diagnostic tests when specific disorders are suspected. All the life processes of the human body are the result of complex biochemical reactions, or of the transport of chemical substances from one part of the body to another by way of the blood stream. Thus, at any time, a wide variety of dissolved chemical substances—glucose, amino acids, enzymes and hormones, to name only a very few—are present in measurable quantities in the blood. But in many illnesses or disorders the relative amounts of these dissolved chemicals are changed from the normal, or substances that are not normally found in the blood stream at all put in an appearance, often providing invaluable clues to the diagnosis of a multitude of illnesses.

Among the most commonly performed of these blood chemistries is the measurement of the level of glucose in the blood—the so-called blood sugar test—and the analysis of the blood for nitrogen-containing waste materials, often an indication of improper kidney function. Ordinarily the blood always contains some glucose, with the level falling off during an overnight fasting period, rising somewhat higher an hour or so after each meal, and then falling back to the fasting level three or four hours later. When a person develops diabetes, however, blood sugar levels remain very high for hours after meals, and some excess sugar may even "spill over" into the urine as it passes through the kidneys' filtering system. In severe, untreated diabetes a number of characteristic symptoms appear to make the diagnosis obvious (*see* table below), but in the early stages of the disease, before any symptoms

begin, the only clue may be abnormally high blood sugar. Since diabetes often appears insidiously, and may be present and doing damage to the body for years before it is detected, a blood sugar test is often performed to screen patients for diabetes in the course of physical examinations. In fact, a refinement of the blood sugar test, called a *glucose tolerance test,* can help identify *potential* diabetics—individuals who do not yet have the disease in active form, but who are on the verge of developing it. Thus, if there is a history of diabetes in a patient's family, the doctor may order a glucose tolerance test as a routine part of a complete physical examination.

Just as a high level of blood sugar suggests the presence of diabetes, an elevated level of nitrogen-containing waste chemicals such as urea in the blood can be an important clue that the kidneys are not working properly to remove these poisons from the blood stream. Similarly, disorders of the thyroid gland can often be detected by measurement of iodine levels in the blood, and a high level of uric acid is characteristically present in persons suffering from gout.

Not all abnormal blood chemistry measurements are related so specifically to individual disorders; some may indicate a wide range of possible diagnoses. For example, the total level of protein in the blood may be decreased significantly in a number of debilitating diseases, and in others the ratio of albumin to globulin may be reversed; the doctor must look further to determine exactly what is causing such a change. Other blood chemistries serve as a general survey or "profile" of the function of the liver in its many complex jobs; while these studies may not pinpoint any *specific* liver disease, they do indicate in general whether the liver is functioning as it should, or whether some aspect of its function is impaired.

Finally, certain blood chemistry studies are designed to detect the appearance in the blood of substances that are normally not there at all, or present only in traces. For example, bile formed in the liver is ordinarily stored in the gall bladder, and then transported into the small intestine through a special bile duct. But if this duct is obstructed for some reason—by a gallstone, for instance, or a tumor—part of the bile backing up behind the obstruction may be absorbed into the blood stream. One of the pigments that gives bile its characteristic yellow-green color, a substance called bilirubin, is normally present in blood only in trace amounts, but when the bile duct is obstructed the amount of bilirubin measurable in the blood serum increases sharply. Indeed, if the level of bilirubin becomes high enough, it may begin to stain tissues throughout the body a distinctive yellowish color, so that the whites of the eyes and the skin turn yellow—a condition known as jaundice. In the old days people incorrectly blamed many illnesses and disorders on an "excess of bile" and spoke of "feeling liverish" or "suffering from biliousness." Today modern blood chemistry has taken folk-lore out of liver disease, and a variety of *liver function tests* help the doctor either exonerate the liver or pinpoint the specific kind of liver malfunction that is present.

There are far too many different kinds of blood chemistries performed today to describe them all in detail. (The accompanying table lists some of the more common of them with a brief note about the purpose of each.) As little as a decade ago, most of these tests had to be done individually, by hand, by trained laboratory chemists using specially prepared reagents and equipment—a slow and costly proposition. Today, thanks to modern automated lab equipment, whole batteries of these tests can be run automatically on a single sample of blood, with no

Common Blood Chemistry Examinations

Procedure	Purpose
Blood sugar (fasting, 2 hours after breakfast, or glucose tolerance test)	Measurements of blood sugar level; diagnosis of diabetes mellitus
Blood urea nitrogen, non-protein nitrogen	Indirect measurements of kidney function
Serum creatinine	Indirect measurement of kidney function
Serum cholesterol, serum triglycerides	Measurement of fat or lipid metabolism
Serum uric acid	Diagnosis of gout
Serum electrolytes (calcium, phosphorus, sodium, potassium, chlorides, magnesium, etc.)	Reflect fluid balance, general metabolic state, presence of acidosis or alkalosis
CO_2 combining power (blood)	Diagnosis and evaluation of diabetic acidosis
Serum bilirubin	Measurement of liver function, evaluation of jaundice
Alkaline phosphatase (a serum enzyme)	Measurement of liver function
Thymol turbidity	Measurement of liver function
Total blood protein, albumin/globulin ratio	A nonspecific measure of health, abnormal in cases of general debilitation, certain renal diseases, anemia, cancer
Acid phosphatase (a serum enzyme)	Diagnosis of prostatic carcinoma, bone-destructive diseases
Serum amylase, serum lipase	Diagnosis of acute pancreatitis
Protein-bound iodine	A measure of thyroid function
Heterophile antibody agglutination	Diagnosis of infectious mononucleosis
C-reactive protein, streptococcus antibody titers	Diagnosis of rheumatic fever
Blood serology	Diagnosis of secondary or tertiary stages of syphilis

possibility of human error, and at a fraction of the former cost, with a chartlike read-out supplied at the end of the line, all in a few minutes.

Of course, these laboratory tests are not by any means an adequate substitute for a careful, periodical medical history and a complete physical examination, but when used to *supplement* the doctor's examination, they are a real step forward toward truly effective preventive health care. Early detection of many disorders and diseases may spell the difference between life and death, continuing good health or permanent disability, and the judicious use of diagnostic laboratory examinations often makes this possible.

Other Laboratory Examinations

In addition to those familiar examinations that are of use not only in diagnosis but also in following the progress of illness during the course of treatment, there are a great many other kinds of lab study that play an important role under special circumstances. For instance, in disorders involving the brain or spinal cord a wealth of diagnostic information can be obtained by an examination of the cerebrospinal fluid—the watery fluid, usually crystal-clear, which bathes the spinal cord, the lower spinal nerves and the brain itself. Samples of this fluid may be obtained by means of a lumbar puncture (LP), sometimes called a "spinal tap." In other kinds of disorders samples of sputum, stool or even digestive fluid from the stomach or upper intestine may be examined. Samples of bone marrow are sometimes needed to diagnose various blood diseases, and abnormal fluid collections in the chest or even surrounding the heart can be tapped, with special techniques, for microscopic examination or chemical analysis.

Other lab tests are designed not to detect abnormalities, but to protect the patient from harm as a result of medicines or other substances that are about to be administered. Some protective antitoxins, for example, are made from horse serum, a foreign protein substance to which many people are allergic. Before administering such an antitoxin, the doctor will invariably inject a tiny drop under the patient's skin, or place a drop of diluted antitoxin in the eye as a test against possible allergic reactions; he knows that some people are so violently allergic to such substances that administration of a full dose might be fatal.

Blood Typing. Another protective lab procedure is the typing and cross-matching of whole blood before it is administered to a patient. The first attempts to transfuse blood from one person to another led to baffling and disappointing results. Sometimes it worked splendidly; other times the same recipient would have a violent *transfusion reaction* almost as soon as the transfusion was begun, break into chills and sweats and even go into shock and die. No one understood why until it was discovered that red cells in the blood may have substances on their surfaces known as *agglutinogens,* while the blood serum may contain *antibodies* that can activate these agglutinogens and cause the red cells bearing them to clump together or "agglutinate" when the red cells of one person come in contact with a different type of antibody in another person's blood. The earliest investigation of this odd state of affairs revealed that two major blood factors seemed to be involved, and they were designated by the capital letters A and B. A donor's blood carrying A-agglutinogens on the red cells could be given to a recipient who had only anti-B antibodies in his serum without any difficulty; but if the same blood were given to a recipient who had anti-A antibodies in his serum, the transfused red cells would begin clumping together, blocking up the tiny capillaries and causing the symptoms of a transfusion reaction. The same reaction would occur if a donor's blood carrying B-agglutinogens on the cells were transfused into a recipient with anti-B antibodies in his serum.

Thus, two major blood groups were described: Group A, containing A-agglutinogens and anti-B antibodies, and Group B, containing B-agglutinogens and anti-A antibodies. However, it was also determined that some people had *neither* A nor B agglutinogens on their red cells; they were therefore designated as Group O, and (at least in theory) could donate blood to either Group A or Group B recipients without danger, and thus became popularly known as "universal donors." A much smaller group of people had *both* A and B agglutinogens on their red cells, and thus could not donate blood to anyone with either anti-A or anti-B antibodies, but could *receive* from either Group A or Group B donors, since the antibodies in these donors' serum would be so rapidly diluted by the recipient's own blood that no clumping of cells could occur. This latter group were called Group AB and became known as "universal recipients."

Because of this disparity in blood groups, it is, of course, imperative that both the recipient's and the donor's blood be typed before a transfusion is attempted. *Blood typing* is a simple laboratory procedure in which red cells from a sample of a patient's blood are mixed with commercially prepared anti-A and anti-B serum on a glass slide, and then examined to see which of the serum antibodies, if any, causes the red cells to agglutinate. A donor's blood is then chosen from the same blood group as the recipient's. Even with this precaution, however, transfusion reactions still occurred from time to time for no apparent reason. As a result, today an additional, more complex procedure called *cross-matching* is carried out whenever a transfusion is planned, wherein donor's cells are mixed with recipient's serum, and recipient's cells are mixed with donor's serum in separate test tubes and incubated at body temperature for an hour or so, then examined under the microscope for any sign of agglutination in either mixture. These precautionary tests are normally done at the hospital or laboratory, in the laboratory of the blood bank, or even both places, and are so effective that transfusion reactions are extremely rare today despite the hundreds of thousands of units of blood that are transfused in this country every year.

Another problem related to blood groups came to light early in this century when it was found that a strange kind of blood disease called *erythroblastosis fetalis* occasionally occurred in newborn babies delivered of mothers who had had blood transfusions for some reason prior to their pregnancies. (*See* p. 833.) The fault lay in a previously unsuspected factor present in the blood of most people, but absent in a small minority. Called the "Rh factor" because it was

first identified in experiments with rhesus monkeys, it had no effect on a baby if the mother carried the Rh-agglutinogen on her red blood cells. But if a woman *without* Rh-agglutinogens—that is, an Rh-negative woman—became pregnant by an Rh-positive father, her baby would be Rh-positive, and anti-Rh antibodies would begin to form in her blood during the pregnancy. If enough of these antibodies were formed, they could then cross the placenta to the baby's blood stream and cause a disease in the baby very similar to a transfusion reaction, in which a great many red blood cells would dissolve and the child might even die at the time of delivery or immediately afterward. This reaction was particularly marked if the Rh-negative woman had, at some earlier time, received a transfusion of Rh-positive blood, so that her body was already "sensitized" to form anti-Rh antibodies the moment Rh-agglutinogens began forming in the unborn baby's blood stream.

Fortunately, blood typing procedures were quickly devised so that Rh-negative women could readily be identified, and care could be taken never to give them transfusions of Rh-positive blood. Alerted ahead of time to possible trouble, obstetricians could be prepared to treat erythroblastosis in a newborn baby of an Rh-negative mother by means of *exchange transfusions* which removed the blood containing anti-Rh antibodies from the baby's body and replaced it with antibody-free blood. Thus, many infant lives were saved by a comparatively simple laboratory test. Today a newly developed "Rh-immune" serum can be administered to Rh-negative women to prevent them from forming anti-Rh-antibodies any time they are exposed to Rh-agglutinogens; as use of this serum becomes more widespread, complete control of "Rh disease" in babies will at last be possible.

Today we know that many other minor blood groups exist in addition to the ABO system and the Rh groups, but for the most part these minor agglutinogens do not stimulate enough antibody formation to cause any trouble. Thus a person's blood type is usually stated only according to the ABO and Rh grouping—"Type A, Rh-positive" or "Type O, Rh-negative," for example. Many people have the mistaken idea that their blood type should be kept somewhere on their person, carried in a wallet or on an identification tag. This may have been a wise precaution during wartime for men on the battlefield, but ordinarily it serves no useful purpose. Any time blood is donated or required for transfusion, it is typed on the spot, regardless of what any identification may say.

Modern Bacteriology. Another important aspect of laboratory work today is the use of bacteriological techniques to stain disease-causing organisms for examination under the microscope, or actually to grow or "culture" bacteria in the laboratory so that they can be identified and their relative sensitivity to various antibiotics tested. Some people assume that the many antibiotic drugs used to fight infection have rendered these bacteriological studies superfluous, but in fact just the opposite is true. Some of the most dangerous bacteria, including the common staphylococcus organisms, rapidly become "immune" to the effects of one antibiotic or another by developing drug-resistant strains. Thus, when treating a staph infection, the only way the doctor can tell which of the many antibiotic drugs available is most likely to be effective is to have the infecting organism cultured and tested against antibiotic samples in the laboratory.

Bacteriological samples may be taken from any source where infection is present: the nose and throat, an infected ear, an abscess, and even from urine when a bladder or kidney infection is suspected. Among the most dangerous of bacterial infections are those in which bacteria are released into the blood stream to produce "blood poisoning" or septicemia. Blood poisoning was once a dreaded killer that could follow virtually any kind of infection; today, by means of careful bacteriological techniques, any bacteria present in samples of blood can be cultured in vials of broth, making swift, specific antibiotic protection against septicemia possible. Similarly, samples of spinal fluid can be cultured to identify the villain when bacteria invade the spinal cord and cause bacterial meningitis. So far, most bacteriological techniques have not been successfully automated, so these lab examinations must still be done by skilled technicians, and thus remain comparatively costly. On the other hand, the information bacteriological studies provide may save days or weeks of debility, hospitalization and time lost at work.

Electrocardiograms. Of all the laboratory studies a patient may encounter in the course of a complete physical examination, none is more widely misunderstood than the electrocardiogram, commonly called "EKG" in America or "ECG" in England. Even patients completely familiar with the procedure sometimes fear that the EKG leads attached to their wrists and ankles are dangerous, and they lie there rigidly, waiting to feel a shock.

Of course, this kind of apprehension is ridiculous; the machine is really nothing more than a highly sensitive *galvanometer,* an instrument designed to detect and record on a paper tape the tiny electrical currents that are produced naturally by the heart's pacemaker—the collection of nerves that regulate the heartbeat—and which then pass down through the heart muscle with each heartbeat in such a way that they can be picked up by EKG leads in contact with the skin. By placing the leads at various places on the body, the technician can thus record tracings of the course these currents follow.

To most laymen, an EKG tracing looks like nothing more than a wiggly black line on a long strip of white graph paper. To the doctor, however, it provides a remarkably clear and detailed "picture" of the structure and function of the heart. From the tracing, for example, he can tell the *rate* of the heartbeat and can determine at a glance even the most subtle disturbance in its rhythm. If such an *arrhythmia* is present, he can also tell just where in the heart the disturbance arises, whether in the thick muscle of the ventricles, in the thin wall of the auricles, or in the pacemaker itself. He can also judge the heart's relative size and position; and finally, since areas of the heart muscle damaged by a coronary attack show characteristic "injury changes" on an EKG tracing soon after the damage has occurred, and may then leave permanent "scar patterns" after an injury has healed, the doctor can often see clear-cut evidence of old coronary disease, or can confirm or rule out a recent coronary attack from a study of one or more EKG tracings taken at daily intervals.

There is no reason to be alarmed if, in the course of a complete physical examination, the doctor orders an EKG tracing even though there have been no symptoms of any heart disease. There is a very sound reason for recording a "healthy" or "normal" electrocardiogram: it provides a *baseline record* of the heart's behavior at a time when it is not impaired in any way. This record then becomes a permanent part of the patient's medical history and can be used for comparison if any heart symptoms develop in the future. Since EKG tracings can be photocopied, or even transmitted electronically from one part of the country to another if necessary, a "healthy" baseline EKG can be retrieved and used for comparison anywhere or any time it is needed.

X-Ray Diagnosis and Treatment

Probably no diagnostic aid has become more controversial in recent times, or more subject to unfounded criticism and scare stories, than the use of X-ray examinations in the modern medical office or clinic. X-rays are dangerous, we are told, and doctors use them far too freely, exposing their patients to excessive amounts of radiation. What the critics rarely mention, however, is that modern X-ray techniques provide one of the most effective diagnostic aids in the medical armamentarium; when used with judgment and discretion they are quite harmless; and without them the doctor would be deprived of one of his major weapons in the fight against disease.

X-rays were first discovered in 1895, more than two-thirds of a century ago, by the German physicist Wilhelm Konrad Roentgen. At first no one knew the nature of these so-called Roentgen rays, but their enormous value in diagnosis was recognized at once. Within four days after news of Roentgen's discovery reached the United States, X-ray pictures were used to help locate a bullet in a patient's leg. Fractured bones could easily be diagnosed by this process, to say nothing of foreign objects in the body, cavities in

teeth, or calcium deposits in arthritic joints. What was more, by filling a soft tissue cavity— the stomach or colon, for example—with a suspension of insoluble metallic salts such as barium chloride, doctors could actually observe the outlines of organs that had previously been beyond the reach of examination. Within a decade doctors who had special training in X-ray diagnosis became the first workers in a completely new branch of medicine known as *roentgenology* or (more commonly) *radiology*.

It soon became apparent, however, that the use of X-rays could involve dangers as well as benefits. Once the phenomenon of natural radioactivity was discovered by Henri Becquerel just a year after Roentgen's discovery of X-rays, it became clear that X-rays were in fact very high-energy *gamma rays,* electromagnetic waves with much shorter wavelength and with far greater energy and penetrating power than waves of visible light. If human tissues were exposed to these rays for too long, or in too large doses, they could cause a scattering of secondary radiation when they struck dense materials such as metal or bone, so that anyone standing in the near vicinity would be irradiated every time an X-ray picture was taken.

In particular, the use of X-rays in those early days proved dangerous to the doctors who were constantly working with X-ray equipment; many pioneering radiologists developed radiation burns and cancer of the skin on their fingers as a result of the common practice of holding X-ray plates in position with unshielded hands. Many others died of bone cancer or leukemia. Also endangered were patients who were examined by *fluoroscopy,* an X-ray technique in which a continuing stream of X-rays was passed through the patient while the radiologist studied a "living X-ray shadow" cast on a fluorescent screen.

As soon as these dangers were discovered, of course, steps were taken to reduce the risk of overirradiation to both doctor and patient. Today these risks have been all but eliminated in three ways: by reducing the amount of exposure necessary to take X-ray pictures; by use of effective shielding so that only the area to be examined is exposed to X-rays; and by judicious

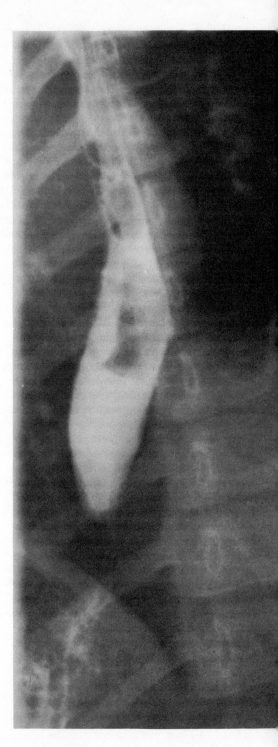

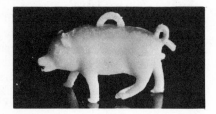

Plate 39
An X-ray curiosity. The patient, a six-year-old child, was brought to the doctor after swallowing a foreign object that seemed "caught in his throat." The careful observer can distinguish the shadow-image of a small, inch-and-one-half long plastic pig lodged in the child's esophagus in this barium swallow X-ray. The pig (see inset, actual size) was subsequently extracted and the child recovered without complications.

restraint on the part of the doctor so that unnecessary X-ray examinations are not performed. For example, modern X-ray machines use *image intensifiers* to help produce better X-ray films with less radiation. Plates of metallic lead, through which X-rays cannot penetrate, or aprons made of lead and rubber, are used to shield both doctor and patient from unnecessary radiation. Fluoroscopy has been abandoned almost completely, except when used for X-ray examination of the stomach or intestines; when it *is* used, the radiologist wears red plastic goggles for fifteen minutes to accommodate his eyes to darkness before entering a pitch-dark X-ray room for the examination. This way his eyes can pick up a very faint, low-radiation image on the fluoroscope, and the patient is exposed to X-rays for only a few brief seconds. Other precautions are also taken; an obstetrician, for example, will guard his pregnant patient against any but emergency X-ray examinations. Thanks to these safeguards, there is little risk of any significant overexposure to X-rays during a physical examination or in the treatment of an illness.

Listed below are a number of X-ray studies that are commonly used in a complete physical examination, depending, of course, on the patient's medical history and the nature of the signs and symptoms specifically under investigation.

Chest X-Ray. Probably the most familiar of all X-ray procedures, chest X-rays are made almost routinely as part of physical examinations, and may be ordered for diagnostic purposes between regular exams. Most useful in detecting early pulmonary tuberculosis, lung cancer or pneumonia, these films have saved innumerable lives. Besides pinpointing disease of the lungs, they also provide valuable information about the size and position of the heart, which is clearly outlined on the film. Most chest X-rays are taken in an *anterior-posterior* (front to back) view, but sometimes a *lateral* (side view) film is also of great value.

How often is a chest X-ray necessary? This depends to some extent upon the health and habits of the patient. Cigarette smokers should have chest X-rays taken at six-month intervals without fail to detect cancer of the lung as early as possible if it develops. Perfectly healthy young people who do not smoke and have had no problem with bronchitis, pneumonia or other upper respiratory infections may need a screening chest film no more often than every two or three years. Again, the best judge of what is of most value to a particular patient is his doctor, but a chest X-ray requires such a minimal exposure to radiation that even frequent films will have no damaging effect, and they should be taken any time there is medical indication.

Flat Plate of the Abdomen. This is another screening X-ray, a single film taken of the abdomen and used either by itself or in combination with other kinds of abdominal X-ray studies for diagnostic purposes. The flat plate can reveal a variety of conditions such as enlargement of the liver or spleen, the presence of calcified gallstones, soft-tissue growths or tumors in the abdomen, or even the presence of a great quantity of constipated stool. When other X-rays of the abdomen are to be taken, the flat plate can reveal collections of intestinal gas, for instance, that might interfere with the proper interpretation of subsequent films.

Upper GI Series. As the name suggests, this is a series of X-ray films made of the upper half of the gastrointestinal (GI) tract when some condition such as a peptic ulcer is suspected. The patient is given a suspension of chalky-tasting but harmless barium chloride to swallow, and the esophagus, stomach, duodenum and upper intestine are examined by the radiologist under a fluoroscope equipped with a device that makes permanent "spot X-ray films" that can be studied later. The whole examination takes only a few moments, and may reveal such various disorders as acute gastritis, ulcer of the stomach or duodenum, cancer of the stomach or pancreas, or the generally benign condition known as hiatus hernia, in which a small defect in the diaphragm allows the upper part of the stomach to protrude into the chest cavity.

Lower GI Series (Barium Enema). These films are taken when some disorder of the lower intestine or colon is suspected, especially rectal polyps or other tumorous growths. A suspension of barium chloride is introduced into the colon by means of an enema, and films are taken both before and after the enema is expelled. Again fluoroscopic examination permits "spot films" of suspicious-looking areas to be taken for careful examination later. Both upper and lower GI series are almost always taken by radiologists because a great deal of skill and experience is needed to perform these examinations and interpret the film.

Intravenous Pyelograms (IVP). These films, which permit the doctor to visualize the interior of the kidneys, ureters and bladder, are possible because of the property of the kidneys to filter certain kinds of foreign chemicals out of the blood stream very rapidly. A special dye containing an iodine compound opaque to X-rays is injected into a vein, and several X-rays of the abdomen are then taken at intervals. Amazingly enough, the kidneys are so efficient that most of the dye is ordinarily filtered out of the blood within some ten minutes after it is injected, and forms a sharply defined shadow of the interior of the kidneys and ureters. This is a comparatively simple X-ray procedure and permits examination of an area that cannot be readily visualized any other way.

Gall Bladder Series. Again an odd physiological property of the body can be used to obtain good X-ray pictures of another organ that would not ordinarily be visible on X-ray. In this case, the patient is given capsules or pills containing an iodine compound to be taken by mouth the night before the examination. This particular compound is one which is incorporated in the bile formed in the liver, and is then concentrated and stored in the gall bladder. Spot X-rays of the gall bladder area taken the next morning reveal a clear image of the interior of the gall bladder (if it is present and functional) and make it possible to see gallstones, often outlined in sharp contrast. After initial films, the patient is given a breakfast with a high-fat content so that the gall bladder is stimulated to empty its bile into the duodenum; subsequent films reveal how effectively the gall bladder is functioning.

Skull Series, Spine Series, and X-Rays of the Extremities. Finally, a number of standardized X-ray series have been developed to permit adequate X-ray visualization of the skull, the upper or lower segments of the spine, the hips, and the extremities. These examinations always require X-rays taken from at least two directions—both anterior-posterior and lateral views—and sometimes at special angles. The procedures are standardized so that films of a patient's lumbar spine, for example, taken by one physician can be readily interpreted by another at a later date. None of these studies is performed routinely with every patient; they are ordered only when some aspect of the history or the physical examination indicates that they will be of real benefit in diagnosis.

Special X-Ray Examinations. There are a number of X-ray procedures that are never done as routine, but provide invaluable information in dealing with specific problems. Certain of these procedures are performed under anesthesia, or even in the course of surgery; others are done only on special indication. For example, *mammography* is a technique to provide X-ray films of the female breasts when a lump in the breast has been found which might prove to be cancerous. Even in early breast cancer, tiny traces of calcium are sometimes deposited in the tumor, evidence of the body's attempt to wall off and isolate the dangerous growth. Before the surgeon undertakes surgical removal of such a lump to determine its nature, he wants all the information he can obtain in advance. Mammography can thus provide an advance clue as to whether a lump may or may not be cancerous.

During gall bladder surgery, especially when gallstones are present, the surgeon's work can sometimes be complicated by the presence of a gallstone wedged tightly in the common bile duct. *Operative cholangiograms* help detect such a hidden danger; the surgeon fills the common duct with an iodine dye during surgery, and X-rays are made and examined on the spot to determine if the common bile duct is free of obstruction, or must be explored with instruments before the surgery is finished. Another kind of X-ray examination done in the operating room under anesthesia is a more detailed examination of the kidney than IVP's make possible. After examining the interior of the patient's bladder with a lighted instrument called a cystoscope, the urologist introduces radio-opaque dye into both ureters from below, under sufficient pressure to fill the urine-collecting cavity of both kidneys. X-rays called *retrograde pyelograms* are then taken in the operating room, and are especially valuable in diagnosing obstructions or tumors of the urinary tract that might be missed by IVP's.

Other even more difficult and specialized X-ray techniques have been developed for examining remote parts of the body. *Myelograms,* for example, are taken to help pinpoint the location of a herniated ("slipped") disk in the spine prior to surgery. *Cerebral angiograms* outlining the arterial blood supply to the brain are made by injecting radio-opaque dye into a carotid artery, and then following the course of the dye in the blood stream by means of a series of rapid-fire X-rays taken in the course of a few seconds. *Angiocardiograms* work in reverse; dye introduced into one of the great veins returning blood to the heart can be followed in its course through the heart chambers, helping detect such heart defects as an abnormal opening between one chamber and another. Perhaps most startling of all the specialized X-ray examinations is the *pneumoencephalogram,* in which cerebrospinal fluid is drained from the spinal canal and replaced with air. Since X-rays pass through air more readily than through watery fluid, these special films provide a shadowy outline of the ventricles of the brain which are normally filled with cerebrospinal fluid, and help identify any obstruction of the spinal canal. After the examination the air is gradually absorbed into the blood stream and the spinal canal is filled once again with naturally forming spinal fluid.

Modern X-Ray Therapy

In addition to their importance in diagnosis, X-rays can also be used in the treatment of a number of disorders. Years ago, before the threat of overexposure was fully recognized, X-rays were used to treat a variety of skin diseases ranging all the way from ringworm infections to adolescent acne. Most such wide-exposure techniques have been abandoned now; the risk is just not worth the possible benefit. But in treating certain deep-seated cancers, for example, X-ray therapy is ideal; X-rays can damage normal, healthy cells if the exposure is great enough, but they seem to damage the abnormal cells of cancer even more. By shielding a patient except for a single small "target zone"—an inoperable cancerous tumor of the lung, for example—huge doses of X-ray irradiation can be focused on the diseased tissue, and cancers exposed in this way often shrink in size, their growth arrested for prolonged intervals. X-ray exposure can also often be used *after* cancer surgery in an effort to destroy any remaining cancer cells that may have seeded in the surrounding area. X-ray therapy can often be combined with, or substituted for, other types of radiation therapy such as exposure to radium, radon, or radioactive cobalt; the radiologist, experienced in using all these substances for treatment, chooses the most effective form of radiation therapy for a given tumor.

In X-ray therapy, of course, the amount of radiation used is far, far greater than that required for any sort of diagnostic X-ray films. In some cases, where cancer is the target of the therapy, exposure to X-rays may be pushed up to the maximum limit the patient can tolerate, and often radiation burns or symptoms of radiation sickness result. Only expert and experienced medical judgment can determine if the potential benefit of the therapy outweighs the dangers and discomforts.

Up until very recently, the use of X-rays and other forms of radiation therapy was restricted to treatment of localized regions—for example, intensive exposure in the area of a lung cancer while shielding the rest of the patient from radiation. Recently, however, there has been experimental use of X-ray and other radiation in smaller doses over longer periods of time to treat such generalized disorders as leukemia. Indeed, one medical center located at Oak Ridge, Tennessee, has recently built an "irradiation chamber" in the form of a comfortably appointed motel room, in which a victim of leukemia can spend two or three days, his whole body receiving a low dosage of radiation the entire time.

X-ray techniques, both for diagnosis and for therapy, are improving and evolving all the time; but all new developments in the use of X-rays are worked out in full awareness of the possible dangers of excessive irradiation. If, however, in the course of diagnostic examination or treatment, a patient becomes concerned about the amount of X-rays he is being exposed to, he should not hesitate to raise the question with his doctor. He should certainly be able to prove, on the basis of expert authority, that his use of X-rays is not even approaching the dangerous level.

Other Special Diagnostic Examinations

Occasionally, during the course of a medical history or a physical examination, something may turn up which demands further investigation beyond the scope of routine diagnostic procedures, and these special studies can be both troublesome and costly. For example, a suspicious spot may appear on a patient's chest X-ray. The doctor may be almost completely convinced that it is the harmless residual of some earlier respiratory disorder, yet he knows it could also be cancer. Additional diagnostic procedures are performed and the patient is subjected to considerable inconvenience and expense only to discover that it was not cancer after all. The question often raised at this point is, "Was it worth it?" The answer must be an emphatic yes. In this case, if the doctor's suspicions had been confirmed and it was cancer, the patient's only hope would have been in early diagnosis and treatment. In short, neither the doctor nor his patient can afford *not* to follow up a suspicious condition whatever the eventual diagnosis, no matter how costly and troublesome it may be. To do otherwise is to gamble with the patient's life.

There are a variety of special examinations designed to identify, or rule out, either cancer of the lung or tuberculosis, the two most threatening causes for the appearance of abnormal spots on a chest X-ray. These tests might include sputum examinations for tubercle bacilli, skin tests to determine if the patient has ever had a tuberculosis infection, other skin tests to help identify various fungus infections of the lung which sometimes masquerade as tuberculosis or cancer, and probably *bronchoscopy,* a procedure in which a long, narrow lighted instrument is used for direct visual examination of the trachea and larger bronchi where cancer often originates. In the course of the same procedure, a saline solution may be used to "wash" the bronchi, and then be recovered by means of a suction device to be examined for cancer cells. It is characteristic of cancerous growths that the malignant cells are not properly glued together as normal cells are, so that some may be broken free by a *bronchial washing* and later appear under the pathologist's microscope as telltale evidence that a cancer is present.

Another type of special examination, the *biopsy,* is very commonly performed to help identify the exact nature of a number of disorders. A biopsy is frequently used to diagnose cancer, but this is not by any means its only use. In fact the procedure, in which a small fragment of tissue is removed from a lesion for microscopic examination by a pathologist, may be helpful in diagnosing noncancerous disorders as far-ranging as boils, warts, cysts, parasitic diseases of various sorts, and menstrual irregularity. Biopsies can be made of practically any part of the body, even of bone marrow, when necessary. Once a bit of biopsied tissue has been removed, it is chemically preserved, hardened and embedded in wax; then slides are made from thin slices of the tissue and stained for microscopic examination. Usually several hours of laboratory preparation are necessary before biopsy slides can be made ready for reading by the pathologist, but when necessary a so-called *frozen section* can be prepared in a few moments and a preliminary examination made by the pathologist while the surgeon and the patient are still in the operating room. (*See* p. 940.) This procedure is particularly helpful when there is a question of cancer and the surgeon does not want to lose even a moment excising it if its presence can be demonstrated.

In less serious situations, of course, the biopsy of such lesions as rectal polyps or subcutaneous cysts can be done in the doctor's office, the specimen preserved and then mailed to the pathologist for a report. Strictly speaking, the commonplace Pap smear examination for early cancer of the cervix is a "biopsy," since cells are scraped from the vulnerable area and then transferred to glass slides for later examination.

The Therapeutic Trial

One additional aid to diagnosis is the perfectly valid, and sometimes even crucial, medical procedure a doctor may choose to follow in unraveling a difficult diagnostic problem. It is simply the prescription of appropriate drugs or medicines on a trial basis in the hope that close observation of their effect on the patient may help confirm or rule out a suspected diagnosis.

This procedure, called a *therapeutic trial,* is not at all the haphazard proposition it might seem to be at first glance. It is rarely used unless the doctor already has strong suspicions of the correct diagnosis and has exhausted other means of confirming it. Even then he will proceed only if he is confident that the "trial medication," whatever it may be, will have no *ill* effect. It is especially valuable when some specific medicine is known to have a clear-cut, readily discernible effect in the case of one given disorder and no other; a favorable response to the medicine, in such a case, becomes a valuable clue to the true nature of the disorder. For example, the pain of angina pectoris, due to impaired circulation of blood to the heart, may be difficult to distinguish, in some cases, from pain due to pleurisy or even peptic ulcer. There is one drug, however—nitroglycerine—which often acts swiftly and specifically to dilate the coronary arteries and relieve the pain of angina pectoris very dramatically, although it has no effect whatever in relieving other kinds of pain. Thus a doctor might prescribe nitroglycerine tentatively as a therapeutic trial, to be used whenever the pain appears. If the pain is quickly and consistently relieved by the medication, the doctor will suspect angina pectoris all the more strongly; but if the medicine fails to relieve the pain, he will know that angina pectoris is unlikely, and look more closely for other causes.

Therapeutic trials of medicine are obviously no substitute for a carefully recorded medical history, a thorough physical examination, laboratory tests, X-ray examinations and other special studies. But in a very practical way they can sometimes be immensely helpful in getting to the source of a patient's problem, and thus play an important role in the modern diagnosis and treatment of illness.

When Diagnosis Fails

The modern doctor has a truly remarkable medical armamentarium to help him diagnose a wide range of health problems. Yet it is still impossible to claim that all these medical resources will invariably lead him to a correct diagnosis of a disorder already present or a condition that may threaten in the future. For all the diagnostic aids available, and for all his knowledge, skill and experience, there are times when a doctor ultimately comes up with no diagnosis at all.

What, then, can you expect a doctor to do if he fails to arrive at a satisfactory diagnosis? First, he may do nothing at all except wait. More than anyone else, he has great respect for the body's remarkable capacity for self-repair, and he knows how often troublesome disorders heal themselves without medical intervention, given time and patience. Alternatively, he may prescribe *symptomatic treatment* to help relieve the discomfort of specific symptoms while he watches and waits. Some doctors scorn the treatment of symptoms as an ineffective stop-gap measure which might even mask the nature of the underlying disorder, but most doctors take a more practical stand. They recognize that the patient seeks, and deserves, relief from pain or other distressing symptoms even as he seeks help in finding the cause of the symptoms. As long as symptomatic treatment is not *substituted* for continuing efforts to diagnose the illness, there is no reason that the patient should be deprived of symptomatic relief whenever possible.

Repeated examinations often unearth the key to a diagnostic puzzle. When a disorder persists, the doctor may order repeated lab tests or X-rays to compare with earlier data. He will almost surely seek consultation with other doctors when he faces a baffling diagnostic problem, and if the patient feels at any time that another doctor's opinion should be obtained, he should have no hesitation about requesting it. Consultation may not bring an answer either, but at least it will help ensure that no stone is left unturned.

Each individual case will dictate the approach to be taken when a satisfactory diagnosis cannot be made. There are cases, for example, in which a conscientious surgeon feels compelled to do an exploratory operation—known as a *laparotomy* —in order to determine a diagnosis; in other cases, apparently similar, the same surgeon may insist upon waiting, watching, and doing nothing. The deciding factors may seem very minor to the patient, but there will always be sound medical judgment behind the decision.

In the long run, most disorders are either diagnosed, at last, or disappear of their own accord. Most grave illnesses do yield to diagnosis, if the search is persistent enough, before they have progressed to a point of no return. The secret is persistent cooperation between doctor and patient, working as a team against a common foe. With the medical resources available today, this kind of teamwork can provide the most effective assurance of continuing good health.

The Doctor's Training

The complex procedure by which a doctor elicits a patient's medical history, performs a physical examination, arrives at one or more tentative diagnoses, and selects laboratory or X-ray studies to help him track down the cause of a patient's complaint obviously requires a great deal of knowledge and experience in observing and treating various kinds of illness. But complex as it is, this procedure follows a completely logical pattern from beginning to end. To many patients, in fact, it may seem to be altogether too automatic. Considering this, might it not be possible for a computer to do a better job than a doctor? Oddly enough, in some respects it would be, and the use of computers as an adjunct to medical diagnosis is already the subject of a great deal of intensive study. There is no question that the computer is going to become as indispensable to tomorrow's physician as skilled laboratory and X-ray personnel are today.

Nevertheless, most of us would feel just a bit uneasy about going to see a computer when we were sick, no matter how reliable and sophisticated it might be. For one thing, a very important part of the doctor-patient relationship is the human element. For another, good judgment is an additional element in the relationship that no computer, no matter how complex, could apply. In the long run, it is *the doctor's judgment* in studying and evaluating a medical problem that we count upon most heavily. And if this is true when we are ill, it is all the more valuable when we try to follow a program of preventive medical care.

Where does the doctor acquire this critical capacity for medical judgment? How does he acquire the necessary knowledge and skill? A century ago training in medicine was far more casual than it is today. In those days a prospective doctor, after a year or two of college, would "read medicine" for another two or three years under the guidance of a local practicing physician. Then he might spend another one to three years studying at a medical college, if he could afford it, learning to examine patients and write case histories in the hospital associated with the school. When he felt adequately prepared, he would take licensure examinations, if any were required in the place where he wanted to practice, and hang out his shingle, sometimes with as little as three years of formal medical training behind him. If he were rich and ambitious enough, he might even spend a few additional years in one of the leading medical centers in Europe, studying under a particular teacher to become a "specialist" in some field of medicine. But one hundred years ago only a very few doctors became specialists; by far the majority went directly from the skimpy basic medical training they had received into the general practice of medicine.

Such a system was informal to say the least. Indeed, by the early 1900s, medical training in America was so haphazard, so variable from one part of the country to another, and so disgracefully inadequate in many areas that it had become a laughingstock to sophisticated physicians in Vienna, Paris and London, and a scandal here at home. Then, in 1910, a stubborn and courageous educator named Abraham Flexner conducted a nationwide study of the sad state of American medical training, pointed out its multiple inadequacies, and scourged the profession for having done nothing to improve it. In addition, he set forth an orderly and sensible blueprint for what modern medical training *ought* to be. Within a decade the Flexner Report had set a new standard for medical education all over the country, and within a very few years thereafter medical training in America was fast becoming the best available in the world, and it remains so to this day.

Today a prospective doctor must spend no less than nine years obtaining his basic medical training anywhere in the United States. First, he has four years of *premedical training* in a college or university, earning a Bachelor of Science or Bachelor of Arts degree. Thereafter, he enters an accredited *medical school* for another four years of intensive study, and upon his graduation spends at least one year in a hospital *internship* before he is qualified to take licensure examinations and enter into general practice. Most young doctors today, however, spend from one to four additional hospital years in *residency training* in some specialized field of medicine, so that it is not uncommon for a doctor to have studied as long as thirteen years or even more before entering practice.

The Premedical Testing Ground

Would-be doctors today come from every region of the country and from all walks of life; many date their interest in medicine from the age of eleven or twelve, and pursue a growing interest in the biological sciences right on into college. Many different courses in high school help guide and develop these interests, with formal introductions to such studies as biology, chemistry and physics. After high school, the premedical courses in college provide not only more advanced scientific studies such as zoology, bacteriology and organic chemistry, but also courses in history, philosophy, literature, the arts and foreign languages, for a good doctor must first of all be a well-educated human being,

capable of dealing effectively with people, not just with illness. At the same time, there are enough scientific challenges to premedicine to test the ability of the would-be doctor to handle the difficult studies that will come later, and to open all sorts of doors for exploration. Many young men and women go on to totally different pursuits after finishing premedical training, but for those who stay with medicine, their four years of college premedicine prepare the ground for the prolonged, intensive study of human illness that begins on the first day of medical school.

Medical School: The Preclinical Years

When a student enters medical school he does not start off at once examining sick people, making hospital rounds and trotting around with a stethoscope sticking out of his pocket. The first two years of medical school are devoted almost entirely to an intensive study of the *basic medical sciences* that underlie virtually everything that is known about human illness and human health today. Obviously no one can hope to understand illness without first knowing what "wellness" is. Thus the first part of medical school training is devoted to learning all about the *normal* structure and function of the human body. This study includes the following subjects:

Anatomy. *The study of the normal structure of the body and its various organ systems.* Much of this study is done in the dissecting laboratory, where medical students spend long hours meticulously dissecting and learning the structure of human cadavers. In addition to his own anatomical dissections, the medical student also studies dissections of particularly complicated parts of the body—the neck, for example, or the hand—especially prepared by doctors taking residency training in surgery, in which a detailed knowledge of anatomy is more important than anywhere else. Because the structure of the brain and nervous system is more complex and difficult than any other part of the body, special attention is paid to the study of *neuroanatomy*. Finally, the student correlates his study of the overall or gross anatomy of the body with the study of the microscopic structure of various body tissues—so-called *microscopic anatomy or histology*. Thus he acquires detailed knowledge both of the structures of the body that can be readily observed and of those too small to be seen without a microscope.

Physiology. *The study of the normal function of the body's different organ systems.* It is in the physiology laboratory that the student learns how blood circulates through the heart and the blood vessels, how the exchange of oxygen and carbon dioxide takes place across the delicate membranes in the lung during respiration, how the digestive system takes in food, digests it and then absorbs the nutrients into the blood stream, and how the kidneys filter waste materials out of the blood. In this laboratory medical students often use each other as "test subjects," measuring changes of blood pressure, while standing or sitting, tracing electrocardiograms to study the function of the heart, measuring the amount of carbon dioxide in exhaled air, and the motility of the stomach before or after eating or while asleep—a long succession of tests and observations, all designed to show what can be expected from the normal human body.

Biochemistry. *The study of the myriads of chemical reactions going on within the cells all over the body.* Virtually all the vital life functions of the body are, in the long run, chemical reactions, and the chemistry of life forms the third leg of the tripod on which the understanding of health and illness is based. Disease can arise from damage to the structure of the body, true, or from the misfunction of an organ system; but it can just as easily result from the breakdown of chemical reactions within the cells. In all three areas the doctor must know the normal in order to recognize and diagnose the abnormal.

Most of the first year of medical school is devoted to these three studies, but the medical student also has some contact with patients by attending special *clinical conferences* at which physician professors present selected patients or case histories as actual examples of the particular aspect of anatomy, physiology or biochemistry the students are studying at the time. One such conference might present a patient with a congenital dislocation of the hip, in order

to illustrate the crippling effect of this anatomical defect. Another day a patient with emphysema might be presented to demonstrate the breakdown of the structure and function of the lung in this disease, while at another conference a patient with diabetes presents a graphic example of a disease caused primarily by a breakdown in one particular biochemical function of the body.

If the first year of medical school is devoted to learning about the *normal* structure and function of the body, the second year is concerned with the *abnormal*—the many diseases that can afflict the human body and how they are detected. The major studies during this year are:

Pathology. *The study of the gross and microscopic changes that take place in the human body in the presence of myriads of different diseases.* The study of pathology is probably the most important of all the basic medical sciences. What, after all, *is* disease? It is the end result of a series of changes from normal that have taken place in the structure or function of the body. Sometimes these changes are caused by an injury, sometimes by the invasion of bacteria or viruses, and sometimes by wear and tear or degeneration of once-healthy tissues. Other changes result from disturbances in the body's normal biochemical reactions, while still others arise from abnormal growth patterns in various cells or tissues, from changes in the hereditary material in germ cells, or from disturbances in the baby's prenatal development which lead to either hereditary or congenital diseases. The medical student, through lectures, laboratory work and the study of textbooks, bit by bit begins to piece together a comprehensive knowledge of the multitudes of pathological changes that can occur in the body, and learns the signs and symptoms that these changes may bring about—the vital clues to the diagnosis of illness.

Bacteriology. *The study of the characteristics of bacteria and viruses that can infect the human body.* There was a time shortly after antibiotics were first discovered when many physicians believed that all types of bacterial diseases would soon be conquered. Nobody today entertains such hopes. Great strides have been made, and many infectious diseases that were once responsible for vast numbers of deaths rarely occur at all any more or can be easily controlled when they do occur; yet there is no single bacterial disease that was known to afflict human beings in 1900 which does not still occur all over the world in spite of the widespread availability of antibiotics. And since bacterial and virus-caused illnesses are still so much with us, a study of the nature of these dangerous invaders and the way they cause illness is a vital part of every medical student's training.

Immunology. *The study of the human body's natural defense mechanisms against bacteria, viruses, and other foreign invaders.* Obviously, this study is closely related to bacteriology. In the case of some infectious illnesses, natural immunity to reinfection occurs so that the same illness can never recur. In the case of other infections, a long-lasting active immunity can be created in the healthy individual by means of vaccination before he ever gets the disease. In addition, although the body's immune reactions are usually considered beneficial, a number of very dangerous illnesses—rheumatic fever, for example, or acute nephritis (kidney inflammation)—can actually be caused by the body's blind overreaction to certain kinds of bacterial infection. Finally, the success of organ transplants depends upon finding ways to suppress normal immune responses that induce the body to reject the transplanted organs. This aspect of immunology is still the subject of intensive research, and when the problem is solved, hopefully not too far in the future, it will open up whole new horizons in medicine. The detailed study of all these immune responses is thus one of the most important parts of the medical student's training.

Pharmacology. *The study of thousands of drugs and other medicinal substances that can have powerful effects on the function of the body, either beneficially in the treatment of illness or deleteriously because of dangerous side effects.* Medicines and drugs have been used to treat illnesses since time immemorial, and a study of the nature and function of these drugs is all the more important considering the vast number of new drugs that are being discovered and used every year. In the past medical students simply memorized thousands of prescriptions that could be used in treating various illnesses, a study known as *materia medica*. Today a student doctor spends hours in the pharmacology laboratory studying the composition and effect of hundreds of potent drugs that are now commonly used in medicine, learning what benefits can be expected from them, and—equally important—what dangers may accompany their use.

Finally, in the second year of medical training, in addition to completing the solid scientific foundation on which his professional skill will be based, the fledgling doctor also begins to learn the rudiments of taking medical histories, completing physical examinations and arriving at tentative diagnoses, the procedures generally known in medicine as "working up the patient." At first students practice on each other, but toward the end of the second medical school year they begin to spend at least some time with patients in the hospital wards acquiring actual experience in these procedures.

Medical School: The Clinical Years

Beginning with the third year in medical school a great change takes place in the training of the would-be doctor. With the solid scientific background of the first two years behind him, the student is now ready to step out into the world of clinical medicine. He must still continue intensive textbook study, but now the texts will be books dealing with medical illness, surgery, obstetrics and pediatrics rather than anatomy and pathology. Even more important, he now spends less time attending didactic lectures, and more time in the actual care of patients in the teaching hospital. This is the year, more than any other, when he begins the long process of "learning by doing" that is so important in medical practice.

This does not, however, mean that the inexperienced student is suddenly handed direct or full responsibility for patients' care in medical or surgical wards. But he does, under the watchful guidance of the attending physicians on the hospital staff, the teaching physicians and the house staff of interns and residents, begin to participate with more experienced doctors in the care of hospitalized patients. Most of the student's time in this third year is divided between the four major areas or "services" into which medical care is traditionally divided: the *medical service,* in which all types of adult illnesses that do not involve surgical correction are diagnosed and treated; the *surgical service,* in which all forms of illness requiring surgical care and attention are treated; the *pediatric service,* in which children's illnesses are treated; and the *obstetrics-gynecology (OB-GYN) service,* in which the student has his first direct contact with maternity patients, labor and delivery room medicine, and the diagnosis and treatment of illnesses, both "medical" and "surgical," that are peculiar to women.

On all of these services the work the medical student does follows a definite pattern. First he becomes acquainted with the patients already hospitalized on the service to which he is assigned, reviewing their hospital charts and case histories and observing their daily care. As new patients are admitted to the service, the medical student undertakes their "hospital admission workups" just as if they were his own patients, duplicating the workup done by the house staff (interns and residents) and reviewed by the attending physicians. These "workups" include eliciting and writing out a detailed medical history, performing a complete physical examination, outlining laboratory and X-ray diagnostic procedures he thinks would help clinch the diagnosis, and listing the differential diagnosis as he sees it. His workups are then reviewed carefully with members of the teaching staff. Anything that has been forgotten or overlooked is picked up; useful suggestions and ideas of merit are noted and may even be incorporated into the patient's care. Then the student proceeds to follow the patient's treatment and recovery, accompanying house doctors and attending physicians on rounds with the patients each day, entering the discussion about the care of all patients that goes on between various physicians acquainted with their progress, meeting with the teaching staff for special formal presentations of particular cases that are being treated, and generally becoming a contributing member of the medical-surgical team of the hospital.

On the surgical service the medical student is, in addition, assigned to assist at various surgical procedures in the operating room—a very low-ranking assistant, to be sure, who is seldom allowed to do more than hold a retractor where the surgeon places it to be held. But he participates at first hand nevertheless, watching the surgical techniques that are being used, actually seeing the surgical lesion just as the surgeon sees it, and learning how routines are performed in the operating room and how emergencies are met. Subsequently, an important part of the surgical service is in following the postoperative care and recovery period of the patients whose surgery he observed.

In the obstetrical service the medical student has his first exposure to the care of maternity patients when they come to the hospital in labor. Ordinarily he does not officiate at the delivery of a baby, although on rare occasions he might if the baby arrives so swiftly that the attending physician or the house staff cannot be reached. Rather he acts as an assistant, learning to recognize the various stages of labor and observing the time-honored procedures, as well as the new techniques, of modern obstetrics. Finally, his time spent in the pediatric service is his first acquaintance with the many diseases peculiar to children. It is during this service that he learns the enormous difference between medical care of weak and fragile children as opposed to strong and hardy adults, and recognizes the other special problems involved in the care of sick children.

Throughout the third year the student also attends a variety of special conferences, lectures in each of the four medical services, the "grand rounds" that are made, usually once a week, on patients in the various services for the specific purpose of teaching not only medical students but experienced physicians as well, X-ray conferences in which he learns to correlate abnormal X-ray findings with the problems of the patients he is treating, and a number of other semiformal and formal teaching procedures. It is at this time, while observing doctors at work among their patients, as well as in clinical conferences and consultations, that he begins to realize that the study of medicine never really comes to an end. Rich in knowledge and experience as the greatest physician may be, there is still much that he can learn, and even he can sometimes be misled, misinformed, or faulty in his judgment.

Nowhere is the fallibility of the physician better demonstrated than at the clinical-pathological conference, a formal exercise in medical study and self-improvement in which virtually all physicians connected with a hospital staff participate. At these conferences a physician ordinarily presents a particularly difficult, baffling or confusing case drawn from his past experience at the hospital with which the other physicians are not familiar. He recounts the presenting complaint of the patient, the history of his illness, the events leading to his hospitalization, the results of his physical examination and the pertinent laboratory or X-ray reports—all without revealing the diagnosis. Then it is up to the other physicians to raise questions about the medical history they would like answered more fully, to suggest further laboratory studies they feel should be done, and then, finally, to attempt to make the correct diagnosis. Ideas and suggestions abound at these meetings, and often strongly conflicting tentative diagnoses are defended by different physicians, because these cases are purposely chosen from among the most difficult and baffling that have ever appeared at the hospital. Not only medical students but interns and residents participate; experienced attending physicians, specialists in all fields, join in the search for diagnosis. Only the presenting physician and the pathologist who has finally determined the true diagnosis from examination of surgical specimens, from biopsies or, in many cases, from post-mortem examinations, know the answer.

It may seem strange that doctors take time from other important duties to play what might appear to be a guessing game, but there is no better way for physicians already in practice to refine their knowledge and for doctors in training to learn the complex byways certain kinds of illness may follow than to match wits in ferreting out difficult diagnoses. Doctors take these conferences with deadly seriousness, for each

one knows that the next patient who walks in his door may present him with precisely such a difficult diagnostic problem, and it may well be that he must either solve that problem or lose the patient—not to another physician but once and for all.

In contrast to the intensely hospital-centered pattern of study and clinical work that the medical student encounters in his third year, the fourth year seems to be far more loose and unstructured. During this last year of medical school more and more of the student's time is devoted not to the study and care of inpatients, but rather to outpatients whose medical problems do not require hospitalization, yet do require medical consultation.

During his inpatient service the third-year medical student has the opportunity to follow many grave or serious illnesses while the patients are hospitalized, but he loses track of their continuing care after they have been discharged from the hospital. During his fourth year he concentrates on this kind of care and experiences precisely the sort of problems the physician in practice must deal with every day in his office. Again his time is divided among the four major medical services; in medical outpatient clinics he becomes acquainted with the long-term continuing care of patients with such afflictions as controlled diabetes, peptic ulcers, arthritis, varicose veins, chronic bronchitis, asthma, emphysema, or a multitude of other conditions which require careful medical supervision but not hospitalization. In the surgical outpatient department, supervised by the teaching and attending staffs of the clinic, he sees both patients who have been referred to the clinic by some other physician for diagnostic consultation and patients who have returned for postoperative checkups and care. In the obstetrical clinic the student has the opportunity to see patients at the beginning of their pregnancies and to follow their maternity care until the time of delivery, thus learning that trouble-free labor and delivery can depend heavily upon the proper preventive care throughout the gestation period. Finally, in the pediatric clinic he not only sees many children with disorders that require outpatient care but also those recently released from the hospital who require convalescent care. In addition, he spends part of his time in a so-called well-baby clinic, in which, with supervision, he learns to examine infants and prepares himself to meet the questions and problems of mothers with babies still in their early years.

It is also during his fourth year that the medical student obtains experience in some of the "specialty services" which are discussed in more detail in the following chapter. For example, he spends time in the ophthalmology clinic observing the kind of problems that present themselves to the specialist in eye diseases. More time will be spent in the ear, nose and throat clinic, the pulmonary function clinic, the orthopedic and fracture clinic, the gynecology clinic, and in clinics devoted to many other medical specialties. The purpose of this kind of training is to acquaint the student with the kinds of problems that require a specialist's attention, so that when he begins his own practice he will be able to judge when consultation is necessary, or when a particular problem should be transferred to the hands of a specialist for the most effective treatment.

The end of the fourth year of medical school is marked by graduation exercises and the conferring of the degree of Doctor of Medicine. It signifies the end of formal classroom teaching for the would-be doctor, and certifies that he has completed the necessary academic work to step into the world of medicine. But with a medical degree, the student does not suddenly become a doctor by any means. Nor is graduation the end of his training, for ahead of him lies a minimum of one year of apprenticeship as an intern in a teaching hospital before he is eligible to take licensure examinations, and in many cases an additional one to four years of residency training in a medical speciality of his own choice.

Internship and Onward

The year of internship, sometimes spoken of as "the fifth year of medical school," is by far the most difficult and demanding of all the years of the medical student's training. It is the year when the graduate doctor becomes a member of the medical staff of a teaching hospital and devotes full time to "learning by doing," with far more responsibility placed in his hands than during any previous period in his training. Thus internship is not only difficult, but is in many ways the richest year of the young doctor's training. His work is still carefully supervised, but now for the first time he has personal responsibility for the diagnosis, care, well-being and progress of patients admitted to the hospital either by private physicians or by the clinics and attending staff physicians of publicly supported hospitals.

Rotating through the four major services once again, the intern is the one who has the first responsibility when a patient is admitted; he takes the first medical history and does the first physical examination, writing up his findings as part of the patient's permanent medical record. Often it is the intern who assigns laboratory studies and writes the initial orders for newly admitted patients. In addition he makes regular rounds with other house physicians and assists in all aspects of the patient's diagnosis, care and treatment. When various special procedures are required, such as a lumbar spinal puncture, intravenous feeding or an emergency electrocardiogram, the intern is the one who is responsible. Much of his work is an endless series of little details and decisions, working closely with residents and staff doctors. During his time spent on the surgical service, the intern becomes a valued assistant at hundreds of surgical operations; during his service on the obstetrical ward, he performs many deliveries and assists at many more. Above all, he enters into the 24-hour-a-day world of medical care, gradually learning the ropes, discovering things that were never taught in medical school, and slowly improving his skill. There is little time for reading or textbook study, yet he is expected as a matter of course to keep up to date on new advances in medicine.

Internship is a crowded, harried and almost unbelievably intense year of service and learning. It is an important part of the process that molds a responsible physician from an interested and capable student, but it lasts only a year,

Where the physician goes from there is up to him. If he wishes to begin his own practice he can do so after passing a lengthy and rigorous qualifying examination. But many young doctors today go on to take residency training in a specialized field of medicine, and the years of residency are in many ways even more demanding than any other aspect of medical education.

The Many Kinds of Doctors

Less than fifty years ago more than 70 percent of all the doctors practicing medicine in America were *general practitioners*—"family doctors" in the broadest sense of the word. Their services covered the whole spectrum of medical care: they treated old and young alike, delivered babies, rendered pediatric care to children, set broken bones or removed diseased gall bladders. It was only in a truly difficult case or an unusual or disastrous situation that the relatively few specialists in one field of medicine or another were called in consultation.

Today the statistics are almost reversed; only some 30 percent of the physicians listed in the registry of the American Medical Association are general practitioners (or *generalists* as some now prefer to be called). Many of the remaining 70 percent never entered general practice at all, but went directly from their medical training into the intensive study of a special field of medicine; others started in general practice but later returned for additional training and started anew as specialists, perhaps discouraged by their limitations as general practitioners or frustrated by the sense that they were "jack of all trades but master of none." And in spite of a renewal of interest in general practice in recent years, a great many patients today regard some medical specialist—an internist (specialist in internal medicine), an obstetrician, a pediatrician, sometimes even a surgeon—as their "family doctor" and their first port of call when illness strikes. Large or small medical clinics staffed by specialists working together have become com-

monplace, and the staffs of most hospitals, whether publicly or privately supported, are dominated by specialists. What is more, with the galloping increase in medical knowledge in the past half-century, innumerable subspecialists have appeared in medicine, with more and more doctors concentrating their attention and efforts in increasingly narrow areas of medicine.

Originally, and still today, the practice of medicine has been divided into three major branches: *internal medicine, surgery* and *obstetrics*—to which a fourth major branch, *pediatrics,* has been added within recent decades. Thus it is appropriate here to review briefly these major medical specialties, the kind of training that each requires, and the capabilities—and limitations—of the medical specialist.

Training of the Internist

Every doctor undergoes at least one year of field training in medical practice as a hospital intern. If his hospital training is in a so-called *rotating internship,* he spends part of his intern year working in each of the four major fields of medicine. The bulk of his year is divided between the medical service and the surgical service, but he also devotes time to the pediatric and the obstetrical services and is assigned to work in the hospital emergency ward, where problems from all four fields of medicine are encountered. At a number of training hospitals, however, doctors-in-training may take a so-called *straight internship,* spending the entire year in the one service in which they wish to become most proficient, as a *medical intern* or a *surgical intern.* Perhaps the best training of all is the two-year rotating internship, in which the young doctor spends six months in each of the four major services.

In any event, after internship, the newly trained doctor takes his licensure examinations in whatever state he wishes to practice and is thus legally qualified as a physician. At this point two alternatives are open to him; he may enter private practice as a *general practitioner,* or he may enter *hospital residency training* in one of the four major fields for further training and experience in a specialty. If he wishes to specialize in internal medicine and become qualified as an *internist* (to be distinguished from an *intern*) he will spend a minimum of three years in residency in internal medicine. Thereafter, restricting his practice to treating patients with purely medical problems, he becomes qualified for special Board examinations in internal medicine and becomes a member of the American Board of Internal Medicine as a formally recognized specialist in internal medicine.

Not all doctors who start residency training in internal medicine (or in any other field) always complete the full residency program. Many, whether training in medicine, surgery or some other specialty, leave residency after a year or two to enter practice, not qualified for specialty Board examinations, but at least better trained in their special field than colleagues who left training after their internships. These men may then, by choice, restrict their practice to their specialty, and may in time, through their practical experience, gain as much proficiency as their colleagues with longer formal training, even if they do not gain formal recognition as specialists.

But internal medicine is an extremely broad field, encompassing all kinds of illnesses that can be treated primarily by means of drugs, medicines or other conservative measures short of surgery. Thus many internists seek to restrict their field of practice still further, entering subspecialties of internal medicine according to their interests and particular skills. Every in-

ternist, for example, must be skilled in the diagnosis of difficult medical puzzles, but some who are particularly attracted to this kind of medical detective work, and are especially skilled at it, become *diagnosticians,* specializing in rooting out the cause of medical troubles, but leaving the problem of treatment to others. Other internists specialize in treatment of diseases of the heart and become *cardiologists;* still others become *gastroenterologists,* concentrating their attention on disorders of the digestive system. Other subspecialists in internal medicine include the following:

Endocrinologists specialize in diagnosis and treatment of disorders of the endocrine or "ductless" glands—the thyroid, the pancreas and the adrenals, among others. Some endocrinologists go even further to specialize in the diagnosis, treatment and care of one particularly difficult and complex glandular disease—diabetes mellitus, for example. There are other examples of one-disease specialists, too; the *rheumatologist,* while treating all kinds of joint diseases, concentrates his attention on rheumatoid arthritis, while some internists subspecialize in the diagnosis and treatment of tuberculosis.

Hematologists devote their attention to diseases of the blood and blood-forming organs—such disorders as leukemia, polycythemia and anemia. *Dermatologists* are specialists in skin diseases of all sorts. Because one disease, syphilis, was so frequently detected because of skin manifestations, dermatologists classically combined their specialty with *syphilology,* and still do, although syphilis has become much less prevalent in its late stages during recent years because of the success of antibiotics in controlling it.

Allergists specialize in another very confusing and difficult medical field, allergic manifestations of all sorts. In a comparatively new specialty, allergists have become extremely valuable as medical consultants as knowledge of these strange disorders increases by leaps and bounds. *Neurologists* are experts in diagnosis and treatment of physical disorders of the nerves, the spinal cord and the brain. Since neurological illnesses have always been among the most baffling of all human disorders, neurologists have a long and respected history among the medical specialists, and a good neurologist even today sometimes seems to be a miracle worker to his colleagues in other branches of medicine. Neurologists often work in close alliance with a surgical subspecialty, *neurosurgery,* in treating neurological disorders.

Specialists in respiratory diseases deal with all sorts of pulmonary disorders, from tuberculosis and bronchiectasis and other lung infections to asthma, emphysema, and other so-called obstructive respiratory diseases. Since many respiratory diseases have been present for years before medical help is sought, these doctors often concentrate on treatment regimens to slow down their progress, and seek to help their patients protect and fully utilize the remaining undiseased lung tissue they still have. In other words, this is one of many medical fields in which swift and dramatic cures are all but impossible; the physician who chooses these specialties must be a crack diagnostician, long on patience and willing to settle for improvement rather than cure.

All of these subspecialists began their training with hospital residency in internal medicine. Some concentrate on the subspecialty in the second and third years of residency training; others complete general medicine residency and then spend one to three additional years training in their subspecialty. A neurologist, for example, trains for three years in neurology *after* three years of general residency have been completed, a total of six years of specialty training after nine years of general medical training. Often doctors training in a specialty are drawn to the hospitals and clinics where world-famous experts in their specialty practice and teach, working as assistants to these men as they train. And some, of course, themselves become top-ranking experts in their own right.

The Special Training of Surgeons

Surgery is technically defined as the branch of medical practice in which disorders are treated by means of surgical intervention—cutting or incising, suturing, instrumental probing, drainage or removal of diseased tissue and other like procedures. And just as general surgery is a broad major medical specialty, there are as many different kinds of surgeon as there are different kinds of internist.

Of course, almost all doctors do a certain amount of minor surgery. In an emergency it does not take a specially trained surgeon to clamp a hemorrhaging artery in order to save a life, nor is a family doctor likely to call in a surgeon consultant to suture a minor laceration or incise and drain a boil. Certain more complex surgical procedures—tonsillectomies, for example, or diagnostic D and C's—have traditionally been performed by general practitioners, and in many areas where trained surgeons are not readily available, the general practitioner may still perform such major procedures as appendectomies or Caesarean sections. But today the great bulk of the surgery done in this country is performed by doctors who have taken special residency training in surgery after their basic medical training and internship have been completed.

The would-be surgeon acquires his training as a surgical resident in a training hospital, spending from one to four or more years seeing surgical patients in the hospital, serving as a house physician on the surgical service, and spending hours daily in the operating rooms, first assisting qualified surgeons and then, as his skill increases, assuming more and more responsibility as a surgeon in his own right, under the watchful eye of the older and more experienced staff surgeons.

The length of surgical residency varies with the individual doctor's personal goals. The doctor who intends to enter general practice, but wants to prepare himself with more surgical experience than his internship alone could provide, may complete just one or two years of surgical residency. If he wants to qualify for the specialty Board examinations given by the American Board of Surgery, in order to enter practice as a specialist in general surgery, he must take a third and fourth year of surgical residency beyond his internship until, as a senior surgical resident, he has acquired experience performing all kinds of surgery, under supervision, that he might expect to meet in practice.

Finally, if he is interested in working in some particular field of surgery, he may be required to take even further training in that surgical sub-specialty. A hundred years ago virtually all specialists in surgery were *general surgeons,* undertaking any and all kinds of surgical problems that might arise. But as surgical procedures became more complex, and as surgical techniques were devised that required extraordinary skill and experience to handle, certain fields of surgery became subspecialties in their own right. Today the skilled general surgeon still undertakes a wide variety of surgical procedures, but he does not hesitate to call on the services of a surgical subspecialist when he encounters a difficult problem, in bone surgery, for example, or surgery of the heart or great blood vessels. Nor will he approach a problem such as brain surgery as long as a skilled neurosurgeon can be consulted.

In addition to specialty training in general surgery, the following are some of the more common surgical subspecialties:

The *orthopedic surgeon* has spent most of his surgical residency gaining extra experience in bone and joint surgery. The orthopedist or "orthopod," as he is commonly called, is qualified to take charge of the care of difficult fractures, the pinning of broken hips, the application of metal plates in the healing of fractures, the construction of artificial joints, and the performance of amputations and their aftercare. The fitting of artificial limbs or *prostheses* also lies in the field of the orthopedic surgeon.

The *thoracic surgeon* specializes in surgery of the lungs or heart—any surgery that requires opening the chest cavity or thorax. Most thoracic surgeons complete their full residency in general surgery and then spend two or more years of further residency training in surgery of the thorax. An even more refined subspecialty of thoracic surgery is *cardiac* or *cardiovascular surgery,* which is usually performed by qualified thoracic surgeons who have extraordinary experience in surgery of the heart and the great blood vessels. This subspecialty has really blossomed only within the last 25 years; although some surgical procedures on the heart were first performed as early as 1909, cardiac surgery has just recently become a great pioneering field in medicine and the object of world-wide publicity and interest. The cardiac surgeon works very closely with the *cardiologist,* a subspecialist in internal medicine, in one of the most effective medical-surgical teams in modern medicine. The cardiologist is responsible for controlling the patient's heart disease, whatever it may be, by medical means, and for signaling the surgeon that the patient will be able to withstand a heart operation before cardiac surgery can be performed.

The *pediatric surgeon* is another surgical specialist who must spend two or more years learning the surgical skills required to perform major surgery on infants or small children after he has finished his full training in general surgery. Again, pediatric surgery is a relatively new surgical specialty; until some 40 years ago surgery on small children was considered a highly risky and dangerous proposition, and there were only a very few pioneers in this field. Today, with the vast improvement in anesthesia techniques, and with the development of a number of excellent children's hospitals in which pediatric surgeons can be trained, almost any medium-sized city in the United States has one or more specialists in this surgical field.

The *plastic surgeon,* or *reconstructive surgeon* as he is more properly called, is too often considered by the layman as primarily a cosmetician who devotes his time and skill to elective procedures designed to improve the appearance, rather than as a serious surgeon. This unfortunate image is thoroughly unfair. True, plastic surgeons do perform cosmetic surgery, but they have also pioneered in the difficult and time-consuming techniques necessary to reconstruct the faces, bodies and limbs of victims of congenital deformities, burns and other serious injuries, as well as patients disfigured in some way as a result of a major surgical procedure. The reconstructive surgeon must have two to three years of special training in his subspecialty after completion of his residency training in general surgery. And today, this subspecialty has achieved the recognition and respect that it so greatly deserves.

The *neurosurgeon* works in one of the most

complex and difficult of all the surgical fields, and must spend more time in training than any other kind of surgeon: from four to five years of residency in neurosurgery after completing a three-year residency in general surgery. The neurosurgeon's work—surgery of the brain, spinal cord or other parts of the nervous system—has been heavily romanticized in popular writing, perhaps because of the aura of mystery or fear that has always surrounded disorders of the brain. But far from being romantic, the work of the neurosurgeon is tedious and difficult; neurosurgical procedures often take many hours to perform, and the neurosurgeon is constantly aware of the extreme delicacy and vulnerability of the part of the body he is operating on. It is also a singularly discouraging field, and one that requires a surgeon of a very stable temperament, since the percentage of failures still far exceeds the percentage of successes. At the turn of the century the greatest teaching centers and the largest number of master surgeons in this field, as in so many other medical specialties, were located in Vienna, and a surgeon aspiring to this subspecialty was practically obliged to go abroad for his final training. Today training of neurosurgeons in America is probably the best available in the world, and aspiring neurosurgeons can obtain their training in any of a dozen or more excellent medical centers across the country.

Training in Medical-Surgical Specialties

In addition to the many purely medical or surgical specialties, there are a number of fields in medicine which involve training in both medical and surgical aspects of the specialty. The *urologist* or *urological surgeon,* for example, is a specialist in the treatment of any kind of disease or disorder of the urogenital system—the kidneys, ureters, bladder, prostate and so forth. Thus the urologist must have special training in both the medical and the surgical techniques required in the treatment of urological problems. Usually he completes at least one and often two years of residency in general surgery after his internship, and then devotes another two to three years to training in urology.

The *otolaryngologist,* sometimes called an ENT (ear, nose and throat) man, also specializes in both medical and surgical treatment of disorders in this field. Although he may spend hours in his office prescribing medical treatment for his patients, he also performs whatever surgery is necessary to correct or cure the disorders that fall within his specialty.

The *ophthalmologist* is another specialist in both medical and surgical treatment, in this case disorders of the eyes. His work involves not only diagnosis and measurement of defects of vision and treatment of such medical eye diseases as glaucoma, but also surgical procedures such as operations for cataracts, transplantations of eye muscles to correct strabismus or cross-eyes, and many other procedures. The would-be ophthalmologist begins his residency in ophthalmology immediately after finishing his internship, or after perhaps one year of general surgical residency, and becomes qualified for specialty Board examinations after three years of concentrated study in his specialty.

Training in Obstetrics, Gynecology and Pediatrics

Technically these fields should also fall under the category of "mixed medical and surgical specialties." The specialist in obstetrics and gynecology (care of pregnancies and care and treatment of female pelvic disorders) takes three to four years of residency training in his specialty after his internship. Much of this training is concerned with prenatal care and the medical problems that may arise during pregnancy, with particular attention paid to the kinds of medical disorder, such as diabetes, syphilis or tuberculosis, which can have a grave effect upon the pregnancy or upon the newborn baby. The other aspect of obstetrics is preparation for the operative procedures that are often necessary in accomplishing difficult or complicated deliveries, in particular, or the performance of Caesarean sections.

Closely related to this field of medicine is the diagnosis and treatment of pelvic disorders of women, again often involving minor or major surgical intervention. Thus the OB-GYN man must be trained as a skillful technician in the delivery room, an astute medical diagnostician and a qualified abdominal surgeon as well. Some areas of general surgery and gynecological surgery overlap; the removal of a diseased ovary, for example, might be performed by a specialist in either field. But even the skillful general surgeon will defer to the gynecologist for consultation in diagnosis, or for the performance of surgery of the female pelvis that promises to be particularly difficult.

The *pediatrician* is trained chiefly in the medical rather than the surgical aspects of his specialty; few pediatricians undertake any surgery more complicated than the removal of tonsils and adenoids. But he must be trained in both medical and surgical diagnosis of the illnesses and disorders of infants and children. The resident in pediatrics spends three to four years learning the special problems encountered by his small patients after his completion of basic medical training and internship. A pediatrician with a particular interest in some aspect of child care—the diagnosis and treatment of children's heart diseases, for example, or the care and treatment of childhood diabetics—may limit his practice to such a subspecialty, much as internists limit their practices to one aspect of internal medicine.

The Auxiliary Medical Specialties

There are a number of fields that defy classification under the four major medical specialties, yet which play an immensely important role in medical practice today.

The *radiologist,* for example, is a specialist in taking and interpreting X-ray films for diagnostic purposes, and in the use of radiation (either from X-rays or from other radioactive materials) in the treatment of a wide variety of disorders. Of course, many general practitioners, orthopedic surgeons, and other medical specialists may take X-rays and read them without the aid of the radiologist. But many X-ray techniques require complex equipment and very specialized knowledge, and the interpretation of X-rays is not by any means a simple matter. Thus most physicians rely on the radiologist for

all but the most routine X-ray techniques and interpretations. As for radiation therapy, this field, too, requires complex equipment and training that is the special province of the radiologist. This medical specialist should not be confused with the X-ray technician, a layman trained in the operation of X-ray equipment. The radiologist is a fully trained physician who follows his internship with three to four years of residency training in radiology to qualify as a specialist.

In quite another field of medicine, the *anesthesiologist* has played an increasingly important role in recent years. Half a century ago chloroform and ether were about the only general anesthetics available, and often were administered by nurses or even lay technicians with the benefit of very little training. Within the past few decades, however, a wide variety of far more satisfactory anesthetics have been discovered, great progress has been made in the techniques of administering them, and it has become clearly apparent that the safety of the patient and the ease with which the surgeon can do his job depend heavily upon the skill and special training of anesthesiologists. Indeed, specialists in anesthesiology have received far too little credit for the enormous strides that have been made in surgery in recent decades. It is precisely *because* of advancing research in this field and the increasing skill of the anesthesiologist as part of the operating room team that many modern surgical procedures have been made possible at all. Not only must the modern anesthesiologist be a fully trained physician with a great deal of experience in all aspects of medicine, he must also be an expert on the physiological effects of various anesthetic agents and skilled in their administration, so that he can choose the safest and most effective anesthetic for any given surgical procedure, and then be fully prepared to deal, on the spot, with any complications of the anesthesia that may arise in the course of surgery.

In the old days, the threat of "anesthesia death" was so great that speed was one of the most important considerations in performing surgery. The man who could remove a diseased appendix in ten minutes was a better surgeon than the one who took twenty minutes and thus subjected his patient to much longer exposure to anesthesia. Today about the only surgical procedure that really depends upon speed is the Caesarean section, because the obstetrician must get the baby out and breathing on its own as quickly as possible in order to avoid exposing him to excessive doses of anesthetic drugs administered to the mother. But aside from this, modern anesthetic drugs and techniques permit long and complex surgical procedures requiring four, five or even twelve or fifteen hours, with relative safety—procedures that surgeons never before dreamed possible. Today the doctor who wishes to become an anesthesiologist begins residency in his specialty immediately after completing internship, and trains for a period of three to four years before he is qualified to take specialty Board examinations.

Pathology is a demanding medical specialty which plays a key role in the modern practice of medicine. Every hospital of any size has at least one *pathologist,* and his main job is to prepare, stain and examine various tissue samples under the microscope and then report what he sees. Part of his function is to provide aid in diagnosis; it is the pathologist who examines Pap smears for evidence of cervical cancer, who administers the clinical laboratory, and who examines and reports on all tissue removed at biopsy in order to establish diagnosis. But it is also the pathologist in the hospital who performs the post-mortem examinations, examines tissue samples removed after death, and provides the "final diagnosis" when the cause of a death is not clearly understood.

It is also the pathologist's job to examine all tissues removed at surgery, and on the basis of what he sees to report *pathological diagnoses* which are then carefully compared with the surgeon's own preoperative and postoperative diagnoses. No surgeon or any other physician is always right 100 percent of the time; but the surgeon who removes too many normal appendixes under the preoperative diagnosis of "acute appendicitis," or performs D and C's with improper indication, or removes too many gall bladders that prove to be perfectly healthy upon pathological examination, will soon be asked to explain the discrepancy between his diagnoses and the pathologist's reports, and directed to correct these abuses or have his surgical privileges in the hospital revoked. Thus the pathologist is in many ways the watchdog of the entire medical community; he is the expert on the nature of disease and its causes, and is often among the best-trained and most highly respected physicians on the hospital staff. Training in pathology begins after a doctor has completed his internship, and involves three to four years of residency in pathology before he is qualified to take Board examinations and become a specialist in pathology.

Perhaps the most mysterious of all the medical specialists, to the average layman, is the *psychiatrist.* It might be easy to overlook the psychiatrist altogether in outlining the medical specialties, for his work tends to be so completely different from any other form of medical practice that it seems unclassifiable. Many people, furthermore, confuse the psychiatrist (who is always first a fully trained physician) with the psychoanalyst (who may or may not be a graduate physician) and the clinical psychologist (who has college training in psychology but does not hold a medical degree). The confusion is understandable; all three of these specialists deal in one way or another with the diagnosis and treatment of mental or emotional disorders. Since these conditions are still only poorly understood, it is not surprising that a variety of approaches to diagnosis and treatment have developed, each requiring its own special kind of training and preparation.

The *psychologist* must earn a degree in psychology, the branch of science which deals with the human mind and human behavior, both normal and abnormal, and then may specialize further in this broad field. Many psychologists engage in research, seeking to learn more about the normals and abnormals of behavior. Others may accept private patients or be employed by schools or other social institutions to assist in identifying the normal from the abnormal in a child's growing mental development, or to help disturbed children or adults adjust more comfortably to the world around them. Still others are specially trained in the administration and interpretation of psychological tests, used either to evaluate intelligence or, in special circumstances, to help diagnose the presence of serious mental imbalances. Many do further graduate study in psychology, *not* medicine, and earn their Ph.D. degrees, thus confusing matters further if they are called "Doctor." In general, however, psychologists who engage in the treatment of mental or emotional disorders confine their practice to relatively minor disturbances of emotional or social behavior, or else work in close conjunction with medically trained psychiatrists. They are not licensed as physicians, and cannot prescribe or administer drugs or medicines except under the supervision of a trained physician.

The psychiatrist *is* a trained physician, studying medicine just like any other medical practitioner through medical school and internship. Following that he enters residency training in psychiatry, usually in a major psychiatric hospital or clinic. There he becomes familiar with the various symptoms of mental illness, and with a wide range of approaches to treatment of mental and emotional disability. These approaches may include the administration of drugs and medicines affecting the patient's mental behavior, and the use of electric shock and the many other forms of therapy. His training also includes intensive experience in the long-term care and maintenance of patients with mental illness. After some four years of such training he is eligible to take Board examinations in psychiatry and to qualify as a specialist in psychiatric diagnosis and treatment.

Many psychiatrists become particularly interested in psychoanalysis, the special form of psychotherapy pioneered by the monumental work of Sigmund Freud and further developed by others. The psychiatrist who wishes to practice psychoanalysis must take additional training in an accredited institute of psychoanalysis after his psychiatric residency is completed, must himself undergo intensive psychoanalysis, and then begins his practice as a "training analyst" under the supervision of the experienced members of the institute. Because of this long and rigorous preparation, relatively few psychiatrists become psychoanalysts, although Freudian insights and therapeutic techniques are an invaluable part of this specialty. Those who do complete special training in psychoanalysis tend to confine their practice to the use of psychoanalysis alone; and while basic medical training is a prerequisite for the practice of psychiatry involving drugs, medications and the many forms of therapy, psychoanalysis itself does *not* necessarily require medical training. Thus psychologists in particular may complete psychoanalytic training and become "lay analysts" qualified to undertake this particular kind of consultative therapy.

The modern psychiatrist is in many respects a pioneer in a relatively unexplored and vastly misunderstood field of medicine. He does indeed have an important place on the medical team, and as more is learned about the function of the mind and about mental illness and disability, an increasing number of young doctors are finding an exciting challenge in this difficult and often maligned field.

The Role of the Specialist in Teaching and Medical Research

Most physicians who train to become qualified specialists enter medical practice in one way or another: in private practice, in association with a hospital, or as a member of a group practice or clinic. Yet in addition to their own practice, or sometimes to its exclusion, there are two other professional activities in which many specialists engage that should not be overlooked: the teaching of medicine and the conducting of medical research.

For most specialists teaching is a part-time occupation, combined with private practice. Even so, it is a demanding job, for as a member of the teaching staff in a school of medicine or in an affiliated hospital, he must deliver clinical lectures, hold rounds and consultations and engage in a multitude of other teaching activities. Unlike many other disciplines, medicine is more than theory, and it can be taught only by physicians who are themselves widely experienced and recognized authorities in the fields they teach. In short, medical students, interns and residents learn their profession not only from lectures and textbooks, but by example.

Often the specialist's remuneration for these teaching functions is minimal; indeed, the vast majority of medical specialists regularly donate time each week to the conducting of free clinics, rounds, or contributions to medical conferences and seminars. Similarly, general practitioners contribute to the training of medical students, interns and residents in the hospitals where they are staff members and where they treat their patients. Throughout medicine there is an unspoken tradition that in addition to his own practice, the doctor has an obligation to teach.

Even less well known is the work that physicians, surgeons and other specialists do in *clinical research* to enlarge the knowledge of diagnosis and treatment of illnesses. New surgical techniques do not appear by magic; they are devised, studied, discussed, and finally tested in the operating room by surgeons seeking new and better ways of handling difficult problems. Ultimately the results of their innovations, whether successful or unsuccessful, are reported at medical meetings and published in medical journals for the guidance of all other physicians working in the same area. Many laymen are horrified at such an idea, assuming that this kind of research involves out-and-out experimentation with the lives and health of patients. But this is far from the truth. Unlike research in other fields, medical research cannot be performed by a simple process of trial and error, for an error may mean the death of a patient. Rather it must be a cautious, painstaking, step-by-step procedure in which the health and survival of the patient are paramount.

The history of medicine is full of examples of how surgical treatment of such illnesses as ulcer disease, gall bladder disease, cancer of the breast, and many others has been gradually improved by skillful research and knowledgeable innovation. Sometimes the advantage or disadvantage of one surgical procedure over another is not immediately clear and easy to establish; it may have to be performed hundreds of times and carefully followed up over a period of years or decades before surgeons can be sure, on the basis of statistics, that it offers a higher percentage of success.

Some specialists devote almost all their time to laboratory research, studying the effects of new drugs and medications on the treatment of certain kinds of illness, for example, or working with laboratory animals to prove the efficacy of new forms of therapy. Other specialists conduct research programs side by side with their regular practice of medicine. The first human heart transplant was not undertaken because a surgeon suddenly was seized with the idea; literally years of tests and experiments were conducted on laboratory animals first, before the surgeon was certain enough of success that he was willing to subject a human patient to the inevitable risks.

Certain risks are, in some cases, unavoidable, but it is important to realize that in any form of medical research involving human patients, the welfare of the patient always comes first. And it is equally important to realize that without the driving search for new and better techniques and methods, for greater understanding of obscure diseases and for better methods of treating them, work that is largely carried out by the medical specialist, the practice of medicine today would still be in the Dark Ages. Past, present and future generations all benefit from the courageous research work which has become part of the tradition of medical practice.

The General Practitioner

With such a variety of doctors engaged in so many different kinds of medical practice, where does the general practitioner fit into the picture? How does a patient know when to consult him or a medical specialist? Many patients regard an internist or a diagnostician as their "family doctor"; women often entrust overall supervision of their health care to their gynecologist or to the obstetrician who delivered their children, even though many of their medical problems may be completely out of his field; mothers may take their children to a pediatrician from the time of infancy onward. But in recent decades people have once again become increasingly aware of the important job the modern general practitioner can do as a true family doctor and first port of call when medical problems arise.

This is a rather abrupt change in attitude, for it was once often said that *no one* could possibly know enough to be a really good general practitioner. General practice was even regarded as a field reserved for those without the interest or ability to pursue a medical specialty. And with an increasing army of specialists available, many men already in general practice began to feel that, in good conscience, they should not handle anything more difficult than a runny nose. In short, the general practitioner was regarded, and even regarded himself, as the low man on the medical totem pole.

But there were, and still are, several things the general practitioner can provide that patients began to find missing in their relations with specialists: an overall knowledge and continuing concern with even the smallest health problems of every member of the family, a ready availability, and a tendency to treat his patients as people rather than abstract illnesses. In addition, there were, and still are, multitudes of small communities or largely rural areas that simply cannot support an army of specialists, and although specialty practitioners can be reached even from remote areas today thanks to various means of rapid transportation, it is the general practitioner who must minister to the everyday health needs of patients in such areas, or even keep them alive until they can reach a specialist. At the same time, those in general practice themselves began to recognize that the good general practitioner had to be one of the sharpest, best-trained and most up-to-date physicians in the entire field of medicine. These changing attitudes and realizations have resulted in the present reawakening of professional interest in general practice and

esteem for the general practitioner. Many patients have come to prefer a "family doctor," and more and more doctors have come to regard general practice in itself as a highly demanding "specialty." There is now a new specialty Board to examine and accredit particularly capable and competent general practitioners who have completed adequate residency training in all fields of medicine in addition to their medical school and internship training. These men can now practice on a professional par with specialists of any sort.

Certainly it is to everyone's advantage to have a single doctor who knows him and his complete health history, lives in the community, is acquainted with others in the family and with their various health problems, and can help not only in diagnosing and treating illness but in supervising programs of preventive health care for the entire family. Such a doctor would probably be a general practitioner or an internist. He may well have had special training in general surgery, or in internal medicine, or in pediatrics or obstetrics, yet prefers to practice general medicine rather than to limit his work to a narrow specialty field. Whatever his training, if he is competent and conscientious, he can, of course, recognize clearly the kinds of problem that require the attention of a specialist, and when referral for special consultation or treatment is necessary, he will work closely with the specialist, teaming his general medical experience with the special skill and experience of the surgeon, the orthopedist, the gynecologist, the dermatologist, the radiologist, or any other medical specialist whose skills are required.

68

Our Modern Hospitals and Auxiliary Medical Services

The doctor, whether he is a general practitioner or a specialist, is obviously the central figure in the provision of health care in this country. Next to the doctor, however, the *sine qua non* of the practice of medicine is the modern hospital with its staff of professional and nonprofessional workers and the wide variety of nursing and technological services they provide. High-quality medical care would be completely impossible without these hospital services; the physician who attempted to practice without them would be virtually handcuffed. No community, however small, can long afford to be without access to first-rate hospital facilities. And despite the fact that the costs of hospital care have spiraled in recent years, the need for well-staffed and well-equipped hospitals will continue to grow in the years to come.

Hospitals have not by any means always played this quintessential role in the provision of health care; it is only within the last hundred years that they have come into their own as useful adjuncts to the diagnosis and treatment of illness. Of course, hospitals of one sort or another have existed for thousands of years, but until the beginning of the last century, they were a far cry from anything we would recognize as a modern hospital. In ancient Egypt and Sumeria, for example, special city quarters were set aside to force the isolation of the diseased and dying from the rest of the population. In biblical times the sufferers of certain forms of disease such as leprosy or mental illness were also isolated in squalid warrens designed more to protect the healthy than to provide any kind of help for the sick. In ancient Greece there were more humane gathering places for the sick, usually at religious sites where oracles were consulted and where physicians ministered to those who came either to convalesce or to die. With the rising dominion of ancient Rome, however, and its later fall, all semblance of humanity vanished. In the waves of plague that swept Europe during the Middle Ages and the early Renaissance, the sheer numbers of dead and dying overwhelmed the few religious sanctuaries that had been established for the ill; the "hospitals" were the streets of the cities. In the centuries that followed, hospitals of a sort were again established, some to survive to the present day and become world famous, yet their essential nature remained as ghastly as before, filthy pesthouses where the sick, the injured or the insane were locked away until they mercifully died.

Gradually, with increasing knowledge of the cause and treatment of disease, and with the awakening of at least a rudimentary form of social conscience, the ill and the insane were cared for with greater compassion. But reform of the hospitals was simply not possible without reform in the abysmal quality of nursing care that prevailed in Europe and America well into the 1800s. As early as 1634 religious orders such as the Sisters of Charity, founded by St. Vincent de Paul (1576–1660), were established to provide nursing care for the sick, but throughout the 1700s the vast majority of "nurses" employed by hospitals were uneducated and ignorant of even the most basic principles of nursing care, often victimizing their patients in rat-infested hospitals and infirmaries, or themselves suffering from various diseases. Then in the early 1800s an important breakthrough in the quality of nursing care occurred when Theodor Fliedner, the young pastor of a Protestant church in the small town of Kaiserswerth in Germany, organized a small body of specially trained women to care for the sick, following the example of the English Quaker philanthropist Elizabeth Fry (1780–1845), who was doing much the same work in England. The nurses at Kaiserswerth were of spotless character and undertook not only all the tasks of hospital maintenance and patient care but also taught nursing, household duties and the management of children and convalescents. It was their example, in part, that formed the background for the monumental work of the well-born English-woman Florence Nightingale (1820–1910), who almost single-handedly undertook to reform the treatment of the sick. Appalled and repelled by the abominable care given the British troops in the Crimean War, Miss Nightingale went to the Crimea and worked vigorously both to improve sanitary conditions and nursing care for wounded soldiers and to train a corps of some 125 nurses. After the war, in England, she battled the British medical establishment to improve hospital conditions there, and she founded the Nightingale School for Nurses at St. Thomas's Hospital in London—a training center that soon became the model for many similar schools. Two major changes of incalculable importance arose as a result of this remarkable woman's work. First, nursing was established once and for all as a highly respected humanitarian profession which required intelligence and character as well as careful preparation and training; and second—certainly of equal importance—a hospital came to be considered not as a place of filth, agony, human degradation and eventual death, but rather a place where patients, no matter how sick, are treated with compassion and the highest quality of professional care.

The Different Kinds of Hospitals

The modern hospital truly embodies the concept of compassionate and highly skilled medical care. Ranging in size from tiny institutions with as few as 20 or 30 beds to mammoth medical centers with beds for 3,000 or more inpatients as well as dozens of outpatient clinics and facilities, there are in this country alone more than 6,500 hospitals of all sorts and descriptions which meet the high standards of accreditation set by the American Hospital Association. The majority of these are *general hospitals* with the personnel and facilities for handling all kinds of illness. In addition, there is a wide variety of *specialty hospitals* which limit their services to the treatment of certain kinds of illnesses. Among these are pediatric hospitals for the treatment of children's diseases, maternity or lying-in hospitals specializing in the care of obstetrical patients, neuropsychiatric hospitals which treat serious mental illness, crippled children's hospitals, orthopedic and fracture hospitals, hospitals that specialize in a particular surgical procedure or in the treatment of a particular disease, and many more.

These many different kinds of hospitals are organized and operated in a wide variety of ways. At one time a large number of hospitals were privately owned by individuals or companies, supported by charges made to the patients and private donations, and operated for profit. Even today many hospitals, including some of major size, are still privately owned and supported without public funding, but very few are operated for profit; most qualify as nonprofit institutions. Of these, many are owned and operated by various religious orders, others by fraternal organizations.

Still another group of hospitals—the majority in existence today—are publicly funded, at least in part, and operated as county, state or federal institutions. Among the latter are the military hospitals concerned with the treatment of armed services personnel and their families; Veterans Administration Hospitals established to provide care for veterans either disabled as a result of their military service or unable to meet the costs of private hospitalization for subsequent illnesses; and United States Public Health Service hospitals. Most tax-supported hospitals were originally intended to provide free medical care for the poor, or those on public relief or welfare rolls, but spiraling hospitalization costs in recent years have forced many of them to institute a sliding scale for their services, charging a given patient according to his ability to pay. Finally, many fine hospitals have been established to serve as adjuncts to the major medical schools, partly supported by private funds and patient charges, with these revenues supplemented in many cases by funds derived from taxation.

The Services of a General Hospital

The major purpose of a general hospital is, of course, to provide diagnostic and treatment facilities, and expert round-the-clock nursing care for patients who cannot be as effectively treated anywhere else. In some cases the patient may be so severely ill, or suffering from an illness that is changing so rapidly, that continuing professional observation of his condition is essential to his treatment and protection—the kind of professional care which simply cannot be provided anywhere but in a hospital. Other patients may be hospitalized to undergo major surgery of some kind, and must then remain until recovery is advanced enough to permit further convalescence at home. Similarly, pregnant women are customarily hospitalized at the beginning of labor and remain in the hospital through delivery of the baby and for a brief recovery period thereafter. Still other patients may be hospitalized in order to receive certain specialized forms of treatment—the administration of intravenous fluids or blood transfusions, for example, or radiation therapy for a cancer, a concentrated period of physical therapy or a brief interval of treatment with an artificial kidney. Many patients come to a hospital emergency room for diagnosis and treatment of an accident or injury or because of the sudden occurrence of some sign or symptom of acute illness that is particularly alarming and requires immediate attention. Finally, some patients are hospitalized so that an intensive diagnostic evaluation can be made, perhaps including numerous X-ray studies and laboratory examinations, with as much speed and economy as possible, since such a diagnostic study might otherwise require weeks of repeated visits to a doctor's office.

In order to handle such a wide variety of demands, the general hospital is ordinarily divided into well-defined treatment units or "services." The *medical service,* for example, has rooms and wards organized to provide continuing observation and nursing care of patients undergoing medical treatment for virtually every kind of illness. On the medical service extensive use is made of the hospital's diagnostic and treatment facilities; the services of the hospital dietician are available to provide any special diets necessary; both routine and special nursing procedures are carried out according to the orders of the patient's doctor; and both the attending physician and house physicians follow the patient's progress closely, greatly aided by observations made by the nursing staff.

The *surgical service* of a general hospital is even more complicated. Since the great majority of surgical patients do not require hospitalization until just prior to their surgery, most of them are received in a preoperative ward or section of the hospital. Here they are interviewed and checked over both by the house doctors and by the attending surgeon and, in most cases, by the anesthesiologist as well. Preoperative patients almost invariably are allowed no food or fluids by mouth for a period of 12 or more hours prior to surgery, and then are given preoperative medication shortly before they are transported to the operating room. In most hospitals the operating suite is a completely separate unit, staffed by specially trained nurses and used exclusively for the performance of surgery. Following surgery the patient is transported to a nearby *recovery room* where extremely close postoperative observation is possible until he has recovered from anesthesia and is considered ready by the surgeon to be returned to his room or to the postoperative surgical ward. Here convalescence can begin under the close observation of nurses experienced in handling postsurgical problems and procedures. Postoperative rounds are made both by the attending surgeon and by house physicians until the first critical hours or days of convalescence are over and the patient can be released to convalesce at home.

The *obstetrical service* operates in much the same way, except that maternity patients are usually isolated on a separate floor or wing of the general hospital, and nurses specially trained in following the progress of labor and assisting at deliveries are on hand to help the patient and her doctor until a baby is safely born and recovery has begun. After delivery the baby is taken to the *newborn nursery,* which is staffed and equipped to handle any problem which may arise during the first few hours or days of his life. Finally, the *pediatric service* of the general hospital is organized much the same as the medical service except that nurses trained in pediatric techniques are on the staff and there are facilities for the treatment, care and observation of sick children of all ages, both medical and surgical.

In addition to these basic major services, most general hospitals have a variety of special service departments designed to handle particular problems. One such department is the *emergency room,* a receiving station staffed with nurses and house physicians prepared to treat victims of injuries, accidents or sudden illnesses at any hour of the day or night with the greatest speed and efficiency possible. The emergency room is always a busy place, with ready and speedy access to diagnostic facilities, medications and the special equipment necessary to handle life-or-death situations as well as comparatively minor problems. A physician on duty in an emergency room may see a man with a broken hip, a woman who arrives by taxicab in the midst of delivering a baby, and a child vomiting blood after eating some automatic dishwashing compound, all within the space of the same half-hour; he and the nurses on duty to assist him must be prepared for literally anything. Some patients who come to the emergency room can be seen, treated, and sent home with referral to follow-up treatment with their own doctor in his office the next day. Another patient may require immediate admission to the hospital for treatment, while a third may die while the doctor tries in vain to treat his injuries from an automobile accident.

Many hospitals operate a hospital ambulance service from the emergency room; others cooperate with community first-aid units, emergency cars or mobile "Medic-One" facilities. More than anywhere else in the hospital the emergency room is the "first port of call," a facility that may spell the difference between life and death, and with that realization many hospitals have extended their emergency services and facilities in two ways—first, by the swift transportation of victims of accidents or sudden illness to the emergency room, sometimes even by helicopter, and second, by equipping emergency vehicles of whatever kind with the personnel and medical facilities necessary to begin definitive treatment of an accident or illness on the scene, even before the victim reaches the hospital emergency room.

Another form of special service that has blossomed in importance in recent years is the *intensive care unit*—a hospital facility, staffed by both house physicians and alert and experienced nurses, that provides minute-by-minute observation and monitoring of patients who are so desperately ill that they require continuing professional help until the crisis is over. These intensive care units maintain constant vigilance over the patient's vital functions and have special equipment such as respirators to sustain breathing and electric defibrillators to jar an arrhythmic heart back into normal rhythm, all available on a moment's notice if they are needed. Accident victims, heart patients, victims of internal hemorrhage and other patients in truly critical condition often owe their lives to the availability of such a service. In one single area alone—the intensive care of victims of severe and massive coronary attacks—these facilities have helped triple and even quadruple the number of those who survive the first critical 48 hours. The cost of intensive care is admittedly high—it has to be—yet there is no better illustration of the way in which modern medical technology and specially organized and trained professional teams have made a major breakthrough in the care of patients who would otherwise certainly die.

Some modern hospitals have created other professional teams for special purposes. Heart surgery, for example, depends heavily upon intensively trained, integrated and coordinated teams of experts—surgeons, cardiologists, anesthesiologists and surgical nurses—who undertake complex operations that would be impossible in any other way. Similar "surgical action teams" have been created to handle major surgery of the vascular system and the lungs. In fact, as the procedures of medical or surgical treatment grow increasingly complex, these expert teams will surely play an even more important role, not only in those few hospitals that are now world famous for some particular specialty, but also in those that aim to provide a full range of modern treatment facilities to their patients.

The Hospital Staff

The professional staff of a typical general hospital—the men and women who make the hospital work—include four groups: the house physicians, the attending or staff physicians, the nursing staff, and those involved in paramedical or auxiliary medical services—physical and occupational therapists, and a variety of technologists and technicians. The *house physicians* are perhaps most intimately in contact with hospitalized patients, and they include both interns and more experienced resident doctors who are paid by the hospital, devote their full time to hospital duties, and serve the needs of the hospital's patients even as they increase their own clinical experience or undergo training in various medical or surgical specialties. (Details of the work and training of house physicians are described in the previous chapter.)

The *attending physicians* constitute the chief medical authority of the hospital. In most hospitals the majority of attending physicians on the staff are doctors—general practitioners or specialists—engaged in active private practice in the community who have been accorded the privileges of admitting patients to the hospital and conducting their treatment there. These doctors are not ordinarily paid by the hospital, but are expected to contribute their time and knowledge to teaching rounds with less experienced doctors, clinical conferences and staff meetings, thus sharing in the responsibility for the pro-

fessional conduct of the hospital's services. In hospitals that are affiliated with medical schools or other medical teaching centers, many of the attending physicians may also be members of the medical school faculty; some may be full-time professors in the medical school who accept supervisory responsibility for the care of patients in the hospital. Furthermore, in most large hospitals certain staff physicians are traditionally employed in full-time hospital service; among these are pathologists, for example, anesthesiologists, radiologists, or the doctors who head up special medical facilities in the hospital such as a department of physical medicine and rehabilitation. On each of the four major services—medical, surgical, obstetrical and pediatric—one particularly capable and experienced physician is customarily appointed Head of Service or Chief of Service and undertakes additional responsibility for the professional conduct of physicians in the particular service he represents.

In addition, the staff physicians of a typical general hospital form a governing body for the hospital, elect from their ranks a chairman and other staff officers and hold regular staff meetings, usually monthly, for discussion and decisions regarding problems in the hospital administration. This governing body has many important duties, and staff meetings are often devoted to educational sessions as well as business, but one of its most important functions is a regular in-depth review of all hospital deaths and of all pathological reports that seem at variance with the attending doctor's diagnosis—one of the most effective forms of self-discipline among practicing physicians. Thus any attending physician who admits patients to the hospital is directly answerable to his colleagues on the hospital staff for his professional competence and for the manner in which he conducts the care of his patients. If a physician cannot or will not meet the high standards required by his colleagues, they may place formal limitations on the kind of cases he can handle, or his privileges to admit and treat patients in the hospital may be completely withdrawn.

The nursing care of patients in a hospital is, of course, the responsibility of the *nursing staff*, which includes supervisory personnel, the registered nurses who provide bedside care and the licensed practical nurses, nurse's aides and volunteers who assist them. Physicians are responsible for determining the direction of every patient's treatment and for giving whatever medical orders are necessary, but in following a physician's orders, directly caring for the patients, observing changes in their condition and staying in continuing communication with the physician, the nursing staff fulfills a professional role without which no hospital could possibly function.

Just as there are many different kinds of physicians, so there are many kinds of nurses on the typical general hospital staff. In earlier decades in this century the vast majority of nurses received their professional training in so-called hospital schools of nursing—training institutions connected with large hospitals in which prospective nurses spent a period of three to four years in general nurse's training, dividing their time between classroom studies and direct on-ward duties of bedside nursing. In recent years, however, as nursing procedures have become more complex and as the inestimable value of expert professional nursing care has become more widely recognized, most of the traditional hospital schools of nursing have given way to a longer formal period of nurse's training that closely resembles the training of physicians. Today the vast majority of young women entering nurse's training enroll in a university program which in most cases involves a minimum of five years of academic study with increasing time spent each year in actual bedside nurse's training in the hospital affiliated with the university. Upon completion of this program, the nurse is awarded a Bachelor of Science degree in nursing as well as the professional Registered Nurse (RN) degree, signifying that she is qualified to undertake general nursing care in any hospital in the country. Nurses who wish to devote their time to a specialized aspect of nursing care—operating room nursing, for example, or pediatric nursing—must take additional years of clinical training in their chosen field, much as resident physicians take additional years of specialty training in hospital service after their "basic" medical training is completed.

Such a pattern of training for nurses has resulted in a steady improvement in the overall quality of nursing care available in our hospitals. But it has also created certain problems. There have never been enough nurses in practice to fulfill the needs of growing numbers of hospitals in the country, and of those who complete the rigorous training, many become nursing specialists while others are soon elevated to supervisory posts on hospital nursing staffs, thus thinning the ranks of the registered nurses necessary for actual bedside care. As a result, a "second rank" of nursing personnel has appeared in increasing numbers on the hospital scene. These are nurses whose training is briefer than that required for the registered nurse and is concentrated largely on the aspects of patient care; their training is undertaken in special schools or in hospitals and leads to formal recognition of the student as a licensed practical nurse (LPN). The LPN can handle a majority of the bedside nursing procedures, and in many hospitals she has become an important mainstay of the nursing staff, but she is answerable to the registered nurse supervising her work and is not qualified to undertake many of the procedures—administration of intravenous medications, for example—that require the broader professional training and experience of the registered nurse.

In many hospitals today a "third rank" of nursing services is provided by nurse's aides, women without professional training who are nevertheless able to help with many of the necessary housekeeping chores of hospital nursing—passing and collecting trays at mealtimes, changing patients' beds, escorting patients to the X-ray, laboratory or physical therapy departments, and so forth. Even with such a variety of people on a typical nursing staff, hospitals today are still short-handed for nursing personnel; after many decades of accepting penurious salaries for the hard work required of them, registered nurses, through their professional organizations, have been demanding and receiving salaries at the professional level that they have so long deserved. Thus there is at last an increasing incentive for young women to make careers in this field, and for trained nurses who have dropped out of active nursing practice in favor of marriage and family to return to their work—a vast reservoir of talent and experience that has only in recent years been recognized, much less utilized.

Finally, *paramedical personnel* complete the picture of the typical hospital staff. These are people, some professionally trained, others not, who fulfill necessary specialty roles in the care of hospital patients. *Physical therapists* and *occupational therapists,* for example, are professionally trained men or women who have completed four or more years of university study, partly devoted to academic work in the liberal arts and biological sciences, and partly to clinical training with specialists who are skilled and experienced in these invaluable forms of treatment; and after graduation additional months are spent in postgraduate clinical training in their specialties before they are qualified. Both physical and occupational therapists work with patients who have physical or mental handicaps to relieve their pain, to restore their strength and—ultimately—to help them achieve the maximum range of function that their capabilities will allow. Victims of strokes or paralyzing spinal cord injuries, for example, benefit immensely from these special forms of therapy; so do victims of arthritis, serious fractures or polio—virtually anyone whose normal physical functions have been temporarily or permanently impaired. The physical therapist treats such conditions by physical means, using light, heat, water, cold, electricity or mechanical agents. The occupational therapist is particularly skilled in directing the patient's everyday activities in order to promote and maintain health, prevent disability, evaluate behavior or treat disfunction.

In addition, there are other professional and semiprofessional men and women who provide a variety of special services on the hospital staff. The *dietician* is trained in nutrition and the preparation of food, and is responsible for directing the hospital's food service and for providing the special diets required by patients. Trained *psychologists* and *social workers* contribute their skills and experience in counseling patients who are forced to make major changes in their way of life outside the hospital as a result of illness or injury. *X-ray technologists*

and *laboratory technicians* are specially trained to perform their jobs and are an indispensable part of the hospital's diagnostic services. *Orderlies* help transport patients and assist the nursing staff with many difficult or physically demanding nursing procedures; and behind the scene, kitchen personnel and the maintenance and janitorial staff also play important roles in the hospital care of patients. Nor should the importance of *hospital volunteers* be underestimated, in most cases women of the community who donate their time and skills to perform a variety of essential hospital services.

No discussion of the staff of a modern hospital would be complete without mention of *hospital administrators,* men or women usually trained in business whose job it is to keep the work of the hospital flowing smoothly on all levels. Hospital administrators, working in concert with the doctors and nurses on the hospital staff, are responsible for maintaining the standards of cleanliness and the quality of medical and nursing services that are necessary for the hospital's accreditation. Further, they are responsible for the proper conduct of the business offices of the hospital, for the orderly admission and discharge of patients, for budgetary problems and for all the complicated paper work that goes along with hospital care, including medical records, insurance claims and bills. Hospital administrators are also responsible for hiring and firing nonmedical personnel, and they constitute an important link between the medical and nonmedical staff and the patients they serve, with the overall objective of keeping the hospital running as effectively and efficiently as possible.

Hospital Admission Procedures

Admission to a hospital can be a confusing and sometimes frightening experience, but the counsel and advice of a doctor is always of enormous help. When hospitalization becomes necessary, the choice of hospital is up to the physician, although he will take the patient's preferences into consideration whenever possible. Sometimes it is not possible, however; a doctor in a city practice may, for example, maintain staff membership and privileges only at certain hospitals, or often the choice of hospital is dictated by the specific medical needs of the patient. The surgeon scheduled to perform a particularly complex or difficult operation may well select the one hospital in the vicinity which he feels will provide the best, most competent and reliable surgical assistance and postoperative care for his patient. Thus if a doctor overrules a patient's preference in selecting a specific hospital, his professional judgment should be accepted. Whatever the hospital chosen, the doctor can often make quite an accurate estimate of the length of time and the costs involved. The patient should recognize, of course, that unexpected complications or unforeseen changes in his medical condition may render such an estimate invalid, but most doctors prefer their patients to have sufficient advance information so that they will not spend their hospital stay worrying about how long it is going to last or how much it will cost.

When a date for hospital admission has been set, the patient should follow the doctor's orders strictly with regard to meals or fluids taken prior to hospitalization, and should make every effort to appear at the hospital admitting office at the appointed time. Part of the hospital admitting procedure involves gathering basic financial data about hospital insurance and the responsibility for payment of costs that are not covered by insurance. Most hospitals also require the entering patient to sign a blanket statement of permission for virtually any kind of treatment that may be necessary. This is not done to permit the doctors or nursing staff to do things the patient does not want done, but rather to provide a broad form of protection for both the patient and the hospital so that emergency measures may be taken if the necessity arises.

The patient is then admitted to a room or ward, and he should remember that from that point on throughout his hospital stay the attending doctor must authorize any medications, special diets, treatment procedures, or diagnostic studies that are necessary, and it is the responsibility of the nursing staff to carry out his orders. Usually one of the house physicians—an intern or a resident or, in some cases, both—visits the patient soon after admission in order to get

acquainted, establish the necessary treatment procedures and ensure the patient's comfort. Every effort is made by everyone on the staff to be as pleasant and thoughtful in the care of the patient as possible. Complaints about treatment should be raised directly with the nurse in charge of the patient's care, or with the patient's doctor, or both, but the patient should bear in mind that hospital personnel must provide care for a large number of patients at the same time, so that unnecessary individual attention may not be possible.

Admission to a hospital is not tantamount to a prison sentence; a patient is not legally bound to remain there if for some reason he categorically does not wish to do so, but he will be asked to sign a waiver releasing the hospital and physician from responsibility if he elects to leave against his doctor's advice. In fact, whether a waiver is signed or not, the act of leaving a hospital against medical advice will automatically absolve the hospital and the attending physician from responsibility for any untoward complications which might arise as a result. In most cases leaving a hospital against a doctor's advice is an extremely foolish step to take, since neither doctor nor hospital has any desire to confine a patient for any longer than necessary. Any grievances which may make a patient wish to leave can usually be ironed out simply by raising the problem with the nursing staff or the doctor or both. Any unresolved complaints should be taken directly to the hospital administrator upon dismissal from the hospital, or to the Grievance Committee of the county medical society, a board of responsible physicians who will undertake an impartial investigation of any serious complaint a patient may have with regard to his treatment by his physician or by a hospital in the community.

Other Community Medical Services

Hospitals are, of course, the major medical facility in most communities for treatment of the seriously ill, on an inpatient basis in the hospital itself, or on an outpatient basis in one or another of the special clinics directly affiliated with the hospital. But in addition *extended care facilities*

—"semihospitals," so to speak—have been established in many communities to care for convalescing patients who do not require full-scale hospitalization but are not yet well enough to continue their convalescence at home. Such facilities have more limited nursing services than hospitals and less direct medical supervision, but they must be fully accredited and can serve an important function in the care of illness at considerably less cost than full-scale hospitalization.

Somewhat similar to extended care facilities are the *nursing homes* which are usually organized for the long-term care of chronically ill patients. Nursing homes in this country range in quality from excellent to abysmal, but governmental regulating organizations are working vigorously to enforce certain necessary minimum standards. The nursing home is not a substitute for a hospital; for the most part these institutions provide only custodial care and nursing supervision. Most nursing homes do have one or more physicians appointed as medical advisers, but the major medical supervision of the patient's care is ordinarily provided by his own doctor.

A final type of medical service that is becoming increasingly common in this country is the *medical clinic,* usually a small- to medium-sized facility in which a group of physicians have their offices, sharing a nursing staff and other personnel and working together as a so-called *group practice.* In some cases such group practices are made up entirely of general practitioners, in other cases entirely of specialists, and in still other cases of general practitioners and specialists together. Even comparatively small clinics of this sort usually have diagnostic facilities— X-ray equipment, for example, clinical laboratory facilities, and even minor surgery facilities —that a single doctor practicing by himself might not be able to provide. Group practices and clinics of this sort have proved to be so sensible and economical for both the patient and the doctor that they are becoming very widespread, particularly in rural or suburban areas where major diagnostic and hospital facilities are not readily available. Not all clinics, however, are small; such nationally recognized medical institutions as the Mayo Clinic in Rochester, Minnesota, the Leahy Clinic in Boston and the

Mason Clinic in Seattle have large numbers of doctors on their staffs qualified for practice in virtually any specialty, all operating in close conjunction with a major hospital and often engaged not only in medical practice but in medical research and teaching as well.

The Pharmacist

One special group of paramedical personnel is often overlooked in a discussion of medical facilities—the pharmacists who play an invaluable role as dispensers of medications not only in hospitals but also at the prescription counters of thousands of drugstores scattered throughout the country. The registered pharmacist is professionally trained in an accredited school of pharmacy and is completely familiar with the thousands of different medications used in the treatment of illness in the dozens of different dosage forms in which these medications are prepared. Professionally licensed by the state in which he practices, the pharmacist is not authorized to prescribe medication—this remains the prerogative of the licensed physician—but he is responsible for accurate and uniform filling of the physician's prescriptions and, indeed, is the only person other than the physician who is legally authorized to dispense prescription medications.

There was a time not too long ago when a great many prescriptions were actually compounded by the pharmacist in his pharmacy according to a doctor's written formula or recipe. Today pharmaceutical manufacturers have, for the most part, taken over this aspect of pharmacy, supplying the vast majority of prescription drugs in already prepared form, such as tablets, capsules, solutions, tinctures, elixirs, drops, suppositories, sterile ampules, etc. Nevertheless, it is the pharmacist's job to know the content and pharmacological action of these drugs, to be aware of possible incompatibilities between medicines that might be taken at the same time, to be fully cognizant of the precautions and contraindications that exist for various medications, to provide a double check against error in the way a given prescription may be written, and to maintain knowledgeable communication with the physician in the case of any prescription that may in some way endanger a patient. In addition to his professional responsibilities, the pharmacist must also be an extremely capable retail merchandiser, maintaining adequate stocks not only of widely used medications but also of drugs that may be called for only infrequently, and constantly checking the expiration dates of any medications that tend to deteriorate with age, so that physician and patient alike can be confident that the drugs he supplies are of full potency and made available at as little expense to the patient as possible.

In actual practice, there are a number of additional ways that the registered pharmacist provides an invaluable service both to physicians and to patients through his knowledge not only of prescription drugs but also of the enormous variety of nonprescription or so-called proprietary ("over the counter") medications carried by most drugstores. The conscientious and ethical pharmacist cannot properly prescribe or recommend treatment for his customers' ills, but his advice and counsel are often sought on an informal basis; he must have the wisdom and experience to recognize the signs or symptoms suggestive enough of serious health problems to know when to refer a customer to a physician, as well as the practical knowledge necessary to recommend suitable nonprescription medicines that may be helpful with minor health problems. Multitudes of people every day benefit from his quiet application of his professional knowledge, and doctors in practice know better than anyone else the invaluable and often much underrated service that he performs in the maintenance of a high quality of health care.

69

Medical Costs and How to Meet Them

Throughout this book there has been a single underlying theme implicit in everything that has been said about health, illness and our modern medical resources: that for any individual, young or old, the maintenance of good health and the prevention of illness is infinitely more desirable than waiting passively for illness to strike. Obviously it is wiser to keep a boat in sailing trim with paint and judicious repairs than to try to save it from sinking at sea. What is more, the maintenance of good health is infinitely less expensive than the treatment of preventable illness when it becomes necessary. The cost of treating any illness today is high, and can become staggering if the illness is difficult, serious or prolonged. The cost of the doctor's or surgeon's services, of X-ray and diagnostic laboratory studies, of drugs and medicines and of even relatively brief hospitalization can swiftly mount up into a significant financial burden, and the loss of income due to missed work can be equally devastating. Even the most generous sick leave arrangement will help ameliorate such an economic loss only during relatively brief illnesses, and is of no help at all when illness strikes nonearning members of the family. Clearly, money budgeted and invested in the maintenance of good health and the prevention of illness is a major bargain considering the remarkable array of medical resources such an investment can command and the long-term benefits that can accrue.

Even with judicious planning, however, the spiraling cost of medical care today, whether preventive or curative, is a matter of great concern to every American family and in recent years has become a major political and social issue throughout the country. Doctors are often blamed for these rising costs, in spite of the fact that some 80 percent of every dollar spent on health care in this country goes not to any physician, but to the hospitals, nursing homes, paramedical personnel, pharmacists and drug manufacturers. And hospitals are similarly accused of driving medical costs higher, even though most hospitals in this country are fighting a desperate battle just to break even in the face of their own rising expenses.

Certainly the cost of medical care is high and steadily moving higher, but whoever or whatever is to blame it is the patient who is ultimately saddled with that cost. Other costs have risen, too, in recent years—television sets, automobiles, home construction and even food—yet these and other expenses are accepted with less bitterness and fewer complaints. A man will cheerfully spend $600 for a color television set but may resent having to pay $500 in surgeon's fees and hospital costs for the repair of a crippling or potentially life-threatening inguinal hernia. A family will think nothing of buying a $3,500 automobile every two years, yet may consider the same amount in hospital and doctors' fees over a much longer period an outrageous hardship. This curious distortion of values is perhaps reflected most clearly and universally in the everyday matter of budgeting family funds. Virtually anyone who owns and operates an automobile in this country knows and accepts with perfect equanimity that some $1,500 a year must be budgeted to meet this expense, year after year. But how many individuals or families budget anything approaching that amount a year to meet the possible cost of necessary medical care? The answer is that very few indeed budget even a third of that amount. Those who do usually figure in only the payment of the premiums on various hospitalization or health insurance plans, which are almost invariably inadequate to meet any but relatively minor demands for care. A great many budget nothing whatsoever, so that *any* medical expense seems extraordinary and oppressive.

Why this sharp difference in attitude toward the cost of health care as compared to other necessary or even luxury expenditures? One reason, beyond doubt, lies in the fact that there are indeed cases in which the cost of medical care is an unexpected and disastrous burden upon the financial resources of an individual or a family. The cost of intensive care for the victim of a succession of coronary thromboses, for example, can go on for months or years and mount up to tens of thousands of dollars. The victim of a kidney disease who requires the use of an artificial kidney machine for the maintenance of life may face costs in excess of $15,000 a year, each and every year, permanently, for as long as he is to survive. Extraordinary medical expenses such as these are seldom a matter of choice but of stark necessity. One *can,* if necessary, survive without a television set or an automobile, but in the face of devastating disease there may be no alternative to the cost of medical care other than death. Fortunately such extreme cases are relatively few, yet the very fact that they can occur at any time, afflicting anyone, is a frightening prospect to contemplate, and the fact that no one (until recent years) could effectively be insured against them made the prospect even more fearful.

Perhaps a more basic reason that the cost of medical care is so universally resented, however, lies in our age-old attitudes toward health and illness. No one really wants to be sick, and it is human nature to take good health for granted. Thus when illness strikes, it is quite naturally

regarded as an unwelcome, painful and distressing burden, unasked for and undeserved. The individual who buys a television set or an automobile is paying for something he wants; the individual confronted with even a relatively small doctor's fee or hospital bill is paying for something he feels he did not really want and did nothing to deserve. And the fact that so many others seem to be spared this undesirable burden merely intensifies the resentment.

Obviously this line of thinking, commonplace as it is, is fallacious. True, most human beings are born with sound bodies in a state of good health. But that wondrous gift does not come with a lifetime guarantee. Good health may be "natural," but then so are the threats of injury and illness. Previous generations were forced to accept these threats fatalistically; there was little that could be done, even by those who could afford it, to prevent or cure illness. Today we have the medical resources to do both. For the first time in history it is within our capability to exercise control over what happens to our bodies —by no means complete control, yet, but an increasing degree of control with each passing year of medical research and discovery. And it is this new element in health care, the capacity not only to cure illness but also to prevent it before it strikes and to add years and possibly even decades of good health to our lives, which makes the resentful attitude toward the cost of modern medical care increasingly irrational. Here, at last, is a pearl of great price, a service that will more than repay the money invested in it. It should not be viewed as a luxury available only to those who can pay for it, nor as an intolerable burden for those who cannot. It is, quite simply, as necessary as life itself. In view of this, a reevaluation of our attitudes toward the cost of health care is long overdue, and every individual or family should make practical provisions, in terms of time and dollars and cents, to institute a regular and continuing program of preventive health care and, insofar as possible, be prepared to deal with serious medical emergencies.

The fact remains, however, that health care in this country *is* expensive. There is little question that in the near future basic social and political decisions will be made affecting the quality and availability of the medical service we will enjoy. But in general there are three approaches to meeting the cost of these services, either today or in the future. First there is the traditional private contract between patient and physician or patient and hospital, with the patient paying from his own resources for whatever medical services he needs if and when he needs them. Second, there is privately purchased health care insurance, whether it is general hospitalization insurance, major medical insurance designed to cover extraordinary medical expenses, Blue Shield-type plans which provide for payment of doctor's fees, or the full coverage of group health insurance plans. These privately purchased health insurance programs in some cases may merely supplement the traditional private payment of medical and hospital expenses; in other cases they may represent the totality of the individual or family's provision for health care. Finally, there are federal or state-sponsored programs designed to meet the cost of medical care for some or all citizens, with the funds necessary to pay for such care accumulated by some form of taxation. Each of these approaches has its advantages, and each has its drawbacks.

The Private Payment Approach

For thousands of years the traditional manner of meeting medical costs has been by means of a private arrangement between the patient and the physician in which a fee was paid for each medical service rendered. This "fee-for-service" arrangement is, of course, still familiar to everyone today. The patient is free to select his own physician and then consult him about his medical problem, whether it be an acute illness or a matter of preventive care. The physician, in turn, undertakes personal and specific responsibility for his patient's care, sets a fee that is generally based upon the amount of time the care requires, the complexity or difficulty of any procedures necessary, and his own evaluation of his qualifications. It is up to the patient to pay this fee when the service has been rendered or, in some cases, at intervals throughout or after the period of treatment. If laboratory and X-ray studies are required, the patient is also charged

for these, and if hospitalization is necessary, the hospital bill is the patient's private obligation as well.

The fee-for-service arrangement has changed little since the days of antiquity. The rules and regulations that have come to surround it in modern times are, in general, designed to protect the patient. Formal licensing procedures have been established to assure patients that only those who can demonstrate adequate medical training, knowledge, experience and skill are permitted to practice the healing arts. It has long been recognized, however, that the physician can at best only aid in the treatment of illness, he cannot command it, so that he is entitled to his fee whether his efforts at treatment are successful or not. On the other hand, physicians themselves have undertaken the obligation to maintain the highest medical standards in their practice, and exert every effort to treat their patients with skill and diligence. Negligence of a patient's needs or welfare is justification for a malpractice action and may even lead to the revoking of a physician's license. Similarly, a patient's failure to pay legitimate medical charges can result in legal action against him.

Finally, it has also been traditional for physicians to scale the charges they made for their services according to their estimation of their patients' ability to pay. Thus for identical services a physician might charge a wealthy patient a high fee, a poorer patient a much more modest fee, and a destitute patient no fee at all. Until quite recently this "sliding scale" was accepted as perfectly proper, even though it meant that the wealthy subsidized, at least to some extent, the health care of the poor. Today, in our more egalitarian society, such a system is generally regarded as grossly inequitable, and most physicians who practice on a fee-for-service basis tend to charge everyone the same fee for the same service, or else make no charge at all in charitable cases.

A private fee-for-service arrangement between doctor and patient has always had, and continues to have, certain obvious advantages and some equally obvious drawbacks. Among the advantages is that the patient is absolutely free to select his own physician, and the physician is equally free to accept or refuse the care of a patient. If he accepts it, the physician assumes personal responsibility for his patient's health and welfare; he becomes "the patient's doctor" in a very specific sense. Of course, if the patient grows dissatisfied with his services, he is free to discharge him, just as the physician, under certain circumstances, can withdraw from a given patient's care, although professional ethics rigidly require that he give the patient ample prior notice and assistance in finding some other physician to provide care. In short, a patient can walk out of a doctor's office without a word in the midst of treatment and never return, but a physician cannot properly abandon a patient.

However, the chief advantage of private medical care is, ideally, the establishment of a continuing and often quite intimate relationship between the doctor and his patient. Armed with detailed knowledge of his patient's health history, personality and background, the physician can, at least theoretically, provide a far higher quality of medical care. Such an arrangement, of course, has one major disadvantage; by and large this kind of high-quality medical care is available only to those who can afford to pay for it, and those less economically fortunate are very often simply out of luck. In earlier times this was an accepted fact of life; the poor were out of luck in a multitude of other ways as well. This is not to say that there was a total lack of compassion with regard to the hardships of illness; pestilence and disease are human conditions that have always crossed social and economic barriers and against which all human beings, rich or poor, share a common dread. Throughout the Middle Ages a variety of charity hospitals and infirmaries were maintained by the Church, for example, for the care of the indigent ill, and from the 1600s on in Europe and later in America, a certain degree of social compassion led to the establishment of workhouses, insane asylums, infirmaries, and lying-in hospitals, although these institutions more closely resembled charnel houses than facilities for the restoration of health.

Then in the late 19th and early 20th centuries the reverberations of a great wave of social reform in Europe and the United States brought about some profound changes in the availability of medical care for many of those who could not afford the cost of private attention. Not only were charity institutions revealed in their true horror, but it was also recognized that the great mass of people did not have access to medical care of any kind. As a result, this same period in history saw the establishment of the first great public hospitals in which a high quality of medical care was made available to those who could not afford private care. In America these institutions included the Massachusetts General Hospital in Boston, Philadelphia General Hospital, Harborview Hospital in Seattle and many, many other state, county and city hospitals throughout the nation, all supported by general taxation and devoted to medical care of the indigent. In addition, the 20th century in America saw the establishment of a large number of Veterans Administration hospitals dedicated to the medical care of veterans of the armed forces who required long-term treatment of illnesses or injuries arising from their military service, or who were unable to meet the cost of treatment for subsequent illnesses.

In many ways these and other public institutions are a remarkable step forward in extending medical care to those who cannot afford it under the private fee-for-service tradition. Many top-ranking American physicians help staff these hospitals with little or no compensation; such institutions are leaders in medical research and experimentation, and they also serve as invaluable training grounds for tens of thousands of fledgling doctors. But perhaps inevitably, many of the benefits of the private fee-for-service tradition are lost. All too often public hospitals are crowded, underfinanced, understaffed, and underequipped, and thus, except in a few extraordinary instances, their quality of care is generally inferior to that available under private auspices. What is more, the quality of care varies enormously from one area of the country to another, from one city to another or even in different areas of the same city. Certain local governments provide generously for the construction and maintenance of these hospitals, others most penuriously. A patient seldom has a choice of public hospital, nor does he have free choice of physician. Finally, there is always the stigma of accepting charity, and the problem of robbing the sick individual of his dignity and damaging his pride. In some cases, this consideration alone is responsible for patients refusing to utilize the services of a public institution that may be first rate in every other way.

Thus it has become obvious in recent years that private medical care for those who can afford it, and publicly supported care for those who cannot, is not the perfect solution to the still-perplexing problems of both the quality and the cost of that care. Private care remains preferable to public care, and costs are rising in both sectors, whoever pays the bill. Further, a long-term, severe or complicated illness, coming unexpectedly and without any budgeting provisions, can still suddenly confront even an affluent family with both an overwhelming economic burden and the necessity for public care.

The Avenue of Medical Insurance

It was undoubtedly to avoid the "lightning bolt" effect of sudden, large and unexpected medical bills that attention was first turned to a second approach to the problem of medical expenses: the concept of hospitalization insurance and prepaid comprehensive group medical plans. By far the most common means by which American families prepare to meet the costs of medical care today involves the purchase of some form of medical insurance, ranging all the way from plans that cover only the most minimal costs of hospitalization, on one hand, to forms of insurance that cover a broad range of medical expenses including hospital charges, the cost of diagnostic studies, doctors' fees, maternity costs, and in some cases even the cost of ambulance service, physical and occupational therapy and other services.

Basically all of these private insurance plans are premium-based programs by which an insurance carrier agrees, in return for the payment of a fixed monthly, semiannual or annual premium, to pay certain fixed amounts against the cost of specified types of medical care when they are required. Since medical insurance programs began evolving in this country in the early 1900s,

they have proliferated in a bewildering variety of coverage plans, differing widely in cost, practicality and actual protective value, and recent statistics indicate that some 70 percent of all American families today have at least some insurance coverage under one or another of these plans.

By far the most common plan today is the private, nonprofit program of hospitalization insurance known as Blue Cross, which varies slightly in its coverage and cost from state to state or region to region, but maintains certain minimum standards on a nationwide basis. Blue Cross programs are administered by hospital and/or physician councils rather than by private profit-making insurance companies, and add only their administrative costs to the medical and hospitalization costs covered in determining the premium to be charged for various services. Nevertheless, Blue Cross programs must survive on their own income rather than on any form of government subsidy, and although they are private programs, they are subject, like other public service companies, to rigid state regulations. Under a typical program, for a fixed annual premium the Blue Cross organization guarantees an individual or family payment of a specified amount per day against the basic cost of hospitalization and maintenance for a specified number of days per year. It also guarantees to pay a certain percentage of laboratory and X-ray fees accrued during hospitalization, to pay a specified amount against maternity care in a hospital, against nursery care for a newborn baby, against hospital operating charges and anesthesia charges, and against the cost of drugs and dressings. In recent years an optional extension of the Blue Cross plan known as Blue Shield provides, in return for an additional premium, for the payment of the physicians' fees in the care of illnesses up to certain limits, both for physicians' services while a patient is hospitalized and for care in the physicians' offices, with a fixed allowance for specific services such as office calls or office procedures, and certain preset amounts paid against the cost of surgical procedures.

The Blue Cross and Blue Shield programs have tremendous advantages for the average individual or family, but they also have some serious disadvantages. Most obvious of the advantages is that a Blue Cross-Blue Shield plan provides an automatic means for an individual or family to budget a certain amount of money per year against the cost of medical care, and also provides a certain basic prepaid protection in the event that illness strikes and medical costs arise. It has the additional advantage of providing relatively greater coverage for less cost than is possible with the insurance plans offered by profit-making insurance companies. Finally, it is a universally recognized and accepted means of covering the bulk of the cost of average hospitalization; for example, any hospital participating in a Blue Cross plan (which includes virtually every hospital of any size in the country) will accept evidence that a patient is a member of Blue Cross (as testified by the possession of a current Blue Cross identification card) as sufficient credentials for admission to the hospital without the necessity of making a cash deposit or any form of prepayment. In recent years, furthermore, Blue Cross programs have been extended (with, of course, an increase in premiums) to cover hospital outpatient care in emergency situations—in other words, emergency room care of acute illnesses or injuries even when hospitalization of the patient is not necessary—so that the cost of emergency situations can be met under most circumstances.

Certain disadvantages, however, continue to plague the Blue Cross programs. First, Blue Cross benefits have always lagged somewhat behind actual hospital costs, so that even a "full coverage" plan may cover only from 60 to 80 percent of a total hospital bill. Second, Blue Cross programs do have limits upon the amount of medical care that will be covered in the course of a given year, and while those limits are relatively generous for the average individual or family, the victim of a prolonged or complex illness may well exhaust his Blue Cross benefits long before his health is restored and thus accrue heavy additional medical costs. Third, most Blue Cross and Blue Shield programs have an age limit, either excluding individuals beyond the age of sixty-five altogether or providing only limited coverage at sharply elevated premiums. This, of

course, is a serious flaw, since it is the aged who are the most likely to require extensive medical care and who at the same time are the least likely to be able to afford it on a private fee-for-service basis. Fourth, certain extremely costly types of medical care—the care of mental illness, for example, or of a long-chronic illness such as tuberculosis—are often either completely excluded from Blue Cross coverage or else the coverage provided is minimal, totally unrealistic, and/or available even in this limited fashion only at a much higher premium.

But the most glaring flaw in virtually all Blue Cross-Blue Shield programs as they commonly exist today lies in the fact that they specifically provide coverage *only for the care of diagnosed illness*. They make little or no provision whatever for the most valuable and the least costly of all forms of medical care; that is, preventive medical care undertaken in the absence of symptomatic illness and directed toward the goal of the maintenance of optimum good health and the prevention, or early diagnosis, of potentially serious illness. Blue Cross-Blue Shield programs do not, for example, provide any coverage for the healthy individual who visits his physician for an annual complete physical examination and diagnostic workup, unless a diagnosis of specific illness is assigned by the doctor. And this flaw flies in the teeth of the single greatest and most invaluable change in attitude toward medical care that has come about in the last five centuries—the attitude that the most important work a physician can do, and the wisest approach to health care that the patient and his family can take, is to seek to prevent, not only to cure, illness.

A final universal shortcoming of Blue Cross and Blue Shield plans is the fact that their coverage falters and fails at precisely those times and in precisely those cases in which adequate coverage is most desperately needed; specifically, those cases that need so-called major medical care—prolonged illnesses requiring long hospitalization, multiple surgical procedures, repeated laboratory and X-ray studies, months or perhaps years of costly follow-up treatment, and thousands of dollars' worth of medications. These, of course, are not "average" cases; the vast majority of families never have to face this kind of true medical disaster, yet when they do occur they can spell economic ruin. Granted, too, that these are cases that *no one* can foresee or be expected to make private provision for, but for that reason alone some form of help should be made available, just as the family who is wiped out by a flood or an earthquake is given public support and assistance to effect recovery. Yet at present there is no program of medical insurance in existence in this country, either private or state-supported, that can or does provide this kind of "disaster insurance" for those who are unfortunate enough to need it.

Of course Blue Cross and Blue Shield programs are not the only forms of private medical insurance protection. There are multitudes of private insurance carriers who offer premium-based insurance against medical costs, some covering hospital costs alone, some including doctors' fees, some providing for outpatient care, some even providing major medical insurance provisions which, at least to some extent, cover extended illnesses and prolonged medical procedures. In many areas of the country, county medical societies sponsor insurance plans that provide extremely broad coverage to enrolled members; these programs usually require significantly higher premiums than the typical Blue Cross-Blue Shield programs, but often individuals or families are enrolled in these programs on a group basis, and major employers in the community participate and pay a part of the premium for their employees as a "fringe benefit" in addition to their regular salary. Finally, in many communities there are broad-based group health cooperative programs in which the sponsoring organization constructs and maintains its own hospitals and outpatient clinics, retains its own panels of physicians on salary, and provides total comprehensive medical care for individuals or families who enroll. Over the years such "closed panel" group health programs have been bitterly opposed by medical societies, which have gone so far as to exclude physicians associated with such programs from membership in various medical organizations, an exclusion which, among other things, has often made it difficult for these physicians to obtain adequate pro-

fessional liability insurance for their own protection. Gradually the opposition of private medicine to these programs has dwindled, and certain of them, such as the Hospital Insurance Plan of New York (HIP) or the Kaiser Permanente Group Health Program in California, have become nationally famous. Unfortunately these programs have their own built-in drawbacks. Usually they do not offer the patient a free choice of physician; the patient is expected to accept whatever doctor is on duty at the time that medical services are needed. Since much of the cost of these programs lies in the cost of maintaining hospital facilities, there is a built-in temptation to avoid hospitalization insofar as possible, or to make it as brief as possible when it is absolutely imperative, whether or not it is in the best interests of the patient. Members of these group health plans often complain of inordinately long waits to see a doctor, and of a lack of real concern on the part of the physicians for their patients. And again, these programs are universally oriented to the treatment of illness, not to the more ideal goal of comprehensive preventive medical care.

Thus the various private medical insurance programs have not, in themselves, proved to be satisfactory solutions to the quality and cost of medical care. The stigma of charity is avoided, but the ideal doctor-patient relationship can also be severely strained. Further, the costs of medical care and insurance adequate to cover them continue to increase in what has often been described as a vicious circle; as medical costs go up, insurance costs must also rise, and with payment for certain medical services guaranteed in advance, the temptation is often to use them, whether they are necessary or not, driving costs up even higher. This is particularly true in regard to hospitalization coverage; patients, doctors and hospitals alike are often guilty of regulating the length of a hospital stay according to the patient's coverage. Overly prolonged hospitalization in Veterans Administration hospitals and tax-supported county hospitals, and hospitalization extended to the limits of a private insurance program or, conversely, terminated when those limits have been reached, are common phenomena equally destructive to the patient's real needs. Hospitalization *must* be based on an impartial professional judgment of the patient's requirements rather than on any economic consideration.

Finally, the concept of preventive medical care aimed at the maintenance of optimum good health must be actively encouraged in light of its immense value, rather than discouraged, as it is under virtually all existing prepaid medical insurance programs, as an "unnecessary luxury." Far from a luxury, it is a pressing *necessity* and must be recognized as such when any plan providing for the cost of medical care is debated. In essence, any truly successful medical plan must meet two vital needs: the need to provide high-quality medical care, including preventive care, to all our citizens, regardless of their ability to pay for it; and the need to protect all our citizens against the rare but economically devastating medical disaster which may strike any family, rich or poor, at any time. Existing medical insurance plans, without exception, fail to fulfill one or another of these necessary criteria.

The State-Sponsored Approach

Faced with the inequities of a purely private doctor-patient fee-for-service arrangement, and with the seemingly inescapable inadequacies of even the most comprehensive private medical insurance plans, it is not surprising that more and more people—and their legislators—have turned their eyes toward the federal government for an ultimate and ideal solution to the problem of medical costs. On the surface it seems so easy, given the apparently unlimited financial resources of the government, and the eagerness with which a great many national leaders urge the government to assume full responsibility in a medical "cradle to grave" program for every citizen. Obviously the problem is not going to go away; obviously it is going to become more and more difficult to solve as the years go by; but is government intervention really the final and best solution?

A precedent for government intervention in the provision of medical care is already deeply entrenched in our society. It began in earnest in the great wave of liberal social legislation that was initiated in the early 1930s when literally millions of Americans were hungry, jobless, economically devastated and utterly unable to afford even the most rudimentary medical care. The establishment of the Social Security system was originally intended to provide the elderly with a minimum basic economic protection after they reached the age when they could no longer retain paying jobs. Beyond that, government intervention continued in the form of state, county and city "relief" programs, later euphemized as welfare programs, which steadily expanded to include provision for tax-supported medical care for the needy as well as income protection and other economic aids. It was further expanded following the Second World War with provisions for the medical care of service veterans, and finally, in recent years, with the establishment of programs funded through the Social Security system to provide medical services for the aged or even for those in younger age groups who became disabled by illness. Gradually, then, sentiment has evolved in favor of a full-scale federally funded health insurance program—"socialized medicine"—which, while it has been debated in various forms and so far defeated, has steadily drawn an increasing number of supporters.

Precedents have also been established in other countries—notably England, Sweden and certain provinces in Canada. They have legislated full and comprehensive programs of National Health Insurance in which general taxes are used to fund medical care for all citizens of all ages regardless of their ability to pay for these services privately. In England medical care on a private fee-for-service basis has not been abolished, but in actual practice the overwhelming majority of medical services are provided to the overwhelming majority of patients under the government-sponsored National Health Insurance plan. With such precedents as these, there is growing public pressure in America to adopt similar comprehensive health insurance programs.

Unfortunately there is sound reason to fear that any such all-inclusive program undertaken in the United States would create more problems than it would solve. Aside from the totally unreasonable objections of many elements of the medical profession who see their professional prerogatives compromised by such a program, there are some very real drawbacks to having the heavy imprint of the government's thumb placed firmly in the middle of the provision of medical care in this country.

One drawback is the simple fact that the single group of people in the country who would be most profoundly affected by a fully comprehensive federal health insurance program—the physicians who would be expected to provide the medical care under such a program—almost universally abhor this degree of federal intervention into the practice of medicine. Contrary to widespread opinion and innuendo, the objection of most doctors to federalized medical programs is *not* based upon the fear that their professional incomes would be adversely affected. It is simply not realistic to imagine that any such program would seriously depress the average physician's income. For such a program to succeed, existing physicians would have to be retained in practice and multitudes of new physicians would have to be attracted to the profession. Far from cutting back doctors' incomes to any degree, income levels would have to be a major means by which the government could attract new recruits into the ranks of medicine. The chief objections doctors have to a federalized medical program are, for the most part, related to professional considerations. They feel that medical decisions regarding the health care of patients can properly be made only by doctors, and they fear that under a federalized medical program many of these decisions would be preempted by a whole new hierarchy of nonmedical administrative personnel who would be in a position to overrule decisions the physicians felt were in their patients' best interests. Doctors also foresee an overwhelming burden of pointless paper work, filling in and filing requests, claims, reports and records in triplicate or quadruplicate, a procedure that can take hours and eventually days away from the actual practice of medicine. Nor are these fears unfounded, for the paper work involved with private insurance programs as well as various local, state and federal medical procedures already in existence is formidable and time-consuming. Doctors also fear that they will be inundated by a wave of trivial medical complaints which will consume even more time at the expense of patients who are in greater need of their attention. Ever jealous of their traditional prerogative as highly respected private professional counselors, vast numbers of doctors abhor the thought of becoming salaried government employees, even though such fears might well prove totally groundless. They also fear that hospital staff appointments, specialty certification, even the renewal of licensure to practice may come to be matters of political expediency rather than a strictly professional concern. And finally, in addition to the threat of lowered professional standards, many doctors predict that the quality of medical care available to the individual patient would also decline.

Beyond doubt at least some of these fears are exaggerated or unwarranted. But if only some of them prove to be real, they could become problems of the greatest nationwide concern. An equally pressing concern is the undeniable fact that the cost of a federal health insurance program would be permanently staggering. The impression that the government will provide "free" medical care could not possibly be further from the truth. The very limited Medicare and Medicaid programs that have been instituted in recent years have already far outstripped their projected cost. We are now faced with the necessity of telling the beneficiaries of these programs—the elderly, the poor and the disabled—that the benefits they were so liberally promised are going to have to be cut back, and that the cost burden to the rest of the nation is even so going to have to be increased.

The fact is that there has never been a single instance in the history of our nation when the federal government has been able to provide a service funded through taxes at a cost lower than or even equal to the cost of the same service provided by private enterprise. It has been estimated, for example, that the provision of medical care by the government will cost the nation anywhere from 15 to 50 percent more for the same services than our present system. And inevitably, it is the taxpayer who will be saddled with these extra costs. In the long run the result may very well be the provision of a vastly poorer quality of medical care at far greater overall cost than even the admittedly imperfect care provided through private hospitalization and medical insurance programs. And perhaps most damaging of all, a federalized medical program would almost certainly mean that the concept of preventive medical care will be lost in the shuffle, and that the brightest hope for health preservation in the future will be permanently buried.

Is there an acceptable alternative? Certainly federal support for the provision of medical care in some segments of our society is going to remain a permanent necessity. Provision to protect our aging population from insupportable medical costs is a necessary obligation. So also is the provision of high-quality medical care to anyone who cannot support the cost himself, without the stigma of charity, a necessary obligation. Massive segments of our population in deprived rural or urban areas must not be denied medical care and health protection. The racial and economic discrimination that still shamefully exists in the provision of medical care must and will be halted. And all individuals or families must have some realistic protection against the truly overwhelming medical costs that do occasionally arise.

With these obligations in mind, the ideal solution to providing high-quality medical care at realistic prices hinges upon three equally important factors. First, the members of the medical profession must come to realize that their obligation to society must extend far beyond mere lip service to the medical needs of the less fortunate. Society subsidizes the education and training of many physicians, provides the doctor with a better than average income for his services, and gives him the opportunity to continue his work, if he so desires, to whatever age he chooses. Society also accords him a degree of respect enjoyed by workers in few other fields. In return, every physician can reasonably be expected to contribute a significant portion of his time, energy and skill to the provision of medical care for the less fortunate in our society to a far greater extent than is actually the case today. Above all, rather than to struggle doggedly to maintain an unrealistic and unacceptable status quo, the physician individually, and through his powerful professional organizations, can search for truly constructive, realistic and dignified solutions to the unresolved problems of providing care for those unable to meet the cost themselves.

Second, the patient—the beneficiary of the high quality of medical care available in this country today—must once and for all divest himself of the notion that medical care should, or ever will, be "free," like the air he breathes or the water he drinks, a service to which he is entitled without any effort or contribution on his part. As long as the present system continues in operation, funds to meet the cost of health care should be budgeted in exactly the same manner as funds to meet the cost of food, shelter or clothing. Health care is primarily the individual's responsibility. He must first do everything within his power to see to it that his requirements for medical care are kept to the barest minimum possible, a goal achievable only through an active and enlightened program of preventive health care. He must also prepare himself to meet at least the average expectable cost of medical care that the maintenance of good health requires. Further, if he is in favor of federally funded medical care, or even if he is indifferent to it, he must realize that he will be the one to benefit or suffer, and either way the money to support it will come out of his pocket. Under these circumstances it is only common sense to make his needs and opinions, whether pro or con, known. Health care is everyone's concern, not only the concern of doctors, medical organizations and legislators, and the way to make that concern felt is through informed action at the community level, and on the state and federal levels through support of those elected officials who will help implement the desired programs.

Finally, the government itself, whether state or federal, must discard medical care as a political issue. Few would disagree that a truly compassionate and civilized society, through its government agencies, must accept responsibility for the health care of the poor, the underprivileged, the unemployed and the abandoned. Means must be found to insure the uninsurable, most notably the aged and infirm who are unable to provide for their own medical care. Means must also be found to protect from financial privation all those faced with prolonged, complicated or permanently debilitating illnesses. What is more, means must be found to fulfill these needs while preserving the individual doctor-patient relationship that plays such an important part in both preventive and curative medical care. But these are *social* issues of the greatest magnitude, not merely planks in a party platform or a means of placating one or another of the powerful legislative lobbies. The government not only serves the people in this country, it *is* the people, and the people must demand that whatever degree of responsibility their government takes in the provision of medical care, at present or in the future, be based upon a realistic and impartial assessment of their own needs. Such a responsibility cannot be met through partisan politics or hasty, ill-conceived political giveaways. It can be fulfilled only through the most careful and knowledgeable long-range planning and research, utilizing the wisdom and experience of the men most qualified in this field before any final plans are implemented.

In the opinion of the majority of qualified professionals in the medical field, the goal of any truly effective health care plan should be twofold: first, the preservation in this country of the very real benefits of the private doctor-patient relationship wherever possible; and second, the availability through government support of high-quality medical care to all those who could not otherwise afford it. This is a large order, yet one that holds greater promise than any current or projected health care program. Such a goal is not unattainable—but its realization must rest squarely on the shoulders of those who will benefit the most: the people.

GLOSSARY

ABORTION: The interruption of an early pregnancy, whether from natural causes or as a result of medical intervention. *Elective abortion:* The interruption of an early pregnancy at the choice of the mother. *Inevitable abortion:* A condition in which the spontaneous or natural disruption of a pregnancy has progressed to such a point that abortion cannot be prevented. *Habitual abortion:* Spontaneous or uncontrollable abortion which occurs in successive pregnancies. *Spontaneous abortion:* The natural and inadvertent loss of an early pregnancy, often for undeterminable reasons. *Therapeutic abortion:* The medical interruption of a pregnancy due to a mortal threat to the mother. *Threatened abortion:* The appearance of signs, notably vaginal bleeding and cramping, suggesting that the spontaneous expulsion of an early pregnancy may be imminent.

ABSCESS: A localized collection of pus in a cavity formed by the death and disintegration of surrounding tissues; *see also* Boil. *Brain abscess:* A lesion within the brain which may occur when bacteria from a superficial lesion are carried through the bloodstream and lodge in the brain. *Lung abscess:* A collection of pus in a cavity within the lung formed by the disintegration of lung tissue. *Peritonsillar abscess (Quinsy):* A pocket of pus deep in the soft tissue of the pharynx in the region around or behind the tonsil. *Peritoneal abscess:* An encysted mass of pus or exudate within the peritoneal cavity of the abdomen.

ACETYLCHOLINE: A chemical that plays an important role in the transmission of a nerve impulse across a synapse or at a myoneural (nerve-muscle) junction.

ACHONDROPLASIA: A congenital disorder of skeletal formation that results in dwarfism.

ACIDOPHILS: Cells in the anterior pituitary gland which secrete growth hormone.

ACIDOSIS: Any condition in which the blood serum or tissue fluids in the body become abnormally acidic. *Diabetic acidosis:* A condition brought on by a breakdown in carbohydrate metabolism due to insulin insufficiency in the diabetic, leading to symptoms of nausea and vomiting, dizziness, deep stertorous breathing and, finally, diabetic coma.

ACINI: Clusters of secretory cells such as those found in the pancreas.

ACROMEGALY: Disproportionate growth of hands, feet, the bones of the skull and the jaw, together with enlargement of the nose and coarsening of facial features due to overproduction of growth hormone by the anterior pituitary gland after physical maturity has been attained.

ACTINOMYCOSIS: An infection resulting from a fungus which often enters the body through infected gums or decayed teeth.

ADDISON'S DISEASE (adrenal insufficiency): An endocrine disorder resulting from underproduction of all the adrenal hormones.

ADENOIDITIS: A bacterial infection of the adenoids.

ADENOIDS: Soft, spongy masses of lymphoid tissue located on the upper surface of the soft palate in the floor of the nasopharynx.

ADENOMA: A benign tumor which develops from glandular or secreting tissue in various organs.

ADRENAL GLANDS: A pair of endocrine (i.e., internally-secreting) glands situated on the upper poles of the kidneys which secrete a variety of hormones necessary to life. The cells in the central core or *adrenal medulla* secrete the hormone epinephrin which helps control the blood pressure and heart rate. Cells in the outer shell or *adrenal cortex* secrete a family of hormones, including *cortisone,* which help control salt and water balance within the body, counteract inflammation, and prepare the body to meet situations of physical or emotional stress.

ADRENALIN: Another name for epinephrin, the hormone produced by the medulla of the adrenal gland.

AEROPHAGIA: Air-swallowing.

AFIBRINOGENEMIA: Total absence of the protein fibrinogen in the blood serum.

AFTERBIRTH: The material, including the placenta, the fetal membranes and the severed umbilical cord, which are expelled from the uterus after the birth of a child.

AGAMMAGLOBULINEMIA: The congenital lack or absence of the protein gamma globulin from the blood serum.

AGGLUTINATION: The clumping together of cells distributed in a fluid.

AGGLUTININS: Sensitizing antibodies which cause agglutination or clumping of cells in a fluid suspension.

AGGLUTINOGENS: Agglutinins attached to the surface of human red blood cells which can be activated by antibodies to cause the cells to clump together or agglutinate in the course of transfusion reactions.

AGRANULOCYTOSIS: A condition in which the bone marrow's capacity to produce white blood cells is markedly reduced or destroyed, often due to extreme sensitivity to certain drugs.

ALBINISM: The complete absence of pigment in the skin, hair or eyes.

ALBUMIN: An important protein in human blood plasma.

ALBUMINURIA: The abnormal appearance of the blood protein albumin in the urine.

ALKALOSIS: Any condition in which the blood serum and tissue fluids of the body become excessively alkaline. *Respiratory alkalosis:* A dangerous condition which arises when too much carbon dioxide has been forced out of the bloodstream by hyperventilation.

ALLERGEN: Any foreign substance not normally present in the body to which the body becomes hypersensitive.

ALLERGY: An acquired excessive sensitivity or hypersensitivity to certain normally harmless foreign substances which find access to the body.

ALOPECIA: Baldness.

ALOPECIA AREATA: Hair loss, temporary or permanent, in which the hair comes out in patches.

ALVEOLI: The tiny clusters of air sacs at the ends of the bronchioles which make up the bulk of lung tissue.

AMEBIASIS (amebic dysentery): A form of diarrheal disease caused by infection with the protozoan organism Endameba histolytica.

AMENORRHEA: Absence or cessation of menstrual flow.

AMNIOCENTESIS: A technique by which a small amount of amniotic fluid is removed from the uterus during gestation for examination and diagnosis of certain congenital defects or diseases prior to the birth of the baby.

AMNIOTIC (amnionic) FLUID: The watery fluid which bathes the fetus within the membranous sac in the uterus.

AMPHETAMINES: A group of drugs which act as powerful cerebral and cardiovascular stimulants and appetite suppressants.

AMYLASE: A pancreatic enzyme which converts dietary starches and complex sugars into simple sugars.

AMYOTROPHIC LACTERAL SCLEROSIS (Lou Gehrig's disease): A fatal nervous system disorder marked by destruction of nerve cells in the spine and brain, leading to progressive muscular weakness, atrophy and paralysis.

ANAPHYLAXIS (anaphylactic shock): A sudden, exaggerated shock-like allergic reaction to foreign substances in the body that may arise as a result of prior sensitization.

ANDROSTERONE: One of the major male sex hormones or androgens.

ANEMIA: Any condition in which the blood is deficient in red cells, or in which the red cells are abnormally small or deficient in hemoglobin content. *Aplastic anemia:* Anemia caused by depression or destruction of the bone marrow's capability to make red cells as a result of chemical poisoning by a toxic agent, allergic manifestations or other reasons. *Folic acid deficiency anemia:* Anemia caused by a deficiency of folic acid in the diet. *Hemolytic anemia:* Anemia caused by abnormal destruction of red cells. *Iron-deficiency anemia:* Anemia resulting from insufficient dietary iron to permit the manufacture of adequate numbers of healthy red cells. *Mediterranean anemia:*

An hereditary anemia in which the red cells are abnormally thin and thus destroyed in excessive numbers in the bloodstream. *Pernicious anemia* (Addison's anemia): Anemia caused by inadequate absorption of dietary vitamin B_{12} (cyancobalamin) into the bloodstream. *Posthemorrhagic anemia:* Anemia resulting from hemorrhage of a torn or injured blood vessel. *Secondary anemia:* Anemia which arises as a secondary effect of some antecedent disease or injury.

ANENCEPHALUS: A congenital deformity in which little or none of the fetal brain develops; an extreme degree of microcephalus.

ANEURYSM: A blood-filled sac formed by the dilatation or stretching of the wall of an artery or vein.

ANGIITIS (arteritis): Inflammation of an artery.

ANGINA PECTORIS: A transitory and severe chest pain associated with inadequate arterial oxygen supply to the heart muscle; a common and recurring symptom of severe arterisoclerotic heart disease.

ANGIOCARDIOGRAM: A sequence of X-ray films visualizing the chambers of the heart taken following the introduction of a radio-opaque dye into one of the great veins returning blood to the heart.

ANGIOGRAPHY: An X-ray examination of the arteries or veins, usually involving the injection of a radio-opaque dye. *Cerebral angiography:* An X-ray examination of the blood vessels within the brain achieved by injecting a carotid artery with a radio-opaque dye.

ANOREXIA NERVOSA: A disorder in which the victim is neurotically or compulsively unable to eat or hold down ingested food.

ANOVULATORY CYCLE: A menstrual cycle in which the ripening and discharge of an ovum does not occur, either due to natural causes or to the medical administration of hormones to suppress ovulation.

ANTABUSE: The proprietary name for a drug used to treat alcoholism.

ANTHRACOSIS (black lung disease, miner's lung): A lung inflammation common among coal miners caused by prolonged exposure to and inhalation of silicate dust; *see also* Silicosis.

ANTIBIOTIC: Any of a group of drugs which combat the growth of bacteria or rickettsia by interfering with their normal growth and development. Antibiotics either kill bacteria directly (bacteriocidal antibiotics) or impair their reproduction (bacteriostatic antibiotics) so that natural body forces can more readily destroy them.

ANTIBODIES: Specific substances produced by the body as a defense against foreign substances or antigens which have found entry into the body. *Heterophile antibodies:* Antibodies which appear in the bloodstream in response to various invading viral organisms, notably the virus of infectious mononucleosis.

ANTIGEN: Any substance that causes the formation of antibodies.

ANTIHISTAMINES: Various drugs which tend to neutralize the effects of histamine released in the body as a result of an allergic reaction, used to help suppress or counteract allergic symptoms.

ANTITOXIN: A substance, often containing naturally produced serum antibodies, which is capable of counteracting specific toxins or poisons that gain entrance to the body. *Polyvalent antitoxin:* A solution or serum containing antitoxins to several separate and distinct toxins in the same preparation.

AORTA: The great artery which carries blood from the left ventricle of the heart to all the major peripheral arteries of the body; rises from the heart (the *ascending aorta*) to form a great *arch* in the chest, then travels downward (the *descending aorta*) through the abdomen until it divides into the right and left *common iliac arteries.*

AORTITIS: Inflammation of the aorta. *Syphilitic aortitis:* Inflammation of a portion of the aorta as a late complication of syphilis.

APGAR RATING: A scale for evaluating the physical condition of a newborn infant, developed by Dr. Virginia Apgar.

APHASIA: Loss or impairment of the ability to use words, usually due to damage or destruction of nerve cells in the brain.

APPENDICITIS: Inflammation of the vermiform appendix.

ARRHYTHMIA: Irregular heartbeat.

ARTERIOLE: Any small arterial branch, especially one just proximal to a capillary.

ARTERIOSCLEROSIS: A generalized disease condition involving thickening and hardening of the arteries throughout the body.

ARTERY: Any of the larger thick-walled blood vessels through which blood is carried from the heart to the peripheral tissues of the body. *Brachial artery:* The great arterial vessel supplying the arm. *Common carotid artery:* One of the paired great arteries carrying blood up the neck to the brain. *Coronary artery:* One of the major arteries carrying blood to the heart muscle. *Femoral artery:* The great artery transporting blood to the leg. *Pulmonary artery:* An artery which carries blood from the right ventricle of the heart to the lungs. *Renal artery:* One of the paired arteries supplying blood to the kidneys, branching from the middle segment of the abdominal aorta on either side.

ARTHRITIS: Inflammation of the joints. *Gonorrheal arthritis:* A bacterial infection of the synovial membranes lining the joint capsules; a late complication of gonorrheal infection. *Infectious arthritis:* Arthritis caused by invasion of a joint by bacteria. *Rheumatoid arthritis:* A chronic disease of the joints, marked by inflammatory changes in the synovial membranes and articular structures of the joints, and by atrophy and rarefaction of the bones in the vicinity of the joints. *Traumatic arthritis:* Inflammation of a joint due to an injury or blow.

ARTIFICIAL RESPIRATION: Any technique by which an individual's respirations are maintained by artificial means; i.e., mouth-to-mouth resuscitation.

ASBESTOSIS: A lung inflammation resulting from prolonged exposure to and inhalation of asbestos dust and fibers.

ASCITES: An abnormal collection of fluid in the abdominal cavity.

ASPHYXIA: A condition marked by deficiency of oxygen and excess of carbon dioxide in the bloodstream, fatal if uncorrected. Commonly associated with choking, strangulation or impaired oxygen-carbon dioxide exchange in the lungs.

ASTHMA: A condition of the upper respiratory tract marked by recurrent attacks of shortness of breath, wheezing, coughing and a sense of constriction in the chest, usually due to spasmodic contraction of the bronchi and often caused by an allergy.

ASTIGMATISM: A visual disturbance due to an irregular curvature of the lens or the cornea of the eye.

ATAXIA: Irregularity of muscle action or severe muscular incoordination, usually due to damage or disease of motor nerve centers in the brain. *Friedreich's ataxia:* A rare hereditary nervous system disease characterized by muscular incoordination.

ATELECTASIS: Collapse of a segment of lung, often due to obstruction of the bronchus leading to the affected segment.

ATHEROMA: A plaque-like deposit of fatty materials and calcium in the wall of an artery.

ATHEROSCLEROSIS: A generalized disorder characterized by formation of atheromas in the walls of the arteries.

ATHETOSIS: A neuromuscular derangement marked by a constant and recurring series of slow wormlike movements of the hands or feet, usually due to disease or damage of motor nerve centers in the brain.

ATRESIA: A congenital absence or narrowing of a tube or channel which is normally open. *Esophageal atresia:* A congenital narrowing of a segment of the esophagus, resulting in pain when food is swallowed.

ATRIA (auricles): The upper chambers of the heart.

ATROPHY: A shrinking or wasting away of a tissue or organ.

AURA: A subjective sensation or phenomenon that sometimes precedes the onset of an epileptic attack or a migraine headache.

AURICLE: The flaring, funnel-shaped portion of the external ear. *Auricles* (atria): The upper chambers of the heart.

AUSCULTATION: The act of listening for sounds within the body with or without a stethoscope.

BABINSKI SIGN: An abnormal reflex in which the toes curl up in response to stimulation of the sole of the foot, usually indicating some disturbance of the motor neurons in the brain.

BACILLI: Long or short rod-shaped bacteria which grow either singly or in chains.

BACTEREMIA: An infection in which bacteria have entered the bloodstream.

BACTERIA: Primitive one-celled plantlike organisms which may invade the body and cause infectious illnesses. Some bacteria (i.e., those normally inhabiting the colon) are normal and beneficial; others are *pathogenic* or disease-producing.

BASAL METABOLISM RATE (BMR): The speed at which biochemical reactions progress throughout the body as measured by the quantity of oxygen consumed by the individual during a measured period of rest.

BARBITURATES: A group of habituating drugs, all derivatives of barbituric acid, which act as profound central nervous system depressants. Under medical direction these drugs are used as sleeping medication or as adjuncts to general anesthesia. Frequently abused as soporifics or "downers."

BASOPHILS: Special cells of the anterior pituitary gland which secrete adrenocorticotrophic hormone (ACTH).

BED SORE: *See* decubitus ulcer.

BELL'S PALSY: A transitory paralysis of the facial nerve.

BERI-BERI: A disease caused by a dietary deficiency of vitamin B$_1$ or thiamin.

BETA CELLS: Clusters of cells in the islets of Langerhans in the pancreas which produce insulin.

BILE: The alkaline digestive secretion manufactured by the liver.

BILE DUCT (common bile duct): The tube carrying bile from the liver and gall bladder into the small intestine.

BILIARY DYSKINESIA: Biliary colic in the absence of gallstones.

BILIRUBIN: The natural body pigment which gives bile its characteristic yellow-green color.

BIOPSY: The surgical removal of a fragment of living tissue for microscopic examination and diagnosis. *Breast biopsy:* The removal and microscopic examination of a fragment of breast tissue for diagnostic purposes. *Scalene node biopsy:* The surgical excision of the lymph glands in the neck above the collarbone for pathological examination.

BLADDER (urinary bladder): A muscular sac in the pelvis which serves as a reservoir for urine. *Neurogenic bladder:* Any disturbance in the normal function of the urinary bladder due to a lesion of the nervous system. *Reflex bladder* (automatic bladder): A condition in which the victim has no sensation of his bladder being full, so that it empties by reflex action when it reaches maximum capacity.

BLASTOMYCOSIS: A chronic infection caused by the fungus Blastomyces dermatitidis.

BLEPHARITIS: An inflammation of the margins of the eyelids.

BLOOD: One of the six basic tissues of the body, a fluid tissue in which the cellular elements (red cells, white cells and platelets) float freely in a liquid medium, the blood plasma. *Blood clot: See* Thrombus; Embolus.

BLOOD COUNT, COMPLETE (CBC): A group of laboratory tests, including enumeration of red and white cells and measurement of hemoglobin content, that are performed on the blood for diagnostic purposes. *Differential blood count:* A microscopic examination of the blood used to determine the relative quantities of various kinds of white cells present.

BLOOD CULTURE: Bacterial culture of a sample of blood for the detection of the presence of bacteria.

BLOOD POISONING: *See* Septicemia.

BLOOD PRESSURE: The force exerted by the blood against the walls of the blood vessels containing it, as measured by a sphygmomanometer. *Diastolic blood pressure:* The point during diastole or relaxation of the heart at which the blood exerts the least pressure against the vessels containing it. *Systolic blood pressure:* The point during systole or contraction of the heart at which the blood exerts the most pressure against the vessels containing it.

BLOOD TYPE: A classification of a person's blood, according to the presence or absence of certain substances that tend to make the red cells *agglutinate* (stick together) used in selecting blood for transfusion. The common blood types are Type O, Type A, Type B and Type AB, and all blood is either Rh Positive or Rh Negative.

BOIL (furuncle): A painful abscess located in the lower layers of the skin or subcutaneous tissue.

BONE: One of the six basic tissues of the body; the material from which the skeleton is composed. *Carpal bones:* The bones of the wrist. *Flat bones:* The bones of the ribs, skull and pelvis. *Long bones:* The bones of the arms and legs. *Short bones:* The bones of the hands, fingers, feet and toes.

BOTULISM: A dangerous disease caused by ingestion of food containing a toxin produced by the bacillus Clostridium botulinum.

BRAIN: The mass of nervous tissue within the cranium; the directing center of the central nervous system. *Brain stem:* The structure at the base of the brain connecting the upper end of the spinal cord with the cerebral hemispheres, and containing both motor and sensory nerve tracts and the cranial nerve nuclei.

BREASTS (mammary glands): Glandular structures on the anterior wall of the chest, relatively undeveloped in the male, which in the female during gestation produce milk to feed the newborn infant. *Breast self-examination:* The procedure performed by the individual to aid in the early identification of possible breast cancer.

BRIGHT'S DISEASE: Any of a variety of malfunctions of the kidney; *see also* Glomerulonephritis.

BRONCHI: The air tubes leading to the lungs formed by the branching of the trachea or windpipe.

BRONCHIECTASIS: Deterioration of the bronchi and bronchioles usually associated with chronic bronchial infection.

BRONCHIOLES: The tiny terminal branches of the bronchi leading to the alveoli.

BRONCHITIS: Inflammation of the bronchi.

BRONCHOSCOPY: The examination of the trachea and the larger bronchi by means of a narrow, lighted tube, the bronchoscope.

BRUCELLOSIS (undulant fever): An infectious disease contracted by man by direct contact with infected animals or by drinking milk products containing the Brucella organism.

BUERGER'S DISEASE (thromboangiitis obliterans): A disorder in which small arteries in the extremities, particularly the toes, become thrombosed or obstructed, often leading to gangrene.

BUNION: An enlargement of the bursa or sac padding the first joint of the great toe, due to chronic pressure, inflammation and scarring.

BURSA: A saclike cavity filled with a viscid fluid and situated over bony prominences to prevent friction.

BURSITIS: Inflammation of a bursa.

CAESAREAN SECTION: The delivery of a fetus by surgical incision of the uterus through the abdominal wall.

CANAL: Any narrow tubelike structure joining one area with another. *Auditory canal:* The tube leading from the external ear to the deeper portions of the ear. *Cervical canal:* The narrow tube which connects the uterine cavity with the vagina. *Root canal:* The continuation of the pulp cavity in the root of a tooth, through which nerves and blood vessels reach the tooth from the jaw. *Semi-circular canals:* Three curved fluid-filled tubules within the inner ear which serve to maintain body equilibrium.

CANCER: A malignant tumor; abnormal and uncontrolled cellular growth, characterized by invasion of surrounding healthy tissue and metastatic spread to distant organs, leading to the formation of secondary growths; *see also* Carcinoma; Sarcoma.

CAPILLARY: Any of the minute blood vessels which connect the arterioles and the venules in the body, forming a closed circulatory network for the blood.

CARBON DIOXIDE: A gas formed in the tissues as a by-product of energy-producing biochemical reactions within the cells and carried by the blood for exhalation from the lungs.

CARBOHYDRATE: One of the three basic food materials used by the body (i.e., carbohydrate, protein and fat) characterized by chemical structure including primarily carbon, hydrogen and oxygen. The most common carbohydrates include sugars, starches and alcohols.

CARBONIC ANHYDRASE: An enzyme which facilitates the transfer of carbon dioxide from tissues to blood and from blood to the alveolar air.

CARCINOMA: A malignant tumor or cancer which develops from epithelial tissue. *Adenocarcinoma:* A cancer which develops from glandular or secreting tissues of the stomach, breast, bronchi or other organs. *Basal-cell carcinoma:* A cancer which develops from the epithelial cells in the deeper layers of the skin. *Bronchogenic carcinoma:* A cancer which develops from the columnar epithelial cells lining the interior of a bronchus. *Carcinoma of the cervix:* A slow-growing cancer which develops from the epithelial cells lining the uterine cervix. *Epithelial carcinoma* (Epithelioma): Any skin cancer which develops from epithelial cells. *Carcinoma in situ:* An early cancerous growth confined to one small surface area without evidence of invasion of deeper cell layers.

CARDIAC ARREST: Interruption of the rhythmic contraction of the heart as a result of injury, chemical irritation or disease.

CARDIAC COMPRESSION (cardiac massage): A means of restoring arrested heartbeat by rhythmic massage or compression of the heart, either externally by compressing the chest wall, or internally through an incision in the chest wall. *External cardiac compression:* A first-aid measure for restoring heartbeat by means of rhythmic pressure on the victim's chest with the hands.

CARDIOSPASM: An irritable spasm of the cardiac sphincter of the stomach.

CARDITIS: Inflammation of the heart.

CARIES: Decay of the teeth or bones.

CARTILAGE: The smooth rubbery tissue or "gristle" usually attached to bones to provide a slippery articulating surface for the joints.

CATARACT: A clouding or opacity of the lens of the eye or its capsule, leading to dimming and blurring of vision.

CATHETER: Any of a variety of narrow tubes inserted through natural body channels to inject or remove fluids or measure pressures as a diagnostic device.

CELIAC DISEASE: A disorder of intestinal absorption of food materials which occurs among children; *see also* Sprue.

CELL: The basic structural unit of all tissues of the body, composed of a cell membrane enclosing a quantity of fluid protoplasm and containing a nucleus which is filled with the genetic material that determined the characteristics of the cell and makes reproduction of the cell possible.

CELLULITIS: Inflammation of the cells, particularly a purulent bacterial infection of loose subcutaneous tissue.

CEMENTUM: The substance which holds a tooth firmly adherent to the bone of the jaw.

CEREBELLUM: The part of the brain concerned with coordination of muscular movements.

CEREBRAL PALSY: Any one of a group of disorders of movement and coordination caused by a prenatal cerebral defect or injury and characterized by varying degrees of paralysis.

CEREBROSPINAL FLUID: The crystal-clear watery liquid that circulates in and around the brain and spinal cord.

CEREBROVASCULAR ACCIDENT (CVA): A disorder within the arteries supplying the brain, including rupture or obstruction which causes impairment of circulation; *see also* Stroke.

CEREBRUM: The two great hemispheres of the brain, containing brain cells that control motion, interpretation of sensation, and mentation.

CERUMEN: A waxy exudate that coats the interior of the external auditory canal.

CERVICITIS: Inflammation of the uterine cervix.

CERVIX: The lower end or mouth of the uterus.

CHALAZION: A small benign tumor of the eyelid.

CHANCROID: A localized venereal infection of the external genitalia caused by a bacillus.

CHEMORECEPTORS: Any sensory nerve endings sensitive to contact with various chemicals; for example, the olfactory receptors in the nose.

CHEMOTHERAPY: The treatment of diseases by administration of chemicals.

CHICKEN POX (varicella). An acute communicable disease, usually of children, caused by a virus and marked by slight fever and an eruption of small water-filled blisters on the skin and mucous membrane.

CHIGGERS (redbugs, harvest mites): Submicroscopic insects which burrow beneath the skin and cause irritable infestations.

CHILBLAINS: A reddening and itching of the skin as a result of recurring mild exposure to damp cold.

CHLOASMA: Pigmented spots, especially on the backs of hands, which appear as a natural part of the aging process.

CHOLANGIOGRAMS: X-ray films of the common bile duct, often taken during surgery.

CHOLECYSTECTOMY: Surgical removal of the gall bladder.

CHOLECYSTITIS: Inflammation or infection of the gall bladder.

CHOLELITHIASIS: Gallstones in the gall bladder or the common bile duct.

CHOLERA: An acute, epidemic infectious disease of the intestine, caused by the Vibrio comma bacillus.

CHOLESTEROL: A natural fatty compound manufactured by the liver and important to the body's metabolism of fatty food materials.

CHOLINESTERASE: An enzyme present in all body tissues which facilitates the transfer of electrochemical messages across synapses between nerve cells or across the junction between nerve cells and muscles.

CHORDAE TENDINEAE: Strands of muscular tissue attached to the heart valves which help control their movement.

CHOREA: A general term used to describe sudden, involuntary muscular movements, usually resulting from irritation or damage to nerve cells. *Huntington's chorea:* A fatal, progressive hereditary nervous system affliction appearing in adult life and marked by progressively severe irregular muscular movements, speech disturbances and dementia. *Sydenham's chorea* (St. Vitus' dance): involuntary purposeless movements of the extremities or trunk as a result of rheumatic fever, usually a transitory symptom.

CHORIOEPITHELIOMA: A rare but violently malignant cancer which develops from fragments of embryonal tissue retained within the uterus following an abortion or miscarriage.

CHROMOSOMES: The genetic templates of the cell nucleus which determine the nature of the cell and the organism of which it is a part.

CHYMOTRYPSIN: A pancreatic enzyme which breaks down protein foods into their component protein molecules and amino acids.

CIRCULATORY SYSTEM: The organ system composed of the heart, the arteries, the capillaries and the veins, through which the blood is continuously circulated to all parts of the body. *Collateral circulation:* A system of secondary or accessory vessels which provides alternative circulation to an area when the normal blood supply is obstructed. *Portal circulation system:* Any circulatory scheme in which blood is carried from a capillary bed into a vein and then into another capillary bed before being returned to the heart; specifically, the hepatic portal circulation system in which venous blood draining the gastrointestinal tract and spleen is conducted by way of the portal vein to the capillary bed of the liver before being returned to the heart. *Pulmonary circulation system:* The portion of the circulatory system through which blood is carried from the right ventricle of the heart to the lungs for oxygenation, then returned to the left ventricle of the heart for distribution to the organs and tissues through the general circulatory system.

CIRCUMCISION: Surgical removal of all or part of the prepuce or foreskin of the penis.

CIRRHOSIS: Literally, "hardening"; a disease of the liver caused by widespread damage to liver tissue which leads to imperfect regeneration and permanent scarring. *Obstructive cirrhosis* (Biliary cirrhosis): Cirrhosis caused by chronic obstruction of the bliary system due to stones, infection of inflammation. *Post-hepatic cirrhosis:* Cirrhosis which may follow a particularly severe infectious hepatitis. *Toxic cirrhosis:* Cirrhosis caused by severe damage to liver cells by some external liver poison such as carbon tetrachloride.

CLAUDICATION: Pain arising from oxygen hunger of tissues, usually the result of obstruction of arterial blood flow. *Intermittent claudication:* A recurring aching pain in the muscles of the legs and feet which occurs during exertion and disappears as soon as the muscles are rested.

CLITORIS: A small sensitive body of erectile tissue situated in the female genital crease above the introitus of the vagina; the female organ corresponding to the male penis.

CLONUS: An abnormal rhythmic tendon reflex that occurs as a response to stretching the Achilles' tendon or the patellar tendon, caused by injury or irritation of certain motor neurons in the brain; also identified as ankle clonus or patellar clonus.

CLOT: A soft, semi-solidified mass of coagulated blood; *see also* Thrombus.

CLUBFOOT: A congenital deformity in which the foot is twisted out of normal anatomical shape or position during gestation.

COAGULATION: A mechanism by which the blood coagulates or clots to form a semisolid mass whenever a blood vessel is torn or injured. *Coagulation (clotting) defects:* Any of a variety of disorders of the coagulation mechanism that cause excessively slow, incomplete or impaired clotting of the blood.

COARCTATION OF THE AORTA: A congenital narrowing or stricture of the aorta, often responsive to surgical correction.

COCCI: Small, spherical or oval shaped bacteria which grow in long chains, pairs or grapelike clusters.

COCCIDIOIDOMYCESIS (valley fever): A fungus infection of the lungs.

COCHLEA: A spiral structure in the inner ear, vital to the transmission of sound.

COITUS: Sexual intercourse. *Coitus interruptus:* An ineffective method of conception control which depends upon male withdrawal during coitus prior to orgasm and ejaculation.

COLCHICINE: A drug derived from chinchona bark used in the treatment of gout.

COLLAGEN: A tough, elastic, somewhat gelatinous material that is a major component of connective tissue. *Collagen diseases:* A family of diseases affecting collagen tissue.

COLIC: Any intermittent, spasmodic and recurring pain; often used in reference to spasmodic abdominal pain which occurs in children following feedings. *Biliary colic:* Spasms or paroxysms of pain due to the presence of gallstones in the gall bladder or bile duct. *Ureteral colic:* Pain due to obstruction or irritation of the ureter.

COLITIS: A chronic ulcerative inflammation of the colon; *also called* ulcerative colitis.

COLOSTOMY: A surgical procedure in which an artificial opening is made into the colon.

COLOSTRUM: A thin milky secretion from the mammary glands during late months of pregnancy in preparation for lactation.

COMA: A profound state of unconsciousness from which the victim cannot be aroused even by painful stimuli.

COMEDONE: Blackhead.

COMPENSATION: The body's capacity to counteract or counterbalance, either naturally or with medical aid, any defect of structure or function.

CONCEPTION: The penetration of a ripened ovum by a viable sperm; fertilization.

CONCUSSION: A jarring injury to the brain.

CONDYLOMATA ACUMINATA (venereal warts): Moist pedunculated growths or warts which form in the anogenital region.

CONGENITAL HEMOLYTIC JAUNDICE: An hereditary anemia in which the red cells absorb excessive amounts of sodium and water and thus are destroyed more readily than normal.

CONJUNCTIVA: The thin, transparent epithelial membrane covering the white of the eye and lining the eyelids.

CONJUNCTIVITIS: An infection or inflammation of the conjunctiva. *Acute conjunctivitis* (Pink-eye): A highly contagious bacterial infection of the conjunctiva. *Gonorrheal conjunctivitis:* A severe inflammation of the conjunctiva in newborn babies caused by infection by gonococci acquired during childbirth.

CONVULSION: A violent involuntary contraction or series of contractions of the skeletal muscles as a result of an abnormal electrical discharge of neurons in the brain. *Febrile convulsion:* Involuntary muscular contractions due to cerebral irritation caused by abnormally high bodily temperature.

CORNEA: The transparent membrane which covers the iris and pupil of the eye.

CORNEAL BLINDNESS: Blindness occurring because of irreparable damage to the cornea.

CORONARY: Referring to the heart, or more particularly to the coronary arteries which supply the heart muscle. *Coronary artery disease:* Atherosclerosis of the coronary arteries. *Coronary insufficiency:* A condition in which the coronary arteries are partially obstructed, thus diminishing the amount of arterial blood available to the heart muscle. *Coronary thrombosis* (coronary occlusion): A condition in which a clot forms or lodges in a branch of one or more coronary arteries, resulting in obstruction of the artery and infarction or death of heart muscle in the area supplied by the vessel; *see also* Heart attack.

CORPUS LUTEUM: A small cluster of hormone-producing cells which forms in the area of the ovary from which a ripened ovum has been released after the ovum has been fertilized; hormones from the corpus luteum help support the implantation and growth of the fertilized ovum in the interior wall of the uterus.

CORTEX: The outer layer of an organ as distinguished from its central portion or medulla.

CORTICOSTEROIDS: A large family of hormones produced in the cortex of the adrenal gland.

CORTISONE (Corticosterone): One of the major hormones produced in the cortex of the adrenal glands.

CRANIOSTENOSIS: Premature closure of the bones of the skull.

CRETINISM: A congenital affliction due to lack of active thyroid hormone and marked by arrested physical and mental development.

CROSSMATCHING: A laboratory procedure used to determine the compatibility of donor blood with the blood of the recipient prior to transfusion.

CROUP: An upper respiratory infection characterized by difficult breathing and a harsh, hoarse barking cough due to inflammation of the vocal cords.

CRYPTORCHIDISM (cryptorchism): Failure of one or both testes to descend into the scrotum.

CURETTAGE: The use of a scraping instrument to remove growths or other matter from the walls of cavities.

CUSHING'S SYNDROME: A group of symptoms generally related to overactivity of the adrenocortical hormones due to a tumor in the pituitary gland.

CYST: An encapsulated nodule, usually filled with fluid. *Baker's cyst:* A cyst of the tendon sheath at the back of the knee filled with synovial fluid. *Corpus luteum cyst:* A cyst of the ovary formed by an accumulation of serum following release of a ripened ovum. *Inflammatory cyst:* A cystic mass formed as a result of a localized inflammation. *Sebaceous cyst:* A collection of oily material from sebaceous glands located in the deeper layers of the skin or subcutaneous tissue.

CYANOSIS: Blueness of the skin as a result of poor oxygenation of the blood.

CYSTIC DUCT: The tube from the gall bladder which joins the hepatic duct from the liver to form the common bile duct.

CYSTIC FIBROSIS (mucoviscidosis): A familial disease characterized by inadequate production of enzymes in the pancreas and disturbances in glandular secretions elsewhere in the body.

CYSTITIS: Infection or inflammation of the urinary bladder.

CYSTOCELE: A herniation or outpouching of the urinary bladder into the vagina.

CYSTOSCOPY: Direct visual examination of the urinary tract by means of a narrow lighted tube inserted into the urethra.

DECORTICATION: A surgical procedure in which lung tissue which is adherent to the wall of the chest is peeled away.

DEFIBRILLATOR: An electrical instrument used to stop fibrillation of the heart muscle and restore normal cardiac rhythm.

DEHYDRATION: Abnormal loss of water from body tissues.

DELIRIUM TREMENS ("D.T.s"): An acute toxic psychosis due to prolonged excessive consumption of alcohol characterized by massive confusion, tremors and hallucinations.

DENGUE FEVER: A viral infection transmitted by the mosquito aedes aegypti.

DENTINE: The main substance of the teeth, which is harder and denser than bone and which underlies the external enamel.

DERMABRASION: A surgical procedure in which the outer layers of skin are abraded to remove superficial scars and other imperfections.

DERMATITIS: A general term to describe all varieties of skin inflammation. *Contact dermatitis:* An inflammatory skin disorder caused by contact of the skin with an allergenic substance. *Seborrheic dermatitis:* Dandruff.

DERMATOMYOSITIS: A generalized inflammatory disease affecting connective tissue in the skin, subcutaneous tissue and underlying muscle.

DERMIS: The layer of skin immediately beneath the epidermis.

DESENSITIZATION: Reducing an individual's sensitivity to various allergens by means of repeated exposure to minute quantities of the allergen.

DESQUAMATION: A flaking or peeling of the outer layers of skin.

DIABETES INSIPIDUS: A pituitary gland disorder characterized by progressively increased excretion of urine combined with excessive thirst.

DIABETES MELLITUS: A complex endocrine disease marked by decreased production of insulin by the pancreas and consequent impairment of carbohydrate metabolism throughout the body.

DIABETIC COMA: A state of profound unconsciousness which results from severe, uncorrected diabetic acidosis. *See* Acidosis, diabetic.

DIALYSIS: The separation of various dissolved or colloidal substances from solution by means of diffusion through a semipermeable membrane; the process by which waste materials are filtered out of the blood into the urine in the kidney.

DIAPHRAGM: The smoothly curving sheet of muscle which separates the thoracic cavity from the abdominal cavity; also a contraceptive device placed in the vagina to cover the mouth of the uterine cervix.

DIGITALIS: A medicine derived from the leaf of the foxglove and used in the treatment of heart ailments.

DIGITOXIN: A sugar-like substance or glycoside which is the medicinally active component of digitalis.

DILATATION AND CURETTEMENT (D & C): A surgical procedure in which the uterine cervix is dilated and the uterine cavity gently scraped with a curette for the purposes of diagnosis or treatment.

DIPHTHERIA: A virulent bacterial throat infection caused by Corynebacterium diphtheriae.

DIPLOCOCCI: Bacteria of the family of cocci which normally grow in pairs and have a characteristic oval shape.

DIPLOPIA: Double vision.

DISLOCATION: An injury in which the bone has been twisted or wrenched out of its normal joint position; also called subluxation. *Congenital hip dislocation:* A condition in which one or both hips are dislocated during gestation or at the time of delivery.

DIURESIS: A marked increase in urination accompanied by reduction in the amount of edema fluid present in the tissues.

DIURETIC: A drug which increases urine production.

DIVERTICULITIS: Inflammation of a diverticulum in the colon.

DIVERTICULUM: A blind pouch or pocket leading from a cavity or tube within the body. *Meckel's diverticulum:* A sac or tubelike outpouching of the ileum derived from an unobliterated embryonic duct.

DORSAL HORN CELLS: Nerve cells located in the posterior portion of the spinal cord which regulate the activity of skeletal muscles.

DOWN'S SYNDROME. *See* Mongolism.

DRACUNCULIASIS: A roundworm infestation transmitted to man by ingestion of infected shellfish.

DRAMAMINE: A non-prescription remedy for motion sickness or mild nausea.

DUCTUS ARTERIOSUS: A channel in the fetus connecting the pulmonary artery directly with the aorta, thus permitting blood to bypass the pulmonary circulation before the lungs are inflated following birth. *Patent ductus arteriosus:* A congenital defect in which the ductus arteriosus, which normally closes and is obliterated soon after the lungs are inflated following birth, remains open, causing progressive strain upon the heart and usually requiring surgical correction.

DYSENTERY: Any of a variety of disorders marked by inflammation of the intestine, especially the colon, and attended by abdominal pain and frequent stools containing blood and mucus. *Amebic dysentery: See* Amebiasis. *Bacillary dysentery* (Shigellosis): An infectious disease caused by bacteria of the Shigella family. *Traveler's dysentery:* Diarrhea and abdominal cramping commonly afflicting people traveling in unfamiliar surroundings.

DYSMENORRHEA (menorrhalgia): Difficult or painful menstruation.

DYSPARUNIA: Difficult or painful sexual intercourse.

DYSPEPSIA: Acid indigestion.

DYSPNEA: Shortness of breath; difficult or labored breathing. *Paroxysmal nocturnal dyspnea:* An acute shortness of breath occurring suddenly during the night, accompanied by a sense of suffocation and oppression.

DYSTOCIA: Difficult labor.

DYSTROPHY: Defective or faulty function.

DYSURIA: Painful urination.

EAR: The organ of hearing, made up of three parts: the *external ear,* including the auricle and the auditory canal, that lies outside the skull; the *middle ear,* immediately behind the tympanic membrane (or eardrum), which contains the auditory ossicles; and the *inner ear,* the fluid-filled innermost chamber of the ear.

ECCHYMOSIS: "Black and blue" discoloration of the skin caused by extravasation of blood; a bruise.

ECLAMPSIA: A toxic disturbance of late pregnancy marked by intermittent convulsions followed by an ever-deepening coma.

ECTODERM: The outermost of the three primitive cell layers of the embryo.

ECZEMA (eczematous dermatitis): An inflammatory skin disease caused by an allergy.

EDEMA: Abnormal quantities of fluid in the intercellular tissue spaces of the body.

EISENMENGER'S COMPLEX: A group of congenital heart defects including stenosis or narrowing of the pulmonary artery, hypertrophy of the right ventricle and overriding of the aorta across the interventricular septum.

EJACULATORY DUCT: The tube which passes from the vas deferens and seminal vesicles to convey semen into the urethra.

ELECTROSHOCK THERAPY: A form of treatment of mental illnesses in which the patient is rendered unconscious and convulsions are induced by carefully controlled electric shocks to the brain.

ELECTROCARDIOGRAM (EKG or ECG): An amplified graphic tracing of the electric current produced by contractions of the heart muscle, used in the diagnosis of heart disease.

ELECTROENCEPHALOGRAM: An amplified graphic recording of electrical activity of the brain.

ELECTROLYTES: Dissolved salts, buffering acids or alkalis normally found in the blood plasma and tissue fluids.

EMBOLISM: The sudden obstruction of an artery or vein by a clot carried by the circulating blood.

EMBOLUS: A blood clot carried through the blood vessels by the current of flowing blood. *Pulmonary embolus:* A blood clot which passes into the lung by way of the pulmonary artery.

EMBRYO: The developing human being from the time of conception to the end of the eighth week of development; thereafter the developing organism is called a *fetus.*

EMESIS: Vomiting; also, the material vomited.

EMETIC: A medication used to induce vomiting; as opposed to antiemetic—a medication used to combat or prevent vomiting.

EMPHYSEMA (pulmonary emphysema): Distention, scarring and fibrosis of lung tissue, usually as a result of chronic inflammatory disease.

EMPYEMA: Pus in the chest cavity.

ENCEPHALITIS (sleeping sickness): Inflammation of the brain.

ENDARTERITIS: Inflammation of the inner lining of the arteries or arterioles.

ENDOCARDITIS: Inflammation of the inner lining of the heart or endocardium. *Acute bacterial endocarditis* (ABE): An acute bacterial infection of the endocardium. *Subacute bacterial endocarditis* (SBE): A more slowly developing and chronic form of bacterial endocarditis.

ENDOCARDIUM: The smooth, satiny inner lining of the heart chambers.

ENDOCRINE: Referring to those glands whose secretions are not carried away by ducts but are absorbed directly into the bloodstream.

ENDODERM: The innermost of the three primitive cell layers of the embryo.

ENDOMETRIOSIS: The implantation and growth of endometrial tissue from the uterus in abnormal locations, notably on the walls of the abdominal cavity.

ENDOMETRITIS: Inflammation of the endometrium.

ENDOMETRIUM: The mucous membrane and glandular tissue that lines the interior cavity of the uterus.

ENTERITIS: Any of a variety of inflammatory disorders of the small intestine.

ENTEROTOXIN: A poisonous substance exuded into the intestine by certain kinds of staphylococcus bacteria growing in contaminated food and stimulating intestinal cramps, distention and diarrhea.

ENURESIS: Bed-wetting.

EPIDERMIS: The outermost and non-vascular layer of the skin.

EPIDIDYMIS: A small oblong mass attached to the upper part of each testicle composed of a long, convoluted tubule.

EPIDIDYMITIS: Inflammation of the epididymis.

EPILEPSY: A chronic or recurring nervous system disorder characterized by convulsive muscular seizures and often loss of consciousness. *Idiopathic epilepsy:* Recurring convulsions wsich cannot be traced to a specific cause.

EPINEPHRIN: A hormone secreted by the medulla of the adrenal gland.

EPISIOTOMY: A surgical incision of the vulva or perineum to facilitate childbirth.

EPISPADIAS: A congenital defect of the male or female urethra.

EPITHELIUM: A membrane-like tissue covering a surface or lining a cavity of the body, consisting of one or more layers of cells with very little intercellular substance.

ERYSIPELAS: A contagious, infectious disease of skin and subcutaneous tissue.

ERYTHEMA NODOSUM ("nodular erythema"): An inflammatory skin disorder characterized by the formation of raised, tender nodules in the skin and connective tissue, usually on the legs.

ERYTHROBLASTOSIS FETALIS (Rh disease): A potentially fatal disease which occurs late in fetal life or soon after birth, characterized by excessive red blood cell destruction and the appearance of immature red cells in the bloodstream, resulting from Rh factor incompatibility with the mother.

ERYTHROBLASTS: Immature nucleated red blood cells, usually confined to the bone marrow.

ERYTHROCYTES: Red blood cells.

ESOPHAGUS: The tubular canal extending from the pharynx to the stomach.

EUSTACHIAN TUBE: A narrow canal extending from the middle ear to the back of the throat which maintains proper air pressure within the ear.

EXANTHEM: Any of a variety of infectious illnesses, most characteristic of childhood, associated with skin rashes or eruptions; also the eruption which characterizes such a disease.

EXOTOXIN: A toxin excreted by an organism into the surrounding medium.

EXPECTORANT: A medicine which loosens and liquefies bronchial secretions so they can be expelled.

FALLOPIAN TUBE (oviduct): The tube down which the ripened ovum is transported from the ovary to the uterus.

FASCICLES: Small bundles or clusters of nerve or muscle fibers.

FEBRILE: Feverish or pertaining to fever.

FECES: The undigested detritus, mixed with bile salts and colon bacilli, which collects in the lower end of the colon for evacuation.

FELON: An infection of the soft tissue in the pad of a finger or thumb.

FETUS: The child in the womb after the end of the eighth week of gestation. *See also* Embryo.

FIBRILLATION: A fast, arrhythmic heartbeat.

FIBRIN: A whitish, insoluble protein substance formed from fibrinogen in the clotting of blood.

FIBRINOGEN: A complex blood protein which is converted into fibrin by the action of thrombin in the process of blood clotting.

FIBROADENOMA: A benign tumor that develops from the fibrous tissue of the breast or from the milk ducts.

FIBROBLAST: A connective tissue cell.

FIBROSARCOMA: A malignant tumor arising from fibrous connective tissue such as tendon or ligament.

FILARIASIS: A roundworm infestation of tropical and subtropical countries.

FISSURE: A cleft or crack. *Anal fissure:* A painful linear ulcer at the margin of the anus.

FISTULA: A deep, sinuous ulcerated channel. *Fistula-in-ano:* An abnormal channel near the anus, which may or may not communicate with the rectum. *Arteriovenous fistula:* An abnormal channel between an artery and a vein. *Bronchopleural fistula:* A channel between the end of a bronchiole and the pleural lining of the chest cavity, caused by the enlargement of a lung abscess. *Tracheo-esophageal fistula:* An abnormal opening between the trachea and the esophagus.

FLAT FOOT (pes planus): A structural deformity in which the heel is rotated outward and the natural bony arch of the foot is flattened due to poor function of supporting ligaments.

FLATUS: Intestinal gases passed per rectum.

FLUOROSCOPY: Examination of the internal organs by means of a fluorescent screen and a roentgen tube.

FOLIC ACID: A vital nutrient, inadequate absorption of which can lead to folic acid deficiency anemia.

FOLLICLE: A very small excretory or secretory duct, sac or gland. *Graafian follicle:* A vesicle in an ovary which contains a developing or potential ovum. *Hair follicle:* The small sac from which a hair grows.

FOLLICULITIS: Small, multiple boils that form due to bacterial growth in hair follicles.

FONTANELLE: The unossified "soft spot" in the cranium of a young infant.

FRACTURE: A crack or break, as of a bone. *Comminuted fracture:* A fracture in which bone fragments are crushed at the site of the break. *Depressed fracture:* A fracture of the skull in which the bony plate is dented inward to exert pressure on part of the brain. *Greenstick fracture:* A crack fracture in which the fractured bone ends are not completely separated. *Open (Compound) fracture:* A fracture in which bone fragments have emerged through the skin and become contaminated with bacteria. *Pathological fracture:* A fracture that occurs through a weakened area of bone in the absence of any fall or blow. *Simple fracture:* A fracture that has not broken skin and in which bone fragments are not shattered.

FRÖHLICH'S SYNDROME: Underdevelopment of the genitals, adiposity of a feminine type, changes in secondary sex characteristics, and metabolic disturbances, all due to underproduction of hormones in the anterior pituitary.

FROZEN SECTION: A technique whereby tissue removed at surgery is quickly frozen, sectioned, and stained for immediate microscopic examination.

FUNDUS: The base or portion of a hollow organ, such as the uterus, which is remotest from its mouth.

FUO: Fever of unknown origin.

GALL BLADDER: A small sacular organ located beneath the liver which serves as a reservoir for bile.

GALLSTONES: Small concretions formed of various insoluble chemicals which may form within the gall bladder.

GAMMA GLOBULINS: Proteins normally occurring in the blood serum which enter into the formation of the body's protective antibodies.

GANGLION: A cluster of nerve tissue that serves as a center of nerve activity; also a cyst which develops in a tendon sheath.

GANGRENE: Massive death or necrosis of tissue due to loss of circulation or bacterial destruction. *Gas gangrene:* Massive death of tissue resulting from dirty, lacerated wounds and infection by gas-producing bacteria.

GASTRECTOMY: Surgical removal of part or all of the stomach. *Sub-total gastrectomy:* Surgical removal of the lower two-thirds of the stomach, usually in treatment of complicated peptic ulcer disease.

GASTRITIS: Inflammation of the stomach lining. *Corrosive gastritis:* A gastritis resulting from ingestion of a poison or corrosive agent.

GASTROENTERITIS: A general term for inflammation of the stomach and intestines.

GASTROJEJUNOSTOMY: An operation in which the stomach is attached to the jejunum, bypassing the duodenum.

GASTROSCOPY: The direct visualization of the interior of the stomach by means of a gastroscope.

GAUCHER'S DISEASE: An hereditary disorder of the lymph nodes and spleen.

GENE: The basic unit controlling the transmission of hereditary characteristics.

GENITALIA: The reproductive organs.

GESTATION: Pregnancy.

GIGANTISM: Excessive growth, usually due to overproduction of growth hormone in individuals who have not yet gained maturity.

GLAND: Any tissue or organ which forms chemical substances within the body and secretes them directly into the bloodstream (endocrine glands) or into ducts which carry them elsewhere (exocrine glands).

GLANDERS: A bacterial disease of horses which is communicable to man.

GLANS PENIS: The head, or terminal end, of the penis.

GLAUCOMA: A disease marked by increased pressure within the eye and progressive blindness when untreated.

GLIAL CELLS: Specialized nerve cells which function to support and nourish adjacent neurons.

GLOBULIN: An important protein in the blood serum.

GLOMERULONEPHRITIS: A dangerous inflammatory disease of the kidney, chiefly affecting the glomeruli. *Acute glomerulonephritis:* The sudden, critical onset of kidney inflammation. *Chronic glomerulonephritis:* An indolent, prolonged form of kidney inflammation.

GLOMERULUS: A tiny convoluted knot of capillary blood vessels contained in the nephron of the kidney.

GLUCAGON: A hormone produced by the alpha cells of the pancreas.

GLUCOSE TOLERANCE TEST: A laboratory test for diabetes mellitus, assessing the capacity of a patient's metabolism to handle or tolerate a large measured dose of ingested glucose.

GLYCOGEN: A complex carbohydrate food material formed and stored in the liver.

GOITER: Enlargement of the thyroid gland. *Exophthalmic goiter* (Graves' disease): Thyroid enlargement associated with abnormal protrusion of the eyeballs, usually due to marked overproduction of thyroid hormone. *Nodular goiter:* Thyroid enlargement with the formation of circumscribed nodules within the gland.

GONAD: A gland which produces a mature germ cell; the ovary or testis.

GONORRHEA: A highly contagious venereal infection caused by Neisseria gonorrheae and transmitted by sexual contact.

GOUT (Gouty arthritis): A metabolic disorder caused by the body's inability to handle purines, with a consequent excess of uric acid in the blood and the formation of chalky deposits in the cartilage of the joints.

GRANULOCYTES: White blood cells formed in the bone marrow.

GRAND MAL SEIZURE: A convulsive disorder marked by sudden loss of consciousness followed by strenuous tonic and clonic contractions of the skeletal muscles; *see also* Epilepsy.

GRANULOMA INGUINALE: A chronic, progressive venereal infection affecting the genitals, anus and surrounding areas.

GRAVES' DISEASE: *See* Exophthalmic goiter.

GUMMA: A soft, destructive inflammatory tumor occurring in tertiary syphilis.

GYNECOMASTIA: Breast enlargement in males.

HALLUCINOGENIC DRUG: A drug or chemical which causes a temporary alteration in mental function or perception.

HAMMER TOE (claw toe): A deformity in which the toe is pulled upward where it joins the foot and bent into severe flexion at the tip.

HAND-SCHÜLLER-CHRISTIAN DISEASE: A rare metabolic disease in children marked by deposits of cholesterol and other fatty materials in bones and lymphoid tissues.

HARELIP: A congenital cleft in the upper lip, usually associated with cleft palate.

HASHIMOTO'S STRUMA: An inflammatory condition of the thyroid gland.

HAY FEVER: An allergic reaction involving mucous membranes of the eyes, nose and upper respiratory tract, usually caused by pollen.

HEART ATTACK: Any sudden painful or arrhythmic affliction of the heart; *see also* Coronary thrombosis.

HEART BLOCK: A condition due to injury, inflammation or scarring that blocks the proper action of the neuromuscular conducting system of the heart.

HEART FAILURE: (congestive heart failure): Any condition in which the heart fails to pump sufficient blood through the general and pulmonary circulatory systems to maintain adequate oxygenation of tissues. *Passive congestion:* A manifestation of congestive heart failure in which the liver and the peripheral soft tissues become congested with edema fluid as a result of poor return of venous blood to the heart.

HEMANGIOMA: A benign tumor of the capillary blood vessels of the skin.

HEMATOMA: A blood clot in the soft tissues of the body due to internal hemorrhage.

HEMATURIA: The presence of red blood cells in the urine.

HEMIANOPIA (half vision): Blindness in one-half the field of vision in one or both eyes.

HEMIPLEGIA: Paralysis of one side of the body.

HEMOGLOBIN: The oxygen-carrying red pigment contained in red blood cells.

HEMOLYSIS: The destruction of red blood cells.

HEMOPHILIA: A severe hereditary disease characterized by delayed clotting of the blood.

HEMOPTYSIS: The spitting up of blood or of blood-stained sputum.

HEMORRHAGE: Bleeding. *Cerebral hemorrhage:* The bursting of a blood vessel in the brain. *Periosteal hemorrhage:* A hemorrhage of the thin, tough, fibrous coating of tissue that overlies the bone. *Post-partum hemorrhage:* Hemorrhage which occurs soon after labor or childbirth. *Subarachnoid hemorrhage:* Hemorrhage due to rupture of one or more blood vessels on the surface of the brain that lies beneath the arachnoid membrane.

HEMORRHOIDS (piles): Varicosed rectal veins. *Thrombosed hemorrhoids:* Varicosed rectal veins in which blood clots have formed, causing pain, inflammation and swelling.

HEPATIC DUCTS: The two ducts draining bile from the liver which join with the cystic duct from the gall bladder to form the common bile duct.

HEPATITIS: Inflammation of the liver. *Infectious hepatitis* (acute infectious jaundice): An acute viral infection of the liver causing jaundice. *Serum hepatitis:* A severe viral infection of the liver transmitted by contaminated instruments or by transfusion of blood infected by the virus.

HERMAPHRODISM: A condition in which both male and female reproductive organs are present in the same individual.

HERNIA: The protrusion of a loop or sac of an organ or tissue through an abnormal opening in the cavity which contains it. *Femoral hernia:* A protrusion of intestine into the femoral canal. *Hiatus hernia* (esophageal hernia, Diaphragmatic hernia): The protrusion of any structure through the esophageal hiatus of the diaphragm. *Incarcerated hernia:* A protruding organ or tissue which has become trapped and cannot return to its normal position. *Inguinal hernia:* A protrusion of intestine into the inguinal canal. *Umbilical hernia:* A protrusion of the intestine at the navel.

HERNIA SAC: A pocket or sac of connective tissue surrounding a hernial defect which contains the protruding organ or tissue.

HERNIORRHAPHY: Surgical repair of a hernia, particularly an inguinal hernia.

HERPES SIMPLEX (cold sore, fever blister): An acute skin inflammation, usually appearing around the mouth, caused by a virus.

HERPES ZOSTER (shingles): An acute viral inflammation of the sensory peripheral nerve cells and ganglia, characterized by painful lesions of the nerve endings beneath the skin.

HIRSCHSPRUNG'S DISEASE (megacolon): A condition in which a segment of bowel congenitally lacks nerve ganglia, thus acting as a barrier to peristalsis, obstructing the normal passage of stool and causing massive enlargement of the colon above the obstruction.

HISTAMINE: An irritating chemical substance released from body cells as part of an allergic reaction.

HISTAMINE HEADACHE: A headache which ordinarily involves just one side of the head, neck, temple and face, thought to be caused by the release of histamine as a result of allergy.

HISTOPLASMOSIS: A severe systemic fungus infection.

HODGKIN'S DISEASE: A chronic, cancer-like disease of the lymph nodes and lymphoid tissue.

HOOKWORM: A parasitic roundworm which attacks man and animals.

HORMONE: A chemical substance secreted into the body fluids by the endocrine glands or other secreting cells which has specific effects on the activities of other organs. *Adrenocorticotrophic hormone* (ACTH): A hormone secreted by the pituitary which stimulates production of hormones by the adrenal cortex. *Androgenic hormones* (androgens): Male sex hormones manufactured by the testes and, to a lesser degree, by the adrenal cortex of both male and female. *Antidiuretic hormone:* The hormone vasopressin, secreted by the posterior pituitary. *Chorionic gonadotropic hormone:* A special hormone produced in the placenta throughout pregnancy. *Estrogenic hormones* (estrogens): Female sex hormones manufactured by the ovaries and, to a lesser extent, by the adrenal cortex, including estriol, estradiol and estrone. *Follicle-stimulating hormone* (FSH): A hormone secreted by the anterior pituitary which stimulates growth and maturation of ova in the ovaries or of sperm in the testes. *Gonadotrophic hormones* (Gonado trophins): A family of hormones produced by the anterior lobe of the pituitary which stimulate certain activities of the gonads. *Growth hormone:* A hormone secreted by the anterior pituitary which controls the rate of skeletal growth and gain of body weight. *Lactogenic hormone:* A gonadotrophin secreted by the pituitary which prepares the female breast for production of milk following delivery. *Thyrotrophic hormone* (TSH): An anterior pituitary hormone which stimulates the manufacture of thyroxin by the thyroid gland.

HYALINE MEMBRANE DISEASE: A disease of newborn infants believed to be the result of inhalation of amniotic fluid by the baby prior to birth which causes the formation of a tenacious "membrane" in the bronchioles preventing normal respiration.

HYDROCELE: A circumscribed collection of fluid within the scrotum.

HYDROCEPHALUS: A condition in which there are abnormal amounts of cerebrospinal fluid in or around the brain.

HYDRONEPHROSIS: A collection of urine in the pelvis of the kidney, usually due to obstruction of the ureter, which causes distention and atrophy of the kidney.

HYDROCORTISONE: One of the hormones produced in the cortex of the adrenal glands.

HYDROPHOBIA: *See* Rabies.

HYDROTHORAX: A collection of edema fluid filling the lower part of the chest cavity outside the lung.

HYMEN (maidenhead): A membranous fold of tissue which partially or wholly covers and occludes the vaginal outlet.

HYPERGLYCEMIA: Abnormally elevated blood sugar.

HYPEROPIA: Far-sightedness.

HYPERPARATHYROIDISM: A disorder caused by overproduction of parathyroid hormone.

HYPERPLASIA: Benign overgrowth of tissue. *Endometrial hyperplasia:* An abnormal but benign overgrowth of the endometrial tissue lining the interior of the uterus, sometimes resulting in abnormal uterine bleeding.

HYPERTENSION: Abnormally high blood pressure.

HYPERTHYROIDISM: A condition brought about by overproduction of thyroxin in the thyroid gland.

HYPERTRICHOSIS: Superfluous hair.

HYPERTROPHY: Abnormal enlargement of an organ or tissue.

HYPOFIBRINOGENEMIA: Deficient levels of fibrinogen in the blood.

HYPOGLYCEMIA: Abnormally low blood sugar.

HYPOGLYCEMIC SHOCK (insulin shock): A shock-like state that arises as a result of an excess of insulin or a deficiency of blood sugar.

HYPOPARATHYROIDISM (parathyroid tetany): A disorder caused by underproduction of parathyroid hormone.

HYPOSPADIAS: A congenital defect in which the urethra is foreshortened and opens on the underside of the penis in the male or into the vagina of the female.

HYPOTENSION: Low blood pressure. *Orthostatic hypotension:* Momentary dizziness caused by a temporary fall in blood pressure due to a change of body position.

HYPOTHYROIDISM: A disorder resulting from deficiency of thyroid activity.

HYSTERECTOMY: Surgical removal of the uterus.

IATROGENIC: Any condition or disorder which arises as a side effect or result of medical intervention.

ILEOSTOMY: A surgical procedure to create an artificial opening into the ileum.

IMMERSION FOOT (trench foot): A condition brought on by prolonged contact with moisture, marked by constriction of blood vessels in the skin and underlying tissue, followed by thrombosis of the veins and an anesthetic gangrene.

IMMUNE REACTION: A post-vaccination reaction which indicates a high degree of immunity.

IMMUNIZATION: Rendering an individual resistant or relatively immune to an infectious disease by stimulating the production of protective antibodies within the body against the causative organism.

IMPACTION: A condition in which a tooth is so embedded in the jaw or beneath already erupted teeth that its eruption is prevented.

IMPETIGO: A contagious, inflammatory skin infection of bacterial origin characterized by isolated pustules.

INCONTINENCE: Inability to control the discharge of urine.

INCUBATION PERIOD: The interval between the time a person is exposed to an infectious illness and the time the first symptoms appear.

INFARCT: An area of tissue destruction due to obstructed circulation.

INFECTION: Any tissue inflammation resulting from the invasion and growth of micro-organisms. *Localized infection:* An infectious inflammation limited to a single or circumscribed area. *Occult infection:* A condition in which either the source or the site of an infection is obscure. *Systemic infection:* An infection involving widespread parts of the body. *Upper respiratory infection* (URI): Any infection which primarily attacks the mucous membrane linings of the nose, throat, larynx or bronchi.

INFLAMMATION: A pathological condition of tissue characterized by pain, swelling, heat and redness.

INFLUENZA (flu): An acute, infectious respiratory disease caused by a virus and marked by widespread systemic symptoms.

INGUINAL CANAL: A tube or canal in the groin through which the infantile testis descends from the abdomen to the scrotum; usually closed or obliterated by the time of birth.

INSULIN: A protein hormone produced by the pancreas which regulates carbohydrate (sugar) metabolism.

INSULIN SHOCK: *See* Hypoglycemic shock.

INSULIN SHOCK THERAPY: A form of treatment for mental illnesses in which sufficient insulin is administered to induce insulin shock and hypoglycemic convulsions in the patient under controlled conditions.

INTERTRIGO: A reddening and maceration of the skin caused by the rubbing together of adjacent moist skin surfaces.

INTERVERTEBRAL DISK: Any of the thick, padded disks of cartilage that lie between the vertebrae, or between the lowest lumbar vertebra and the sacrum.

INTESTINE: The long, tubelike section of the digestive tract extending from the lower end of the stomach to the anus. The intestine is generally divided into the small intestine, composed of the duodenum (the first portion of the small intestine), the jejunum (the middle portion) and the ileum (the lower one-third of the small intestine), and the large intestine made up of the cecum (the dilated intestinal pouch which forms the beginning of the large intestine, site of the vermiform appendix), the colon (the large intestine from the cecum to the rectum) and the rectum or rectal canal, the lower few inches of the colon terminating in the anal orifice.

INTRAUTERINE DEVICE (IUD): A small shaped bit of plastic inserted into the cervical entrance to the uterus to prevent contraception.

INTUSSUSCEPTION: A condition in which a portion of the intestine telescopes on itself and can, if not released, cause strangulation of that segment of the bowel.

IN UTERO: Within the uterus.

INVOLUTE: Return to normal size after enlargement.

IPECAC (syrup of ipecac): Medication which stimulates vomiting.

IRIS: The circular pigmented membrane behind the cornea in the eye, perforated by the pupil.

ISCHEMIA: Local deficiency of blood to a tissue area, chiefly due to contraction, compression or destruction of the arterial blood supply. *Mycocardial ischemia:* Starvation of the heart for oxygen due to acute or chronic deficiency of circulation to the heart muscle.

ISLETS OF LANGERHANS: The nests of cells in the pancreas which secrete insulin.

JACKSONIAN SEIZURE: A convulsive disorder triggered by irritation of a single focal point or area in the brain and often first involving muscular contractions in a single portion of the body before progressing to generalized convulsion.

JAUNDICE: A yellowish discoloration of the tissues of the body, whites of the eyes, skin and mucous membranes, usually resulting from the presence of bile or free hemoglobin pigments in the blood serum.

JEJUNOSTOMY: A surgical procedure to create an opening into the jejunum.

KELOID: An abnormally large, thickened scar.

KERATITIS: Inflammation of the cornea.

KERATOSIS: A horny growth of the skin such as a wart or callus. *Seborrheic keratoses:* Benign, brownish wart-like growths formed from epithelial cells; primarily signs of aging skin. *Senile keratoses:* Flat, warty skin lesions with a dry scaly surface; a precancerous skin disorder.

KOPLIK'S SPOTS: Small, white cottony-looking spots inside the cheeks, a diagnostic sign of measles (rubeola).

KWASHIORKOR: Cirrhosis of the liver, prevalent in many parts of the world due to protein-deficient starvation level diets, especially common among children.

KIDNEYS: Small, bean-shaped paired organs located against the posterior abdominal wall at the level of the small of the back but outside the peritoneal cavity; the major filtering organs of the urinary system, vital for the excretion of dissolved waste materials from the bloodstream. *Artificial kidney:* A mechanical filtering device which can be connected to a patient's bloodstream and is used as a temporary substitute for kidney function when the natural organs are diseased or impaired. *Kidney failure* (renal failure): Any condition in which the natural kidneys' function is impaired sufficiently that the kidneys cannot adequately perform their excretory function. *Kidney stones* (calculi): Stonelike concretions of insoluble chemicals which can form in the kidneys and occasionally are passed from the kidney pelvis into the ureters or urinary bladder. *Kidney pelvis:* The cavity of the kidney into which urine drains and which connects with the ureter.

LABIA: Lips.

LABIA MAJORA: The hairy folds of skin on either side of the vulvar crease.

LABIA MINORA: The folds of mucous membrane on either side of the vulvar crease within the labia majora.

LABOR: The period of uterine contractions at the end of gestation during which the baby is expelled from the uterus and transported down the birth canal. The final stage of labor involves delivery of the child followed by expulsion of the afterbirth (placenta and fetal membranes).

LACERATION: A wound made by tearing or cutting.

LACRIMAL DUCT: The tube which drains tears from the eye into the nasal passages.

LACRIMAL GLANDS (tear glands): Glands in the soft tissue surrounding the eye which produce tears.

LACTATION: The secretion of milk during the post partum period, or the interval during which it takes place.

LAPAROSCOPY: The exploratory examination of the interior of the abdominal cavity made possible by insertion of a thin, lighted viewingscope, the laparoscope, through a small abdominal incision.

LAPAROTOMY: A surgical incision, usually of the abdomen, done for purposes of exploration and diagnosis.

LARYNGITIS: Inflammation of the larynx.

LARYNGOSCOPY: Direct inspection of the inside of the larynx and the vocal cords by means of a lighted instrument, the laryngoscope.

LARYNGOTRACHEOBRONCHITIS: An acute bacterial infection of the larynx, trachea and bronchi.

LARYNX: The voice box, an organ composed of cartilage and muscle located in the throat and containing the vocal cords.

LEGG-CALVÉ-PERTHES DISEASE: A degenerative disease of the ball of the hip bone or femur.

LEISHMANIASIS: A protozoan infection transmitted by the bite of sand flies.

LENS: The transparent crystalline structure of the eye which focuses light on the retina.

LEPROSY (Hansen's disease): A chronic, destructive bacterial infection primarily affecting the skin, mucous membranes, subcutaneous tissues and peripheral nerves.

LESION: Any localized pathological process. *Pre-cancerous lesion:* An abnormal sore, ulcer or other localized pathological process which tends to be transformed at some point into a cancer. *Primary lesion:* The initial growth of a malignant neoplasm. *Secondary (metastatic) lesion:* The multiple malignant tumors that result from spread of cancerous cells from a primary lesion to distant parts of the body by way of the bloodstream or lymphatics.

LEUCOCYTES: White blood cells. *Granulocytic leucocytes* (granulocytes): Leucocytes with multi-lobed nuclei which are formed in the bone marrow. *Mononuclear leucocytes:* Leucocytes with single-lobed nuclei which are formed in the bone marrow. *Lymphocytic leucocytes:* Leucocytes with single-lobed nuclei which are formed in the lymph glands.

LEUKEMIA: A malignant disease of the blood-forming organs in which greatly increased numbers of immature leucocytes are formed and released into the circulating blood. *Lymphocytic leukemia:* A leukemia marked by a preponderant overproduction of lymphocytic leucocytes. *Granulocytic leukemia:* A leukemia marked by excessive formation of granulocytic leucocytes in the bone marrow.

LEUKOPLAKIA: A whitish, plaque-like lesion of mucous membrane which is often pre-cancerous.

LEUKORRHEA: A whitish, viscid vaginal discharge.

LEVIN TUBE: A narrow rubber or plastic tube which is passed down the esophagus into the stomach.

LICHEN PLANUS: An itchy inflammatory eruption of the skin characterized by somewhat violet-colored, irregular lesions with a sheen.

LIGAMENT: Any tough, fibrous band which connects bones or supports organs.

LIGATION: Tying off or blocking by means of a ligature. *Tubal ligation:* The tying off and cutting of the Fallopian tubes; a means of voluntary sterilization in the female.

LIPASE: A pancreatic enzyme which acts upon fats to break them down into fatty acids.

LIPOMA: A benign growth of fatty tissue in the breast or other subcutaneous tissues.

LIVER: The large, dome-shaped glandular organ in the upper right part of the abdominal cavity which produces bile, converts sugars into glycogen, and performs many other vital body functions.

LOBE: A rounded or circumscribed portion of an organ, especially one marked off by a fissure. *Frontal lobes:* The cerebral lobes of the brain located in the forehead which form the nerve centers controlling mentation and judgment. *Parietal lobes:* The cerebral lobes of the brain at the top of the head containing nerve centers controlling voluntary motion of the limbs and moderating certain sensory impulses. *Temporal lobes:* The cerebral lobes located at the sides of the brain containing the nerve centers controlling sensory interpretations. *Occipital lobes:* The cerebral lobes at the posterior base of the brain containing the nerve centers controlling interpretation of visual images.

LOCHIA: The vaginal discharge that takes place during the first week or two after childbirth.

LORDOSIS: An exaggerated curvature of the spine.

LUMBAGO: Muscular aching in the lower or lumbar region of the back.

LUNGS: Large, spongy paired organs which fill the chest cavity on either side of the midline and which inflate and deflate with air during breathing to permit intake of oxygen and exhalation of carbon dioxide; the major organs of respiration.

LUPUS ERYTHEMATOSUS: A degenerative collagen disease marked by the appearance of a characteristic red skin rash on the cheeks and nose and elsewhere on the body.

LYMPH: Extracellular body fluid, mostly water, containing body salts, nutriments and lymphocytes.

LYMPH GLANDS: Patches of tissue that form at the juncture of lymph channels.

LYMPH NODES: Glandlike structures arranged in groups interposed throughout the lymphatic system which filter lymph and manufacture lymphocytes.

LYMPHATICS (lymph channels): The loosely connected vessels or channels conveying lymphatic fluid from one area of the body to another.

LYMPHOCYTES (lymphocytic leucocytes): White blood cells which are formed in the lymph glands and make their way into the bloodstream by way of the lymph channels.

LYMPHOGRANULOMA VENEREUM: A venereal disease caused by a virus and characterized by large swollen lymph glands in the groin or around the rectum.

LYMPHOMA: Any of a variety of tumors, usually malignant, involving lymphoid tissues.

LYMPHOSARCOMA: A malignant tumor arising in the lymph nodes.

MACERATION: Crushing or grinding tissue to a degree that the normal tissue architecture is destroyed.

MALARIA: A severe protozoan infection transmitted to man by the bite of infected Anopheles mosquitoes and characterized by intermittent episodes of fever and chills.

MALOCCLUSION: Abnormal closure or contact of the teeth of the upper and lower jaw.

MAMMOGRAPHY: A special X-ray technique for examination of the breast.

MARROW: The tissue making up the interior of bones. *Red Marrow:* The spongy blood-enriched marrow of developing bone, of the ribs, vertebrae and many of the smaller bones; the site of the manufacture of red blood cells and of the granulocytic white cells. *Yellow marrow:* The fatty bone marrow material found in the interior of the shafts of long bones.

MASSETERS: The muscles which clamp the jaws together and make chewing possible.

MASTECTOMY: Surgical removal of the breast. *Radical mastectomy:* An extensive surgical procedure involving the excision of the entire breast, the muscle layers covering the ribs beneath the breast and all of the lymph nodes in the axilla on the affected side, often performed as treatment of cancer of the breast. *Simple mastectomy:* Surgical excision of the glandular tissue of the breast alone, sometimes performed as treatment of cancer or other breast diseases.

MASTITIS: Inflammation of the breast. *Septic mastitis:* Bacterial invasion and infection of the breast.

MASTOIDECTOMY: Surgical excision of infected mastoid bone which lies in the skull behind the ear.

McBURNEY'S POINT: An area in the middle of the right lower quadrant of the abdomen which is often the point of special tenderness in acute appendicitis.

MEASLES: (rubeola, "red measles," "hard measles," "ten-day measles"): A contagious febrile virus infection marked by a characteristic red rash.

MEATUS: Any small natural passage or opening, particularly to the urethra.

MECONIUM ILEUS: Obstruction of the bowel of the newborn with thick meconium, the material which collects there prior to birth.

MEDIASTINUM: The area within the thorax that lies between the lungs laterally and extends from the breastbone to the spine in which the heart, the trachea and mainstem bronchi, the pulmonary arteries and veins, the aorta and the vena cava are located.

MEDULLA: The central portion of an organ as distinguished from its outer layer or cortex.

MEDULLA OBLONGATA: That part of the brain stem where the spinal cord fuses with the brain.

MEGACOLON: *See* Hirschsprung's disease.

MEGAKARYOCYTES: The giant cells in the bone marrow which produce the blood platelets.

MEIOSIS: The process by which germ cells divide reducing the number of chromosomes from the normal full complement to half complement.

MELANIN: A brown or brownish-black pigment of the skin and hair.

MELANOMA (malignant melanoma): A highly malignant tumor of the skin, usually developing from a pigmented nevus or mole.

MENARCHE: The onset of menstruation.

MÉNIÈRE'S SYNDROME: A collection of symptoms including ringing in the ears, vertigo and hearing impairment, related to disease or disorder of the inner ear.

MENINGES: The three delicate membrane layers that envelop the brain and spinal cord: the outer layer (dura mater), the middle, vascular layer (the arachnoid membrane), and the inner layer (pia mater).

MENINGISMUS: Acute pain and distress at the back of the skull and along the spinal cord upon flexion of the neck and back, indicative of meningeal irritation due to infection or inflammation.

MENINGITIS: Inflammation of the meninges.

MENINGOCOCCAL MENINGITIS: A bacterial infection of the meninges caused by Micrococcus meningitidis.

MENINGOCELE: Hernial protrusion of the meninges, usually due to a congenital developmental defect.

MENINGOCOCCUS (Micrococcus meningitidis): A virulent microorganism, specifically a gram-negative diplococcus, which causes meningococcal meningitis and/or meningococcemia.

MENOPAUSE: The cessation of menstruation; the so-called "change of life."

MENORRHAGIA: Excessive menstrual flow.

MESENTERY: The thin double layer of peritoneum securing the intestines to the rear wall of the abdomen.

MESODERM: The middle of the three primative cell layers of the embryo.

METABOLISM: The sum of all the physical and chemical processes by which living tissue is produced and maintained.

METASTASIS: The spread of a disease or a disease process, specifically cancer, from its original focus to surrounding tissue and more distant tissues and organs.

MICROCEPHALUS: A rare congenital condition in which many of the higher brain centers in the cerebrum fail to develop.

MID-BRAIN: That part of the brain above and surrounding the brain stem containing nerve centers which monitor emotions, pains and pleasure sensations and the libido.

MIGRAINE HEADACHE: A syndrome characterized by periodic severe headaches, often accompanied by nausea, vomiting and various sensory disturbances.

MILIARIA (heat rash; prickly heat): A mild inflammatory skin rash due to obstruction of sweat glands.

MITOSIS: The process by which cells divide forming daughter cells with the normal full complement of chromosomes.

MONGOLISM (Down's syndrome): A non-hereditary congenital defect marked by retardation of both physical and mental development.

MONILIASIS: A fungus infection caused by Candida albicans; see also Thrush.

MONOCYTES: White blood cells with single-lobed nuclei, formed in the bone marrow.

MONONUCLEOSIS (infectious mononucleosis, glandular fever): An acute infectious disease, believed to be viral in origin, characterized by abnormal numbers of lymphocytes in the blood.

MORBIDITY: The capacity of a disease or condition to cause distressing and/or disabling symptoms.

MOTOR END-PLATE: The flattened terminal end of a motor nerve fiber upon a muscle fiber.

MUCOUS MEMBRANE (mucosa): A membrane composed of epithelial cells, usually lining internal tunnels or canals of the body (i.e., the mouth, the gastrointestinal tract, the vagina, etc.) and normally kept moist by secretions of a slightly sticky substance, mucus, produced by special glands in the epithelium.

MULTIPLE SCLEROSIS (MS): A severe, progressive degenerative disease of the peripheral nervous system.

MUMPS (acute parotitis): A virus infection which causes painful inflammation and swelling of the parotid and other salivary glands. *Mumps orchitis:* Acute inflammation of the testicles or ovaries in the course of an acute infection by the mumps virus. *Mumps pancreatitis:* Inflammation of the pancreas during an acute infection by the mumps virus.

MUSCLE: One of the six basic forms of tissue making up the body, composed of bundles or fascicles of long, narrow cells which have the power to contract or shorten in response to nervous or chemical stimulation. *Skeletal muscle* (voluntary muscle): Striated muscle tissue attached to bone which responds to voluntary nerve impulses, so that its action is under conscious, willful control. *Smooth muscle* (involuntary muscle): Nonstriated muscle which forms the walls of the blood vessels, the stomach, the intestines and many tubes and ducts within the body, which responds to involuntary nerve impulses and thus cannot be consciously or willfully controlled.

MUSCULAR DYSTROPHY: An hereditary disease characterized by progressive shrinking or wasting of skeletal muscle.

MYASTHENIA GRAVIS: A muscle disease marked by progressive exhaustion or paralysis of muscles without sensory disturbance or atrophy.

MYCOSIS: Any infestation or infection caused by a fungus.

MYELOBLASTS: The so-called precursor cells of granulocytes normally found in the bone marrow, but which may appear in large numbers in the circulating blood in the presence of certain forms of leukemia.

MYELOCELE: A protrusion or herniation of the spinal cord.

MYELOMA (multiple myeloma): A cancerous growth which usually originates in multiple areas of bone or bone marrow throughout the body.

MYOGLOBIN: The hemoglobin-like pigment in striated muscle cells.

MYELIN: A waxy coating which normally ensheaths individual nerve fibrils and plays a vital role in the transmission of nerve impulses.

MYELOGRAM: Diagnostic X-ray of the spinal cord.

MYOCARDITIS: Inflammation of the myocardium or heart muscle. *Diphtheria myocarditis:* A toxic myocarditis caused by the toxin produced by the diphtheria organism during a diphtheria infection. *Fiedler's myocarditis:* A severe inflammatory disorder of the heart muscle of unknown origin. *Viral myocarditis:* Inflammation of the myocardium caused by a virus.

MYOCARDIUM: The thick muscular wall of the heart.

MYOMA: A noncancerous fibrous tumor of muscle tissue. *Uterine myoma* (fibroid tumor): A tumor that develops from the muscular elements of the uterine wall.

MYONEURAL JUNCTION: The area of junction or contact between a motor nerve ending and the muscle to which it is distributed.

MYOPIA: Near-sightedness.

MYOSARCOMA: A malignant tumor arising in smooth muscle.

MYOSITIS (fibrositis): Inflammation of the skeletal muscles. *Over-use myositis:* Inflammation of the muscles caused by unusual or prolonged use.

MYRINGOTOMY: A surgical incision to open the tympanic membrane (eardrum).

MYXEDEMA: A condition resulting from extremely low thyroid production.

NASOPHARYNX: The back of the throat above the soft palate.

NECK DISSECTION: A surgical procedure often used for the treatment of cancer of the throat, larynx or thyroid, which involves excision of the primary lesion along with adjacent lymph nodes and muscle and subcutaneous tissue.

NECROSIS: The death of tissue cells.

NEOPLASM: Literally "new growth," a mass or tumor of new tissue which grows independently of its surrounding structures and has no physiological use.

NEPHRITIS: Inflammation of the kidney.

NEPHRON: The basic filtering unit within the kidney.

NEPHROSIS: A noninflammatory degenerative condition of the kidney.

NEPHROTIC SYNDROME: A collection of symptoms including edema, decreased serum albumin and albuminuria resulting from a degenerative disorder of the kidneys.

NEPHROTOXIC: Destructive to kidney tissue.

NERVE: A cell or bundle of cells or fibrils along which electrochemical nerve impulses are conducted. *Acoustic nerve:* The cranial nerve which mediates the sense of hearing. *Afferent nerve:* Any nerve which transmits impulses from the periphery inward, usually sensory data to the brain. *Cranial nerve:* Any of twelve pairs of peripheral nerves that arise from nuclei in the brain stem and in general provide sensory and motor innervation to the structures of the head. *Efferent nerve:* Any nerve which transmits impulses toward the periphery usually motor impulses from the brain or spinal cord. *Facial nerve:* The cranial nerve which, together with the trigeminal nerve, controls most of the muscles of expression in the face. *Glossopharyngeal nerve:* The cranial nerve which, together with the hypoglossal nerve, controls swallowing and the movement of the tongue. *Hypoglossal nerve:* The cranial nerve which, together with the glossopharyngeal nerve, controls swallowing and movement of the tongue. *Motor nerves:* Nerve cells which transmit the impulses from the brain to the skeletal muscles. *Occulomotor nerve:* The cranial nerve which helps control the movement of the eyes in their sockets. *Olfactory nerve:* The cranial nerve which mediates the sense of smell. *Optic nerve:* The cranial nerve which mediates vision. *Sciatic nerve:* The peripheral nerve which provides innervation to the entire leg. *Sensory (receptor) nerves:* Nerve cells which transmit impulses from the skin to the spinal cord and thence to the cerebral cortex. *Trigeminal nerve:* A cranial nerve which, together with the facial nerve, controls most of the muscles of expression in the face. *Ulnar nerve:* The peripheral nerve carrying motor nerve fibers to the ring finger and little finger. *Vagus nerve:* The cranial nerve which extends from the brain stem to the stomach and helps control the secretion of acid gastric juice.

NERVOUS SYSTEM: The complex system composed primarily of nerve cells, one of the basic body tissues, spreading throughout the body for the transmission of electrochemical nerve impulses between the brain and the spinal cord on the one hand and distant parts of the body on the other. The central nervous system includes all the nerve cells in the brain and the spinal cord which receive sensory nerve impulses from the skin and other distant organs and transmit them to the higher brain centers, and transmit motor impulses originating in the brain or spinal cord to

muscle cells in all parts of the body; the peripheral nervous system is composed of the spinal nerves originating in the spinal cord and the cranial nerves originating in the brain stem and traveling to all peripheral parts of the body. The autonomic nervous system is a separate system of nerve cells and ganglia which supplies the glands, the heart and the smooth muscles with involuntary sensory and motor innervation.

NEURALGIA: Paroxysms of pain along the distribution of a single sensory nerve. *Glossopharyngeal neuralgia:* Recurrent attacks of acute pain in the back of the throat, tongue and middle ear due to irritation of the glossopharyngeal nerve.

NEURITIS: Inflammation of a nerve or nerve tissue. *Peripheral neuritis:* Inflammation of the nerve endings or of terminal nerves.

NEUROFIBROMATA: Soft, white "dangling moles" which hang from the skin by short, narrow pedicles.

NEUROGENIC JOINT DISEASE (Charcot's joints): Any disorder of the articulating joints of the musculoskeletal system caused by a dysfunction of the nervous system.

NEUROMA: A new growth or tumor of nerve cells. *Acoustic neuroma:* A benign but space-taking tumor of the acoustic nerve, the cranial nerve which mediates hearing.

NEURONS (neurones): Nerve cells.

NEVUS (mole): a nest of cells, usually pigmented, in or beneath the skin.

NIEMANN-PICK'S DISEASE: A disorder in which certain fatty materials are stored in the lymphoid tissues.

NOCTURIA: Excessive urination at night.

NOREPINEPHRIN: A hormone similar to epinephrin or adrenalin which is produced at the myoneural junctions all over the body and works in concert with epinephrin in the body's "fight-flight" reaction to stress.

NUCLEIC ACID: A complex protein substance found in the nuclei of cells and intimately involved, in the form of ribonucleic acid (RNA) or desoxyribose nucleic acid (DNA), in the genetic determination of cellular characteristics.

NUCLEUS: A spheroid body within a cell, forming the essential and vital part.

NYSTAGMUS: An involuntary rhythmic jerking motion of the eyes when they are turned sharply to the right or left, observed in certain nervous system disorders.

OCCLUSION: Obstruction; also closure or contact of the teeth of the upper and lower jaw. *Coronary occlusion:* Obstruction of a coronary artery by a blood clot or an atheromatous plaque.

ONYCHOMYCOSIS: A fungus disease of the nails of the fingers and toes.

OPTHALMOSCOPE: A small lighted instrument with which a doctor examines the interior of the eye.

OPTIC CHIASMA: The X-shaped crossing of optic nerve bundles that occurs between the eyes and the brain, accounting for the transmission of visual images from each eye to both sides of the visual cortex.

ORCHITIS: Inflammation of a testis.

ORTHODONTIA: The field of dentistry that deals with the prevention and correction of irregularities and malocclusion of the teeth.

ORTHOPNEA: Shortness of breath or difficulty in breathing associated with the physical position of the body.

OSGOOD-SCHLATTER DISEASE: A traumatic and inflammatory disorder of the anterior growth center of the upper end of the tibia, usually seen in adolescent children.

OSSICLES: The three tiny bones (the malleus, the incus and the stapes) within the middle ear.

OSTEITIS FIBROSA CYSTICA: A generalized decalcification of the entire skeleton resulting from overactivity of the parathyroid glands.

OSTEOARTHRITIS (degenerative joint disease): A form of chronic joint inflammation occurring chiefly in elderly people and marked by degeneration of bone and cartilage and thickening of the synovial membrane.

OSTEOBLASTS: The bone-making cells within the cartilage.

OSTEOCHONDROSIS: A disease of one or more of the growth or ossification centers in children.

OSTEOCLASTS: Cells concerned with the absorption and removal of bone.

OSTEOMALACIA: Softening of bone due to lack of calcium and phosphorus.

OSTEOMA: An overgrowth or tumor of bone.

OSTEOGENESIS IMPERFECTA: An hereditary bone disease involving general weakness of bone throughout the body with marked decrease in the deposit of calcium.

OSTEOMYELITIS: Infection of the bone.

OSTEOPOROSIS: A degenerative process of aging in which bones became brittle due to a decrease in calcium.

OTITIS MEDIA: A bacterial or viral infection of the middle ear.

OTOSCLEROSIS: A disorder in which the ossicles of the middle ear become frozen together and lose their function.

OVARY: The female reproductive gland in which the ova are formed.

OXYTOCIN: A hormone secreted by the posterior pituitary gland which has a potent effect on uterine contraction during labor.

PACEMAKER: The sino-auricular node; the neurological focus in the right auricle of the heart which triggers and "paces" the heartbeat. *Electronic pacemaker* (cardiac pacemaker): A mechanical device implanted in the chest wall or the heart to substitute for damaged or destroyed sino-articular node.

PAGET'S DISEASE (Osteitis deformans): A chronic disorder characterized by decalcification of weight-bearing bones, with deformities in the new bone generated in the decalcified areas.

PALATE: The partition of bone, cartilage and soft tissue which separates the oral cavity from the nasal cavity. *Cleft palate:* A congenital defect in which the bone and/or cartilage of the palate is imperfectly closed.

PALSY: Paralysis.

PANCREAS: A glandular organ located behind the stomach which manufactures enzymes to aid in digestion and produces the hormone insulin.

PANCREATIC DUCT: The excretory duct which carries digestive enzymes from the pancreas into the duodenum.

PAPILLA: A small, nipple-shaped elevation.

PAPILLARY MUSCLE: The tiny muscles which act to raise up body hairs in their follicles.

PAPILLOMA: A form of epithelial tumor. *Intraductal papilloma:* A benign tumor of the breast which grows from the milk ducts.

PARALYSIS: Temporary or permanent impairment of muscular function due to a nervous system disorder.

PARALYTIC ILEUS: A condition in which the smooth muscle in the ileum becomes inactive, causing stasis of intestinal motion through the ileum.

PARAPLEGIA: Paralysis of both legs from the hips down.

PARATHORMONE: The hormone secreted by the parathyroid glands which regulates the metabolism of calcium and phosphorus within the body.

PARATHYROID GLANDS: Small endocrine glands located in two groups on the posterior surface of the thyroid gland.

PARATHYROID ADENOMA: A benign tumor of one of the parathyroid glands.

PARATYPHOID (Salmonella infection): A bacterial intestinal infection caused by bacilli of the Salmonella family, similar to but not identical to, nor as serious as, typhoid infection.

PARESIS: A slight or incomplete paralysis. *General paresis:* A chronic syphilitic meningoencephalitis, characterized by progressive dementia and a generalized paralysis which is ultimately fatal.

PARKINSON'S DISEASE (paralysis agitans): A chronic disorder of the motor control and reflex centers of the brain.

PARONYCHIA: A bacterial infection in the region around the fingernails or toenails.

PARTURITION: The act or process of childbirth.

PEDICULOSIS: Infestation with lice.

PELLAGRA: A condition resulting from niacin deficiency in the diet which causes a sore, red, swollen tongue and generalized dermatitis.

PELVIC INFLAMMATORY DISEASE (PID): A widespread bacterial infection of the female reproductive organs, usually as a result of gonorrhea.

PEMPHIGUS: A potentially fatal disease of the skin characterized by the appearance of giant water blisters (bullae).

PENICILLIN: An important antibiotic formed by the common mold Penicillium notatum and capable of destroying many disease-causing bacteria.

PEPSIN: A gastric enzyme in the stomach which aids in the digestion of protein.

PEPTIC ULCER. An ulcer on the mucous membrane of the esophagus, stomach or duodenum, caused by the action of the acid gastric juice.

PERIARTERITIS NODOSA: A rare collagen disease in which elastic connective tissue in the walls of smaller arteries tends to degenerate.

PERICARDITIS: Inflammation of the pericardium. *Chronic constrictive pericarditis:* A condition in which the heart is slowly and progressively compressed by the thickening of the pericardium as a result of inflammation, healing and scarring.

PERICARDIUM: The fibrous sac surrounding and enclosing the heart.

PERIOSTEUM: The thin, tough, fibrous coating of tissue that overlies the bone and is rich in nerve endings.

PERISTALSIS: The gentle contraction of smooth muscle which propels food down the intestinal tract.

PERITONEAL IRRITATION: A condition in which the peritoneum becomes extremely sensitive to touch or pressure as a result of chemical irritation or inflammation.

PERITONEUM: The serous membrane lining the abdominal wall and surrounding and covering the abdominal organs.

PERITONITIS: Inflammation of the peritoneum. *Chemical peritonitis:* Inflammation of the peritoneum due to chemical irritation. *Infected or septic peritonitis:* Inflammation of the peritoneum due to contamination by infectious organisms.

PESSARY: A device placed in the vagina to support the uterus; also a contraceptive diaphragm.

PETECHIAE: Small capillary hemorrhages that are visible under the skin.

PETIT MAL SEIZURE: A convulsive disorder characterized by sudden brief periods of unconsciousness with immediate recovery; a form of epilepsy.

PHAGOCYTOSIS: The engulfing of microorganisms and other cells and substances by phagocytes (white blood cells).

PHARYNGEAL SPEECH: A method of speech substituted for natural speech by those whose voice boxes have been surgically removed.

PHARYNGITIS: Inflammation of the pharynx.

PHARYNX: The structure which extends from the back of the mouth to the larynx; also called the throat.

PHENYLKETONURIA (PKU): A congenital metabolic defect which, if untreated, leads to progressive mental degeneration and early death.

PHENYLPYRUVIC ACID: A chemical breakdown product normally excreted in the urine.

PHEOCHROMOCYTOMA: A hormone-producing tumor of the adrenal gland, often responsible for an exaggerated hypertension.

PHIMOSIS: A condition in which a tight, inelastic foreskin constricts the end of the penis making erection impossible or extremely painful.

PHLEBITIS: Inflammation of the veins.

PHLEBOTOMY: A surgical procedure in which a vein is opened to remove blood; blood-letting.

PHOCOMELIA: A condition in which a fetus has imperfectly or incompletely formed upper and lower extremities.

PHOSPHOLIPIDS: A group of fatty substances, some of which play a critical role in the structure and function of nervous tissue.

PINEAL GLAND: A small glandular body of unknown function located in the center of the brain, occasionally subject to tumor formation or cancerous degeneration.

PINWORM: A small roundworm, Enterobius vermicularis, which is a common and relatively harmless parasite in man.

PITUITARY GLAND: A tiny endocrine gland located in a pocket in the base of the skull, composed of an anterior and a posterior portion.

PITYRIASIS ROSEA: An inflammatory disease, probably viral in origin, characterized by rosy-colored oval patches on the skin, usually on the back, trunk or arms.

PLACENTA: The round, flat organ within the uterus through which the fetus is nourished during gestation. *Abruptio placenta:* The premature separation of a portion of a normally implanted placenta from the wall of the uterus. *Placenta praevia:* A placenta which develops in the lower portion of the uterus so that it partially or completely covers the cervical opening.

PLATELETS: Small colorless corpuscles in the blood which are concerned with coagulation.

PLEOMORPHISM: The assumption of various distinct forms by a single organism or tissue.

PLEURA (pleural membrane): A epithelial membrane lining the lungs and the inside of the chest cavity.

PLEURAL FRICTION RUB: A squeaky sound heard through the stethoscope when pleuritis is present due to rubbing together of two pleural surfaces.

PLEURISY (pleuritis): Inflammation of the pleura or the pain associated with it.

PLEUROPNEUMONIA: An infectious disease of cattle.

PLEXUS: A network. *Carotid plexus:* A gathering of nerve cells on the surface of the carotid artery in the neck. *Solar plexus:* A network of autonomic nerves located high in the abdomen.

PNEUMOCONEOSIS: A chronic fibrous reaction in the lungs to the inhalation of dust.

PNEUMONECTOMY: Surgical removal of all or part of a lung.

PNEUMOENCEPHALOGRAM: An X-ray technique for examination of the brain in which cerebrospinal fluid is drained and replaced by air as a contrast medium.

PNEUMONIA: Any bacterial, viral or chemical inflammation of lung tissue. *Aspiration pneumonia:* A pneumonia caused by the inhalation of regurgitated stomach contents. *Bronchial pneumonia:* Bacterial infection of lung tissue surrounding the smaller bronchi and bronchioles. *Chemical pneumonia:* Pneumonia caused by the inhalation of various irritative or poisonous chemicals. *Hypostatic pneumonia* (stasis pneumonia): Pneumonia which results from prolonged periods of shallow breathing in which the lungs never adequately fill with air. *Lobar pneumonia:* Bacterial infection of one or more lobes of the lung. *Oil pneumonia:* A chemical pneumonia caused by the aspiration of oil or oily products. *Viral pneumonia:* A diffuse viral infection of lung tissue.

PNEUMOTHORAX: A condition in which air enters the chest cavity outside the lung, spontaneously or as a result of an injury or a surgical procedure, resulting in partial or complete collapse of the lung. *Pressure pneumothorax:* A condition in which air enters the chest cavity outside the lung under high pressure, effecting complete collapse of the lung.

POLIOMYELITIS (infantile paralysis): An acute infectious virus disease affecting the gastrointestinal tract and, in some cases, nerve cells in the spinal cord or brain stem, attended by destruction of motor nerve cells and resulting in paralysis and muscular atrophy. *Bulbar poliomyelitis:* An extremely dangerous and often fatal form of poliomyelitis in which the virus attacks nerve cells at the base of the brain.

POLYCYSTIC DISEASE: An uncommon hereditary condition in which much of the tissue of both kidneys is replaced by cysts.

POLYCYTHEMIA: A condition caused by the presence of too many red cells in the bloodstream.

POLYP: An overgrowth of mucous membrane.

PONS: The "bridge" of nerve fibers attaching the brain stem to higher brain centers.

POSTURAL DRAINAGE: A home-care procedure in which the body is inverted so that the thorax is lower than the hips to allow gravity to effect drainage of bronchial secretions.

PPLO (pleuro-pneumonia-like organisms): Infectious microorganisms in a class apart from bacteria, rickettsiae or viruses.

PREECLAMPSIA: A toxic condition of late pregnancy characterized by fluid retention, elevation of blood pressure and kidney malfunction.

PREGNANCY: The condition of having a developing embryo or fetus in the body. *Ectopic pregnancy:* An extra-uterine pregnancy. *Tubal pregnancy:* An ectopic pregnancy in which the fertilized ovum lodges in a Fallopian tube rather than in the uterus.

PRESBYOPIA: Hardening of the lenses of the eyes due to advancing age, which causes the near point of distinct vision to recede progressively.

PRESENTATION: The manner or position in which the fetus enters or becomes engaged in the birth canal at the beginning of labor. *Breech presentation:* A buttocks-first or feet-first presentation. *Face presentation:* A face-first presentation. *Transverse presentation:* A condition in which the baby lies crosswise in the pelvis at the time labor begins. *Vertex presentation:* A head-first presentation.

PRIAPISM: An abnormally persistent erection of the penis.

PROCTOSCOPY: The technique for direct visualization of the lower 10 inches of the colon by the use of a lighted instrument, the proctoscope.

PROGESTERONE: A sex hormone which prepares the uterus for the reception and development of the fertilized ovum.

PROLAPSE: A falling down or downward displacement. *Prolapse of the cord:* A condition in which the umbilical cord emerges from the uterine cervix ahead of the presenting part of the baby at the beginning of labor. *Prolapse of the uterus:* A protrusion of the uterus into the vaginal cavity or even the vaginal orifice.

PROPHYLAXIS: Preventive treatment.

PROSTATE GLAND: A male gland that produces a sticky fluid in which sperm are carried out through the penis during ejaculation.

PROSTATISM (benign prostatic hypertrophy): A benign overgrowth or enlargement of the prostate gland, or the symptom complex that arises from such a condition.

PROSTATITIS: Inflammation of the prostate gland.

PROSTHESIS: Any artificial organ or part, such as an artificial eye, leg or denture.

PROTEIN: Any of a group of complex nitrogen-containing carbon compounds which form the principal building blocks of cell protoplasm. Proteins are essentially complex combinations of amino acids and their derivatives.

PROTEIN-BOUND IODINE TEST (PBI): Measurement of the amount of iodine bound up with proteins in the blood serum; an accurate means of measuring thyroid function.

PROTHROMBIN: A chemical agent in blood plasma which is the precursor of thrombin, necessary for blood coagulation.

PROTOPLASM: The only known form of matter in which life is manifested—a jelly-like fluid containing proteins, lipids, carbohydrates and inorganic salts with water.

PRURITIS ANI: Inflammation of the anal orifice accompanied by intense itching.

PSITTACOSIS (parrot fever): A pneumonia-like infection caused by a virus transmitted by infected birds.

PSORIASIS: A disfiguring skin disease of unknown cause marked by thickened red plaques, usually covered with whitish scale, and usually itching.

PSYCHOMOTOR SEIZURE: A convulsive manifestation in which the victim becomes temporarily disoriented and engaged in physical motion which he cannot later remember.

PSYCHONEUROSES: Mild to moderately severe mental disfunctions characterized by exaggerated defenses against unresolved emotional conflict.

PSYCHOSES: Severe, profound and often prolonged mental disfunctions characterized by disintegration of the personality and a distorted concept of reality.

PTOSIS: Drooping of an eyelid.

PTYALIN: An enzyme occurring in the saliva which converts starch into maltose and dextrose.

PUDENDAL BLOCK: A local anesthetic technique to anesthetize the pudendal nerves serving the lower genital tract and vaginal outlet during labor.

PUERPERAL SEPSIS (childbed fever): A streptococcus infection of the uterus which follows childbirth.

PULMONARY: Pertaining to the lungs.

PULP CAVITY: The interior of a tooth, composed of soft tissue and containing nerves, blood vessels and connective tissue.

PUPIL: An aperture in the center of the iris which permits light to enter.

PURPURA: A condition characterized by minute hemorrhages under the skin or in other organs as a result of rupture of capillary blood vessels. *Thrombocytopenic purpura:* Purpura due to a deficiency of platelets in the blood leading to extraordinary spontaneous bruising and pinpoint hemorrhages.

PYELITIS: Any inflammation of the kidney.

PYELOGRAM (intravenous pyelogram or IVP): X-ray studies in which the interior of the kidneys, ureters and bladder are outlined by means of a radio-opaque dye injected into the bloodstream and concentrated in the kidneys. *Retrograde pyelogram:* An X-ray examination of the interior of the kidneys and ureters accomplished by injecting a radio-opaque dye up the ureter under pressure.

PYELONEPHRITIS: A bacterial infection of the kidney characterized by inflammation.

PYLORIS (pyloric sphincter): The narrow muscular canal between the stomach and the duodenum which opens and closes to allow food to pass.

PYORRHEA (gingurtis): A chronic inflammation of the gums and tissues surrounding the teeth.

Q FEVER: A pneumonia-like rickettsial disease.

QUADRIPLEGIA: Paralysis of all four extremities.

QUINIDINE: A potent drug used in treatment of heart ailments.

RABIES (hydrophobia): An acute, infectious viral disease communicated to man by the bite of an infected animal.

RAYNAUD'S DISEASE: A form of arteritis in which arteries to the extremities go into periods of spasm, causing attacks of pain and cyanosis due to reduced blood flow.

RECTOCELE: A hernial protrusion of the wall of the rectum through the posterior wall of the vagina.

REFRACTORY PERIOD: The brief period of relaxation of cardiac muscle.

RELAPSING FEVER: An infection caused by spirochetes which is transmitted to man by lice or ticks.

REMISSION: A diminution or abatement of the symptoms of a disease. *Spontaneous remission:* A remission of symptoms that cannot be accounted for by medical treatment.

RENAL: Pertaining to the kidney.

RENIN: An enzyme liberated by ischemia of the kidney.

RESPIRATORY MEMBRANE: A layer of epithelial cells one cell layer thick, which forms a lining around the alveoli within the lungs.

REST: A fragment of embryonic tissue that has been retained within the adult organism.

RETICULOCYTES: Young red blood cells which still retain fragments or shreds of a disintegrated nucleus.

RETICULO-ENDOTHELIAL TISSUE (lymphoid tissue): The tissue of which the lymph glands are composed and which is found in the spleen, liver and other organs, comprising a system to maintain and cleanse the blood.

RETINA: The membrane of light-sensitive cells lining the interior of the back of the eye which receives images and transmits them to the optic nerve centers. *Retinal detachment:* A condition in which the visual lining of the inside of the eye becomes detached from the layer of tissue behind it.

RETINOBLASTOMA: A malignant tumor of the retina.

RETROFLEXION (of the uterus): The bending backward of the body of the uterus upon the cervix.

RETROLENTAL FIBROPLASIA: A form of blindness in the newborn arising from the use of excessively high concentrations of oxygen for resuscitation during the neonatal period.

RETROVERSION (of the uterus): A backward displacement of the entire uterus in relation to the pelvic axis.

RHABDOMYOSARCOMA: A rare, malignant tumor developing in large skeletal muscles.

RHEUMATIC FEVER: An inflammatory disease attacking connective tissue in the body and often causing permanent damage to the heart valves.

RHEUMATIC HEART DISEASE: Disease of the heart muscle or valves caused by rheumatic fever.

RHEUMATISM: A generalized layman's term for aching of the joints, often associated with but not necessarily limited to rheumatoid arthritis.

RH DISEASE. *See* Erythroblastosis fetalis.

RH FACTOR: A protein substance or agglutinin, transmitted as a genetic dominant, which is normally present in the blood in most individuals thus known as "Rh-positive," but absent in a small minority, who are thus known as "Rh-negative."

RHINOPHYMA: A coarsening and thickening of the skin of the nose.

RICKETS: A condition caused by deficiency of vitamin D, especially in children, which prevents normal development of bones and teeth.

RICKETTSIA: A group of pathogenic microorganisms intermediate in size and natural properties between bacteria and viruses and transmitted to man by infected insects.

RIEDEL'S STRUMA: A thyroid condition characterized by the development of a small, hard fibrous goiter.

RINGWORM INFECTION: A highly contagious fungus growth so called because of the circular skin lesions it causes.

ROCKY MOUNTAIN SPOTTED FEVER: A rickettsial disease spread by wood ticks.

ROSACEA: A disease affecting the skin of the nose, forehead and cheeks, marked by flushing, followed by red coloration due to dilatation of the capillaries with acne-like pustules.

ROSEOLA INFANTUM (exanthem subitum): A childhood rash disease marked by high remittent fever followed by a fine red rash on the trunk.

RUBELLA ("German measles," "Three-day measles"): An acute febrile childhood rash disease caused by a virus, marked by a characteristic skin rash of a few days' duration.

RUBEOLA. *See* Measles.

SALMONELLA: A family name of a group of rod-shaped bacilli which infect the intestinal tract and are responsible for such diseases as typhoid fever and the less severe paratyphoid infections commonly known as "salmonella food poisoning."

SALPINGITIS: Inflammation or infection of the Fallopian tubes. *Gonorrheal salpingitis:* Gonorrheal infection of the Fallopian tubes.

SARCOMA: A malignant tumor developing from connective tissue, bone or muscle. *Chondrosarcoma:* A cancer that originates in cartilage at the end of a bone. *Ewing's sarcoma:* A highly malignant cancer that develops in the shafts of long bones, particularly in children. *Osteogenic sarcoma:* A primary cancer of bone. *Uterine sarcoma:* A cancer arising from muscle or fibrous tissue in the wall of the uterus.

SCABIES: A skin disease caused by infestation of the itch mite, Sarcoptes scabiei, which bores beneath the skin.

SCARLET FEVER: A contagious, febrile throat infection caused by a streptococcus.

SCHISTOSOMIASIS: A flatworm infestation transmitted to man by certain fresh-water snails.

SCIATICA: A neurological syndrome characterized by pain and other symptoms in the distribution of the sciatic nerve to the leg.

SCLERA: The tough white supporting tunic of the eyeball, covering it entirely except for the cornea.

SCLERODERMA: A disease marked by slowly progressive, diffuse thickening and rigidity of the skin and subcutaneous tissues, often affecting the joints and tendons as well as internal organs.

SCLEROSIS: Hardening, thickening or scarring.

SCOLIOSIS: A lateral or side-to-side S-curve deformity of the spine.

SCRUB TYPHUS FEVER: A milder form of typhus fever, spread by itch mites or chiggers.

SCROTUM: The external pouch which contains the testicles and their accessory organs.

SCURVY: A disease caused by a deficiency of vitamin C in the diet.

SEBACEOUS GLANDS: Glands located in the outer layers of the skin, which secrete an oily substance known as sebum.

SEDIMENTATION RATE: The measurement of the speed with which red cells settle to the bottom of a tube of blood that has been mixed with an anticoagulant.

SEMEN: The fluid produced by the prostate gland which carries sperm out of the urethral canal during ejaculation.

SEMINAL VESICLES: Saclike organs adjacent to the prostate gland which store sperm from the testes.

SEMINOMA: A cancer of the testis or ovary.

SENILITY (senile dementia): Progressive and irreversible deterioration of brain function in old age due to impaired circulation to the brain.

SENSITIZATION: Contact with an allergen which renders the body hypersensitive or vulnerable to an allergic reaction upon repeated contact.

SEPSIS: A generalized poisoning or toxicity of the body arising from bacterial infection.

SEPTICEMIA (blood poisoning): Invasion of the bloodstream by an infectious organism.

SEPTUM: Any separating partition within the body.

SEQUESTRUM: A chunk of infected dead bone covered by thick layers of newly deposited living bone not yet attacked by infection.

SEROLOGICAL TEST FOR SYPHILIS (STS): Any of a variety of diagnostic blood tests for syphilis.

SHOCK: The sequence of physiological changes, often overwhelming, that the body undergoes in response to blood loss, impairment of circulation, severe pain or emotional trauma.

SICKLE-CELL DISEASE (sickle-cell anemia): An anemia primarily affecting Negroes which results from a hereditary abnormality in the structure of the hemoglobin in the red cells.

SILICOSIS: A widespread lung inflammation resulting from prolonged exposure to and inhalation of silicon-containing dust.

SIMMOND'S DISEASE: A profound endocrine disturbance resulting from massive pituitary gland destruction due to hemorrhage or tumor.

SINUS: An opening or hollow enclosed space, in particular one of several air-filled cavities in the head communicating with the nose.

SINO-AURICULAR NODE (sino-atrial or SA node): A small nodule of autonomic nerve cells located in the wall of the right auricle of the heart. *See also* Pacemaker.

SMALLPOX (variola): An acute, infectious, epidemic disease caused by the virus Borreliota variolae.

SPASTIC: Hypertonic or contracted, so that the muscles are stiff and the movements awkward.

SPECULUM: An instrument for opening to view a passage or cavity of the body.

SPERM: The male reproductive cell produced in the testes.

SPERMATOCELE: A cystic or sacular distention of the epididymis.

SPHINCTER: A circular "purse-string" muscle which opens and closes in valve-like fashion to allow food or other substances to pass; for example, the cardiac sphincter, a muscle at the top of the stomach which opens and closes to allow food to pass into the stomach from the esophagus; or the anal sphincter, the circular muscle of the anus which permits control over evacuation of feces.

SPHYGMOMANOMETER: An instrument used to measure blood pressure.

SPINA BIFIDA: A congenital cleft or splitting of the vertebral column with meningeal protrusion.

SPINAL CORD: The part of the central nervous system which is lodged in the vertebral column.

SPIROCHETES: A family of bacteria that are comparatively large and spiral-shaped.

SPLANCHNICECTOMY: The surgical removal of the autonomic nerve ganglia that lie along both sides of the spine on the back wall of the abdomen.

SPLEEN: A small oval organ located in the left upper quadrant of the abdomen which aids in the storage of blood and the destruction of aging red blood cells and platelets.

SPLEENECTOMY: The surgical removal of the spleen.

SPONTANEOUS DELIVERY: Delivery of a child without the use of forceps.

SPRAIN: A twisting or wrenching injury to a joint which stretches or tears the supporting ligaments.

SPRUE: A disorder of intestinal absorption.

SPUTUM: The sticky, mucoid secretion that forms within the bronchi and bronchioles and is expelled by coughing.

STAPHYLOCOCCUS: A genus of small, spherical, gram-positive bacteria which grow in clusters.

STASIS: Any stoppage of normal flow or motion in the body, as of the circulating blood, the flow of other fluids, or the passage of food down the intestine. *Urinary stasis:* A stoppage of the flow of urine or the pooling of urine behind an obstruction.

STATUS ASTHMATICUS: A continuous and aggravated asthmatic state which persists to the point of exhaustion and collapse of the victim.

STATUS EPILEPTICUS: A condition in which the victim has repeated grand mal seizures at rapid intervals.

STENOSIS: A narrowing, hardening or stricturing of a duct or canal. *Aortic stenosis:* A narrowing and hardening of the leaflets of the aortic valve of the heart. *Mitral stenosis:* A narrowing and hardening of the mitral valve of the heart. *Pulmonic stenosis:* A narrowing and hardening of the pulmonic valve of the heart. *Pyloric stenosis:* A condition, often congenital, in which the pyloric canal leading from stomach to duodenum is hardened and constricted due to overgrowth of muscular tissue.

STERNUM: The breastbone.

STEROID: Any of a wide variety of chemical substances, natural or artificial, with the characteristic structure of (and often used synonymously for) the cortisone-like hormones.

STETHOSCOPE: An instrument used for detecting normal and abnormal sounds within the body.

STONE BRUISE: An injury due to a hard blow on the under surface of the heel which leads to bursitis or inflammation of the bony lining of the heel.

STRABISMUS: A condition in which the eyes do not converge properly on an image, leading to such disorders as crosseye (medial stabismus) or walleye (lateral strabismus).

STRAIN: An injury that occurs to muscle or tendon due to overuse or stretching.

STREPTOCOCCUS: A genus of small, spherical, gram-positive bacteria which grow in chains.

STRIA: "Stretch marks" or lines on the skin caused by distention, particularly in obesity or pregnancy.

STROKE (apoplexy): A cerebrovascular accident in which brain tissue is damaged because of hemorrhage or rupture of a blood vessel within the brain, or as a result of an obstructive blood clot in the cerebral circulation.

STY: Inflammation or infection of one or more of the sebaceous glands of the eyelids.

SUBDURAL HEMATOMA: Bleeding between the dural and arachnoid membranes of the brain resulting in formation of a hematoma just beneath the outer meningeal membrane.

SUNSTROKE (heat hyperpyrexia): A dangerous condition marked by elevated body temperature, coma and sometimes convulsions, produced by prolonged exposure to the sun.

SUPPOSITORY: A medication suspended in an oily or waxy coating with a low melting point, intended for introduction into the rectum, vagina or urethra.

SYMPTOM: Any subjective indication of disease or disorder of the body, such as pain, nausea, insomnia, etc.

SYNAPSE: The region of contact between fibrils of two adjacent neurons, forming the place where a nerve impulse is transmitted from one neuron to another.

SYNDROME: A group or cluster of symptoms which characteristically occur together.

SYNOVIAL FLUID: A viscid fluid resembling the white of an egg, which is secreted by the synovial membrane and contained in joint cavities, bursae and tendon sheaths.

SYNOVIAL MEMBRANE: A slippery, lubricated connective tissue membrane which lines joint cavities, bursae and tendon sheaths and is the source of synovial fluid.

SYNTHESIS: The building up of a chemical compound by the union of less complex component elements.

SYPHILIS: A contagious venereal disease. *Congenital syphilis:* Syphilis existing in a child at birth as a result of the infection crossing the placenta from mother to fetus.

SYRINGOMYELIA: A progressive congenital disease of the spinal cord arising from unknown causes.

TABES DORSALIS (locomotor ataxia): A degeneration of the dorsal nerves of the spinal cord as a result of tertiary syphilis, with loss or disorganization of the normal functions of the lower extremities.

TACHYCARDIA: Extreme rapidity of heartbeat.

TAMPONADE (cardiac tamponade): Compression of the heart due to the presence of blood or other fluid within the pericardium.

TAPEWORM: A flatworm which is parasitic in man, transmitted by ingestion of poorly cooked infested meat or fish.

TARTAR (calculus): The chalky incrustation that forms on neglected teeth.

TAY-SACHS DISEASE: A degenerative disorder of the brain.

TENDON: The fibrous cord of connective tissue by which a muscle is attached to a bone or other structure.

TENDONITIS: Inflammation of a tendon or tendons.

TENOSYNOVITIS: Inflammation of a tendon involving the synovial membrane canal through which the tendon moves.

TERATOMA (teratocarcinoma): A tumor, usually malignant, arising from embryonic rests or fetal material congenitally included in an otherwise normal fetus.

TESTES (testicles): The twin reproductive glands in the scrotum of a male which produce sperm.

TESTOSTERONE: A sex hormone manufactured in the testes.

TETANUS (lockjaw): An acute infectious disease caused by a toxin produced in the body by the Clostridium tetani and marked by spasms of the muscles of the jaw and back.

TETANUS TOXOID: Tetanus toxin which has been neutralized with a weak solution of formaldehyde, for use as a vaccine.

TETANY: A syndrome manifested by sharp flexion of the wrist and ankle joints, muscle twitchings, cramps and convulsions.

TETRALOGY OF FALLOT: A group of congenital cardiac defects including pulmonic stenosis, interventricular septal defects, dextroposition of the aorta so that it receives blood from the right as well as from the left ventricle, and hypertrophy of right ventricle, all of which can occur simultaneously.

THORACENTESIS: A procedure in which blood or fluid in the chest is drawn off with a syringe and needle.

THORACIC DUCT: A thin-walled tube in the chest which collects lymph from the major lymphatic channels and drains it into the superior vena cava.

THORACOPLASTY: The permanent collapse of a lung by surgical removal of ribs.

THORAX: The chest cavity.

THROMBOANGIITIS OBLITERANS. *See* Buerger's disease.

THROMBOCYTES: Blood platelets.

THROMBOENDARTERECTOMY: A surgical procedure to remove a thrombus from a major vessel.

THROMBOPHLEBITIS: Inflammation of the wall of a vein, with formation of a thrombus.

THROMBOSIS: The formation, development or presence of a thrombus or blood clot within a blood vessel.

THROMBUS: A blood clot that has formed within a blood vessel.

THRUSH (moniliasis): A fungus infection, often occurring in the mouth in children, caused by the fungus organism Candida albicans.

THYMUS GLAND: A glandular structure located high in the chest in front of the trachea. The thymus is large in infants and children, then atrophies markedly with the approach of maturity and is believed to play an important role in the body's immune defenses.

THYROGLOBULIN: A combination of thyroid hormone and large proteins known as globulins, which are stored in the thyroid gland.

THYROID GLAND: A large endocrine or ductless gland located in front of and on either side of the trachea.

THYROIDECTOMY: Surgical removal of a large portion of the thyroid gland.

THYROIDITIS: Inflammation of the thyroid.

THYROTOXICOSIS: A disease condition caused by excessive production of thyroid hormone by the thyroid gland.

THYROXIN: A hormone produced by the thyroid gland.

TIC DOULOUREUX: An exceedingly painful spasm of muscles on one side of the face or jaw that results from irritation of a branch of the trigeminal nerve.

TINEA: A family of fungus organisms which attack skin, scalp or nails. *Tinea capitis:* Ringworm of the scalp. *Tinea corporis:* Ringworm of the body. *Tinea pedis:* Athlete's foot.

TINNITUS: Ringing in the ears.

TITER: The quantity of a substance required to produce a reaction with a given volume of another substance, or the amount of one substance required to correspond with a given amount of another substance.

TOMOGRAM: A technique for X-ray examination of deep tissues and organs within the body.

TONGUE TIE: A thin membrane of tissue extending from the midline of the under surface of the tongue to the floor of the mouth, restricting free movement of the tongue.

TONOMETER: An instrument for measuring tension, especially the tension or pressure of fluid within the eye.

TONSILLITIS: A bacterial infection of the tonsils.

TONSILS: Soft, spongy lymphoid tissue masses on either side of the throat, visible below the soft palate.

T & A (tonsillectomy and adenoidectomy): The surgical removal of tonsils and adenoids.

TOPHI: Chalky nodules of uric acid in crystal form, often found in the joints with gout.

TORSION: The act or condition of being twisted.

TORTICOLLIS: Stiff neck; wry neck.

TOURNIQUET: Any band or ligature applied around a limb for the purpose of constricting blood flow or controlling hemorrhage.

TOXIN: A poisonous substance of microbic, vegetable or animal origin.

TOXOPLASMOSIS: A severe disease of the nervous system caused by a protozoan parasite.

TRACHEA: The windpipe.

TRACHEITIS: Inflammation of the trachea.

TRACHEOBRONCHITIS: Inflammation of the trachea and mainstem bronchi.

TRACHEOSTOMY: A surgical opening of the trachea below the level of the larynx to permit insertion of a breathing tube.

TRACHOMA: A serious inflammatory viral infection of the eye.

TRANSFUSION: The infusion of a donor's blood or packed red cells into the veins of a recipient. *Exchange transfusion:* The simultaneous transfusion of a donor's blood and withdrawal of an infant's blood in treatment of erythroblastosis fetalis (Rh disease). *Transfusion reaction:* A condition characterized by chills, sweats and shock induced by the transfusion of improperly matched blood.

TRANSPOSITION OF THE GREAT VESSELS: A congenital abnormality of the cardiovascular system in which the aorta and the pulmonary artery develop in transposed position.

TREMOR: A gross or fine persisting involuntary movement of one or more parts of the body, usually an extremity. *Athetoid tremor:* A slow, undulating or wormlike involuntary movement of an extremity; *see* Athetosis. *Intention tremor:* A tremor which is not evident when the involved part is at rest, but which begins as soon as it is put into purposeful motion. *Tremor at rest:* A tremor which is apparent only when the involved part is relaxed and which disappears as soon as voluntary motion begins.

TREPHINE: A rounded saw blade or crown saw for the removal of a circular disk of bone, chiefly from the skull.

TRICHINIASIS (Trichinosis): A roundworm infestation of skeletal muscle, usually contrasted by eating infested and undercooked pork.

TRICHOTILLOMANIA: A nervous habit of twisting, pulling out, or chewing one's hair.

TRIGLYCERIDES: Fatty compounds biochemically manufactured by the liver and important to the body's metabolism of fatty food materials.

TRYPANOSOMIASIS (African sleeping sickness): A central nervous system disease caused by a protozoan parasite transmitted by the bite of the tsetse fly.

TRYPSIN: A pancreatic enzyme which breaks down protein foods into their component protein molecules.

TUBERCULOSIS: A chronic infectious disease caused by Mycobacterium tuberculosis, which chiefly afflicts the lung, but may also involve bone, larynx, subcutaneous tissues, kidney or virtually any other organ or tissue of the body.

TUBULE: A small tube or duct. *Seminiferous tubule:* One of the microscopically small, folded ducts which make up most of the substance of the testis and in which the sperm are formed.

TULAREMIA (rabbit fever): An acute and severe infection, a disease of rodents resembling plague, which is transmitted to man by the bites of insects or the handling of infected animals.

TUMOR: A swelling, morbid enlargement, new growth or neoplasm. *Benign tumor:* A localized tumor not given to invasion of surrounding tissues or metastasis and hence not malignant; favorable for recovery. *Cystic tumor:* A tumor that is not solid but more or less hollow or filled with fluid. *Functioning tumor:* A tumor, usually a carcinoma, which continues to produce the secretions from the gland or tissue in which it develops. *Malignant tumor:* A neoplasm which is given to invasion of surrounding tissues and the tendency to seed to distant areas; hence, virulent and ultimately fatal unless checked by treatment; a cancer. *Non-functioning tumor:* A carcinoma which does not have the ability to produce the secretions from the gland or tissue in which it develops. *Secondary tumor* (metastatic tumor): A tumor which develops from cells from a primary cancer spread by way of the bloodstream or lymphatics.

TYMPANIC MEMBRANE (eardrum): The tightly stretched oval of fibrous tissue separating the external auditory canal from the middle ear.

TYPHOID FEVER (enteric fever): An acute generalized infection caused by bacteria of the Salmonella family.

TYPHUS FEVER: A rickettsial disease transmitted by body lice, itch mites (chiggers) or rat fleas. *Murine typhus fever:* A rickettsial disease transmitted by rat fleas.

ULCER: A sore or break in the surface of the skin or internal body tisssues. *Corneal ulcer:* An ulcer that forms on the surface of the cornea. *Decubitus ulcer* (bed sore, pressure sore): A deep, ulcerating sore which develops on soft tissue of the body due to continuing pressure. *Peptic ulcer:* An ulcer that forms in the stomach or duodenum.

ULNAR NERVE PALSY: Paralysis of the little finger and ring finger as a result of injury to the ulnar nerve.

UMBILICAL CORD: The flexible tube connecting the umbilicus of the fetus with the placenta in the uterus.

UREA: A nitrogen-containing waste chemical excreted in the urine.

UREMIA: A toxic condition related to failure of kidney function to eliminate urea and other waste materials from the bloodstream.

URETER: The tube which conveys urine from the kidney to the bladder.

URETHROCELE: A sacular pocket formed by an outpouching of the urethra through a muscular defect in the vaginal wall.

URETHRA: The tube which carries urine from the bladder to the outside.

URI: Upper respiratory infection.

URINE: The fluid excretion produced by the kidneys as a means of flushing soluble waste materials out of the body.

URTICARIA (hives): Raised, red, itching patches which occur on the surface of the skin as an allergic reaction.

UTERUS: The womb.

UVULA: The tag of tisssue hanging from the soft palate above the root of the tongue.

VACCINATION: Inoculation with vaccinia virus as a means of inducing immunity to smallpox; more generally, a term used by laymen to describe any immunization procedure involving injection or inoculation.

VAGINA: The canal in the female, extending from the vulva to the cervix, which receives the penis during sexual intercourse.

VALVE: A small fibrous structure which regulates the flow of body fluids, in particular the cardiac valves of the heart or the valves within the veins.

VALVULITIS: Inflammation of the cardiac valves.

VARICELLA: *See* Chickenpox.

VARICES (varicose veins, varicosities): Enlarged, stretched and tortuous veins. *Esophageal varices:* Enlarged veins of the esophagus which have been stretched because of excessive pressure within the portal vein. *Varicocele:* Varicose veins of the spermatic cord and scrotum.

VARICOSE ULCER: An ulcer caused by the breakdown of skin tissue in cases of advanced varices.

VAS DEFERENS: The narrow vessel through which sperm pass from the testes to the seminal vesicles.

VASECTOMY: Surgical ligation and cutting of the vas deferens; a means of voluntary sterilization in the male.

VASOPRESSIN: One of the hormones secreted by the posterior lobe of the pituitary gland.

VEIN: A vessel which conveys the blood to or toward the heart. *Portal vein:* The large abdominal vein which is central to the hepatic portal circulatory system. *Vena cava:* The great vein which drains blood from the area below the heart (inferior vena cava) and the area above the heart (superior vena cava) into the right auricle.

VENEREAL DISEASE (VD): Any of a variety of infectious diseases primarily transmitted by means of sexual intercourse or sexual contact of any kind; for example, syphilis and gonorrhea.

VENTRICLE: Any small cavity, especially either of the two lower cavities or pumping chambers of the heart, or any one of several fluid-filled cavities of the brain.

VERMIFORM APPENDIX: A wormlike appendage of the cecum.

VERNIX: A waxy material which covers the skin of the fetus.

VERTEBRAE: The chunky bones of the spine. *Cervical vertebrae:* The upper seven vertebrae. *Dorsal vertebrae:* The fifteen vertebrae immediately below the cervical vertebrae. *Lumbar vertebrae:* The five vertebrae immediately below the dorsal vertebra. *Sacral vertebrae:* The fused vertebral segments forming the sacrum adjoining and below the fifth lumbar vertebra.

VERTIGO: Dizziness.

VILLI: The microscopically small threadlike projections covering the interior mucosa of the small intestine.

VINCENT'S DISEASE (trench mouth): An acute, painful ulcerative infection of the gums caused by two symbiotic bacteria.

VIREMIA: The presence of virus in the blood.

VIRUS: A parasitic microorganism, smaller than most bacteria and capable of multiplication only within a living susceptible host cell.

VITAL CAPACITY: The maximum amount of air that can be sucked into the lungs in a forced respiration.

VITILIGO: The loss of pigmentation in various irregular and sharply demarcated patches of skin.

VOCAL CORDS: Two thin, semicircular membranes in the larynx which vibrate as air passes, making vocal sounds possible.

VOLVULUS: Intestinal obstruction due to a knotting and twisting of the bowel.

VULVA: The creaselike structure that forms the external portion of the female genital organs.

VULVOVAGINITIS: Inflammation of the vulva and the vagina.

WARTS (verrucae): Benign tumors of the skin, believed to be viral in origin. *Plantar warts:* Painful warts which occur on the soles of the feet. *Venereal warts: See* Condylomata acuminata.

WEN: A cystic lesion that forms within the skin, filled with an odorless, waxy material.

WHOOPING COUGH (pertussis): A bacterial infection of the respiratory tract characterized by peculiar paroxysms of coughing which end in a whooping respiration.

WILMS' TUMOR: A childhood cancer arising from changes in foci of primitive cells remaining in the kidney after its development is complete.

XANTHOMA: A small, flat, yellow-colored plaque on the skin due to deposits of lipoids.

YAWS: A highly contagious nonvenereal infection of the superficial tissues caused by a spirochete similar to that of syphilis and limited to the tropical regions.

YELLOW FEVER: An acute infectious virus disease transmitted by mosquitoes.

INDEX

Boldface numbers indicate the principal discussion of a subject.

A-B-C-D procedure in resuscitation, **111,** 118, 119
Abdomen: physical examination, 965; wounds, 138; X-rays, diagnostic, 977
Abdominal pain: laxatives avoided, 135, 641; persistent, 627; stomach ache, 135
Abortion, **921–923;** childbed fever in, 753; elective, 921–923; gas gangrene from, 222; habitual, 818; illegal, 753, 758, 921, 922; inevitable, 819; spontaneous, *see* Miscarriage; therapeutic, 823, 921; threatened, 818–819
Abrasions, 124
Abruptio placentae, 829, **831–832,** 845, 846
Abscesses, 126, 206–207, **209;** amebic, 259–260; lung, 465, 470, **484;** peritoneal, 645; peritonsillar, 473
Acetylcholine, 52, 54
Achilles tendon reflex, 347
Achondroplasia (chondrodystrophy), **307–308,** 708
Acid-base balance, 79
Acidophils, 707
Acini, 660
Acne, 59, 206–208, **393–396,** 901; false beliefs on, 394–395; treatment, 395–396
Acoustic holography, 449
Acoustic nerve, *see* Auditory nerve
Acoustic neuroma, 437
Acromegaly, 708
Acrophobia, 780
Adam's apple, 456
Addison, Thomas, 517, 682, 704
Addison's disease (adrenal insufficiency), 392, 682, **704–705**
Adenocarcinoma, 938; of breast, 448
Adenoidectomy, tonsillectomy and (T and A), **193–195,** 197, 438, 535

Adenoids, **193,** 456, 471, 473
Adenoma, parathyroid, 695, 696
Adolescence, **899–908;** breast development, 444–445; communication with parents, 907–908; drug abuse, 796–797, 799–800; emotional problems, 775, 901–902; generation gap, 899–900, 907–908; marijuana use, 796; mental health, 806; parental authority, 905–907; puberty, problems of, 900–902; *see also* Puberty; sex education, 903–905
Adoption, 916
Adrenal cortex, 73, **684–685,** 704; overactivity, disorders, 705–706; sex hormones produced, 685; *see also* Adrenal hormones; Corticosteroids
Adrenal exhaustion, 73
Adrenal gland disorders, **704–707;** Addison's disease, 392, 682, **704–705;** adrenogenital syndrome, 705, 706; Cushing's syndrome, 392, **705–706,** 708; hypoglycemia and, 703; pheochromocytoma, 585, 587, **706–707;** skin in, 392; tumors, 706–707
Adrenal glands, 73, **684–685;** in breast cancer, 450; *see also* Adrenal cortex; Adrenal medulla
Adrenal hormones, 73, **684–685,** 704, 707, 708, 716, 735; *see also* Corticosteroids
Adrenalin (epinephrine), 73, 492–493, **684,** 704, 706–707
Adrenal insufficiency (Addison's disease), 392, 682, **704–705**
Adrenal medulla, 73, **684,** 704, 706
Adrenocorticotropic hormone (ACTH), 74, 316, 491, 685, **688,** 706–708
Adrenogenital syndrome, 705, 706
Aedes aegypti, 234–236

Aerophagia (air swallowing), 456, 615, 620
Afibrinogenemia, 531
Afterbirth, 818
Agammaglobulinemia, 532
Aged, the, **944–958;** families, living with, 944–945, 955–956; fractured hip, 295, 952; fractures, 32, 295, 307, 948–949, 952; health care, 945, 947; home nursing care, **160–161,** 956; housing for, 945; increasing number of, 944; Medicare, 945, 1019; nursing homes, 370, 945, **955–957,** 1009; physical changes, 947–955; retirement, 946–947; retirement communities, 945; senility, **367, 370,** 950; Social Security, 945, 1018; *see also* Aging
Agglutinins, 77
Agglutinogens, 972
Aging, 98, 592, **944–958;** bone changes, 31–32, 307, 948–949; cardiovascular system, 953–954; digestive system, 954; eyes, 951; infectious diseases, 947–948; nervous system disorders, 949–950; physical changes, 947–955; respiratory system disorders, 948, 952–953; sexual activity, 955; skin and hair changes, 400–402, 407, 950–951; teeth, 951; urinary tract disorders, 949, 954–955
Agoraphobia, 780
Agranulocytosis, 532
Air: inhaled and exhaled, 461–462; swallowed, 456, 615, 620, 855, 856; vital capacity, 461, 952
Air pollution, 504, 505
Airway device, 108
Albinos, 60, **401**
Albumin, 79; in urine, 723–725, 727
Alcohol, 790–791; barbiturates and, 342, 794; diabetes and, 702; digestion of, 666; drinking habits, 924,

1047

Alcohol (*cont'd*)
927; gastric dilatation and, 620; gastritis and, 630, 631, 790; impotence and, 744; in weight reduction, 930
Alcoholics Anonymous, 792–793
Alcoholic stupor, 114–115, **341–342**
Alcoholism, **790–793;** anemia in, 517, 518; aspiration pneumonia in, 488; brain damage in, 371; cirrhosis and, 90, 666–667, 791; cure and treatment, 791–793; habits leading to, 924; pancreatitis and, 662
Alcohol psychosis (delirium tremens), 371, 790
Alexandria, Egypt, medical school, 6
Alimentary canal, 609; *see also* Digestive tract
Alkalosis, 79; respiratory, 64
Allergens, 387–388, 391–392, 492–493, 561
Allergies, 97–98, **387–392,** 490, 923; anaphylactic shock and, 139–140, 388; to beestings, 139–140, **389;** to cosmetics, 390, 413–414; to drugs (medicinal), 390–391; emergency kit for, 140, 389; emotional factors in, 388, 490, 493; food, of babies, 864–865; inflammation and, 556; sinusitis, allergic, 472; skin disorders, 61, **387–392;** skin tests, 391, 491; treatment, 391–392; to vaccine, 972; *see also* Asthma; Hay fever
Allergist, 992
Alopecia (baldness), **40–41,** 950–951
Alopecia areata, 411
Alpha cells, 696
Alveoli, 63, 64, 455, 457, 460; in asthma, 494; in emphysema, 494
Amebiasis (amebic dysentery), 176, **259–260**
Amenorrhea, 761
American Academy of Pediatrics, 190
American Arthritis and Rheumatism Foundation, 315, 331
American Board of Internal Medicine, 992
American Board of Surgery, 993
American Cancer Society, 331
American Heart Association, 562
American Hospital Association, 1002
American Medical Association, 329, 991
Amino acids, 79, 86, 90, 93, 660, 888
Aminophylline, 493
Ammonia in blood, 669
Amnesia, 359–360; retrograde, 360
Amniocentesis, 376, 880
Amniotic fluid, 829, 835
Amobarbital (Amytal), 886
Amphetamines, 794; for weight control, 931
Amphotericin B, 276
Amylase, 86, 660–662
Amyotrophic lateral sclerosis, 53, 293, **372–373**
Anal canal, 612, 646; *see also* Anus

Anal disorders, *see* Anorectal disorders
Anaphylactic shock, **139–140,** 388
Anatomy, study of, 8, 984–985
Androgen (androgens), 394, 395, 446, **685–686,** 735; in adrenogenital syndrome, 705; in breast cancer, 450, 842
Androsterone, 685, 735
Anemia, 77, **515–521;** aplastic, 520; in cancer, 521, 657; congenital hemolytic jaundice, 519–520; drugs causing, 32, 520; folic acid deficiency, 517, 518, 628; heart failure and, 574; hemolytic, 77, **518–520;** hemoplastic, 77; iron-deficiency, 77, **515–516,** 518, 890; in kidney disorders, 521, 588; in leukemia, 78, 524; in lymphosarcoma, 528; Mediterranean, 519; pernicious, 77, 392, **516–518,** 631, 891; posthemorrhagic, 515, 534; in pregnancy, 515, 518, **821–822;** secondary, 520–521; self-treatment, danger of, 521; sickle-cell, 518–520
Anencephalus, 373
Anesthesia in childbirth, 835–836, **838–839;** caudal (subspinal), 839; inhalation, 838; local, 838; spinal (saddle block), 838–841
Anesthesiologist, 996–997
Aneurysm, 83; stroke and, 361; subarachnoid hemorrhage and, 364
Angiitis, 565
Angina pectoris, 579, 593, **595–597, 600;** early knowledge of, 4; exercise and, 597; pain in digestive disorders compared with, 595, 623; treatment, 596–597, 600
Angiogram: cerebral, 350, 365, 979; of heart, 552, 555, 565, 979
Animals, domestic: fleas, 269; infection spread by, 266, 269, 274–275; rabies shots, 240
Animals, wild: bites, 142, 240–241; plague transmitted by, 274
Ankles: edema, 576, 580; fractures, 299; reflexes, 347; sprains, **130–131,** 304
Anorectal disorders, **645–647;** anal fissure, 638, **646;** anal pruritus, 647; fistula-in-ano, 646–647; hemorrhoids, *see* Hemorrhoids
Anorexia nervosa, 785
Anoxia, 64
Antabuse, 792
Antepar (piperazine), 226, 267
Anthracosis (black lung disease), 485, 487
Anthrax, 274–275
Antibiotics: for colds, caution on, 227; discovery of, 12
Antibodies, 76, 97, **174,** 387, 972–973; heterophile, 198
Antidiuretic hormone, 709, 716
Antidotes for poisons, 117
Antigens, 387

Antihemophilic globulin factor, 531
Antihistamines, 61; for allergies, 391–392, 491; for colds, 227; for insect bites and stings, 139, 140; for sinusitis, 472
Antitoxin, polyvalent, 222; *see also* Immunization
Anus, 612, 635; anal fissure, 638, **646;** fistula-in-ano, 646–647; imperforate, 877; pruritus, 647
Anxiety, **771–774,** 778, 785, 870
Anxiety panic state, 779, 781
Anxiety reaction, 779
Aorta, 81, 543, 552; aneurysm, 245, 565, 566; coarctation of, 547; in malposition of great vessels, 550; syphilis in, 245, 565, 566; in transposition of great vessels, 547–548
Aortic commisurotomy, 563
Aortic stenosis, 548–550, 561–562
Aortic valve, 544
Apgar, Virginia, 843
Apgar rating scale, 843, 874–875
Aphasia, 46
Aplastic anemia, 520
Apoplexy, *see* Stroke
Appendicitis, **638–642;** "chronic," 639; diagnosis, 640; laxatives, warning on, 135, 641; pain resembling, 623, 632–633, 640, 662; pinworm as cause, 267; surgery, 640–641; white cell count in, 78, 639
Appendix, vermiform, 612, 639
Aqueous humor, 426
Arachnoid membrane, 47
Areola, 444, 445
Arms: artificial, 302; bones, 27; fractured, 128, 295–296
Arteries, **81–83,** 542–543; bleeding, control of, 104–107; congenital abnormalities, 546–549; grafts, 83, 547, 552, 565, 568, 600, 605; hardening of, *see* Arteriosclerosis; Atherosclerosis; in hypertension, 583, 585, 588, 589; inflammatory disorders, 565–568; malposition of great vessels, 550; transposition of great vessels, 547–548, 550; veins compared with, 568; *see also* Cardiovascular system; *entries under* Coronary; names of arteries
Arterioles, 81, 543; in hypertension, 583, 585, 588
Arteriosclerosis, 360, 367, 592, 943, 953; *see also* Atherosclerosis
Arteriovenous fistula, 878
Arteriovenous shunts, 546, 548
Arteritis, 565
Arthritis, 32, **310–320;** gonorrheal, 249, 312, 723; gouty, 319–320; infectious (septic), 311–312; osteoarthritis, **317–319;** 948; in rheumatic fever, 561, 562; rheumatoid, 40, 73, **312–317,** 520, 560, 561; syphilitic, 312; traumatic, 310, 311, 320–321; tuberculous, 312
Artificial heart, 605

Artificial insemination, 742
Artificial kidney machine, 65, 69, **725–727,** 728–729, 1012
Artificial respiration, **107–110;** mouth-to-mouth, **107–108,** 111, 113, 114, 116, 118, 129, 461, 468; mouth-to-nose, 107, 108, 111, 113; prone-pressure, 108–109; spine arm-lift (Sylvester method), 109
Asbestosis, 485
Ascaris infection, 266
Ascaris lumbricoides, 265, 266
Ascites (ascitic fluid), 666, 667
Ascorbic acid, *see* Vitamin C
Asklepios, 5
Asphyxia (respiratory failure), 103–104, **107–110;** carbon monoxide poisoning, 115–116; choking, 64, 107, **114,** 469
Aspirin: for children, 155, 181; esophageal burn from, 615; poisoning from, 116, 155, 863; in pregnancy, caution on, 823
Asthma, bronchial, 64, 468, **491–494;** allergies and, 388, 492; chronic, 494; emotional factors in, 493; treatment, 391–392, 492–493
Astigmatism, 95–96, 427
Atabrine (quinacrine hydrochloride), 264, 268
Ataxia, 882
Atelectasis, 64, 463, 469, 489
Atheroma, 592–593
Atherosclerosis, 39, 53, 81–83, **592–594,** 604–605, 943; aging and, 367, 943, 953; cholesterol and, 604; contributing factors, 594; in coronary artery disease, 593–596, 598–599; diabetes and, 594, 698; hypertension and, 588, 594, 597; polyunsaturated fats and, 890; stroke and, 360
Athetosis (athetoid tremor), 882
Athlete's foot, 176, **399**
Atlas (neck vertebra), 30
Atresia, 550
Atria (auricles), 82, 543–544, 551
Atrial septal defects, 551
Auditory canal, 433–434
Auditory nerve (acoustic nerve), 44, 347, 438; streptomycin damage, 53
Aureomycin, 175
Auricle (of ear), 433
Auricles (of heart, atria), 82, 543–544, 551
Auricular fibrillation, 579
Australoid race, 60
Autonomic nervous system, 43, **48–49,** 52, 86, 544, 684, 784
Autosuggestion, 681
Avicenna, 7–8
Axis (neck vertebra), 30

Babinski sign, 348
Baby (babies), **850–866;** allergies, food, 864–865; bathing, 858–859; bed, 862; behavior development, 852–853, 866; birth (delivery), 840–

Baby (babies) (*cont'd*)
846; *see also* Childbirth; "blue," 65, **548–551,** 876; bones, 31, 852, 868; bottle feeding, 855–857; breast feeding, 847–848, **853–855;** burping, 856, 857, 864; care of, planning, 850–852; clothing, 862; colds, 862, **863;** colic, **864,** 865; congenital defects and disorders, 874–880; danger signals and emergencies, 862–863; deformed, and drugs in pregnancy, 822–823; demand schedule of feeding, 853, 856; diapers, 860–861; diarrhea, 865; emotional conflicts, 774; examination at birth, Apgar rating scale, 842–843; foods, solid, 858, 864–865; hair, 409; head (skull), 27, 841, 844–845, 852, 857, 878; newborn nursery, 1004; parental relationships and, 849; plastic pants, 860–861; premature, 828–829, 897; Rh disease, *see* Rh disease and Rh factor; room for, 861; skin irritations, 859, 860, 865; sleeping, 861; sudden death syndrome, 897–898; thrush, 176, 647, 859, **863–864**
Baby fat, 852, 866, 867
Bacillary dysentery (shigellosis), 258–259, 312
Bacilli, 171
Back pain, *see* Low back pain
Bacteria, 170–172; bacilli, 171; cocci, 171; discovery of, 169–170; gram-negative and gram-positive, 170; spirochetes, 170, 171
Bacterial endocarditis, 558–560; acute (ABE) and subacute (SBE), 558
Bacterial folliculitis, 396–397
Bacteriology, 985–986; laboratory studies, 974
Bad breath (halitosis), 419, 420, 423
Bailey, Charles, 41, 563
Baker's cyst, 288
Balance, abnormalities, 347
Baldness (alopecia), **410–411,** 950–951
Banting, Frederick Grant, 72–73
Barbiturates: alcohol and, 342, 794; habitual use, 794–795; overdosage, 794; poisoning, 342
Bartholin's glands, 747, 753–754
Basal metabolism rate (BMR), 683, 692
"Baseball finger," 296–297
Basle, University, 8
Basophils, 707, 708
Bathing: baby, 858–859; in home nursing, 162–163
Battered child syndrome, 896–897
Beaumont, William, 84
Beck, Claude S., 38
Becquerel, Henri, 975
Bed: for baby, 862; for home nursing, 162
Bedbugs, 270
Bedsores (decubitus ulcers), 386–387
Bed-wetting (enuresis), 869–871

Beestings, 139–140; allergic reaction to, 139–140, **389**
Bee venom, 139
Bell's palsy, 344
Benadryl, 139
Benzedrine, 794
Beriberi, 574, 891
Berthold, Arnold, 682
Best, Charles Herbert, 72–73
Beta cells, 72, 661, 663, 683, 696, 703
Bile, 87, 611, 672; in jaundice, 665, 971
Bile duct, common, 611, 662, **672,** 674, 970
Bile ducts, 664, 665, 672, 676
Bile salts, 86, 664
Biliary colic (gall bladder attack), 673–674, 676
Biliary dyskinesia, 673
Biliary system: cancer, 676–677; disorders, 672; in pancreatitis, 662
Bilirubin, 672, 971
Biopsy, 447, 449, 980–981; for cancer, 448–449, **940–941;** frozen section, 940–941, 980
Birth, *see* Childbirth; Labor
Birth control, *see* Contraception
Birthmarks, 59, **400–401,** 896
Black Death (bubonic plague), 273–274
Black eye, 127, **429,** 534
Blackheads (comedones), 59, **394–395**
Black lung disease (anthracosis), 485, 487
Black water fever, 264
Black widow spider, 140
Bladder, urinary, *see* Urinary bladder
Bladder control, 869–871
Blalock, Alfred, 41
Blastomycosis, 276
Bleeding, control of, **104–107;** chest injuries, 468; direct pressure, 105–106; hemorrhage, 533–537, *see also* Hemorrhage; lacerations, 124, 125, 127; tourniquet, 105–106; wounds, 138
Blepharitis, 429
Blindness, 430–431, 433; congenital, from gonorrhea, 249, 880; corneal, 430; retrolental fibroplasia, 880–881
Blister, 58, **134,** 557
Blood, 20, **75–81,** 511–515; ammonia in, 669; arterial, 62, 543–544; in bowel movement, 538, 650, 658, 667, 940, 954; carbon dioxide in, 62, 63, 459–460; circulation, **80–81,** 83, 511–512; circulation, discovery of, 5, 8, 75, 81, 512, 583; clotting, 76, 78–79, 533; clotting disorders, 529–532; clotting test, 969–970; collateral circulation, 83; flow, adjustment of, 542–545; glucose in (blood sugar), 696–698, 702, 703; in kidneys, 65, 68, 69, 714–716; laboratory examinations, 732, **969–974;** loss, tolerance of, 534; from lungs, 538, 939; oxygen in, 76–77;

Blood (*cont'd*)
 oxygen exchange in lungs, 62, 82; proteins, 79, 512–513, 714, 717; sedimentation rate, 969; types, *see* Blood groups; in urine, 717, 720–725, 730–731; venous, 62, 543–544; vomiting (coffee-grounds vomit), 535, 538, 650, 954
Blood banks, 540–541
Blood cells, red (erythrocytes), 32, 76–78, 513–514; in anemia, 515–516, 518–521; count, 969; packed, 540; in polycythemia, 521–523; sedimentation rate, 969; in urine, 717, 720, 721, 723, 724, 730–731
Blood cells, white (leucocytes), 22, 32, 78, 97, 513, 514; agranulocytosis, 532; in anemia, 520; in appendicitis, 78, 639; count, 969; granulocytes, 514, 525, 969; in infections, 153, 172, 311; in leukemia, 78, 524–526, 969; lymphocytes, *see* Lymphocytes; monocytes, 514, 969; in urine, 720, 721
Blood count, complete, 969
Blood disorders, **515–532;** coagulation and clotting defects, 529–532; *see also* Anemia; Leukemia; other disorders
Blood donors, 540–541, 973
Blood groups, 77, **539–540;** typing, 972–974
Bloodletting, 681; in heart failure, 581; in polycythemia vera, 523
Blood platelets, 32, 78, 79, 513, 514, 524, 529, 530
Blood poisoning (sepsis, septicemia), 172, **206–208,** 515, 974
Blood pressure, 542–543, **582–584;** diastolic, 583; epinephrine and, 73; high, *see* Hypertension; low (hypotension), 584; normal and abnormal, 583–584; measurement, 582–583, 964; systolic, 583
Blood sugar (glucose), 696–698, 702, 703
Blood sugar test, 970
Blood transfusion, 75–78, **539–541;** aplastic anemia and, 520; blood groups, 540, 972–973; donors, 540–541, 973; exchange, 834, 973; hemolytic anemia and, 518, 519; in hemophilia, 531; hepatitis and, 540; reactions to, 540, 972; Rh factor and, 833–834, 973–974
"Blue babies," 65, **548–551,** 876
Blue Cross and Blue Shield programs, 1015–1017
Blushing, 59
Body: as energy-producing organism, 84–85; as functioning unit, 19–20; healing mechanism, 97; self-regulating mechanisms, 97–98
Body odor, 57, **413**
Boils, 61, **208,** 394; bacterial folliculitis, 396–397
Bologna, University, 8

Bone, 20, 23, **25–32,** 294; archaeological study of, 32; cells, 21–22; in detective work, 32; flat bones, 294; fractures, *see* Fractures; grafts, 302; growth and changes, 31–32, 868; long bones, 294; marrow, *see* Marrow; short bones, 294
Bone disorders, **304–309;** anemia in, 520; arthritis, *see* Arthritis; cancer, 306–307; infections, 32, 305; osteomyelitis, 27, 29, 209–210, **304–306;** osteoporosis, 309, 948; tuberculosis, 214, **305–306,** 328; tumors, benign, 306
Bottle feeding, 855–857; equipment, list, 856–857; formula, 857
Botulism, 219, **260–261**
Bowel control, 869
Bowels, *see* Colon; Intestine, small
Boy Scouts, 145
Brachial artery, 83
Brain, **42–47;** blood supply, 53; cerebellum, 44; cerebral cortex (gray matter), 45; cerebrum, 44–45; embryonic development, 58; frontal lobes, 45–46; ganglia, 45; hemisphere dominance, 46, 362; hemispheres, 43–46; hypothalamus, 45, 687; *see also* Pituitary gland; medulla oblongata, 43–44; meninges (meningeal membranes), 43, 46–47; midbrain, 43–44; nervous impulses in, 52; neuroglia (glial cells), 43; occipital lobes, 46; parietal lobes, 46; pineal gland, 46; pons, 43–44; prefrontal lobes, 45–46; structure and function, studies of, 49; temporal lobes, 46; thalamus, 45; ventricles, 47; visual cortex, 46; white matter, 45
Brain disorders, 46, 53; abscess, 209; alcoholism and, 371; cerebrovascular accidents, 342, **360–365,** 588; *see also* Stroke; congenital defects, 373, 375–377; convulsions, 342–343, **883–884;** examination, 349–351; fever and, 156; headache in, 339, 365, 366; Parkinson's disease, 45, 344, **365–366;** respiration and, 463; syphilitic (general paresis), 245, 345; tremor in, 345; tumors, 53, **366–367,** 368–369, 440, 463, 937; unconsciousness in, 342; *see also* Mental disorders
Brain fever, *see* Encephalitis
Brain injury, 46, **358–359;** amnesia and, 46; concussion, 297, 359
Brain stem, 43–45, 54
Breastbone (sternum), 457, 464
Breast disorders, 444, **446–450;** cancer, **446–450,** 940–942, 955; cancer symptoms, 939, 940; cystic disease (mammary dysplasia), 447; hypertrophy (abnormal enlargement), 446; mastitis, acute, 446–447; tumors, benign, 447–448
Breast feeding, 847–848, **853–855**

Breast pump, 854
Breasts, **444–452;** development in puberty, 444–445; as erogenous zones in nursing, 854–855; mammography, 449, 940, 978; milk, 847, 848, 853–854, 864, 892; normal changes, 444–445; in pregnancy, 445, 817, 830; self-examination, **450–451,** 939, 967
Breast surgery: biopsy, 447, 449, **940–941;** cosmetic, 451–452; mastectomy, radical, 449; mastectomy, simple, 447; silastic implants, 447, 452
Breathing, 457, 459–460; control of, 459–460; *see also* Dyspnea; Respiration
Breathing devices, positive pressure, 121
Bright, Richard, 723
Bright's disease, 723
Broca, Pierre Paul, 49
Bronchi, 63, 457, 460, 461; choking, 64, 469; drainage, 953; obstruction, 64, 469–470; washing, 980
Bronchial asthma, 468, **491–494;** *see also* Asthma
Bronchial pneumonia (bronchiolar), 64, 217, 482
Bronchiectasis, 64, 457, **476–477,** 478–479, 495, 895, 896, 952
Bronchioles, 63, 64, 457, 460, 461, 476–477
Bronchitis, 64, 470, **475–476;** acute, 475–476; chronic, 475, 476, 494–495; emphysema and, 494–495; 952; virus, 228; whooping cough and, 187
Bronchogenic carcinoma, 498, 503, 504
Bronchopleural fistula, 484
Bronchoscope, 121, 470, 504, 980
Brucellosis (undulant fever), 275
Bruises, 127
Buboes, 250, 273
Bubonic plague, 273–274, 874
Buerger's disease (thromboangiitis obliterans), 565
Bulla, 403
Bullous emphysema (disappearing lung disease), 64, **494–497**
Bunion, 322–323
Burns, 61, **119–122;** electrical, 118; emergency care, 119–120; esophageal, 615; gastric, 630; hospital treatment, 121–122
Bursa, 310, 322
Bursitis, 311, **322**

Caesarean section, 756, 831, 832, 834, 835, 844, 845, **846,** 847, 997
Calamine lotion, 139, 142
Calcium: in bone, 26–27, 31–32; deficiency, 890; in gallstones, 672; in kidney stones, 718, 719; in parathyroid disorders, 694–695
Calluses, 386
Calories, 928

Camping, minimal pack equipment, 137

Cancer, **936–943**; adenocarcinoma, 448, 938; anemia in, 521, 657; basal-cell carcinoma, 405–406; biopsy for, 498–499, **940–941**; of bone, 306–307; in brain, metastatic, 367; of breast, **446–450**, 939–942, 955; bronchogenic carcinoma, 498, 503, 504; cells in, 93, 937–938; of cervix, 754–755, 966; in children, 896; of colon, 657–659; danger signs, 939–940; diagnosis, 940–941; of digestive system, 613, **655–659**; drug therapy for, 505, 520, 523, 528, 942; of esophagus, 657; of female genital system, 96, **754–759**; of gall bladder, 676–677; growth of, 937–939; of kidney, 730–731; of larynx, 475, **499–500**; leukemia, *see* Leukemia; of lip, 499; of liver, 665, **669**; of lung, 367, 457, **500–507**, 924, 939; lymphosarcoma, 527–528; of male genital system, 740–741; menopause and, 935; metastasis of, 937–938; of mouth, **499**, 657; of muscle, 292; of ovaries, 758–759; of pancreas, 87, 567, **664**, 676; Pap test for, 754–755, 966, 980; peptic ulcer associated with, 650, 651, 655, 657; primary and secondary lesions, 938; of prostate, 411, **741**, 942, 955; from radiation injury, 975; radiation treatment, 499, 500, 505, 507, 730, 740, 755, 757, 759, 941–942, 979; of rectum, 645, **658–659**; research on, 942; of respiratory tract, 498–500; sarcoma, 938; *see also* Sarcoma; skin, *see* Skin cancer; smoking and, 406, 457, 504, 505, 924, 977; squamous-cell (epithelial) carcinoma, 405–406, 938; of stomach, 631, 650, 651, **655–657**; symptoms, warning signs, 939–940; of throat, 499–500; of thyroid, 693; treatment, general, 941–942; of urinary system, 730–731; of uterus, 754–757, 820, 966

Candida albicans, 176, 647, 753, 863–864

Cannabis sativa, 795

Capillaries, 77, 79, 81, 543; in digestive system, 86, 87, 90; in kidneys, 68; in liver, 90; in lungs, 63, 460; peripheral capillary bed, 76; in portal circulation system, 83; in skin, 59

Carbohydrates, **888–889**; in diet, 929; digestion of, 86; metabolism in diabetes, 696–697, 702

Carbon dioxide, 79; in blood, 62, 63, 459–460; deficiency (respiratory alkalosis), 63–64; in lungs, 63–64; in respiration, 455–456, 459–461

Carbonic anhydrase, 460

Carbon monoxide poisoning, 65, **115–116,** 342

Carbon tetrachloride poisoning, 668, 800

Carbuncle, 209

Carcinoma, *see* Cancer

Cardiac arrest, 38–39, **110–111,** 114

Cardiac catheterization, 554, 555

Cardiac compression, external, **110–111,** 114, 116, 118, 468

Cardiac defibrillator (shock box), 38–39, 121

Cardiac output, 573

Cardiac sphincter, 611; spasm (cardiospasm), 615–616

Cardiac tamponade, 564

Cardiac valves, *see* Heart valves

Cardiologist, 992, 994

Cardiorespiratory system, 461

Cardiospasm, 615–616

Cardiovascular system, 23, **75–83,** 511–512; in respiration, 455–456, 460–461; *see also* Blood; Circulatory system; Heart

Cardiovascular system disorders, 83, **511–605;** aging and, 953–954; blood, 515–532; congenital abnormalities of great vessels, 545–549; inflammatory diseases, 556–558, 564–572; shunts, arteriovenous, 546, 548; *see also* Heart disorders; names of disorders

Carditis, meningococcal, 560

Caries, 419–420

Carotene, 891

Carotid artery, 110; bleeding from, 104–105; common, 83

Carotid endarterectomy, 362

Carotid plexus, 544

Carpal bones, 296

Cartilage, 25, 27, 31, 294, 310; of knee, 321; in osteoarthritis, 317–318

Carville, La., hospital for leprosy, 272

Cataracts, **430,** 699, 951

Catheter, in-dwelling, 160

Catheterization, cardiac, 554, 555

Caucasoid race, skin and hair, 57, 60

Cauda equina, 47

Cecum, 612

Celiac syndrome (celiac disease), 628, **893–894**

Cells, **20–22;** in cancer, 93, 937–938; division and reproduction, **92–95,** 937; haploid, 94, 95; structure, 21; wall, 21

Cellulitis, 172, **206–208**

Central nervous system, **42–47;** *see also* Brain; Spinal cord

Cerebellum, 44

Cerebral angiogram, 350, 365, 979

Cerebral arteries: atherosclerosis 593; obstruction, 53, 360, 361

Cerebral cortex, 45

Cerebral hemorrhage, 588; *see also* Cerebrovascular accidents

Cerebral palsy, 293, 344, **882–883**

Cerebral thrombosis, 360, 361

Cerebral ventriculogram, 351

Cerebrospinal fluid, 972

Cerebrovascular accidents, 342, **360–365,** 588; stroke, 53, 115, 156, **360–364,** 532, 588, 593, 950; subarachnoid hemorrhage, 364–365; subdural hematoma, 365, 882

Cerebrum, 44–45

Cervical canal, 746

Cervical nerves, 48

Cervical rib, 458

Cervicitis, 754

Cervix of uterus, 746, 749, 750, 752, 754, 918; cancer, 754–755, 966; in childbirth, 829, 836, 837; physical examination, 966; in pregnancy, 831

Cesarean section, *see* Caesarean section

Cestoda, 177

Chafing (intertrigo), 385

Chagas' disease, 278

Chalazion, 430

Chancre, 244–245

Chancroid, 250

Chapping, 386

Charcot joint, 322

Charity institutions and services, 1014–1015

Charley horse, 38, 131, **284**

Chemical peritonitis, 644

Chemical pneumonia, 218, **487–488**

Chemicals: anemia from, 520; skin irritation from, 556

Chemoreceptors, 440

Chest injuries, **464–465, 468;** first aid, 468; flail chest, 297, 465; fractures, 464–465; *see also* Fractures, ribs; medical treatment, 468; respiration and, 462

Chest wounds, penetrating, **125–126,** 138, 465, 468

Chest X-ray, 213, 214, 504, 505, 578, 939, **977,** 980

Chewing, 610–611

Chicken pox (varicella), **182–183,** 471

Chiggers (harvest mites, redbugs), 269; typhus carried by, 238–239

Chilblain, 384

Childbed fever, 207, **753,** 847

Childbirth, **834–846;** arm or shoulder presentation, 844; breech presentation, 843–844; Caesarean section, 756, 831, 832, 834, 835, 844, 845, **846,** 847, 997; complications, 843–846; delivery, 840–846; face presentation, 844; forceps in, 842; hemorrhage in, 39, 831, 846; hospital arrangements, 830, 837, 848; natural, 839–840; post-partum period, 846–847; premature, 828–829, 897; preparations for, 830; stillbirth, 828–829; transverse presentation, 844; *see also* Labor

Childhood diseases, **191–203;** preventable, 185–190

"Childhood rash" diseases, **178–184,** 471; chicken pox, **182–183,** 471; measles-type, 178–182; *see also*

"Childhood rash diseases (*cont'd*)
German measles; Measles; roseola
infantum, 181; scarlet fever, **183–
184,** 471
Children, **867–898;** baby, new, as
problem, 849, 866; battered child
syndrome, 896–897; bone growth,
31, 868; congenital abnormalities
of great vessels, 545–549; congenital disorders, 874–880; congenital heart malformations, 65,
82–83, **549–555;** discipline and permissiveness with, 871–872; emotional conflicts, 774–775; emotional
development, 870–872; growth and
development, physical, 867–870;
home nursing care, 158–159; immunizations (table), 873–874; intestinal absorption disorders, 893–
896; mental health, 806–807; nutrition and nutritional disorders, 887–
893; parental responsibility for,
915–917; punishment of, 871, 897;
sexual curiosity, 872; sibling rivalry,
870; toilet training, 869; vitamin
deficiency disorders, 891–893
Chills, fever and, 149
Chiropractic, 330–331
Chloasma, 400
Chlorine gas, 487
Chlorine in water, 487
Choking, 64, 107, **114,** 469
Cholangiogram, operative, 674, 675,
978
Cholecystectomy, 90, 672, 674
Cholecystitis, 672, 676
Cholelithiasis (gallstones), 90, 662,
670–676
Cholera, **258,** 621; immunization, 258,
874
Cholesterol, 592, 664, 889; in athero-
sclerosis, 604; in gallstones, 672
Choline, 666, 889
Cholinesterase, 52, 54
Chondrodystrophy (achondroplasia),
307–308, 708
Chondrosarcoma, 307
Chordae tendineae, 561
Chorea: Huntington's, 373; in rheu-
matic fever (Sydenham's), 45, 344
Chorioepithelioma: of testes, 740; of
uterus, 756–757, 820
Chorionic gonadotrophin, 689, 813
Chromosomes, 21, 94, 95; Phila-
delphia (Ph₁) in leukemia, 525;
typing, sex determination by, 750
Chymotrypsin, 85–86
Cigarettes, *see* Smoking
Cilia, 457, 746
Cimex lectularius (bedbug), 270
Circle of Willis, 83
Circulatory failure, 103–104, **110–111,**
external cardiac compression, **110–
111,** 114, 116, 118, 468; heart-lung
resuscitation, 111
Circulatory system, **75–83,** 511–512;
blood flow, 542–545; portal, 664–

Circulatory system (*cont'd*)
665; pulmonary, 62, 82, 461, 511;
in respiration, 455–456, 460–461;
see also Cardiovascular system;
Heart
Circumcision, 736, **737,** 738, 848–849,
859–860
Cirrhosis, 90, 569, **666–668,** 669; al-
coholism and, 90, 666–667, 791;
obstructive (biliary), 668; post-
hepatitis, 202, 668; toxic, 668;
treatment, 667–668
Claustrophobia, 780
Clawtoe (hammertoe), 323
Cleft palate, 441, 875
Clinics, group practice, 1009
Clitoris, 747
Clostridium, 171, 219
Clostridium botulinum, 260
Clostridium perfringens, 221
Clostridium tetani, 219
Clubbing of fingers and toes, 477, 522
Clubfoot, 878
Coarctation of aorta, 547
Cobalt, radioactive, cancer therapy,
941
Cocaine, 793, 797, 798
Cocci, 171
Coccidioidomycosis, 276
Coccygeal nerves, 48
Cochlea, 434, 435
Codeine, 798
Coitus interruptus, 918
Colchicine, 320
Cold, common, **225–228,** 470–471; of
the aged, 948; air passages in, 64;
of babies, 862, 863; treatment, 226–
227; vaccine (cold shots), 227, 948
Cold sore (herpes simplex), 230–231
Colic, **864,** 865
Colitis, ulcerative, **634–638,** 644
Collagen, 560, 561
Collagen diseases, 40–41, 291, 313,
403, 560, 567
Collarbone, fracture, 297, 464, 465
Collip, James Bertram, 72–73
Colon, 86, 88, 609, 610, 612; cancer,
657–659; congenital defects, 877;
congenital megacolon, 86, 89, 622;
diverticulitis, 640, **642–644;** irritable
(spastic), 623–624; motility disorders, 621–624; muscles, 39;
proctoscopic examination, 966;
rectocele, 751; surgery, 637–638;
ulcerative colitis, **634–638,** 644
Colostrum, 445, 847
Coma, 115, 341; diabetic, 103, 114–
115, 342, **698–699;** hepatic, 668–
669
Comedones (blackheads), 59, **394–
395**
Common bile duct, 611, 662, **672,**
674, 970
Common cold, *see* Cold, common
Compensation (defense mechanism),
776

Computers: as diagnostic aids, 968,
971–972, 983; nervous system compared to, 42
Conception (fertilization), 94, **747–
748,** 811–812
Concussion, 297, **359**
Condylomata acuminata, 398
Congenital disorders, **874–880;** of
brain and nervous system, 373–377;
of cardiovascular system, 545–549;
of digestive system, 876–878; of
female genital system, 749–752; of
heart, 65, 82–83, **549–555,** 876; of
kidneys, 729; of male genital system, 736–738
Congenital fibrocystic disease of pancreas, 661
Congenital hemolytic jaundice, 519–
520
Congenital megacolon, 86, 89, 622
Conjunctiva, 425, 429, 430
Conjunctivitis, acute (pinkeye), **205–
206,** 429
Connective tissue, 20, 23, 33, 40–41;
cells, 22; disorders, 40–41, **403–405;**
in nervous system, 49
Constipation, **622–623;** hypertonic
(irritable colon), 623–624; mistaken ideas on, 614, 622, in pregnancy, 824, 827; rectocele and, 751
Contact lenses, 432–433
Contraception, **917–921;** coitus inter-
ruptus, 918; condom, 918; dia-
phragm, 918–919; intrauterine
device (IUD), 919; Pill, *see* Pill,
the; rhythm method, 917–918;
spermicidal preparations, 918–919;
sterilization, 920–921
Contracture, muscular, 283
Contusions, 124, **127–128**
Conversion reaction (conversion hys-
teria), 781
Convulsions, febrile, **151–152,** 885
Convulsive disorders, 115, 342–343,
883–887; *see also* Epilepsy
Cornea, 426, 428, 429
Corneal blindness, 430
Corneal transplant, 430
Corneal ulcer, 428
Corns, 386
Coronary arteries, 82; infarction, 39,
82; surgery, 600, 605
Coronary artery disease, 588, **594–
605;** angina pectoris in, 593, **595–
597, 600;** atherosclerosis, 594–596,
598–599; treatment, experiments in,
605
Coronary insufficiency, **595,** 600
Coronary occlusion, 114, 600
Coronary thrombosis (heart attack),
103, 532, 588, 592, 593, 596, **600–
604,** 943; acute coronary care unit,
603; early knowledge of, 4, 19; occurrence, factors in, 600; prevention, 603; symptoms, 601; treatment, 602–603
Corpus luteum cyst, 758

Corticosteroids, 41, 73, 404, **684–685,** 704; for Addison's disease, 704–705; allergies and, 388; hair growth and, 410; for Hodgkin's disease, 528; for leukemia, 526; for rheumatic fever, 73, 562; for rheumatoid arthritis, 73, 316; synthetic, 73

Cortisone, 41, 73, **685,** 704, 705; for thrombocytopenic purpura, 530

Cortisone-like hormones, 705, 706; for allergies, 391–392, 491, 493; for rheumatic fever, 562; for skin disorders, 395, 402, 403; for ulcerative colitis, 637

Corynebacterium diphtheriae, 171, 185, 471, 560

Cosmetics, allergy to, 390, 413–414

Cosmetic surgery, 951

Cost of medical care, *see* Medical costs

Coué, Émile, 681

Coughing, 64; as cancer symptom, warning, 939; mechanism of, 462

Cough syrups, 226–228

Cradle cap, 859

Cranial nerves, 44, 47–48, 347, 425, 967

Craniostenosis, 878

Cretinism, 376, 683, 691, 693

Crohn's disease (regional enteritis), 632–634

Cross eyes, 427, 852

Croup (acute laryngotracheobronchitis), 477, 480

Cryptorchidism (undescended testicles), **737–738,** 875

Curare, 54

Cushing's syndrome, 392, **705–706,** 708

Cutaneous system, 55–61; *see also* Skin

Cuts (lacerations), 124–127

Cyanide poisoning, 65

Cyanocobalamin, *see* Vitamin B₁₂

Cyanosis, 215; of babies, 548, 549

Cycloid personality, 786–787, 804

Cystic disease of breast (mammary dysplasia), 447

Cystic duct, 669, 672, 674

Cystic fibrosis of pancreas, 661, 877, **893–896**

Cystic tumors of ovary, 758

Cystitis, **721–723,** 731, 826

Cystocele, 722, 751, 948

Cystoscope, 719, 731, 733

Cysts: ovarian, 757–759; sebaceous, 394, 401

D and C (dilatation and curettage of uterus), 721, 753, **754–755,** 756–758, 760, 820, 922

Dandruff (seborrheic dermatitis), 58, **411–412,** 429

Darwin, Charles, 95

DDT, poisoning by, 520

Deafness, 438–439; conductive, 438; congenital, 438–439; perceptive, 439

Death, 945, **957–958;** sudden death syndrome, 897–898

Decortication of lung, 482

Decubitus ulcers (bedsores), 386–387

Defense mechanisms, **775–777,** 778–779

Defibrillator, cardiac (shock box), 38–39, 121

Dehydration, 621, 622, 728, **887–888;** control of, 155; polycythemia and, 521

Delirium tremens, 371, 790

Delusions, 800, 801

Dementia praecox, *see* Schizophrenia

Demerol (meperidine), 798

Demyelinating diseases, 54

Dengue fever, 236–237

Denis, Jean Baptiste, 77

Dental care and treatment, **418–423;** of adults, 924; in childhood, 868

Dentures, 421, 951

Deoxyribonucleic acid (DNA), **93–94,** 174, 525

Depilatories, 410

Depressive reaction, 780–781, **935–936**

Dermabrasion, 396

Dermatitis, 61; contact, 390; eczematous, 389–390; neurodermatitis, 393; seborrheic (dandruff), 58, **411–412,** 429

Dermatologist, 992

Dermatology, 381

Dermatomyositis, 61, **291–292**

Dermis, 59

De Vries, Hugo, 95

Dexedrine, 794

Dextran, 539

Diabetes (diabetes mellitus), 87, **696–703;** acidosis in, 79, 698, 699; adult, 72, 699; atherosclerosis and, 594, 698; blood sugar test, 970; brittle diabetics, 700–701; carcinoma of pancreas and, 87; in Cushing's syndrome, 706; glucose in urine, 68, 696–698; heredity of, 96, 661, 696; insulin production and, 696–700; insulin shock, 103, 360, 663, **700–701,** 703; insulin treatment, 72–73; 699–702; juvenile, 72, 699–701; medication, substitutes for insulin, 702; nephrotic syndrome in, 727; occurrence, 696; in pregnancy, 701–702, 826; primary, 661; secondary (sugar diabetes), 661; symptoms, 698–699; xanthoma in, 392

Diabetes insipidus, 709

Diabetic coma, 103, 114–115, 342, **698–699**

Diagnostic aids, **968–982;** laboratory studies, 968–975; special examinations, 980; therapeutic trial, 981; X-rays, 975–979; *see also* Laboratory studies; X-rays, diagnostic

Diagnostician, 992

Dial 911, emergency service, 123

Dialysis, 726

Diaper rash, 860, 861

Diapers, 860–861

Diaphragm: muscle, 39; in respiration, 459

Diaphragm (contraceptive), 918–919

Diaphragmatic hernia (hiatus hernia), **616–619,** 650–651

Diarrhea, **621–622;** infantile, 865; suppressant medicines, 621–622; travelers', **255–256,** 621

Diet: aging and, 951, 953, 954; fads and crash diets, 928–929; in pregnancy, 825; for weight control, 928–930; *see also* Weight control

Digestion, **84–91,** 610–612

Digestive juices, 86, 87, 610, 611, 613, 616, 620, 660, 661; in peptic ulcer, 648–649, 651, 654

Digestive system, 609–612

Digestive system disorders, 87, **612–647;** aging and, 954; cancer, *see* Cancer; congenital, 876–878; gastritis, 630–632; gastroenteritis, 253–256; infections, bacterial and parasitic, 253–261; intestinal, *see* Intestinal disorders; malabsorption, 613, 627–629, 893–896; motility, 614–624; obstructive, 624–627; in pernicious anemia, 516, 517; psychosomatic and emotional aspects, 613–614, 623, 629, 632, 634–635, 637, 784–785; *see also* names of disorders

Digitalis: for heart disease, 82, **578–579,** 581; poisoning from plant, 143

Digitoxin, 578–579

Dilantin (diphenylhydantoin), 886

Dilatation and curettement, *see* D and C

Dilaudid (dihydromorphinone), 798

Diphtheria, **185–186,** 471, 473; bacteria in, 172; immunization (DPT vaccine), **186–188,** 221, 873–874; Schick test, 186

Diphtheria myocarditis, 560

Diplococcus pneumoniae, 215, 482

Diplopia, 290, 426–427

Disappearing lung disease (bullous emphysema), 64, **495–497**

Dislocations, 295, **303–304;** finger, 296–297; first aid, 130; hip, 303–304; hip, congenital, 309

Dissociative reaction, 781

Diuresis, 578

Diuretics, 578, 580, 591, 709, 717, 825, 832

Diverticulitis, 640, **642–644**

Dizziness (vertigo), **345,** 435, 437

DNA (deoxyribonucleic acid), **93–94,** 174, 525

Doctors: death of patient, decisions on, 957–958; in early 20th century, 12–13; general practitioners, 991, 992, 999–1000; government medical programs opposed, 1019; group practice, 1009; in hospitals, 984, 992, 993, 1005; modern, 13–14;

Doctors (*cont'd*)
  patient's relationship with, 961–963, 967, 983; payment for services, *see* Medical costs; specialists in teaching and research, 998–999; training, 983–998; *see also* Medical education
Dog bites, 141–142; rabies from, 141–142, **239–241**
Dogs: *Ascaris* infection, 266; fleas, 269; ticks, 238
Dolophine (methadone), 798, 799
Dorsal horn cells, 245
Down's syndrome (mongolism), 96, 376, 377, **879–880**
DPT vaccine (diphtheria, pertussis, tetanus), **186–188**, 221, 873–874
Dracunculiasis, 277–278
Dramamine, 135, 256, 345, 437
Drinking, *see* Alcohol
Dropsy, *see* Edema
Drug abuse, **793–800**; amphetamines, 794; barbiturates, 794–795; combinations of drugs, 794, 795; depressant drugs, 794; hallucinogenic drugs, **795–797**, 807; LSD, 797; marijuana, 795–796; narcotics, addictive, 793, 794, **797–799**; serum hepatitis and, 203; stimulating drugs, 794; therapy, 799; withdrawal symptoms, 343–345, 798
Drugs (medicinal): agranulocytosis from, 532; allergy to, 390–391; anemia from, 32; liver damage from, 668; as poisons, 800, 863; in pregnancy, and deformed babies, 822–823; storage and disposal of, 165
Ductus arteriosus, 546–548; patent, **546–547**, 552
Dumping syndrome, 654
Duodenum, 85, 87, 611, 620, 665; cancer, 657; functions, 660; ulcer, *see* Peptic ulcer
Dura mater, 46–47
Dwarfism: achondroplasia, **307–308**, 708; pituitary (midget), 308, 708
Dysentery: amebic, 259–260; bacillary, 258–259, 312; traveler's, **255–256**, 621
Dysmenorrhea, 761
Dyspareunia, 764
Dyspnea (difficult breathing): in heart failure, 574, 576; orthopnea, 576; paroxysmal nocturnal, 576
Dystocia, 844
Dysuria, 722

Earache: otitis media, **196–197**, 437, 471; treatment, 134–135
Ear disorders, **435–439**; aging and, 952; congenital hearing defect, 878; deafness and hearing loss, **438–439**, 952; infections, **196–197**, 436–437; physical abnormalities, 435–436; ringing (tinnitus), 437
Eardrum (tympanic membrane), 434; ruptured, 196, **436**

Ears, **433–439**; care of, 439; foreign bodies in, **132**, 436; physical examination, 963; piercing for earrings, 439; structure and function, 433–435; wax in, 434–436, 438, 439
Ebers, Georg Moritz, Papyrus, 4–5
Ecchymosis (black-and-blue mark), 127–128, 284
Eclampsia, 832
Ectoderm, 22, 58
Ectopic pregnancy, *see* Tubal pregnancy
Eczema (eczematous dermatitis), 389–390; infantile, 865
EDC (expected date of confinement), 815
Edema (swelling), 79, 82; in glomerulonephritis, 723, 724; in heart disease, 576, 578; in myxedema, 691; in nephrotic syndrome, 727; in pregnancy, 824, 832; premenstrual, 762
Ego, **774**, 778
Ehrlich, Paul, 247
Eisenmenger's complex, 551
Ejaculatory duct, 735
Elbow: "funny bone," 50; joint, 30–31
Electrical appliances, safety, 118
Electrical shock, 117–119; *see also* Electroshock therapy
Electrocardiogram (EKG), 578, 596–597, **974–975**; in coronary thrombosis, 601–602
Electroencephalogram, 349
Electrolysis, 410
Electrolytes, 714; in plasma, 79, 512
Electroshock therapy, 360, 783, **803**, 805, 936
Elks Therapy Program for Children, 331
Embolus (emboli), 83, 532; bacterial, 558–559; pulmonary, 65, 83, 532, 567; stroke and, 361, 532
Embryo, 95, 812, **815–816**, 818; development, 22, 58; implantation, 812
Embryonal rests: in ovary, 758; in scrotum, 740
Emergencies, **124–147**; animal bites, 141–142; of babies, 862–863; burns, 119–122; carbon monoxide intoxication, 115–116; chest wounds, penetrating, **125–126**, 138, 465, 468; circulatory failure, 103–104, **110–111**; dislocations, sprains, and strains, 130–131; dog bites, 141–142; do's and don'ts, 144–145; electrical shock, 117–119; exposure, 137–138; foreign bodies, 131–133; fractures, 128–130; frostbite, 136–137; heat exhaustion, 135–136; hemorrhage, 103, **104–107**, 533–539; hospital treatment, 120–122; insect bites and stings, 139–140; lacerations, abrasions, and contusions, 124–128; minor, 133–135; order of priority in treatment, **103–104**, 144; plant poisons, 142–143; poisoning,

Emergencies (*cont'd*)
  116–117; radiation injuries, 143–144, respiratory failure, 103–104, **107–111**; serious, 103–123; shock, 103–104, **111–113**; snakebites, 140–141; sunstroke, 136; trench foot, 137; wounds, **124–127**, 138
Emergency services, 122–123, 146
Emergency telephone numbers, 146
Emetics, 116–117
Emotional disorders, **769–777**; anxiety, **771–774**, 778, 779; conflict, life stages, 774–775; defense mechanisms, 775–777; depressive reaction, 780–781, **935–936**; *see also* Mental disorders
Emotional problems (tension), 769, 774–775; in adolescence, 775, 901–902; allergies and, 388, 490, 493; in digestive disorders, 613–614, 623–624, 629, 632, 634–635, 637, 784–785; hypertension and, 588, 590–591, 784; in marriage, 912; in menopause, 934; muscular disorders and, 286–287, 784; peptic ulcer and, 613, 649–650, 654–655; premenstrual tension, **762–763**, 923, 934; skin disorders and, 388, 393, 784
Emphysema, pulmonary, 64, 463, 476, 485, **494–495**, 896, 952; bullous (disappearing lung disease), 64, **495–497**; whooping cough and, 187
Empyema, 465, 482–484
Encephalitis (brain fever), 885; measles and, 180; in mononucleosis, 198; mumps, 192–193; tic and, 344; viral, 53
Endarteritis, 557
Endocarditis, 557; bacterial, 558–560
Endocardium, 557–558
Endocrine gland disorders, 74, **690–709**; adrenal, 704–707; in childhood, 868; parathyroid, 694–696; pituitary, 707–709; thyroid, 690–694; *see also* separate entries, e.g., Thyroid gland disorders; names of disorders
Endocrine glands, 69–74, **681–689**; adrenals, 73, **684–685**; gonads, 73, 93–96, **685–686**, 734; hormones, *see* Hormones; parathyroid, 683, **694–696**; pineal, 46, **689**; pituitary, 45, 73–74, **686–689**; thymus, 290–291, **689**; thyroid, 69, 72, **682–683**; *see also* Endocrine gland disorders *and* separate entries, e.g., Thyroid gland
Endocrinologist, 992
Endocrinology, 682, 706
Endoderm, 22, 58
Endometriosis, 759–761
Endometrium, 746, 748; cancer, 756; in menstruation, 748, 812–813
Enema: in abdominal pain, warning on, 641; Fleet, 135, 641; oil retention, 623
Enteritis, regional, 632–634

Enterobius vermicularis, 266
Enuresis (bed-wetting), 869–871
Enzymes, 660–661, 715, 888; in digestion, 85–87, 90; "intrinsic factor," 517
Ephedrine, 226, 535
Epidermis, 58
Epididymis, 735
Epididymitis, acute, 738
Epiglottis, 456, 611
Epilepsy, 342–343, **883–887;** early knowledge of, 4, 19; first aid, 887; grand mal, 342, 343, 360, **883–884,** 886, 887; idiopathic, 343, 885; Jacksonian seizure, 342–343, 884; petit mal, 342, 884, 886; psychomotor seizure, 342, 884, 886; status epilepticus, 884
Epinephrine (adrenalin), 73, 492–493, **684,** 704, 706–707
Episiotomy, 842, 843
Epispadias, 737
Epithelioma (epithelial carcinoma), 405–406, 938
Epithelium (epithelial tissue), 20, 23, 62; in blood vessels, 81; cells, 22; in digestive system, 86–87; in endocrine glands, 69, 72, 74; exchange function, 62, 65, 81; filtration function, 65, 68; in intestines, 86–87; in kidneys, 65, 68; in lungs, 62–65; secretion function, 69; in skin, 58
Equilibrium: control of, 44; disorders of, 437–438
Erectile tissue, 736
Erection of penis, 736, 737; impotence, 743–744; priapism, 741
Ergostrate, 843
Erysipelas, 206
Erythema nodosum, 405
Erythroblastosis fetalis (Rh disease), 514, 828, **833–834,** 882, 973
Erythroblasts, 513–514
Erythrocytes, *see* Blood cells, red
Eskimos, 60, 214
Esophageal atresia, 615
Esophageal hernia (hiatus hernia), **616–619,** 650–651
Esophageal spasm, 615
Esophageal varices, 81, 569, **572,** 667
Esophagoscopy, 617, 657
Esophagus, 85, 456, 610, 611, 615–617; burns, 615, 630; cancer, 657; foreign bodies in, 133, 977; muscles, 38; in poisoning, hospital treatment, 121
Esters, 90
Estradiol, 685
Estriol, 685
Estrogen (estrogens), 395, **685–686,** 747–748, 760, 812; breast development and, 444, 446; in cancer, 448, 450, 942, 955; in menopause, 934
Estrone, 685
Estrus, 734
Eustachian tubes, 196, 197, **434,** 438
Ewing's sarcoma, 307

Exanthem subitum (roseola infantum), 181
Exercise: myositis caused by, 39, 131, **284–286;** overexertion and, 931–933; programs of, 286, 932–933, 949
Exhibitionism, 789
Exophthalmic goiter, 690, 691
Exotoxin, 185
Expected date of confinement (EDC), 815
Expectorants, 64, 187, 227
Exposure, 137–138
Extended care facilities, 163–164, 1008–1009
External cardiac compression, **110–111,** 114, 116, 118, 468
Extracellular fluid space, 80
Extraocular muscles, 425, 427
Eye banks, 430
Eye disorders, **427–431;** acute conjunctivitis (pinkeye), **205–206,** 429; black eye, 127, **429,** 534; cataracts, **430,** 699, 951; corneal blindness, 430; in diabetes, 699; flashburn, 382, **428–429;** glaucoma, **430–431,** 951; gonorrhea, babies' eyes protected from, 249, 842, 880; in herpes simplex, 231; in herpes zoster, 206, 430; in hypertension, 585, 588; infections, 429–430; injuries, 428–429; in myasthenia gravis, 290; retinal detachment, 431, 881; retinoblastoma, 431, 896; retrolental fibroplasia, 880–881; scleral hemorrhage, 535–536; snow blindness, 382, 428–429; structural defects, 427–428; trachoma, **232,** 429; tumors, 431; of vision, 346, **426–427;** vitamin A deficiency and, 891
Eyedrops, 432
Eyeglasses, 431–432, 925
Eyes, 50, **424–433;** aging and, 951; of baby, 852; brain and nerves in control of, 44, 46; care, 431–433, 925; foreign bodies in, **132,** 428; injuries, 428–429; nervous system injuries, 53; physical examination, 963–964; structure and function, 425–427; tests for hay fever, 491
Eyestrain, 431–432

Facial nerves, 44, 347
Fainting, 115, **341,** 584
Faith healing, 331
Fallopian tubes, 640, **746–747,** 748, 811; abnormalities, 749; cysts, 758; pregnancy in, *see* Tubal pregnancy; tubal ligation, 920–921
Fallot, tetralogy of, 549–550
Familial spastic paralysis, 375
Family planning, 916, 917; *see also* Contraception
Fascia, 40
Fats, 86, **889–890;** in body, 889; in diet, 929; polyunsaturated, 890; saturated and unsaturated, 889–890

Fatty acids, 86, 90
Febrile convulsions, **151–152,** 885
Fecal impaction, 623
Feet, *see* Foot
Felon, 126, **207**
Femoral artery, 83, 104–105, 110
Femoral nerve, 48
Femur, 27; fractures, 26, 34–35
Fertilization, *see* Ova, fertilization
Fetishism, 789
Fetus: bone formation, 31; cardiovascular system, 545–546; development, 22, 816–817, 824; heartbeat, 824; movements, 824
Fever, **148–156;** chills and, 149; control of, 154–156; crisis, 149, 216; home nursing care, 158; inflammation and, 557; persistent, as cancer symptom, 940; recurring low-grade, 153, 940; of unknown origin (FUO), **153–154,** 558
Fever blister (herpes simplex), 230–231
Fibrillation, 38, 121, 601; auricular, 579; ventricular, 118, 121
Fibrin, 79, 287
Fibrinogen, 79, 531
Fibroadenoma of breast, 447–448
Fibroblast, 557
Fibroid tumors, 292; of uterus, 755–757
Fibrosarcoma, 292
Fibrositis, 286–287
Fibrothorax, 465
Fiedler's myocarditis, 564
Filariasis, 277
Fingernails, *see* Nails
Fingers: dislocations, 296–297; felon, 126; fractures, 296–297; joints, 30; lacerations, 125; numbness, 346
Finlay, Carlos Juan, 235
First aid, **103–147;** artificial respiration, **107–110,** 111, 113, 114, 116, 118, 129, 461, 468; books (manuals), 145; burns, 119–120; carbon monoxide poisoning, 115–116; chest injuries, 468; circulatory failure, 103–104, **110–111;** dislocations, 130; do's and don'ts in, 144–145; electrical shock, 117–119; epilepsy, 887; external cardiac compression, **110–111,** 114, 116, 118, 468; fractures, **128–130,** 300; heart-lung resuscitation, **111,** 118; heat exhaustion, 135–136; hemorrhage, 103, **104–107;** lacerations, 124–127; order of priority in, **103–104,** 144; poisoning, 116–117; respiratory failure, 103–104, **107–111;** shock, 103–104, **111–113;** snakebites, 140–141; sprains, 130–131; strains, 131; sunstroke, 136; training programs, 145; unconsciousness, 113–115; wounds, **124–127,** 138
First-aid kit, 145–146
Fish hook in skin, 126

Fistulas, 209; arteriovenous, 878; in-ano, 646–647; intestinal, 632; tracheoesophageal, 876–877
Flail chest, 297, 465
Flashburn (of eyes), 382, **428–429**
Flatfoot, 322
Fleas, 269; plague transmitted by, 273; typhus transmitted by, 175, 238–239
Fleming, Sir Alexander, 12
Flexner, Abraham, 984
Fliedner, Theodor, 1002
Flu, *see* Influenza
Fluoride, tooth decay and, 420
Fluoroscopy, 975, 977
Folic acid, 894; deficiency, 891
Folic acid deficiency anemia, 517, 518, 628
Follicle-stimulating hormone (FSH), 74, **688–689**, 735, 748
Follicular cyst, 758
Folliculitis, bacterial, 396–397
Fontanelles, 852
Food poisoning: botulism, 219, **260–261**; staphylococcal, 253–254
Foot: bunion, 322–323; care, 924–925; corns and calluses, 386; flatfoot, 322; fractures, 299; hammertoe (clawtoe), 323; joints, 31; plantar wart, 397; reflexes, 347–348; stone bruising, 323
Forceps in childbirth, 842
Foreign bodies, **131–133**; in ear, 132, 436; in esophagus, 133, 977; in eye, 132, 428; in lungs, 64, 133; in nose, 132–133, 441–442; in rectum, 133; in respiratory tract, 64, 133, 462, **468–470**; in skin or soft tissues, 132; swallowed, 133, 862, 977; in throat, 107, **114**, 121, 133, 456; in vagina, 133; in wounds, 126
Foreskin (prepuce), 735–738
Fractures, 32, 128–130, **294–303**; aging and, 32, 295, 307, 948–949, 952; ankle or foot, 299; arm or leg (long bones), 128, **295–296**, 302; chest injuries, 464–465; in childhood, 868; collarbone, 297; comminuted, 295; femur (thighbone), 26, 34–35, **295–296**; finger, 296–297; first aid, **128–130**, 300; healing, 97, 300–301; hip (upper end of femur), **295–296**, 952; identification of, 128, 299; jaw, 297; Küntscher nails for, 26; neck, 53, 128, **298**, 354–355, 357; open (compound), 294–295; pathological, 306, 307, 527–528, 695; pelvis, 129, **298–299**, 730; ribs, 128–129, 297, 462, **464–467**; simple, 294; skull, 128, **297**, 302, 359; treatment, 300–303; vertebrae (spine), 128, **298**, 302, 356–357; wrist, 296; X-ray diagnosis, 300
Freckles, 57, **400**
Freud, Sigmund, 772, 782, 806, 998
Freudian psychology, 772–774
Friction rub, 40, 484, 563, 965

Friedländer's bacillus, 217, 482, 484
Friedreich's ataxia, 375
Frigidity, sexual, 764
Fritsch, Gustav, 49
Fröhlich's syndrome, 708
Frostbite, 383–384; treatment, 136–137, 384
Fry, Elizabeth, 1002
Fungus infections, 176; internal (systemic), 276; skin, 385, **398–399**
FUO (fever of unknown origin), **153–154**, 558
Furuncles (boils), 61, **208**

Gag reflex, 614
Gait, abnormalities, 346
Galen, 6–8, 81
Gall bladder, 87, 609–611, 631, 650, 660, 662, 665, **669–677**; cancer, 676–677; cholecystitis, 672, 676; cholelithiasis (gallstones), 90, 662, **670–676**; diet for disorders, 676; removal (cholecystectomy), 90, 672, 674; ruptured, 674, 676; X-rays, 672–674, 978
Gall bladder attack (biliary colic), 673–674, 676
Gallstones, 90, 662, **670–676**
Gamma globulin, 79; agammaglobulinemia, 532; for infectious hepatitis, 202; with measles vaccine, 179, 180
Gamma rays, 975
Ganglia: basal, 45; brain, 45; nerve, 49
Ganglion (tendon disorders), 287–288
Gangrene, 221, 565, 593, 625, 673, 674, 676; gas, 221–222
Gas (gases): intestinal, 615, 620, 628; poisonous, 487
Gas gangrene, 221–222
Gastrectomy: subtotal, 654; total, 863
Gastric dilatation, acute, 617, 620
Gastric juices, 86, 87, 610, 611, 613, 616, 620, 648–649, 661
Gastric ulcer, *see* Peptic ulcer
Gastritis: acute, 630–631; alcohol and, 630, 631, 790; chronic, 631–632; corrosive, 631; peptic ulcer resembling, 650
Gastroenteritis, 253–256; nonspecific, 256; treatment, 256
Gastroenterologist, 992
Gastrointestinal tract, **84–91**; disorders, *see* Digestive system disorders; X-rays, *see* X-rays, diagnostic
Gastrojejunostomy, 654
Gastroscopy, 651, 657
Gastrostomy, 121
Gaucher's disease, 528–529
General paresis, 245
General practitioners, 991, 992, 999–1000
Generation gap, 899–900, 907–908
Genes, 94
Genetic code, 93–94
Genetics, 95–96

Genital system, female, 94–96, 713, **745–785**; anatomy and functions, 745–749; cancer, tumors, and cysts, 754–759; congenital anomalies and defects, 749–752; infections and inflammations, 752–754; infertility, 742, **763–764**; physical examination (pelvic), 966; *see also* Childbirth; Menstruation; Pregnancy
Genital system, male, 94–96, 713, **734–744**; anatomy, 734–736; cancer, 740–741; congenital anomalies and defects, 736–738; impotence, 743–744; infections and inflammations, nonvenereal, 738–740; infertility, 192, 738, **741–743**; physical examination, 966; tuberculosis, 740
Geriatrics, 945
Geriatrist, 945
German measles, **180–181**, 375, 435, 545–546; congenital heart defects from, 549, 555; in pregnancy, 181, 375, 435, 549, 555, 814, **823–824**; vaccination, 181, 555, 823–824, 873
Germ cells (sex cells), 93–95
Germ theory of disease, 169, 172–173
Gestation, *see* Pregnancy
Giant cell tumor, 306
Gigantism, pituitary, 707–708
Gingivitis, 420–421
Girl Scouts, 145
Glanders, 275
Glandular fever (infectious mononucleosis), **197–199**, 514
Glans penis, 735–736
Glasses, 432, 925; dark, 431–432
Glaucoma, 430–431, 951
Glial cells (neuroglia), 43, 50
Globulins, 79
Glomeruli, 68, 715, 717
Glomerulonephritis, 69, **723–726**, 728; acute, 184, 210, 560, 724–726; chronic, 724–726; corticosteroids in, 73; streptococcal infections and, 184, 724
Glossopharyngeal nerves, 347
Glossopharyngeal neuralgia, 356
Glucagon, 696–697
Glucose, 79, 90, 696–697, 888; in blood (blood sugar), 696–698, 702, 703; insulin and, 72, 697–698; kidney filtration of, 714; in urine, 68, 696–698
Glucose tolerance test, 697, 977
Glue sniffing, 800
Gluten, 894
Glycogen, 87, 90, 664, 684, 696, 697, 888
Goiter, 72, 683, **690–693**; exophthalmic, 690, 691; nodular, 692
Goldblatt, Harry, 69
Goldblatt kidney (Goldblatt hypertension), 585
Gold compounds for arthritis, 315–316
Gonadotrophic hormones, 688–689

Gonads, 94, **685–686**, 734; hormones, 73, 95, 96, 685–686; *see also* Ovaries; Testicles
Gonococci, 171, 248, 250
Gonorrhea, **248–250**; arthritis in, 249, 312, 723; baby's eyes protected from, 842, 880; blindness, congenital, from, 249, 880; in female, 723, 752, 758; in male, 723; protection and treatment, 249–250; salpingitis in, 249; urethritis in, 723
"Goose pimples," 57
Gorgas, William, 236
Gout (gouty arthritis), 319–320
Government programs for medical care, 1018–1021
Graafian follicle, rupture, 640
Gram, Hans Christian, 170
Gram-negative and gram-positive bacteria, 170
Grand mal, *see* Epilepsy
Granulocytes (granulocytic leucocytes), 514, 525, 969
Granuloma inguinale, 251
Graves, Robert, 691
Graves' disease, 691
Grippe, *see* Influenza
Griseofulvin, 399, 408
Group therapy, 783, 793, 799
Growth hormone, 31, 74, **687**, 707–708
Guilt feelings, 773, 805
Gummas, 246
Gums, 415; care, 422–423; diseases, 420–421
Gut, 609–610
Gynecomastia, 395, 446

Hair, **409–414**; aging and, 950–951; baldness, 410–411, 950–951; on body, 57, 409–410; care, 412–414; color, 60; gray or white, 409–410; growth patterns, 409–410; racial characteristics, 60; superfluous (hirsutism), 410
Hair follicles, 56, 57, 59, 409
Haldane, John Scott, 63–64
Halitosis (bad breath), 419, 420, 423
Hallucinations, 800, 801
Hallucinogenic drugs, 794, **795–797**, 807
Hammertoe (clawtoe), 323
Hand: lacerations, 125; numbness, 346; *see also* Fingers
Hand-Schüller-Christian disease, 529
Handicapped, the: agencies and services for, 331; home nursing care, 159
Hangnail, 407–408
Hangover, 338, 790
Hansen, Gerhardt Henrik, 272
Hansen's disease (leprosy), 61, **271–272**
Haploid cells, 94, 95
Harborview Hospital, Seattle, 1014
Harelip, 441, 875
Harvey, William, 5, 8, 81, 512, 583, 681

Hashimoto's struma, 694
Hashish, 795
Hay fever, 388, 490–491; treatment, 391–392
Headache, 338–340; cerebrospinal fluid balance and, 47; histamine, 340; in hypertension, 339, 585; migraine, 339–340, 923; sinus, 225, 472
Head injuries, **358–359**; intracranial hemorrhage, 103; unconsciousness and, 342
Healing, mechanism of, 97
Health care, 7–16, 925; for the aged, 945, 947; attitudes toward, 13–14; costs, 14–15, 1011; *see also* Medical costs; goal of, 15–16; history, 7–9, 11–16; in middle age, 926–927; preventive, 15–16, 1016, 1018; services, 3–4, 1008–1009
Hearing, **434–435**; bone conduction, 435; disorders and loss of, 346, **438–439**, 925, 952
Hearing aids, 438–439, 952
Heart, **80–83**; anatomy, 543–545; artificial, 605; cardiac defibrillator (shock box), 38–39; cardiac output, 573; in circulation, 80–83, 542–545; connective tissue, 40; early knowledge of, 75; endocardium, mesocardium, and pericardium, 557–558; external cardiac compression, **110–111**, 114, 116, 118, 468; massage, 38; muscle, 38, 39, 81–82, 544–545; pacemaker, 81, 545; pacemaker, electronic, 545; physical examination, 964–965; valves, *see* Heart valves; as vital organ, 25; *see also* entries under Cardiac
Heart attack, *see* Coronary thrombosis
Heartbeat, 511–512, 573, 583; of fetus, 824; rapid (tachycardia), 576
Heart block, 545
Heartburn, 630, 631; angina pectoris distinguished from, 595, 623; coronary thrombosis distinguished from, 516, 601; in hiatus hernia, 516; in peptic ulcer, 650
Heart disorders: in anemia, 516; cardiac arrest, 38–39, 110, 114, 121; congenital malformations, 65, 82–83, **549–555**, 876; fibrillation, 38, 118, 121; heart block, 545; heart failure, *see* Heart failure; inflammatory diseases, 556–564; kidney disease, hypertension and, 69; in polycythemia, 522; rheumatic, *see* Rheumatic fever
Heart failure, **573–581**; in aortic stenosis, 549; of babies, 548; causes, 573–574; congestive, *see* Heart failure, congestive *below;* crisis, 580–581; definition, 573; digitalis for, 82, 578–579, 581; examination for, 577–578; in pulmonic stenosis, 548; in rheumatic

Heart failure (*cont'd*)
fever, 562; in septal defects, 551; symptoms, 574, 576–577; treatment, 577–580
Heart failure, congestive, 82, **574–581**, 953; in bacterial endocarditis, 559; crisis, 580–581; definition, 574; in dermatomyositis, 291; hypertension and, 588; liver disorders and, 576–577, 665; in myocarditis, 564; treatment, 577–580
Heart-lung by-pass machine, 121, 461, **552**
Heart-lung resuscitation, **111**, 118
Heart murmurs, 965; in aortic stenosis, 549; in patent ductus arteriosus, 547; in pulmonic stenosis, 548; in rheumatic heart disease, 561
Heart rhythm, 965; arrythmias, 579, 974; gallop, 965; in rheumatic heart disease, 561
Heart sounds (tones), 965
Heart surgery, 41, 121, **552–555**, 994, 1004–1005; bacterial endocarditis after, 558; catheterization, 554, 555; commissurotomy, mitral or aortic, 563; decision for, 552, 555; heart valves, 41, 548, 549, 552, 553, 563; for patent ductus arteriosus, 547; for pericarditis, 564; for transposition of great vessels, 548
Heart transplants, 41, 605, 999
Heart valves, 82, **543–544**; aortic, 544; aortic stenosis, 548–549, 561–562; artificial, 41, 548, 549; in bacterial endocarditis, 559; commissurotomy, mitral or aortic, 563; congenital defects, 549–550; mitral, 544; mitral stenosis, 550, 561; pulmonic, 544; pulmonic stenosis, 548–549; in rheumatic fever, 560, 563; surgery, 41, 548, 549, 552, 553, 563; tricuspid, 544; valvulitis, 557
Heat exhaustion, 115, **135–136**, 156
Heat rash (miliaria, prickly heat), 59, **384–385**
Heat stroke (sunstroke), 115, **136**, 156
Heberden's nodes, 318
Hemangioma, 400, 896
Hematologist, 992
Hematoma, 127, **533–534**, 831; brain, 297, 365; subdural, 365, 882
Hematuria, *see* Blood, in urine
Hemianopia, 426
Hemiplegia, 360
Hemoglobin, 63, 76–77, 460, 513, 888; S (sickle-cell trait), 519
Hemolysis, 222, 513, 518–519
Hemolytic anemia, 77, **518–520**
Hemolytic crisis, 519
Hemophilia, 96, **530–531**
Hemophilus influenzae, 200, 217, 482
Hemophilus pertussis, 471
Hemoptysis, 538
Hemorrhage, 77, 78, 103, 529, **533–539**; arterial, 104–107; in bacterial endocarditis (small localized), 559;

Hemorrhage (*cont'd*)
as cancer symptom, warning, 939–940; cerebral, *see* Cerebrovascular accidents; in childbirth, 39, 831, 846; in cirrhosis, 667; control of, 104–107, **533–537;** *see also* Bleeding, control of; from esophageal varices, 569; in hemophilia, 531; internal, 533, 537–538; intracranial, 103; menstrual, 537, 756–757; periosteal, 295; petechial, 559; posthemorrhagic anemia, **515,** 534; rectal, 536–537; scleral, 535–536; shock and, 533, 534, 538–539; subarachnoid, 364–365; from tonsillectomy and adenoidectomy, 535; from varicose veins, 536; vomiting blood, 535, 538, 939–940
Hemorrhoids, 81, 569, **570–572,** 635, 645–646; bleeding, 536, 571; in pregnancy, 826, 827; thrombosed, 569, 571–572, 638
Hepatic artery, 664–665
Hepatic coma, 668–669
Hepatic ducts, 611, 669, 672
Hepatic failure, 668–669
Hepatitis, infectious (acute infectious jaundice), 90, 159, **200–202,** 569, 668, 874
Hepatitis, serum, **202–203,** 668; blood transfusion and, 540
Heredity, 95–96; of diabetes, 96, 661, 696; of hemophilia, 530
Hermaphroditism, 96, 750
Hernia, **624–626;** femoral, 625; hiatus (esophageal, diaphragmatic), **616–619,** 650–651; incarcerated, 625–626; inguinal, 624–626, 738, **875;** intervertebral disk, slipped, 325, 824, 979; strangulated, 625; surgery for, 617, 626; trusses for, 626; umbilical, 624, **875–876**
Herniorrhaphy, 626
Heroin, 793, **798–799**
Herpes simplex (cold sore, fever blister), **230–231,** 383
Herpes zoster (shingles), **231–232,** 358; eye disorders in, 206, 430
Hewson, William, 79
Hiatus hernia, **616–619,** 650–651
Hiccups (singultus), 345–346, 462
High blood pressure, *see* Hypertension
Hiking, minimal pack equipment for, 137
Hip: dislocation, 303–304; dislocation, congenital, 309; fracture (upper end of femur), 295–296, 952; joint, 27, 30
Hippocrates, 5–6
Hippocratic Oath, 6
Hirschsprung, Harold, 86
Hirschsprung's disease (congenital megacolon), 86, 89, 622, 877
Hirsutism, 410
Histamine, 61, 388
Histoplasmosis, 276
Hitzig, Eduard, 49

Hives (urticaria), 61, **388–389,** 490; from insect bites and stings, 389
Hoarseness, 473, 475, 498, 499; cancer symptom, 939
Hodgkin, Thomas, 528
Hodgkin's disease, 502, 504, 526, **528**
Holography, acoustic, 449
Home nursing care, **157–165;** of the aged, **160–161,** 956; bathing, 162–163; bed, 162; bedpan and urinal, 163; bedsores, 386–387; in childhood rash diseases, 179–180, 182–184; of children, 158–159; feeding, 163; of the handicapped or chronically ill, 159–160; medical supplies, list, 164–165; nurse's attitude, 161–162; patient's room, 162; professional services, 163–164, 956
Homosexuality, 787–789
Hookworm disease, 177, **264–266**
Hormones, 69, 72–74, **681–682;** adrenal, 73, **684–685,** 704, 707, 708, 716, 735; *see also* Corticosteroids; discovery of, 681–682; gonadotrophic, 688–689; growth, 31, 74, **687;** in menopause, 934; parathyroid, 694–695; pituitary, 74, 683, **686–689,** 735, 747–748; in pregnancy, 812–813; sex, *see* Sex hormones; thyroid, 72, 74, 604, **683**
Hornets, 139
Hospital Insurance Plan of New York (HIP), 1017
Hospitals, **1001–1008;** administrators, 1007; admission procedures, 1007–1008; attitudes toward, 13–14, 961; childbirth in, 830, 837, 1004; cost of care, *see* Medical costs; emergency services, 122, 146, 1003, 1004; extended care facilities, 163–164, 1008–1009; history of, 1001–1002, 1014; intensive care unit, 1004; kinds of, 1002–1003; medical service, 1003; obstetrical service, 1004; paramedical personnel, 1007; pediatric service, 1004; physicians, 984, 992, 993, 1005; public, 1014–1015; rooming in, after childbirth, 848; semiprofessional and specialized workers, 1007; services, 1003–1005; staff, 1005–1007; statistics on, 3; surgical service, 1003; volunteers and nurses' aides, 1006, 1007
Hospitals, neuropsychiatric, 770, 783, 790, 805, 807; for drug addiction, 799; for schizophrenia, 802–803
Humerus, 30
Hunchback, 309; Pott's disease, 214, 306
Hunger, 614
Huntington's chorea, 373
Hyaline membrane disease, 881
Hydrocarbons, chlorinated as poisons, 668, 800
Hydrocele, 740
Hydrocephalus, **375,** 377, 878

Hydrochloric acid, 85, 660; in gastritis, 631; in peptic ulcer, 648, 651; in pernicious anemia, 517
Hydrocortisone, 73, 316
Hydrolysis, 85
Hydronephrosis, 729–731
Hydrophobia, *see* Rabies
Hydrothorax (hydropneumothorax), 482, 483
Hymen (maidenhead), 747, 749, 913, 966
Hyperopia, 427
Hyperpyrexia (sunstroke), 115, **136,** 156
Hypersensitivity, 387
Hypertension, 82, **582–591,** 923; aging and, 953; atherosclerosis and, 588, 594, 597; benign essential, 582, 589; causes, 585, 588; in coarctation of aorta, 547; complications, 588–589; in Cushing's syndrome, 706; definition, 583; emotional tension and, 588, 590–591, 784; headache in, 339, 585; heart failure and, 574, 582; kidney disorders and, 69, 585, 586, 588–589, 723–725; liver disorders and, 585; malignant, 582, 584, 589; onset, 584–585; in pheochromocytoma, 706–707; in pregnancy, 832; prevention, 589–591; smoking and, 590; stroke and, 362, 364, 588; treatment, 591; weight control in, 589–590
Hyperthyroidism, 72, 683, **691–693,** 707
Hypertrichosis (superfluous hair), 410
Hypnotism, 681, 783
Hypofibrinogenemia, 531
Hypoglossal nerves, 347
Hypoglycemia, 663, 683, **703–704**
Hypoglycemic shock, *see* Insulin shock
Hypoparathyroidism (parathyroid tetany), 694–695
Hypospadias, 737
Hypotension, 584; orthostatic, 584
Hypothalamus, 45, 687
Hypothyroidism (myxedema), 72, 392, 604, 683, **691–692**
Hysterectomy, 752, 755–757, 761

Id, **773–774,** 778
Idiots, 377
Ileocecal valve, 612
Ileostomy, 638
Ileum, 86, 626, 632
Ileus, paralytic, 620–621
Imbeciles, 377
Immersion foot (trench foot), 137, **384**
Immune reactions, 97, 387–388, 527
Immunization: in childhood (table), 873–874; cholera, 258, 874; DPT (diphtheria, pertussis, tetanus), **186–188,** 220, 873–874; paratyphoid, 255, 257–258, 874; plague, 274, 874;

Immunization: in childhood (cont'd)
poliomyelitis, 175, **188, 190,** 873;
Rocky Mountain spotted fever, 238;
smallpox, 174–175, 231, **233–234,**
874; tetanus, 126, **220–221;** typhoid,
255, 257–258, 874; typhus, 239; yellow fever, **235–236,** 874
Impetigo, 204–205
Impotence, male, 743–744
Incontinence, 731; stress, 751
Incus, 434
Indians, American: skin and hair, 60;
smallpox, 232; tuberculosis, 214
Indigestion, see Gastritis; Gastroenteritis
Indomethacin, 320
Infantile paralysis, see Poliomyelitis
Infarct, 559
Infection, **169–177;** bacteria, 170–172;
fungi, 176; parasites (worms), 176–
177; pleural pneumonia-like or-
ganisms (PPLO), 175–176; proto-
zoa, 176–177; rickettsiae, 175;
viruses, 172–175, **224–237**
Infectious diseases: fever and, 151,
153–154; home nursing care, 159
Infectious hepatitis (acute infectious
jaundice), 90, **200–202,** 569, 874;
home nursing care, 159, 201
Infectious mononucleosis (glandular
fever), **197–199,** 514
Infertility, female, 742, **763–764**
Infertility, male, **741–743;** mumps as
cause of, 192, 738
Inflammation, 40, **556–558**
Influenza, 224, **228–230,** 471; of the
aged, 948; Asian flu, 224, 229;
Hong Kong flu, 224, 229; intestinal
flu, 229, 621; pneumonia and, 217,
230; stomach flu, 229, 253, 254;
vaccine, 230, 948
Inguinal hernia, 624–626, 738, **875**
Insanity, see Mental disorders; Psychoses
Insect bites and stings, **139–140,** 385–
386; allergic reactions, 139–140,
389; rickettsial infections from, 175;
skin disorders from, 61, **268–270,**
399–400
Insecticides, 139; anemia from, 520
Insect repellents, 139
Insemination, artificial, 742
Insulin, 72–73; diabetes and produc-
tion of, 696–700; diabetes treatment
with, 72–73, **699–702;** hunger sensa-
tions caused by, 86; for pancreatitis,
663; secretion by pancreas, 72, 87,
661, 683, **696–698**
Insulin shock, 103, 360, 663, **700–701,**
703
Insulin shock therapy, 803
Insurance, health, see Medical costs
Intelligence quotient (IQ), 377
Intensive care unit, 1004
Intercostal muscles, 459
Intermittent claudication, 565, 593
Internal medicine, 991

Internist, 991–993
Internship, 984, 989–992
Interstitial cell fluid, 55
Intertrigo (chafing), 385
Intervertebral disks: disk syndrome,
325–326; disorders, 325–326;
slipped (herniated), 325, 824, 979
Intestinal disorders, 87, **253–261;** diverticulitis, 640, **642–644;** gastrointestinal infections, 253–256;
lymphosarcoma as obstruction, 527;
malabsorption, 613, **627–629,** 893–
896; motility, 620–624; obstruction,
624–627; regional enteritis, 632–
634; ulcerative colitis, **634–638,** 644;
see also Digestive system disorders
Intestinal flu, 38, 229, 621
Intestinal gas, 615, 620, 628
Intestine, large, see Colon
Intestine, small, 85–87, **609–612,** 660;
cancer, 657; motility disorders, 620–
621; see also Duodenum; Ileum;
Jejunum
Intracellular fluid space, 80
Intracranial hemorrhage, 103
Intrauterine device (IUD), 919
Intravascular fluid space, 80
Intravenous pyelogram (IVP), 68,
70–71, 732–733, **978**
"Intrinsic factor" in pernicious ane-
mia, 517
Introitus, 747
Introjection (defense mechanism),
776
Intussusception, 626–627
Involutional melancholia, **805,** 935
Iodine: in blood, 72; protein-bound,
test (PBI), 692; in salt, 890; in
thyroid disorders, 690–691, 693
Iodine, radioactive (I¹³¹), 693; up-
take test, 692
Ions in plasma, 79
Ipecac, syrup of, 116–117
IQ (intelligence quotient), 377
Iris (of eye), 426
Iron deficiency, 890
Iron-deficiency anemia, 77, **515–516,**
518, 890
Iron lung, 463
Irritable colon (irritable bowel syn-
drome, spastic colon), 623–624
Ischemia, 82, 284
Islet cell tumor, 663, 703
Islets of Langerhans, 663, 683, 696,
699, 706
Isoniazid for tuberculosis, 213–214,
312, 721
Itch mites, 268–269; see also Chiggers
IUD (intrauterine device), 919
Ivanovski, Dmitri Iosifovich, 173

Jacksonian seizure, 342–343, 884
Jaundice, 90, 392, **665–666,** 971; in
cancer of pancreas, 664; in cirrhosis, 667; congenital hemolytic, 519–
520; in gall bladder attack, 673,

Jaundice (cont'd)
676; in infectious hepatitis, 201,
202; in mononucleosis, 198
Jaw: dislocation, 304; fracture, 297;
muscles, 33, 85; teeth and, 417–419
Jejunum, 86, 617, 620
Jenner, Edward, 9, 233
Jogging, 933
Joint disorders, 40–41, **310–331;**
neurogenic, 321–322; treatment,
agencies and organizations, 331;
treatment, specialists in, 328–331;
see also Arthritis; Low back pain
Joint mice, 318, 321
Joint prostheses, 302
Joints, 25, 27, 30–31, 294, 310; connective tissue, 40; dislocations, 130,
303–304; fractures, 295–296; injuries, 32, **130–131;** sprains, 130–131

Kaiser Permanente Group Health
Program, 1017
Kaiserswerth, nurses' training, 1002
Kala-azar, 278
Keloids, 401
Kerasin, 528
Keratitis, 429–430
Keratosis: seborrheic, 401–402;
senile, 407
Kidney disorders, 68–69, **717–733;**
anemia in, 521, 588; appendicitis
resembling, 640; bacterial emboli
in, 559; cancer, 730–731; congenital
defects, 729; diabetes insipidus,
709; diagnostic examinations, 731–
733; glomerulonephritis, 69, 73,
184, 210, 560, **723–725,** 728; Goldblatt kidney, 585; headache in, 339;
hydronephrosis, **729–730,** 731; hypertension and, 69, 585, 586, 588–
589, 723–725; injuries, 69, 730;
kidney colic, 695; nephrosis, 723,
727; nephrotic syndrome, 69, 723,
727–728; polycystic disease, 729; in
pregnancy, 826, 832; pyelitis, 720–
721; pyelonephritis, 720–721; renal
failure, 69, 723–727, **728–729;**
stones, see Kidney stones; toxemia
of pregnancy, 728, 826, **832;** tuberculosis, 68–69, 214, 721; uremia,
588–589, 717–718, 720, 725
Kidneys, **65–69,** 70–71, 713–718; artificial, 65, 69, **725–727,** 728–729,
1012; bifid, 729; blood in, 65, 68,
69, 714–716; differential barrier
membrane, 68; floating (fallen),
729; functions, 68, 713–716; glomeruli, 68, 715, 717; nephrons,
715, 716; pelvis, 715; transplants,
65, 726–727; tubules, 68, 715; as
vital organs, 25, 65
Kidney stones (calculi), 71, **718–720,**
721; parathyroid disorders and, 695;
in ureter (ureteral colic), 69, 718–
719
Knee, 30; Charcot joint, 322; locking,
321; reflexes, 347

Knidos, medical school, 5
Koch, Robert, 8, 170, 212
Kolff, William J., 726
Koplik's spots, 179
Kos, medical school, 5
Kouwenhoven, William B., 38
Küntscher nails, 26
Kwashiorkor, 666–668

Labia majora, 747
Labia minora, 747
Labor, **834–846;** anesthesia in, 835–836, **838–839;** approach of, 834–835; complications, 843–846; false, 836–837; fluid discharge, 829, 835; induced, 837; prelabor contractions, 836; premature, 828–829; terminal, and delivery, 840–842; uterine contractions, 39, 834–838, 840–841, 843; uterine inertia, 845
Laboratory studies, **968–975;** bacteriological, 974; blood chemistry, 732; blood-clotting test, 969–970; blood count, complete, 969; blood typing, 972–974; electrocardiogram, *see* Electrocardiogram; urinalysis, 732, 969
Lacerations, **124–127;** face, 125; fingers, hand, or wrist, 125; lip, 125; scalp, 125
Lacrimal ducts, 426
Lacrimal glands, 426
Lactation, 445
Lactogenic hormone, 689
Laënnec, René, 212
Landsteiner, Carl, 77, 78, 539–540
Laparoscopy, 821
Laparotomy, 627, 634, 982
Laryngitis, 473, 475
Laryngoscopy, 475, 499
Laryngotracheobronchitis, acute (croup), 477, 480
Larynx, 456–457, 471; cancer, 475, **499–500;** polyps, 475, 499–500; speech without, after surgery, 500; tuberculosis, 475
Laxatives, 622; in pregnancy, caution on, 827
Laxatives, avoiding, 623; with abdominal pain, 135, 641; for babies, 860; with diarrhea, 256; with swallowed objects, 133
Lazy eye syndrome, 428
L-dopa, 366
Leahy Clinic, Boston, 1009
Leeuwenhoek, Anton van, 8, 21
Leg (legs): artificial, 302; in Buerger's disease, 565; fractured, 128, **295–296,** 302; varicose veins, 568–570
Legg-Calvé-Perthes disease, 308
Leishmania donovani, 177
Leishmaniasis, 278
Leonardo da Vinci, 8
Leprosy (Hansen's disease), 61, **271–272**
Leptospira icteroides, 236
Leucocytes, *see* Blood cells, white

Leukemia, 32, 504, **523–526;** anemia in, 78, 524; lymphatic, 896; lymphocytic and granulocytic, 525, 526; polycythemia vera and, 522, 523; treatment, 526, 942, 979; white blood cells in, 78, 524–526, 969
Leukoplakia, 499
Leukorrhea, 752
Levin tube, 620
Libido, 685, 743
Lice, 139, **269,** 275; typhus transmitted by, 175, 238–239
Lichen planus, 397
Life expectancy: increase in, 944; racial factors in, 944
Ligaments, 25, 282, 294
Lightning, 117, **119**
Liniments, 285
Lip: cancer, 499; lacerations, 125
Lipase, 86, 661, 662
Lipids, 79, 593, 604, 727, 889
Lipoma of breast, 448
Lipoproteins, 79
Lister, Joseph, 9
Liver, 86, 87, 90, 609–611, **664–669,** 681; circulatory system, 83, **664–665;** functions, 87, 90, 664; function tests, 971; secretions, 85–87, 611, 660; transplants, 669; as vital organ, 25
Liver disorders, 90, **664–669;** abscess, 209, 260; cancer, 665, **669;** cirrhosis, 90, 569, **666–668,** 669, 791; congestion, passive, 665; in heart failure, 576–577, 665; hepatic coma, 668–669; in hypertension, 585; infectious hepatitis, 90, 159, **200–202,** 569, 668; kwashiorkor, 666–668; liver failure, 668–669; lymphosarcoma, 527; serum hepatitis, 202–203
Liver failure, 668–669
Liver spots (skin), 950
Live wires, 117–119
Lochia, 847
Lockjaw, *see* Tetanus
Lordosis, 328
Low back pain, **323–326;** disorders causing, 323–324; intervertebral disk abnormalities, 325–326; mechanical defects causing, 324–325; psychosomatic, 324
Lower respiratory infections, 470
LSD (lysergic acid diethylamide), **797;** in schizophrenia, 802–803
Lues, *see* Syphilis
Lumbago, 285
Lumbar nerves, 48
Lumbar puncture (spinal tap), 47, 154, **348–349,** 972
Lumbosacral joint, 324; sprain, 324, 325
Lumbosacral syndrome, 324
Lung cancer, 367, 457, **500–507,** 924, 939; metastatic, 500, 501, 504; primary, 500, 504; smoking and, 504, 505, 924, 977

Lung disorders, 64–65, **480–489;** abscess, 465, 470, **484;** bleeding from, 538; in bronchiectasis, 477; cancer, *see* Lung cancer; fibrosis, 485, 953; lower respiratory infections, 470; polycythemia and, 78, 522; rib fractures and, 464–465; silicosis, 485–487; *see also* Pneumonia; Tuberculosis; other disorders
Lungs, **62–65,** 66–67; anatomy, 62–63; blood circulation in, 62, 82; in chest wounds, 138; foreign bodies in, 64, 133; inhalation of foreign matter, 485; physical examination, 964–965; in respiration, 455, 457, 460–461
Lupus erythematosus, 40, 61, 383, **403–404,** 560; chronic discoid, 404; disseminated (systemic), 404
Luteinizing hormone, 688, 689
Lymph, 80, 527
Lymphatic leukemia, 526
Lymphatics (lymph vessels), 80, 86, 527
Lymphatic system, 526–527
Lymph nodes, 80, **526–527;** in breast cancer, 449; in Hodgkin's disease, 528; in larynx cancer, 500; in leukemia, 524; in lymphosarcoma, 527; in mastitis, 446; in mononucleosis, 197, 198; physical examination, 964; in thyroid cancer, 693
Lymphocytes (lymphocytic leucocytes), 514, 527, 969; in leukemia, 525, 526, 969; in mononucleosis, 197, 198, 514
Lymphogranuloma venereum, 250–251
Lymphoid tissue, 78, 438, 526, 527; disorders, 526–529; in pharyngitis, 472; in upper respiratory infections, 193
Lymphoma, 526–529
Lymphosarcoma, 526–528

McBurney's point, 640
McDowell, Ephraim, 757
Macleod, J. J. R., 72
Maidenhead (hymen), 747, 749, 913, 966
Malaria, 176, **262–264,** 268; control, 264; hemolytic anemia in, 518
Malignant melanoma, 59, 400, 406, 431
Malleus, 434
Malnutrition: in childhood, 868; skin in, 392
Malpighi, Marcello, 8
Malta fever (brucellosis), 275
Mammary dysplasia (cystic disease of breast), 447
Mammary glands, 58
Mammography, X-ray, 449, 940, 978
Manic-depressive psychosis, 804–805
March of Dimes (National Foundation), 331
Marijuana, 795–796
Marriage, **911–915;** decision for, 912–913; physical examination before,

Marriage (cont'd)
913; psychological compatibility, 912, 914–915; sexual compatibility, 913–914

Marrow, 77, 78, 513, 514; agranulocytosis, 532; in anemia, 520; in leukemia, 78, 524–526; in lymphosarcoma, 527; in polycythemia, 521; red, 31, 32; transplants, 520; yellow, 31

Marsupialization, 753

Masculinization: adrenogenital syndrome, 705; tumors, 410, 685–686

Masochism, 789

Mason Clinic, Seattle, 1009

Massachusetts General Hospital, Boston, 1014

Masseter muscles, 33, 85

Mastectomy: radical, 449; simple, 447

Mastitis, acute (septic), 446–447

Mastoidectomy, 196

Mastoiditis, 196, 437

Masturbation, 736, 743, 902–903

Maturity, 909–925; emotional conflicts, 775, 912; habits, harmful, 923–924; illnesses, common, 923–925; sexual, 909–911

Mayo Clinic, Rochester, Minn., 1009

Measles (rubeola), 178–180, 471; encephalitis and, 180; vaccine, 180, 181, 873–874

Measles, German, see German measles

Measles-type diseases, 178–182

Meatus, 736

Meckel's diverticulum, 642–644

Meconium ileus, 877, 894–895

Mediastinum, 457, 459

Medic I unit, 103, 1004

Medicaid, 1019

Medical costs, 14–15, 1011–1021; Blue Cross and Blue Shield programs, 1015–1017; charity services, 1014–1015; government plans and programs, 1018–1021; group health programs, 1017; insurance, private plans, 1015–1018; National Health Insurance (British and Swedish), 1018; private payment to physician, 1013–1015

Medical education, 983–998; anatomy, 984–985; bacteriology, 985–986; biochemistry, 985; clinical work, 986–989; degree, 989; immunology, 986; internship, 984, 989–992; obstetrics and gynecology, 995–996; pathology, 985; pediatrics, 996; pharmacology, 986; physiology, 985; premedical, 984; residency training, 984, 992, 993, 1005; surgeons, 993–995

Medical history (of patient), 961–963

Medical insurance, see Medical costs

Medical research, clinical, 999

Medical schools, 984; history of, 5–8; see also Medical education

Medical Self-Help program, first-aid training, 145

Medical service (care), 987, 1003

Medical supplies: first-aid kit, 145–146; for home nursing, list, 164–165

Medical textbooks, history of: Avicenna, 7–8; Galen, 7; Hippocrates, 6; Papyrus of Ebers, 4–5; Rhazes, 7

Medicare, 945, 1019

Medicine, history of, 4–10; Arabic and Persian, 7–8; Egyptian, 4–5; Greek, 5–6; infection, knowledge of, 169–170; Middle Ages and Renaissance, 7–8; modern discoveries, 8–12, 24; Roman (Galen), 6–7

Mediterranean anemia, 519

Medulla oblongata, 43–44

Megacolon, congenital, 86, 89, 877

Megakaryocytes, 78, 514

Meiosis, 93–95

Melancholia, involutional, 805, 935

Melanin, 56–57, 59

Melanoma, malignant, 59, 400, 406, 431

Memory: amnesia, 359–360; blocking, 360, 776; Freud's theories of, 772; in schizophrenia, 801

Menarche, 748, 900–901

Mendel, Gregor Johann, 95

Ménière's syndrome, 345, 437–438

Meninges, 43, 46–47, 199; arachnoid membrane, 47; dura mater, 46–47; pia mater, 47

Meningioma, 366, 937

Meningismus, 199

Meningitis, 154, 358, 885; headache in, 339; meningococcal (epidemic spinal), 199–200, 358; in mononucleosis, 198; mumps and, 192–193

Meningocele, 373, 375, 878

Meningococcal carditis, 560

Meningococci, 171, 199, 200

Menopause, 94, 95, 686, 692, 748–749, 763, 926, 933–935; breasts in, 445; cancer and, 935; involutional melancholia in, 805; male, 686, 743; menopausal syndrome, 763, 933–935; vaginal bleeding after, 756–757

Menorrhagia, 537, 761

Menstruation, 94, 748–749; in adolescence, 900–901; amenorrhea (missing), 761; anemia and, 515–516; breast feeding and, 848; breast symptoms, 445, 447; discomfort (dysmenorrhea), 761; disorders, 756–758, 761–763; endometriosis and, 760; excessive bleeding, 537, 756–757, 761; the Pill and, 537; in pregnancy, stopped, 748, 812–813; premenstrual tension, 762–763, 923; resumed after childbirth, 847; sexual intercourse and, 748, 918

Mental disorders, 769–771, 778–808; changing attitudes toward, 806–808; chemotherapy, 803–804; early attitudes toward, 9, 770; institutional care, see Hospitals, neuropsychiatric; involutional melancholia, 805, 935; manic-depressive psycho-

Mental disorders (cont'd)
sis, 804–805; paranoia, 804; in pernicious anemia, 516; personality disorders, 773, 777, 785–787, 800–801; psychoneuroses, 770–771, 776, 777, 779–784; psychoses, 770, 777, 797, 800–805; psychosomatic, 770, 777, 784–785; see also Psychosomatic disorders; psychotherapy, 782–784; psychosurgery, 803; schizophrenia, 800–804, 805, 807–808; senility, 367, 370, 950; shock therapy, 360, 783, 803, 805, 936; treatment, 9, 782–784, 802–808

Mental illness, 769–771; definition of terms, 769–770

Mental retardation, 376–377; cerebral palsy and, 882; mongolism, 96, 376, 377, 879–880; phenylketonuria, 96, 376–377, 878–879

Meperidine (Demerol), 798

Mescaline, 797

Mesenchyme, 644

Mesmer, F. A., 681

Mesoderm, 22, 58

Metabolic cycles, 90

Metabolic defects, inborn (congenital), 96

Metabolism, 62, 85, 90–91, 455; basal metabolism rate, 689, 692; cellular (intermediary), 90; corticosteroids in, 73; weight gain and, 927

Methadone (Dolophine), 798; for heroin addiction, 799

Methamphetamine, 794

Methionine, 666

Methyl-dopa, 591

Methylphenidate (Ritalin), 794, 936

Michelangelo, 8

Microcephalus, 373, 375

Microscope, early use of, 8

Micturition, see Urination

Midbrain, 43

Middle age, 926–943; cancer in, see Cancer; depressive reaction, 780–781, 935–936; exercise in, 931–933; health hazards, general, 943; menopause, see Menopause; weight control in, 927–931

Midget, 308, 708

Migraine headache, 339–340, 923

Miliaria (heat rash, prickly heat), 59, 384–385

Milk: allergy to, 864–865; ascorbic acid in, 892; vitamin D enriched, 892

Milk, mother's, 847, 848, 853–854, 864, 892

Minerals in nutrition, 890

Miner's lung, 485–487

Miscarriage (spontaneous abortion), 818–820; midterm, 828–829; uterine tumors and, 756

Mitosis, 92–95

Mitral commisurotomy, 563

Mitral stenosis, 550, 561–562

Mitral valve, 544

Moles, 59, **400**, 406; changes in, as cancer symptoms, 940
Mongolism (Down's syndrome), 96, 376, 377, **879–880**
Mongoloid race, skin and hair, 60
Monilia (vaginitis), 753
Moniliasis (thrush), 176, 859, **863–864**
Monocytes, 514, 969
Mononucleosis, infectious, **197–199**, 514
Montgomery's glands, 445
Montpelier, University, 8
Morbidity, definition, 470
Morning sickness, 817–818
Morons, 377
Morphine, 793, 798; for heart failure, 580, 581
Mortality, definition, 470
Mosquitoes: anopheles, 262–263, 269; bites, 139; dengue fever transmitted by, 236–237; malaria transmitted by, 262–263, 268; yellow fever transmitted by, 234–236
Motion sickness, **135**, 345, 435, 437
Motor nerve end plates, 50, 52
Motor nerves, 47–50, 54; examination, 347; injuries, 353
Mountain sickness, 522
Mouth, 610; cancer, **499**, 657
Mouth breathing, 443
Mouth-to-mouth resuscitation, **107–108**, 113, 116, 129, 461; in chest injuries, 468; in choking, 114; in circulatory failure, 111; in electrical shock, 118
Mouth-to-nose resuscitation, **107–108**, 111, 113
Mucous membranes, 56
Mucus, 64
Multiple myeloma, 307
Multiple sclerosis, 54, 293, **371–372**
Mumps (acute parotitis), **191–193**, 471; vaccine, 192, 873
Mumps orchitis, 192, 738
Mumps pancreatitis, 661–662
Murine typhus, 239
Muscle, 20, 22–23, 25, **32–40**; atrophy, 33, 282–283; cells, 22–23; fascicles, 282; flexors and extensors, 283; hypertrophy, 33, 282–283; insertion, 282; origin, 282; skeletal (voluntary or striated), 33, **281–283**; smooth (involuntary), 33, 38, 48, 86, 281, 544; spasm, 38; tics, 292, **343–344**; tremors, 292, **343–345**
Muscle disorders and injuries, 39–40, **281–293**; cancer, 292; contracture, 283; fatigue, 284; generalized myositis, 286–287; major, 288–292; minor, 283–287; overuse myositis, 39, 131, **284–285**; sprains, **130–131**, 282, 304; strains, **131**, 282; tumors, benign, 292
Muscular dystrophy, **288–289**, 880
Muscular Dystrophy Association, 880

Musculoskeletal system, **25–41**; of the aged, 948–949; disorders, 26, 948
Mushrooms, poisonous, 143
Myasthenia gravis, 40, 54, **289–291**, 689
Mycobacterium leprae, 272
Mycobacterium tuberculosis, 211, 480
Myelin, 50
Myeloblasts, 514
Myelocele, 878
Myelogram, 979
Myeloma, multiple, 307
Myocardial infarction, acute, *see* Coronary thrombosis
Myocardial ischemia, 595
Myocarditis, 557, **564**; diphtheria, 560; Fiedler's, 564; viral, 560
Myocardium, 557–558
Myoglobin, 282
Myoma, 292, 755–756
Myoneural junction, 52, 54
Myopia, 427
Myosarcoma, 292
Myositis: generalized, 286–287; overuse, 39, 131, **284–285**
Myringotomy, 196
Myxedema (hypothyroidism), 72, 392, 604, 683, **691–692**

Nails, 58, **407–409**; biting, 393; care, 413; hangnail, 407–408; ingrown, 408; injuries, 407–408; onychomycosis, 176, **408**; paronychia, 126–127, **408**; ringworm, 176, **408**; splinter hemorrhages under, 536, 559; thin or brittle, 408–409
Narcotics, addictive, 793, 794, **797–799**
Nasopharynx, 456, 470, 472; pharyngitis, 472–473
National Foundation (March of Dimes), 331
National Health Insurance (British and Swedish), 1018
Natural childbirth, 839–840
Naturopath, 331
Neck: fractures, 53, 128, **298**, 354–355, 357; stiff or wry (torticollis), 285–286; vertebrae, 30; whiplash injury, 326–328
Necrosis, 557
Negroes: polycythemia vera, 522; sickle-cell anemia, 518–520; skin and hair, 57, 60; skin disorders, 400–402
Nembutal (pentobarbital), 886
Neoplasm: definition, 937; *see also* Cancer; Tumors
Neo-Synephrine (phenylephrine), 226, 535
Nephrons, 715, 716
Nephrosis, 723, 727
Nephrotic syndrome, 69, 723, **727–728**
Nerve cells, *see* Neurons
Nerve endings: motor end plates, 50, 52; sensory receptors, 50–52; in skin, 50, 51, 57, 59; synapses, 50

Nerves: cranial, 44, 47–48; fibers, 50; ganglia, 49; motor (efferent), 47–50, 54; plexuses, 49; sensory (afferent), 47–50, 54; transmission of impulses, 50–52; trunks, 48, 50
Nervous breakdown, 781
Nervous system, **42–54**, 511; autonomic, 43, **48–49**, 52, 86, 544, 684, 784; central (brain and spinal cord), 42–47; injuries, 53–54; neurological examination, 346–349; peripheral, 43, **47–48**, 53, 352–353, 356; physical examination, 966–967; structure and function, study of, 49
Nervous system disorders, 53–54, **355–377**; aging and, 949–950; congenital and hereditary, 373–377; peripheral nerves, 352–353, 356; spinal cord, 53, 54, **356–358**; symptoms, 335–349; syphilitic, 54, 245; *see also* Brain disorders; Brain injury
Nettles, stinging, 143, 385
Neuralgia, 353, 356, 950; glossopharyngeal, 356; tic douloureux, 344, 356
Neuritis, 353, 356; peripheral, in alcoholism, 791
Neurofibroma, 400
Neurogenic bladder, 731
Neuroglia (glial cells), 43, 50
Neurohumeral reactions, 684
Neurologist, 329, 967, 992–993
Neuroma, 366–367
Neurons (nerve cells), 20, 49–51; control, 50; motor, 49–50; sensory (receptor), 49–51; transmitter, 50
Neuropsychiatric hospitals, *see* Hospitals, neuropsychiatric
Neuroses, 769–771; *see also* Psychoneuroses
Neurosurgeon, 329, 993–995
Nevus, pigmented, *see* Mole
Niacin (nicotinic acid), 891
Niemann-Pick disease, 529
Night blindness, 427, 891
Nightingale, Florence, 1002
Nipples (for bottles), 855, 857
Nipples (of breasts), 444–445, 817; supernumerary, 444
Nitroglycerine: for angina pectoris, 596, 597; for heart failure, 579
Nocturia, 722
Norepinephrine (noradrenalin), 73, 684
Nose, **439–443**; broken, 441; care of, 442–443; defects and injuries, 441–443; foreign bodies in, **132–133**, 441–442; infections, 442; physical examination, 963; plastic surgery, 443; polyps, 442, 472, 498; rhinophyma (rum nose), 396; septum, misplaced, 443
Nosebleed, 134, 442, 534–535; in cirrhosis, 667; first aid, **134**, 535; in hemophilia, 531
Nose drops, 226, **443**, 535
Nostrils (nares), 440, 441

Nuclear wall, 21
Nucleic acids, 79, 174
Nurses: hospital staff, 1005–1006; licensed practical (LPN), 1006; Registered (RN), 1006; training, 1006
Nurse's aides, 1006
Nursing, history of, 1002
Nursing homes, 370, 945, **955–957**, 1009
Nursing services: extended care, 163–164, 1008–1009; home, professional, 163–164, 956; see also Home nursing care; public health, 164
Nutritional disorders, **887–893**; vitamin deficiencies, 891–893
Nutrition in childhood, 887–893
Nymphomania, 789
Nystagmus, 437

Oak Ridge, Tenn., radiation center, 979
Obesity, **927–931**; diabetes and, 696, 702; habits leading to, 923–924, 927–928; pituitary hormones in, 687, 708; see also Weight control
Obstetrician, 811, 814
Obstetrics, 991, 995–996; hospital service, 1004
Obstetrics-gynecology service, 987, 995–996
Occupational therapist, 330, 1007
Oculomotor nerves, 44, 347
Old age, see Aged, the; Aging
Olfactory nerves, 44, 347, 440
Olfactory receptors, 440
Onychomycosis, 176, **408**
Ophthalmologist, 432, 995
Opium derivatives, 793, **797–798**
Optic chiasma, 425
Optician, 432
Optic nerves, 44, 347, 425
Optometrist, 423
Orchitis, acute, 738; in mumps, 192, 738
Orgasm, 736, 747
Orthodontia, 418, 422
Orthopedic surgeon, 329, 994
Orthopnea, 576
Osgood-Schlatter disease, 308
Osmosis, 63, 68
Osmotic pressure balance, 79
Ossicles, 434, 438, 952
Osteitis deformans (Paget's disease), 308
Osteitis fibrosa cystica, 308
Osteoarthritis, **317–319**, 948, 950
Osteoblasts, 31
Osteochondrosis, 308
Osteoclasts, 31
Osteogenesis imperfecta, 307
Osteogenic sarcoma, 307
Osteoma (bone cyst), 306
Osteomalacia, 307
Osteomyelitis, 27, 29, 209–210, **304–306**

Osteopathic physician, 329–330
Osteoporosis, 307, 948
Otitis media, **196–197**, 437, 471
Otolaryngologist, 437, 438, 995
Otosclerosis, 438, 952
Otoscope, 436, 963
Ova (ovum), 94, 95, 685, 686, 734, **746–748**; cyst formation and, 758; fertilization, 94, 736, 742, 746–747, 811–812; gonadotrophic hormones affecting, 688–689; in multiple births, 746, 827–828
Ovaries, 94, 685, **746–747**; abnormalities, 749; in breast cancer, 450; cancer, 758–759; cysts and tumors, 757–759; in endometriosis, 759–761; hormones, 73, **685–686**, 747–748; in mumps, 192
Oviducts, see Fallopian tubes
Ovulation, 94, 747, 748, 811–812; end of, in menopause, 933; resumed after childbirth, 847; and rhythm method of contraception, 917–918; temperature and, 764, 812, 917
Oxygen, 455; anoxia, 64; asphyxia and, 107; in blood, 76–77; in brain, 53; in lungs, 62–65, 82; nerve cells using, 50; "poisoning," 63–64; polycythemia and, 521–522; in respiration, 46, 455–457, 460–462; therapeutic, for babies, danger of, 881
Oxytocin, 687, 837

Pacemaker, cardiac, 81, **544–545**; electronic, 545
Packed red cells, 540
Paget, Sir James, 308
Paget's disease (osteitis deformans), 308
Pain, referred, 337, 595
Pain threshold, 337–338
Palate: cancer, 657; cleft, 441; hard, 440; soft, 440
Palmer, Daniel David, 330
Palsy, 353; Bell's, 344, 353; cerebral, 293, 344, **882–883**; ulnar nerve, 353
Pancreas, 86, 610, **660–664**; cancer, 87, 567, **664**, 676; congenital fibrocystic disease (cystic fibrosis), 661, 877, **893–896**; insulin secretion, 72, 87, 661, 683, **696–698**; secretions, 85–87, 611, 660–662, 682; tumors, benign, 663
Pancreatic duct, 611, 660, 662, 682
Pancreatitis, 87; acute, 662–663; chronic, 663; mumps, 661–662
Papanicolaou, George N., 754
Papillary muscle, 57
Papilloma: intraductal, 448; in urinary bladder, 731
Pap smear (Pap test), 754–755, 966, 980
Para-amino benzoic acid (PABA), 721
Para-amino salicylic acid (PAS), 214
Paracelsus, 7, 8

Paralysis: paraplegia, 25, 356, 358; quadriplegia, 357, 358; spastic type, 375; from stroke, 360–361
Paralysis agitans, see Parkinson's disease
Paralytic ileus, 620–621
Paranoia, 804
Paranoid personality, 787, 804
Paranoid schizophrenia, 802
Paraplegia, 25, 356, 358; progressive spastic, 375
Parasitic infections, 176–177; insects, 61, **268–270**; worms, 177, **264–268**
Parathyroid glands, 683, **694–696**; adenoma, 695, 696; hyperparathyroidism, 695–696; hypoparathyroidism (parathyroid tetany), 694–695
Parathyroid hormone, 694–695
Paritonsillar abscess, 473
Paratyphoid (salmonella) infections, 254–255; immunization, 255, 257–258, 874
Paré, Ambroise, 9
Parenthood, **915–917**; adolescents and parents, 899–909; baby and, 849; planned, 916, 917
Paresis, general, 245
Parkinson, James, 366
Parkinson's disease (Parkinsonism, paralysis agitans), **365–366**; muscles in, 45; tremor in, 344
Paronychia (nailbed infection), 126–127, **408**
Parotid glands, 610
Parotitis, acute, see Mumps
Paroxysmal nocturnal dyspnea, 576
Parrot fever (psittacosis), 275–276
Passive-dependent personality, 786, 795, 798
Pasteur, Louis, 8, 169, 241, 242
Pasteurella pestis, 171, 273, 482
Pasteurella tularensis, 275
Patellar clonus, 347
Patent ductus arteriosus, **546–547**, 552
Pathologist, 997
Pectoral muscles, 459
Pediatrician, 851–852, 996
Pediatrics, 991
Pediatric service, 987, 1004
Pediatric surgeon, 994
Pediculosis (lice), 269
Pellagra, 392, 891
Pelvic examination, 966
Pelvic girdle, 745
Pelvic inflammatory disease (PID), 249, **753**
Pelvic organs, see Genital system, female
Pelvis, 27, 30, 36–37; fracture, 129, **298–299**, 730
Pemphigus, 403
Penicillin: for bacterial endocarditis, 559; discovery of, 12; for gonorrhea, 248–250; for pneumonia, 216; for rheumatic fever, 561–563; for scarlet fever, 184; for syphilis, 247

Penis, 713, 717, **735–736;** cancer, 740; congenital abnormalities, 736–737; erection, 736, 737, 741, 743–744
Pepsin, 85, 611, 648
Peptic ulcer, 87, 631, **648–655,** 662, 673, 923; bleeding from, 538, 650, 654; cancer and, 650, 651, 655, 657; diet, 651, 654; emotional tension (stress) and, 613, 649–650, 654–655; freezing of stomach as treatment, 655; medical treatment, 651, 654; occurrence, 649; pancreatic tumor, ulcerogenic, 663; parathyroid disorders and, 695; perforation, 644–645, 654; peritonitis from, 644–645; surgery, 654–655; symptoms and diagnosis, 650–651
Peptides, 660
Periarteritis nodosa, 565, 567
Pericarditis, 557, **563–564;** chronic constrictive, 564; in mononucleosis, 198
Pericardium, **557–558,** 560, 644
Periodontal tissues, 415
Periosteal hemorrhage, 295
Periosteum, 27, 40
Peristalsis, 38, 86, 613; disorders of, 614–615
Peritoneum, 40, 644, 745; abscesses, 645; in hernia, 625, 626
Peritonitis, 40, **644–645;** in appendicitis, 640, 644; chemical, 644; in gall bladder attack, 674, 676; infected, 644; in ulcerative colitis, 635, 644
Pernicious anemia, 77, 392, **516–518,** 631, 891
Personality: cycloid, 786–787, 804; dual, 800; Freud's theories on, 772–774; inadequate (passive-dependent), 786, 795, 798; paranoid, 786, 804; psychopathic, 787; schizoid, 786, 801
Personality disorders, 770, 773, 777, **785–787,** 800–801, 804
Perspiration, 57, 149
Pertussis (whooping cough), **187–188,** 471
Pessary, 751
Petechiae, 529
Petechial hemorrhage, 559
Petit mal, *see* Epilepsy
Peyote, 797
Pfeiffer, Emil, 197
Phagocytosis, 78
Pharmacist, 1009–1010
Pharyngeal speech (without larynx), 500
Pharyngitis, 472–473
Pharynx, 456, 471, 610
Phenylalanine, 879
Phenylbutasone, 316, 318
Phenylketonuria (PKU), 96, 376–377, **878–879**
Phenylpyruvic acid, 879
Pheochromocytoma, 585, 587, **706–707**

Philadelphia chromosome (Ph₁), 525
Philadelphia General Hospital, 1014
Phimosis, 737
Phlebitis, 565, **567–568,** 569
Phlebotomy, 581
Phobias (phobic reaction), 779–780
Phobophobia, 780
Phocomelia, 822
Phospholipids, 604, 889
Phosphorus: in nutrition, 890; radioactive, *see* Radioactive phosphorus
Physiatrist, 329
Physical examination, **963–967;** abdomen, 965; blood pressure, 964; diagnostic aids, 968–982; ears, nose, and throat, 963; eyes, 963–964; genital system, 966; heart and lungs, 964–965; lymph glands, 964; neurological, **346–349,** 967; rectal and proctoscopic, 966; skin, 963; temperature, pulse, and respiration (TPR), 964; thyroid gland, 964
Physical therapist, 330, 1007
Physical therapy: for musculoskeletal disorders, 330; after stroke, 363–364
Pia mater, 47
Pica, 265
PID (pelvic inflammatory disease), 249, **753**
Piles, *see* Hemorrhoids
Pill, the, 742, 760, 764, 819, **919–920;** menstrual irregularity and, 537; progesterone in, 688–689; side effects, 919–920
Pimples (acne), 59, 206–208, **393–396**
Pineal gland, 46, **689**
Pinealoma, 46, 689
Pinkeye (acute conjunctivitis), **205–206,** 429
Pinworm infections, 177, **266–268;** anal pruritus from, 647
Piperazine (Antepar), 266, 267
Pitocin, 837, 839, 843, 845
Pituitary gland, 45, 73–74, **686–689;** posterior and anterior lobes, 686–687
Pituitary gland disorders, **707–709;** acromegaly, 708; diabetes insipidus, 709; dwarfism, 307–308, 708; Fröhlich's syndrome, 708; gigantism, 707–708; hypoglycemia in, 703; obesity in, 687, 708; Simmonds' disease, 708; tumor, 707–709
Pituitary hormones, 74, 683, **686–689,** 704, 735, 747–748; ACTH, *see* Adrenocorticotropic hormone; gonadotrophic, 688–689; growth hormone, 31, 74, **687;** *see also* Sex hormones
Pityriasis rosea, 397
Placenta, 748, 816, 818, 819, 821; abruptio placentae, 829, **831–832,** 845; expelled after birth, 843; placenta previa, 829, **831–832,** 845, 846

Plague: bubonic, 273–274, 874; pneumonic, 273
Plants, poisonous, 142–143, 390
Plasma, 76, 79–80, 90, 512–513, 540; freeze-dried, 121; in hemophilia, 531; proteins in, 79–80; in shock, 539
Plasma expanders, 121, 539
Plastic surgeon, 994
Plastic surgery: of breasts, 451–452; cosmetic, 951; of nose, 443
Platelets, blood, 32, 78, 79, 513, 514, 524, 529, 530
Play therapy, 783
Pleomorphism, 171
Pleura, 40, 464, 465, 644
Pleural pneumonia-like organisms (PPLO), 175–176
Pleuritis (pleurisy), 40, 463, **484**
Pneumococci, 171, 215
Pneumoconioses, 485, 487
Pneumoencephalogram, 349, 351, 979
Pneumonectomy, 213, 505
Pneumonia, 64–65, **214–218,** 480, 482; arthritis in, 312; aspiration, 120, 218, **487–488;** bronchial (bronchiolar), 64, 217, 482; bronchiectasis and, 477; bronchitis and, 476; chemical, 218, **487–488;** cystic fibrosis and, 895; Hippocrates' description of, 6; hydrothorax in, 482, 483; hypostatic (stasis), 218, **488–489;** influenza and, 217, 230; lobar, 64, 67, **215–216,** 312, 482; lung abscess in, 484; oil, 218, 226, 442, **488;** pleurisy in, 484; viral, 64, 228, 482; whooping cough and, 187
Pneumonic plague, 273
Pneumothorax: artificial, 213; pressure, 465; spontaneous, 64, 463, 465, **497**
Poison Control Centers, **116, 117,** 143
Poisoning, **116–117;** anemia from chemical agents, 520; antidotes, 117; babies, harmful substances swallowed, 863; barbiturates, 342; botulism, 219, **260–261;** carbon monoxide, 65, **115–116,** 342; carbon tetrachloride, **668,** 800; cirrhosis, toxic, 668; containers, safety in, 117; corrosive gastritis, 631; cyanide, 65; drugs, medicinal, 800; food, staphylococcal poisoning, 253–254; hospital treatment, 121; plant poisons, 142–143, 390
Poison ivy, 142, **390;** vaccine, 142
Poison oak, 142, 390
Poison sumac, 142–143, 390
Poliomyelitis, **188–190,** 292, 358; bone disorders and, 308–309; bulbar, 189; epidemics, 188; immunization, 175, **188, 190,** 873; motor neurons in, 39–40, 51, 54; muscles in, 39–40; respiration and, 463
Polycystic disease, 729
Polycythemia, 78, **521–523;** relative, 521; secondary, 522

Polycythemia vera, 522–523
Polyps: laryngeal, 475, 498–499; nasal, 442, 472, 498; rectal or intestinal, 659, 938; sinus, 472, 474; urinary bladder, 731, 948; uterine, 757, 760
Pons, 43–44
Portal circulation system, 664–665
Portal vein, 83, 665, 667
Port wine stain (birthmark), 59, 401, 896
Positive pressure breathing devices, 121
Potassium in nutrition, 890
Pott's disease (tuberculosis of spine), 214, 306
PPLO (pleural pneumonia-like organisms), 175–176
Precursor cells, 32
Preeclampsia (toxemia of pregnancy), 728, 826, **832**
Pregnancy, 94–95, **811–835;** amniocentesis in, 376; anemia in, 515, 518, **821–822;** breast feeding and, 848; breasts in, 445, 817, 830; constipation in, 824, 827; diabetes in, 701–702, 826; doctor-patient relationship, 814–815; expected date of confinement (EDC), 815; first trimester, 815–824; fluid retention, 824–825, 831, 832; German measles (rubella) in, 181, 375, 435, 549, 555, 814, **823–824;** gonadotrophic hormones in, 689; hemorrhoids in, 826, 827; medications in, and deformed babies, 822–823; menstruation stopped, 748, 812–813; miscarriage, 818–820, 828–829; *see also* Abortion; morning sickness, 817–818; multiple, 827–828; Rh disease, *see* Rh disease and Rh factor; second trimester, 824–829; tests, 813–814; third trimester, 829–835; thrombophlebitis in, 567; toxemia of, 728, 826, **832;** tubal (ectopic), 640, 644, 748, **820–821;** unwanted, 910, 911, 915; urinary system infections, 721, 825–826; uterus in, 39, 747, 815–817, 824–826; varicose veins, 568–570, **826–827;** weight control, 824–825, 831
Preludin, 794
Premature birth, **828–829,** 897
Premedical training, 984
Premenstrual tension, **762–763,** 923
Prepuce (foreskin), 735–738
Presbyopia, 427
Pressor drugs, 539
Pressure sores (bedsores), 386–387
Priapism, 741
Prickly heat (miliaria, heat rash), 59, **384–385,** 865
Prime years, *see* Maturity
Probenecid, 320
Proctoscope, 623, 658–659, 966
Progesterone, 688, 748, 812; in endometriosis, 760; in the Pill, 688–689
Progressive spastic paraplegia, 375

Projection (defense mechanism), 776
Prone-pressure artificial respiration, 108–109
Prostate gland, 717, 735, 740; benign hypertrophy (prostatism), 739–740, 948; cancer, 411, **741,** 942, 955; infection (prostatitis), 738, **739;** urinary obstruction, 723
Prostheses (artificial limbs and joints), 302
Protein-bound iodine test (PBI), 692
Proteins, **888–889;** in blood, 79, 512–513, 714, 717; deficiency, 888–889; in diet, 929; digestion of, 86, 660; in plasma, 79–80, 90; in urine, 68, 727, 826, 832
Proteoses, 660
Prothrombin, 90, 664; vitamin K and, 532
Protoplasm, 21
Protozoan infections, 176–177, 278
Prowazek, Stanislav von, 175
Pruritus, anal, 647
Pseudohermaphroditism, 750
Psittacosis (parrot fever), 275–276
Psoriasis, 61, **402–403,** 411–412
Psychiatrist, 782–784, 806–807, 997–998
Psychiatry, 770–771
Psychic energizers (drugs), 936
Psychoanalysis, 770, 782–783, 998
Psychoanalyst, 997–998
Psychologist, 997–998
Psychology, Freud's theories, 772–774
Psychomotor seizures, 342
Psychoneuroses, 770–771, 776, 777, **779–784;** anxiety reaction, 779; conversion reaction, 781; counseling for, 782–783; depressive reaction, 780–781, **935–936;** dissociative reaction, 781; phobic reaction (phobias), 779–780; treatment, 782–784
Psychoneurotic skin abuse, 393
Psychopathic personality, 787
Psychoses, 770, 777, **800–805;** involutional melancholia, **805,** 935; LSD and, 797, 802–803; manic-depressive, 804–805; paranoia, 804; schizophrenia, **800–804,** 805, 807–808
Psychosomatic disorders, 770, 777, **784–785;** of digestive system, 613–614, 623, 629, 632, 634–635, 637
Psychosurgery, 803
Psychotherapy, **782–784,** 803; directive and nondirective, 783; group, 783, 793, 799; play, 783; tranquilizers, 783
Psychotic break, 801
Ptyalin, 610
Puberty, **900–903;** breast development, 444–445; growth in, 867, 900; emotional problems, 775, 901–902; secondary sex characteristics, 685, 747, 900; sex in, 900–901, 909
Public health, history of, 7, 9
Public health nursing services, 164

Public Health Service, 14, 230, 246, 271, 331, 562; hospitals, 1003; immunization, 186, 235, 255–256, 274; tuberculosis prevention, 214; vaccination rules, 234
Public Welfare, 14
Puerperal sepsis, 207, **753,** 847
Pulmonary artery, 63; septal defects, 551; in transposition of great vessels, 547–548
Pulmonary circulatory system, 62, 82, 461, 511
Pulmonary embolus, 65, 83, 463, 532, 567, 601
Pulmonary emphysema, *see* Emphysema, pulmonary
Pulmonary fibrosis, 485, 953
Pulmonic stenosis, 548, 550
Pulmonic valve, 544, 548
Pulse, 542, 964
Puncture wounds, **126,** 219–220, 222
Pupil (of eye), 426
Purpura, 514, **529–530;** thrombocytopenic, 529–530
Pus, 172, 557, 826
Pyelitis, 720–721
Pyelogram: intravenous, 68, 70–71, 732–733, **978;** retrograde, 730–732, 979
Pyelonephritis, 720–721; tuberculous, 721
Pyloric sphincter, 611
Pyloric stenosis, 877–878
Pyloroplasty, 654
Pylorus, 648, 654
Pyorrhea, 420–421

Q fever, 175, **276**
Quacks, 330–331
Quadriplegia, 357, 358
Quinacrine hydrochloride (Atabrine) 264, 268, 397
Quinidine, 579
Quinine, 263
Quinsy sore throat, 473

Rabbit fever (tularemia), 275
Rabies, 141–142, **239–242;** treatment, 241–242; vaccine, 240–242
Race: life expectancy and, 944; skin and hair characteristics, 59–60
Rachitic rosary, 892
Radiation, cancer treatment with, 499, 500, 505, 507, 730, 740, 757, 941–942, 979
Radiation injury, 51–52, **143–144,** 975, 979
Radiation sickness, 143–144; agranulocytosis in, 532; anemia in, 520
Radical neck dissection, 500
Radioactive iodine (I^{131}), 693; uptake test, 692
Radioactive phosphorus (P^{32}), 520, 523; for leukemia, 526; for polycythemia vera, 523
Radiologist, 996
Radiology (roentgenology), 975

Radium: cancer treatment with, 499, 730, 740, 755, 757, 941; injury from, 520

Radius, 27, 30

Radon, cancer treatment with, 499, 730, 941

Raphael, 8

Rationalization (defense mechanism), 776

Rats, plague spread by, 273

Rattlesnake venom, 518

Raynaud's disease, 565

Reaction formations, 776

Read, Grantly Dick, 839

Rectocele, 751

Rectum, 612; cancer, 645, **658–659;** foreign bodies in, 133; hemorrhage from, 536–537, 570–571; hemorrhoids, *see* Hemorrhoids; physical examination, 966; polyps, 659, 938

Red blood cells, *see* Blood cells, red

Red Cross, first-aid training, 145

Reed, Walter, 235

Reflexes, 347–348, 966–967

Regional enteritis, 632–634

Rehabilitative medicine, 309, 329

Relapsing fever, 275

Renal arteries, 68, 714, 729; obstruction, 585, 586

Renal failure, 69, 723–727, **728–729**

Renal veins, 715

Renin, 85, 716

Repression (defense mechanism), 776

Reproduction, 92–96

Respiration, **455–463;** artificial, *see* Artificial respiration; brain in control of, 46, 456, 459–460; breathing, mechanics of, 457, 459–460; circulation and, 455–456, 460–461; rate of, 461; shallow (guarded), 468; vital capacity, 461, 952

Respiratory alkalosis, 64

Respiratory center, 459–460, 463

Respiratory failure (asphyxia), 103–104, **107–110;** hospital treatment, 121

Respiratory membrane, 63, 64, 455, 457, 460, 462, 470

Respiratory tract disorders, 462–463; aging and, 948, 952–953; of babies, newborn, 881, 882; cancer, 498–500; common cold, 64, **225–228;** foreign bodies, 64, 133, 462, **468–470;** influenza, 224, **228–230;** pneumonia, *see* Pneumonia; specialists in, 993; upper respiratory infections (URI's), 193–196, **470–480,** 863

Respiratory tree, 456–457

Reticulocytes, 77

Retina, 425, 426, 699; detachment, 431, 881

Retinoblastoma, 431, 896

Retirement, 946–947

Retirement communities, 945

Retrograde pyelogram, 730–732, 979

Retrolental fibroplasia, 880–881

Reversal (defense mechanism), 776

Rhabdomyosarcoma, 292

Rhazes, 7

Rh disease and Rh factor, 514, 518, 540, 814, 820, 828, **833–834,** 882, 973–974

Rheumatic fever, 40–41, 97, 210, 313, **560–563,** 564, 574; anemia in, 520; chorea in (Sydenham's), 45, 344; corticosteroids in, 73, 562; scarlet fever and, 184; surgery (commissurotomy), 563; treatment, 562–563

Rheumatic heart disease, 41, **560–563,** 574

Rheumatism, 313, 561

Rheumatoid arthritis, 40, **312–317,** 560, 561; corticosteroids in, 73, 316; key symptoms, 315; treatment, 315–317

Rheumatologist, 329, 992

Rh factor, *see* Rh disease and Rh factor

Rhinophyma, 396

Riboflavin (vitamin B₂) deficiency, 891

Ribonucleic acid (RNA), 174, 525

Ribs, 27, 30; cervical, 458; floating, 459; fractures, 128–129, 297, 462, **464–467;** in respiration, 457–459

Rickets, 308, 422, **892**

Ricketts, Howard Taylor, 175

Rickettsiae, 175, 224

Rickettsial infections, 224–225, 237–239, 268, 276

Riedel's struma, 694

Ringworm, 176, **398–399;** of nail (onychomycosis), 176, **408**

Ritalin (methylphenidate), 794, 936

RNA (ribonucleic acid), 174, 525

Rocky Mountain spotted fever, 175, **237–238,** 268, 270

Roentgen, Wilhelm Konrad, 975

Roentgenology (radiology), 975

Rosacea, 396

Roseola infantum (exanthem subitum), 181

Rubella, *see* German measles

Rubeola, *see* Measles

Rubin test, 760

Rush, Benjamin, 9, 235

S-A node (sino-atrial node), 545

Sabin, Albert, 188

Sabin vaccine, 188, 190

Sacral nerves, 48

Sacroiliac syndrome, 324, 325

Sadism, 789

St. Martin, Alexis, 84

St. Vitus' dance (Sydenham's chorea), 45, 344

Salerno medical school, 7

Salicylic acid, 312

Salivary glands, **610–611,** 682

Salk, Jonas, 188

Salk vaccine, 188, 190

Salmonella, 171, 256; bone infections, 305

Salmonella (paratyphoid) infections, 254–255; immunization, 255, 257–258

Salpingitis, 640; gonorrheal, 249

Salt (sodium chloride), 890; in body, 714; restriction, 580, 590

Sanger, Frederick, 697

Sarcoma, 938; Ewing's, 307; osteogenic, 307; uterine, 757

Satyrism, 789

Scabies, 268–269

Scalp: disorders, 411–412; hemorrhage from wound, 536; lacerations, 125; ringworm, 398

Scarlet fever (scarlatina), **183–184,** 471

Scars, 58, 557; keloids, 401

Schaudinn, Fritz, 246

Schick test, 186

Schistosomiasis, 278

Schizoid personality, 786, 801

Schizophrenia, **800–804,** 805, 807–808; catatonic, 802; hebephrenic, 802; paranoid, 802; treatment, 802–804

Sciatica, 325, 356

Sciatic nerve, 48, 356

Sclera, 426, 429

Sclera hemorrhage, 535–536

Scleroderma, 61, **403–405,** 560

Scoliosis, 309, **328,** 880

Scorpion strings, 140

Scrotum, 734, 735, 738; benign growths in, 740; embryonal rests, 740; hydrocele, 740; spermatocele, 740; varicocele, 740

Scrub typhus (tsutsugamushi disease), 175, **239**

Scurvy, 392, **529,** 891–892

Sebaceous cysts, 394, 401

Sebaceous glands, 56, 59; acne and, 393–395; hair and, 409

Seborrheic dermatitis (dandruff), 58, **411–412,** 429

Seborrheic keratoses, 401–402

Sebum, 56, 59

Seconal (secobarbital), 886

Secondary sex characteristics, 685, 747, 900

Semen, 717, 735

Semicircular canal, 435

Seminal vesicles, 717, 735, 740

Seminiferous tubules, 735

Seminoma, 740

Semmelweis, Ignatz, 207

Senile keratosis, 407

Senility (senile dementia), **367, 370** 950

Sensory nerve endings (receptors), 50–52

Sensory nerves, **47–51,** injuries, 353; neurological examination, 347

Septicemia (sepsis, blood poisoning), 172, **206–208,** 515, 974

Serological test for syphilis (STS), 246

Serum hepatitis, *see* Hepatitis, serum

Sex: aging and, 955; behavior, standards of, 910–911; of child, pre-

Sex: aging and (cont'd)
determination, 916; children's curiosity about, 872, 900; compatibility in marriage, 913–914; in puberty, 900–901, 909; sexual maturity, 909–911
Sex cells (germ cells), 93–95
Sex characteristics, secondary, 685, 747, 900
Sex education, **903–905;** in early childhood, 872; in venereal disease control, 251–252, 904
Sex hormones, 73, 95, 96, 682, **685–686,** 735, 747–748, 812; aging and, 955; cancer and, 942, 955; masculinizing and feminizing changes, 685–686; in menopause, 934; pituitary, 686, 688–689, 747–748
Sexual deviation, 787–790
Sexual intercourse, 94–95, 734, 736, 747; aging and, 955; health and, 736; menstrual cycle and, 748, 918; miscarriage and, 819–820; moral standards and, 910–911; in post-partum period, 847; in pregnancy, 830
Sherrington, Sir Charles Scott, 49
Shigella, 258–259
Shigellosis (bacillary dysentery), 258–259
Shingles (herpes zoster), 206, **231–232,** 358
Shock, 103–104, **111–113,** 116, 533, 538–539; amnesia and, 360; anaphylactic, **139–140,** 388; from bee-stings, 139–140; electrical, 117–119; first aid, 111–113; in fractures, 129, 130; hemorrhage and, 533, 534, 538–539; insulin, *see* Insulin shock; post-partum, 846; renal failure in, 728; from wounds, 138
Shock therapy, 360, 783, **803,** 805, 936
Shoulder blade, fracture, 464, 465
Shoulder joint, 30
Shriners' Hospitals for Crippled Children, 331
Sickle-cell anemia (sickling disease), 518–520
Silicosis, 485–487
Simmonds' disease, 708
Singer, Charles, 235
Singultus, *see* Hiccups
Sino-atrial node (S-A node), 545
Sinuses: maxillary, 472; paranasal, 472; supraorbital, 472
Sinusitis, **471–472;** allergic, 472; chronic, 472; headache, 225, 472; polyps, 472, 474
Skene's glands, 747, 753–754
Skin, **55–61;** aging and, 950; capillaries, 59; care, 412–413; color, 56–57, 59–60; dermabrasion treatment, 396; dermis, 59; elastic tissue, 56; epidermis, 58; fat under, 56; foreign bodies in, 132; functions, 56–58; inflammation, 556–557;

Skin (cont'd)
melanin pigment, 56–57, 59; nerve endings, 50, 51, 57, 59; pain and temperature receptors, 50, 51, 57; physical examination, 963; structure, 58–59
Skin abuse, psychoneurotic, 393
Skin cancer, **405–407,** 938; basal-cell carcinoma, 405–406; moles and, 59, 400, 406; precancerous lesions, 406–407; squamous-cell carcinoma, 406, 938
Skin disorders, 60–61, **381–407;** acne, 59, 206–208, **393–396,** 901; allergies, 61, **387–392;** of baby, 859, 860, 865; cancer, *see* Skin cancer; chafing and chapping, 385–386; chemical irritations, 385–386; emotional factors in, 388, 393, 784; from external factors, 382–387; fungus infections, 385, **398–399;** infections, viral and bacterial, 204–205, 230–232; insect parasites, 61, **268–270,** 399–400; malnutrition and, 392; metabolic and glandular, 392; pigmentation, 400–402; serious, 402–405; in tuberculosis, 61
Skull, 27, 46; of baby, 27, 841, 844–845, 852, 857, 878; fractures, 128, **297,** 302, 359; sutures, 27
Sleep, **340–341;** of baby, 861; in childhood, 868–869
Sleeping sickness, African (trypanosomiasis), 177, **278**
Slotin, Louis, 51–52
Smallpox (variola), 232–234; vaccination, 9, 174–175, 231, **233–234,** 874
Smell, sense of, 346, **439–440,** 951
Smoke inhalation, 487
Smoking: angina pectoris and, 597; atherosclerosis and, 594; bronchitis and, 476; Buerger's disease and, 565; cancer and, 406, 457; cancer of lung and, 504, 505, 924, 977; cancer of respiratory tract and, 498, 499; coronary artery disease and, 603; emphysema and, 495; hypertension and, 590; respiratory disorders and, 457; stopping, 505, 590, 924
Snakebite kit, 141
Snakebites, 140, 141
Snakes, 140–141
Sneezing, mechanism, 462
Snow blindness, 382, **428–429**
Social Security, 14, 945, 1018
Society for Crippled Children and Adults, 331
Sodium chloride, *see* Salt
Sodium cyanide poisoning, 65
Solar plexus, 49
Somatotrophic hormone, *see* Growth hormone
Sore throat, 471; in diphtheria, 185–186; pharyngitis, 472–473; quinsy, 473; in tonsillitis, 193

Sound receptors, 50, 434
Sound waves, frequencies, 434–435
Spastic gait, 882
Spastic paralysis, 375; familial, 375
Spastic paraplegia, progressive, 375
Speculum, 754, 963, 966
Speech: in cerebral palsy, 882, 883; learning to talk, 869; pharyngeal, after removal of larynx, 500
Speed (drug), 794
Sperm, 94, 685, 686, 689, 717, **734–736;** ejaculation, 736, 743, 744; in fertilization, *see* Ova, fertilization; infertility, 741–742
Spermatocele, 740
Sphingomyelin, 529
Sphygmomanometer, 583
Spider bites, 140
Spider nevi, 667
Spina bifida, **373–375,** 878
Spinal cord, 43, **47–50,** 52, 353; disorders, 53, 54, 356–358; embryonic development, 58; injuries, 53; syphilis in, 245; tumor, 358
Spinal curvature, 328
Spinal nerves, 47–48, 353
Spinal reflex arc, 47
Spinal tap (lumbar puncture), 47, 154, **348–349,** 972
Spine, *see* Vertebrae
Spirochetes, 170, 171
Splanchnicectomy, 591
Spleen: bacterial emboli in, 559; blood platelets in, 514; in hemolytic anemia, 519–520; in infectious mononucleosis, 198; in leukemia, 525; in lymphoid disorders, 527–529; lymphoid tissue in, 527; in polycythemia vera, 523; rupture, 644
Splenectomy: in hemolytic anemia, 520; in Hodgkin's disease, 528; in thrombocytopenic purpura, 530
Splinters, 132
Splints, 129
Spotted fever (epidemic spinal meningitis), 199–200; *see also* Rocky Mountain spotted fever
Sprains, **130–131,** 282, 295, 304; intervertebral, 324, 325; lumbosacral, 324–325
Sprue, 517, **628–629,** 891
Squamous-cell carcinoma, 405–406, 938
Squint (strabismus), 290, **427–428**
Stanley, Wendell M., 173
Stapes, 434
Staphylococci, 171
Staphylococcus albus, 204
Staphylococcus aureus, 171, 204
Staphylococcus infections, **204–210;** arthritis, 311, 312; boils and carbuncles, 61, **208–209;** bone, 305; food poisoning, 253–254; paritonsillar abscess, 473
Status asthmaticus, 492
Status epilepticus, 884

Stenosis, 550
Sterility, *see* Infertility
Sterilization, male and female, 920–921
Steroid hormones, *see* Corticosteroids
Sternum (breastbone), 457, 464
Stethoscope, 964–965
Still, Andrew Taylor, 329
Stockings, supportive, 570, 827
Stokes, Adrian, 236
Stomach, 85, **609–611;** burns, 630; cancer, 631, 650, 651, **655–657;** freezing for ulcer treatment, 655; gastric dilatation, acute, 617, 620; in poisoning, hospital treatment, 121; secretions, *see* Gastric juices; surgery, 654, 663; ulcer, *see* Peptic ulcer
Stomach ache, 135; *see also* Abdominal pain
Stomach flu, 229, 253, 254
Stomach pump, 121, 620
Stone bruising, 323
Strabismus (squint), 290, **427–428**
Strains, muscle, 131
Strawberry birthmark, 400–401
Streptococci, 171; Group A beta-hemolytic, 183
Streptococcus infections, **204–210;** arthritis, 311, 312; bone, 305; glomerulonephritis and, 184, 724; paritonsillar abscess, 473; scarlet fever, **183–184,** 471; strep-sensitivity diseases, 210
Streptococcus viridans, 558; in rheumatic fever, 561–563
Streptomycin: auditory nerve damage from, 53; for tuberculosis, 213–214, 312, 721
Stroke, 53, 115, 360–364, 532, 588, 593, 950; care of patient, 362–364; little, 364; repeated attacks, 364
STS (serological test for syphilis), 246
Sty, 429
Subarachnoid hemorrhage, 364–365
Subdural hematoma, 365, 882
Sublimation (defense mechanism), 776
Sublingual glands, 610
Submaxillary glands, 610
Subsonic waves, 434–435
Subtotal gastrectomy, 654
Subtotal thyroidectomy, 693
Sudden death syndrome, 897–898
Sugar: in blood (glucose), 696–698, 702, 703; in urine in diabetes, 696–698, 700
Sugars, digestion of, 86, 888
Sulfinpyrazone, 320
Sunburn, 58, 135, **382–383,** 401
Sunstroke (hyperpyrexia), 115, **136,** 156
Superego, **773–774,** 776, 778
Supportive hose, 570, 827
Suprarenal glands, *see* Adrenal glands

Surgeons: general, 994; neurosurgeon, 329, 993–995; orthopedic, 329, 994; pediatric, 994; plastic (reconstructive), 994; thoracic, 994; training of, 993–995
Surgery, 991; history of, 6, 9
Surgical service, 987, 1003–1004
Sutton, Richard L., Jr., 411
Swallowing: difficulty in, 614–615, 939; muscles in, 38
Sweat glands, 57, 59
Sydenham, Thomas, 9
Sydenham's chorea (St. Vitus' dance), 45, 344
Sylvester method (supine arm-lift), artificial respiration, 109
Synapses, 50
Synovial fluid, 40, 310, 311, 317, 318, 321
Synovial membrane, 287, 310
Syphilis, **243–248;** aneurysm of aorta from, 245, 565, 566; arthritis in, 312; brain disorders, 245, 345; congenital, 246, 880; control and treatment, 246–248; in female, 752; joint disorders in, 312, 321–322; malaria infection as cure for, 263; nervous system disorders, 54, 245; premarital examination as protection, 913; primary, 244–245; secondary, 245; spirochete, *Treponema pallidum,* 170, 171, 244, 247, 250; tertiary, 245; tests for, 246
Syphilology, 992
Syringomelia, 358

T and A, *see* Tonsillectomy and adenoidectomy
Tabes dorsalis, 54, **245**
Tachycardia, 576
Tamponade, cardiac, 564
Tanning, 57, 383
Tapeworms, 177, **268**
Tartar, 420
Taste, sense of, 346
Taste buds, 610, 611
Taussig, Helen, 41
Tay-Sachs disease, 375–377
Tear gas, 487
Teeth, **415–423;** abnormalities of development, 417–418; aging and, 951; bicuspids, 416–417; canines, 416–417; care, *see* Dental care and treatment; caries, 419–420; decidual (baby), 416–418, 868; dentures, 421, 951; extra or missing, 417–418; fluorides for protection of, 420; impaction, 418; incisors, 416–417; injury, 419; malocclusion, 418–419; molars, 416–418; occlusion, 416; permanent, 416–418, 868; structure, 415–416; wisdom, 418
Teething, 416
Telephone numbers, emergency, 146

Temperature (body): Centigrade and Fahrenheit, 150; measurement with thermometer, 150; normal, 149; ovulation and, 764, 812, 917; variation and regulation, 148–149
Temperature, pulse, and respiration (TPR), 964
Tendonitis, 40, 287
Tendons, 25, 33, 40, 282, 287–288; reflexes, 347–348, 967
Tenosynovitis, 287
Teratoma (teratocarcinoma) of testes, 740
Testes (testicles), 94, 734–735, 740; cancer, 740; descent of, 625, 708; hormones, 73, **685–686,** 735, *see also* Sex hormones; nerves, 49; orchitis, acute, 738; orchitis in mumps, 192, 738; torsion, 739; undescended (cryptorchidism), **737–378,** 875
Testosterone, 685, 735; for baldness, 411; for impotence, caution on, 744, 955
Tetanus (lockjaw), 11–12, **219–221;** dog bites and, 141; immunization, 126, **220–221;** puncture wounds and, 126; toxin, 172, 220; toxoid, 220
Tetany, 63–64, 890
Tetracyclines in pregnancy, dangers of, 822
Tetralogy of Fallot, 549–550
Thalamus, 45
Thalidomide, 822
Therapeutic trial, 981
Thermometer (fever), 150
Thiamine (vitamin B₁), 891
Thirst, 614–615
Thoracentesis, 468, 482
Thoracic duct, 527
Thoracic nerves, 48
Thoracic surgeon, 994
Thoracoplasty, 213
Thorax, 457, 459
Throat: foreign bodies in, 107, **114,** 121, 133; physical examination, 963; sore, *see* Sore throat
Thromboangiitis obliterans (Buerger's disease), 565
Thrombocytes, 32, 78, 79, 513; *see also* Platelets, blood
Thromboendarterectomy, 568
Thrombophlebitis, 532, **567–568,** 569, 664
Thrombosis, 532, 574; coronary, *see* Coronary thrombosis; stroke and, 360, 532
Thrombus (thrombi), 83, 513, 514, 532; in aterosclerosis, 593; in phlebitis (thrombophlebitis), 567–569; in polycythemia, 521, 523; saddle, 567–568; in sickle-cell anemia, 519
Thrush (moniliasis), 176, 647, 859, 863–864
Thymoma, 689

Thymus gland, 290–291, 689
Thyroglobulin, 692
Thyroidectomy, subtotal, 693
Thyroid extract, 72, 693, 694
Thyroid gland, 69, 72, **682–683;** physical examination, 964
Thyroid gland disorders, 690–694; cancer, 693; goiter, 72, 683, **690–693;** heart failure and, 574; hyperthyroidism, 72, 683, **691–693,** 707; hypothyroidism (myxedema), 72, 392, 604, 683, 691–692; surgery, 693, 694; thyroiditis, 691, 693–694; thyroid storm (thyroid crisis), 691, 693; tremor, 345; tumors, 585, 692, 693
Thyroid hormone (thyroxin), 72, 74, **683,** 687, 692; in atherosclerosis, 604; iodine and, 690–691, 693; synthetic, 693, 694
Thyroiditis, 691, 693–694; chronic, 694
Thyroid-stimulating (thyrotrophic) hormone (TSH), 74, **687**
Thyroid storm, 691, 693
Thyrotoxicosis, 691
Tic, 292, **343–344**
Tic douloureux, 344, 356
Tick paralysis, 270
Ticks, 139, 275; removal of, 238, 269–270; rickettsial diseases transmitted by, 175, **237–238,** 268
Tinea, 176
Tinea capitis, 176, 398
Tinea corporis, 176, 398
Tinea cruris, 398
Tinea pedis, 176, 399
Tinnitus, 437
Tissues, 20, 22–23
Tobacco mosaic virus, 173
Toenails, see Nails
Toilet training, 869
Tomogram, 504
Tongue, 611; in artificial respiration, 107–109; cancer, 657
Tongue-tie, 876
Tonometer, 431
Tonsillectomy and adenoidectomy (T and A), **193–195,** 197, 438; bleeding after, 535
Tonsillitis, **193–194,** 471
Tonsils, **193,** 456, 473
Toothache, **134,** 423
Toothbrushes, 422
Toothpaste, 420, 422
Tophi, 320
Torticollis (wry neck, stiff neck), 285–286
Total gastrectomy, 663
Tourniquet, 105–106
Toxemia of pregnancy (preeclampsia), 728, 826, 832
Toxoplasmosis, 278
Trachea, 63, 456; foreign bodies in, 107, **114,** 133, 456
Tracheitis, 475
Tracheobronchitis, 475

Tracheoesophageal fistula, 876–877
Tracheostomy, **114,** 121, 186, 480
Trachoma, **232,** 429
Trampoline, dangers of, 357
Tranquilizers in psychotherapy, 783, 803, 805
Transfusion, see Blood transfusion
Transplants: bone marrow, 520; cornea, 430; heart, 41, 605, 999; kidney, 65, 726–727; liver, 669; rejection reaction, 98, 520, 726
Transposition of great vessels, 547–548
Trauma, 533
Travelers' diarrhea, **255–256,** 621
Tremor, 292, **343–345;** athetoid, 882
Trench fever, 175
Trench foot (immersion foot), 137, **384**
Trench mouth (Vincent's infection, Vincent's angina), 171, **218–219,** 421
Treponema pallidum, 170, 171, 244, 247, 250
Trichinella, 117, 277, 292
Trichiniasis (trichinosis), 177, **276–277,** 292
Trichomonas vaginalis, 177, 278, **752–753**
Trichotillomania, 393
Tricuspid valve, 544, 550
Trigeminal nerves, 44, 344, 347
Triglycerides, 592–593, 604, 664
Trusses, 626
Trypanosomiasis (African sleeping sickness), 177, **278**
Trypsin, 85–86, 660
Tsetse fly, 177, 278
Tsutsugamushi disease, 175, **239**
Tubal ligation, 920–921
Tubal pregnancy, 640, 644, 748, **820–821**
Tuberculosis, 65, 97, **211–214,** 480, 481; anemia in, 520; arthritis in, 312; of bone, 214, 305–306, 328; chest X-rays for detection, 213, 214; of kidneys, 68–69, 214, 721; of larynx, 475; of male genital system, 740; pulmonary, **211–214,** 480, 481; skin in, 61; skin tests for, 214; of spine (Pott's disease), 214, 306; surgery for, 213; treatment, 213–214
Tularemia (rabbit fever), 275
Tumors: adrenal glands, 706–707; brain, 53, **366–367,** 368–369, 440, 463, 937; definition, 937; eye, 431; masculinizing and feminizing changes, 410, 685–686; nose, 442; ovarian, 757–759; pituitary, 707–709; precancerous, 938; spinal cord, 358; thyroid, 585, 692, 693; ureter obstructed by, 69; see also Cancer
Tumors, benign, 937; adrenal glands, 585, 587; bone, 306; brain, 366–367, 937; breast, 447–448; muscle,

Tumors, benign (cont'd)
292; pancreas, 663; parathyroid, 695, 696; respiratory tract, 498–499; uterus, 755–756
Twins: fraternal, 746, 828; identical, 746, 827–828
Tympanic membrane, see Eardrum
Typhoid fever, **256–258,** 312; carriers, 257; gall bladder disease and, 676; immunization, 255, 257–258, 874
"Typhoid Mary," 257
Typhus, **238–239;** insect bites and, 175, 238–239; murine, 239; scrub, 175, 239

Ulcer: corneal, 428; decubitus (bedsore), 386–387; oriental or tropical (leishmaniasis), 278; peptic, see Peptic ulcer; varicose, 570
Ulcerative colitis, **634–638,** 644; surgery, 637–638
Ulna, 27, 30
Ulnar nerve, 50, 353
Ulnar nerve palsy, 353
Ultrasonic waves, 434–435, 438
Umbilical cord, 816, 842, 859; in birth canal, 845–846
Umbilical hernia, 624, **875–876**
Unconscious, the, Freud's theories on, 772–774, 782–783
Unconsciousness, 113–115, **340–342;** circulatory failure, 103–104, **110–111;** fainting, 115, **341;** in head injuries, 359
Undulant fever (brucellosis), 275
United Cerebral Palsy Association, 331
Upper respiratory infections (URI's), **470–480;** of babies, 863; in childhood, 193–196
Urea, 68, 79, 718
Uremia, 588–589, 717–718, 720, 725
Ureter, 68, 715, 717; atresia, 878; cancer, 730–731; injuries, 730; kidney stone in, 69, 718–719; obstruction, 69
Ureteral colic, 719
Urethra, 68, 717; cancer, 730; female, 745; injuries, 730; male, abnormalities and disorders, 736–737, 740; in pelvic fracture, 299
Urethritis, 721, 723
Urethrocele, 722
Uric acid, 68, 79; gout and, 319–320
Urinalysis, 732, 969
Urinary bladder, 68, 713, 715, 716; bladder control, 869–871; cancer, 730–731; cystitis, **721–723,** 731, 826; diverticuli, 948; injuries, 730; muscles, 38; neurogenic, 731; polyps or papillomas, 731, 948; in pregnancy, 826; rupture, 644; stones in, 718; vaginal defects and, 751
Urinary stasis, 719, 722

Urinary system, 713–718; *see also* Kidneys; Ureter; Urethra; Urinary bladder
Urinary system disorders, 538, **717–733**; aging and, 949, 954–955; in pregnancy, 721, 825–826
Urination, 713, 716–717; aging and, 948, 955; of babies, 860; bladder control, 869–871; in cystitis, 721–722; in diabetes, 698, 699; in diabetes insipidus, 709; enuresis (bedwetting), 869–871; incontinence, 731, 751; neurogenic bladder, 731; nocturia, 722; painful (dysuria), 721, 722; in pregnancy, 824, 826; in prostate disorders, 739, 741
Urine, **713–717**; albumin in, 723–725, 727; blood in, 717, 720–725, 730–731; in cystitis, 721–722; in diabetes, 696–698, 700; dyes in, 722; formation in kidneys, 68, 713–716; in glomerulonephritis, 723–724; glucose in, 68, 696–698, 700; output, 24-hour, 717, 728; phenylpyruvic acid in, 879; pregnancy tests, 813–814; protein in, 68, 727, 826, 832; pus in, 68, 720, 721, 826; in pyelitis and pyelonephritis, 720; in renal failure, 728; sugar in, 696–698, 700
Urologist, 718, 995
Urticaria (hives), 61, **388–389**, 490
Uterus, 94, **746–748**, 812; abnormalities, 749–752; cancer, 754–757, 820; cervix, *see* Cervix of uterus; contractions in childbirth, 39, 747, 834–838, 840–841, 843; in endometriosis, 759, 761; fibroid tumors (myomata), 755–756; gangrenous infection, 222; hyperplasia, 757; hysterectomy, 752, 755–757, 761; lining, *see* Endometrium; muscles, 39; physical examination, 966; polyps, 757, 760; in pregnancy, 39, 747, 815–817, 824–826; prolapse, 752; retrodisplacement, 750–751, 760; rupture, 845; shrinkage after childbirth, 847; uterine inertia in labor, 845
Uvula, 611

Vaccine: allergy to, 972; cold, 227, 948; German measles (rubella), 181, 555, 823–824; influenza, 230, 938; measles, 180, 181, 873–874; mumps, 192; poliomyelitis, 175, 188, 190, 873; rabies, 240–242; smallpox, 9, 174–175, 231, **233–234**; *see also* Immunization
Vagina, 747; abnormalities, 749, 751–752; aging and, 955; bleeding from, abnormal, 756, 757, 761–762, 818, 831–832; douche, 918; foreign bodies in, 133; inflammation (vaginitis), 133, **752–753**
Vaginal plastics operation, 751
Vagotomy, 654

Vagus nerve, 49, 347, 654
Valvulitis, 557
Vaporizers, 476
Varicella (chicken pox), **182–183**, 471
Varices, **568–572**; esophageal, 569, 572; rectal, *see* Hemorrhoids
Varicocele, 740
Varicose veins, 81, **568–572**; bleeding from, 536, 569–570; in legs, 568–570; in pregnancy, 568–570, **826–827**; surgery for, 570; ulcers in, 570
Variola, *see* Smallpox
Vas deferens, 735, 920–921
Vasectomy, 735, 920–921
Vasopressin, 686–687, 709
Veins, 81, 542–543; arteries compared with, 568; bleeding, control of, 105–106; disorders, 564–572; *see also* Cardiovascular system; Varicose veins
Vena cava, 68, 527, 542–544, 715; inferior, 81; superior, 81
Venereal diseases, 96, **243–252**; education in control of, 251–252, 904; minor, 250–251; in youth, 243, 247–248, 251–252; *see also* Gonorrhea; Syphilis
Ventricles, 82, 543–544, 547; in tetralogy of Fallot, 549–550
Ventricular fibrillation, 118, 121
Ventricular septal defects, 550–551
Ventriculogram, cerebral, 351
Venules, 81, 543
Vernix, 842
Verrucae (warts), 397–398
Vertebrae, 294; aging and, 948, 950, 952; disks, *see* Intervertebral disks; dislocations, 130; fractures, 128, **298**, 302, 356–357; fractures, compression, 528; intervertebral sprain, 324, 325; joints between, 31; low back pain, 324–326; spinal cord in, 47, 50; spinal curvature, 328; spinal nerves and, 47, 48; tuberculosis of, 306
Vertigo (dizziness), **345**, 435, 437
Vesalius, Andreas, 8, 81
Veterans Administration Hospitals, 1002–1003, 1014, 1017
Villi, 86, 611
Vincent, J. Henri, 218
Vincent de Paul, St., 1001
Vincent's infection (Vincent's angina, trench mouth), 171, **218–219**, 421
Virchow, Rudolf, 95
Viremia, 178
Viruses, 172–175
Virus infections, 172–175, **224–237**
Vision, 426–427; disorders of, 346, 426–427; peripheral, 426
Visiting nurses, 164
Visual cortex, 46
Vital capacity (respiration), 461, 952
Vital signs (temperature, pulse, and respiration), 964

Vitamin A, 628, 894; deficiency, 392, 891; excess, 893
Vitamin B, deficiency, 392, 891
Vitamin B₁ (thiamine), 891
Vitamin B₂ (riboflavin), deficiency, 891
Vitamin B₁₂ (cyanocobalamin), 77, 517, 518, 628, 891, 894
Vitamin C (ascorbic acid), 517, 890; in bone growth, 31; for cold prevention, 228; deficiency, 891–892
Vitamin D, 628, 890, 894; in bone growth, 31; deficiency, 892; excess, 893
Vitamin K, 612; deficiency, 628, 892–893; prothrombin and, 532
Vitamins, **890–893**; in alcoholism, deficiency, 791; for babies, 857; deficiency disorders, 891–893; discovery of, 681; excess of, 893; fat-soluble, 628; synthesis in liver, 90; teeth and, 422
Vitiligo, 383, **401**
Vitreous humor, 426
Vocal cords, 456–457, 473, 475
Volunteers of America, 331
Volvak, Simeon, 175
Volvulus, 627
Vomiting, mechanism of, 615
Voyeurism, 789
Vulva, 747
Vulvovaginitis, 752

Waksman, Selman, 213
Walter, Carl, 726
Warts (verrucae), 397–398; plantar, 397; venereal, 398
Wasps, 139
Wasserman test for syphilis, 246
Water: for babies, 856; drinking, 856; fluoridation of, 420; loss from body, 79, 856, 887–888; retention in pregnancy, 824–825, 831, 832
Water in body, 79–80, 714; retention in pregnancy, 824–825, 831, 832
Weight control, **927–931**; in angina pectoris, 597; in arthritis, 318; in coronary artery disease, 603; diet, 928–930; drugs for, 931; fads and crash diets, 928–929; in heart failure, 580; in hypertension, 589–590; organizations for, 931; in pregnancy, 824–825, 831
Weight loss as cancer symptom, 940
Weight Watchers, Incorporated, 931
Welch, William Henry, 222
Wen, 401
Whiplash injury of neck, 326–328
White blood cells, *see* Blood cells, white
Whooping cough (pertussis), **187–188**, 471; immunization (DPT vaccine), **186–188**, 221, 873–874
Wild animal bites, 142; rabies from, 240–241
Wilms's tumor, 730, 896
Withering, William, 82, 578

Woodbury, R. A., 39

Worms, 117, **264–268;** *Ascaris,* 266; dracunculiasis, 277–278; filariasis, 277; hookworm, 177, 264–266; pinworm, 177, 266–268; schistosomiasis, 278; tapeworm, 177, 268; trichinosis, **276–277,** 292

Wounds, **124–127;** chest, penetrating, **125–126,** 138, 465, 468; foreign bodies in, 126; gunshot, 138; puncture, **126,** 219–220, 222; stab, 138

Wrist: fracture (Colles'), 296; joints, 31; lacerations, 125; tendons, 40; tenosynovitis, 287

Xanthoma, 392

X-rays: danger of, 143, 975; discovery of, 975; protection from, 975–977; radiologist's interpretation of, 996

X-rays, diagnostic, **975–979;** abdomen, 977; for cancer, 504, 505, 940; chest, 213, 214, 504, 505, 578, 939, **977,** 980; dental, 421; fractures, 300; gall bladder, 672–674, 978; gastrointestinal tract (GI), 617, 623, 626, 634, 642, 650–651, 657, 658, **977–978;** heart, 552, 555, 565; intravenous pyelogram, 68, 70–71, 732–733, **978;** kidneys, 729, 731–733; for lung cancer, 504, 505; mammography, 449, 940, 978;

X-rays, diagnostic (*cont'd*) neurological examination, 348; specialized, 978–979; swallowed object, 977

X-ray therapy, 979–980; cancer, 450, 505, 507, 730, 757, 759, 941, 979; Hodgkin's disease, 528; leukemia, 526, 979; lymphoid disorders, 528, 529; skin disorders, 395, 402

Yawning, mechanism, 462

Yaws, 275

Yellow fever, **234–236,** 874

Zuelzer, Georg, 72

73 74 75 76 77 10 9 8 7 6 5 4 3 2 1